HUMAN FILARIASIS

HUMAN FILARIASIS

A Global Survey of Epidemiology and Control

Manabu Sasa

UNIVERSITY PARK PRESS
Baltimore • London • Tokyo

UNIVERSITY PARK PRESS
Baltimore · London · Tokyo

Library of Congress Cataloging in Publication Data

Sasa, Manabu, 1916–
    Human filariasis.

    1. Filariasis. 2. Filariasis—Prevention. I. Title. [DNLM:
1. Filariasis—Occurrence. 2. Filariasis—Prevention and control.
WC880 S252h]
RA644.F5S27   614.5′5′52   76-26204
ISBN 0–8391–0957–1

Originally published by
UNIVERSITY OF TOKYO PRESS

CONTENTS

v

PREFACE

While engaged in field and laboratory works in epidemiology and control of filariasis, I recognized the necessity for a textbook on human filariasis as a guideline for research. This book has been compiled in order to fill such a need for field and laboratory workers as well as medical students interested in the problems of human filariology. It has taken me nearly five years, to complete the manuscript and for various reasons, it was not an easy task to complete such a monograph within such a short period.

Most of the work of collecting references as well as reviewing literature was conducted while the author was staying at Stone House of the U.S. National Institute of Health as Fogarty Scholar during the five months in 1971 and three months in 1973 while on leave from the Institute of Medical Science, University of Tokyo. Special thanks are due to Dr. James, F. Haggerty, Dr. Robert Omata and associates at the Fogarty International Center, NIH, for their kind assistance.

English is not my mother tongue, and I hope the text of this book would be understandable, though it may not be grammatically perfect. Before submitting the manuscript to the publisher, the draft was read and revised by Mrs. Phylis Ogawa, an American, who kindly spent most of her time reading the manuscript after her arrival in Japan. Many thanks are due also to Dr. Hiroshi Tanaka, Dr. Akiko Shirasaka, Miss Fumiko Ebisawa and other members of the Department of Parasitology, Institute of Medical Science, University of Tokyo, to Dr. M. Yasuno and his colleagues at the National Institute for Environmental Studies, Tsukuba, and to Ms. Etsuko Hamao and members of the University of Tokyo Press for their assistance in preparing the manuscript.

Research for this book was supported by a grant from the World Health Organization (Division of Malaria and Other Parasitic Diseases). It was also carried out as a project of the Japan-United States Cooperative Medical Science Program (Parasitic Diseases Panel). Publication of this book was subsidized by the Grant-in-Aid for Scientific Research of the Japanese Ministry of Education, Science and Culture.

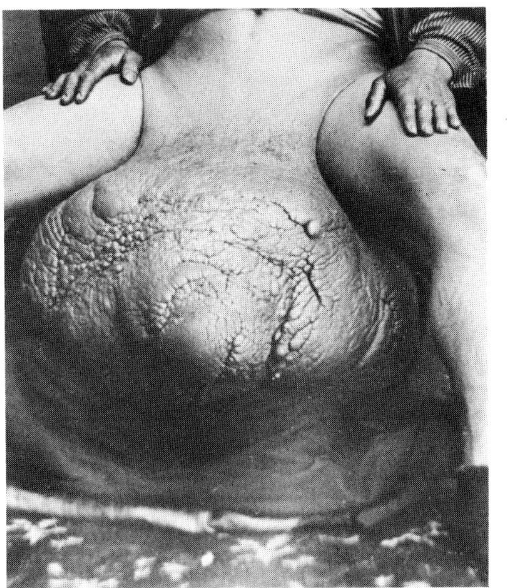

1A

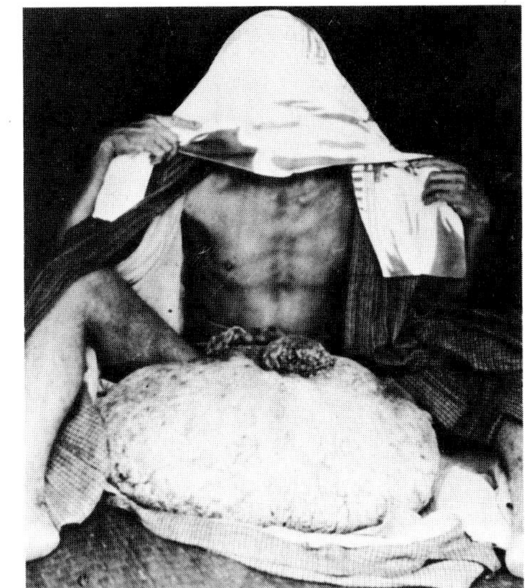

1B

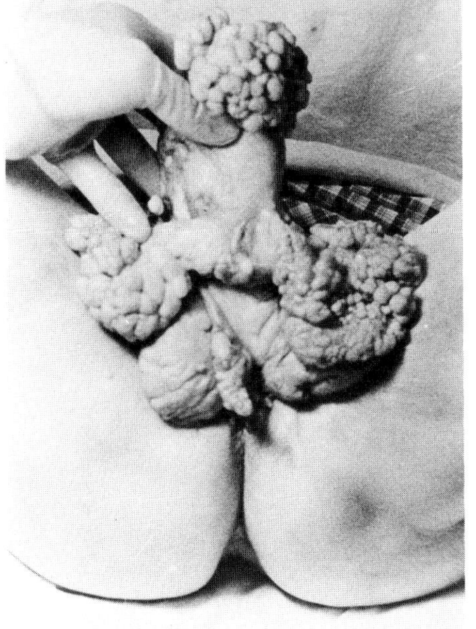

1C

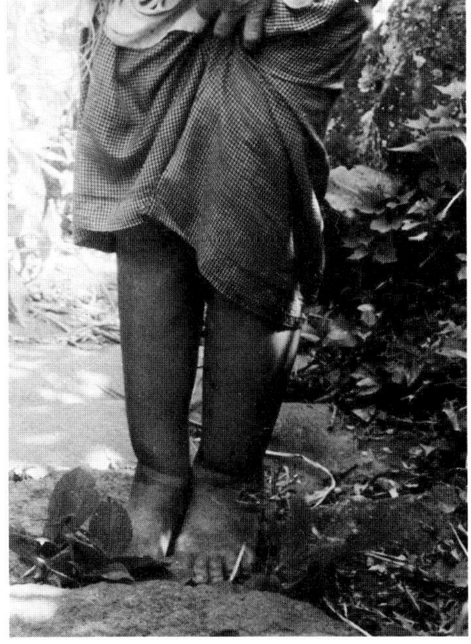

1D

Plate 2

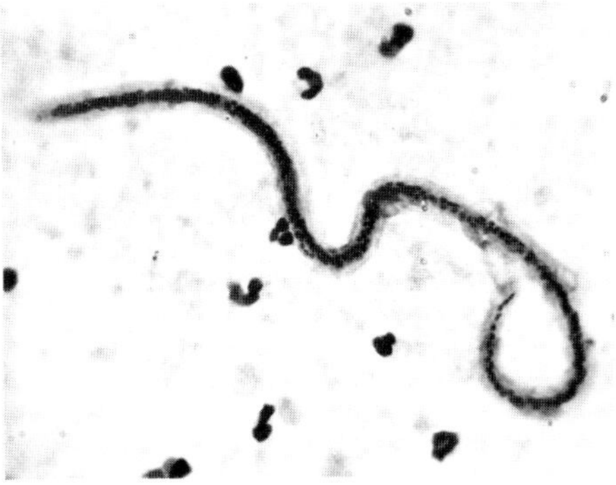

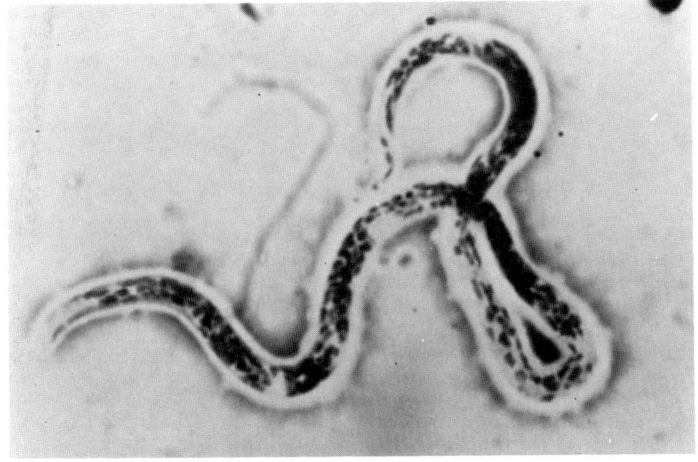

2A

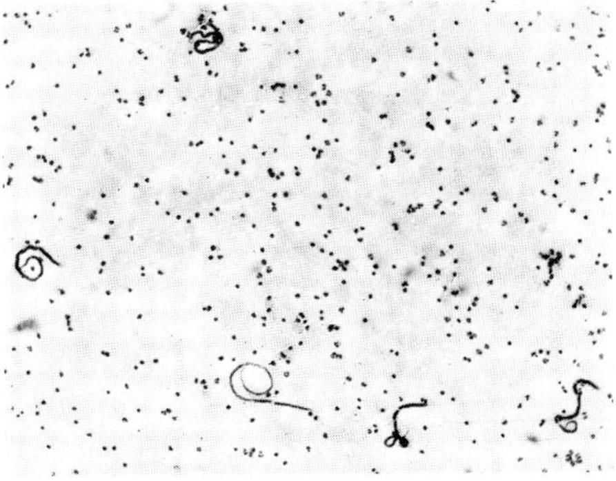

2B

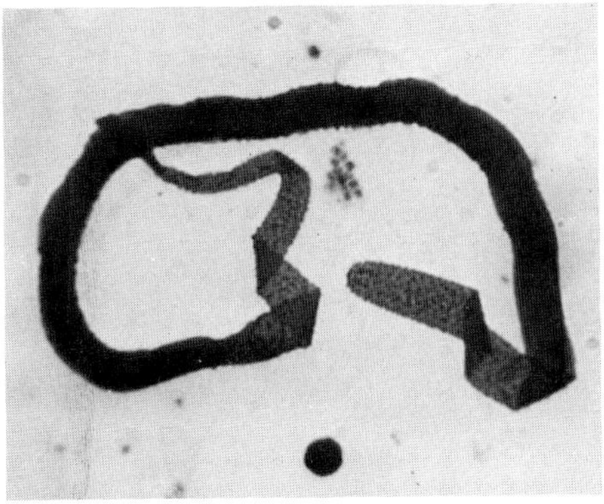

2C

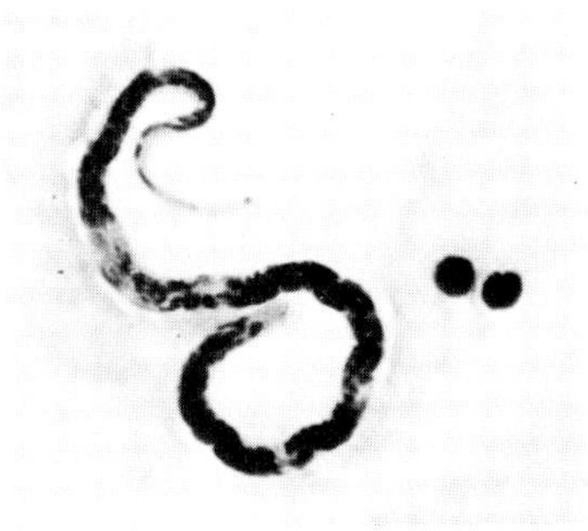

2D

2E

Plate 2. Microfilariae of *Wuchereria bancrofti*, *Brugia malayi* and the Timor-filaria

2A. *W. bancrofti*, hematoxylin staining; blood smear of a case from Amami, southern Japan

2B. Mixed infection of *W. bancrofti* (one slender and longer microfilaria) and *B. malayi* (five other thicker and shorter microfilariae); blood smear of a case from Hachijo-Koshima Japan

2C. Microfilaria (with sheath) of *B. malayi*; Giemsa staining; blood smear of a case from Hachijo-Koshima

2D. *B. malayi*; hematoxylin staining; blood smear of a case from Hachijo-Koshima (2A–2D. photo by Mr. Seigo Noda)

2E. Timor-filaria; hematoxylin staining; blood smear of a case from Indonesian Timor (photo by Dr. Tozo Kanda)

Plate 3

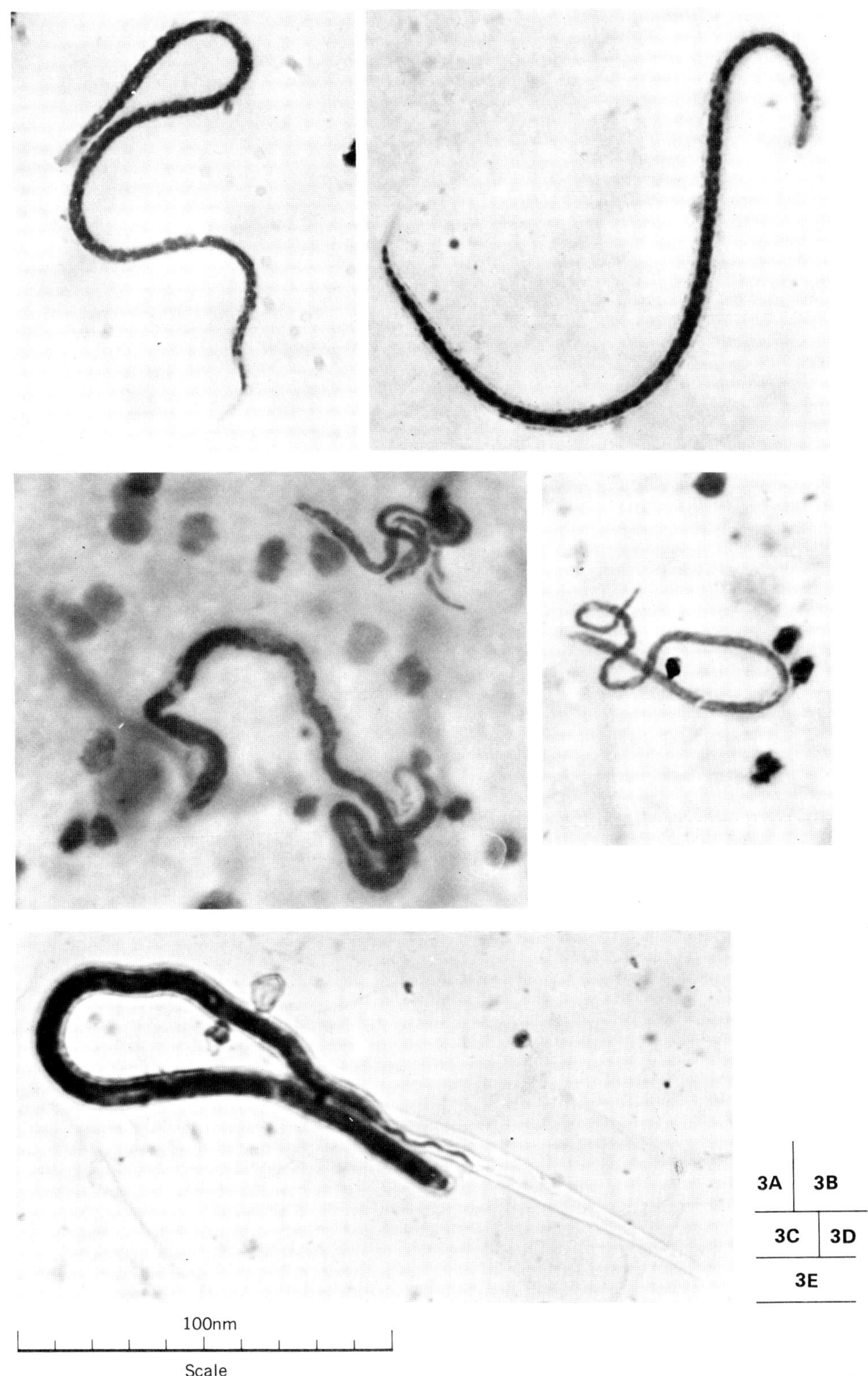

Plate 3.   Microfilariae of African filarial species (all from cases from the Central African Republic; Giemsa staining; photo by Dr. Shigeo Hayashi)

3A.   and 3B.   *Onchocerca volvulus* in skin snips

3C.   A mixed infection of *Loa loa* and *Dipetalonema perstans* (below) in a blood smear

3D.   *Dipetalonema perstans* in a blood smear

3E.   *Loa loa* in a blood smear

HUMAN FILARIASIS

INTRODUCTION

The Antifilariasis Campaign: Its History and Future Prospects

The nematodes generally called "filariae" include several hundred species of worms parasitic in the tissues of various vertebrate hosts, and at least several species among them are known to be the causative agents of serious diseases in man. STOLL (1947) estimated that of the 3,000 million people estimated to populate the world, the number of people infected with *Wuchereria bancrofti* was 189 million while 13 million were infected with *Loa loa*, 27 million with *Dipetalonema perstans*, 20 million with *Onchocerca volvulus*, and 7 million with *Mansonella ozzardi*.

Before the end of World War II, and until the discovery of diethylcarbamazine (DEC) as a filaricide, no effective measures had been available in controlling filariasis except for some general sanitary measures for reducing the population density of the mosquito vectors. In Egypt, for example, filariasis due to *Wuchereria bancrofti* was highly prevalent in eastern parts of the Nile Delta, and large numbers of people were suffering from elephantiasis, hydrocele, and other filarial infections. Experimental studies and epidemiological investigations conducted from 1930 to 1936 showed that an urban mosquito, *Culex pipiens*, was the principal vector, and that the mosquito breeds mainly in wells in the villages. A campaign was begun to construct pipe lines or irrigation ditches for water supply, and to fill up the wells. Later, a country-wide survey of filariasis, reported in 1946, indicated that remarkable reductions in microfilaremia rates were achieved in areas where wells were abolished. Whereas the rates were still high in villages where the people still depended on wells for the water supply (BAZ. 1946).

Bancroftian filariasis was introduced and became endemic in certain areas in the northwestern parts of Australia, and in the city of Charleston in the southern United States. Relatively high incidences of microfilaremia cases were reported from these areas until about 1920. However, the disease disappeared rather spontaneously from Australia and the United States before World War II, presumably due to the reduction of the vector mosquito, *Culex pipiens*, resulting from improvements in general sanitary conditions. A similar phenomenon was also observed on the mainland of Japan, where endemic foci of bancroftian filariasis were recorded, throughout Kyushu, Shikoku, and Honshu. However, the results of blood surveys conducted from 1958 to 1964 under the national filariasis control program of Japan demonstrated that the disease had disappeared spontaneously from most of these areas before applying any specific control measure.

We cannot, however, be too optimistic about the future eradication of filariasis as a world health problem. Recent investigations on the epidemiology of filariasis have shown that the problems are much more complex and difficult than previously thought, so that spontaneous reduction or eradication through the improvement in general sanitary measures can be expected probably only in the temperate zones, where the transmission season is short, and where the reduction of the vector populations significantly affects the intensity of transmission necessary to maintain the infection. As demonstrated in Sri Lanka, the transmission of filariasis in tropical countries can be maintained or increased by the presence of extremely low vector population densities (see Section 8A. 4). In such countries, where the climate is so favorable for transmission, the disease probably cannot be effectively controlled by larval control measures alone.

The discovery of diethylcarbamazine (DEC) by HEWITT *et al.* (1947) as an effective filaricide brought about a revolution in the history of the antifilariasis campaign. Before this, antimony compounds were practically the only drugs effective against filarial infections, but these could not be used extensively in mass treatment campaigns because of their toxicity and relative inefficacy. Some arsenicals were found to be effective, especially on adult filariae, at almost the same time as DEC was discovered, but these compounds, and some of their improved forms, were too toxic for general use. On the other hand, the successful results reported by KESSEL (1957) and his associates in the South Pacific on the effective control of filariasis due to diurnally subperiodic *W. bancrofti* encouraged later workers to undertake mass drug administration campaigns against other filarial species and forms endemic elsewhere in the world.

It was fortunate that Hewitt and his co-workers tested the antifilarial activity of DEC with *Litomosoides carinii* infection in cotton rats. If they had tested the drug with other laboratory animal systems, such as *Dipetalonema witei* infection in gerbiles, or *Dirofilaria immitis* in dogs, the drug might have been judged to be ineffective. It was also lucky that the original authors did not conduct the *in vitro* tests. As demonstrated by HAWKING *et al.* (1950), DEC has no direct *in vitro* filaricidal effects. When administered to dogs infected with *Dirofilaria immitis,* DEC was shown to be not only ineffective as a filaricide, but it also frequently caused fatal side effects due to shock. However, such dangerous reactions have never been encountered in the treatment of human cases infected with various forms of *Wuchereria* or *Brugia* filariae, though millions of people have already received the full course of DEC treatments. DEC was demonstrated by later workers to be effective against all forms and species of human filariae, though its efficacy and side reactions differed considerably according to the species of the parasites.

As an example of a filariasis control program which turned out to be more or less successful, reference should be made to the outline of the results obtained in Japan (see Section 8C.5). Before the country-wide filariasis control project was initiated in 1962, basic research and pilot studies were conducted by several groups of Japanese workers for about ten years, accumulating information necessary to develop effective and efficient methods of control, with special reference to microfilaria survey methods and drug administration schemes. It was recommended, first, to conduct blood examinations of whole populations by taking measured blood samples (three linear smears of 10 mm^3 each), and to record the number of microfilariae found in each of the smears. Secondly, since it was not clear what dosage regimens were most effective, safe, and economic, pilot drug administration experiments were designed to observe the results obtained after administration of various doses of DEC at different time intervals (daily, weekly, or monthly), and for various periods. These experiments were conducted mainly in the Amami Islands, where people were living in large numbers of small villages isolated from each other by mountain and sea, and where the microfilaremia rates were from 10 to 20% throughout the area. After several years of comparative studies, it became clear that, in the treatment of *W. bancrofti* infection with DEC, the maximum single dose tolerated is about 8 mg per kg of the body weight, and at least 70 mg per kg of DEC should be administered in total in order to achieve effective control of the parasite. As the standard method, it was recommended to give the drug at a dose of about 6 mg per kg, once a day, for 12 times, totaling 72 mg per kg per person. Since no significant differences were observed between the groups administered by the daily, the weekly, and the monthly doses, it was recommended to give the drug once every day in order to complete the course within shortest period. The cure rates of microfilaria carriers were found to be highly correlated with the total dose administered, such as only 30% with 20 mg per kg, 50% with 40 mg per kg, 80% with 70 mg per kg, and 95% with 140 mg per kg.

The most important problem encountered in the drug administration program was its side effects. Because of the severe fever reactions frequently encountered soon after the initial dose of DEC is administered, the anti-filariasis campaigns initiated in many regions of the world failed when the people refused to take additional doses of the drug. However, statistical analysis of the attack rates of various side effects encountered in the Amami Islands in treatments with various DEC dosage schemes showed two important aspects of its nature. First, DEC has its own toxic effect, though never dangerous, of causing nausea or vomiting, which starts a few minutes after being swallowed; the severity of this type of adverse effect is independent of whether the person is infected or not. This adverse side effect is solely dependent on the amount of the drug, and thus can be avoided by reducing the dose to a certain level, such as 6 mg per kg of the body weight. The second type of adverse effect is a fever reaction accompanied by dizziness. This was found to be highly correlated with the microfilarial load of individual cases and rather independent of the dose of the drug. Because the fever reaction starts not immediately after the drug was taken, but usually about ten hours thereafter, it is assumed that the reaction is caused by the release of a pyrogen from the microfilariae killed by the drug. This type of side effect has never been found to be dangerous, and it subsides within a few hours to a few days even when additional doses of DEC are administered. The fever reaction never occurs after most of the microfilariae are destroyed.

One of the main reasons that the filariasis control program in Japan was effective was the success of the health education of the people, especially their understanding about the nature of the febrile reaction. Before administering the drug to the people, they were informed about the likelihood of a fever reaction, and the expected severity (since these can be predicted from the results of blood examination). As a rule, those who have over 1 microfilaria per 1 mm^3 of blood are expected to have a relatively severe fever reaction with a probability of some 80%; the probability is roughly 40%, and the reaction is usually less severe in those with 0.1 to 1.0 microfilaria per 1 mm^3; and it is lower than 10% in those with less than 0.1 per 1 mm^3. The health workers gave special care to those with high microfilarial loads, and congratulated them when the fever occurred as predicted because it is the initial sign of cure of the disease. Further encouragement was then given to take additional doses in order to kill the parasite completely. Those persons who refused to take additional doses of the drug because of the fear of the fever reaction, of course, could not be cured.

The national filariasis control program for the mainland of Japan began its activity in 1962 in six prefectures, under financial and technical support from the Ministry of Health and Welfare. The program was expanded to cover nine prefectures in 1964. The filariasis control program of the Ryukyu Islands was started in 1964, with the Miyako region as the initial target. It was expanded, in 1967, to cover also the Yaeyama region, and the main island of Okinawa in 1969. The details of the results achieved were published in several reports which were partly reviewed by Sasa *et al.* (1967, 1970). In all of these prefectures or regions, it was intended to examine the blood of whole populations of villages suspected to be in the endemic areas of filariasis, and to treat only the positive microfilaria cases with the standard course of DEC administration. Such procedures were to be repeatedly applied to the same areas on an annual or biannual basis until no more microfilaremia cases could be found. Co-operation of the people with this project was excellent especially in the Miyako and Yaeyama regions of Okinawa, where almost 100% of the inhabitants received the blood examinations every year. Nearly all persons found to be harboring microfilariae were treated with the full course of the drug administration. The control of vector mosquitoes with general environmental sanitation measures, as well as the use of insecticides was initiated in all of these target areas. Large numbers of scientific reports were made on the taxonomy, biology, ecology, vectorial capacity and insecticide resistance of the filariasis vectors (mainly the *Culex pipiens* complex), in connection with the progress of the filariasis control project in Japan.

It should be pointed out here that the work done by the filariasis control teams organized in Japan was, in most cases, far from the comprehensive program originally planned. For various reasons, the budgets supporting these projects from national sources were terminated by 1970 except for certain areas in Okinawa. However, interestingly enough, sporadic reports from the former endemic areas in the mainland of Japan suggest that the disease is disappearing even though the control measures applied were more or less incomplete.

Filariasis has been noted to be highly prevalent in some of the islands in the South Pacific, notably Tahiti, Samoa, Tonga, and Fiji. Although these islands are free from malaria because of the absence of anopheline mosquitoes, filariasis has been a serious health hazard to the inhabitants. The microfilaremia and elephantiasis rates observed in these regions are among the highest recorded in the world. The parasite found in this area is peculiar, in that the microfilariae exhibit almost no periodicity, and the larval development takes place in day-biting mosquitoes of the *Aedes polynesiensis* complex.

The first successful result in the control of filariasis in this region by the mass treatment of the populations with DEC was reported by KESSEL (1957) from Tahiti. Similar control projects are also in progress in American Samoa, Western Samoa, and Fiji. In these regions, effective control of vector mosquitoes is impracticable because their breeding places are unlimited and widely scattered. The control scheme, therefore, depends solely on the drug. In Western Samoa, DEC was administered to the whole island at doses of 5 mg per kg, once a week, for six times, followed by the same doses at monthly intervals for 12 times. In both cases, the total dosage was 90 mg per kg of the body weight. Some 80% of the whole population was estimated to have taken at least 12 doses. The microfilaremia rate observed with sample populations was about 20% in the pretreatment survey conducted in 1964–65, but dropped to 1.63% in the posttreatment survey in 1967. The geometric mean of the microfilarial density per 20 mm³ blood samples (taken from positive cases) likewise dropped from 27 to 2.7. After this, a second round of mass drug administration was completed in 1971, with the dosage scheme of 6 mg per kg, once a month, for 12 times. The surveillance is still in progress to determine whether these treatments interrupted the transmission of filariasis, or whether the transmission would resume in future, despite such intensive treatments of the whole population.

The author has quoted here two examples of filariasis control programs which were very promising, in view of the eradication of the disease from an area. There are a number of other filariasis control projects in progress in other regions of the world. Some of them have been reported to be quite effective while many others have turned out to be rather disappointing.

It should be pointed out that there still exist large areas, especially in Africa and South Asia, where various kinds of filariasis are known to be endemic, but no control activity has ever been practiced or planned. Moreover, there are a number of regions in the world where filariasis is suspected to be endemic, but which have never been surveyed by professional workers. As for the future prospect for the eradication of filariasis from the world, we are still far from the goal.

The complexity of epidemiology

There are a number of problems to be considered in planning a filariasis control program. First of all, it should be remembered that the mode of transmission and the epidemiology of filariasis differ greatly in the various filarial species and forms, and by the localities. Human filarial species of the genera *Wuchereria* and *Brugia* are transmitted by mosquitoes (Culicidae), *Dipetalonema* and *Mansonella* by *Culicoides* (Ceratopogonidae), *Loa* by *Chrysops* (Tabanidae), and *Onchocerca* by *Simulium* (Simuliidae). The bionomics and geographic distribution of these insect vectors differ greatly among the families, and even among different species of the same families. Filariasis caused by the same species of the parasite may exhibit quite different epidemiological features because of the differences in the local vector species. This is frequently the case in *Wuchereria bancrofti* or *Brugia malayi* infections. The occurrence of physiological races within the same parasite species has been noted in *Wuchereria*, *Brugia* and *Loa*, especially in the pattern of the microfilarial periodicity. In planning a control program for an endemic region, it is essential to accumulate basic information on the characters of the parasite, and the vector.

Vector control or drug treatment?

In planning control programs for vector-borne diseases, it is always a problem to determine whether the treatment of the vector populations, or that of the human reservoirs would be more effective and economic for the reduction or interruption of transmission. In the control of malaria, for example, it has been shown that the reduction of infective mosquitoes by an indoor spray of residual insecticides is the most effective measure, and also that interruption of transmission of the parasite from an endemic area is difficult to achieve by mass administration of chemotherapeutics only. In filariasis, however, the situation has been shown to be reversed, in general. The effective control of the vectors of filariasis by the use of insecticides or other measures is usually more difficult than those of malaria. Even when the vectors could be almost completely eradicated from an endemic area, as achieved by OMORI *et al.* (1972) from a small isolated village in Japan, it takes more than ten years of continuous effort to reduce the number of human microfilaria carriers to near zero.

On the other hand, the treatment of the majority of parasite carriers among the human populations with diethylcarbamazine has been demonstrated to be effective in reducing the microfilaria carriers (infective sources) to a minimum level for certain long periods, thus relieving the people from episodes of acute symptoms, even in areas (such as the South Pacific) where no effective vector control measures are available.

It is the author's opinion, however, that efforts to reduce the vector population by all available means are valuable and effective, especially when combined with a drug treatment project. In the present stage of our knowledge, complete eradication of parasite carriers from human populations will never be achieved by the use of a drug alone; when the vector population is reduced below a certain critical level simultaneously, it appears that the disease dies out spontaneously by the combined effects. This was probably the case in most of the former filariasis endemic areas in Japan where neither the drug administration, nor the vector control was complete in effect and coverage; however, the integrated control program was effective.

Mass drug administration or selective treatment of microfilaria cases?

Theoretically, it is obvious that mass administration of DEC to the whole population is more efficient in reducing the parasite carriers than the treatment of only the positive microfilaremia cases, especially in endemic areas with high prevalence rates. In the latter method, it is necessary to conduct blood examinations of the whole people repeatedly, at certain time intervals, such as once every year, in order to detect the cases to be treated. In the former, sample blood surveys are usually sufficient for evaluation of the results, and they are easier to practice in regions where professional medical workers are scarce. The mass drug administration program has been shown to be especially effective in the South Pacific, where the disease is prevalent among the isolated populations.

On the other hand, the methods of selective treatment of positive cases after mass blood examination have been adopted, with more or less successful results, in Japan, Sri Lanka, Brazil, etc. In these countries, the endemic areas are widely distributed, with varying prevalence rates, and it is difficult to delimit them from the nonendemic areas. The nonselective mass drug administration program requires tremendous amounts of the drug, in order to cover the whole populations suspected to be infected. In areas where the microfilaremia rates are relatively low, the selective treatment method is more economic and efficient, in view of the cost of drugs, and it is superior for the better care of individual cases. It should be pointed out that there always exist large numbers of "occult parasite carriers" among the people who were apparently negative at a single blood examination, therefore, blood surveys should be made repeatedly on the same population, in order to achieve satisfactory results.

Problems in vector control

As pointed out previously, efforts to reduce the vector population are necessary, even though their effects are slow and less conspicuous than those expected from the mass drug administration. Previous research has shown that large numbers of bloodsucking arthropod species are involved in the transmission of filariasis endemic in various regions of the world, and effective control measures should be developed for each species and for each region. In the control of *Culex pipiens fatigans*, the principal vector of the nocturnally periodic *Wuchereria bancrofti* found in most of the tropical and subtropical countries, an indoor spray of DDT which is usually very effective in the control of malaria vectors has been shown to be almost in-effective in the control of filariasis because of the development of insecti-cide resistance. The larvae also developed resistance to various chlorinated insecticides, including DDT and BHC. On the other hand, some organo-phosphorous insecticides are effective against its larvae, while being low in toxicity to man, and biologically degradable. Promising results have been reported in the use of indoor spraying of fenitrothion, an organophos-phorous compound, against the adults of *C. p. fatigans*.

In most endemic areas, the clearing of breeding places by general sani-tary measures is effective in reducing the vector population. Since the *C. p. fatigan* larvae develop in artificial sewage pools, the installment of a water supply system to replace water containers, and a sewage system to drain polluted waters, are effective measures in the case of *fatigans*-borne filariasis.

Promising results have been reported recently on the use of a viviparous fish, *Poecilia reticulata*, in the biological control of *C. p. fatigans* (SASA *et al.*, 1965; SASA, 1972). The fish is a native of tropical South America, and is highly adapted to breed in polluted waters, and to eradicate mos-quito larvae after they reach a certain population density. Many per-manent sewage pools can be made free from mosquito larvae more effi-ciently by the use of this fish than with insecticides. It has also been shown recently that the combined use of the fish and certain low-toxicity insec-ticides (such as 0.1 ppm of fenitrothion) is more efficient than the single use of either the fish or the insecticide. It usually requires several months before the fish population increases to levels effective to kill all the mos-quito larvae, while repeated applications is required in order to maintain the pools free from mosquito larvae by insecticide alone. When both are introduced simultaneously, the large numbers of mosquito larvae are killed immediately by the insecticide, and the relatively small numbers of fish eat all the mosquito eggs subsequently laid on the pools (a fish can eat only about 20 mature mosquito larvae per day, but can consume several hundred mosquito eggs per day).

As shown in the above examples, there are a number of new and promis-ing techniques for the effective and economic control of various filariasis vectors. However, the methods now available for the control of filariasis are obviously far from ideal, and most of the present workers admit that it is difficult to achieve eradication of the disease from the vast endemic areas now existing by the present day methods. Solutions can only be found through basic research directed to the various aspects of the dynamics of transmission of filariasis.

Part 1 | **The Parasites, the Disease, and the Vectors**

1 | Filaria and Filariasis

1.1 Definition of Filaria and Filariasis

FILARIASIS is a group of human and animal infectious diseases caused by nematode parasites of the Order Filariidea, commonly called "filariae". According to YAMAGUTI (1961), the Order contains three families: Filariidae, Stephanofilariidae, and Dipetalonematidae. Within the families, 39 genera and 229 species are parasitic in mammals, 43 genera and 255 species are parasitic in birds, 12 genera and 30 species are parasitic in reptiles, and 3 genera and 23 species are parasitic in amphibians. The adult filarial worms live in vessels, tissues, or body cavities of the vertebrate hosts. The females produce embryos called microfilariae. The larval development takes place in certain bloodsucking invertebrate intermediate hosts.

The filarial parasites may be classified into the three main groups by the habitat of the adult worms, i.e., the cutaneous group (including *L. loa*, *O. volvulus* and *D. streptocerca*), the lymphatic group (including *W. bancrofti* and *B. malayi*) and the body cavity group (including *D. perstans* and *M. ozzardi*). The life cycle of various species and forms of filariae in view of the definitive and intermediate hosts and the development sites of larvae and adult worms was reviewed by SCHACHER (1973).

The adult worms are cylindrical, very thin and long, usually measuring several centimeters in length. The mouth is simple, circular, or somewhat dorsoventrally elongated, and is surrounded by papillae; lips are absent, and the buccal cavity is rudimentary. The esophagus is thin, and not muscular. Males have spicules, both with and without caudal alae. The microfilariae are snakelike organisms measuring one-fifth to one-third of a millimeter. Some species produce "sheathed microfilariae", in which the egg membrane lengthens to enclose the elongated embryo; while in others, the egg membrane ruptures, and sets free a naked larva called the "unsheathed microfilaria". The microfilariae do not develop further in the vertebrate hosts, but when ingested by an appropriate intermediate host, they invade certain organs or body cavities, increasing in size, and develop into "infective larvae".

It usually takes at least one week to ten days for the microfilariae to develop into infective larvae in the intermediate hosts. Various blood sucking arthropods, such as mosquitoes (Culicidae), black flies (Simuliidae), biting midges (*Culicoides*: Ceratopogoniidae), fleas, mites, and ticks are known to serve as intermediate hosts of different filarial species. Each filarial species is quite host-specific, i.e., a given filaria will develop only in certain species of vertebrates, and blood-sucking arthropods. Transmission of the parasite to a new vertebrate host is effected by bites of the insects or mites that harbor the infective larvae.

Various filarial parasites are known to cause diseases in man and animals. In the field of veterinary medicine, filariasis is often a serious health hazard to dogs, horses, sheep, goats, and cattle. The dog heartworm, *Dirofilaria immitis*, is among the wellknown filarial parasites of domestic animals. *Setaria cervi* of cattle often causes damage to the central nervous system in sheep, goats, and horses. Various filarial species are known to cause skin diseases in cattle and horses.

The term "filaria" is not a scientific name, but a common name for the parasite of the Order Filariidea. The generic name *Filaria* was often used by classical workers as the scientific name of human filariae, such as *Filaria bancrofti*, or *Filaria malayi*. In the present concept of taxonomy, the genus *Filaria* Mueller, 1787, in strict sense, includes only a few species parasitic in some small mammals, with *Filaria martis* Gmelin, 1870, as the genotype.

1.2 Taxonomy of the parasite

1.2.1 Species of filariae

At present, seven filarial species have been recognized to be normally parasitic in man. They all belong to the Family Dipetalonematidae of the Order Filariidea. The taxonomic status of these species is shown in Table 1-1, and their geographic distribution, pathogenicity, site of infection of adult worms, characteristics of the microfilariae, and vectors are summarized in Table 1-2.

Wuchereria bancrofti (Wb), the causative agent of Bancroft's filariasis or filariasis bancrofti, is widely distributed throughout most of the warm regions of the world. The adults live in the lymphatics, and produce sheathed microfilariae which appear in the peripheral blood. Various species of mosquitoes serve as the intermediate hosts.

Brugia malayi (Bm) causing malayan filariasis or filariasis malayi is restricted in its geographic distribution to South and East Asia. The adults also live in lymph canals or nodules, and microfilariae are sheathed. The intermediate hosts are mosquitoes of the genera *Mansonia*, *Anopheles*, and *Aedes*.

Table 1-1.   Taxonomic position of human filariae.

Order FILARIIDEA Yamaguti, 1961
  Family Filariidae Claus 1885
  Family Stephanofilariidae Wehr, 1935
  Family Dipetalonematidae Wehr, 1935
    Subfamily Dipetalonematidae Wehr, 1935
      Genus *Dipetalonema* Diesing, 1861
        Dipetalonema perstans (Manson, 1891)
        Dipetalonema streptocerca (Macfie et Corson, 1922)
      Genus *Wuchereria* Silva Araujo, 1877
        Wuchereria bancrofti (Cobbold, 1877)
      Genus *Brugia* Buckley, 1960
        Brugia malayi (Lichtenstein, 1927)
      Genus *Mansonella* Faust, 1929
        Mansonella ozzardi (Manson, 1897)
    Subfamily Dirofilariinae Wehr, 1935
      Genus *Loa* Stiles, 1905
        Loa loa (Guyot, 1778)
    Subfamily Oncocercinae Yamaguti, 1961
      Genus *Oncocerca* Creplin, 1846 (= *Onchocerca* Diesing, 1841)
        Oncocerca volvulus (Leuckart, 1893)

"Timor filaria," was described, from research done on Timor Island by
DAVID & EDESON (1965), as a new species, but to which no scientific name
has yet been given. The microfilariae resemble those of *B. malayi*, but are
larger, with longer cephalic space. They have a sheath which is difficult to
stain with Giemsa. The adults are still unknown. The parasite causes elephantiasis, and is presumably transmitted by mosquitoes.

Dipetalonema perstans and *D. streptocerca* are the filarial parasites transmitted by biting midges of the genus *Culicoides*, family Ceratopogoniidae.
They are endemic among the people in tropical Africa. *D. perstans* is also
endemic in South America.

FAIN (1974) described a new species, *Dipetalonema semiclarum*; the
microfilariae were found in the blood and skin of people from Equateur
Province, Zaire (see Section 4B).

Mansonella ozzardi is another human filaria transmitted by the *Culicoides* species, and is distributed only in the New World. The adult worms
of these species are found in body cavities, or subcutaneous tissues of man.
The microfilariae are unsheathed, and show little periodicity.

Loa loa is another tropical African species, and is transmitted by tabanid
flies of the genus *Chrysops*. The adults normally live in subcutaneous tissue,
frequently provoking painful swellings. The microfilariae are sheathed,
and have a diurnal periodicity.

Onchocerca volvulus is widely distributed in tropical Africa and Middle
America, with black flies of the genus *Simulium* as vectors. The adults live
in subcutaneous tissue, causing skin nodules. Ocular complications which

Table 1-2. Comparison of the main human filaria species.

Species	Geographic distribution	Pathogenicity	Adults (site of infection)	Microfilariae (characteristics)	Vector
Wuchereria bancrofti	Asia, Pacific, tropical Africa and the Americas	lymphangitis, fever, elephantiasis hydrocele, chyluria	lymphatics	found in blood, sheathed, periodicity variable	Culicidae (mosquitoes)
Brugia malayi	South and East Asia	lymphangitis, fever elephantiasis	lymphatics	found in blood, sheathed, nocturnally periodic or subperiodic	Culicidae (mosquitoes)
Dipetalonema perstans	Africa and South America	no definite pathogenicity	peritoneal & pleural cavity	found in blood, unsheathed, nocturnally subperiodic	*Culicoides* (biting midges)
Dipetalonema streptocerca	Africa (Ghana and Congo)	cutaneous edema, elephantiasis	subcutaneous tissues	found in skin, unsheathed nonperiodic	*Culicoides*
Mansonella ozzardi	Central and South America	no definite pathogenicity	peritoneal cavity	found in blood, unsheathed, nonperiodic	*Culicoides*
Loa loa	tropical Africa	skin swellings allergic reactions	subcutaneous tissues	found in blood, sheathed, diurnally periodic	*Chrysops* (Tabanidae, or horse fly)
Onchocerca volvulus	Africa, Central and South America	skin nodules ocular complications (blindness)	subcutaneous tissues	found in skin, unsheathed, nonperiodic	*Similium* (black fly)

often end in blindness are important symptoms. The microfilariae are unsheathed; they are found mainly in the skin, rarely in the circulating blood. STOLL (1947) gave the following estimates of the numbers of people infected with the respective filarial species:

W. bancrofti: 157 million in Asia, 22 million in Africa, 9 million in Central and South America, 1 million in Oceania.

Loa loa: 13 million in Africa.

O. volvulus: 19 million in Africa, 1 million in Central and South America.

D. perstans: 19 million in Africa, 1 million in Oceania, 7 million in Central and South America.

M. ozzardi: 7 million in Central and South America.

1.2.2 Different populations within the species

1.2.2.1 The concept of infraspecific taxonomy

In the classical concept of taxonomy, a population of animals or plants has been recognized as a species only when it is morphologically distinct from other related populations, when it has certain physiological characteristics different from others, and when it is ecologically and reproductively isolated from other populations. However, there are a variety of forms or populations which do not satisfy all of these requirements. In such cases, it is safer not to treat them as a valid species, but rather to include these forms within a known species. Most modern taxonomists recognize a population as a distinct species when they are certain that it is "reproductively isolated" from others, even when it lacks morphological or physiological evidence for the differentiation.

With regard to our present knowledge, at least the above seven kinds of human filariae, called by different scientific names, are considered here to represent distinct species, i.e., they differ from each other in morphological structures, and also in certain physiological characteristics, and their reproductive isolation is probably complete. In the course of evolution, they must have separated before they became parasitic in man, since there are a number of closely related filarial species of the same genera parasitic in animals other than man. The genera *Brugia*, *Dipetalonema*, and *Onchocerca*, in particular, have a number of species parasitic in animals and closely related to that in man, but differing in certain morphological and physiological characteristics.

On the other hand, the existence of various populations which exhibit different physiological or ecological characteristics within the apparently same species of human filariae has also been noted. When they lack distinct morphological characteristics for the differentiation, they have been treated by various names, such as races, forms, or types. This will be discussed in detail in the following chapters. It is assumed that various grades of isolation and characterizations are involved among these infraspecific populations. These populations have possibly achieved a partial evolution in establishing a more distinctive specific status in future. Various factors are acting as the forces of natural selection for the evolution, among which, the most powerful seems to be the adaptation to the behavior of local vectors. The difference in the pattern of the microfilarial periodicity is an example of this type of adaptation.

In order to clarify the evolutional status of the various recognized infraspecific populations for human filarial species, they are divided into the following categories: 1) physiological races, in reference to the microfilarial periodicity; 2) ecological types, in reference to the adaptation to local vector mosquitoes; and 3) other forms.

In this context, the term "race" means a population with genetically uniform physiological or morphological characteristics by which it can be differentiated from other populations of the same species. A race is usually isolated from other populations either geographically or ecologically, and thus, can be regarded as synonymous with the taxonomic concept of a subspecies. It is expected that, at least in some combinations, hybrids can be produced, and will be reproductive for further generations if individuals from two different races of the same species are experimentally mated. If hybrids cannot be produced, or they are completely incapable of producing F_2 and further offsprings, the two populations tentatively designated as different "races" should be regarded as different "species," even when they are morphologically indistinguishable. However, since it is usually difficult to confirm that two morphologically indistinguishable natural populations are completely isolated in reproductivity, it is safer to consider that they belong to different races or subspecies, rather than to treat them as different species, using different scientific names for such populations.

The term "type" is used in this text to differentiate filariasis due to the same species of a parasite, but exhibiting different ecological or epidemiological characteristics, in connection with the behavior of the local vector species. For example, *B. malayi* infection in Hachijo-Koshima of Japan, or Chejudo of Korea, is a disease associated with a rocky seacoast, while the same disease in southern Asia occurs in swamp areas, or in villages surrounded by rice paddies. The parasite may be the same in physiological and genetical characters, but the environment of the endemic areas is quite different, leading to a difference in the breeding habitat of the vector mosquitoes. If the two parasite populations can also be differentiated by their physiological and genetical characters in compatibility of development in different intermediate host species, they can be regarded as different physiological races.

The word "form" is used as a general term for differentiating various populations associated with specialized characters, especially when it is not clear whether they differ from each other at the level of species, subspecies, race, or other minor categories.

1.2.2.2. Physiological races

One of the most remarkable aspects in the problems of infraspecific taxonomy of human filariae is the occurrence of some clearly defined races, each characterized by the pattern of the microfilarial periodicity. Methods for the statistical analysis of such a characteristic are described in Section 11F; a more detailed explanation of these races is given for each parasite in the following chapters.

In *W. bancrofti*, three races differing in the microfilarial periodicity have been recognized: a nocturnally periodic race distributed widely throughout tropical and subtropical zones of the world (with the exception of the Polynesian subregion); a nonperiodic, or more precisely, diurnally sub-periodic race restricted to the Polynesian subregion; and a nocturnally subperiodic race reported in a jungle area in West Thailand. These races take different groups of mosquitoes as the intermediate hosts, and the microfilarial periodicity of each race coincides with the circadian rhythm of the biting activity of the principal vector mosquitoes.

In *B. malayi*, the occurrence of two distinct races, a nocturnally periodic race and a nocturnally subperiodic race, was reported first from Malaya. The endemic areas are geographically isolated, and each takes different mosquito vectors. Some morphological differences have also been pointed out, though these were not absolutely distinctive. Both races were later recorded from a number of areas in southern and eastern Asia.

The microfilariae of *L. loa* in human hosts are diurnally periodic, and are transmitted by a day-biting horse fly species of the genus *Chrysops*. A similar parasite is found in some monkeys dwelling in the same tropical forest areas in Africa. This parasite was shown to be nocturnally periodic, and transmitted by a crepuscular-biting species of *Chrysops*. They are also slightly different in morphological character, such as the size of the micro-filariae. Both races were found to develop well in simian hosts when in-oculated experimentally, and each exhibits its own pattern of microfilarial periodicity in the experimental hosts. Thus, they were found to be geneti-cally different in the periodicity of microfilariae, but not in their affinity for the hosts. Hybrids between the two races could be produced experiment-ally, and they were fully reproductive for further generations. Therefore, these two parasite populations were shown not to be different species in the strict sense, but populations established as different physiological races through natural selection by the behavior of the intermediate and the final hosts.

1.2.2.3. Ecological types

Endemic areas of filariasis are established when the parasite is intro-duced in an area where transmission can be maintained by the presence of sufficient numbers of both the intermediate and final hosts. It has been shown that the same filarial race can develop in different species of inter-mediate hosts which may be ecologically and physiologically quite differ-ent. In such cases, filariasis due to the same species and races occurs in areas associated with different environmental backgrounds.

The nocturnally periodic race of *B. malayi* in southern Asia occurs most frequently in swampy areas, where large numbers of *Mansonioides* mos-quitoes breed. On the other hand, apparently the same race of the parasite is endemic on volcanic islands in East Asia, where another intermediate host, *Aedes togoi*, can find its own breeding place in rock pools on the seacoast. The same parasite is endemic in rice paddy areas in East Asia, where it finds *Anopheles sinensis* as another intermediate host.

Similar but more complicated evidence has been found for the nocturnally periodic *W. bancrofti*. In many areas in the world, this race of the parasite develops in the house mosquito, *Culex pipiens*, which breeds in sewage pools and artificial containers around houses, and thus, is an urban disease. However, this race of filaria also develops very well in many *Anopheles* species, which are usually found in rural areas. Such a rural type of *W. bancrofti* infection is more common than the urban type in Africa and in many regions of Southeast Asia. In the Philippines, this type of filariasis is endemic in many abaca-growing areas. The parasite is mainly transmitted by *Aedes poecilus*, whose larvae breed in leaf axils of the abaca plant.

It should be noted that in at least some of these cases, the parasites which exhibit the same pattern of microfilarial periodicity, but which are transmitted by different species of mosquitoes were shown to be physiologically and genetically different in their adaptation for development in the intermediate hosts. In Africa and Malaya, for example, the *W. bancrofti* race transmitted by *Anopheles* species was shown to be less efficient in developing in *Culex pipiens* than the urban race of *W. bancrofti*. In all of these experimental studies, the differences were of a quantitative nature and thus, they are mostly "incompletely defined races" rather than being completely defined races, such as those based on the microfilarial periodicity.

It is assumed that the parasites have undergone various grades of speciations during the course of evolution. Some of them, such as the two races of *B. malayi* or those of the nocturnally periodic and the nonperiodic races of *W. bancrofti*, are considered to have reached a status of nearly different species. On the other hand, the nocturnally periodic *B. malayi* endemic in Hachijo-Koshima of Japan and Chejudo of Korea, is probably a recent introduction because it is transmitted by a day-biting mosquito, *Aedes togoi*. If the parasite continues to breed many years from now, it may possibly evolve to a diurnally subperiodic race, such as seen in Polynesia.

1.3 Differential diagnosis of filariasis and filariae

Filariasis caused by different species of parasites may be differentiated by the clinical signs, so long as these are characteristic to each type of filariasis. However, the more reliable measure is the detection and identification of the microfilariae. No specific immunological methods have yet been developed with which the infections from different filarial species can be diagnosed.

1.3.1 Differential diagnosis by clinical signs

Filariasis due to *W. bancrofti* and *B. malayi* differs from other types of filariasis in that the adult worms reside in the lymphatic systems and cause various symptoms resulting from acute or chronic inflammation and the blockage of lymph canals. In *W. bancrofti* infection, these appear in the forms of elephantiasis of the legs or hands, hydrocele, and chyluria. In *B. malayi* infection, the urinary and genital systems are rarely affected, though elephantiasis is common. Therefore, it can be roughly stated that the common occurrence of hydrocele or chyluria in an area is a sign of the prevalence of *W. bancrofti* infection, while symptoms of only elephantiasis, but not other clinical lesions, indicate that the disease is due to *B. malayi*. (For details, see Chapter 2.)

For onchocerciasis, there are some typical skin and eye lesions by which the disease can be diagnosed (see Chapter 5). The common occurrence of blindness in villages near rivers and streams is indicative of the endemic areas of onchocerciasis in tropical Africa and the Americas.

Loa loa infection causes a typical skin lesion called "Calabar swelling," and also an eye disease caused by the migration of the adult worm into the conjunctiva. (see Chapter 3.)

In *Dipetalonema perstans*, *D. streptocerca*, and *Mansonella ozzardi* infections, characteristic clinical symptoms have not been recognized. Most workers have considered these parasites to be usually nonpathogenic, while some workers have noticed certain nonspecific and allergic symptoms associated with the infections.

1.3.2 Differential diagnosis by the adult worms

The morphological characteristics of the adult worms are the most important features for determining the taxonomic status of a filarial parasite. Detailed studies have been carried out on the structure of the adult worms of various human filarial parasites so long as the materials were available. However, the adult worms of human filariae are usually difficult to recover from human patients, except in certain specialized cases. The adult worms of human filariae are classified into the following groups by their normal habitat in the human tissues:

(1) In the lymphatics: *W. bancrofti, B. malayi*
(2) In the subcutaneous tissues: *L. loa, O. volvulus, D. streptocerca*
(3) In the body cavity: *D. perstans, M. ozzardi*

Of the above seven species of human filariae, the adult worms of *O. volvulus* have been frequently recovered from skin nodules, especially in areas where the surgical extirpation has been a routine procedure for the treatment. Those of *L. loa* have also been recovered surgically from eye lesions or skin swellings. Those lodging in the lymphatics have been recovered only in specialized studies or on autopsy. The adults of *D. perstans* and *M. ozzardi* are poorly known because they have been found in only one or two autopsy cases. The adults of *D. streptocerca* have not yet been recovered from human hosts.

The above seven species of human filariae all belong to the Family Dipetalonematidae Wehr, 1935, but fall into three different subfamilies: Dipetalonematinae (*W. bancrofti, B. malayi, D. streptocerca* and *D. perstans*), Dirofilariinae (*L. loa*), and Onchocerciinae (*O. volvulus*). (See Table 1-1.) Their adults show morphological characters corresponding to these subfamilies and to their own genera and species.

The genus *Onchocerca* is especially characterized by the structure of the cuticula, which has distinct transverse striations and spiral thickenings. The skin of the adults of all other human filarial species is smooth. The adult Onchocerciinae have short tails, but the tail of the adult Dipetalonematinae is long and more than twice as long as wide at the position of the anus. In the subfamily Dirofilariinae, the caudal alae of the male is well developed, the esophagus is divided into two parts, and the tail is short (YAMAGUTI, 1961).

The morphological characters of the adult of each species are described in following sections. For the differential diagnosis of *Wuchereria* and *Brugia*, see Section 2A.2.2.

1.3.3 Differential diagnosis by the microfilariae

At the present time, the positive diagnosis of a filarial infection can be made only when the microfilariae are detected and identified. There have been a number of studies made on the morphology of the microfilariae, one of the most basic and comprehensive made by FÜLLEBORN (1913). The information along this line was extended by BRUG (1928) and FENG (1933b) for differential diagnosis of the microfilariae of *W. bancrofti* and *B. malayi*. The main characteristics used for the identification are shown in Table 1-3 and Fig 1-1.

Abbreviations: *W.b.* (*Wuchereria bancrofti*); *B.m.* (*Brugia malayi*); *T.f.* (Timor filaria); *L.l* (*Loa loa*); *M.o.* (*Mansonella ozzardi*); *D.p.* (*Dipetalonema perstans*); *D.s.* (*Dipetalonema streptocerca*); *O.v.* (*Onchocerca volvulus*)

Main habitat: the microfilariae of *W.b. B.m, T.f., L.l., M.o.*, and *D.p* are found mainly in the blood, while those of *D.s.* and *O.v.* are mainly in the skin. This difference however, is not absolute; the microfilariae of the former group may be found in skin snips if it contains blood. In rare cases, the skin dwelling microfilariae may be found in blood samples. *W.b.* microfilariae are frequently found in hydrocele fluid or chylous urine. Other microfilariae, especially those of *O.v.*, are found also in urine, hydrocele fluid and lymph nodes. The distribution and density of *D.s.* microfilariae and *O.v.* microfilariae in the skin differs according to the body site; this will be discussed in Chapter 5.

Table 1-3.   Comparison of microfilariae in man.

Species	*Wuchereria bancrofti*	*Brugia malayi*	Timor filaria	*Loa loa*	*Mansonella ozzardi*	*Dipetalonema perstans*	*Dipetalonema streptocerca*	*Onchocerca volvulus*	
Main habitat:	blood, hydrocele fluid	blood	blood	blood	blood	blood	skin	skin	
Periodicity:	nocturnally periodic or diurnally subperiodic	nocturnally periodic or subperiodic	nocturnally periodic	diurnally periodic	non-periodic	non-periodic	non-periodic	non-periodic	
Sheath:	present	present	present	present	absent	absent	absent	absent	
Length:								Small	Large
mean (μ)	260	220	287	275	200	195	210	254	332
range (μ)	244–296	177–230	265–323	250–300	173–240	190–200	180–240	221–287	295–358
Tail shape:	tapers to point	tapers, swollen at caudal nuclei	tapers, swollen at caudal nuclei	blunt truncated end	blunt rounded end	blunt truncated end	bent like a fishhook	tapers to point	
Caudal nuclei:	absent	present (isolated)	present (isolated)	present (terminal)	absent	present (terminal)	present (terminal)	absent	

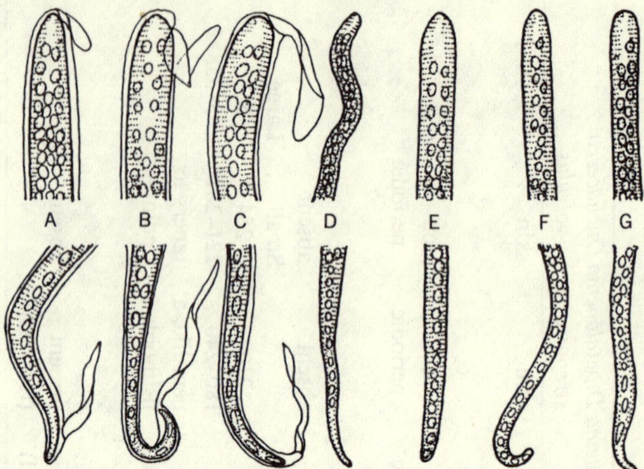

Fig. 1-1. Differential characteristics of head and tail ends of the microfilariae of A. *Wuchereria bancrofti*; B. *Brugia malayi*; C. *Loa loa*; D. *Onchocerca volvulus*; E. *Dipetalonema perstans*, F. *D. streptocerca* and G. *Mansonella ozzardi* (quoted from "Craig & Faust: Clinical Parasitology," 1970, by permission of the publisher: Lea & Fiebiger Co.).

Microfilarial periodicity: the density of microfilariae in the circulating blood may differ greatly according to the hour of day and by the species and race. Those of the nonperiodic or subperiodic races may be detected at any time of day, but in the periodic races, it is necessary to examine the blood during the peak hours. In West Africa, for example, *D.p.* may be detected at any time of day, but it is necessary to take blood at night for the detection of *W.b.*, and at around noon for the diagnosis of *L.l.* For details of the microfilarial periodicity, see Section 11F.

Presence or absence of the sheath: The sheath of microfilariae is a thin and elongated egg shell. The microfilariae of *W.b.*, *B.m.*, *T.f.*, and *L.l.* are encapsulated by a sheath, while those of the other species have no sheath. The presence or absence of the sheath can be clearly seen in fresh specimens. In Giemsa-stained blood smears, the sheath of *W.b.* and *T.f.* is hardly visible, because it does not take the dye, while that of *B.m.* is usually well stained. The sheath of the former group of microfilariae can be demonstrated more clearly when stained with hematoxylin (see Section 10 B,2.3). It should also be noted that the sheathed microfilariae often escape from the sheath while being dessicated in thick blood smears, and thus, the sheath and the naked microfilariae are seen closely set. The percentage of such ex-sheathed microfilariae is usually higher in the periodic race than in the subperiodic race of *B.malayi*; this can be used for differentiating the two races (WILSON *et al.*, 1958).

Body size: The size of microfilariae is sometimes an important and easily distinguished character for differentiating species. For example, the microfilariae of *W.b.* and *D.p.* can be easily recognized in thick blood smears by the size, the former being much longer than the latter. Those of *M.o.* are also very small. *O.v.* and *D.s.* in the skin can be differentiated, also very easily, by the size and shape of the tail. In Asia, the microfilariae of *W.b.* and *B.m.* are sometimes found in the same areas and in the same blood samples, but can be differentiated since the former is longer and more slender. The Timor microfilariae were first recognized as different from those of *B.m.* by being much larger.

However, microfilariae are originally soft-bodied creatures and can lengthen or shorten their bodies while actively moving. Their length and thichness vary considerably according to the method of making preparations. FÜLLEBORN (1913), for example, measured the length of the microfilariae of *Dirofilaria immitis* in the same dog, under various conditions, and gave the following average length: 323.1μ, in fresh blood, stored for 16 days in icebox and examined wet; 314.4μ when fixed in 5% formalin, and the sediment is examined wet; 297.0μ, when fixed in 5% acetic acid and examined wet; 260.0μ, in fresh blood and measured by photography; 258.0μ, in dried thick blood smear; 236.5μ, when fixed in hot alcohol; 149.3μ, when centrifuged in distilled water and dried. Because it was found that the size of microfilariae varies greatly in thick blood smears, depending upon the method of drying, he recommended measuring the length of microfilariae in wet specimens fixed in 5% formalin (see Section 10 B.2.2).

The problem of determing the length and thickness of microfilariae in thick blood smears is especially important. For example, Fülleborn (1908, 1913) pointed out that microfilariae become shorter and thicker when thick blood smears are more slowly dessicated, and thus, recommended prompt drying of the smears. It is, therefore, routine procedure in Japan to dry blood smears with a fan when it is necessary to make a detailed study of the structure.

There have been a number of discussions made on the size of microfilariae examined by the thick smear method, but special care should be taken for the evaluation of the results. GALLIARD & BRYGOO (1955) described a new variety of microfilariae, *Microfilaria bancrofti* var. *vaucelli*, found in thick smears, collected from people on the southeast coast of Madagascar. These microfilariae were similar in structure to *W.b.* microfilariae, but were shorter, thicker, and kinky, similar to those of *B.m.* This was later raised to a specific rank by GALLIARD (1959). However, SCHACHER (1969) conducted detailed morphological studies of these and other microfilariae from various regions of the world, and concluded that the characteristics found by the above workers were probably caused by protracted drying of the blood films, and that the proposed new species was a synonym of *W. bancrofti* (see Chapter 2).

According to the measurements by FENG (1933) of the formalin-fixed specimens, the average, minimum, and maximum lengths of 14 specimens of the microfilariae of *B. malayi* was 269.90μ, 240μ, and 298μ, while those of 23 specimens of *W. bancrofti* were 298.43μ, 274.6μ, and 317.3μ, respectively. In wet smears fixed with hot 70% alcohol and stained in hemalum, the average, minimum, and maximum lengths of the microfilariae of *B. malayi* were 209.84μ, 177.7μ, and 230.8μ, while those of *W. bancrofti* were 269.82μ, 244.6μ, and 296.2μ, respectively. The alcohol-fixed specimens were much shorter than the formalin-fixed ones, and in both methods, the microfilariae of *B. malayi* were significantly shorter than those of *W. bancrofti*, though the difference in length was not an absolute measure for identification. FENG (1933) also stated that if thick smears are slowly dried, or they are too old before they are dehemoglobinized, or the ordinary dry fixation method is employed, the microfilariae in many cases are shrunk; thus, the length of both species of microfilaria may be reduced to half or less than half the length of properly prepared specimens.

The body shape and general appearance: Besides the length and width of the microfilariae, their body shape is sometimes a character useful for identification of the species. For example, as pointed out by BRUG (1927) in his original description, the microfilariae of *W.b.* in ordinary thick blood smears usually show graceful curves, while those of *B.m.* have secondary waves and are kinky in general appearance. In properly prepared smears, such a difference is so characteristic, that the two microfilariae can be recognized at a glance. The same may be said of the difference between the microfilariae of *W.b.* and *L.l.*, but as pointed out by FÜLLEBORN (1914), those of *W. b.* may appear similar to *L.l.* and *B.m.* if the smears are dried too slowly.

The tail: the shape of the tail end of microfilariae is characteristic to each species. For example, the microfilariae of *D.s.* recovered from the skin of people in tropical Africa can be differentiated easily from those of *O.v.* since the former are more slender in diameter and have a curved (fishhook shaped), blunt tail, in contrast to the latter, whose body is thicker, and have a tail which is slender and tapers to a sharp end. This was recognized by MACFIE & CORSON (1922) in their original description of *D.s.*

The microfilariae of *M.o.* and *D.p.* sometimes coexist in the blood of people in the Guianas (South America). MANSON (1897) differentiated the two species by the shape of the tail, the former being sharply pointed, while the latter is blunt.

In the stained blood smears, the microfilariae of *B.m.* have a very slender tail containing two (rarely three) small caudal nuclei. The presence of the caudal nuclei is the most characteristic structure of this species, differing from all other human filariae. *W.b.* microfilariae are devoid of nuclei in the tail end, while those of *L.l.* have nuclei at the tail end.

External structures: As in other nematode embryos or larvae, microfilariae are relatively simple in external structures and lacking in characteristics useful for the identification of the species. Because of the transparency of the cuticle and the small size of some of the appendages, it has been difficult to observe the detailed external structure of microfilariae with ordinary microscopes, but recent developments in the use of scanning electron microscopes have greatly facilitated the demonstration of their true surface structures. The following are the external structures of microfilariae described by previous workers through observations with optical microscopes:

(a) Mouth parts:
FÜLLEBORN (1913) stated that the presence of a mouth and the structure of the surrounding "preputial apparatus", as well as a refractile stilet, were discussed by a number of early workers; however, the drawings made from optical microscopes were, in general, poor and imperfect.

(b) The cuticle:
Early workers pointed out that the cuticles of microfilariae have numerous, fine, transverse striae when naked specimens are examined under high power magnification. BRUG (1927) noted that striation is more conspicuous in the microfilariae of *B.m.* than in those of *W.b.* The size and shape of these striae are clearly demonstrated by electron microscopy.

(c) The tail apparatus:
FÜLLEBORN (1913) described a pair of structures named Schwanzgebilde, stained dark red by eosin and situated at about the junction of the single and double row of the nuclear column of the posterior part of microfilariae of *W.b.* and *L.l.* These were found by FENG (1933) to be larger and more marked in *B.m.* than in *W.b.*

Internal structures: Microfilariae have various internal structures which become visible when properly stained with certain dyes. Their position, size, and shape are characteristic to each species. There are numerous, closely set nuclei through the entire length of the body except for the anterior part (cephalic space), at the position of nerve ring, and near the tail in certain species. The general appearance of the nuclear column differs considerably according to the species. In *W.b.*, for example, the nuclei are generally round and well separated from each other, while in *B.m.* they are oval, overlapping, and difficult to distinguish.

The basic structure of microfilariae for various species of human filariae has been investigated by a number of workers. A standard method for description and measurement of various specialized structures of microfilariae was proposed by FÜLLEBORN (1913) and was followed by most later workers. Certain "fixed points" were designated, and their relative position in percentages to the total length were found to be stable figures for each species, regardless of the variations in the size. The following are the main characteristics useful for the identification of species: (see Fig 1-2).

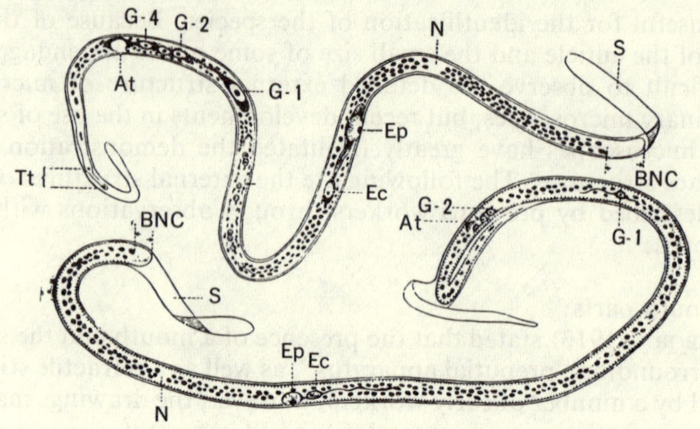

Fig. 1-2. A schematic drawing of the microfilariae of *Brugia malayi* (above) and *Wuchereria bancrofti* (below); from Sasa & Hayashi (1953). AP: anal pore; BNC: cephalic space, and begining of nuclear column; EC: excretory cell; EP: excretory pore; G-1 to G-4: the G-cells; N: nerve ring; S: sheath; TN: terminal or caudal nuclei

(a) The cephalic space:

This is the most anterior part of a microfilaria devoid of any nuclei. The percentage of this space to the total length, as well as the ratio of length to width, sometimes differs greatly among the filarial species. For example, BRUG (1927) noticed a difference in relative length of the cephalic space which was 3.18% average in *B.m.*, about twice as long as that of *W.b.*, which was 1.58% average. Further the cephalic space is longer in the Timor microfilaria, being 4.5% of the total length; moreover, the ratio of length to width is about 3:1, in contrast to 2:1 in *B.m.*, as reported by DAVID & EDESON (1965).

(b) The nerve ring:

This is a part of microfilariae seen in stained specimens as a clear band, lacking nuclei. In the microfilariae of *W.b.* and *B.m.*, it lies at about 20% of the total length, and there are no significant differences in the position.

(c) The excretory pore and excretory cell:

The excretory pore is a structure situated at about 30% of the body length of the microfilariae of *W.b.* and *B.m.* It is seen as an oval body devoid of nuclei in stained specimens. In methylgreen-pyronin stain, the pore stains pink and appears very distinct. In azur II and eosin stain, the wall stains blue and the contents red. The excretory cell is connected to it with a fine tube, situated close to the excretory pore at about 31% of the total body length in *W.b.* In *B.m.*, the cell lies far behind it, at about 37%.

(d) The inner body:

The inner body, or "Innenkörper" of FÜLLEBORN (1908), is a structure

seen most distinctly in formalin-fixed specimens of *W.b.* and *B.m.*, being
more marked in the latter; only rarely is it visible in *L.l.*, *D.p.*, and *M.o.*
It may be clearly demonstrated in fresh specimens vitally stained with neutral red, but less conspicuous in hematoxilin or Giemsa-stained smears.
It is situated at about 40% of the body length, near the G-1 cell, and is assumed to consist of food materials.

(e) The G cells:
The G cells are a group of four cells G-1 to G-4 designated by RODEN-
WALDT (1908) to be the origins of a genital organ. Their relative size and position are characteristic to each species. They are most clearly seen in azur
II-eosin or methylgreen pyronin-stained specimens, but are often difficult
to differentiate from other nuclei in hematoxilin or Giemsa-stained specimens. In the microfilariae of *B.m.*, the G-1 cell is a very large, elongated,
prominent structure, rich in cytoplasm. It has a big nucleus, 8.79μ in average length (Feng, 1933), and its width is more than half the width of the
body; its center is situated at a point averaging 68.33% of total length. The
G-2, G-3, and G-4 cells of *B.m.* microfilariae are also larger than those of
W.b. and about half the size of G-1. They are closely connected to each
other; the distance between G-1 and G-2 is much shorter in *B.m.* than in
W.b. Their positions, on the average, are 73.82%, 76.02%, and 78.42% of
total body length, respectively.

In *W.b.* microfilariae, the G-1 cell is much smaller than that of *B.m.*,
about one-third the width of the body; it has very little cytoplasm. The
G-2, G-3, and G-4 cells in *W.b.* microfilariae are situated farther from
G-1 than they are in *B.m.*; they almost as large as G-1, but smaller than
those of *B.m.*, and well differentiated from each other. Their relative positions are 70.14%, 79.50%, 80.74% and 81.99%, respectively (Feng, 1933)

In *L.l.* microfilariae, the G-1 cell is a large, oval structure, as in *B.m.*,
and sometimes occupies the entire width of the body. Its center is situated
at 68.9% of total body length (FÜLLEBORN, 1913).

(f) The anal pore:
This round or oval-shaped structure is situated at about 82% of total body
length, both in *W.b.* and *B.m.* It is much larger in *B.m.* than in *W.b.* It is
best seen in azur II-eosin or hemalum-stained specimens, and the reaction
is similar to that of the excretory pore. In *B.m.*, both excretory and anal
pores occupy more than half, or nearly the entire width of the body, while
those of *W.b.* are usually about one-third of the body width. In *B.m.*, the
anal pore is situated well behind the G-4 cell, while in *W.b.*, it lies at about
the same position as G-4.

(g) Caudal nuclei:
As stated previously, the difference in the shape of the tail end of microfilariae is an important and sometimes easily recognizable characteristic
for species identification. The presence or absence of nuclei in the tail part,
and if present, their size and shape are sometimes identifying structures

for the species. Among the sheathed microfilariae found in the circulating blood, *B.m.* microfilariae have very narrow tails containing two or three small caudal nuclei, which are situated far apart from the nuclear column. The tail parts of *W.b.* microfilariae are tapering and not as thin as in *B.m.*, they are sharply pointed and devoid of nuclei. On the other hand, *L.l.* microfilariae have a nuclear column continuous to the tail end, and there is a large nucleus situated at the posterior extremity of the body.

Of the unsheathed microfilariae found in the circulating blood, those of *D.p.* are blunt tailed and have nuclei almost to the tail end, while those of *M.o.* are sharp tailed and have no nuclei in the tail part. In the unsheathed microfilariae found in the skin, those of *D.s.* have a curved tail like a fish-hook, with nuclei to near the tip. The tail end of *O.v.* microfilariae are tapered and lacking in nuclei, as illustrated by FAUST *et al.* (1970).

1.3.4 Differential diagnosis by the larval stage filariae

Filarial parasites pass three larval stages while developing in an intermediate host. The fully developed third stage larvae are called "mature" or "infective" larvae. The species or species-groups of larval filariae may be identified by the morphology, by the species of intermediate hosts, and by the site of development in the intermediate host.

According to NELSON (1960), at least 150 species of filariae are known; however, the life cycle had been studied in only 38 species. Of these, 23 were shown to complete their development in mosquitoes. Among the human filariae, *W. bancrofti*, *B. malayi*, and probably the Timor filaria develop in mosquitoes. *L. loa* develops in *Chrysops*; *O. volvulus* in *Simulium*; and *D. perstans*, *D. streptocerca* and *M. ozzardi* in *Culicoides*.

The mode of development and the morphology of various developmental stages of filarial larvae can be studied by experimental infections in adequate intermediate hosts. On the other hand, it is necessary to identify the filarial species found in naturally caught intermediate hosts in order to determine natural vectors of a filarial species. Methods for identification and differential diagnosis of filarial larvae are described in the following sections:

In mosquitoes: see	Section 2A.2.4
In *Chrysops*: see	Section 3.3.3
In *Simulium*: see	Section 5.3.3
In *Culicoides*: see	Sections 4A.3.3, 4B.3.3, 4C.3.3

The metamorphosis of filarial larvae developing in the body of intermediate hosts has been investigated thoroughly by a number of workers for various species.

In the case of *W. bancrofti* or *B. malayi* larvae developing in mosquito intermediate hosts, the microfilariae ingested with the blood lose the sheath in a few hours, and the first stage larvae penetrate the wall of the midgut and reach the thoracic muscle in the course of several hours. During the next two days they transform into short, sausage-shaped organisms measuring from 125 to 250μ in length by 10 to 17μ in diameter.

By the fifth or sixth day, the tail atrophies to a mere stump, and the intestinal tract and body cavity become differentiated, though the genital premordia are still inconspicuous. Then, the larvae shed their skin and enter the second stage, where they measure from 200 to 300μ in length and 15 to 30μ in diameter. The second ecdysis takes place, under optimal conditions, on the tenth or eleventh day, and the worms rapidly elongate into the filiform third stage larvae, measuring approximately 1,400μ by 20μ. The course of such a metamorphosis was studied in detail by KOBAYASHI (1940, 1941) for *W. bancrofti* and by FENG (1936) for *B. malayi*.

1.4 Vectors of human filariasis

The known vectors of human filariae are bloodsucking insects of the Order Diptera, belonging to the following four families:

> Culicidae (mosquitoes): *Wuchereria bancrofti* and *Brugia malayi* (see Chapter 2)
> Simuliidae (black flies): *Onchocerca volvulus* (see Chapter 5)
> Certopogonidae (biting midges): *Dipetalonema perstans* and *D. streptocerca* (see Chapter 4)
> Tabanidae (horse flies): *Loa loa* (see Chapter 3)

It should be noted that the above groups of bloodsucking insects may also serve as vectors of animal filariae; thus, filarial larvae found in naturally caught specimens are not necessarily of human origin. Some animal filariae are known to be transmitted by insects other than the above four families, or by acarines.; for example, fleas are the vectors of *Dirofilaria repens* of dogs, the tropical rat mite is the vector of *Litomsoides carinii* in cotton rats, and the soft tick, *Ornithodoros* spp., is the vector of *Dipetalonema witei* in gerbiles.

2 | Filariasis Due to *Wuchereria* and *Brugia*

2A. The Genera *Wuchereria* and *Brugia*

2A.1 Taxonomic status

As stated before, the filarial parasites of the genus *Wuchereria* and *Brugia* are closely related and share a number of important characteristics. They can be easily differentiated from other human filariae by their morphology, physiology, and pathogenicity. Their adults usually live in the lymphatics; the microfilariae are sheathed, appear in the peripheral blood, exhibit nocturnal periodicity (except in the South Pacific), and the larval development takes place in mosquitoes. The clinical signs caused by the parasites are also similar: recurrent attacks of lymphangitis, fever in the acute stage, and lymphoedema or elephantiasis in the chronic stage. The effect of diethylcarbamazine (DEC) in *Wuchereria* and *Brugia* infections has also been shown to be quite similar.

The taxonomic status of the human parasite described by BRUG (1927), based mainly on the morphology of microfilariae, by the scientific name of *Filaria malayi*, remained uncertain until RAO & MAPLESTONE (1940) discovered the adults in a cyst of a human case in India. The authors placed the two species into the genus *Wuchereria*, because they considered the adults to be very similar to those of *bancrofti*.

Much more information has since been added to the taxonomy of the *malayi*-group of filariae. BUCKLEY & EDESON (1956) gave a comprehensive description of the adult morphology of *malayi* with materials collected from animals in Malaya. An additional two species of the *malayi*-group were discovered from animals: *pahangi* from Malaya and *patei* from Africa. Based on the study of these materials, BUCKLEY (1960) created a new genus, *Brugia*, for the *malayi*-group of filariae.

In our present concept, the genus *Wuchereria* contains only a single species, *bancrofti*, which is exclusively parasitic in man. On the other hand, a number of species parasitic in animals which fall in the genus *Brugia*, have since been recorded (see Section 2C.4.4). The decision as to whether a filarial parasite belongs to the genus *Wuchereria* or *Brugia* can be made, as a rule, by studying the morphology of adults, microfilariae, and infective larvae in mosquitoes; identification of the species within the genus *Brugia* is based usually on adult morphology.

In creating the genus *Brugia* with the separation of the three species from *Wuchereria*, BUCKLEY (1960) pointed out the following characteristics:

1) The microfilariae of *Brugia malayi*, *B. pahangi*, and *B. patei* are all alike, and it is difficult to differentiate them. All three are morphologically quite distinct from the microfilariae of *W. bancrofti*.

2) The left spicule in the three species of *Brugia* is characterized by a rather complex center section; in *Wuchereria*, it is a simple structure.

3) The caudal papillae in the three species of *Brugia* are relatively few in number. In the anal region, there is typically a total of 11, comprised of: four pairs of ventrolaterals, two postanals, and one large preanal papilla. In *Wuchereria*, the anal papillae number about 24, consisting of: 9 to 12 ventrolaterals on each side, two postanals, and one preanal papilla. In addition to the group of anal papillae, there are two papillae (typically in *Brugia* and about four in *Wuchereria* situated between the anal papillae and the tip of the tail.

4) The three species of *Brugia* are relatively small in size. The maximum length of a female is about 60 mm, and the maximum width is 190μ; males grow to about 25 mm in length and are less than 100μ in width. In *W. bancrofti*, the females attain 100 mm in length and 300μ in width; males grow up to 40 mm long and about 190μ wide

2A.2 Differential diagnosis

2A.2.1 Clinical Signs

Results of clinical surveys from all previous workers have agreed that clinical lesions in *B. malayi* infection are confined to the limbs and appear in forms of lymphoedema or elephantiasis of the legs or hands. The involvement of genital or urinary organs, such as hydrocele, funiculitis, or chyluria, are typical to *W. bancrofti* cases; they are only rarely or never encountered in *B. malayi* cases. Lymphangitis and lymphadenitis, accompanied by fever, are very common in *B. malayi* infection, especially in its acute stage; they are usually more severe and frequent than in the *W. bancrofti* infection. The febrile reaction, which appears in microfilaria carriers after administration of the first dose of DEC, is generally more acute and severe in *Brugia* cases than that seen in *Wuchereria* cases.

2A.2.2 Adults

As stated in the previous section, the adults of *Brugia* spp. can be differentiated from those of *W. bancrofti* by the morphological characters. In males, the structure of the left spicules, as well as the numbers and arrangements of caudal and anal papillae, are characteristic to each species. In females, the genus can be identified by the structure of microfilariae in the uterus and vulva (see also Sections 2A.1, 2B.3.1 and 2C.3.1).

2A.2.3 Microfilariae

Since BRUG (1927) described *Filaria malayi* as a new species, the differential diagnosis of its infection from that of *bancrofti* has been made chiefly by the morphology of the microfilariae. Detailed studies on the comparative anatomies of the microfilariae of the two species were made subsequently by BRUG (1931) in Indonesia, FENG (1933) in China, and HAYASHI *et al.* (1951) and SASA *et al.* (1952) in Japan. For routine identification, the two microfilariae can be rather easily differentiated in blood smears stained simply with Giemsa or azur II solution, but for detailed study of various anatomical structures, special staining agents, such as hematoxylin or methylgreen pyronin dyes are recommended (see Section 10B.2.3). The characteristics which were pointed out by these workers for differentiation of the microfilariae were shown in Fig. 1-2 and Section 1.3.3.)

The comparative measurements of the fixed points presented by FENG (1933) and HAYASHI *et al.* (1951) are shown in Table 2-1.

Table 2-1. Comparison of the relative position (percentage of the total body length) of the fixed points of the microfilariae of *B. malayi* and *W. bancrofti* (for abbreviations, see Fig. 1-2).

Fixed points	*W. bancrofti* (China)*	*B. malayi* (China)*	*B. malayi* (Japan)**
BNC	1.58	3.18	3.82
N	18.77	20.72	22.62
EP	28.95	30.09	31.42
EC	30.75	37.07	37.99
G-1	70.14	68.33	67.17
G-2	79.50	73.82	74.17
G-3	80.74	76.02	76.89
G-4	81.99	78.42	78.83
AP	82.48	82.28	81.64

*From FENG (1933); **From HAYASHI *et al.* (1951)

2A.2.4 Mosquito stage larvae

According to NELSON (1960), at least 23 species of filariae are known to complete their development in mosquitoes. In order to determine the natural vectors of wuchereriasis or brugiasis, it is, therefore, necessary to differentiate the larvae of *W. bancrofti* and *B. malayi* from those of animal filariae which might be found in mosquitoes caught in endemic areas of human filariasis. Comprehensive studies were made on the differential diagnosis of mosquito stage larvae by NELSON (1959, 1960) in Kenya, and by WHARTON (1962) in Malaya (Table 2-2).

Table 2-2. A key to the identification of mature filaria larvae in mosquitoes (after NELSON, 1959, modified by RAMACHANDRAN, 1970).

(1) Caudal papillae or protuberances present	(2)
No caudal papillae	(9)
(2) Length more than 1100μ	(3)
Length less than 1100μ	(6)
(3) Three equal bubble like caudal papillae	*W. bancrofti*
Three caudal papillae of various shapes and sizes	(4)
(4) Terminal or dorsal papilla prominent	(5)
All three papillae poorly developed; anal ratio less than 4.5:	*B. malayi; B. pahangi.*
(5) Terminal dorsal papilla "dog's nose" shape; lateral papillae poorly developed; larva narrows between anus and extremity; anal ratio averages 4.5	*B. patei.*
Terminal papilla large and central; two small lateral sub-terminal alae; anal ratio less than 3	*Setaria equina*
(6) Anus more than 50μ from extremity	(8)
Anus less than 50μ from extremity	(7)
(7) Three small terminal papillae	*Dirofilaria corynodes*
One small terminal papilla with or without two very small subterminal papillae	*Dirofilaria immitis* or *D. repens*
One conspicuous terminal papilla and a pair of smaller less conspicuous subventral papillae	*B. tupaiae*
(8) Three prominent terminal papillae	*D. arbuta*
Two prominent earlike lateral papillae	*Breinlia sergenti*
(9) Length usually less than 1100μ; anus less than 50μ from extremity	*Foleyella* spp.
Length 1000μ-1250μ; anus more than 50μ from extremity	*C. flavescens*

The immature larvae of *W. bancrofti* and *B. malayi* develop in the thoracic muscle of mosquitoes, as do those of *Setaria* spp. On the other hand, *Dirofilaria immitis*, *D. repens*, and *D. magnilarvatum* spend the immature stage in the Malpighian tubules, while *Dirofilaria corinodes*, *Dipetalonema arbuta*, and *Foleyella* spp. develop in the fat body cells of mosquitoes. The third stage larvae of these species can be found in any part of the mosquito body cavity.

In general, it is difficult to identify filarial species by immature larvae. On the other hand, species differentiation can usually be made with mature larvae, except between closely related species, such as *B. malayi* and *B.*

pahangi. The characteristics which have proven valuable in differentiation are:

Body length: The mature larvae of *W. bancrofti* and *B. malayi*, as well as those of *Setaria* spp. are more than 1,100μ in length and can be readily distinguished from those of *Dirofilaria* spp., which are shorter in length.

The position of the anus: The anus is much nearer the caudal extremity in *Dirofilaria* spp. than in *W. bancrofti, Brugia* spp., or *Dipetalonema* spp. The "anal ratio" was defined by WHARTON (1957) as the distance from the anus to the caudal extremity, divided by the breadth of the larvae halfway from the anus to the caudal extremity. In *Dirofilaria* spp., this ratio averages approximately 2, while it is about 4.5 in *W. bancrofti*, and about 4 in *Brugia* spp.

The shape of the caudal extremity: The most characteristic feature for diagnosis is the structure of the caudal extremity. The mature larvae of most filarial species found in mosquitoes are provided with three caudal papillae, though these are lacking in some animal filariae. In *W. bancrofti*, these papillae are conspicuous, subequal in size, and bubblelike. In *B. malayi* and *B. pahangi*, they are ill defined, with broad bases, and only slightly elevated. In *B. patei* of East Africa, the terminal or dorsal papilla is prominent and shaped like a dog's nose, while the lateral papillae are poorly developed. In *Setaria equina*, the terminal papilla is prominent, conical in shape; the lateral papillae are smaller, but well defined. The structures of the caudal part of mature larvae recovered from mosquitoes from the Kenya coast were described by NELSON (1959, 1960), and those from Malaya were illustrated by WHARTON (1962) (Fig. 2-1).

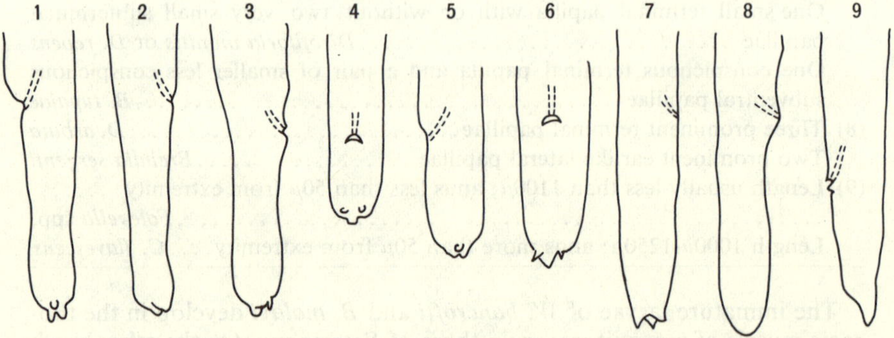

Fig. 2-1.   The shape of the caudal extremities of mature larvae (redrawn from Nelson, 1960).
1. *W. bancrofti* (1175 to 1550μ); 2. *Brugia* spp. (1280 to 1720μ); 3. *Setaria equina* (1280 to 1720μ); 4. *Dirofilaria repens* (640 to 1080μ); 5. *D. corinoides* (680 to 1000μ); 6. *D. magnilarvatum* (960 to 1095μ); 7. *Dipetalonema arbuta* (880 to 1160μ); 8. *Conispiculum guindiensis* (1000 to 1250μ); 9. *Folleyella* spp. (640 to 840μ).

WHARTON (1962) gave accounts on the filaria larvae found in mosquitoes collected in an endemic area of *B. malayi* (subperiodic form), in the swamp forest area of East Pahang. At least eight species of filaria larvae were identified in naturally caught mosquitoes: *B. malayi* and *B. pahangi*, which could not be distinguished morphologically and could be identified only by adult worms recovered after inoculating them into experimental animals; *Dirofilaria magnilarvata* in monkeys; *D. repens* in civets and domestic cats; Types I, II, III, and IV of unknown species, among which I and II are probably *Setaria* species. The biometrical values of these filaria larvae are shown in Table 2-3.

A method for differentiating *B. pahangi* larvae from *B. malayi* larvae was described by BECKETT & MACDONALD (1971). When the infected mosquitoes (*Aedes aegypti* and *Mansonia uniformis*) are examined between five and nine days after being fed on cats harboring the microfilariae of either of the species, the rectal plug of the developing larvae provided a means of distinguishing the two species. In *B. malayi*, it forms a large protuberance and is situated closer to the posterior end of the larvae than in the case of *B. pahangi*. The difference is very marked at five days, but becomes less well defined as the larvae grow older.

2A.3 Physiological races and ecological types

As described in Section 1.2.2, and will be discussed for each filarial species, various physiological races and ecological types have been recognized both in *W. bancrofti* and *B. malayi*. These are summarized in Table 2-4 (also see Sections 2B.3 and 2C.3).

2B. *Wuchereria bancrofti* (Cobbold,1877)

This is the most widespread and common species among human filariae. As stated previously, the adult worms reside in the lymph canals and nodes of man. Frequently, they cause fever and lymphangitis in the acute stage, elephantiasis, hydrocele, chyluria, and other symptoms due to the blockage of lymph systems in the chronic stage. The disease is a serious health hazard and public health problem in many countries in the tropics.

The microfilariae of *W. bancrofti* are found in the circulating blood, hydrocele fluid, chylous urine, lymph nodes, etc. Three physiological races, differing in the pattern of the microfilarial periodicity, have been noted; various ecological types have been differentiated according to the endemic foci, as shown in Table 2-4. Several groups of mosquitoes have been incriminated as important and principal vectors of each ecological type of wuchereriasis.

Table 2-3.   Filarial larvae encountered in mosquitoes from swamp forest areas of East Pahang, Malaya, and their mosquito hosts in nature (after wharton, 1962).

Species (no. measured)	Length Mean (range)	Maximum width Mean (range)	Anal ratio Mean (range)	Terminal papillae	Hosts in nature
B. malayi (88)	1560 (1235–2000)	25 (22–29)	3•9 (3•1–4•7)	Three indistinct and variable	*M. dives, M. annulata, M. bonneae, M. uniformis*
B. pahangi (68)	1520 (1275–1905)	23 (21–27)	4•0 (3•3–4•9)	Three indistinct and variable	*M. dives, M. annulata*
W. bancrofti (22)	1560 (1150–1770)	22 (21–24)	4•5 (3•6–5•0)	Three clear, rounded	*A. leifer*
D. immitis (29)	1020 (860–1150)	28 (27–29)	1•8 (1•5–2•2)	One central terminal knob	*M. dives, M. bounneae, M. annulata, M.(C.) aureosquammata, M. nigrosignata, Aed. (Aed.) hirsutipleura, Aed. butleri, C. annulus*
D. magnilarvata (9)	1025 (960–1110)	25 (24–26)	2•1 (2•0–2•2)	Two subterminal, one terminal pointed	*M. bonneae, M. annulata*
D. repens (12)	990 (825–1110)	24 (22–26)	2•0 (1•8–2•2)	Two lateral, indistinct	*M. dives, M. bonneae, M. annulata, M. nigrosignata*
Type I (20)	1990 (1550–2310)	32 (25–36)	2•6 (2•0–3•0)	One central terminal hook	*M. uniformis, M. dives/bonneae, M. crassipes, M. nigrosignata, A. umbrosus, A. indiensis*
Type II (21)	2495 (2200–2750)	37 (34–47)	2•7 (2•3–3•0)	One central terminal bulbous	*M. uniformis, M. dives/bonneae, M. dives, M. annulata, M. nigrosignata, A. indiensis*
Type III (10)	1235 (1080–1390)	21 (18–24)	5•5 (4•3–7•0)	Two prominent lateral earlike	*C.(Neo.) simplicicornis, C. gelidus, C. bitaeniorgynchus*
Type IV (21)	1675 (1525–1940)	35 (25–42)	2•9 (2•5–3•3)	Two lateral rounded	*M. nigrosignata, M. hodgkini*

Table 2-4. Physiological races and main ecological types of *W. bancrofti* and *B. malayi*.

Species	Physiological race	Main vector	Ecological features	Geographic distribution
Wuchereria bancrofti	Nocturnally periodic	*Culex pipiens* s. 1.	urban or semiurban	nearly cosmopolitan
		Anopheles spp.	rural	Tropical Africa Southeast Asia Papuan region
		Aedes poecilus	abaca-growing area	Philippines
	Diurnally subperiodic	*Aedes (Stegomyia) polynesiensis*-group	semiurban and rural	South Pacific islands (Polynesian region)
		Aedes (Ochlerotatus) vigilax	swampy coast area	New Caledonia
	Nocturnally subperiodic	*Aedes (Finlaya) niveus*	forest villages	Thailand
Brugia malayi	Nocturnally periodic	*Mansonia* spp. *Anopheles* spp. *Aedes (Finlaya) togoi*	open swamp area rice paddy or swamp area rocky coast area	South and Southeast Asia East and Southeast Asia East Asia
	Nocturnally subperiodic	*Mansonia* spp.	swamp forest area	Southeast Asia

A number of national or regional program for the control of *W. bancrofti* infection are in progress. The drug DEC is effective against both microfilariae and adult worms if administered by adequate dosage schemes and in sufficient doses. Its side effects are relatively mild and never dangerous in a *W. bancrofti* infection. Antimosquito measures are also sometimes effective, under certain environmental conditions. Successful results in the control of wuchereriasis have been reported from some South Pacific islands, Japan, and several other countries and regions.

2B.1 Historical notes

The dramatic symptoms caused by the infection of *W. bancrofti*, especially the enormous swelling of legs or scrotum, were recorded in much of the old and ancient medical literature of India, Persia, China, Japan, etc.; they were often referred to as symptoms of *elephantiasis arabicum* by the Western physicians

The embryonic form of the parasite was first discovered and described by DEMARQUAY (1863) in Paris, from hydrocele fluid of patients from Havana, Cuba. The worms were actively moving, and by the absence of internal organs, they were designated as embryos. Three years later, WUCHERER (1866) in Bahia, Brazil, discovered the microfilariae in urine of a patient suspected of suffering from urinary bilharziasis. The same parasite was found by DA SILVA (1868) from hematuria of a Brazilian patient.

The discovery of the microfilariae in the peripheral blood was reported by LEWIS (1872), from a Hindu in Calcutta, India. The parasite was ruled out as being a species of the nematode family Filariidae by BUSK, and the term "*Filaria sanguinis hominis*" was proposed for this parasite.

The adult worm of this parasite had remained unknown until BANCROFT in Brisbane, Australia, found it in a lymphatic abscess on the arm of a Chinese patient on 21 December 1876. The first worm was dead, but later, four live worms, all females, were obtained by him from the spermatic cord of a hydrocele patient.

COBBOLD (1877), in London, received and examined these specimens, and made a short report in a form of "Correspondence to the Editor," which appeared in the 14 July 1877 issue of *Lancet*. In this paper, Cobbold proposed the scientific name *Filaria bancrofti* to this parasite. As for the morphology of this parasite, he only stated: "The worm is about the thickness of a human hair, and is from three to four inches long. By two loops from the centre of its body it emits the filariae described by Carter in immense numbers." Therefore, it is doubtful whether this constitutes a valid description of *Filaria bancrofti* as a scientific nomenclature, even if the paper would have antidated all other scientific names proposed for this parasite. Actually, LEWIS (1877), in the 29 September issue of *Lancet*, gave a comprehensive description with beautiful illustrations of adult worms he recovered in Calcutta on 8 August from a patient of elephantiasis of the scrotum. In this paper, Lewis also claimed that he had already used a scientific name, *Filaria sanguinis hominis*, in describing the microfilariae in his previous papers. Subsequent discoveries of female worms were made in the same year by DA SILVA ARAUJO & DOS SANTOS (1877) in Brazil. The first male was described by BROWNE (1888), with a specimen found in India by SIBTHERPE. The generic name *Wuchereria* was created by DA SILVA ARAUJO, in 1878, when he described the microfilariae found in the blood of patients in Rio de Janeiro, Brazil.

In the meantime, two important facts about filariasis, i.e., the discovery of the mosquito transmission of the parasite, and of the periodicity of microfilariae, were discovered by MANSON (1877, 1879), who was working in Amoy, South China, as a medical officer. His comprehensive reports on filariasis in South China appeared every year beginning 1872 in "China Maritime Customs Medical Reports," published by the Inspectorate General of Customs in Shanghai. His famous report on "The Mosquito Found to be the Nurse" appeared in the 14th issue of this series containing reports for the half year ending on 30 September 1877. By admitting that "the development of filaria cannot progress far in the host containing the parent worms," and that "the embryos must escape from the original host," he considered that the mosquito might be the "nurse" of larval filaria. To test this idea, he procured mosquitoes that had fed on the patient's blood; examining the expressed contents of their abdomens daily with a microscope, he found that his idea was correct, and that the hematozoon, after passing through a series of highly interesting metamorphoses, much increased in size, possessed an alimentary canal, and were otherwise suited for an independent existence.

However, he could not keep the mosquitoes alive for many days, and most of them died about the fourth or fifth day after feeding. In hundreds of mosquitoes he watched, he was successful in finding the last stage filariae in only four instances. Most mosquitoes were found drowned and decayed in water. Thus, for the future history of the filaria, he stated:

> "There can be little doubt as to the subsequent history of the filaria; or that escaping into the water in which mosquito died, it is through the medium of this fluid brought into contact with the tissues of man, and then either piercing the integument, or, what is more probable, being swallowed, it works its way through the alimentary canal to its final residing place. Arrived there its development is perfected, fecundation is effected, and finally the embryo filariae we meet with in the blood are discharged in successive swarms and in countless numbers. In this way the genetic cycle is completed."

Another important discovery made by Manson at almost the same time was the nocturnal periodicity of microfilariae. MANSON (1879) stated:

> "Two years ago, writing on the habits of *filaria sanguinis hominis* (*filaria Bancrofti*), I remarked that in filarial patients the embryos were frequently temporarily absent from the blood. I was not aware at that time of any law governing this. My examinations were usually made in the

early evening or late in the evening, and of the two assistants I employed one worked during the day, the other after 6 o'clock in the evening. I remarked that the former made very few finds in comparison to the latter, but attributed this to accident. Several months ago I gave directions for a filarious patient's blood to be examined daily, and a register to be kept of the examinations. On some day there appeared to be great abundance of filariae, on the other days none, or very few. I noticed that when they were abundant the examination was made on busy days, when there was much work to be done in the hospital, and extra work of this sort had to be got through in the evening; and that when they were absent, the examination was made during the day. Recollecting the different results obtained by my assistants according as they worked during the day or after dark, and suspecting now that this was not altogether accident, I made a series of systematic examinations every four hours in this patient and in others, with the view of ascertaining if this periodicity was maintained in every case. I examined a number of patients in this way, with the results of finding that unless there is some disturbance, filaria embryos invariably begin to appear in the circulation at sunset, their numbers gradually increase till about midnight, during the early morning they become fewer by degrees, and by 9 or 10 o'clock in the forenoon it is a very rare thing to find one in the blood. Till sunset they appear to have completely deserted the circulation, but with the evening they come back again, to disappear in the morning, and so on with the utmost regularity every day and from day to day. The circle is completed every 24 hours, and there are no longer spells of absence, as I at one time supposed, than from morning to evening."

Later, MANSON (1881) published the pattern of microfilarial periodicity in two cases by recording the microfilarial counts at three hour intervals for a period of as long as 23 days, and demonstrated the above stated periodicity in a beautiful chart.

MANSON (1882) made continuous observations of the periodicity of microfilariae in the circulating blood for a 16 day period in one case, 26 days in another case, and for 20 days in the third case. He demonstrated that the periodicity could be converted to the appearance during daytime and disappearance during nighttime by keeping the patients awake during nighttime and allowing them to sleep from morning to afternoon.

The mode of transmission of filarial larvae from mosquito to man was later clarified by experimental studies conducted in Brisbane, by younger BANCROFT (THOMAS LABE) and LOW. BANCROFT (1899) traced the development of filarial larvae in the thorax of mosquitoes; he observed that the development took place efficiently in *Culex ciliaris* (= *C. pipiens fatigans*), but not in *C. notoscriptus* or *C. annulirostris*. He gained the idea that mature larvae in mosquitoes would enter into the human host in the act of biting, such as demonstrated by Ross for malaria. Low was dispatched from London to Australia, in order to confirm the presence of filarial larvae in the proboscises of mosquitoes. By sectioning them in celloidin, it was proved, in one of the first specimens sectioned, that larvae did exist.

The result was published by Low (1900) in his paper "A recent Observation on *Filaria nocturna* in *Culex* and Probable Infection in Man." About this time, Captain JAMES in Travancore, India, was also undertaking research on the metamorphosis of filaria in mosquitoes, and in April 1900, he succeeded in finding larval filariae in the proboscis of *Anopheles rossi* and other species of genus *Anopheles*.

The filarial parasite investigated in these days, by various workers in China, Australia, India, Brazil, etc., was all nocturnally periodic; in fact, Manson called it *Filaria nocturna*. However, occurrence of another form which exhibited no microfilarial periodicity was reported by Surgeon THORPE (1896) from the South Pacific islands. Although the prevalence of elephantiasis in this region had been well noted, its etiology had been almost uninvestigated. The possibility that the parasite found in the blood of natives might not be *Filaria nocturna* was pointed out by MANSON (1894) in his paper on *elephantiasis arabicum* in the South Sea Islands (*British Medical Journal*, 2 June 1894). Thorpe, in Tonga or the Friendly Islands, examined 214 adults during the period from August to December, 1895. In his report, Thorpe stated,

> "At first, the examinations were made at night only, but in October, considering it expedient to make a few control observations in the daytime, I found to my astonishment, that the filariae exhibited no periodicity, but were swarming in the blood practically in as great numbers as at night. The parasite moreover possessed a well-marked sheath, and in general appearance resembled *F. nocturna*. Ninety-six natives were examined both day and night, and with two exceptions, all those with filariae in the blood at night exhibited them in the daytime in equal numbers, and *vice versa*."

After submitting the stained specimens to Manson, they came to the conclusion that no sufficient grounds existed for regarding this filaria as a new species. In a discussion, Thorpe assumed that the periodicity had been altered by habits of the natives of the Tonga Islands, as they "employ themselves in conversation, not only at any time during the day, but also at night; if one wakens, and is not disposed to sleep again, he wakes his neighbour to have some talk."

The occurrence of the "nonperiodic" form of filaria in other islands in the South Pacific, and the fact that its nonperiodic character was independent of the sleeping habits of the Polynesians, but rather dependent on the biting habit of the local vector mosquitoes, were confirmed by later workers. However, as far as wuchereriasis and *W. bancrofti* were concerned, most of the essential facts, except for the discovery of effective measures in the treatment, were elucidated by these pioneer workers before the end of last century. The history referring to these early contributions was described in detail by MANSON-BAHR (1959) in a series of papers entitled "The Story of Filaria bancrofti," (*Journal of Tropical Medicine and Hygiene*, Vol. 62, Parts 1 to 5).

There were remarkable contributions made to the epidemiology and control of filariasis bancrofti after World War II, as summarized in the 'Introduction' of this book. The discovery of diethylcarbamazine (DEC) as a filaricide in animal experiments conducted by HEWITT *et al.* (1947), followed by successful results in the treatment of *W. bancrofti* infections in man by SANTIAGO-STEVENSON *et al.* (1947), were revolutionary events in the history of filariasis research. HAWKING *et al.* (1950) demonstrated a peculiar aspect of the mode of action of DEC on the filarial parasites, i.e., the drug has no direct effect on the parasite *in vitro*, but exhibits an opsonin-like activity in the infected animals.

The first promising results in the control of filariasis bancrofti by mass administration of DEC were reported by KESSEL (1957) from a small island in the South Pacific, where a group of people received the drug once a month for periods of one to two years; remarkable reductions in the microfilaria rates were observed. Through subsequent studies by a number of workers in various endemic foci of the disease, it has become clear that effective control of the infection could be achieved if DEC is administered to the infected populations under adequate dosage schemes, as will be discussed later (see Section 2B.5.3). Remarkable progress has also been made in the methods for epidemiological survey and analysis of the survey data (see Chapter 11).

2B.2 Geographic distribution

W. bancrofti infection in man has been recorded in nearly all countries or territories in the tropical and subtropical zones of the world, with the exceptions of the desert or very dry areas. The disease has been noted also from some temperate zone districts, such as the mainland of Japan, middle China, and some European countries. In Japan, endemic foci have been found to occur up to the snow countries in Aomori, northern Honshu, to a latitude of 42°N.

The following are countries or territories where *W. bancrofti* infection has been reported in the medical literature: (*by clinical signs only)

American Region:
North and Central Americas: United States, *Mexico, *Guatemala, Costa Rica
West Indies: Puerto Rico, Cuba, Virgin Islands, St. Kitts, *Montserrat, Guadeloupe, *Dominica, Martinique, *St. Lucia, Barbados, *Trinidad
South America: *Colombia, Venezuela, Guyana, Surinam, French Guiana, Brazil

African Region:
North Africa: Egypt, Tunisia, Algeria
West Africa: Senegal, Gambia, Guinea Bissau, Cape Verde

Islands, Guinea, Mali, Sierra Leone, Liberia, Ivory Coast, Upper Volta, Dahomey

Central Africa: Niger, Chad, Nigeria, Cameroon, São Tomé, and Principe, Zaire

East Africa: Mozambique, Rhodesia, Zambia, Malawi, Tanzania, Kenya, Uganda, Ethiopia, Sudan

Indian Ocean islands: Madagascar, Comores, Mauritius, Reunion, Seychelles, Chagos

European Region: Italy (Sicily), Yugoslavia (Macedonia), Turkey, Hungary

Asian Region:

South Asia: India, Nepal, Sri Lanka, Maldives, Bangladesh, Burma

Southeast Asia: Thailand, Laos, Khmer, North Vietnam, South Vietnam, Philippines, Malaysia, Singapore, Indonesia, Portuguese Timor

East Asia: China, Hong Kong, Korea, Japan

South Pacific Region:

Australian Subregion (NPWb): Australia

Micronesian Subregion (NPWb): Marianas, Guam, Carolines, Marshalls, Gilberts, Nauru, Ocean

Papuan Subregion (NPWb): Irian Barat, Papua New Guinea, Bismarck Islands, Solomon Islands, New Hebrides

New Caledonian Subregion (DSWb): New Caledonia, Loyalty Islands

Polynesian Subregion: (DSWb) Fiji, Tonga, Rotuma, Ellice Islands, Tokelau Islands, Wallis and Hoorn Islands, Western Samoa, American Samoa, Niue, Cook Islands, Society Islands, Tubuai Islands, Tuamotu Archipelago, Marquesas Islands, Pitcairn

Note:

* known only by clinical cases and lacking in parasitological evidence.

Of the three main physiological races of *W. bancrofti*, the diurnally subperiodic race (DSWb) occurs only in the New Caledonian and the Polynesian subregion, while the race distributed to all other geographical zones is nocturnally periodic (NPWb). The nocturnally subperiodic race (NSWb) has been recorded in a forest tribe in Thailand.

2B.3 The Parasite

The adult worms of *W. bancrofti* live in the lymph canals and lymph nodes of man. The microfilariae produced by female worms appear in the circulating blood, or occasionally in hydrocele fluid or chylous urine. The microfilariae, when ingested by mosquito intermediate hosts, lose their sheaths and penetrate the midgut into the body cavity within a few hours; reaching the thoracic muscle, they develop to the mature larvae in about two weeks. The infection takes place when the mosquitoes containing mature larvae bite a human. It is assumed that about one year is required for the larvae to grow into adult worms, mate, and produce microfilariae in human hosts.

2B.3.1 Adults (also see Section 2A. 1, 2A.2.2)

The adult male worms measure about 40 mm in length and 0.1 mm in diameter, while females measure 80 to 100 mm in length and 0.24 to 0.3 mm in diameter (FAUST *et al.*, 1970). They are creamy white, threadlike worms, with a smooth cuticula. The head has two rings of small sessile papillae. The mouth is unarmed, and lacks the buccal vestibule. The caudal extremity of the male is curved. There are a maximum of 12 pairs (eight preanal and four postanal) of perianal papillae and three pairs of caudal papillae. The copulatory spicules are unequal and dissimilar. The gubernaculum is crescent shaped. Caudal alae are absent. The female vulva opens at the cervical position.

2B.3.2 Microfilariae

Morphology (see Section 1.3.3)
Physiology (see Section 2B.4.3)

2B.3.3 Mosquito stage larvae (see 2A.2.4)

The larvae of *W. bancrofti* pass three stages in a mosquito intermediate host. After being ingested with the blood meal by an appropriate mosquito host, the microfilariae lose their sheaths (or egg shell), penetrate the wall of midgut into the body cavity, and reach the thoracic muscle in several hours to half a day. During the next two days, the larvae metamorphose into a short and thick sausagelike form measuring 125 to 250μ in length and 10 to 17μ in diameter. The development and differentiation of various organs proceed rapidly thereafter, and the first larval skin is shed after five to six days. The second stage larvae, at this point, measure 225 to 300μ in length and 15 to 30μ in diameter. The intestinal canal has become well differentiated, while the genital premordia are still inconspicuous. The second ecdysis occurs on about the tenth day. The worm rapidly elongates into a snakelike mature larva, which measures 1,200 to $1,600\mu$ in length and 18 to 23μ in diameter. The mature larvae leave the thoracic muscle and may be found in any part of the mosquito body cavity (e.g., proboscis, head, thorax, abdomen, legs). When the mosquito takes a blood meal, the infective larvae make their way through the proboscis and enter the skin through the puncture wound.

2B.4 Taxonomic problems

As partly discussed in the previous sections, there have been a number of problems raised in reference to the nomenclature and classification of *Wuchereria bancrofti*. These problems are classified and briefly summarized below.

2B.4.1 Important synonyms

Filaria sanguinis hominis of BUSK (1872), or of LEWIS (1872); a name proposed for the embryonic form (microfilaria) discovered by Lewis in the blood of a patient in Calcutta, India. Description of the adult female worm by the same scientific name was made by LEWIS (1877).

Filaria bancrofti Cobbold, 1877; a scientific name created for the adult worm discovered by Joseph Bancroft in a Chinese patient in Australia.

Filaria nocturna Manson, 1891; a common name used by Manson and other later authors for the nocturnally periodic microfilariae, in contrast to *Filaria diurna* Manson, 1891, which refers to the diurnally periodic microfilariae of *Loa loa*.

Filaria philippinensis Ashburn & Craig, 1906; These authors considered a filaria they found among prisoners in the Philippines as new species, mainly because the microfilariae did not show nocturnal periodicity, and the parasite was apparently nonpathogenic. (This scientific name is now considered a synonym of *W. bancrofti* because all later workers have demonstrated that the microfilariae in man in the same regions of the Philippines are the nocturnally periodic type, the same type as seen in other areas in Southeast Asia. For details, see Section 8B. 6.)

Wuchereria pacifica Manson-Bahr, 1941; the scientific name proposed for the nonperiodic type of *Wuchereria* in the South Pacific region. (To create a scientific name based simply on the difference in the periodicity of microfilariae, and without any morphological evidence, was debated by other workers; see next section).

Microfilaria bancrofti var. *vauceli* Galliard et Brygoo, 1955, and *Wuchereria vauceli* Galliard, 1959; names proposed for microfilariae in man in the southeastern coastal region of Madagascar (see next section).

2B.4.2 Morphological forms

Various morphological forms have been reported to be varieties or sibling species of *W. bancrofti*. These are:

1. *Microfilaria bancrofti* var. *vauceli* Galliard et Brygoo, 1955; from the southeast coast of Madagascar.

2. "Typic form, Type Y, and Type Z" of the microfilariae of *W. bancrofti* were reported by Carvalho (1955) from Recife, Brazil.

3. *Wuchereria lewisi* Schacher, 1969, from Recife, Brazil.

GALLIARD & BRYGOO (1955) described a new variety of microfilariae, *Microfilaria bancrofti* var. *vauceli*, found in thick blood smears collected from the people on the southeast coast of Madagascar (in Manakara, Fort Carnot, Laforano, and Ifaho). These were similar in general appearance to the microfilariae of *Brugia malayi*, and smaller in size than those of *W. bancrofti*. The body was irregularly curved, with secondary waves, but had no caudal nuclei. The authors presented the differential diagnosis of the three forms. This form was later raised to full species status, *Wuchereria vauceli*, by GALLIARD (1959).

SCHACHER & GEDDAWI (1969) and SCHACHER (1969) conducted morphometric and nuclear count studies of materials collected from microfilaria carriers in one of the original type localities of *W. vauceli* in Madagascar; they found no essential difference from specimens of *W. bancrofti* obtained from other regions of the world. SCHACHER (1969) considered that the secondary kinked attitude, described as one of the characteristic features of *W. vauceli* microfilariae, was possibly a result of shrinking caused by protracted drying of the blood film, or delay in dehemoglobinization, and in the light of the overall morphological similarity, *W. vauceli* should be a synonym of *W. bancrofti*.

DE CARVALHO (1955), while conducting epidemiological surveys of filariasis in Recife, Brazil, recognized three different forms of microfilariae of *W. bancrofti*, which differed primarily in the characteristics listed in the following table (Table 2–5). He considered two possibilities: one, the form Y and Z were microfilariae of a new species of filariae, or varieties of *bancrofti*; or two, they could be simple morphological variations of the same species of *bancrofti*.

Table 2-5. Characters for differentiating the three forms of the microfilariae of *W. bancrofti* in Recife, Brazil (after CARVALHO, 1955).

Characters	Typic form	Type Y	Type Z
Ratio between the width and length of the cephalic space	1.10	0.60	0.73
Intermediate width (microns)	7.10	5.65	8.29
Average length (microns)	295.50	316.96	316.21
Average distance between anticedent part and the nerve ring (microns)	53.89	60.07	60.22

SCHACHER *et al.* (1967) and SCHACHER & GEDDAWI (1969) made analyses of the speciation and evolution in *W. bancrofti* by comparing the numbers of nuclei in microfilariae collected from various endemic regions of the world. The mean number and the standard deviation of nuclei between the cephalic space and nerve ring varied from 98.3 ± 3.3 for those from Selangor, Malaya, to 70.1 ± 4.4 for Brazil-y. The specimens from Selangor and Thailand, on the one hand, and from Brazil (subcategory designated "Brazil-y"), on the other, were considered as at least subspecifically different from the remaining groups. Later, SCHACHER (1969) made more detailed comparative studies of the microfilariae from various geographic regions, and created a new species, *Wuchereria lewisi*, for the microfilariae obtained from a man in Recife, Brazil. This corresponded to microfilariae designated as Brazil-y by CARVALHO (1955) and SCHACHER & GEDDAWI (1969). This species was described on a purely morphometric basis, and no account was taken of physiological, ecological, pathological or other biological aspects.

According to the original description of *W. lewisi* by SCHACHER (1969), the microfilariae are nocturnally periodic, sheathed, lying in graceful coils; moreover, the coils are less marked than those of *W. bancrofti* microfilariae and are without secondary kinking (such as seen in *B. malayi*). The somatic nuclei are discrete, oval, overlapping where crowded, but with distinct borders; they are countable; furthermore, the nuclear column stops before the tip of the tail. The mean body dimensions and their standard deviations are: length, 224 ± 18.37μ; cephalic space length, 4.33 ± 0.66μ; cephalic space width, 3.18 ± 0.39μ; body width at nerve ring level, 3.64 ± 0.21μ. The number of nuclei between the end of cephalic space and the nerve ring is 70.06 ± 0.63; the number between the nerve ring and excretory pore is 42.16 ± 0.60. All of these values were found to be significantly smaller than those of *W. bancrofti* microfilariae; however, the measurement data by the "fixed points method" (distance of various organs behind the head expressed as a percentage of total length) did not clearly differentiate the microfilariae of *W. bancrofti* from those of *W. lewisi*. SCHACHER (1969) also concluded, on the basis of studies with both nuclear numbers and morphometric methods, that both *W. pacifica* Manson-Bahr, 1941 and *W. vauceli* (Galliard et Brygoo, 1955) were synonyms of *W. bancrofti*.

2B.4.3 Physiological races

There has been evidence demonstrated of the occurrence of various races within *W. bancrofti* which differ in physiological or genetical characters, but lack morphological characteristics for differentiation. These are generally treated as races in this text, but at least some of them may be regarded as distinct subspecies.

2B.4.3.1 Periodicity of microfilariae

As shown by SASA & TANAKA (1972, 1974; also see Section 11F), the *W. bancrofti* now known to be endemic in the world can be classified into three physiological races by the pattern of the microfilarial periodicity, namely, (1) the nocturnally periodic race found almost all over the tropical and subtropical regions of the world (with the exception of the Polynesian and New Caledonian regions), (2) the nonperiodic (or "a slightly diurnally periodic") race endemic in the Polynesian and the New Caledonian regions, and (3) the nocturnally subperiodic race reported by HARINASUTA *et al.* (1970) from West Thailand.

As stated previously, the nocturnal periodicity of the appearance (or the increase in density) of microfilariae in the circulating blood of hosts was demonstrated first by MANSON (1879) in Amoy, South China. The same phenomenon has been confirmed by later workers from various regions of the world as to be a common character of *W. bancrofti* microfilariae. In the meantime, THORPE (1896) reported that the microfilariae in man in some South Pacific islands could be found in the day blood in almost the same numbers as were found in the night blood of the same patients, and thus lacked periodicity. Later investigators have shown that the same "nonperiodic" form of *W. bancrofti* is endemic in many islands in the South Pacific, and is transmitted mainly by the day-biting mosquitoes of the *Aedes* (*Stegomyia*) *polynesiensis* group (in the Polyneisan region) or *Aedes* (*Ochlerotatus*) *vigilax* (in the New Caledonian region).

The physiological and genetic entity of this form of parasite, as well as its geographical isolation from the periodic form of *W. bancrofti*, has been well established, thus MANSON-BAHR (1941) proposed a new name, *Wuchereria pacifica*, for this nonperiodic form. However, this idea was strongly opposed by LOW (1941), LANE (1942), and BAYLIS (1942) because it was based purely on physiological characteristics and lacked morphological evidence. MANSON-BAHR & MUGGLETON (1952) later designated it as *W. bancrofti* var. *pacifica*.

According to BUCKLEY (1952), the specimens of the adult worms of the nonperiodic form from Fiji and the Pacific islands were smaller than those of the nocturnally periodic form; the average length of six females was 58.6 mm and that of six males was 27.7 mm in these areas, while 16 females from Guyana, the Congo, the Philippines, and Australia were 77.5 mm long in average, and the males were 32.9 mm long in average. It was also noticed that the tail of immature females of the Fijian specimens lacked the bulbous swelling which seemed to characterize females from British Guiana, and the head of the nonperiodic worms *en face* was oval, in contrast to that of the periodic form being subcircular. However, GALLIARD & CHABAUD (1953) compared these findings with a male and female from Tahiti, where filariasis is nonperiodic, and found that the male had a length of 31.5 mm and the female 76.5 mm; furthermore, the tail of female had a bulbous swelling and viewing *en face*, the head was subcircular, not oval. The studies of adult worms by FAIN (1951) and BUCKLEY & SINGH (1965) were also unable to distinguish between the two forms.

Filaria philippinensis Ashburn et Craig, 1906, described as a new species, is almost certainly a synonym of *W. bancrofti*. ASHBURN & CRAIG (1906, 1907) found microfilariae in the blood of four prisoners from Ambos Camarines, Luzon Island. They considered the parasite to be different from

Filaria nocturna (= *W. bancrofti*) in the absence of nocturnal periodicity and by lack of any pathogenicity. However, all later workers in the Philippines have shown that *W. bancrofti* in the same and other regions in this country is nocturnally periodic. It cannot be concluded that the microfilariae observed by these authors were nonperiodic, because the examinations were made with unmeasured blood samples, and only the presence or absence of microfilariae in day and night blood smears were observed. (See Section 8B. 6.)

The occurrence of a nocturnally subperiodic form of *W. bancrofti* was reported by HARINASUTA *et al.* (1970) from Kanchanaburi Province in West Thailand. The endemic area was isolated from other more civilized areas by mountains and jungle, and a species of forest mosquito of the *Aedes niveus* group was attributed to be the vector. By statistical analysis of the microfilaria periodicity survey data reported by the original authors, SASA & TANAKA (1972) estimated that this form represents a population distinct from the previously reported nocturnally periodic type of *W. bancrofti*. (See Section 11F. 5.)

This author suspects that a form of *W. bancrofti* reported by CANET (1950) from an aboriginal race, "Stieng," in a mountainous region in South Vietnam might possibly be the same nocturnally subperiodic form as reported from the forest region of West Thailand, because a positive rate of 30.9% (30 positives out of 97 persons examined) was observed in day blood examinations, in contrast to a rate of 40.9% (47 of 115) in night blood examinations of the same population.

It should also be noted here that the result of a nuclear count study conducted by SCHACHER & GEDDAWI (1969) showed statistically significant differences between the Thai microfilariae and the other groups of *W. bancrofti*.

2B.4.3.2 Compatibility with vectors

Evidence has also been shown for the presence of physiological forms within the *W. bancrofti* complex which differ in their susceptibility for development in vector mosquitoes. In Malaya, WHARTON (1960a) reported that a rural form of *W. bancrofti* in Pahang was about 20 times less efficient in its development in *Culex fatigans* than the urban race of *W. bancrofti* tested at the same time, and that *Anopheles whartoni* was acting as the principal vector of the former race (see Section 8B. 7).

It has been observed by a number of workers in Africa that *W. bancrofti* in rural areas, though being nocturnally periodic, is highly adapted for development in anopheline mosquitoes, but less so in *Culex fatigans* (see Section 2E and 7B, C).

The diurnally subperiodic form of *W. bancrofti* in the South Pacific islands is transmitted mainly by the day-biting mosquitoes of the genus *Aedes*, especially by *Aedes polynesiensis* and related species of the subgenus *Stegomyia*, which are all extremely poor vectors of the nocturnally periodic *W. bancrofti*. MANSON-BAHR & MUGGLETON (1952) found that

Culex fatigans was a poor or incompatible host to the South Pacific form of *W. bancrofti*.

2B.4.3.3 Pathogenesis

There have been some reports suggesting that a race of *W. bancrofti* in certain regions might be lower or higher in pathogenicity. For example, CANET (1950) found relatively high microfilarial rates among the mountain people in South Vietnam, but saw almost no patients showing clinical symptoms. He suggested that this filarial race might be different from the previously known *W. bancrofti* in its pathogenicity (see Section 8B. 5). However, this and similar reports need to be further investigated in order to clarify whether the absence or scarcity of clinical cases is due to the physiological character of the parasite race or to the intensity of infection among the populations.

On the other hand, it is a fairly well-established fact that the ratios and the patterns of the various clinical signs in *W. bancrofti* infections differ between the tropical and the Temperate Zones. It has been shown in a number of reports from the South Pacific islands, India, Sri Lanka and other tropical zones that elephantiasis of the legs is the most common clinical manifestation, while chyluria is extremely rare. On the other hand, reports from Japan and continental China suggest that elephantiasis is rather rare, especially in the Temperate Zone, and chyluria is one of the most commonly encountered symptoms. It is, however, not clear whether such a difference in the pathogenicity originated from the difference in the physiological character of the parasite, or from other factors related to the behavior of the vectors or the human hosts.

2B.4.4 Ecological types

As stated previously (Section 1.2.2.3), *W. bancrofti* has been shown to complete the larval development in various mosquito species. On the other hand, each mosquito species exhibits ecological and physiological characters different from other species, and can maintain its population only in areas where environmental conditions are suitable for its breeding. Therefore, the epidemiological or ecological features differ greatly among the endemic areas according to the species of the main vectors. In the case of *W. bancrofti* infection, the following types have been recognized. More detailed descriptions of the ecology of each mosquito species are given in Section 2E.3.

(a) The *Culex fatigans* type

The nocturnally periodic race of *W. bancrofti* transmitted by mosquitoes of the *Culex pipiens* complex (including the races *pipiens*, *pallens*, *fatigans*, and *molestus*) is the most widely distributed ecological type, and has often been referred to as the "*urban type*" by various authors in contrast to the "*rural type*" of *W. bancrofti* infections transmitted by other more rural mosquito species. *Culex pipiens* (in the wider sense) is a highly domestic mosquito; it breeds mainly in sewage pools and other polluted waters found near human dwellings. The adults bite man mainly inside houses. Its biting habit is a highly nocturnal type. Endemic foci of this type of *W. bancrofti* have been found from almost all over the tropical and subtropical regions, as well as from certain regions in the Temperate Zone (see Section 2B.2; Table 2-4).

(b) The *Anopheles* types

The mosquito genus *Anopheles* contains a large number of species with different behaviors and ecological characters. Some of them are known to be important vectors of human malaria and also of some human and animal filariae. The *W. bancrofti* found in the following regions have been demonstrated to be mainly or partly transmitted by certain species or species-groups of *Anopheles*. It should be noted that in most of these areas, the same anopheline species act as the vectors of both malaria and filariasis, though the geographic distribution of malaria is usually wider than that of filariasis. Because most of the breeding places of anopheline mosquitoes are located in rural environments, this type of filariasis has been referred as "rural filariasis" by various workers.

In tropical Africa: *Anopheles gambiae, An. funestus*, and related species are the principal vectors of *W. bancrofti* in rural areas (see Section 2E.5).

In China: *Feng* (1931) demonstrated that *An. sinensis* was the main vector of *W. bancrofti* in Woosung. This is a species widely distributed in the Orient, and the larvae breed mainly in rice paddies and swamps (see Section 8C.1).

In Malaya: *An. maculatus, An. whartoni*, and several other anophelines were shown to be the vectors of the rural type of filariasis bancrofti (see Section 8B.7).

In the Philippines: *An. minimus flavirostris* was shown to be the main vector of *W. bancrofti* in Mountain Province of Luzon and in Palawan (see Section 8B.6).

In the Papua-New Guinea region: mosquitoes of the *An. punctulatus* group are the principal vectors of *W. bancrofti* (see Section 9C).

(c) The *Aedes* (*Finlaya*) *poecilus* type

The nocturnally periodic *W. bancrofti* endemic in the abaca-growing areas in the Philippines are transmitted mainly by *Aedes* (*Finlaya*) *poecilus*, whose larvae breed in the leaf axils of abaca plant (see Section 8B.6). Mosquitoes of the same subgenus and with similar breeding habits, called "the *Aedes* (*Finlaya*) *kochi* group," have also been proved to be efficient vectors of the diurnally subperiodic race of *W. bancrofti* in the Polynesian zone (see Sections 9E and 2E.3).

(d) The *Aedes* (*Ochlerotatus*) *vigilax* type

Breeding in brackish water swamps a day-biting mosquito called *Aedes*

(*Ochlerotatus*) *vigilax* has been shown to be the main vector of the diurnally subperiodic race of *W. bancrofti* endemic in the New Caledonian zone (see Section 9D).

(e) The *Aedes* (*Stegomyia*) *polynesiensis* type

The mosquitoes of the subgenus *Stegomyia*, genus *Aedes*, are small, active, day-biting species, and those of the *Aedes polynesiensis* group are the principal vectors of the nonperiodic (or diurnally subperiodic) form of *W. bancrofti* in the Polynesian Region. Some other species of the same subgenus, such as *Ae. aegypti* and *Ae. albopictus*, are widely distributed in other regions of the world. Though voracious human biters, they are usually incompatible or poor hosts for the nocturnally periodic *W. bancrofti*.

2B.5 Filariasis due to *W. bancrofti*

2B.5.1 Pathology and symptomatology

The sequential development of filariasis bancrofti may be classified into the following stages:

(a) The biological incubation period (the period from the time of infection to the appearance of microfilariae in the circulating blood): It has been estimated to require a year or more for the *W. bancrofti* larvae introduced in man by mosquito bites to mature in the lymphatics and produce microfilariae. In native populations exposed continuously to the infection by the bites of vector mosquitoes, the youngest age at which the microfilariae may be detected in the circulating blood is usually older than two years, even in the most heavily infested endemic areas.

(b) The patent but symptomless period:
When blood surveys are made on native populations in endemic areas of *W. bancrofti*, there usually exist considerable numbers of people, especially in young age groups, who are completely symptomless, though microfilariae are found in the circulating blood, often in enormous numbers. It is estimated that in such a patent, the symptomless period may last several years, or even throughout life in native populations. For example, a 14-year-old girl examined by the author in Miyako, Okinawa, had over 400 microfilariae per 10 mm³ blood, but was apparently completely healthy and had no enlarged or palpable lymph nodes.

(c) The acute stage:
This is the stage in which frequent attacks of "filarial fever" occur, usually associated with lymphangitis or lymphadenitis, due to inflammatory or allergic reactions to adult worms, or to the microfilariae. Such reactions usually occur on legs, hands, and scrotum. These fever attack and acute

inflammations occur at irregular intervals, and usually become less frequent as the disease becomes more chronic. At the same time, the permanent lesions caused by lymphatic obstructions, such as the swelling of lymph nodes and the thickening of lymph vessels, become more and more evident.

(d) The chronic stage:

The most conspicuous features of clinical symptoms caused as a result of *W. bancrofti* infection are noted in the chronic stage. Such syndromes are called elephantiasis, hydrocele, and chyluria. These lesions are considered to be caused mainly by the blockage of the lymphatics. If the obstruction occurs in the extremities, it results in lymphoedema and then further to elephantiasis of the legs or arms. The blockage of lymphatics leading to the male genital organs causes hydrocele and other acute or chronic inflammations in the scrotum. More serious clinical effects may be caused by the blockage of the abdominal or thoracic lymph vessels, which eventually cause chyluria or hematochyluria of a chronic and often incurable nature. It should also be noted here that, although certain drugs such as DEC might be effective in killing the parasite, the chronic lesions resulting from the infection are mostly incurable.

MANSON-BAHR (1953a) discussed the pathological and clinical aspects of filariasis, based mainly on experiences in the South Pacific. He classified the pathological changes into the following stages:

(a) Incubation period:

The period between the infection and the development of symptoms observed in American soldiers by DICKSON *et al.* (1943), FLYNN *et al.* (1944), KING *et al.* (1944), and Wartman (1947) usually lies between three and 18 months, but can be as short as one month.

(b) The primary or allergic stage:

The earliest lesions described are in glands and subcutaneous tissue where there is edema and eosinophilic infiltration of the tissue surrounding young adult worms. This causes lymphangitis, fever, funiculitis, and orchitis, which are the earliest clinical or allergic manifestations. Later, death of the worm can occur when necrosis is found with an infiltration of the tissue with plasma cells, lymphocytes, and macrophages. Later still, epithelioid cells appear with the formation of pseudotubercles, which contain fibroblasts, macrophages, endothelial cells, and even giant cells.

(c) The secondary or carrier stage:

According to NEUMANN (1944), in Samoa microfilariae are not found in the blood until seven years after the first possible infection. In the case of American soldiers infected during the war, MICHAEL (1944) showed that microfilariae were not found in the blood in any of the several thousand examinations. MANSON-BAHR (1953a) considered that it required from two to seven years for the worm to mature, become fertilized, and for the microfilariae to appear in the blood stream.

(d) The tertiary or obstructive stage:

The pathological changes of the later stages of filariasis are caused by the destruction of the lymphatic filter of the lymph glands, with consequent blocking and dilatation of the lymphatics. There is a granulomatous inflammation of the endothelium lining of the lymphatics with eventual occlusion. This has been called obliterative endolymphangitis by BAHR (1912) and has also been described by MICHAEL (1945).

A reaction around the adult worm lying in the lymphatics was shown to be a cause of lymphatic obstruction by BAHR (1912). This lymphatic obstruction can produce extensive lymphatic varices, and when the thoracic duct is blocked, the dilated lymphatics of the bladder and pelvis may rupture with the production of chyluria. As a result of lymphatic obstruction, microfilariae can no longer reach the blood stream, so they remain in the glands. These pathological changes cause elephantiasis, lymph scrotum, varicose groin, and enlargement of epitrochlear glands. A filarial abscess may also develop when infection occurs around a dead filarial worm.

MANSON-BAHR (1953a) classified the clinical manifestations of filariasis bancrofti into the following categories:

Lymphangitis and filarial (elephantoid) fever: These are the earliest symptoms of filariasis. They are represented by fever (associated with lymphangitis) called "mumu" in Samoa, "wanganga" in Fiji, and "kusafurui" in Japan. The fever last several days, is accompanied by rigors and general malaise, then terminates abruptly with profuse sweating. Lymphangitis spreads centrifugally, as a hard cord-like swelling or red superficial streak from the lymph glands, where the adult worms lie. These attacks recur at varying intervals, usually becoming less frequent as the disease becomes more chronic.

Endemic funiculitis and orchitis: These are due to lymphangitis of the spermatic cord and are early symptoms of filariasis. They were the most common clinical manifestations among the American soldiers exposed to the infection in the South Pacific during World War II.

Filarial glandular enlargements: Soft glandular enlargements were the first abnormality noted by THOMSON *et al.* (1945) in soldiers in World War II, and are the most common and earliest sign of the tertiary stage. The most common site is the groin, followed by the epitrochlear region. However, glandular enlargement is not a specific sign of filariasis, and must be differentiated from similar affections due to other causes.

Lympth scrotum: This is a very common manifestation of filariasis bancrofiti, and is a result of lymphatic obstructions in the scrotum formed in the tertiary stage of the disease. The scrotum enlarges and shows a number of varices.

Elephantiasis: This is a manifestation of hypertrophy of the connective tissues, followed by edematous swellings. It most frequently affects the leg, but may also occur in the arms, breast, scrotum, vulva, or any other body part. In general, elephantiasis occurs more frequently in endemic areas of heavy infection, such as in Tahiti and Samoa, rather than in areas with lighter infection. In endemic areas in the Temperate Zone, elephantiasis is usually very rare, in contrast to the common occurrence of hydrocele and chyluria.

The disease starts, at first, with slight enlargement of one leg or arm. The limb increases in size with recurrent attacks of filarial or elephantoid fever. Gradually, the affected part swells and the edema disappears to be replaced by the characteristic rough, elephantlike skin.

Chyluria: This is presumably manifestation of the blockage of the thoracic duct, and is characterized by the discharge of milky or bloody-milky urine, containing fat droplets and protein. The urine often contains a large amount of fibrin and coagulates in the urethra or in the bladder. Chyluria or hematochyluria in filariasis patients often appear suddenly, without previous history of other filarial affections, usually preceded by lumbago or abdominal pains. Chyluria usually disappears spontaneously, but recurs at varying intervals.

Chyluria is, as a rule, a rare clinical manifestation in endemic areas of *W. bancrofti* in tropical regions. For example, MANSON-BAHR (1953a) states, "I have seen two proven cases in Fiji; however, this manifestation is uncommon in Fiji." In Sri Lanka, ABDULCADER & SASA (1966) reported that among 3,407 filariasis cases examined in the filaria clincis, 2,983 had elephantiasis (including lymphoedema), and 422 had hydrocele, while chyluria was found in only two cases. On the other hand, chyluria is generally the most important and frequent clinical manifestation of *W. bancrofti* filariasis in the Temperate Zone; among 111 cases of clinical fiarilasis reported by SHIMONO (1961) from Ehime, Japan, 103 (92.8%) showed chyluria, while there were only 4 cases with hydrocele, and another 4 with elephantiasis.

Ocular filariasis bancrofti:
The inflammation of the eye, associated with the occurrence of adult *W. bancrofti* in the anterior eye chamber, has been described by FERNANDO (1934), WRIGHT (1934), and CHATTERJEE (1954).

The acute symptoms associated with the *W. bancrofti* infection in American soldiers who were exposed to heavy infections during a short period in hyperendemic areas of nonperiodic *W. bancrofti* in the Samoa-Ellice-Wallis areas have been elaborately studied by HUNTINGTON *et al.*, 1944; WARTMAN & KING, 1944; WARTMAN, 1947; and TRENT, 1963. The main symptoms were lymphangitis of an extremity, lymphadenitis proximal to the involved lymphangitis, and acute inflammation of the scrotum and its contents. In no instances were microfilariae found in the circulating blood, within a period of two years after exposure to the infection.

The chronic lesions occurring in the male genital organ such as funiculo-epididymitis, periorchitis, and hydrocele, as a result of the infection with *W. bancrofti*, were studied especially in Puerto Rico by LICHTERBERG & MEDINA (1957), JACHOWSKI *et al.* (1962), and GALINDO *et al.* (1962).

2B.5.2 Diagnosis

The diagnosis of *W. bancrofti* infection in man may theoretically be made by the following techniques

    (a) By clinical signs (see Section 2B.5.1)

    (b) By demonstration of parasite, i.e., microfilaria or adult worm (see Section 10A.2)

    (c) By immunological signs.

The details of procedures, and discussions of the reliability of each method are described separately, as indicated above. In general, it can be stated that each diagnostic method has both merits and demerits, in view of sensitivity and specificity.

2B.5.3 Treatment and control

The methods for treatment and control of *W. bancrofti* filariasis may be classified into the three categories: (a) symptomatic treatment of clinical filariasis cases; (b) chemotherapy of human parasite carriers to treat or prevent clinical attacks, and the prevention of infection of mosquitoes, and (c) the reduction of infections in man by vector control. Operations in all these categories are usually necessary in every filariasis control program.

2B.5.3.1 Symptomatic treatment

Most signs of acute filariasis stages, such as the fever attacks, acute lymphangitis and lymphadenitis, acute hydrocele or funiculitis, and lymphoedema of the limbs in early stages, may be cured by chemotherapy for the clearance of the parasite, for example, the administration of DEC at daily doses of 6 mg per kg, several times at daily or weekly intervals. It is, however, necessary to give 12 or more doses of DEC in order to expect a radical cure through the complete clearance of adult worms. Signs of the chronic filariasis stages, such as elephantiasis of the limbs, chronic hydrocele or elephantiasis of the scrotum, chronic discharging sinuses, chyluria or hematochyluria, are usually unaffected or only incompletely cured by chemotherapeutic means, and it sometimes becomes necessary to apply surgical or other symptomatic treatments to relieve the suffering of the patients. Various symptomatic treatments of filariasis have been described in textbooks of clinical tropical medicine such as ADAMS & MAEGRAITH (1964).

(a) Surgical treatment of hydrocele or elephantiasis of the scrotum:
This is often necessary and usually effective with good prognosis. Hydro-

cele sacks are removed together with local lymph varices. During the operation, care must be taken not to hurt the cords or damage the testes, which are usually functional and tied down to the posterior aspect of the tumor. Details of surgical procedures can be found in the appropriate texts.

(b) Treatment of elephantiasis of the legs or hands:
Surgical removal of elephantoid tissues and drainage of lymph, such as by a modified Kondoleon operation, has been practiced by various workers. The results of such surgery have not always been satisfactory; there is sometimes difficulty in closing the skin incisions. On the other hand, a method of treatment of elephantiasis of the lower limbs by pressure banding, such as described by KNOTT (1938), has proved to be effective and is widely practiced in the South Pacific.

(c) Treatment of chyluria:
Chyluria of filarial origin should be treated, first of all, by administration of intensive doses of DEC, such as 6 mg per kg, once a day for a period of three weeks, in order to remove adult worms which might possibly cause obstruction of the lymph canals. In chyluria cases, the microfilariae are usually negative in an examination of the circulating blood, but they are frequently found in the chylous urine. DEC usually has no side effect on chyluria cases, and the fever reaction which frequently occurs in microfilaria carriers is usually not a problem in the treatment of chyluria.

In most patients, the occurrence of chyluria is not continuous, but shows intermittent remission. In other words, the spontaneous disappearance of chyluria or hematochyluria for periods of several weeks to several months, and its reccurrence, is a common episode. Therefore, it is usually difficult to judge whether a treatment was really effective, or it accidentally coincided with the spontaneous cure. Ingestion of large amounts of fat often provokes chyluria, and thus, the patients are generally advised to avoid eating too much fatty food at one time.

The introduction of certain chemicals for the purpose of pyelography has been shown by WOOD (1929, quoted by KITAMURA & KATAMINE, 1953) to be occasionally effective in chylous urine. In reviews by FUTAGAMI *et al.* (1940) and KITAMURA & KATAMINE (1953), the treatment of chyluria patients by injection of 15 to 25% sodium iodide, 15 to 20% sodium bromide, or 1 to 3% silver nitrate into the renal pelvis by catheter has been widely practiced by Japanese urologists. In this technique, a diagnosis by cystoscopy is first made to determine which side of the ureter discharges the chylous urine; then the solution is injected into the renal pelvis by a catheter (No. 5 or 6) with gentle pressure, starting with about 20 ml for the first dose. The treatment is repeated at intervals of two or three days for about ten times, until the chylous urine disappears at least for a certain period. In a statistical study by FUTAGAMI *et al.* (1940) on 368 chyluria cases at Nagasaki University Hospital, 51.5% of the patients treated with this method were judged to have been cured.

Chyluria may be a troublesome, often painful or disabling affliction for its victims, but is usually not an acute fatal disease; therefore, nonsurgical, symptomatic treatment methods are generally recommended. However, in cases with severe symptoms, surgical operations for a radical cure of chyluria or hematochyluria have been practiced in the university hospitals of Nagasaki and Kagoshima, in southwestern Japan. The procedures of the surgical operation and the results were described in detail by KITAMURA & KATAMINE (1953), KITAMINE (1953), and OKAMOTO *et al.* (1956). Because chyluria and hematochyluria is caused by the discharge of lymph fluid into the renal pelvis, as a result of obstruction of the trunk lymph canals in the abdominal and thoracic cavities by the adult filarial worms, surgical removal and clearance of collateral lymph vessels discharging into the renal pelvis, by cutting the surrounding soft tissues, have proved to be effective in most cases, at least for certain periods.

2B.5.3.2 Chemotherapy

There have been three major groups of compounds used in the chemotherapy of *W. bancrofti* filariasis, i.e., diethylcarbamazine (DEC), antimonials, and arsenicals. Since the efficacy and relative safety of DEC in treating various filarial parasites was established both by experimental and field studies, this compound has been used extensively in both the chemotherapy of microfilaria carriers and the mass treatment of the infected human populations. Some arsenical and antimonial compounds were demonstrated to be highly effective against the adult filarial parasites, but these are not recommended for general use because of their toxicity (see Section 10E.1).

(a) Diethylcarbamazine (DEC)

This compound was discovered as an effective filaricide by HEWITT *et al.* (1947) in experimental studies with *Litomosoides carinii* infection in cotton rats, and was also shown to be effective in the treatment of *W. bancrofti* filariasis in man by SANTIAGO-STEVENSON *et al.* (1947). An excellent study was made by HAWKING *et al.* (1950) on the mode of action of DEC on filarial worms. DEC has been used extensively in the chemotherapy of *W. bancrofti* infection, especially after KESSEL (1957) and his colleagues demonstrated that it could be used safely, and was highly effective in mass treatment. Various dosage regimens have been proposed for the effective and safe use of this compound under various conditions. The compound causes febrile reactions when administered to parasite carriers harboring many microfilariae, and this is the main reason that DEC has not yet been able to be used widely in some countries, such as in India. However, such side effects were shown to be caused by the death of the parasite, especially microfilariae; they are not dangerous in the treatment of *Wuchereria* and *Brugia* infections.

Dosage regimens of DEC administration:
Various dosage regimens have been proposed and practiced in the mass

treatment of *W. bancrofti* carriers. In general, excellent results in the control of *W. bancrofti* have been reported from areas where the drug is administered to microfilaria cases or to all the people by single doses of about 6 mg per kg, once a day for 12 times or more. The drug was administered once every day (Japan, Ceylon, Brazil, etc.), once every week (Malaya, some Pacific Islands, etc.) and once every month (Tahiti, American Samoa, Western Samoa, etc.). The cure rate of microfilaria carriers has been generally poor in areas where only small total doses were administered (such as 4 mg per kg, daily, five days, 20 mg per kg in total: India). In comparative studies of the curative effects of DEC administered at various dosage regimens conducted in the Amami Islands, SASA (1963), YAMAMOTO (1965), and KANDA & ISHII (1966) concluded that the most important factor was the total dose to be administered to the individual cases. In order to obtain 80% or higher cure rates, this dose should be at least 72 mg per kg. The effects were not very different for the different intervals between the single doses, whether these intervals were daily, weekly, or monthly. The drug was also shown to be effective when administered in small doses for long periods after mixed in food, drinks, or cooking salt, in reports by KANDA *et al.* (1967) from Japan, HAWKING & MARQUES (1967) from Brazil, and ICMR (1971) from India.

Large, single dose treatment method:

The treatment of *W. bancrofti* and *B. malayi* carriers by the administration of a large, single dose of DEC, such as 1.0 g (20 mg per kg) in adults, has been widely practiced in China and was reported to be easily practicable and effective (see Section 8C.1). For example, CH'EN TZU-TA *et al.* (1959a) in Nanking Army Hospital treated 372 filaria carriers (330 with *W. bancrofti*, 31 with *B. malayi*, and 5 with both) with DEC given by seven different dosage schemes. The largest dosage was 3.0 g a day, and 3.0 g in two days, while the smallest dosage was 1.5 g in ten hours. More or less satisfactory results in reducing microfilaremia were obtained with these regimens. However, more gastrointestinal symptoms, mainly nausea and vomiting, occurred in patients given a large single dose, such as 1 g at a time, while those treated with single doses of 0.5 g or less tolerated the drug well.

CH'EN TZU-TA *et al.* (1959b) further reported that one to two-day intensive DEC treatment, such as four 0.5 g doses given in two days, or four 0.4 g doses given in ten hours, was sufficient to kill adult worms of *W. bancrofti* and *B. malayi*, and render the blood free from microfilariae in most cases.

Single dose DEC treatment was also reported by the EPIDEMIC PREVENTION DEPARTMENT OF FUKIEN (1959). Four treatment schedules were used: one dose of 1.0 g at night, one dose of 1.0 g after lunch, two doses during the day and night (1.0 g before bedtime, and 0.5 g the next morning), and two doses in two nights (1.0 g the first night, and 0.5 g the second night). Among these, the single dose treatment at night was most successful. Of 144 cases thus treated and re-examined, 133 (90%) became negative in microfilaria examinations. Patients with initial microfilaria counts of less than 100 per 20 mm³ showed a higher clearance rate than those with more microfilariae. The single dose treatment given at night was practiced in the Nanp'ing Special Administrative Region on 15,914 *B. malayi* cases; it was not only effective, but also easily accepted by the public. The microfilariae disappeared from over 92% of the cases thus treated, and the microfilariae was reduced by over 97%. In Minch'ing, the microfilariae disappeared from the blood immediately after the treatment in 93.4% of the cases, and three months later, in 96.6% of 90 cases re-examined.

HSIEH *et al.* (1960) reported the results of large single dose DEC treatments conducted on *B. malayi* and *W. bancrofti* carriers in Shanghai (also see Section 8C.1). DEC was given to microfilaria carriers by a single dose of 1.0 g to adults (20 mg per kg in children) at 9 to 10 p.m. The patients were persuaded to sleep after taking the drug, as complete rest could make them tolerate the drug better. Of 186 cases with *B. malayi* re-examined after the treatment, 154 (82.8%) were found negative. Those with lower initial microfilaria counts showed a better clearance rate. Of 1,052 cases with *W. bancrofti* re-examined, 708 (60.4%) turned negative. In this group, those with initial counts of 1 to 5 per 40 mm³ showed a clearance rate of 69%, while for those with initial counts over ten, only 33% became negative. The reactions encountered after the treatment were mainly fever, bone ache, general malaise, nausea, and vomiting. The incidence of those with fever was 86% (295 of 341) in *B. malayi* carriers, and 28% (141 of 505) in *W. bancrofti* carriers, while those with nausea were 39.3% (154 of 341) for *B. malayi* cases and 21.5% (175 of 505) in the *W. bancrofti* group. Other reactions were painless nodules in the scrotum in *W. bancrofti* cases, and erysipelatoid inflammatory indurations in the inguinal region or thigh in cases with *B. malayi*.

The filaricidal effects of DEC on adult worms:
These were described by CH'EN (1964), in China. This action was seen by the appearance of nodules in the lymph vessels. In bancroftian filariasis, these nodules were mainly found in the lymph vessels of the spermatic cords, and less frequently in those of the extremities, while in malayan filariasis they mainly appeared in the lymph vessels of the lower and the upper extremities, especially the inner portions of the thigh and arm, near the inguinal and axillary regions. Occasionally, they could also be seen in the lymph vessels of the trunk. The percentages of nodular reactions after various dosage schedules of DEC averaged 81.3% in bancroftian filariasis and 54.8% in malayan filariasis. The nodules usually appear on the second to seventh day after the first dose for bancroftian filariasis, and on the fourth to fourteenth day in malayan filariasis. They varied in size from 0.3, by 0.5 cm up to 4.0 cm by 5.0 cm, generally about 1 cm by 2 cm. Of 116 nodules surgically removed and dissected, 99 were found to contain from one to twelve (usually three or four) adult worms, both males and females. These nodular formations were shown to be a reaction to

dead adult worms. The nodules were usually absorbed completely in a few months, but occasionally remained as small firm nodules for as long as six months. Very rarely did they result in filarial abscesses. If the amount of DEC was sufficient to kill all the adult worms, there was no nodular reaction after a second course of treatment conducted several months after the first course.

Side effects of DEC:
Since it was used for the first time in *W. bancrofti* cases by SANTIAGO-STEVENSON *et al.* (1947), DEC has been found to cause various side effects or adverse reactions in man when administered for the purpose of treating filariasis. These include general reactions associated with fever, and also gastrointestinal irritation, such as nausea and vomiting. The frequent occurrence of these adverse reactions among the people treated with the drug has been the main reason that the control of filariasis with DEC has not been practiced in some countries, including the world's largest endemic areas in India.

As will be discussed in Section 10E.1, DEC is a compound extremely low in toxicity in itself, and oral LD-50 is 560 mg per kg in mice and 400 mg per kg in rats. HAWKING (1973) stated that it is remarkably safe when given to man, and although hundreds of thousands of people have been treated, no case of death proved to be due to DEC has been reported; the untoward reactions in man may be annoying, but they are never dangerous. In Japan alone, over 100,000 persons carrying the microfilariae of *W. bancrofti* were treated with DEC with no fatal or dangerous case reported.

As clearly demonstrated in a field study conducted in the endemic areas of *W. bancrofti* filariasis in the Amami Islands by SASA *et al.* (1963; see Table 2-6 and Fig. 2-2 and 2-3), the adverse effects of DEC take two essentially different forms each with different origins, i.e., the symptoms caused by the toxic effect of the drug itself, and those caused as a result of destruction of the parasite, especially the microfilariae. The toxic effect results mainly in nausea, vomiting, and other symptoms of gastric irritation; its severity is dependent upon the amount of drug administered at one time, but independent of whether the person is infected with filaria or not. Such symptoms rarely appear in doses such as 0.3 g (6 mg per kg, in adults) of DEC citrate at one time, but occur in most of people when a larger dose, such as 1.0 g is swallowed at one time. On the other hand, the general symptoms, represented mainly by fever and dizziness, occur only in persons carrying filaria; furthermore the attack rate and severity of such reactions are highly correlated to the microfilarial load of patients at the time of the drug administration. The rise of body temperature in persons carrying many microfilariae begins about ten hours after the initial dose of the drug is swallowed, but not immediately after taking the drug. Such a febrile reaction lasts for a few hours to a few days, and subsides gradually, even when subsequent doses are continuously administered. The severity of the fever is rather independent from the amount of the drug taken by the in-

Table 2-6. The attack rate of side reactions after administration of different doses of diethylcarbamazine as classified by the microfilarial densities of the carriers (after Sasa *et al.*, 1963).

Group A. 2mg/kg, Group B. 8mg/kg, Group C. 16mg/kg.

Mf. density for 30mm²	No. of cases observed			NAUSEA AND VOMITING			CHILLI-NESS			BEDRID-DEN		NO COM-PLAINTS	
	A	B	C	A	B	C	A	B	A	B	A	B
				%	%	%	%	%	%	%	%	%
100 & over	17	9	2	23.6	0.0	50.0	53.0	55.6	64.7	66.7	11.8	11.1
50–99	17	5	8	17.7	20.0	75.0	64.7	40.0	59.9	40.0	11.8	29.0
30–49	20	6	9	15.0	33.3	77.8	60.0	50.0	45.0	33.3	10.0	16.7
20–29	13	11	2	0.0	27.2	50.0	23.0	27.2	23.0	36.4	53.9	27.2
10–19	11	16	6	9.1	18.7	66.7	36.4	25.0	18.2	18.7	36.4	56.4
0–9	40	49	31	2.5	12.2	80.6	5.0	14.3	12.5	0.0	87.5	49.0
TOTAL	118	96	58	9.3	15.6	75.9	39.8	25.0	33.9	17.7	44.0	40.6

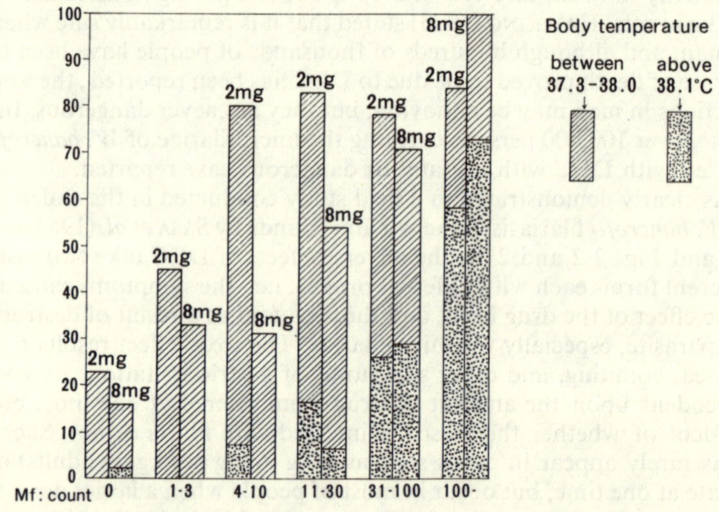

Fig. 2-2. Relationship between the microfilarial counts of the carriers and the fever attack rate after diethylcarbamazine administrations of daily doses of 2 mg per kg (left) and 8 mg per kg (right). (After Sasa *et al.*, 1963).

dividual cases, and occurs even in persons to whom small doses such as 2 mg per kg are administered at one time. Since this is a predictable, transient reaction and never dangerous, it can be easily accepted and tolerated when a thorough health education program is presented to the people in the endemic areas. The persons who carry many microfilariae,

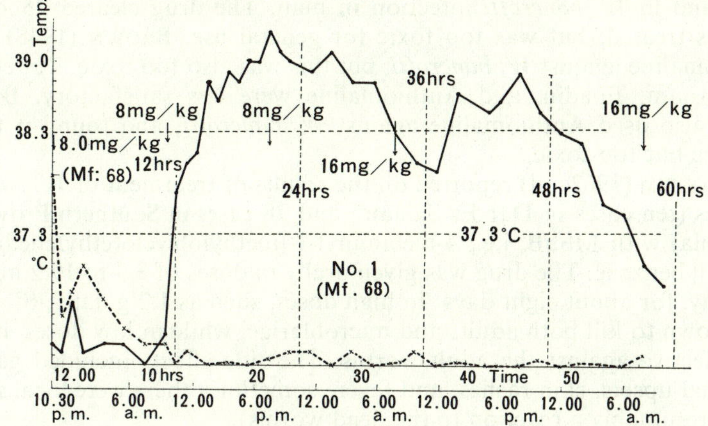

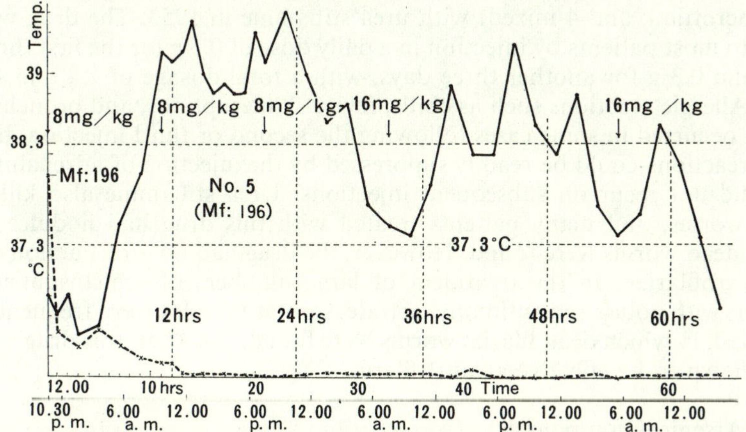

Fig. 2-3. The body temperature and microfilaria density curves in two cases of high density microfilaria carriers during the first three days of intensive treatment with DEC (*W. bancrofti* cases in the Amami Islands; from SASA *et al.*, 1963).

●——● body temperature; ×–––––× relative microfilarial count

such as above 1.0 per mm³ of night blood, should be taken under special care and should be informed that the fever reaction is a sign of cure for them.

(b) Antimonial compounds:

The antifilarial action of antimonials was demonstrated as early as in 1920 by ROGERS, who showed that tartar emetic was effective against *W. bancrofti*. CULBERTSON (1947, 1948) reported the effects of Neostibosan and related antimonials in the chemotherapy of filariasis in experimental animals, and in *W. bancrofti* infection in man. The drug cleared 25 of 35 patients treated, but was too toxic for general use. BROWN (1948) used Anthiomaline against *W. bancrofti*, but this was also too toxic. The effects of Neostam, Fuadin, and Anthiomaline were less satisfactory. Brown (1948) also used Anthiomaline against *W. bancrofti*, and found it to be effective but too toxic.

FRIEDHEIM (1962c, d) reported on the results of treatment of *W. bancrofti* cases (ten cases in Dar Es Salaam, and 78 cases in Southern Province, Tanzania) with MSbB, i.e., 4-melaminyl-1-[methylolcyclo(ethylenedithiastibina)] benzene. The drug was given orally in doses of 8.4 to 19.2 mg per kg a day, for about eight days. In high doses, such as 1.2 g daily, the drug was shown to kill both adults and microfilariae, while in low doses, it was still effective against the adult worms. The side effects included gastrointestinal upsets, skin rashes, and fever; sometimes there were local swellings (presumably a reaction to the dead worms).

CH'EN TZU-TA (1964), in China, treated 40 cases of filariasis (20 malayan, 16 bancroftian, and 4 mixed) with urea stibamine in 1953. The drug was given to most patients by injection in a daily dose of 0.5 g for the first three days and 0.3 g for another three days, with a total dosage of 2.4 g in six days. Allergic reactions such as chills, fever, skin eruptions, and bronchial spasm occurred in some cases following the second or third injection, but these reactions could be readily suppressed by the injection of adrenaline; they did not recur on subsequent injections. Urea stibamine also killed adult worms, and many patients treated with this drug had nodules in which dead worms were found. However, the drug had no direct action on the microfilariae. In the treatment of large numbers of schistosomiasis patients with potassium antimony tartrate, scrotal nodules were frequently observed, in which dead filarial worms were found, and thus, this drug was also shown to be effective against filaria.

(c) Arsenical compounds:

The phenylarsenoxides (such as Sarvarsan) introduced by early workers showed the first successes in the chemotherapy of syphilis and trypanosomiases. OTTO & MAREN (1947, 1949) studied the filaricidal action of a large number of arsenical compounds upon *Litomosoides carinii* in cotton rats and *Dirofilaria immitis* in dogs; they obtained the most promising results with "arsenamide" or (p-carbamylphenylarsylenedithio) diacetic acid.

Treatment of human *W. bancrofti* patients with arsenamide was carried out by various workers (THETFORD *et al.*, 1948; OTTO *et al.*, 1952, 1953; MCFADZEAN & HAWKING, 1954). It was demonstrated that if the compound was given intravenously in doses of 1 mg per kg for 15 days, both the adults and the microfilariae were killed. This treatment was usually tolerated, but toxic effects on the liver were seen in some patients.

Promising results have also been obtained with the melarsen derivatives. FRIEDHEIM (1962a) developed a soluble compound called Mel W (melarsenoxide potassium dimercaptosuccinate), and treated 35 cases infected with

W. bancrofti by intramuscular injection of one to five doses of 10 mg per kg. The compound was shown to be effective against the adult worms, and 28 patients became free of microfilariae within nine months. More extensive use of Mel W was made by McCarthy *et al.* (1962) in the Pacific, and by Van Dijk (1963) in New Guinea.

In all of these reports, it was confirmed that Mel W had excellent macrofilaricidal effects and could cure *W. bancrofti* infection, even with a single intramuscular injection in most cases treated. However, sporadic reports were made by various workers on the serious toxic effect of the compound. For example, Hawking (1973) reported a fatal case. In South America, 150 young male adults carrying microfilariae of *W. bancrofti* were treated with a single dose of Mel W intramuscularly. Half the patients received 7.6 to 9.4 mg per kg (ceiling for total dose was 500 mg). These doses were well tolerated with respect to the immediate reaction. But six days after the injection, one young man began to develop fever, headache, vomiting, and hallucinations. He relapsed into a coma, and died 14 days after the injection. At the post-mortem examination, many areas of petechial hemorrhage were found in the white central substance of the cerebrum and cellebellum, especially in the corpus callosum and occipital lobes.

Mel W was also shown to be effective as a macrofilaricide against *Onchocerca volvulus*, but the occurrence of arsenical encephalopathy has also been encountered (see Section 5.4.4b.3).

According to Ch'en (1964), 23 cases of filariasis were treated in China, in 1953, by intravenous injection of chloroarsen, 0.068 g every three days up to 0.68 g for ten injections. Reaction to the treatment was generally mild; only few patients had high fever and skin rashes, and one patient had bronchial spasms, which was relieved promptly by the subcutaneous injection of adrenaline. Nodules (formed as a result of the death of adult worms) appeared in 16 of 23 cases, and of ten nodules removed, nine contained adult worms.

Subsequently, in August 1953, carbarsone was tried in ten cases of bancroftian filariasis. The dose was 0.5 g, twice daily for ten days. No reaction of any kind was observed in the first six days, but from the seventh day onward until one or two days after the cessation of treatment, nodules appeared in nine cases. When four scrotal nodules were removed and dissected, many adult worms were found. Satisfactory results were also obtained in ten malayan cases. Later, a large scale experiment was carried out on 69 cases (19 malayan, 30 bancroftian, and 20 patients without microfilariae in the blood). The total dosage in ten days was 10 g in 53 cases, 15 g in 9 cases, and 5 g in 7 cases. No toxic reaction was observed. As none of the cases treated with 5 g schedule had nodules, and the number of nodules found in the cases treated with 15 g was not higher than that in the 10 g group, the 10 g dose was considered sufficient for killing adult worms. Between 1953 and 1954, more than 700 cases of filariasis were treated, in China, with 0.5 g of carbarsone and 0.05 g of DEC twice a day for ten days. The results of the combined treatment were satisfactory.

2B.5.3.3 Vector control

The effectiveness of the prevention of infection with *W. bancrofti* in endemic areas by vector control measures has been noted to differ greatly according to the species of vectors involved in the transmission, and also by the environmental and social conditions. In general, the effects of reduction of the population density, longevity, and infectivity of the vector upon the prevalence of filariasis in human populations is much less marked than in the case of malaria, where the control of adult mosquitoes by indoor applications of residual insecticides has caused acute drops in the prevalence and incidence of the disease. OMORI *et al.* (1972), for example, conducted an experimental study on the effects of vector control on the microfilarial rate of people on a small island where no drug treatment had been performed. The microfilarial rate in 1961, before start of the vector control work, was 14.0% (81 positives of 577 persons examined). The rate was shown to drop gradually every year, and it took ten years until the number of microfilaria cases were reduced to only 2 out of 430 villagers examined in 1970 (Table 2-7).

Table 2-7. The reductions in the microfilarial rate and the density from examination of 60 mm^3 blood samples of all people in Nagate Village, Nagasaki, during a ten-year period of continuous vector control, starting in 1961 (after OMORI *et al.* 1972).

Year	1961	1962	1963	1964	1965	1966	1967	1968	1969	1970
No. of persons examined (A)	577	571	567	541	493	515	491	441	447	430
No. of mf. positives (B)	81	71	62	53	39	31	20	9	5	2
% mf. positives	14.0	12.4	10.9	9.8	7.9	6.0	4.1	2.0	1.1	0.5
Total No. of mf. (C)	6,408	4,794	3,851	1,761	1,057	889	402	142	37	24
Mean No. of mf. (C)/(B)	79.1	67.5	62.1	33.1	27.1	28.7	20.1	15.8	7.4	12.0
(C)/(A)	11.11	8.40	6.79	3.26	2.14	1.73	0.82	0.32	0.08	0.06

Spontaneous decreases and natural disappearance of *W. bancrofti* filariasis have occurred in some emdemic areas in the United States, Australia, Egypt, Europe, and mainland Japan, presumably due to the reduction in vector density as a result of improvements in environmental sanitation. However, in humid tropical areas where the transmission season is longer, and the survival rate of vectors is higher than in the above Temperate zone endemic areas, it is much more difficult to expect such an effect from vector control alone. Previous trials for the control of filariasis by indoor spraying of DDT and other residual insecticides have generally proved to be ineffective for various reasons. The control of mosquito larvae by insecticides, such as is practiced extensively in India and Sri Lanka, is also doubtful in its effectiveness in the reduction of *W. bancrofti* filariasis (see Section 10D.3.2).

In our experiences with the control of *W. bancrofti* filariasis, there has been no country in the tropical zones where successful results have been obtained by vector control alone. The extensive use of DEC in the mass treatment of infected human populations has been shown to be a more efficient measure. In general, the vector control activities are considered valuable as a secondary step, assisting the mass drug administration campaigns.

2C. *Brugia malayi* (Lichtenstein, 1927)

Filariasis caused by *Brugia malayi* (LICHTENSTEIN, 1927) is widespread in South and East Asia, but had been confused with filariasis bancrofti until recently. LICHTENSTEIN (1927) and BRUG (1927) reported that the microfilariae found in blood smears collected from humans in a village in Sumatra were morphologically different from those of *W. bancrofti*. They named the parasite *Filaria malayi*. The same form of microfilariae was found to be widely spread in South and East Asia by later workers. The adult form was discovered in a patient in India and described by RAO & MAPLESTONE (1940). The parasite was placed into the genus *Brugia* erected by BUCKLEY (1960) for this, and related filarial parasites found in animals.

The clinical signs associated with filariasis malayi are similar to those found in filariasis bancrofti, but are generally more acute. Fever attacks and elephantiasis of limbs are common, but the involvement of genital and urinary organs is usually absent. *B. malayi* is more susceptible to diethylcarbamazine (DEC) than *W. bancrofti*, but the fever reaction of the host is more severe. The vectors are mosquitoes of genera *Mansonia*, *Anopheles*, and *Aedes*.

2C.1 Historical notes

LICHTENSTEIN (1927), while engaged in studies on epidemiology and transmission of filariasis at Bireuen, North Sumatra, obtained the unexpected result that the microfilariae ingested by *Culex fatigans* did not develop in this mosquito. Filariasis was prevalent in this region, and microfilariae were found in 13 of 57 persons examined at Samalanga, 13 of 23 examined at Garoegoe, 10 of 16 examined at Leuboe, 8 of 12 examined at M. Gloempang Doea, and 26 of 67 examined at Bireuen. The specimens of microfilariae collected at Bireuen were sent to Brug, in Jakarta, for identification. BRUG (1927) examined the microfilariae in thick blood smears and discovered that they differed morphologically from those of *W. bancrofti*, at least by the presence of two or three isolated nuclei in the tail part, and also, that the anal pore was situated farther forward. The parasite was recognized as a new species, distinct from *W. bancrofti* by the morphological characters, by the incompatibility of *C. fatigans* as the vector, and also by the absence of clinical manifestations other than elephantiasis. A scientific name, *Filaria malayi*, was proposed by Brug.

There have been some misunderstandings and confusions about the type locality and the original author of this species. Many people believe that the type locality of *B. malayi* is the Celebes because it is stated in *Craig & Faust's Clinical Parasitology*, "This filaria was first observed by Lichtenstein in its microfilaria stage in blood films of natives of the Celebes and was described by BRUG (1927) as a new species." (1970, 8th ed. p. 376). However, as stated previously, the place where Lichtenstein collected the blood smear was Aceh, North Sumatra.

Another more important problem is the authorship of this scientific name. The papers describing *Filaria malayi* by Lichtenstein and by Brug appeared in *Geneeskundig Tijdschrift voor Nederlandsch-Indië*, 1927, Vol. 67, the former paper in pages 742 to 749, and the latter in pages 750 to 755. Although it has been generally accepted that it was Brug who first proposed the scientific name *Filaria malayi*, this name had been used already by Lichtenstein in the preceding pages, with morphological descriptions of the microfilariae sufficient for differentiation from those of *W. bancrofti*. Therefore, the credit, as the original author of the term *Filaria malayi* should be given to LICHTENSTEIN (1927) in place of BRUG (1927).

As a summary in his original paper describing *Filaria malayi*, LICHTENSTEIN (1927) states:

> (1) It was not successful to infect *Culex fatigans* with the microfilariae occurring in Bireuen; (2) the microfilariae occurring in Bireuen differ from those of *Filaria bancrofti* by the presence of two or three isolated nuclei in the tail end and by the anal pore being situated more anteriorly; (3) the filaria discovered in Bireuen is named, henceforth, *Filaria malayi*; (4) the distribution of filaria in Bireuen, on the northern coast of Atjeh, is very uneven, being scarce in Samalanga but numerous in Peusangan and Gloempang Doea; (5) the filaria in Bireuen does not cause acute filarial disease; (6) elephantiasis occurs very commonly in Bireuen; its distribution is the same as that of the filaria; however, no microfilariae were found in examinations of night blood of 20 elephantiasis patients; (7) only elephantiasis of the leg is observed.

More comprehensive studies on the morphology of the microfilariae and the geographic distribution of this new filaria were conducted by BRUG (1928), BRUG & DE ROOK (1930), and BRUG (1931a, b). Thick blood smears containing microfilariae were collected from various localities of

Indonesia, and *B. malayi* was shown to be widely distributed in Sumatra, Java, Kalimantan, Sulawesi, and a number of small islands of the Indonesian Archipelago, with the exception of Irian (New Guinea). BRUG & DE ROOK (1930), in Sumatra, found that *Mansonia* (*Mansonioides*) mosquitoes were the efficient vectors of this new filaria. The absence of clinical lesions other than elephantiasis of limbs was noted in most endemic areas of *Filaria malayi*.

On the other hand, KORKE (1927–9) in his surveys of filariasis in Bihar and Orissa, India, also recognized the occurrence of an "atypical form" of microfilariae besides the typical *bancrofti* form. In 1929, he reported that this atypical form closely resembled *Microfilaria malayi* as described by BRUG (1927). IYENGER (1932) further observed that the type of filaria occurring in coastal areas of Travancore was different from *W. bancrofti* in other areas of India in the morphology of the microfilariae; also, the chief vector of the Travancore filaria was *Mansonia annulifera* and not *Culex fatigans*. He concluded that the parasite was probably identical with the *Filaria malayi* of BRUG. The occurrence of the same form of filariasis in many other districts of India was confirmed by later workers.

FENG (1933a) conducted a blood survey of prisoners in Amoy, and found *Microfilaria malayi* in a carrier who had come from Chekian Province, China. FENG (1933b) further reported that *Microfilaria malayi* had been found frequently from filariasis cases in this province. He made comprehensive studies on the morphological structures of the microfilariae of *malayi* and *bancrofti*. FENG (1934) demonstrated that *Anopheles sinensis* and *Mansonia uniformis* were the efficient vectors.

The occurrence of *Filaria malayi* was recorded by STRAHAN & NORRIS (1934) from Malaya, and by GALLIARD (1936) from Tonkin, North Vietnam.

Endemic foci of *B. malayi* filariasis were discovered and described by SENOO (1943) and SENOO & LINCICOME (1951) from southern Korea. A small and isolated endemic focus of a periodic form of *B. malayi* was found by HAYASHI *et al.* (1951) and SASA *et al.* (1951, 1952) from Hachijo-Koshima Island, for the first time in Japan. Incidentally, *B. malayi* filariasis on this island was shown to be a new ecological type being transmitted by *Aedes* (*Finlaya*) *togoi*, whose larvae breed mainly in rock pools on the beach. This type of *Aedes togoi*-borne malayan filariasis has been reported to occur also in coastal villages in continental China (GUN, 1960), and also in coastal villages on Cheju Island in southern Korea (Kim & Seo, 1968).

In the Philippines, CABRERA & ROZEBOOM (1964) discovered endemic foci of a subperiodic form of *B. malayi* in Palawan. CABRERA and his associates discovered additional endemic foci from several other islands in the Philippines (see Section 8B. 6).

The adult worm of *Filaria malayi* was first discovered and described by RAO & MAPLESTONE (1940), in India. The authors recovered two males and two females from a cyst on the right forearm of a patient in the Shertalai area in North Travancore, where IYENGER (1938) reported the occurrence of malayan filariasis in large numbers of people. The patient had micro-filariae of *malayi* in the blood, and the fluid of the cyst also contained many microfilariae. The authors found that the adult worms were quite similar to that of *W. bancrofti*, and that the females were practically identical, but recognized slight difference between the two species in the structure of spicules and caudal papillae in the males. They stated: "This worm is practically identical with *W. bancrofti*. The females were quite indistinguishable. In the case of males, when seen side by side, it is obvious that those of the new species are much more delicate than those of *W. bancrofti* and they also lack the distinct transverse corrugations on the stout part of spicules seen in *W. bancrofti*." These authors, therefore, considered that this species should be placed into the same genus as *bancrofti*, and thus proposed to call it *Wuchereria malayi* (BRUG, 1927) RAO & MAPLESTONE, 1940. The adult worms of *malayi* were also recovered and described by BONNE *et al.* (1941) from a human autopsy case in Jakarta, Indonesia.

A series of important contributions to the knowledge of *malayi* and related filarial species were made by workers in Malaya. TURNER & EDESON (1957) and WILSON *et al.* (1958) reported on the occurrence of two distinct patterns of microfilarial periodicity in *malayi* infections, one being nocturnally periodic, and another nocturnally subperiodic. The former is endemic in open rice fields or swamp areas and is transmitted mainly by *Anopheles*; the latter is endemic among inhabitants of forest areas and is transmitted by certain *Mansonia* mosquitoes. Subsequent studies by EDESON & WHARTON (1957–8) and by LAING *et al.* (1960) have shown that the subperiodic form is a zoonosis which also occurs in wild and domestic animals; it can be transmitted experimentally from man to cats and *vice versa*. Another filarial species closely related to *malayi*, and now called *Brugia pahangi* (BUCKLEY & EDESON, 1956), was recovered from cats and dogs in the same endemic areas. EDESON *et al.* (1960) demonstrated this species to be capable of developing into mature adults when inoculated into human volunteers.

The taxonomic status of this group of filarial parasites were revised after the discovery of a number of species parasitic in animals. BUCKLEY & EDESON (1956) provided a detailed description of the adult of *malayi* recovered from a Kra monkey naturally infected in Malaya, and BUCKLEY (1960) created a genus, *Brugia*, for this and two other related species, *B. pahangi* and *B. patei*. Several other species for this genus, from Asia and elsewhere, were later described. (See 2C.4.4)

2C.2 Geographic distribution

Malayan filariasis is a disease endemic exclusively in South and East Asia. Its occurrence has been reported from India, Ceylon, Burma, Thailand, North Vietnam, the Philippines, Malaysia, Indonesia, China, South Korea, and Japan (Table 2-8). The endemic areas extend westward to about 75°E (Kerala, India), northward to 37°N (South Korea), southward to 8°S (Sumba Island, Indonesia), and eastward to 139°E (Hachijo-Koshima, Japan) in East Asia, and to 131°E (Ceram Island, Indonesia) in South Asia. The spread of Malayan filariasis has been apparently barricaded to the north and west by the desert zone, extending from West Pakistan to Mongolia. The temperature is probably another factor that has restricted its distribution northwards beyond the southern parts of Japan, Korea, and China. The borderline of its distribution in southeastern Asia is situated between the Moluccas Islands and New Guinea, as shown in Fig. 2-4, roughly corresponding to the Weber line, which separates the Oriental region from the Papuan region.

Table 2-8. Geographic distribution of the two races of *Brugia malayi* (NPBm: the nocturnally periodic race; NSBm: the nocturnally subperiodic race).

India: Kerala, Andhra Pradesh, Assam, Orissa, Madhya Pradesh, West Bengal; NPBm only
Sri Lanka: NPBm only
Bangladesh: NPBm only
Thailand: southern provinces-both NPBm and NSBm
West Malaysia (Malaya): both NPBm and NSBm
East Malaysia (North Borneo): probably NSBm
Indonesia: Sumatra, Kalimantan, Sulawesi and Ceram; both NPBm and NSBm
Philippines: Palawan, Sulu, Mindanao, and Samar; mainly NSBm
North Vietnam: only NPBm
China: Kiangsu, Anhwei, Chekiang, Fukien, Hunan, Hupeh, Honan, Kwangsi, Kweichow, Szechwan; NPBm only
Korea: Cheju Island and southern districts; NPBm only
Japan: Hachijo Koshima; NPBm only

2C.3 The parasite

2C.3.1 Adults

As stated previously, the adult worms of *B. malayi* in man were first described by RAO & MAPLESTONE (1940) in India, and in the following year by BONNE *et al.* (1941) from Indonesia. A much more complete description was provided by BUCKLEY & EDESON (1956), from a natural infection of a Kra monkey in Malaysia.

The adults of *B. malayi* usually dwell in the dilated lymphatics. According to FAUST *et al.* (1970), mature females vary in length from 43.5 to 55 mm and in breadth from 0.130 to 0.170 mm, while mature males vary in length from 13.5 to 23.3 mm and in breadth from 0.07 to 0.08 mm.

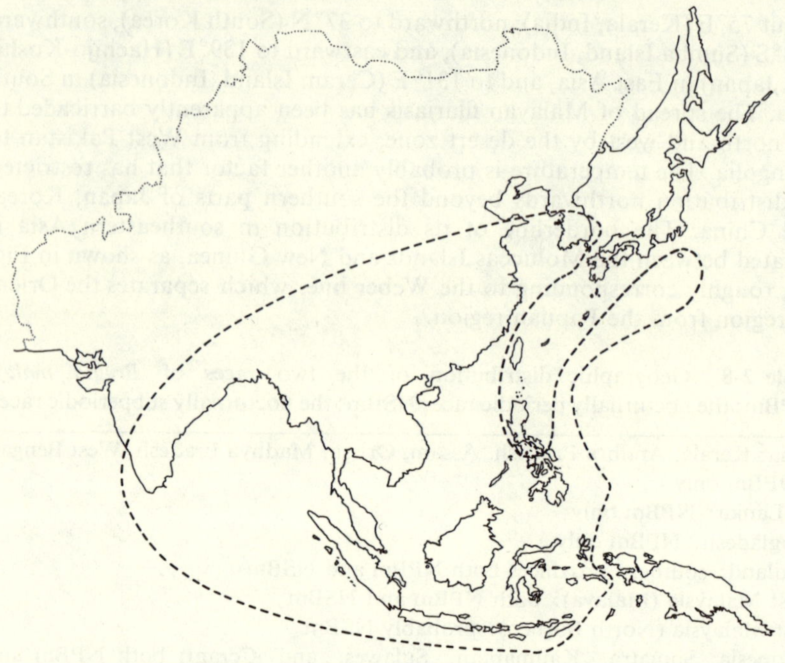

Fig. 2-4. Geographic distribution of endemic foci of *Brugia malayi*.

According to BUCKLEY (1960), in *W. bancrofti*, the female attains 100 mm in length and 0.30 mm in breadth, and the males grow to 40 mm long and 0.19 mm wide.

The anterior end of the adult worm of *B. malayi* has a nonlabiate mouth surrounded by two rows of minute papillae, an inner row of six and an outer row of four, just as *W. bancrofti*; however, larger and more prominent than in *W. bancrofti*.

The female vulva is cervical in position and consists of a transverse slit. The ovejector is folded, and the vagina is a long, double-walled tube with a narrow lumen. The uterus is bifurcated, except for its distal portion. The microfilariae are crowded together in coiled masses within the uterus and the vagina.

The caudal part of the male is coiled, and has certain specialized structures. There are typically 11 papillae in the anal region (four pairs of ventrolaterals, two postanals, and one large preanal); in *W. bancrofti*, these are usually 24 in number. At the tip of the tail, there are four to six small papillae. Midway between the tail end and the adanal papillae, there are usually two papillae (these usually number four in *W. bancrofti*).

Of the two copulatory spicules, the long left one is a complex structure, consisting of three parts, i.e., a proximal tubular portion having a pitted appearance, a short, median, nontubular portion, and a distal, solid, curved rod which extends through the anogenital opening. In *W. bancrofti*, this left spicule is a simple structure. The right spicule is much shorter, curved ventrally, and consists of a proximal tubular half and a narrower, cylindrical, distal portion through which the left spicule runs. There is a crescentic gubernaculum, as in *W. bancrofti*. (For adult morphology also see Section 2A.1.)

2C.3.2 The microfilariae

For morphology: see 2A.2.3
For physiology: see 2C.4.2

2C.3.3 Mosquito stage larvae

The complete development of *B. malayi* larvae from microfilaria to mature stage was observed first by BRUG & DE ROOK (1930) in the *Mansonia* (*Mansonioides*) species. The first comprehensive study of the development and metamorphosis was carried out by FENG (1936), in China, by using *Anopheles sinensis* as the experimental intermediate host. At a room temperature of 29 to 32°C, the microfilariae begin to leave the mosquito midgut and appear in the body cavity about three hours after the infective meal. The migration of the larvae from the midgut to the thoracic muscle is completed in about ten hours, and the larvae reach the mature stage in six to six and one-half days. The development of the larvae includes a shortening of the body from the eighth hour to the 36th hour, and an elongation of the body thereafter to the sixth day. During this time, the larvae pass the first, second, and third stages. Descriptions of the morphology of these developmental stages, as well as the changes in the structures of various organs in the course of development, were beautifully illustrated in the article by FENG (1936).

2C.4 Taxonomic problems

2C.4.1 Important synonyms

The scientific name of this parasite has generally been referred to as *Filaria malayi* Brug, 1927, or *Brugia malayi* (Brug, 1927). However, for the reasons stated in Section 2C.1, the scientific name "*Filaria malayi* Lichtenstein, 1927" evidently has priority over *Filaria malayi* Brug, 1927.

The microfilariae found in humans in Kerala, India, and called by KORKE (1927) the "atypical form," were later shown by IYENGAR (1932) to be identical with the *Filaria malayi* of BRUG (1927).

RAO & MAPLESTONE (1940) proposed, when they first discovered the adult worms in human in India, to place this species in the genus *Wuchereria* because of its similarity in adult morphology to that of *Wuchereria bancrofti* (Cobbold, 1877). However, BUCKLEY (1960) created a new generic name, *Brugia*, with *malayi* as the genotype, and pointed out the presence of essential morphological differences between the adults of *W. bancrofti* and those of the *malayi*-group. Since then, the scientific name *Brugia malayi* (Brug, 1927) has generally been used for this parasite.

2C.4.2 Physiological races

As in *W. bancrofti*, two distinct races, differing in the microfilarial periodicity, are known in *B. malayi* in man, i.e., a nocturnally periodic and a nocturnally subperiodic race. They can be further classified into ecological types according to the principal vector species.

The occurrence of two forms of *B. malayi* differing in the feature of the microfilarial periodicity was first described by TURNER & EDESON (1957), and further by WILSON *et al.* (1958), in Malaya. These workers observed that the microfilariae in the blood of patients from Penang were markedly nocturnal and rarely found during day, while those in patients from Pahang showed some nocturnal rise but were found at nearly all times. The former was highly infective to *Anopheles barbirostris* but not to *Mansonia dives*, while the relation was reversed in the latter. EDESON & WHARTON (1958) further demonstrated that the latter (subperiodic form) could be easily transmitted to some monkeys, cats, and dogs; however, the former (periodic form) did not develop well in animals. In other words, the two forms were found to differ not only in their microfilarial periodicity, but also in their infectivity to mosquitoes and to vertebrate hosts.

According to our present knowledge, the nocturnally periodic form of *B. malayi* is more widespread than the nocturnally subperiodic form. The latter has been recorded to be endemic only from certain swamp forest areas of Malaysia, Thailand, Indonesia, and the Philippines, with the *Mansonia dives/bonneae* group as the principal vector. As a result of statistical analysis of the microfilarial periodicity survey data recorded by previous workers, SASA & TANAKA (1972, 1974) have indicated that the two forms can be clearly differentiated by the values of the "periodicity index." The index is around 90 in the periodic form, in contrast to values as low as about 30 in the subperiodic form (see Section 11F.4).

The main characteristics for differential diagnosis of the two physiological races of *B. malayi* are shown in Table 2-9. The differences in the compatibility of various mosquito species in Malaya to the two races of *B. malayi* and to *B. pahangi* are summarized in Table 2-10.

It has been shown by EDESON & WHARTON (1957, 1958) that the nocturnally subperiodic race of *B. malayi* can be transmitted by mosquitoes from man to various laboratory and wild animals. Cats and some monkeys, especially, were found to be highly susceptible as the hosts of this filarial race. LAING *et al.* (1961) further demonstrated that the subperiodic *B.*

Table 2-9. Summary of the differences between the two races of *Brugia malayi* (after WILSON *et al.*, 1958).

Feature	Periodic form.	Semi-periodic form
Microfilarial periodicity	Markedly nocturnal; micro- filariae rarely found during day.	Some nocturnal rise, but microfilariae readily found at all times.
Microfilarial appearances in Giemsa-stained blood films.	Empty sheaths common; few microfilariae still enclosed in sheath.	Empty sheaths very rare; many microfilariae still enclosed in sheath.
Formalin-fixed microfilariae.	Greater mean length.	Shorter mean length.
Experimental mosquito infections.	Highly infective to *Anopheles barbirostris*; does not develop readily in *Mansonia longipalpis*.	Does not develop readily in *A. barbirostris*; highly infective to *M. longipalpis*.
Natural vectors	*A. barbirostris, hyrcanus*	*M. longipalpis, annulatus, uniformis.*
Experimental infections in cats.	Does not develop well; microfilaria count remains low.	Infections readily established with high microfilaria counts.
Natural infections in cats	Rare	Common
Terrain	Coastal rice fields and open swamps.	Fresh water, swamp forest.

malayi race could be successfully transmitted to golden hamsters, dogs, white rats, and leaf monkeys, by subcutaneous inoculation of infective larvae, and could be maintained for successive generations in these laboratory animals. On the other hand, the periodic race of *B. malayi* was less adapted for development in animal hosts, and its transmission to cats was always characterized by long prepatent periods (95 to 175 days), light or scant microfilaremia, and calcified worms at post-mortem examination. Transmission of the periodic form to hamsters and rats was unsuccessful, but rhesus and leaf-monkeys were found to be relatively good hosts.

From these and other studies conducted by previous workers, it has become clear that the two races of *B. malayi* can be clearly differentiated by various physiological characters; furthermore, the two races are apparently isolated from each other as distinct populations. Although there has been no morphological evidence available for the distinction of the two races, these populations seem to represent at least different "subspecies" in the concept of modern taxonomy.

In this connection, a question arises as to which of the two races represents the type subspecies described first by LICHTENSTEIN (1927) and BRUG (1927) from Bireuen, North Sumatra. BRUG (1928) stated that the periodicity of the microfilariae of '*malayi*' was less conspicuous than that of *bancrofti*, but all the periodicity studies by this and later workers in Indonesia were conducted in endemic areas other than the type locality. Therefore, an expedition for the resurvey of the type locality of *B. malayi* was conducted recently by a joint team of Indonesian and Japanese workers. Altogether five *B. malayi* carriers and one *W. bancrofti* carriers were examined, in August 1974, at Bireuen, by taking 60 mm³ blood samples at two-hour intervals over a period of 24 hours. The microfilariae of *B. malayi* and *W. bancrofti* studied on this occasion were both shown to be the nocturnally periodic types.

2C.4.3 Ecological types

There have been at least three ecological types of *B. malayi* infections known to occur in East and South Asia; each is characterized by the breeding habits of the main vector species. Of the two physiological races of *B. malayi*, the nocturnally subperiodic race is apparently represented only by the swamp forest type transmitted by the *Mansonia dives/bonneae* group. The periodic form falls into at least two distinct types: the open swamp or rice paddy type transmitted by *Mansonia* and *Anopheles*, and the rocky beach type transmitted by *Aedes togoi*.

(a) The *Mansonia dives/bonneae* type (forest swamp type)

The subperiodic race of *B. malayi* infection has been confirmed to be endemic in West Malaysia, Indonesia, and the Philippines. Most of these endemic areas are the villages in or near swamp forests, where *Mansonia* (*Mansonioides*) *bonneae* and *M. dives* (= *M. longipalpis*) breed abundantly. Natural infections of these species with *B. malayi* were demonstrated in Malaya (WILSON *et al.*, 1958; WHARTON, 1962), and in the Philippines (CABRERA & ROZEBOOM, 1964).

(b) The *Mansonia uniformis* type (open swamp type)

Many of the endemic areas of the nocturnally periodic type of *B. malayi* in South and Southeast Asia have been found to be in open swamp areas where *Mansonia* (*Mansonioides*) *uniformis* and related species (*M. indiana*, *M. annulifera*) breed abundantly and act as the main vectors. This type of endemic foci is usually located in villages surrounded by open swamps and rice paddies; consequently, this type is sometimes indistinguishable from the *Anepheles* type of endemic foci. They are, however, quite distinct from those of the subperiodic race which are usually found in jungle or forest villages.

M. uniformis and related open swamp mosquitoes were shown to act as vectors of the nocturnally periodic *B. malayi* in Penang and Kedah, Malaysia (WILSON & REID, 1951); in Kerala, India (IYENGAR, 1938); in Ceylon (CARTER, 1950); and in China (FENG, 1934).

(c) The *Anopheles* type. (rice paddy type)

Various species of *Anopheles* mosquitoes, which breed mainly in rice paddies, open swamps, and ponds, have been incriminated as the main or secondary vectors of the periodic race of *B. malayi*. In some endemic areas, both *Mansonioides* spp. and *Anopheles* spp. were shown to be acting as the natural vectors, though their relative importance seemed to differ according to the areas and the seasons.

In Perak, West Malaysia, *Anopheles campestris* was shown to be the vector of the periodic race of *B. malayi* in the coastal rice field areas (REID, 1962). Two other species of the *Anopheles barbirostris* group, i.e., *An. barbirostris* and *An. donaldi*, were shown to be good hosts for periodic *B. malayi* (WHARTON, 1962).

Table 2-10. Comparison of the susceptibility of various mosquito species in Malaya for the development of the three races of *Brugia* (summarized from WHARTON, 1962).

Mosquito species	*B. malayi* periodic race	*B. malayi* subperiodic race	*Brugia pahangi*
Mansonia			
dives	poor	good	poor
bonneae	none	good	none
annulata	poor	good	good
uniformis	good	good	poor
Armigeres			
subalbatus	none	none	good
Anopheles			
campestris	good	none	good
barbirostrus	good	none	good
donaldi	good	none	good

An. barbirostris was also shown to be the vector of periodic *B. malayi* in Indonesia by TESCH (1937) and PARTONO *et al.* (1972).

An. sinensis was reported to be the main vector of periodic *B. malayi* in the rice paddy areas of China (FENG, 1934; MIAO & LIU, 1962), and also in the inland rice paddy areas of southern Korea (KANDA *et al.*, 1974).

(d) The *Aedes togoi* type (rocky beach type)

Aedes togoi (THEOBALD, 1907), a mosquito species which breeds in rock pools on the beach in East Asia, was incriminated as the vector of the nocturnally periodic *B. malayi* in Hachijo-Koshima, Japan (SASA *et al.*, 1952). Endemic areas of *B. malayi* with similar ecological backgrounds have been reported from Cheju Island, South Korea (Kim & Seo, 1968), and from continental China (GUN, 1960). Filariasis malayi of this type is endemic in villages near the coast where large numbers of rock pools exist on the beach.

2C.4.4 Brugia species in man and animals

When the genus *Brugia* was created by BUCKLEY (1960) for separating the *malayi*-group of filariae from *Wuchereria bancrofti*, three species were included in this new genus: *malayi*, *pahangi*, and *patei*. Several additional species (discussed in the following paragraphs) with closely related structures have been discovered and described as members of *Brugia*. They are very similar or indistinguishable in the morphology of the microfilariae. They have been differentiated usually by adult morphology, especially by the structure of male genitalia.

1) *B. malayi* (Lichtenstein, 1927): (Original description in Geneesk. Tijdschr. Nederlandsch-Indie, Volume 67, pp.742–749). Described by the microfilariae in thick blood smears from man in northern Sumatra, and is now known to be widely endemic in South and East Asia. The subperiodic race has been found also in domestic and wild animals in Malaysia.

2) *B. pahangi* (Buckley et Edeson, 1956): (Original description in *J. Helminthol*, Vol. 30, pp. 1–20). Occurs naturally in a wide range of animals in Malaya. It has been experimentally transmitted to a number of animal species, and also to man.

3) *B. patei* (Buckley, Nelson et Heisch, 1958): (Original description in *J. Helminthol*, Vol. 32, pp. 73–80). Found in the lymphatics of cats, dogs, and genet cats on Pate Island, Kenya.

4) *B. buckleyi* Dissanaike et Panamanthan, 1962.: (Original description in *J. Helminthol.*, Vol. 35, pp. 209–220). Found in heart and blood vessels of the hare in Sri Lanka.

5) *B. ceylonensis* Jayewardene, 1962: (Original description in *J. Helminthol.* Vol. 36, pp. 269–280). Found in the lymphatics of dogs in Sri Lanka.

6) *B. guyanensis* Orihel, 1964: (Original description in *J. Parasitol.*, Vol. 50, pp. 115–118). Found in lymphatics of coatimundi in Guyana, South America.

7) *B. beaveri* Ash et Little, 1964: (Original description in *J. Parasit.*, Vol. 50, pp. 119–123). Found in the lymphatics of the raccoon, *Procyon lotor*, in Louisiana, U.S.A.

8) *B. tupaiae* Orihel, 1966: (Original description in *J. Parasitol.*, Vol. 52, pp. 162–165). Found in the lymphatics of the tree shrew, *Tupaia glis*, in Malaysia. The development in the intermediate and the definitive hosts were studied by ORIHEL (1967). MANNING *et al.* (1972) studied *B. tupaiae* in Thailand.

2C.5 Filariasis due to *B. malayi*

2C.5.1 Pathology and symptomatology

Human filariasis due to *B. malayi* has been noted by conspicuous clinical manifestations, which are sometimes similar but basically different from those caused by the *W. bancrofti* infection. In general, the occurrence of acute symptoms, such as fever attacks and lymphangitis, is more frequently encountered in the endemic areas of *B. malayi* than in those of *W. bancrofti*. Lymphoedema and elephantiasis of the legs and hands are common to both, but the absence of involvement in the genitourinary organs, such as funiculitis, hydrocele, and chyluria (common in *W. bancrofti* filariasis), is a characteristic feature of *B. malayi* filariasis.

The course of development of filariasis due to *B. malayi* may be classified as follows:

    (a) Subclinical filariasis
        (a.1) The prepatent period
        (a.2) Patent phase with microfilaremia
    (b) Clinical filariasis
        (b.1) Recurrent adenolymphangitis
        (b.2) Elephantiasis

(a.1) The prepatent period: i.e., the period from infection by the bite of mosquito vectors to the development of microfilaremia, has been determined experimentally to be 76 to 80 days in cats by EDESON & WHARTON (1957). These findings correspond to the age of the youngest microfilaria carrier (three and one-half months) found among the population of endemic areas of *B. malayi* filariasis. Under natural conditions, however, the prepatent period is assumed to be longer because of the various factors which reduce the chance of successful mating of the adult worms (TURNER, 1959).

(a.2) The microfilaremia stage: A proportion of persons exposed to infection with *B. malayi* begin to show microfilariae in circulating blood after some time. These microfilaria carriers are probably symptomless at first, and at least a part of them become spontaneously negative for microfilariae even without developing any clinical symptoms or signs. However, especially in heavy endemic areas, many of them begin to show acute symptoms, and later may develop chronic signs, such as irreversible elephantiasis of the limbs. The microfilariae become, for the most part, undetectable after some years, especially after the patients have developed chronic signs.

WILSON & RAMACHANDRAN (1971) conducted long-term observations on microfilaremia in man and animals infected with the subperiodic *B. malayi*, in East Pahang, Malaysia. A village was selected as the site of a pilot control experiment, and dieldrin house spraying was conducted twice a year from 1955 to 1960. Blood examinations of the villagers were conducted every year from 1953 to 1960. In subjects examined at yearly intervals, the rise to a peak count often took three to four years, while the subsequent decline to a low level or to zero would take five to six years (see Sections 8B.7 and 10A.3).

(b) Clinical filariasis

The course of development of clinical filariasis in *B. malayi* infection may be classified into the two stages: recurrent adenolymphangitis in the acute stage, and elephantiasis of limbs in the chronic stage.

(b.1) The acute stage: recurrent adenolymphangitis

Recurrent episodes of fever with acute inflammation of the superficial lymph nodes and their associated lymphatics are characteristic features of filariasis due to *B. malayi*, as noted by POYNTON & HODGKIN (1938), WILSON & REID (1951), TURNER (1959) from Malaya, RAO (1936, 1940, 1945), J. SINGH *et al.* (1956c) from India, DASSANAYAKE (1938, 1939) from Sri Lanka, IYENGAR (1953), from Southern Thailand, and SASA *et al.* (1952) from Japan. As described in detail by TURNER (1959), the first symptom is usually a painful and tender enlargement of the superficial inguinal nodes of one side, accompanied by fever. After some hours, pain and tenderness, and later, bandlike streaks of redness of the skin, in the line of the lymphatics, spread down the limb. There is sometimes an induration, under the reddened skin, about three inches long and one-half inch wide. Fever and constitutional symptoms usually persist for three to five days, before ending by rapid lysis with heavy sweating. The signs of adenitis and lymphangitis resolve gradually during next six or seven days. Swelling of the distal part of the limb may occur at about the third day. At first, the swelling is slight and tends to regress completely after the episode has ended, but after repeated attacks, the swelling does not subside and develops to elephantiasis.

Enlargement of lymph nodes (especially of groin, epitrochlear, and cubital) has been described as a typical syndrome of *B. malayi* infection by a number of workers (VAN SLEE, 1930; TESCH, 1937; POYNTON & HODGKIN, 1938; RAO, 1942). However, as pointed out by WILSON & REID (1951), a number of microfilaria carriers of *B. malayi* have no palpable glands, while EDESON (1959) found that the incidence of enlarged glands among children is also high in nonfilarial areas, and thus cannot be taken as a characteristic feature of filariasis.

Abscess formation around the enlarged nodes or along the lymphatics, especially in the inguinal region, has been noted to be common in *B. malayi* filariasis by a number of workers (VAN SLEE, 1930; DASSANAYAKE, 1938; POYNTON & HODGKIN, 1938; TURNER, 1959).

The acute symptoms resulting from infection of *B. malayi* which occurred among French and North African soldiers in North Vietnam were described by GALLIARD (1957; see Section 8B.4). The typical syndrome that occurred among the servicemen exposed to heavy infection for short periods was apparently different from that seen among the native people, and eosinophilia, enlargement of lymph nodes, and bronchitis with attacks of asthma were the three principal symptoms.

Three reports have so far been made on the observations of clinical manifestations produced after experimental infection of *B. malayi* in man. BUCKLEY (1958) inoculated a human volunteer with about 20 infective larvae of *B. malayi* (?) from a naturally infected monkey, *Macaca irus*. Aside from mild swellings of regional (inguinal) lymph nodes seven months after inoculation, the clinical findings were mainly respiratory, accompanied by blood eosinophilia. EDESON *et al.* (1960) inoculated two volunteers (one had a pre-existing, apparently natural *B. malayi* infection) with subperiodic *B. malayi*. Both volunteers experienced regional lymph node enlargement, lymphangitis, and transient swellings of the inoculated arms, beginning about one month after inoculation. Two other subjects inoculated with *B. pahangi* had similar clinical pictures. No fever was mentioned (also see Section 8B.7). DONDERO *et al.* (1972) inoculated each of three volunteers with about 50 infective larvae of subperiodic *B. malayi*, dissected from *Aedes togoi*. The injections were made subcutaneously into the forearm. Recurrent and transient lymphadenitis, lymphangitis, and nodular skin swellings, unaccompanied by fever, appeared in all of the three subjects, from about four weeks after the inoculation. Microfilaremia was found only in one case (subject A), from 17 weeks after the inoculation, and it remained detectable until treatment with DEC. The pattern and level of blood eosinophilia varied markedly from host to host; subject A had no appreciable change following infection until DEC was administered, whereupon, he showed the typical rapid plunge and then quick rise; subject B, starting with a baseline eosinophilia of 12%, experienced a steady decline; only subject C showed a higher level than baseline after infection.

(b.2) The chronic stage: elephantiasis

The permanent swelling of a part of the body, called elephantiasis, is a common sign of filariasis due to *W. bancrofti* and *B. malayi* in their chronic stages. In the latter, the involvement of body parts other than limbs, such as genital organs and breast, is extremely rare or practically absent. The upper extremities are much less frequently affected than the legs. Statistical studies on the incidence of elephantiasis and other clinical signs due to *B. malayi* infection were reported by BRUG (1931) from Indonesia, MOON (1937) from Korea, POYNTON & HODGKIN (1938) and TURNER (1959) from Malaya, DASSANAYAKE (1938, 1939) from Sri Lanka, RAGHAVAN & KRISHNAN (1949) and J. SINGH *et al.* (1956c) from India.

On Sri Kotta Island, Madras, India, for example, 89 elephantiasis cases due to *B. malayi* infection were examined by RAGHAVAN & KRISHNAN (1949). Of these, 56 (62.9%) showed the manifestation on only one leg, 21 (23.6%) on both legs, 7 (7.9%) on a hand only, and 5 (5.6%) on both hand and leg. In Penang, Malaysia, TURNER (1959) examined 37 cases of elephantiasis, of whom 22 (59%) had signs on one leg only, 11 (30%) on both legs, 3 (8%) on both leg and hand, and 1 (3%) on the scrotum.

In Shertalai Taluk, Kerala, India, JASWANT SINGH *et al.* (1956c) examined 8,463 persons (covering 3.3% of the total population) for microfilaremia and disease signs. They found 1,776 (20.9%) *B. malayi* microfilaria carriers and 16 *W. bancrofti* carriers. A total of 2,011 cases had clinical signs. The disease manifestations were elephantiasis of the leg in 1,298 cases, elephantiasis of the hand in 44, elephantiasis of both leg and hand in 142, fever and lymphangitis in 516 cases, and filarial scrotum (presumably due to *W. bancrofti* infection) in 11 cases.

One of the characteristic features of clinical manifestations of *B. malayi* infection is the absence of urogenital lesions and chylous symptoms, which are so characteristic of bancroftian filariasis. In the first report on the occurrence of a new species of human filaria (*Filaria malayi*) in North Sumatra by LICHTENSTEIN (1927), it was pointed out that elephantiasis of the legs was the main feature of the disease and urogenital manifestations were absent. KORKE (1929), in Bihar and Orissa, also recognized that the occurrence of his "atypical form" of microfilariae (determined to be identical with *B. malayi* by later workers) was associated with elephantiasis of legs but not with urogenital lesions. RAO (1940), for example, conducted an epidemiological survey of Ratnapur in the Central Province of India. The filaria infection consisted entirely of *B. malayi*. Out of the total population of 4,950 in the town, 2,000 persons were examined clinically by house-to-house visit; 78 had elephantiasis of the leg or arm; among them, 35 had elephantiasis of one leg, 42 had elephantiasis of both legs, and one had elephantiasis of one arm. Elephantiasis of the genitals, hydrocele, and chyluria were entirely absent. The absence of genital syndromes (hydrocele, funiculitis, elephantiasis of the scrotum, etc.) and of urinary symptoms (chyluria, hematochyluria) in *B. malayi* cases have been noted also by a number of later workers in various regions, such as in India by IYENGAR (1932), NAIR & ROY (1958), NAIR *et al.* (1959), in Sri Lanka by DASSANA-YAKE (1938, 1939), in Korea by MOON (1939), in Malaya by POYNTON & HODGKIN (1938), TURNER (1959), and in Japan by SASA *et al.* (1952).

"Infection of *B. malayi* adult worms in the human eye."

JOON-WAH *et al.* (1974) reported on a case of *B. malayi* infection of the conjunctiva where an adult male and a gravid female were recovered in perfect condition. The patient was a 23-year-old female rubber tapper from Johore, West Malaysia, and had complaints of pain, redness and watery discharge of the right eye. There was a cyst under the lower bulbar conjunctiva, from which a complete male and a gravid female of *B. malayi* were recovered. The patient had microfilariae of *B. malayi* in her blood.

2C.5.2 Diagnosis

2C.5.2.1 Clinical diagnosis

As stated in the previous section, the frequent occurrence of filarial fever cases and of elephantiasis of the limbs without involvement of the genital and urinary organs is a characteristic sign of filariasis due to *B. malayi*.

2C.5.2.2 Parasitological diagnosis

As in the case of *W. bancrofti* infection, the detection of the microfilariae from the peripheral blood is at present the only practicable and reliable diagnostic method of *B. malayi* infection, though it is usually successful in only a part of the infected populations.

> Methods for examination of microfilariae in the blood (see Section 10B.2.2)
>
> Methods for identification of the microfilariae (see Section 1.3.3)
>
> The efficiency of detection of microfilariae in blood samples (see Section 11D).
>
> The daytime provocation of the microfilariae by DEC administration (see Section 10B.2.2.d)

2C.5.2.3 Immunological diagnosis

Only a few references are available on the immunological tests for *B. malayi* infection; little information is available on the significance of various test methods, or their practical usefulness.

WILSON (1961), in a review of filariasis in Malaya, concluded that immunological tests were not satisfactory because most published accounts of diagnostic methods other than the blood examination for the microfilariae, such as skin reactions and complement fixation tests, indicate that they are not sufficiently specific, and that false negatives are common."

In the past, skin tests were conducted by POYNTON & HODGKIN (1938) in Malaya, and by KATAMINE *et al.* (1973), with *Dirofilaria* FPT antigen, in Cheju Island, Korea. Complement fixation tests were reported by HUSSON & SCHNEIDER (1958) for various filarial species including *B. malayi*, and DANARAJ *et al.* (1959) for *Brugia* infection and eosinophilic lung.

2C.5.3 Treatment

Previous studies by a number of workers in various endemic areas of *B. malayi* have shown that DEC is highly effective against the parasite when sufficient doses are administered.

As in the treatment of *W. bancrofti* cases, the drug is administered usually in a dose of some 6 mg per kg of body weight, once a day, for ten times, at daily, weekly, or sometimes monthly intervals, the total dose of 60 mg per kg is used as a standard. *B. malayi* is more susceptible to the treatment with DEC than *W. bancrofti*, but the febrile reactions that may occur after administration of the initial dose are definitely more severe than those encountered in the treatment of *W. bancrofti* cases. The frequent occurrence of such severe febrile reactions is the main reason that mass treatment of *B. malayi* carriers has been difficult to accomplish in many endemic areas.

A preliminary experiment of the use of DEC in *B. malayi* infection was conducted first by WILSON (1950), in Malaya. Twenty microfilaria carriers without clinical symptoms, eight cases of clinical filariasis without microfilaremia, and one with both were treated with varying doses of DEC. The drug was shown to be highly effective, but most of the patients developed severe reactions associated with high fever (see Section 8B.7). HAYASHI *et al.* (1951) and SASA *et al.* (1952) also conducted trial experiments of the treatment of *B. malayi* cases, in Hachijo-Koshima, and reported that microfilaria carriers who received total doses of 60 mg per kg or more became permanently negative for microfilariae. These authors also noted the occurrence of severe reactions in most of those who were treated with DEC (see Section 8C.4).

By analyzing these and later observations, it has become evident that effective control and treatment of *B. malayi* filariasis can be made by careful use of DEC, and that the side reactions are usually transient and not dangerous.

TURNER (1959) and TURNER & SODHY (1959) conducted trial mass treatment of *B. malayi* cases in Malaya with single daily doses, while EDESON & WHARTON (1958) described the results of single doses given at weekly or monthly intervals to *B. malayi* cases in Malaya.

TURNER (1959), treated a total of 70 filariasis patients (mostly microfilaria carriers) from an endemic area of the periodic form of *B. malayi* in Penang, Malaysia, with DEC, given in different doses once per day. There was much variation in the effects of smaller dosages against the microfilariae, and although as little as 0.25 mg per kg per day reduced the microfilaria count by 63% over a five-day period, the effect was too slow. Larger doses were more rapidly and more regularly effective. The febrile reactions, often quite severe, occurred in 54 of 55 microfilaria carriers when the dosage was high enough to remove microfilariae from the blood. Febrile reactions did not occur in patients with negative blood films (60 mm³). After the febrile reaction had subsided, large increases in dosage never provoked a recurrence of the febrile symptoms. Minor local reactions (lymphadenitis and lymphangitis) occurred in 15 patients, irrespective of the presence of microfilariae in the blood.

TURNER & SODHY (1959) conducted a trial mass treatment of *B. malayi* filariasis with single daily doses of DEC. A rural village on Penang Island, Malaysia, with a population of 156 and a microfilaria rate of 27% (39 positives of 144) was selected. DEC was administered to all the people starting with small doses (0.5 mg per kg to those with 30 or more microfilariae per 20 mm³; 1.0 mg per kg to those with less than 30 microfilariae per 20 mm³; 2.0 mg per kg to those with no microfilaria). The dosage was increased later; it was aimed at giving at least 60 mg per kg in total. When the trial ended after 48 days, 86% (134 of 156) had received total dosages of more than 40 mg per kg, and satisfactory reductions of microfilaremia were obtained at later blood surveys. However, febrile reactions occurred in all the known microfilaria carriers and also in 19 % (20 of 105) of persons with negative blood films. Many of the people were unable to tolerate such large doses of the drug; therefore, it was concluded that mass treatment of *B. malayi* filariasis needed to be carefully supervised because of the high incidence of the febrile reaction, and simpler DEC schedules were preferable.

EDESON & WHARTON (1958) conducted treatment of *B. malayi* carriers with monthly or weekly doses of DEC. The carriers were from the endemic areas of the subperiodic form of *B. malayi* in the lower reaches of the Pahang and Kuantan rivers who had been admitted to the District Hospital. Doses were: (a) 1, 2, 4, or 6 mg per kg given once a month for six months, (b) 5 mg per kg given once a week for six weeks, and (c) an initial dose of 0.5 mg per kg followed by increasing monthly or weekly doses to a final dose of 8 mg per kg. At the end of the treatment, all dosage regimens had reduced the microfilarial counts by at least 93 %; doses of 4.5 mg or 6 mg per kg had reduced the counts by 99 %. Most patients reported a reduction in the number of filarial attacks following the treatment. Practically all the patients suffered a sharp febrile reaction within 24 hours of the first dose, and the use of a small initial dose did not eliminate the reaction completely. Very few patients suffered any reaction after the second and subsequent doses, despite the occasional persistence of numbers of microfilariae. The results suggested that mass administration of DEC at doses of about 5 mg per kg by weekly or monthly intervals should be successful in reducing the human microfilaria carriers to a very low level.

EDESON & LAING (1959) demonstrated that in cats experimentally infected with *B. malayi* and *B. pahangi*, DEC administered either orally or intraperitoneally can kill the adult worms of the two filarial species. However, its effect on the microfilariae in cats was much slower and less satisfactory than in man.

In China, treatment of large numbers of *B. malayi* carriers was conducted after 1952 with various dosage regimens of DEC, especially by administration of a large single dose, as described in the previous section (2B.5.2). According to HSIEH *et al.* (1960), for example, 186 *B. malayi* carriers were treated with a single dose of 1 g of DEC; of these, 154 (82.8 %) were found negative when re-examined, while in the *W. bancrofti* carriers only 708 (60.4%) of 1,052 cases treated with the same method turned negative. The attack rate of the fever reaction in *B. malayi* cases was 86.5 % (295 of 341) and was much higher than that in *W. bancrofti* cases (27.9 % or 141 of 505). CH'EN (1964) reviewed the results of mass drug treatments of *B. malayi* and *W. bancrofti* cases in China. He demonstrated that dead adult worms of *B. malayi* and *W. bancrofti* formed in nodules after administration of DEC, or certain antimony and arsenic preparations (see also Section 2B.5.3.2).

Clinical observations were also made by CABRERA (1966a) on the malayan filariasis cases treated with diethylcarbamazine (DEC) in Palawan. A total of 44 cases from Quezon municipality were examined and treated. The majority of the cases had enlargement of epitrochlear and inguinal lymph nodes; five had elephantiasis of either leg or scrotum, and about one-third showed no physical signs. DEC was administered at daily doses of 6 mg per kg body weight for 12 days, with a total dose of 72 mg per kg. Microfilarial densities were directly related to the rise of temperature, the higher the density, the higher the temperature. Approximately 95% of them had fever ranging from 37.3 to 40.6°C, and 89% had fever from four to nine hours after the drug administration. Fever appeared earlier in those with high microfilarial counts. The average duration of fever was about three days. The microfilariae disappeared from the treated cases from a few hours after the drug intake to as long as nine days after, with the exception of a case who had 165 microfilariae at the start of treatment and remained positive even after the termination of the treatment. The time required for the clearance of microfilariae was also directly related to the initial microfilarial count.

NAIR (1968) in Kerala, India, carried out an analytical study on the clinical reactions in asymptomatic *B. malayi* carriers caused by DEC therapy. In general, their reactions were very severe; many of them were completely prostrated and had to rest in bed during the reaction period. Common symptoms were high fever accompanied by chills, rigors, severe headache, and body ache. Anorexia was common, and nausea and vomiting occurred in many cases. These reactions occurred within six to 12 hours and reached the maximum in 24 to 36 hours after the initial dose. There was delirium in one case, and convulsion in another. These severe reactions subsided in two to four days, and nothing untoward occurred. There was a significant correlation between the microfilarial density and the intensity of reactions among 77 carriers who received a single dose of 6 mg per kg. (See Section 8A.2.)

Note: Surgery and other symptomatic treatments are usually not necessary in filariasis malayi, because it does not affect genitourinary organs. Elephantiasis due to *B. malayi* infection does not reach the enormous sizes often seen in filariasis bancrofti, and surgical treatment is usually a contraindication. However, the treatment of secondary bacterial infection, such as with antibiotics, is often necessary in patients with elephantiasis of the limbs.

2C.5.4 Vector control

Experiments for the prevention of infection of *B. malayi* by the control of either the larvae or adult mosquito vectors have been reported by several workers.

In Malaysia, a pilot control experiment was initiated in 1954, in a small village, Kampong Ubai, in East Pahang. All the houses were sprayed with dieldrin emulsion at 1.0 g per m² every six months beginning in 1954. Blood surveys were conducted every year from 1953 to 1960. However, the efficacy of this control measure was not satisfactory, and the microfilaria rate, which was 40% before the insecticide application, still remained at 19% in 1960 (WHARTON *et al.*, 1958; WILSON, 1961; WILSON & RAMACHANDRAN, 1971).

In Sri Lanka, *B. malayi* was shown to be widely endemic in the surveys conducted from 1937 to 1939; the microfilaria rate was 6.8% (405 positives of 5,922 examined) in Southern Province, 29.8% (1,153 of 3,871) in North-western Province, 10.4% (111 of 1,063) in Eastern Province, and 11.3% (15 of 133) in North-Central Province. (DASSANAYAKE, 1938, 1939). *B. malayi* was also confirmed to be widely endemic in surveys conducted in 1947. However, *B. malayi* carriers were shown to have completely disappeared from the country in the country-wide blood survey program conducted during a period from 1959 to 1965 (ABDULCADER & SASA, 1966). Clearance of *Pistia* (the host plant of *Mansonia* spp., the vector mosquitoes) was recommended by Dassanayake, but this was never widely practiced. The only possible explanation for this disappearance of the parasite was the effect of DDT house spraying, practiced extensively in this country for the purpose of malaria control. This spraying also covered the endemic areas of *B. malayi* filariasis in the above provinces.

In India, IYENGAR (1938) conducted detailed studies on the epidemiology and control of filariasis in Travancore, Kerala State. *Mansonia* (*Mansonioides*) *annulifera* and related species were shown to be the main vectors of *B. malayi*, highly prevalent in this region. The larvae and pupae of these mosquito vectors were shown to breed in swamps and pools with a water plant *Pistia* as the main host. A pilot control program of *Mansonioides* mosquitoes was started in 1934 with the removal of *Pistia* plant from tanks and pools in an area of some 25 square miles in Shertalai. This was reported to have effected a striking reduction in the incidence of *Mansonia* mosquitoes.

JOSEPH *et al.* (1960) conducted pilot studies for the control of *B. malayi* filariasis in Kerala. The following four measures were tested: (a) *Mansonioides* control by indoor residual spraying of dieldrin, 50 mg per square foot, from May to June, 1958 and January 1959; (b) *Mansonioides* control, as above, accompanied by mass therapy with DEC in doses of 200 mg for adults per day for five days; (c) *Mansonioides* control through *Pistia* clearance by manual removal; and (d) *Pistia* clearance combined with DEC mass therapy. The indoor application of dieldrin reduced the density of *M. annulifera* to practically zero for at least six months, but its effect on *M. uniformis* lasted only two months, and led to a remarkable increase in the prevalence of dieldrin-resistant *Culex fatigans*. (see section 8A.2, India, Kerala.)

In the small endemic focus of *B. malayi* filariasis on Hachijo-Koshima Island, Japan, epidemiological surveys, treatment of the patients with DEC, and the control of vectors by various measures were practiced since the disease was discovered in 1950. The main vector was determined to be

Aedes togoi, which bred both in natural rock pools on the beach and in artificial water containers in the villages. The mosquito larvae breeding in large concrete tanks was effectively controlled by the release of 'medaka' (*Oryzias latipes*), or goldfish. Larviciding with applications of DDT dust by helicopter on the rock pools, and residual house spraying of DDT emulsion were tried once in 1956. DDT indoor spraying was conducted in 1958 and 1963. HAYASHI (1959) made analytical studies on the effectiveness of the drug treatments and the vector control measures from results of repeated blood surveys. The island was free from *B. malayi* carriers when the villages were surveyed for the last time in 1968 (SASA *et al.* 1970).

2D. The Timor filaria

This is a human filaria first reported by DAVID & EDESON (1964, 1965) from Portuguese Timor. It is known to be endemic only in Timor and the Flores Islands of the Indonesian Archipelago. The adults are still unknown. The microfilariae are closely related to those of *B. malayi*, but are definitely larger in size; the cephalic space is more slender in the Timor microfilariae (length to width ratio of 1:3) than in *B. malayi* microfilariae (length to width ratio of 1:2); the sheath of *B. malayi* stains well with Giemsa, but that of the Timor microfilariae remains almost unstained in the Giemsa solution (like the sheath of *W. bancrofti*).

The microfilariae were found to be nocturnally periodic. The vector is still unknown, and no animal reservoirs have yet been found.

This type of microfilariae were reported also from the Indonesian part of Timor by OEMIJATI & TJOEN (1966) and OEMIJATI & PARTONO (1971), and from the Flores by KURIHARA & OEMIJATI (1975).

For morphological characters, see Table 2-11.

For epidemiological data, see 9B. 10 (Timor).

2E. Mosquito vectors of human filariasis

2E.1 Host-parasite relationship

2E.1.1 Culicidae, or mosquitoes

Mosquitoes or insects of the family Culicidae belong to the suborder Nematocera of the order Diptera. Over 2,000 species are classified into some 30 genera and three subfamilies. Some members of this family are known to act as the vectors of human and animal filariasis, human and animal malaria, and human and animal viral diseases (such as yellow fever, dengue fever, and certain viral encephalitides).

Table 2-11. Differences between the microfilariae of the Timor-filaria, and *Brugia malayi* (two races) from Malaya (re-arranged from data by DAVID & EDESON, 1965; average measurements in μ).

	Timor-microfilaria	B. malayi (periodic)	B. malayi (subperiodic)
Formalin-fixed specimens			
No. measured	20	100	190
length	357.9	265.5	256.1
Air-dried specimens			
No. measured	16	36	25
length	287.0	234.1	199.0
width at 1st nucleus	4.4	4.2	4.0
Cephalic space:length:	12.8(4.5%)	8.3(3.6%)	8.1(4.0%)
ratio, length:width	3:1	2:1	2:1
Head to: nerve ring	63.8(22.3%)	50.8(21.7%)	45.4(22.6%)
excretory pore	84.4(29.4%)	71.5(30.6%)	62.3(31.2%)
Innenkörper	145.3(50.6%)	123.6(52.8%)	105.5(52.8%)
Innenkörper end	197.7(68.9%)	154.1(66.8%)	133.9(67.1%)
anus	238.0(82.9%)	189.4(81.2%)	162.2(81.2%)
Staining of sheath:			
with haemalum	+	+	+
with Giemsa	−	++	++

It should be noted that not all mosquitoes can serve as vectors of these diseases; in fact, certain disease agents can develop to the infective stage only when ingested by certain species or species-groups of the mosquitoes. For example, the vectors of malaria are restricted to members of the genus *Anopheles*, and usually to a few species within this genus. The main vectors of urban yellow fever and dengue fever are a few species of the subgenus *Stegomyia*. In East and South Asia, only *Culex tritaeniorhynchus* and a few other related species act as the vectors of Japanese encephalitis.

As stated elsewhere, the mosquitoes which serve as vectors of human filariasis are also limited to certain groups of species. However, filariasis vectors differ from other disease vectors in that they may include members of entirely different genera, not taxonomically related to each other. So far, the known vectors of human filariasis have been recorded from four main genera: *Anopheles, Aedes, Culex,* and *Mansonia.* The capacity of mosquito species or strains to serve as intermediate hosts of a filaria species is not of the all-or-none type; there seem to exist various grades of compatibility between the vectors and the parasites.

There have been large numbers of studies conducted in the past on the taxonomy, bionomics, and control of mosquitoes. The classical monographs on mosquitoes of the world compiled by THEOBALD (1910–13) and EDWARDS (1932) are still useful and important literature for their classification. A synoptic catalogue, extremely useful for the classification of mosquitoes, was published by STONE *et al.* (1959). MATTINGLY (1973) gave accounts on the taxonomy and biology of mosquitoes, with a key to genera and some important species. Reviews were made by the following authors in relation to the transmission of human filariasis by mosquitoes in various regions of the world.

> EDWARDS (1922): vector, general
> VEVERS (1924): list of filaria carriers
> RAGHAVAN (1956): *Anopheles* as filaria vectors
> MANSON-BAHR (1959): vectors of *W. bancrofti*
> KESSEL (1961): list of mosquito vectors
> RAGHAVAN (1961): vectors of *W. bancrofti* and *B. malayi*
> IYENGAR (1960, 1965): Pacific region
> BELKIN (1962): mosquitoes of the South Pacific
> WHARTON (1963): adaptation of *Wuchereria* and *Brugia* to mosquitoes
> EDESON & WILSON (1964): review of epidemiology
> MOUCHET *et al.* (1965): African region
> HAMON *et al.* (1967): African region
> RAMALINGAM *et al.* (1969): Southeast Asia
> MATTINGLY (1969): general
> RAMALINGAM (1973): Southeast Asia
> CHOW (1973): the Western Pacific region

2E.1.2 Determination of mosquito vectors

In order to determine a mosquito vector in an endemic area of filariasis, it is necessary to confirm the following evidence for a species of mosquito: (a) naturally caught specimens of a species of mosquito contain infective stage larvae of a filarial form, (b) the same form of infective larvae develop in a laboratory-bred, clean colony of the same mosquito species after being fed on a microfilaria carrier, and (c) that the same mosquito species feed on the blood of humans in this endemic area.

The efficiency of a mosquito species or race as a vector of filariasis is dependent further on various factors which will be discussed in the next section.

(a) Investigation of the natural infection of mosquitoes

In this procedure, wild mosquitoes are collected with various methods (collection with human or animal bait, or with various mosquito traps; see Section 10C.2.3), and are dissected individually for examination of filarial infection. If filaria larvae are discovered, it is necessary to identify the species and the stage by the method explained in Sectin 2A.4.2. Only the mosquito species which have been shown to harbor the third stage larvae of a given filarial species may be regarded as natural vectors. The results are usually reported by the number of each species of mosquito dissected, and the numbers and percentages of the specimens found to be infected with all stages of larvae and with mature larvae. It is also recommended that the frequency distribution of the numbers of mature and immature stage larvae found per mosquito be presented.

(b) Experimental infection study

The vectorial capability of a mosquito species can also be estimated by an experimental infection study, in which laboratory-bred or naturally caught mosquitoes are fed on a microfilaria carrier, then dissected after certain intervals for examination of the filaria larvae in various body parts. In room temperatures of 25 to 30°C, found in the tropics, it usually requires 11 to 13 days in the case of *W. bancrofti* and 7 to 10 days in the case of *B. malayi* for the development from microfilariae to the infective stage larvae in the body of mosquitoes. The methods for keeping the infected mosquitoes in the laboratory and for the dissection of mosquitoes are described in Section 10C.1. Methods for the identification of the filaria larvae in the mosquitoes are shown in Section 2A.2.4.

In the field studies in endemic areas of filariasis, a method employed by BRUG & DE ROOK (1930) is useful for rapid determination of the local filaria vectors. These authors exposed a microfilaria carrier to mosquito bites at a certain time of the day, and as soon as a mosquito had inserted its proboscis into the skin, a test tube was put carefully over it and held in position until the mosquito became fully engorged and flew into the test tube. The mosquitoes in the test tubes were kept in a humid chamber as long as they survived. They were dissected as soon as they were found dead. By this method, these authors could determine not only the species of the mosquito vectors of *B. malayi*, but also the relative abundance and biting time of various mosquito species in the endemic areas of Sumatra (see Section 8B.9).

2E.1.3 Efficiency of various mosquito species as filaria vectors

As previously discussed, not all mosquito species serve as vectors of *W. bancrofti* or *B. malayi*, and the efficiency of a mosquito population as a vector of certain filarial race differs greatly according to the species or race. Previous studies conducted by various workers in different endemic areas of filariasis have shown that although large numbers of mosquito species may be found, the species which actually transmit the parasite are usually restricted to only a few species, or perhaps only one among them. The species or species-complex which serve most efficiently in the transmission is called the major (principal, or primary) vector. Those which play less significant roles in the transmission are called the secondary or minor vectors.

Various factors are involved in determining the efficiency of a mosquito population in the transmission of filariasis. This is discussed quantitatively in Sections 10A.2 and 10C.2. For example, some species cannot be vectors of human filariae, simply because they do not bite man, i.e., they are either autogenous, or feed exclusively on animals other than man. In general, there are big differences in the anthropophilic characters among mosquito species. Also, some mosquito species do not transmit the parasite because they do not allow the development of filaria larvae. Under natural environments, some species may be poor vectors because the population density is low, or the average life span is too short.

Among the various factors which are involved in determining the efficiency of a mosquito species in the transmission of filariasis in an endemic area, the following are considered to be important: (1) the efficiency in ingesting microfilariae when taking a blood meal from a filaria carrier, (2) compatibility with the filaria larvae for their development to the infective stage, (3) the survival rate during the period required for the full development of the filaria larvae, (4) the anthropophilic index, or the percentage of the mosquito species attacking a human host and taking a blood meal, and (5) the population density in an endemic area throughout the year.

The efficiency of filaria larvae to develop in various mosquito species has been investigated by many workers in various regions of the world with different races of *W. bancrofti* and *B. malayi*. For example, YAMADA (1927) fed 24 species of Japanese mosquitoes on a carrier of the nocturnally periodic race of *W. bancrofti*, and classified the results into the following categories, according to the compatibility:

a. Species in which no larval development takes place;
- a.1. Species in which the larvae cannot penetrate the midgut: *Tripteroides bambusa*
- a.2. Species in which the larvae die after penetrating into the body cavity: *Aedes koreicus, Aedes vexans nipponii, Aedes sticticus., Aedes imprimens*
- a.3. Species in which the larvae partly reach the thoracic muscle, but die without making further growth: *Aedes esoensis, Aedes japonicus, Aedes dorsalis, Anopheles sineroides*

b. Species in which the larval development stops without reaching the mature stage;
- b.1. Species in which the development stops at the first stage: *Culex annulus, Aedes yamadai, Aedes albopictus. Aedes albolataralis, Aedes galloisi*
- b.2. Species in which the development stops at the second stage: *Aedes chemulpoensis, Culex bitaeniorhynchus*
- b.3. Species in which the development stops at the early third stage: *Armigeres subalbatus*

c. Species in which the larvae develop to the mature stage.
- c.1. Species in which only a small number can reach the mature stage larvae: *Anopheles sinensis, Culex tritaeniorhynchus, Culex sinensis*
- c.2. Species in which the majority of larvae reach the mature

stage, namely, the most efficient intermediate hosts: *Culex whitmorei, Culex vagans, Culex pipiens pallens, Aedes togoi*

There have been important contributions made to understanding the role played by *Ae. aegypti* as an experimental intermediate host of the subperiodic race of *B. malayi*, referring to the genetics of mosquitoes in the susceptibility for the development of filarial larvae. RAMACHANDRAN *et al.* (1960), in search for laboratory vectors of *B. malayi* which would be easier to maintain than *Mansonioides* mosquitoes, showed that a colony of *Aedes aegypti* which came originally from West Africa and was maintained at the Liverpool School of Tropical Medicine was a moderately susceptible host for both the nocturnally subperiodic and periodic races of *B. malayi*. Some 30% (98 out of 316) of this colony were shown to harbor infective filarial larvae when dissected ten or more days after being fed on a cat infected with the subperiodic race of *B. malayi*.

MACDONALD (1962a) conducted a laboratory experiment for selecting a strain of *Ae. aegypti* from the above colony which was more susceptible for the development of *B. malayi*. By mating the males and the females reared from eggs produced by mothers in which mature filaria larvae were found to have developed, a susceptible strain was established and maintained through 15 generations.

MACDONALD (1962b) further carried out experimental studies on the genetical basis of the susceptibility in *Ae. aegypti* to infection with *B. malayi*. A series of crosses and backcrosses was made between the susceptible and the refractory strains from Rangoon, Malaya, and Trinidad. The offsprings of the crosses were tested for the susceptibility to infection with *B. malayi*. The results showed that it was controlled by a sex-linked recessive gene, which was designated f^m.

MACDONALD (1963) reported that the strain of *Ae. aegypti* selected for susceptibility to infection with the subperiodic *B. malayi* race still failed to support the development of the parasite at a rate of 15.2% through generations F_1 to F_{15}. The progeny of a series of phenotypically refractory mosquitoes in generations F_{15}, F_{16}, F_{18}, and F_{19} were tested to show whether they were genotypically refractory. Thirty-two of 33 progeny test confirmed that the refractory parents had been homozygous for the gene controlling the susceptibility.

2E.2 Filarial races and main mosquito vectors

As stated previously, several species or species-groups of mosquitoes have been incriminated as the major or minor vectors of various physiological races of the parasites. Both filariasis bancrofti and malayi can be classified into different epidemiological types according to the differences in the ecological features of the major vector mosquitoes. The main types are as follows:

(a.1) Nocturnally periodic *W. bancrofti* (NPWb)

    (a.1.1) The *Culex fatigans* type: urban or semiurban in distribution, transmitted mainly by the house mosquito of the *Culex pipiens* complex; widely distributed throughout the subtropical and tropical zones of the world.

    (a.1.2) The *Anopheles* type: The types transmitted by various species of *Anopheles* found in large areas of tropical Africa, certain rural areas of South and East Asia, and the Pacific islands. The species of mosquitoes involved and their ecology are quite different according to the region they inhabit. Malaria and filariasis are frequently transmitted by the same mosquito species within a given region.

    (a.1.3) The *Aedes (Finlaya) poecilus* type: commonly found in the abaca-growing regions in the Philippines.

    (a.1.4) The *Mansonioides* type: in certain swampy areas of Papua, where *B. malayi* is absent, NPWb was shown to be transmitted by *Mansonioides* mosquitoes (VAN DIJK, 1958). In Narsapur, Madras, India, SOMASUNDARAM (1949) reported *Mansonioides* to be the main vector of *W. bancrofti* endemic in this delta area.

(a.2) Diurnally subperiodic *W. bancrofti* (DSWb)

    (a.2.1) The *Aedes (Stegomyia) polynesiensis* type: the type widely distributed throughout islands of the Polynesian region, with the day-biting mosquitoes of the *Ae. polynesiensis* group as the primary vectors.

    (a.2.2) The *Aedes (Finlaya) fijiensis* type: several night-biting *Finlaya* species with spotted wings (the *kochi* group) have been shown to act as efficient vectors of the DSWb race in certain Polynesian islands, and are of possible importance as vectors in the inland regions of the islands. They generally breed in the leaf axils of plants.

    (a.2.3) The *Aedes (Ochlerotatus) vigilax* types: in New Caledonia and the Loyalty Islands, where mosquitoes of the *Aedes polynesiensis* group are completely absent, this day-biting mosquito, which belongs to a different subgenus and breeds in open, brackish marshes near the coast, is the major vector.

(a.3) Nocturnally subperiodic *W. bancrofti* (NSWb)

    (a.3.1) The *Aedes (Finlaya) niveus* type: a species of the *Aedes niveus* group, it is the only mosquito found naturally infected in the endemic area in West Thailand.

(b.1) Nocturnally periodic *B. malayi* (NPBm)

    (b.1.1) The *Mansonia (Mansonioides) uniformis* type: an ecological type endemic to open, swampy areas in South and East Asia, where several species of open swamp mosquitoes of the *M. uniformis* group act as the main vectors.

(b.1.2) The *Anopheles* (*Anopheles*) *barbirostris* type: an ecological type endemic to rice paddy areas in South and East Asia, where *An. barbirostris, An. hyrcanus,* and related species of the subgenus *Anopheles* serve as the major vectors.

(b.1.3) The *Aedes* (*Finlaya*) *togoi* type; a type endemic to villages near rocky beachs, where the major vector, *Ae. togoi,* breeds in brackish water pools.

(b.2) Nocturnally subperiodic *B. malayi* (NSBm)

(b.2.1) The *Mansonia* (*Mansonioides*) *dives/bonneae* type: the only known ecological type of this race of *B. malayi* is that transmitted mainly by the *M. dives/bonneae* groups of mosquitoes which breed in swamp forests in Southeast Asia.

2E.3 The main mosquito vectors involved in the transmission of human filariasis

According to the classification proposed by STONE *et al.* (1959), the family Culicidae is divided into three subfamilies, Anophelinae (includes three genera), Toxorhynchitinae (one genus), and Culicinae (27 genera); it includes 110 valid genera and subgenera, and 2,426 valid species. A number of new species were described later, but the basic structure of the taxonomy of Culicidae has remained unchanged since then.

Both *W. bancrofti* and *B. malayi* are unique among the various arthropod-transmitted parasites in that larval development can take place in several quite taxonomically independent groups of intermediate hosts. Of the more than 30 genera and 110 subgenera of the family Culicidae, the important vectors of human filariasis fall into the following taxa:

(A) Subfamily Anophelinae

(A.1) Genus *Anopheles* Meigen, 1818

This genus, notorious as the vector of human malaria, also includes some species important as vectors of *W. bancrofti* and *B. malayi* in certain rural regions in the Pacific, South America, tropical Africa, and Asia. The following are main species groups which include important vectors of filariasis.

(A.1.a) Subgenus *Anopheles* Meigen, 1818

(1) *An. hyrcanus* group: NPWb and NPBm in East Asia

(2) *An. barbirostris* group: NPBm in Southeast Asia

  (3) *An. bancroftii* group: NPWb in the Papuan region
  (4) *An. umbrosus* group: NPWb in Southeast Asia

(A.1.b) Subgenus *Cellia* Theobald, 1902
  (1) *An. gambiae* group: NPWb in tropical Africa
  (2) *An. punctulatus* group: NPWb in the Papuan region
  (3) *Cellia*-species: NPWb in South and Southeast Asia
(A.1.c) New World anophelines as secondary or accidental vectors
  of NPWb
  (1) Subgenus *Nyssorhynchus* Blanchard, 1902
  (2) Subgenus *Kerteszia* Theobald, 1905

(A.1.a) Subgenus *Anopheles* Meigen, 1818

In the adults, the vein "costa" (anterior margin of the wing) is completely dark, or divided by pale spots into not more than three dark marks. This is in contrast to those of *Cellia*, in which the costa is divided by pale spots into four or more dark marks involving both the costa and vein I. In the larvae, the bases of inner clypeal hairs are closely set, and the antennal shaft hair is often large and branched.

(A.1.a.1) *Anopheles* (*Anopheles*) *hyrcanus* group

This group of species is characterized by having two white spots on the costa, and a tuft of dark scales on the abdominal sternite VIII and on each side of the clypeus. This group of mosquitoes is distributed widely in South and East Asia, and includes over ten closely related forms, which are sometimes difficult to be morphologically differentiated. However, there seem to exist remarkable differences in the behavior and affinity to various pathogens among these forms. Excellent reviews and revisions were made by RIED (1953, 1968) on the *An. sinensis* group of Southeast Asia. The following species have been reported to be involved in the transmission of human filariasis.

Anopheles (*Anopheles*) *sinensis* Wiedemann, 1828

A species widely distributed to East and South Asia; there seem to exist various physiological races, especially in reference to anthropophily. In China, FENG (1931) found this species to be the main vector of *W. bancrofti* in the Woosung district. FENG (1936) and WU (1959) further demonstrated that *An. sinensis* was also the principal vector of *B. malayi* endemic in the rice-growing areas in middle China. In Korea, this species was also shown to be acting as the vector of *B. malayi* in the rice paddy areas in Kyungpook (KANDA *et al.*, 1974).

Anopheles (*Anopheles*) *nigerrimus* Giles, 1900

This species was reported to be infected with filaria larvae in endemic areas of *B. malayi* in Sri Lanka by CARTER (1948), with an infection rate of the mature larvae of 1.9%; in southern Thailand by LYENGAR (1953), with a rate of 3.7% for all stages; and in Contai, West Bengal, India, by SEN (1957, quoted by RAGHAVAN, 1961). In experimental infections with

W. bancrofti, RAO & IYENGAR (1932) demonstrated that 55.5% of *An. nigerrimus* tested developed mature larvae.

(A.1.a.2) *Anopheles* (*Anopheles*) *barbirostris* group

This group of at least ten species of mosquitoes of the series *Myzorhynchus*, in the subgenus *Anopheles*, all closely related morphologically, had been generally confused as "*barbirostris*", until recently. REID (1962) conducted detailed studies on the taxonomy of this group of mosquitoes in Southeast Asia, and separated the group into some ten species, including five new species. These are:

An. barbirostris van der Wulp, 1884; *An. campestris* Reid, 1962; *An. donaldi* Reid, 1962; *An. hodgkini* Reid, 1962; *An. pollicaris* Reid, 1962; *An. franciscoi* Reid, 1962; *An. barbumbrosus* Strickland & Chowdhury, 1927; *An. vanus* Walher, 1859; *An. manalangi* Mendoza, 1940; *An. ahomi* Chowdhury, 1929; and "Ceylon species" (*pseudoscutellaris* of CARTER, 1925). There seem to exist remarkable differences among these closely related species in their capability to be the vectors of filariasis and malaria.

In Sulawesi, JURGENS (1932), BRUG (1937) and PARTONO *et al.* (1972) found "*barbirostris*" to be the principal natural vector of *B. malayi*.

In southeast Kalimantan, KARIADI (1938) reported natural (two out of 29) and experimental (seven out of seven) infections with *B. malayi*, presumably in *An. donaldi*.

In Malaya, POYNTON & HODGKIN (1938) found "*barbirostris*" refractory to infection with the subperiodic race of *B. malayi* in Pahang. WHARTON (1960) also demonstrated that the subperiodic race of *B. malayi* does not develop in *barbirostris*, *campestris*, or *donaldi*. On the other hand, REID (1962) reported that the periodic race of *B. malayi* develops readily in these three species of mosquitoes, and also that *An. campestris* is the main vector of the periodic race of *B. malayi* in northwest Malaya (Wellesley, Penang, and Krian provinces).

In the southern region of Thailand, IYENGAR (1953) examined mosquitoes in an endemic area of *B. malayi*, found infections with filarial larvae in ten mosquito species; among them were *An. barbirostris* (11.7%, or 42 positives of 358), *An. niggerimus* (3.7%, or 3 of 81), *An. sinensis* (3.6%, or 3 of 83), *An. albotaeniatus* (4.0%, or 1 of 25) and *An. umbrosus* (3.3%, or 1 of 30). Infected mosquitoes were also found in four species of *Mansonia* (see Section 9:B.1).

In an endemic area of *B. malayi* in Kerala, India, IYENGAR (1938) found natural infection with filaria larvae in eight species of mosquitoes, among which *An. barbirostris* had larvae in three of 205 specimens (see Section 9A.2).

(A.1.a.3) *Anopheles* (*Anopheles*) *bancroftii* group

This group, closely related to the *An. barbirostris* group, being large dark mosquitoes with very shaggy, black palps, have wings with areas of mixed, broad, black and white scales, giving a finely speckled appearance.

The *bancroftii*-group is differentiated from the *barbirostris*-group by the speckled legs, and by the position of the wing fringe. This group is distributed mainly in the Papuan region. REID (1962) recognized the following three forms:

Anopheles (*Anopheles*) *bancroftii* Giles, 1902: Australia, New Guinea, Bismarck Archipelago

Anopheles barbirostris var. *barbiventris* Brug, 1938: Sulawesi

Anopeles (*Anopheles*) *pseudobarbirostris* Ludlow, 1902: Philippines, Sulawesi, Moluccas, (New Guinea).

As for the relationship to filariasis, ELSBACH (1937a, b) conducted an epidemiological study on *W. bancrofti* infection at Tanah Merah, in Boven Digoer, West Irian, and obtained a natural infection rate with filarial larvae of 10.9% (72 of 655) and an experimental infection rate of 49% (22 of 45) in *Anopheles barbirostris bancroftii*.

(A.1.a.4) *Anopheles* (*Anopheles*) *umbrosus* group

The most characteristic feature of this group is the absence of developed palmate hairs on the abdomen of the larva. The adult is without a pale fringe spot on the hind margin of the wing, the basal half of the costa is without pale scales, and there are no scales on the abdominal sternites. About a dozen species are known; all breed in shady areas and are characteristic of the evergreen tropical rain forests of Southeast Asia. The following species have been reported to be involved in the transmission of filariasis.

Anopheles (*Anopheles*) *letifer* Sandosham, 1944

A species closely related to *An. umbrosus* (Theobald, 1903); for detailed differential diagnosis refer to REID (1968). WHARTON *et al.* (1963) in a study of malaria and filariasis among the aborigines in Selangor and Pahang, West Malaysia, found this species to be the main vector of malaria and *W. bancrofti* infection in lowland settlements in Selangor.

Anopheles (*Anopheles*) *whartoni* Reid, 1963

A species very close to *An. letifer*, and known only in the lowland parts of East Pahang, Malaysia. In a village in East Pahang, both *W. bancrofti* and *B. malayi* were found to be endemic, and *An. whartoni* was incriminated as the main vector of *W. bancrofti* based on epidemiological evidence and the results of experimental infection studies (WHARTON, 1960; REID, 1963).

(A.1.b) Subgenus *Cellia* Theobald, 1902

A subgenus of *Anopheles* containing over 150 species distributed mainly in the Oriental and the Ethiopian regions. This subgenus includes a number of important species which serve as vectors of malaria and filariasis. In the females, mosquitoes of this subgenus have the costa of the wing divided by pale spots into four or more dark marks involving both the costa and vein I. In the larva, the bases of inner clypeal hairs are wide apart, and the antennal shaft hair is minute and simple.

The subgenus *Cellia* is further classified into six series, according to REID (1968), namely *Neomyzomyia, Myzomyia, Neocellia, Cellia, Pyretophorus,* and *Paramyzomyia.* The species known to be important vectors of malaria and filariasis are scattered among these six series. There has been no evidence reported that members of this subgenus are involved in the transmission of *B. malayi. W. bancrofti,* on the other hand, is apparently well adapted for development in mosquitoes of this group, and at least in tropical Africa and in the Papuan region, mosquitoes of this subgenus have been confirmed to be the major vectors of *W. bancrofti.*

Species of *Cellia* are discussed in this text according to three zoogeographical groups: (1) *An. gambiae* group in Africa (2) *An. punctulatus* group in the Papuan zone, and (3) miscellaneous *Cellia* species in South Asia.

(A.1.b.1) *Anopheles (Cellia) gambiae-funestus* groups

Mosquitoes of the *gambiae* and the *funestus* groups of the genus *Anopheles,* subgenus *Cellia,* are the main vectors of malaria and filariasis bancrofti in the tropical and subtropical regions of Africa. In this connection, many reports are available describing the taxonomy, biology, and disease transmission of these groups of mosquitoes, such as HOLSTEIN (1954), HORSEFALL (1955), MACDONALD (1957), MUCHET *et al.* (1965), HAMON *et al.* (1967) BRENGUES *et al.* (1968), SERVICE (1970), and GREEN (1972).

According to MACDONALD (1957), both *An. gambiae* Giles, 1902 and *An. funestus* Giles, 1900 are widely distributed in Africa; *An. gambiae* is catholic in its choice of breeding place with a bias towards sunlit, open pools, and *An. funestus* is associated with vegetated swamps, grassy riversides, and suchlike water. In most instances, both species in the equatorial zone are highly anthropophilic, with the daily mortality lying between three and seven percent in *An. gambiae,* and slightly higher in *An. funestus.* They are, therefore, one of the most efficient vectors of malaria in the world. As will be discussed in detail in Chapter 7, these two species also act as the main vectors of *W. bancrofti* in most endemic areas of tropical Africa.

The *Anopheles gambiae* complex has been shown to comprise several physiological races, or sibling species. By mating experiments among different colonies of this group of mosquitoes, DAVIDSON & JACKSON (1962), DAVIDSON (1964), and PATERSON (1964) revealed that what was formerly referred to as *An. gambiae* Giles, 1902, is composed of at least five sibling species: three freshwater forms, A, B, and C; and two brackish water species, *An. merus* Dönitz, 1902 and *An. melas* Theobald, 1903. Attempts for separating these forms by external morphology have been only partially successful. However, COLUZZI & SABATINI (1967) succeeded in separating the species A and B by the chromosome structure of the larval salivary glands. COLUZZI (1968) further discovered that the polytene chromosomes of the ovarian nurse cells of half-gravid females could be used as a direct and quick means for identification of the adult *An. gambiae.* By utilizing this technique, SERVICE (1970) showed that species A was predominant over species B in all but one of 13 villages in northern Nigeria. No significant differences were seen between the two species in host preference, or sporozoite rate.

GREEN (1972) presented maps of the XR chromosomes of the ovarian nurse cells of species A, B, and C. In this study, freshly blood-fed females were kept in individual tubes at 15°C for 48 hours. Ovaries dissected from the half-gravid females were preserved in fresh Carnoi's fluid overnight; these were transferred to 50% proprionic acid for about 15 minutes, until they became gelatinous. They were then macerated in a drop of lactoacetic orcein for about five minutes; the materials were washed in 50% proprionic acid, and were squashed in acid under a siliconized cover slip. In the chromosome maps, the position of the dilatation at 3D-4B in species C, and at 4C-5A in species B was shown to be a reliable diagnostic feature for the two species, while the most obvious features distinguishing species A were the homologous dilatation occurring between 1C and 2A, and the heavy double band at 3D (the homologous bands occur at 1D in species B and C).

Previous studies by various workers in West Africa have shown that *An. gambiae* s.1., *An. melas* and *An. funestus* are the main vectors of *W. bancrofti*, while in the coastal areas of East Africa *C. fatigans* was shown also to be involved in the transmission besides *An. gambiae* and *An. funestus*.

In West Africa, for example, *An. gambiae* s.1. was shown to be naturally infected with *W. bancrofti* by ANNETT *et al.* (1901) and TAYLOR (1930) in Nigeria, by HICKS (1932) and GORDON *et al.* (1932) in Sierra Leone, by KARTMAN (1946) in Senegal, by BARBER *et al.* (1932), DILLER (1947) and GELFAND (1955) in Liberia, by BRENGUES *et al.* (1968) in Upper Volta, by FERREIRA *et al.* (1948) in Guinea, by MUIRHEAD-THOMPSOM (1954) in Ghana, by BERTRAM *et al.* (1958) in Gambia, and by HAMON *et al.* (1962), BRENGUES *et al.* (1965, 1968) and SUBRA *et al.* (1967) in Ivory Coast.

An. funestus was shown to be the natural vector of *W. bancrofti* by TAILOR (1930) in Nigeria, by GORDON *et al.* (1932) in Sierra Leone, by KARTMAN (1946) in Senegal, by GELFAND (1955) in Liberia, by BRENGUES *et al.* (1968) in Upper Volta, and by BERNER (quated by JORDAN, 1960) in Ghana.

An. melas was demonstrated to be naturally infected with *W. bancrofti* by GELFAND (1955) in Liberia, by TOUMANOFF (1958) in Guinea, by BERTRAM *et al.* (1958) in Gambia, and by SUBRA & COZ (quoted by BRENGUES *et al.*, 1968) from Ivory Coast.

An. welcomei was shown by BRENGUES *et al.* (1968) to be also naturally infected with *W. bancrofti* in Upper Volta.

In East Africa, for example, NELSON *et al.* (1962) conducted a comprehensive study on Kenya coast on the transmission of human and animal filariasis by various mosquitoes (see also Section 7D.6). *W. bancrofti* infection in mosquitoes was seen mainly in *An. gambiae*, *An. funestus* and *C. fatigans*. Filaria larvae found in other mosquito species were mostly those of animal filariae.

WHITE (1971a, b) conducted studies on the transmission of *W. bancrofti* in three contrasting endemic areas in north-eastern Tanzania. As the results, it was estimated that the transmission was due 54% to *An. gambiae* (mainly species B) and 46% to *An. funestus* in an inland village, Gonja. In rural district around Muhenza, the transmission was due 52% to *An. funestus*, 40% to *An. gambiae*, and 8% to *C. fatigans*. In the urban part of Tanga City, the only significant vector of *W. bancrofti* was *C. fatigans* (see Section 7D.5).

SMITH (1955a, b, c, d) found in his study on the transmission of *W. bancrofti* on Ukara Island on Lake Victoria, Tanzania, that both *An. gambiae* and *An. funestus* were the sole vectors, though a little transmission might take place by *An. pharoensis* (See Section 7D.5).

An. gambiae and *An. funestus* were also shown to be the main vectors of *W. bancrofti* in Malagesi (Madagascar), and were more efficient vectors of local *W. bancrofti* than *C. fatigans*. However, *C. fatigans* was demonstrated to be the main vector of *W. bancrofti* endemic on other Indian Ocean islands, such as Mauritius, the Comores, the Seychelles, and the Maldives (see Section 7E).

(A.1.b.2) *Anopheles* (*Cellia*) *punctulatus* group

This species group in the subgenus *Cellia* is indigenous to the Papuan region, and is notorious as an efficient vector of malaria and filariasis. ROZEBOOM & KNIGHT (1946) made a comprehensive study on the systematics of this group, and came to the conclusion that it consists of four distinct species:

> *An. punctulatus* Doenitz, 1901
> *An. farauti* Laveran, 1902
> *An. koliensis* Owen, 1945
> *An. clowi* Rozeboom et Knight, 1946.

The second and the third species correspond to the *An. punctulatus* noted by various authors. As for the systematics, distribution, and biology of this group, BELKIN (1962) gave detailed accounts. The first three species are the principal vectors of the nocturnally periodic *W. bancrofti* in the Papuan region. *An. farauti* has a wide range of distribution throughout West Irian, Papua, New Guinea, the Bismarck Archipelago, the Solomon Islands, New Hebrides, Australia, the Moluccas Islands, and the Banda Islands. *An. farauti* and *An. koliensis* are restricted to New Guinea, the Bismarck Archipelago, and the Solomon Islands (see Section 9C).

(A.1.b.3) Miscellaneous *Cellia* species in South Asia

A large number of *Cellia* species are endemic in South and Southeast Asia, and some of them have been noted to be highly anthropophilic, acting as important vectors or malaria. They are usually suitable hosts of *W. bancrofti*; certain species among them have been shown to be the primary vectors in the rural endemic areas in Malaysia, the Philippines, India, etc. Some additional *Cellia* species have given indications of being secondary or suspected vectors in a number of localities.

Anopheles (*Cellia*) *maculatus* Theobald, 1901

This species, widely distributed in South and Southeast Asia, is a major vector of malaria in Malaysia.

In Pulau Aur, an offshore island of West Malaysia, CHEONG & ABU HASSAN (1965) found 30 of 208 *An. maculatus* to be infected with filaria larvae, and five of them to be carrying mature larvae of *W. bancrofti*, thus incriminating this species as the principal vector. In Pulau Tioman, BALA-SINGAM *et al.* (1967) found the similar situation (see Section 9B.7).

Anopheles (*Cellia*) *minimus* Theobald, 1901

This species is widely distributed in Southeast Asia, and is a notorious vector of malaria in the hilly regions of Thailand, Indochina, South China, Taiwan, and the Yaeyama Islands.

In Hong Kong, JACKSON (1936) conducted epidemiological studies on *W. bancrofti* infection, and found natural infections with filarial larvae in 59 of 2432 *An. minimus*, 5 of 165 *An. jeyporiensis candinensis* Koizumi, 1924, and 6 of 442 *Culex fatigans* (see Section 8C.3).

In a mountain district of Hainan Island, South China, WANG (1959) reported that infective larvae of *W. bancrofti* were found in *An. minimus*, *An. jeyporiensis* var. *candinensis*, and *An. leucosphyrus*. *An. minimus* consti-tuted about 90 % of all mosquitoes found inside houses (see Section 8C.1).

Anopheles (*Cellia*) *minimus flavirostris* (Ludlow, 1914)

This subspecies of *minimus* is known mainly in the Philippines and Bor-neo, and is the principal vector of malaria in the Philippines. Two ecologi-cal types of *W. bancrofti* infection have been noted from the Philippines: one transmitted chiefly by *Aedes poecilus* in the abaca-growing areas, and another transmitted by *An. minimus flavirostris* in certain rural areas. The latter type of endemic areas were reported by ROSEBOOM & CABRERA (1963, 1964) from Mountain Province of Luzon, where 5 of 321 *An. minimus fla-virostris* were infected and 4 of them had mature larvae of *W. bancrofti*. In Palawan, ROZEBOOM & CABRERA (1965b) indicated that this species was also the major vector of *W. bancrofti*.

Anopheles (*Cellia*) *philippinensis* Ludlow, 1902

This species is widely distributed in South and Southeast Asia. It has been noted to be the principal vector of malaria in Bengal, India, and Bangladesh. In the Birbhum District of Bengal, IYENGAR (1941) reported high rates of natural infections of *An. philippinensis* with malaria sporozo-ites and mature larvae of *W. bancrofti*. This indicated that the main vector of *W. bancrofti* in this rural area was not *Culex fatigans* but *An. philippin-ensis*.

Anopheles (*Cellia*) *tesselatus* Theobald, 1901

This species is widely distributed in South and Southeast Asia, the Mo-luccas, and New Guinea. In the Maldives, IYENGAR (1952) showed that *Culex fatigans* is the main vector of *W. bancrofti*; however, 4 of 22 *An. tesselatus* he dissected were infected with filarial larvae (see Section 8A.5).

(A.1.c) Subgenus *Nyssorhynchus* Blanchard, 1902

This is a subgenus of *Anopheles* indigenous to the New World. The following species were reported to be involved in the transmission of *W. bancrofti* in South America and the Antilles.

Anopheles (*Nyssorhynchus*) *albimanus* Wiedemann, 1821: (i.e., *tarsimaculatus* Goeldi, 1905)

This species is found widely in the Antilles, the United States, Mexico, and Central and South America. O'CONNOR & BEATTY (1938) in St. Croix found 1 out of 10 *An. albimanus* to be naturally infected, but they considered this species to be a minor vector because its distribution is rather limited.

In Belém, Brazil, DAVIS (1935) obtained a sample of proboscis infection of mature larvae of *W. bancrofti* in *An. tarsimaculatus* infected experimentally.

Anopheles (*Nyssorhynchus*) *aquasalis* Curry, 1932

In Belém, Brazil, CAUSEY *et al.* (1945) found the infection with mature larvae in 1 of 332 *An. aquasalis* dissected. In Guyana, BURTON (1964, 1967) reported that *An. aquasalis* and *Mansonia titillans* were the secondary vectors of *W. bancrofti*, while *C. fatigans* acted as the primary vector.

Anopheles (*Nyssorhynchus*) *darlingi* Root, 1926

In Belém, Brazil, DAVIS (1931) reported 7% of 200 *An. darlingi* dissected were infected. CAUSEY *et al.* (1945) found three *An. darlingi* out of 563 examined were infected, and one had mature larvae. In Guyana, GIGLIOLI (1948) found at Lodge Village, in the suburbs of Georgetown, that 22 *An. darlingi* out of 515 examined were infected, and two among them had mature larvae; the author concluded that *An. darlingi* was as efficient as *C. fatigans* in the transmission of *W. bancrofti* in this region.

(A.1.d) Subgenus *Kerteszia* Theobald, 1905

This is also a New World subgenus of *Anopheles*. The only one record of the involvement of this member in the transmission of human filariasis is as follows.

Anopheles (*Kerteszia*) *bellator* Dyar et Knab, 1906

In Ponta Grossa, Brazil, RACHOU *et al.* (1955b) found one of three specimens of *An. bellator* to be infected with first stage larvae.

(B) Subfamily Culicinae

(B.1) Genus *Mansonia* Blanchard, 1901

One of the characteristics of the mosquitoes of the genus *Mansonia* is the structure of the siphon of the larvae, which is modified for piercing subaquatic plant tissues with sclerosed, saw-toothed processes at the tip. The trumpets of the pupae are also modified for piercing plant tissues. The *Mansonia* mosquitoes, therefore, breed in swamps and ponds, attached to roots or stems of aquatic plants throughout the larval and pupal stages.

The genus is divided into four subgenera, i.e., *Mansonia*, *Mansonioides*, *Coquillettidia*, and *Rhynchotaenia*. Of these, the subgenus *Mansonioides* includes important vectors of *B. malayi* in South and East Asia. Sporadic reports are also available on the natural infection of subgenera *Mansonioides*, *Mansonia*, and *Rhynchotaenia* with nocturnally periodic *W. bancrofti*.

(Further investigations are necessary, in most of these cases, to confirm whether the filaria larvae in *Mansonia* were really those of *W. bancrofti*, or were misdiagnoses of animal filaria larvae.)

An excellent review was made by WHARTON (1962) on the biology of *Mansonia* mosquitoes in relation to the transmission of filariasis in Southeast Asia.

(B.1.a) Subgenus *Mansonioides* Theobald, 1907

Some ten species have been recorded as members of this subgenus, among which six are indigenous to the Oriental region, three to the Papuan region, and one to the Ethiopian region. This subgenus includes important vectors of both the periodic and the subperiodic races of *B. malayi* in South and East Asia. Sporadic reports have been made also on the infection of *Mansonioides* species with *W. bancrofti* larvae. Adult mosquitoes of this subgenus are mostly dark colored, with ornamentations characteristic to each species on the scutum of thorax, and white bands or spots on legs. The wing has large, broad scales, often of asymmetrical shape.

It should be noted that species within this subgenus are not equally suitable for development of the periodic and the subperiodic race of *B. malayi*. The environmental requirements of their breeding places are also not the same. For example, the *M. dives* and *M. bonneae* groups breed in swamp forests, serve as efficient vectors of the subperiodic race, but are poor vectors of the periodic race of *B. malayi*. On the other hand, natural vectors of the periodic race of *B. malayi* are mostly open swamp breeders, such as *M. uniformis* and *M. annulifera*.

Mosquitoes of the subgenus *Mansonioides* have also been incriminated as the vector of the nocturnally periodic race of *W. bancrofti* in the Bangkla area of New Guinea by VAN DIJK (1958) and by DE ROOK & VAN DIJK (1959), and in Palacole, Tamil Nadu, India, by SOMASUNDARAM (1949).

(B.1.a.1) The *dives-bonneae* group

Mansonia (*Mansonioides*) *dives* (Schneider, 1868) and *Mansonia* (*Mansonioides*) *bonneae* Edwards, 1930 are two closely related species difficult to be distinguished morphologically. They have been confused by most previous workers to be a single species, and were often referred to as *M. annulipes* Walker, 1857 or *M. longipalpis* Walker, 1857. *M. dives* has a wide distribution in India, Thailand, Malaysia, Indonesia, the Philippines, New Guinea, and Australia. *M. bonneae* have been recorded from Malaysia, Borneo, Thailand, and the Philippines.

BRUG & DE ROOK (1930) conducted field studies in Benkoelen, Sumatra. *B. malayi* (presumably the subperiodic race) was the only human filaria in this region, and cases infected with *W. bancrofti* were absent. *M. annulipes* (now *M. dives*) and *M. annulata* were the most abundant mosquitoes. They were shown to be naturally infected, and to serve as efficient hosts when infected experimentally. This was the first report that *Mansonioides* mosquitoes were involved in the transmission of human filariae.

In Malaya, POYNTON & HODGKIN (1939) showed that *M. longipalpis* (now *M. dives/bonneae* complex) is the vector of *B. malayi* in the swamp forest areas in Perak, Pahang, and Sabak Bernam. Detailed studies on the transmission of the subperiodic race of *B. malayi* in Pahang by *dives/bonneae* group were conducted by WHARTON (1957, 1962). This group of mosquitoes was shown to be the vector of subperiodic *B. malayi* in Sabah by BARCLAY (1969), in southern Thailand by GUPTAVINAJ *et al.* (1971), and in the Philippines by CABRERA & ROZEBOOM (1964) and CABRERA (1966b).

Experimentally, *M. bonneae* is a poor vector of the periodic race of *B. malayi*, but WHARTON *et al.* (1963) indicated that *M. dives* could transmit the periodic race of *B. malayi* in West Malaysia.

(B.1.a.2)   The *uniformis-annulifera* group
Mansonia (*Mansonioides*) *annulata* Leicester, 1908
M. annulata occurs in West Malaysia, Thailand, Sumatra, Borneo, and the Philippines. It breeds in swamps on the forest fringe. This species was shown to be the vector of *B. malayi* in Sumatra by BRUG & DE ROOK (1930) and REES *et al.* (1958; quoted by Lie, 1970), in Kalimantan by KLOKKE (1961), in West Malaysia by WHARTON (1962), and in Thailand by HARINASUTA *et al.* (1970a).
Mansonia (*Mansonioides*) *annulifera* (Theobald, 1901)
This mosquito has a wide range of distribution in the Oriental region (India, Sri Lanka, Indochina, Thailand, Malaysia, Indonesia, the Philippines), and New Guinea. A very domestic mosquito, it breeds in small pools and ponds around houses where *Pistia* and other water plants, suitable for the attachment of larvae, are available.
This species was shown to be an efficient vector of periodic *B. malayi* in Kerala, India (IYENGAR, 1938, PAL *et al.* 1960), and to some extent in Sri Lanka (CARTER, 1933), Thailand (IYENGAR, 1953) and Kalimantan (KARIADI, 1938). Detailed studies on the bionomics were conducted by PAL *et al.* (1960).
Mansonia (*Mansonioides*) *uniformis* (Theobald, 1901)
This species occurs extensively in the Oriental region northward up to Japan, westward to large parts of tropical Africa, and eastward to the Papuan region. Larvae and pupae breed in open swamps and ponds, attaching to water plants, such as *Eichhornia crassipes* (water hyacinth), *Pistia stratiotes* (water cabbage), etc. The biology of this and related species in India was investigated extensively by BURTON (1959, 1960). The females of *M. uniformis* were shown to prefer to feed on cattle and have a very low anthropophilic index; being 2.8% in India (PAL *et al.*, 1960), and 2.0% in West Malaysia (WHARTON, 1962).
Since it is a common mosquito in open swamp areas, *M. uniformis* has been incriminated as an important vector of periodic *B. malayi* in Kerala, India (IYENGAR, 1938; PAL *et al.*, 1960), in Thailand (IYENGAR, 1953; HARINASUTA *et al.*, 1970a), Malaya (HODGKIN, 1938, 1940, quoted by WHARTON,

1962; REID *et al.* 1962; WHARTON, 1962), and in Kalimantan (KARIADI, 1938).

M. uniformis has also been shown to transmit a subperiodic race of *B. malayi* in Malaya (WHARTON, 1962; RAMACHANDRAN *et al.*, 1970), and in southern Thailand (GUPTAVANIJ *et al.*, 1971).

In the Bamgi-Ia area of the southwestern plain of West Irian, *M. uniformis* and possibly *M. papuensis* Tayler, 1914, were incriminated as the vectors of nocturnally periodic *W. bancrofti* by VAN DIJK (1958), and DE ROOK & VAN DIJK (1959). However, BRUNHES *et al.* (1972) demonstrated that *M. uniformis* in Malagesi (Madagascar) was refractory to the development of *W. bancrofti* larvae, and also that none of *M. uniformis* specimens were naturally infected with third stage larvae of *W. bancrofti*, though it harbored those of animal filariae (see Section 7E.1).

Mansonia (*Mansonioides*) *indiana* Edwards, 1930

This species also has a wide distribution in South Asia: India, Sri Lanka, Thailand, Malaysia, Indonesia, and New Guinea. The larvae breed in open swamps, attaching to water plants, such as the water hyacinth, *Eichhornia crassipes*.

M. indiana has been incriminated as a minor vector of *B. malayi* in India (IYENGAR, 1938), in Sri Lanka (DASSANAYAKE, 1938) in southern Thailand (IYENGAR, 1953; HARINASUTA *et al.* 1970a), and in Java (LIE *et al.*, 1960).

(B.1.c) Subgenus *Rhynchotaenia* Brethes, 1910

Mansonia (*Rhynchotaenia*) *juxtamansonia* (Chagas, 1907)

In an experimental study of infection in various mosquito species in Belém, Brazil, DAVIS (1935) reported that proboscis infection with mature larvae of *W. bancrofti* was obtained in *M. juxtamansonia*.

(B.1.d) Subgenus *Mansonia* Blanchard, 1901

Mansonia (*Mansonia*) *titillans* (Walker, 1848)

A secondary vector of nocturnally periodic *W. bancrofti* in Guyana, South America (BURTON 1964; 1967).

(B.2) Genus *Aedes* Meigen, 1818

This is the largest genus in the family Culicidae, and comprises 23 subgenera and some several hundred species. They are mostly blackish mosquitoes and usually daytime biters, though some members bite man during the nighttime and may transmit nocturnally periodic filariae. The subgenera containing important vectors of human filariasis are *Ochlerotatus*, *Finlaya*, and *Stegomyia*.

(B.2.a) Subgenus *Ochlerotatus* Lynch Arribalzaga, 1891

Aedes (*Ochlerotatus*) *vigilax* (Skuse, 1889)

This species has a wide distribution in Australia, New Guinea, New Hebrides, New Caledonia, Indonesia, Thailand, and Indochina. It was shown to be the main vector of the nonperiodic race of *W. bancrofti* in the New Caledonian zone by IYENGAR (1954). Detailed studies on the bionomics of this mosquito in New Caledonia were reported by IYENGAR (1965; see section 9D).

The larvae of *Ae. vigilax* breed in open stagnant pools containing saline water, and thus its distribution is restricted to areas near the coast. The females are day-time biters and exophilous (*i.e.* usually stay outdoors). In coastal villages in New Caledonia, IYENGAR (1954a) observed an infection rate of 5%, and LACOUR & RAGEAU (1957) found 2.2% to be infected with filaria larvae. High infection rates with *W. bancrofti* larvae were recorded in experimental infections in New Caledonia (IYENGAR, 1954a; IYENGAR & MENON, 1956: BACKHOUSE & WOODHILL, 1956).

Aedes (*Ochlerotatus*) *edgari* Stone et Rosen, 1952

A species indigenous to the Society Islands, Polynesia. This was shown to be an efficient laboratory vector of the diurnally subperiodic race of *W. bancrofti* in Tahiti by STONE & ROSEN (1952).

Aedes (*Ochlerotatus*) *scapularis* (Rondani, 1848)

A New World species. RACHOU *et al.* (1955b) reported natural infection of *Ae. scapularis* with nocturnally periodic *W. bancrofti* at Santa Catarina, Brazil.

Aedes (*Ochlerotatus*) *taeniorhynchus* (Wiedemann, 1821)

This species is found on coasts and inland saline areas in the Americas, *i.e.*, from Massachusetts to Brazil, California to Peru, and the West Indies.

In St. Croix, the Virgin Islands, O'CONNOR & BEATTY (1938) made a study of the infection of mosquitoes with *W. bancrofti* larvae and found an infection rate of 25.1% and an infective rate of 2.3% in 5,000 C. *fatigans* dissected. Infections with immature larvae in *Ae. taeniorhynchus* were also found by these anthors.

(B.2.b) Subgenus *Finlaya* Theobald, 1903

This is a large subgenus within the genus *Aedes*, and includes over 180 recognized species as of 1959. The subgenus is characterized by the presence of well-developed claspettes, by the absence of a prominent basal lobe in the male genitalia, by the development of a large, only slightly retracted abdominal segment VIII, and by a short cercus in the female.

The subgenus is further classified into several groups, each with distinct characters. Some members of this subgenus have been noted to be highly adapted for the development of various filarial larvae, or to be actually playing an important role in the transmission of human filariasis.

The taxonomy of various groups of *Finlaya* was developed extensively by Knight and his co-workers from 1946 to 1952. KNIGHT & MARKS (1952) published a checklist of *Finlaya*. MARKS (1947) gave a key to the *kochi* group of the Australasian region. Descriptions of *Finlaya* in the South Pacific were published by *Belkin* (1962).

(B.2.b.1) *Aedes* (*Finlaya*) *togoi* (Theobald, 1907)

This species is known to occur in Japan, Korea, China, Taiwan, Siberia, and also in Okinawa, Ogasawara, and Marcus Island. It was reported recently by RAMALINGAM (1969) to occur in Vietnam, Thailand, and West

Malaysia. The adults are dark-colored mosquitoes with peculiar longitudinal stripes on the mesonotum and white bands on most of the leg joints; the wing is not speckled. The larvae are dark colored, with a short siphon, and numerous combs on the eighth abdominal segment. The larvae breed mainly near the beach in rock pools containing saline water.

Ae. togoi was found to be the principal vector of the nocturnally periodic race of *B. malayi* in Hachijo-Koshima Island, Japan (SASA *et al.*, 1952). The same species was reported to be the vector of *B. malayi* in coastal regions of continental China by LI (1959b) and GUN (1960), and also from Cheju Island, South Korea by KIM & SEO (1968), LEE (1969) and WADA *et al.* (1973).

Ae. togoi is also an excellent intermediate host of nocturnally periodic *W. bancrofti* when experimentally infected (MOCHIZUKI, 1913; YAMADA, 1927; OMORI, 1962). It was shown to be a secondary vector of *W. bancrofti* in fishing villages in Nagasaki (OMORI, 1962).

RAMACHANDRAN *et al.* (1963) showed that *Ae. togoi* is an excellent experimental intermediate host of various filarial species, including the periodic and subperiodic races of *B. malayi*. The rural strain of *W. bancrofti* in Malaya, *B. pahangi*, *B. patei*, *Dirofilaria immitis* of dogs, *Breinlia* sp., and *Setaria* spp. also develop very well in this mosquito. *Ae. togoi* is a large mosquito, easily bred in laboratories and allows the development of large numbers of infective larvae.

(B.2.b.2) *Aedes* (*Finlaya*) *niveus* (Ludlow, 1903)

Mosquitoes of the *Ae. niveus* group includes a number of closely related species with a pair of white patches on the shoulder parts of mesothorax. Taxonomic accounts on this group of mosquitoes were made by KNIGHT (1946) and COLLES (1959).

In West Thailand, HARINASUTA *et al.* (1970) incriminated the *Ae. niveus* group as the vector of a nocturnally subperiodic form of *W. bancrofti*. In an endemic area in the Sankla-buri district, a total of 9,303 mosquitoes were collected on human bait from May 1965 to June 1966, among which the most abundant (2,775) were of the *Ae. niveus* group mosquitoes. Of 2,724 specimens of this group dissected, 6 (0.22%) contained mature larvae of *W. bancrofti*, and 22 (0.81%) were found infected with filaria larvae. No infection with the mature larvae was found in other mosquito species (see Section 8B.1).

Ae. niveus was shown to be a secondary vector of nocturnally periodic *W. bancrofti* in Mountain Province of Luzon, Philippines, by ROZEBOOM & CABRERA (1963, 1964). Of 43 *Ae. niveus* naturally caught and dissected, 11 had filaria larvae and 2 had mature larvae (see Section 8B.6).

(B.2.b.3) The *kochi* group

Mosquitoes of the *kochi* group of *Finlaya* are characterized by spotted wings with bands of dark and light scales, and thus can be easily differentiated from other *Finlaya* species which are all dark scaled. Most members of this group breed in the leaf axils of various plants, such as banana, taro, pandanus, etc.

Two important subgroups of vectors are included here: *Ae. poecilus*, the principal vector of nocturnally periodic *W. bancrofti* in abaca-growing areas in the Philippines, and *Ae. fijiensis* and related species which serve as secondary vectors of the nonperiodic *W. bancrofti* in the Polynesian region.

Important references for the *kochi* group are:

KNIGHT & LAFFOON (1946): keys to the Oriental *kochi* group;

MARKS (1947): descriptions of the Australasian *kochi* group;

BELKIN (1962): descriptions of the *kochi* group in the South Pacific;

RAMALINGAM (1968): the *kochi* group of Samoa.

(B.2.b.3a) *Aedes* (*Finlaya*) *poecilus* (Theobald, 1903)

A species of the *kochi* group widely distributed in South and Southeast Asia, i.e., from India through Burma, Thailand, Malaysia, Indonesia, and the Philippines.

The occurrence of endemic areas of nocturnally periodic *W. bancrofti* transmitted chiefly by *Ae. poecilus* has been noted only from the Philippines (CABRERA & TUBANGUI, 1951; ROZEBOOM & CABRERA, 1956). This is due to the extensive growing of the abaca plant in certain regions of the Philippines. (See Section 7B.6.)

(B.2.b.3b) The *fijiensis* subgroup

The following are important species of the *kochi* group in the Polynesian region which serve as potential or secondary vectors of nonperiodic *W. bancrofti* next to the *Aedes* (*Stegomyia*) *polynesiensis* group of mosquitoes.

In Fiji:

Aedes (*Finlaya*) *fijiensis* Marks, 1947

A species known only from Fiji. Natural infections with filarial larvae were recorded by SYMES (1955) and BURNETT (1960), but according to IYENGAR (1965), this mosquito is not an important vector because its distribution is limited. The larvae breeds exclusively in the leaf axils of *Pandanus*.

In Samoa:

The following three species have been noted to breed in Western Samoa and American Samoa. According to RAMALINGAM (1968), all three species are suited for the development of the nonperiodic race of *W. bancrofti*, and may be important vectors in the inland villages. Their larval breeding places are in the leaf axils of *Pandanus*, taro, *Freycinetia*, etc.

Aedes (*Finlaya*) *samoanus* (Grunberg, 1913)

Aedes (*Finlaya*) *oceanicus* Belkin, 1962

Aedes (*Finlaya*) *tutuilae* Ramalingam et Belkin, 1965

(B.2.c) Subgenus *Stegomyia* Theobald, 1901

This subgenus of *Aedes*, containing about 100 species, includes important vectors of dengue fever, yellow fever, and certain forms of human or animal filariasis. The adults are small, blackish, but ornamented with peculiar white markings on the thorax and legs. The females are usually voracious human biters. The biting activity takes place during the day-time, and generally outdoors. Larvae breed in small rainwater containers such as coconut shells, tree and bamboo holes, empty cans, jars, and barrels.

(B.2.c.1) *Aedes* (*Stegomyia*) *aegypti* (Linnaeus, 1762)
This is a species notorious as the vector of yellow fever and dengue fever. It has a very wide distribution throughout the tropical zones of the world.

Ae. aegypti are usually refractory to infection with *W. bancrofti* (both periodic and nonperiodic races), and have never been shown to be impor-tant natural vectors. However, sporadic reports are available on the dis-covery of developmental stage or more rarely, mature stage filarial larvae in naturally caught *Ae. aegypti*. It has never been shown to act as a natural vector of *B. malayi*, but under experimental conditions, certain races of *Ae. aegypti* are susceptible to infection with the subperiodic race, and have been used in the laboratory transmission of the parasite (see Section 2E.1.3).

(B.2.c.2) The *Aedes* (*Stegomyia*) *scutellaris* group
A group of *Stegomyia* with a median longitudinal white stripe on the mesonotum, and three continuous stripes of white scales on the pleura of the thorax. Members of this taxonomic group in the Polynesian region, especially *Ae. polynesiensis* and allied species, are the principal vectors of the nonperiodic, or the diurnally subperiodic race of *W. bancrofti*. Details of the taxonomy and epidemiology of the *Ae. scutellaris* group in the South Pacific can be found in reports by: MARKS (1951), STONE *et al.* (1959), BELKIN (1962), IYENGAR (1965), RAMALINGAM & BELKIN (1964), and RA-MALINGAM (1968). The following are the species recognized to be the vec-tors in each of the Polynesian islands or island groups:
Aedes (*Stegomyia*) *polynesiensis* Marks, 1951
Distribution: Fiji, Horne Islands (Hoorn, Futuna), Wallis Islands, Ellice Islands, Tokelau Islands, Samoa Islands, northern and southern Cook Islands, Society Islands, Austral Islands, Marquesas Islands, Tua-motu Archipelago, and Pitcairn Islands (after BELKIN, 1962).

This is the most important vector of the nonperiodic race of *W. bancrofti* in the Polynesian region wherever it occurs. The females are exophilic, day-biting, voracious human biters, and highly adapted for the development of the larvae of the nonperiodic Polynesian race of *W. bancrofti*. The larvae breed in all types of artificial and natural containers of rainwater around houses, and sometimes even in the crab holes made in sandy beaches. It has been considered, therefore, difficult to interrupt the transmission of *W. bancrofti* filariasis in Polynesia by the control of these mosquito vectors.

Aedes (*Stegomyia*) *pseudoscutellaris* (Theobald, 1910)

A species known only from Fiji. Because of the similarities in the morphology, this species had been confused with *Ae. polynesiensia* until MARKS (1951) created a new species for the more widely distributed form. According to IYENGAR (1965), both *Ae. pseudoscutellaris* and *Ae. polynesinensis* are the important vectors of the nonperiodic *W. bancrofti*. MATAIKA *et al.* (1970) reported that the latter is more abundant and important as the vector in the populated coastal areas, while *Ae. pseudoscutellaris* is more common in the inland areas.

Aedes (*Stegomyia*) *tongae* Edwards, 1926; and *Aedes* (*Stegomyia*) *tabu* Ramalingam et Belkin, 1965

According to RAMALINGAM & BELKIN (1965) and RAMALINGAM (1968), two species of the *Ae. scutellaris* group occur in the Tonga Islands, *Ae. tongae* and *Ae. tabu*. The former is distributed on the Haapai and the Vavau groups, while *Ae. tabu* occurs on the Tongatapu and Haapai groups.

RAMALINGAM & BELKIN (1964, 1965) and RAMALINGAM (1968) conducted comprehensive entomological and epidemiological studies in Tongatapu, and found *Ae. tabu* to be the main vector of the nonperiodic *W. bancrofti* in this region.

Aedes (*Stegomyia*) *upolensis* Marks, 1957

A species indigenous to the Samoa Islands. RAMALINGAM (1968) found that in American Samoa 9% were positive for all stages of the larvae and 1.8% were positive for the mature larvae. However, SUZUKI & SONE (1974) considered this species to be of minor importance in the transmission of filariasis in Western Samoa because the population density was much lower than *Ae. polynesiensis*.

Aedes (*Stegomyia*) *cooki* Belkin, 1962

This was assumed by IYENGAR (1965) to be the vector of nonperiodic *W. bancrofti* in Niue (not Cook Islands!) because this was the only species of the *Ae. scutellaris* group found on this island.

Aedes (*Stegomyia*) *rotumae* Belkin, 1962

A species recorded from Rotuma Island (see Section 6E.3). Because this is the only species of *Ae. scutellaris* group found on this island, IYENGAR (1965) assumed it to be the vector of nonperiodic *W. bancrofti*.

Aedes (*Stegomyia*) *futunae* Belkin, 1962

A species recorded by Belkin (1962) from Alofi Island of the Hoorn Islands (Alofi and Futuna); it is assumed to occur also on Futuna Island, which is only several km from Alofi. Belkin also considered this species to be the probable main vector of filariasis in the Futuna group because it was apparently more abundant than *Ae. polynesiensis*.

(B.3) The genus *Culex* Linnaeus, 1758

This is a large genus comprising 16 subgenera and several hundred species. The most important subgenus among them is *Culex*, in which STONE *et al.* (1959) listed 182 species and a number of subspecies. Adults of *Culex* are usually reddish brown to brown in color, and are active during the nighttime. They can be differentiated from adults of other genera by the presence of well-developed pulvillia near the end of the tarsi. The larvae are generally characterized by a long and slender siphon.

Several species of the subgenus *Culex* have been noted to be the vectors of *W. bancrofti* (nocturnally periodic race), among which *Culex pipiens* is by far the important vector in many urban endemic areas. Other species have been noted to be minor or secondary vectors in certain rural endemic areas.

(B.3.a) The *Culex pipiens* complex

Culex (*Culex*) *pipiens* Linnaeus, 1758, is a mosquito species highly domestic and widely distributed throughout the world. The females are night-biters, usually highly anthropophilic, and excellent intermediate hosts of *W. bancrofti*. However, they are sometimes less adapted than certain anopheline species for the development of certain rural strains of *W. bancrofti*, and only poorly adapted for the development of the Pacific (diurnally subperiodic) race of *W. bancrofti*. The larvae of this species breed usually in open ditches, sewage pools, and artificial containers of polluted water.

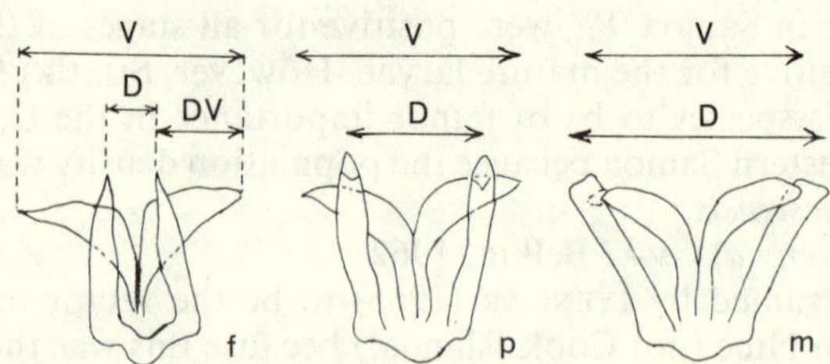

Fig. 2-5.   Diagram of dorsal and ventral arms of the phallosome of male genitalia; f: *fatigans*, p: *pallens*, m: *moletus* (Sasa *et al.*, 1967)

Mosquitoes of the *Culex pipiens* complex are further classified into several geographical or physiological subspecies, among which the following are of practical importance. The geographic distribution, morphological and genetical characters, and the crossing experiments among these subspecies in East and South Asia were reported by SASA *et al.* (1966, 1967; see Table 2-12 and Fig. 2-5, 2-6).

(i) *Culex pipiens pipiens* Linnaeus, 1758: This subspecies is considered to be found in Europe and northern parts of North America. It has a D/V ratio (see Fig. 2-5) of about 1.0; physiologically not autogenous and not stenogamous (see 'Note'); difficult to be bred in cages.

(ii) *Culex pipiens fatigans* Wiedemann, 1828 (= *Culex quinquefasciatus* Say, 1823): This subspecies is found in the tropical and subtropical zones of the world. It is an excellent intermediate host of *W. bancrofti*. The D/V

Table 2-12. The averages and standard deviations of D/V values (in percentages) of various colonies of the *Culex pipiens* complex collected from South Asia and Japan (SASA *et al.*, 1967).

Form & Code No.	Locality of collection		Latitude of the locality (in degress)	Number examined	Average D/V	Standard deviation
fatigans						
RGf	Rangoon		16.8 N	220	33.0	3.15
PJf	Kuala Lumpur		3.2 N	100	29.2	4.38
BKf	Bangkok		14.0 N	100	36.2	4.51
SBf	Lahad Datu	(Sabah)	5.0 N	100	31.6	5.22
TAf	Taketomi	(Okinawa)	24.4 N	102	29.1	8.90
MKf	Miyako	(Okinawa)	24.8 N	101	32.8	2.87
NHf	Nahr	(Okinawa)	26.1 N	113	32.1	2.96
KOf	Koniya	(Amami)	28.2 N	100	35.2	6.37
pallens						
KGAp	Kagoshima	(Kyushu)	31.5 N	100	49.1	5.37
KGBp	Kagoshima	(Kyushu)	31.5 N	107	42.4	8.17
SKp	Sakito	(Kyushu)	33.0 N	80	57.4	4.88
KTp	Kyoto	(Honshu)	35.0 N	103	73.1	7.32
NGp	Nogoya	(Honshu)	35.2 N	119	62.8	6.04
HRp	Kawasaki	(Honshu)	35.5 N	107	80.0	9.35
DAp	Tokyo	(Honshu)	35.6 N	102	69.1	8.18
DBp	Tokyo	(Honshu)	35.6 N	103	72.8	6.05
SDp	Sendai	(Honshu)	38.3 N	98	81.3	6.36
SRAp	Sapporo	(Hokkaido)	43.0 N	110	90.2	5.67
SRBp	Sapporo	(Hokkaido)	43.0 N	41	88.5	7.35
ASp	Ashibetsu	(Hokkaido)	43.5 N	29	74.8	7.87
molestus						
KWm	Kawasaki	(Honshu)	35.5 N	105	123.2	8.86
ORm	Tokyo	(Honshu)	35.6 N	120	125.2	7.23
TSm	Tokyo	(Honshu)	35.6 N	109	124.0	7.81
IRm	Teharan	(Iran)	35.5 N	100	132.5	12.58

ratio is approximately 0.3. It is neither autogenous nor stenogamous, but is easily bred in cages.

(iii) *Culex pipiens pallens* Coquillette, 1898: This is a form showing intermediate characters between the two extreme populations, *i.e.*, between *pipiens* s. str., and *fatigans*. The value of D/V varies from 0.3 to 1.0, and is correlated with the latitude of the locality of collection (see Fig. 2-6). It is neither autogenous nor stenogamous. This is also a main vector of *W. bancrofti* in the Temperate zone, such as in Japan and China.

(iv) *Culex pipiens molestus* Forskal, 1775: This subspecific name has

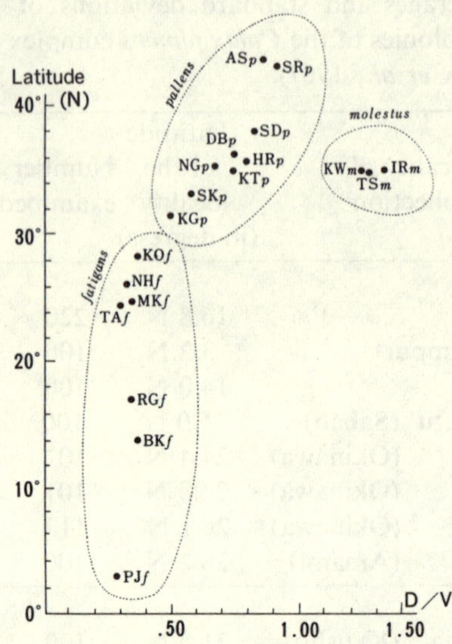

Fig. 2-6.   Correlation between latitude of the locality of collection and the average D/V ratio of male genitalia of the *Culex pipiens* complex (Sasa *et al.*, 1967).

been attributed to the autogenous and stenogamous race found in Egypt, the Middle East, Japan, and North America. It has the largest D/V ratio, 1.2, of all the subspecies. Eggs are usually deposited on sewage water in dark basements of concrete buildings. This race was also shown to be susceptible to the development of *W. bancrofti* larvae by FUJISAKI (1958).

Note: Autogeny is the genetic characteristic of female mosquitoes which allows them to produce eggs without first taking a blood meal. On the other hand, females of most mosquito species (or races) require a blood meal for producing eggs, otherwise, the ovaries remain undeveloped. The autogenous mosquitoes may take blood meals after they have deposited the first batch of eggs. Stenogamy is another physiological characteristic of *molestus* races, describing the ability of the male and female to copulate in a small space, such as in a test tube. They are capable of mating even in completely dark spaces, such as the basements of buildings. For details of the characteristic, refer to SASA *et al.* (1967).

Since MANSON (1877) demonstrated for the first time the development of the larvae of *W. bancrofti* in *C. fatigans* in Amoy, South China, large numbers of reports have been made from various regions of the world on the role played by this species in the transmission of human filariasis. Mosquitoes of the *C. pipiens* complex are the principal vectors of nocturnally periodic *W. bancrofti* in many parts of the tropical, subtropical, and Temperate Zones, including most countries in South and East Asia, coastal and urbanized areas in Africa, the West Indies, South America, and Micronesia. The form of *W. bancrofti* transmitted by *C. pipiens* complex is often referred to as the urban type in contrast to the more rural nature of that transmitted by *Anopheles* and *Aedes* mosquitoes.

Mosquitoes of the *Culex pipiens* complex (either *fatigans* or *pallens*) have been reported to be important vectors of nocturnally periodic *W. bancrofti* endemic in the following regions and countries:

American Region: North and Central America (the United States, Costa Rica), West Indies (many islands, see Section 6B), South America (the Guianas and Brazil)

African Region: certain urban areas in East and West Africa, Egypt.

Asian Region: South Asia (India, Sri Lanka, the Maldives, Bangladesh, and Burma), Southeast Asia (urban areas in South Vietnam, Singapore, and Indonesia), East Asia (China, the Pescadores, Hong Kong, and Japan)

Pacific Region: Micronesia (see Section 9B)

Since the mosquitoes of this complex are the major vector of *W. bancrofti* and the most common pest mosquitoes throughout the world, a large amount of literature is available on the taxonomy, bionomics, and vectorial capacity of this species. Some important references on the bionomics of the *Culex pipiens* complex are: ABDULCADER (1965, 1967: Sri Lanka). BURTON (1956, 1960: India; 1964, 1967: Gayana), CHOW (1957: Sri Lanka; 1959: Jakarta), DeMEILLON *et al.* (1967: Rangoon), FENG (1933a: Amoy), HEIDOR (1931: Queensland), HU (1935: Shanghai), IKESHOJI (1971: attractants), McMILLAN (1960: New Guinea), NAGATOMO (1960: Nagasaki, Japan), OMORI (1962 a,b, 1966, 1967, 1968, 1970: Japan), PARTONO (1970: Jakarta), LAVEN (1957: genetics), RAO & IYENGAR (1929: India), SAMARAWICKREMA (1967: Sri Lanka), SASA *et al.* (1964, 1965 a,b,c, 1966, 1967, Japan & Asia), SINHA (1967, 1968: global review), SUBRAMANYAM & Tampa (1958: Madras, India), SINGH *et al.* (1963 b,c: India), WATTAL & KARLA (1960, 1961: India), TADANO (1969; insecticide resistance), UMINO (1965 a, b, c, 1966: genetics and insecticide resistance), SUZUKI (1971: Insecticide resistance, review).

Although *Culex pipiens fatigans* has been shown to serve as an excellent intermediate host for the urban form of *W. bancrofti*, the species was demonstrated to be less efficient than *Anopheles* spp. for the larval development of some rural races of *W. bancrofti* in Africa (Maasch, 1973) and also in Malaya (WHARTON, 1960). This species was also shown to be refractory to *B. malayi* in Sumatra by LICHTENSTEIN (1927), and in India by IYENGAR (1932) and RAGHAVAN & KRISHNAN (1949b).

(B.3.b) The *Culex bitaeniorhynchus* groups

This is a species group within the subgenus *Culex*, with the following common morphological characteristics:

Adults: Large mosquitoes with yellowish white scales on the anterior half of the mesonotum. There are no leaflike bristles on the subapical lobe of male genitalia.

Larvae: The respiratory siphon is very long and slender, with only a few small pecten scales on the base of the siphon, and with only a few comb scales on eighth abdominal segment. The larvae usually breed in swamps and rice paddies, and are often associated with the green algae, *Spirogyra*.

Culex (*Culex*) *bitaeniorhynchus* Giles, 1901

This is a species widely distributed in East and South Asia. Natural infection with nocturnally periodic *W. bancrofti* was recorded by IYENGAR (1938) from Travancore, India, and by DE ROOK (1957a) from Berau, West Irian. The infection rate was 0.3% with all stages of the larvae in the former, and 19.7% with all stages of the larvae, and 2.1% with mature larvae, in the latter. DE ROOK (1957a) also reported that infective larvae were recovered from 87.0% of *C. bitaeniorhynchus* experimentally infected with *W. bancrofti* at Berau, West Irian. However, YAMADA (1927), in Japan, observed in experimental infection that the larvae of *W. bancrofti* ceased their development in *C. bitaeniorhynchus* at the second stage.

(B.3.c) The *gelidus-sitiens* group

Mosquitoes of this group belong to the subgenus *Culex*. They include important human biters and disease vectors, for example, *Culex tritaeniorhynchus*, the main vector of Japanese encephalitis in East and Southeast Asia. Adults of this group are generally small mosquitoes with a white band on the middle part of proboscis, and white rings on most leg joints. There are leaflike bristles on the subapical lobe of the male genitalia. The larvae have long and slender respiratory siphons, and numerous comb scales on eighth abdominal segment. Several species of this group have also been noted to be infected with filaria larvae, or to carry infective stage larvae of *W. bancrofti* in rural endemic areas in South Asia and the Pacific, though their role is usually secondary or minor in the transmission of filariasis.

Culex (*Culex*) *annulirostris* Skuse, 1889

DE ROOK (1957a) at Berau, West Irian, found 25.5% to be infected with all stages of larvae and 1.6% with infective larvae of *W. bancrofti*. On Pam Island, West Irian, DE ROOK (1957b) reported 6.8% (3 of 44) to be infected and 2.3% (1 of 44) to be containing mature larvae of *W. bancrofti* (In both areas, *An. farauti* was the main vector of *W. bancrofti* but three other species of mosquitoes, including *C. annulirostris*, were also found to contain mature larvae).

Culex (*Culex*) *gelidus* Theobald, 1901

In Travancore, India, IYENGAR (1938, quoted by RAGHAVAN, 1961) reported 0.1% being infected with filaria larvae.

Culex (*Culex*) *sitiens* Wiedemann, 1828

A species widely distributed in South Asia, North Australia, the Pacific islands, and Africa. The larvae breed in pools of brackish water. Filaria infection was reported by IYENGAR (1938) from Tranvancore, India, by GALLIARD *et al.* (1949) in Tahiti, by CARTER (1948) in Sri Lanka (*B. malayi*), and by IYENGAR (1952) in the Maldives.

Culex (Culex) whitmorei (Giles, 1904)

YAMADA (1927), in an experimental infection study, showed that excellent development of *W. bancrofti* to the infective stage took place in this mosquito.

The *Culex tritaeniorhynchus-pseudovishnui* subgroup

The adults of mosquitoes of this subgroup are morphologically closely related and often difficult to separate in field studies. A revision of the taxonomy of this group in Southeast Asia was published by COLLESS (1957). *Culex tritaeniorhynchus* is also famous as the main vector of Japanese encephalitis in East and South Asia. YAMADA (1927) found no development of *W. bancrofti* larvae beyond the first stage in *C. annulus* (= *pseudovishnui*), and only a small number could reach the mature stage in *C. tritaeniorhynchus*. IYENGAR (1938) in Travancore, India, reported natural infection in 3 of 3,237 *C. vishnui* caught in an endemic area of *B. malayi*. CARTER (1948), in endemic areas of *B. malayi* in Sri Lanka, observed 1.16% of naturally caught *C. tritaeniorhynchus* to be infected with mature larvae. WOLFE & ASLAMKHAN (1972) conducted a mosquito infection study in endemic areas of *W. bancrofti* in Bangladesh; they observed 12 of 5,569 *C. vishnui* complex mosquitoes (composed probably of *C. annulus. C. pseudovishnui*, and *C. tritaeniorhynchus*) to be infected with all stages of the larvae, of which 2 had mature larvae. In the same area, 3,454 *C. fatigans* were dissected; 373 (10.5%) were infected and 40 (1.1%) contained mature larvae.

2E.4 Control of mosquito vectors

In control programs of filariasis due to *W. bancrofti* or *B. malayi*, the operations are directed usually to the control of both parasites and the vectors. In most cases, the parasite control operations such as by administration of DEC to the whole population or to microfilaria carriers are more dramatic in the effects than those to the control of vector mosquitoes. As shown by OMORI *et al.* (1972), it takes at least 10 years for the spontaneous disappearance of microfilariae from people in endemic areas of filariasis by application of vector control operations alone. Nevertheless, if vector control operations are effectively pursued simultaneously with the drug treatment of human populations, the effective control or eradication of filariasis is considered to be achieved much more efficiently than by the use of the drug alone (see Section 10D.3.2).

3

Filariasis due to *Loa loa*

3.1 Historical notes

Because the adult worms of *Loa loa* are frequently found in the eyes of patients, the parasite has attracted the attention of physicians for many years. It was described under various names, such as *Filaria loa Guyot*, 1778, *Filaria oculi humani* Dujardin, 1845, *F. lacrimalis* Dubini, 1850, *F. oculi* Gervais et van Beneden, 1859, and *F. subconjunctivalis* Guyon, 1864. The embryos in the circulating blood are diurnally periodic, and have often been referred to as *Microfilaria diurna* Manson, 1891.

According to FAUST *et al.* (1970, *Clinical Parasitology*), there were a series of case reports on "eye worm" infections among West African slaves imported into the Neotropical region, from 1770, when Mongin extracted this worm from the eye of a Negro woman in St. Domingo, West Indies. In Africa, the first record of this worm was made by GUYOT in 1777 from Angola.

Later investigators showed that endemic areas of *L. loa* infection are confined to the rain-forest belt of West and Central Africa, and equatorial Sudan. STOLL (1947) estimated the world incidence of *L. loa* infection to be 13 million cases.

3.2 Geographic distribution

Human and simian infections with *L. loa* have been recorded only from the African region, and from the limited regions covered mainly by tropical rain forests, where the *Chrysops* vectors can easily find breeding places. *L. loa* infection in man has been recorded in the medical literature from the following countries and territories:

West Africa: Senegal, Guinea, Mali, Dahomey, Niger, Chad, Nigéria
Central Africa: Cameroons, Ubangui-Shari, Zaire, Gabon, Angola
East Africa: Zambia, Malawi, Uganda, Sudan

3.3 The parasite

3.3.1 Adult

According to Looss (1904), who first made a detailed study on the adults of *L. loa*, the males measure 30 to 34 mm in length and 0.35 to 0.43 mm in diameter; the females measure from 50 to 70 mm in length and 0.5 mm in diameter. The cuticula is ornamented with small bosses. The mouth is provided with one pair of lateral papillae and two pairs of submedian papillae, all sessile and small. The caudal end of the male curves ventrally and has narrow wings. There are about eight pairs of perianal papillae, five pairs of large preanal and three pairs of small postanal papillae. The pair of copulatory spicules are unequal in size and dissimilar in shape. The female vulva opens in the cervical region. The structure of adult *L. loa* was illustrated by York & Maplestone (1926) in their textbook "The Nematode parasites of Vertebrates" (Fig. 286, p. 418).

3.3.2 Microfilariae

See Section 1.3.3

3.3.3 Larval stages in vectors

The larval development of *L. loa* takes place in certain horse fly species of the genus *Chrysops*. In West Africa, *C. silacea* has been incriminated as the principal vector of human loiasis. The larval stages developing in the vector were described by CONNAL & CONNAL (1922), and more precisely by LAVOIPIERRE (1958a) and WILLIAMS (1960, 1961a). At a temperature between 82.6°F and 86.6°F, the microfilariae after being ingested by *C. silacea* develop to the infective larvae in seven days, molt twice, and pass three larval stages, as in other filarial larvae. The larvae develop in the fat body tissues of the fly, mainly in that of the abdomen; they move to the head after they have completed the second ecdysis.

The day-to-day development and the morphology of each stage of the larvae were described in detail by WILLIAMS (1960). The third stage larvae in the fly (on the seventh day) were $2,019 \pm 144\ \mu$ in length and 30 ± 2 μ in width (average of 14 specimens), with an average tail length of 51μ. Three prominent papillalike structures were at the tip of the tail, one in a dorsal position and the others paired in lateroventral positions. They were rounded, fleshy structures, each containing a narrow lumen which opened through a minute pore at the tip. There were also a pair of subterminal papillae longer and more cylindrical than the terminal three.

3.3.4 Physiological races

In the rain forest zone of West Cameroon, where about 30% of the human population was infected with *L. loa*, GORDON *et al.* (1950) found that three species of monkeys most common in the forest adjoining human habitat (*i.e.*, the drill, or *Mandrillus leucophaeus*, the putty-nosed quenon, or *Circopithecus mona mona*,) were infected with a form of *Loa* morphologically indistinguishable from that in man except for their larger size. DUKE & WIJERS (1958) and DUKE (1960a, b), in a series of experimental studies on loiasis in monkeys, demonstrated that the microfilariae of *Loa* in monkeys were nocturnally periodic, but that the drill could be infected experimentally with the diurnally periodic human strain, as well as with its natural nocturnally periodic strain, by inoculation with infective larvae collected from *Chrysops*. When the infective larvae of human origin came to maturity in the drill, after a prepatent interval of four to five months, the microfilariae were found to have a typically diurnal periodicity, exactly as in man. The vectors of simian *Loa* were determined to be the crepuscular canopy-dwelling *Chrysops langi* and *C. centurionis*. These authors concluded that the transmission of *Loa* from man to monkeys would probably be extremely rare under natural conditions.

DUKE (1964) conducted experiments for hybridization between the diurnally periodic human strain of *Loa* (DD) and the nocturnally periodic simian strain (NN) in the drill host, *Mandrillus leucophaeus*. He allowed young, virgin females of each strain to mate with males of the opposite strain. The females fertilized by heterologous males produced microfilariae, but were not highly fecund. The F-1 hybrid microfilariae thus produced were intermediate in length between those of the parent strains. They showed a periodicity which was predominantly diurnal. After ingestion by *Chrysops*, these microfilariae developed normally to infective larvae which, when inoculated into clean drills, produced fertile hybrid adult worms (DN). The hybrid adults were of large size, approximating the NN parents. They mated among themselves, producing microfilariae of complex periodicity. Studies of the length and periodicity of the F-2 microfilariae, and the results of backcrossing DN hybrid males with virgin females of parent strains suggested that the two strains were segregating along simple Mendelian lines with respect to somatic size and periodicity. Under experimental conditions, some hybrid matings did take place in drills when infective larvae of the two strains were inoculated simultaneously; however, such hybridization and propagation of hybrid strains probably do not occur in nature.

3.4 Human loiasis

3.4.1 Symptomatology

The adult worms of *Loa* normally live in and move around the subcutaneous tissues, often provoking a temporary inflammation commonly called "Calabar swelling" or "fugitive swelling". According to Duke (1973), it is usually a "hen's egg" or Wasp sting type" of fugitive edema, lasting two to three days; the swellings, however, may sometimes involve the whole limb, usually the arm. In some patients the swelling may start as reddish lumps about three cm across; they then extend circumferentially with an ever widening red ring at the periphery reaching a diameter as large as 20 cm.

The adult worms often enter the front of the eye ball causing severe conjunctivitis; they can be seen moving under the conjunctiva.

Eosinophilia:

It has been noted by many workers that *L. loa* can produce high eosinophilia. DUKE (1973) states that it often produces an eosinophilia rate of 60 to 90% with otherwise-normal white blood cell counts; totals of 20,000 to 50,000 or even more white blood cells per mm³, may give rise, at first glance, to fears of leukemia.

Albuminuria:

It has also been noted that albuminuria is often accompanied by *L. loa* infection in man. (SNIJDERS, 1935; GENTILINI *et al.*, 1963). Treatment with DEC may cause an increase in albuminuria before clearing it.

Meningo-encephalitis:

A syndrome of meningoencephalitis has been reported in connection with *L. loa* infection, especially when DEC is given to persons harboring very high concentrations of microfilariae in their peripheral blood. KIVITS (1952), in the Kangu region of Zaire, where loiasis was hyperendemic, reported on the occurrence of fatal or seriously ill cases of encephalitis caused by the invasion of *Loa* microfilariae in the cerebrospinal fluid. DOWNIE (1966) stated that prolonged coma may result from blockage of the cerebral capillaries by moribund microfilariae after administration of DEC, and in some cases that recovered there was permanent cerebral damage. BRUMPT *et al.* (1969) state that patients showing over 2,500 microfilariae per 50 mm³ blood were at high risk of such reactions, and they have recorded persons with as many as 12,500 microfilariae per 50 mm³. FAIN (1969) reported that such meningoencephalitis cases were not rare in any of the hospitals in the Kangu region of Zaire, especially in children from 5 to 12 years of age. Most of these cases had the symptoms soon after they took DEC, which was sold freely in the pharmacies.

Other symptoms reported to be associated with *Loa* infection:

TOUSSAINT & DANIS (1965) reported on the finding of retinal hemorrhages and exudate associated with high microfilaria concentrations of *L. loa* in a white patient, who died of meningoencephalitis.

IVE *et al.* (1967) reported on endomyocardial fibrosis in Nigeria which was associated with eosinophilia, fever, swelling of the face, and irritation of the skin; its geographical distribution was similar to that of *L. loa*.

3.4.2 Diagnosis

The only reliable means of diagnosis of *Loa* infection in man at present is demonstration of either the microfilariae in the blood or the adults in the tissues. There have been no immunological methods yet established for a sure diagnosis of loiasis.

Because the microfilariae in the circulating blood of human hosts exhibit conspicuous diurnal periodicity with a peak density at about noon, the collection of blood samples for the diagnosis of *Loa* infection should be made during the daytime. Because the *L. loa* microfilariae are sheathed, special attention should be paid to attempt to differentiate them from those of *W. bancrofti* by their morphological characters (see Section 1.3.3).

The adult filariae recovered from under the skin or from the eye should also be examined morphologically for identification of the species (see Section 3.3.1).

3.4.3 Treatment

LAGRANGE (1949) and WANSON (1949), in Zaire, demonstrated that DEC in relatively low dosages was effective in clearing the microfilariae of *L. loa* and curing the skin swellings. Trial treatments of human loiasis with DEC were reported also by MURGATROYD & WOODRUFF(1949), SHOOKHOFF & DWORK (1949), GERMAIN *et al.* (1950) and HECKENROTH *et al.* (1950). WOODRUFF (1951) observed that relatively small doses of DEC could eliminate the microfilariae from the human blood stream and bring about their destruction in the liver, while high and prolonged doses of the drug caused death of the adult worms in the tissues. KERSHAW *et al.* (1955) conducted an experiment to eliminate the human microfilarial reservoirs by administration of DEC, and to see its effect on the infection rates of vector populations. In two small villages in the rain forest of Cameroon, where monkeys infected with *L. loa* were common, no marked reduction in the infection rates of the flies was obtained, while on a rubber estate at Sapele, Nigeria, where monkeys were relatively rare, the infection rate among man-biting *Chrysops* showed a remarkable drop. In Sapele, northern Nigeria, DUKE & MOORE (1961) conducted mass treatments of microfilaria carriers with an adult dosage of three tablets (200 mg of DEC citrate each) per day for 20 days. They found that 89.4% (286 of 320) of the previously positive cases became negative in the posttreatment examination conducted one month after completion of the treatment. These authors state that the drug could be safely administered to the parasite carriers, and was effective in reducing the microfilariae to extremely low levels. However, the infection rate of *C. silacea* was reduced to only about one-half of the pretreatment level (6.1% in the pretreatment survey and 3.1% in the posttreatment survey), probably because about one-third of the human population refused to co-operate with the study.

As stated before, the occurrence of severe side reactions after administration of DEC has been noted in hyperendemic areas of loiasis, such as the Kangu region of Zaire. Duke (1973) states that in patients with high densities of microfilariae, it is safer to begin the treatment with low doses, such as 1 mg per kg of body weight, three times a day. Duke further recommended that steroid be administered simultaneously, at least during the first two or three days when the main load of microfilariae is being destroyed.

Duke (1973) demonstrated that DEC is also effective in killing adult worms of *L. loa*; in fact, reactions attributable to dying adult worms occur during the first five to seven days of full dose treatment. DEC treatment is especially effective in lightly parasitized persons, who often suffer the most from the presence of the parasite, and exhibit the greatest number of signs and symptoms. In heavily parasitized persons, on the other hand, some of the adult worms may well resist several courses of treatment.

3.4.4 Chemoprophylaxis

DEC was demonstrated by Duke (1961, 1963) to be effective against the immature stages of *L. loa* developing in monkeys and in man, and useful as a prophylactic drug. Infective larvae of *L. loa* were collected from *Chrysops silacea* and *C. dimidiata* previously fed on parasite carriers; they were then inoculated into young drills, which were subsequently treated with various compounds, including antimonials, arsenicals, suramin, and DEC. When autopsied three to six months later, all the untreated animals, as well as those treated with the drugs (except for DEC), were found to harbor the adults of *Loa* at rates of about one-third of the inoculated numbers. In animals treated with DEC, complete clearance of the parasite was observed in those which received relatively high doses, such as over 100 mg per kg in total; over 90% of the parasites were killed by daily administrations of as low as 5 mg per kg. In later experiments with human volunteers, it was also demonstrated that 5 mg per kg of DEC taken daily for three days, once a month, or larger doses, could give complete prophylaxis against *L. loa* infection. Development of a peculiar papular skin reaction due to the death of the parasites in the skin was noted in those treated with DEC.

3.5 Vectors

3.5.1 The horse-fly genus *Chrysops*

Tabanidae, or horse flies, belong to the Suborder Brachycera of the Order Diptera. They are stoutly built flies, and differ from members of the suborder Nematocera (for example mosquitoes, black flies, and biting midges) in that the antennae are short and consist usually of only three distinct segments. According to OLDROYD (1973), there are over 3,000 species in the world. Medically important horse flies belong to one of the following three genera: *Chrysops*, with banded wings and spotted eyes, often called "deer flies"; *Hematopota*, with speckled wings, and eyes marked with zig-zag bands; or *Tabanus*, a very large and complex genus, usually with clear wings and with eyes either uniformly colored or with one or more horizontal bands.

The life history of horse flies consist of egg, larval, pupal and adult stages. Only females suck blood. The larval habitat is usually in the wet mud at the edges of streams, ponds, swamps, rice paddies, lakes, and rivers. Most larvae of *Chrysops* feed on vegetable debris, while those of *Hematopota* and *Tabanus* are carnivorous and feed on other insects, worms, and even their own species.

The vectors of *Loa loa* are species of *Chrysops* living in the canopy in tropical Africa, and four species are concerned. DUKE (1955, 1960) found that *C. silacea* and *C. dimidiata* are active by day and transmit human loiasis, the microfilariae of which appear in the peripheral blood by day. On the other hand, *C. centurionis* and *C. langi* are mainly crepuscular and nocturnal biters, feeding upon monkeys sleeping in the treetops whose peripheral blood contains the microfilariae of *Loa* at night.

The complete development of the microfilariae of *L. loa* up to mature larvae was shown by LEIPER (1912, quoted by DUKE, 1955) and later by CONNAL & CONNAL (1922) to take place in *Chrysops silacea* and *C. dimidiata*, the two horse-fly species commonly biting man at Sapele, in southern Nigeria. These authors also showed that wild horse-flies were naturally infected, and were, without doubt, the two main vectors of loiasis, in West Africa. These two species were also found to be the principal vectors of loiasis in Zaire (FAIN, 1969). In southern Sudan, where some 15% of the population showed microfilariae in the blood, WOODMAN & BOKHARI (1941) observed slow development of *L. loa* in *Chrysops distinctipennis*, and considered it to be the local vector. WOODMAN (1949) further recorded its partial development in *C. longicornis*.

3.5.2 Host-parasite relationship

KERSHAW *et al.* (1953, 1954a, b, c, 1955a, b, 1956, 1957) and NICHOLAS & KERSHAW (1954, Pt. 3) conducted studies on the intake of various species of microfilariae by their insect vectors, their survival in the vectors, and their effect on the survival of the vectors. As for the intake of *L. loa* by *Chrysops*, KERSHAW *et al.* (1954a, pt. 2) demonstrated that the actual intake showed a wide variation; most of the flies took fewer microfilariae than might have been expected considering the microfilarial density of the peripheral blood, and the amount of blood ingested by the flies. KERSHAW *et al.* (1954b, Pt. 4) further showed that the longevity of the fly population was not significantly influenced by the development of larvae of *L. loa*, though high mortalities were seen in a logarithmic rate proportional to the age in naturally caught flies under the laboratory conditions. KERSHAW *et al.* (1954c, Pt. 5) reported that the number of infective forms found in the flies which survived long enough to support the development of the infective forms was almost the same to the number of microfilariae taken in.

KERSHAW *et al.* (1955a, Pt. 6) conducted further observations on the intake of the microfilariae of *L. loa* and *D. perstans* by *Chrysops silacea* under laboratory conditions. It was shown that the actual intake, the expected intake, the population exposed, and the population at risk in the conditions of the experiment were all related.

KERSHAW *et al.* (1956, Pt. 8) determined the amount of blood ingested by *C. silacea* and *C. dimidiata* under natural and laboratory conditions. In laboratory conditions at Kumba, the weight of unfed *C. silacea* was 15.3 mg on the average, with a standard deviation of 2.7 mg; the size of the average blood meal ingested was 35.4 mm^3, with a standard deviation of 11.6 mm^3. In the natural conditions at Sapele, the average weight and standard deviation of unfed *C. silacea* was 12.9 mg and 2.8 mg, respectively, and the amount of blood ingested was 24.2 mm^3 on the average, with a standard deviation of 9.7 mm^3; the average weight and standard deviation of unfed *C. dimidiata* was 10.5 mg and 2.3 mg, respectively, while the amount of blood ingested was 19.7 mm^3 on the average, with a standard deviation of 11.2 mm^3. In all of these cases, the size of blood meal ingested to repletion by the horse flies was about twice the weight of the unfed flies.

KERSHAW *et al.* (1957, Pt. 9) studied the pattern of the frequency of the blood meals taken in by *C. silacea*, and the survival of the fly in natural conditions in the rain forest of the British Cameroons, and on a rubber estate in the Niger Delta. The length of that interval was deduced from the stage of development of the larvae of *L. loa* in infected flies. The flies which came to bite man were made up of two groups: (a) those which feed three or four days after an infecting meal, and again in the last three or four days, and which, when coming to bite and transmit the infection, contain infective larvae at least ten days old; and (b) a population which feeds about the fifth day and comes in again about the tenth day, when the infective larvae have only just completed their development. The survival rate of the flies was also assessed from the ratios of flies containing various developmental stages of *L. loa* larvae, by empirically fitting different rates of mortality to the two groups and comparing the predicted number of survivors with the observed data.

DUKE *et al.* (1956) conducted observations on the relationship between the size of the blood meal taken in by *Chrysops silacea*, the development of the fly's ovaries, and the development of the *L. loa* microfilariae taken in with the blood meal. It was shown that the stimulus leading to the development of the ovaries of wild *C. silacea* tends to be of the "all-or-none" type, that is, no fly showed development of the ovaries after a blood meal of less than 3.6 mg, nor did any fly fail to show normal development of the ovaries after a blood meal of more than 14.2 mg. The microfilariae of *L.*

loa developed normally irrespective of the size of the blood meal and regardless of whether or not the ovaries developed.

3.5.3 Bionomics of *Chrysops* vectors

The ecology and biology of the various species of *Chrysops* were investigated extensively by workers in the British Cameroons; it was shown that the problems of loiasis and its transmission by various species of horse flies were more complex than previously considered. According to the record of the Helminthiasis Research Unit at Kumba, four species of *Chrysops* were caught on the wing. Of these, *C. silacea* constituted the majority of the population which bit man, *C. dimidiata* less than 0.5%, *C. langi* only three specimens, and *C. centurionis* only one specimen (WILLIAMS, 1960). On the other hand, the species composition of *Chrysops* collected as larvae and pupae from their breeding places in streams and swamps was shown to be quite different; in fact, *C. longicornis* constituted 30% of all, *C. langi* 29%, and *C. silacea* 26% (CREWE, 1955). Altogether, eight species of *Chrysops*, seven species of *Tabanus*, and a species of *Hematopota* were reared and identified from their breeding places (WILLIAMS, 1961b, 1962). OLDROYD (1957) recorded 38 species of *Chrysops* to be existing in the Ethiopian region alone.

DUKE (1955b, c, d, e; 1958, 1959, 1960) conducted a series of studies on the biting habits of *Chrysops* in the British Cameroons, and obtained the following results:

(1). Observations were made on the biting density and biting cycle of *C. silacea* in the rain forest near Kumba at various heights from the ground level, *i.e.*, above the canopy (130 feet), in the canopy (92 feet), in the open layer (28 feet), and on the forest floor. The numbers of the flies caught in a 24-hour-catch were 28, 169, 151, and 72, respectively. The biting activity was highest, in general, between 1 to 2 p.m. or 2 to 3 p.m.; almost no biting was done at night, though the biting cycle varied considerably from one level to another (DUKE, 1955b).

(2). The biting density of *C. silacea* at ground level in the rain forest was increased more than six times when catches were made in the presence of a wood fire. The flies released at canopy level were attracted down to ground level by the smell of wood smoke (DUKE, 1955c).

(3). More *C. silacea* per man per hour were caught by groups of eight or 16 persons at ground level of the forest than by a single person. When a group of persons moved, the biting density became lower, but it increased when the group took a rest (DUKE, 1955d).

(4). In a study of the flight range of *C. silacea* in the Kumba area, it was shown that the biting density measured in the presence of a wood fire in a clearing bordered by a rain forest diminished logarithmically as the distance between the catching station and the forest increased. The biting density fell to one-tenth of the forest value at 530 yards from the forest in a cleared area planted with rubber saplings 10 to 12 feet high, and at 100 yards in a still clearer area planted with rubber saplings 1.5 to 2 feet high (DUKE, 1955e).

(5). A series of 24-hour catches was made by DUKE (1958) on a canopy platform erected in the rain forest of Bombe, about 20 miles from Kumba, where drills and other monkeys infected with *Loa* were plentiful. In contrast to *C. silacea* and *C. dimidiata*, which showed a diurnal biting activity with morning and afternoon peaks, *C. langi* and *C. centrionis* were found to be crepuscular biters, showing a single sharp peak of biting activity at about sunset. The incidence of infection with *Loa* was found to be higher in the latter two species than in the former two. DUKE (1958) believed that *C. langi* and *C. centurionis* probably obtained their blood meals almost entirely from monkeys, and considered them to be the natural vectors of the simian *Loa* parasite.

(6). A comparison was made by DUKE (1959) between the biting habits of *Chrysops silacea* and *C. dimidiata* (Bombe form) in the rain forest at Kumba. In the absence of a wood fire, *C. dimidiata* was more efficient than *C. silacea* in finding stationary human bait on the forest floor. The annual cycles of biting density of the two species were markedly different; *C. silacea* was most active from April to December, while *C. dimidiata* showed two peaks, one from November to January and the other from March to May, its biting density dropping nearly to zero from June to October. In observations on the infective biting densities over 27 months, a peak was found regularly in the months of April, May, and June.

(7). According to DUKE (1960), the parous females of *C. silacea* and *C. dimidiata* could be differentiated from the nulliparous flies by the presence of follicular relics in ovarioles as in other bloodsucking Diptera flies using the method described by DETINOVA (1962; see Section 10c.2.4): The biting density of the nulliparous *Chrysops* shows a peak in the morning, while that of the parous ones became highest in the afternoon, thus exhibiting two biting density peaks every day. Only parous females were found to be infected with *L. loa* larvae.

Further extensive studies on the bionomics of *Chrysops* spp. in relation to the transmission of loiasis in the southern Cameroons were reported by WILLIAMS (1960, 1961a, b, 1963a, b, c), CREWE (1961a, b), and CREWE & WILLIAMS (1961).

3.5.4 Control of vectors

DUKE (1973) pointed out that in rain forest areas, normal village development automatically produces a degree of control of loiasis transmission. As the village enlarges and the adjacent forest is cleared for farmland, the breeding sites of *Chrysops* in the forest mud tend to be drained and cleared of the vegetation suitable for the deposition of egg masses. The fact that this process of village development alone can have a marked effect is evident from studies of the prevalence rates of the infection in villages at different stages of development.

Duke also states that some developments of the environment may increase transmission. Notably, this occurs when rubber plantations are established adjacent to *Chrysops* breeding sites in swamp forests, as at Sapele, in southern Nigeria. The mature rubber plantation provides a perfect, shaded canopy, under which *Chrysops* can hunt the rubber tappers.

The spraying of *Chrysops* breeding sites with insecticides is a possible control measure, and application of dieldrin at about 380 mg per m^2 of the active ingredient was shown to maintain the sites free from larvae for as long as two-and-one-half years (DUKE, 1973). However, the practical application of this, or safer insecticides, in the control of horse flies is considered to be extremely difficult in view of the cost, manpower, and effectiveness.

4 | Filariasis due to *Dipetalonema* and *Mansonella*

4 | Filariasis due to *Dipetalonema* and *Mansonella*

4A. *Dipetalonema perstans* (Manson, 1891)

4A.1 Historical notes

In November 1890, MANSON, at the invitation of Dr. Stephen Mackenzie of London Hospital, examined the blood of an African Negro who was suffering from sleeping sickness. He found two filarial embryos; one of them was the ordinary *Filaria bancrofti*, but the other was a smaller parasite which he, in January 1891, proposed to call "*Filaria sanguinis hominis perstans*, and shortly after that to *Filaria perstans*, to comply with binary zoological nomenclature.

In 1895, Firket confirmed Manson's original observation that the "minor" embryos existed in two size; one measuring 160 to 180 μ the other measuring 80 to 90 μ.

In 1897, Manson found two forms of microfilariae in blood smears sent by Ozzard from Guyana; the one with a sharp tail was named *Filaria ozzardi*, and the other, with a blunt tail, was later confirmed to be identical with *Filaria perstans*.

The adult form of *F. perstans* was collected from the mesentery of an aboriginal Indian in Guyana and described in 1898 by Daniels.

RAILLIET, HENRY & LANGERON (1912) placed "*perstans*" in the genus *Acanthocheilonema* Cobbold, 1870, because the adult form of this species was shown to be very similar to its type species, *Acanthocheilonema dracunculoides* Cobbold, 1870. However, YORKE & MAPLESTONE (1926) considered *Acanthocheilonema* as a synonym of *Dipetalonema* Diesing, 1861. YEH (1957) placed this filaria in the genus *Tetrapetalonema* Faust, 1935; DUNN & LAMBRECHT (1963) were in favor of this idea. CHAUBAUD & ANDERSON (1959) and NELSON (1965) considered that *perstans* should be placed in the genus *Dipetalonema*, because the grounds for splitting *Dipetalonema* into several genera were insufficient.

D. perstans has been cited in a number of textbooks and a good deal literature to be present in New Guinea. For example, SHARP (1928) stated that it was found in New Guinea by Manson. In the 16th edition (1966) of "Manson's Tropical Diseases" by MANSON-BAHR, it is stated that *D. perstans* occurs "probably also in New Guinea" (p. 987). This probably originated from the following short note described by MANSON (1897) in a footnote to his report "On Certain New Species of Nematode Haematozoa occurring in America," (Brit. Med. J., 25 December 1897, p. 1838): "Since the foregoing was written I have found in blood from a native of New Guinea (northeast coast), a small, sharp-tailed, sheathless filaria closely resembling, if not identical with, filaria Demarquayi."

However, there have been no later reports from New Guinea confirming the occurrence of *D. perstans*, and the only human filaria reported to be endemic on this large island so far has been *Wuchereria bancrofti*.

4A.2 Geographic distribution

Dipetalonema perstans infection in man has been recorded from the following countries or territories in South America, and Africa:

    South America: (see Table 6-1, Chapter 6)

        Trinidad, Guyana (British Guiana), Surinam (Dutch Guiana)

    Africa: (see Table 7-1, Chapter 7)

        Northern Africa: Tunisia, Algeria

        Western Africa: Senegal, Gambia, Guinea, Mali, Sierra Leone, Liberia, Ivory Coast, Upper Volta, Dahomey, Niger, Chad, Nigeria

        Central Africa: Cameroons, Ubangui-Shari, São Tomé, Principe, Gabon, Zaire, Angola

        Eastern Africa: Rhodesia, Zambia, Tanzania, Kenya, Uganda, Sudan

4A.3 The parasite

4A.3.1 Adults

Although *D. perstans* is a parasite widely distributed among the people in the tropical Americas and tropical Africa, its adults have been recovered on only a few occasions, and its structure is only poorly known. According to FAUST *et al.* (1970), they are creamy white, elongated, cylindroid filariae with a smooth cuticula, a bluntly rounded, unarmed anterior end, surmounted by a shield having a pair of large lateral and two pairs of submedian papillae. The caudal extremity is curved ventrally in both sexes, and bifurcated forming a pair of triangular, nonmuscular flaps. The males measure about 45 mm by 60 μ, the females 70 to 80 mm by 60 μ. The posterior end of the male is distinguished by having four preanal pairs of papillae and one postanal pair, and very unequal, rodlike copulatory spicules. The vulva of the female lies in the cervical region.

4A.3.2 Microfilariae

The microfilariae of *D. perstans* appear in the circulating blood of human carriers at all hours of day, not showing the nocturnal or the diurnal periodicity found in *W. bancrofti* and *L. loa* in the same regions of Africa. (The name "*perstans*" comes from the persistent appearance of the microfilariae.) Although they are commonly found in the blood of natives in Africa, there have been no detailed descriptions published on their morphology, such as worked out by FENG (1933) with the microfilariae of *W. bancrofti* and *B. malayi* in China. Only poor illustrations, such as prepared by CRAIG & FAUST in their textbook on *Clinical Parasitology* (1970, 8th ed. p. 391), are available.

MANSON (1897) recognized at least four forms of microfilariae in man by the morphology, i.e., *Filaria nocturna* (= *W. bancrofti*), *Filaria diurna* (*L. loa*), *Filaria perstans*, and *Filaria demarquai* (= *M. ozzardi*). The former two are sheathed, and the latter two are unsheathed. The latter two were differentiated by the shape of the tail, which is blunt in *perstans* and sharp in *ozzardi*.

According to FROS (1956), the microfilariae of *D. perstans* in Surinam are 152 to 207 μ (average being 185 μ) in length in alcohol-fixed blood smears; they contain nuclei to the very end of the tail, where the body is thickened like a drumstick around the last nucleus. On the other hand, those of *M. ozzardi* are 110 to 232 μ (average being 163 μ) in body length in alcohol-fixed blood smears; the tail is slender and tapering to a point at the end and devoid of nuclei.

4A.3.3 Larval stages in vectors

The development of the larvae of *D. perstans* in the *Culicoides* intermediate hosts were studied by several workers, as described in Section 4A.5, but no detailed description of the developing and mature larvae has been published.

4A.4 Pathogenesis

Since it is so widely distributed among the natives in tropical Africa and does not cause significant signs of disease, it has been generally accepted, in most textbooks, that *D. perstans* is a parasite harmless to its hosts.

However, there have been a number of recent reports made on the possible link between this parasite and various clinical illness.

ROSS (1937) and BOURGUIGNON (1937) were two of the earliest workers to suggest the possible cause-effect relationship between the infection of *D. perstans* and clinical illness. ROSS (1937) reported, from the Lower Gwelo area of Rhodesia, five cases of general ill health and fugitive swellings. BOURGUIGNON (1937) referred to an African soldier showing *D. perstans* infection who died of hepatitis following upper abdominal colic, biliousness, and vomiting; upon autopsy, the liver showed areas of necrosis associated with numerous microfilariae. Additional case reports were made by TEISCHLER (1938), MOSLER (1939), and GARRATT (1945).

More recently, FOSTER (1956) reported a case from the Cameroons of a 20-year-old male African who died of pericarditis with effusion; microfilariae were found in the fluid before death. STROHSCHNEIDER (1956) examined 152 cases of *D. perstans* infection among African workers in Uganda. He found that 39 of them had clinical symptoms, such as giddiness, aching limbs, periodic itching, and abdominal or pectoral pains; seven cases among these were unusually severe and had developed edema of the lower limbs or scrotum. GELFAND & BERNBERG (1959) found, in Rhodesia, a European patient with microfilaremia, eosinophilia, fever, and joint swelling. GELFAND & WESSELS (1964) further reported from Rhodesia on a European female patient carrying the microfilariae of *D. perstans*; she had a marked tiredness, epigastric discomfort, headache, swollen ankles, and subsequently, liver lesions, ascites, and cardiac changes.

Additional case reports were made by a number of workers in Rhodesia. WISEMAN (1967) examined 40 Europeans and 8 Africans infected with *D. perstans*; he found that 77% of them had pruritus or rashes, transient swellings, and pain over the liver, and 69% had eosinophilia. DUKES *et al.* (1968) reported on a European soldier who was taken ill in the Zambesi Valley; at first, he was suspected of having cerebral malaria, but the malaria parasite was negative, and he continued to deteriorate on antimalarial treatment. Subsequently, microfilariae of *D. perstans* were found in his spinal fluid on three occasions. Microfilariae of *D. perstans* were also found in the spinal fluid of an African patient who had mild, nonspecific symptoms. HOLMES *et al.* (1969) investigated 50 cases of *D. perstans* carriers in Rhodesia and stated that joint pains were the most significant finding in the study; there was eosinophilia in 80%, mostly mild to moderate in degree. CLARKE *et al.* (1971) gave a comprehensive review of the problems of *D. perstans* infections in Rhodesia (see Section 7D. 2).

Studies on the diagnosis and treatment of *D. perstans* filariasis were made by ADOLPH *et al.* (1962) on 61 cases who had come back to the United States after spending from four months to 30 or more years in endemic areas of *D. perstans* in Africa; 34 among them were positive for microfilariae of *D. perstans*, but these were detected mostly only by Knott's concentration method (see Section 10B.2.2.3). Serologic tests of bentonite flocculation and hemagglutination were also performed with extracts from adult *Dirofilaria immitis* as the antigen. Seventeen among the microfilaria positive cases exhibited symptoms which were believed to be attributable to *D. perstans*. Fourteen who were symptomatic had no microfilariae in the blood, but 12 of 13 tested were positive by the serologic tests.

ADOLPH *et al.* (1962) selected the following symptoms as associated with *D. perstans* infection:

a. Swelling in forearms, hands, and face which usually recedes in about three or four days, often recurring, resembling "Calabar swellings" in loiasis

b. Itching of skin (with or without rash or ulceration)

c. Pain or ache in the bursae and joint synovia

d. Pain or ache in serous cavities

e. Pain or ache in the liver region

f. Neurological and psychic symptoms

g. Extreme exhaustion, not otherwise accounted for

4A.5 Treatment

There have been a number of reports made on the results of trail treatments of *D. perstans* infections with DEC (JURGATROYD & WOODRUFF, 1949; SHOOKOFF & DWORK, 1949; WANSON, 1949; GERMAIN *et al.*, 1950; Heckenroth *et al.*, 1950; ALMEIDA, 1952; McGREGOR *et al.*, 1952; STROHSCHNEIDER, 1956). The oral administration of DEC was effective in reducing or clearing the microfilariae of *D. perstans* from the peripheral blood, but the effects were usually only temporary and in most cases the microfilariae reappeared in the blood after the treatment was suspended. STROHSCHNEIDER (1956) conducted intraperitoneal injection of DEC solution in two cases of *D. perstans* patients; the microfilaremia relapsed in one case but the blood remained negative for seven months in another case. ADOLPH *et al.* (1962) carried out intensive DEC treatment of confirmed or suspected cases of *D. perstans* filariasis who had come back from Africa to Chicago; the drug was given orally on the basis of 2 mg per kg four times a day for 10 successive days, and 8 or 9 courses of such treatments were repeated at intervals of three weeks. In some cases provocation of symptoms and initial appearance of microfilariae in the blood were observed when the treatment started. However, resolution of symptoms and apparent recovery followed in most instances, together with permanent disappearance of the microfilariae.

4A.6 Vectors

The mode of transmission of *D. perstans* remained unknown for many years. LOW (1903) tested various species of mosquitoes, fleas, and lice and obtained some larval development in a mosquito, *Taeniorhynchus fusco-pennatus*. FÜLLEBORN (1908) observed considerable development in *Anopheles maculipennis*. However, these and later experiments with mosquitoes never yielded full development to the mature form. FELDMANN (1904, 1905a, b) suspected an argasid tick (probably *Ornithodoros moubata*) as the intermediate host, but this idea was eventually disproved.

A successful result in the search for the vector was obtained first by SHARP (1928), who found, at Mamfe, British Cameroon, that larvae of *D. perstans* underwent complete metamorphoses in *Culicoides milnei* (= *austeni*) under experimental conditions; moreover, Sharp found that 7% of wild-caught *C. milnei* were infected in the same area where 92% of the people showed microfilariae of *D. perstans*. He also stated that *C. grahami* would probably be another natural vector (see Section 7C.4).

CHARDOME & PEEL (1949), while making an epidemiological study of filariasis in the region around Mbandaka, Zaire, observed that the microfilariae of *D. streptocerca* were ingested by a biting midge, *Culicoides grahami*, and completed their development in the fly; however, the microfilariae of *D. perstans* in the blood were not ingested by the fly. HENRARD & PEEL (1949) conducted the experimental feeding of *C. grahami* on the microfilarial carriers of *D. perstans* and *D. streptocerca*, obtaining similar results. On these grounds, these authors suggested that since one of Sharp's subjects was also infected with *D. streptocerca*, Sharp had observed the development of *D. streptocerca* and not *D. perstans*.

The observations of these authors in Zaire concerning the inability of *C. grahami* to ingest the microfilariae of *D. perstans* were later disproved by NICHOLAS *et al.* (1952) in the British Cameroons, who demonstrated that the microfilariae of both *D. perstans* and *L. loa* were taken up by *C. grahami*; moreover, the number of the microfilariae found in the blood meal corresponded well with that expected from the density in the circulating blood of the donor.

HOPKINS & NICHOLAS (1952) further showed that the microfilariae of *D. perstans* ingested by *C. milnei* and *C. grahami* would develop to mature larvae; however, while the number of those found in the former species was approximately what was expected, those in the latter species were much fewer than expected from the estimated number of the microfilariae ingested by the fly. NICHOLAS & KERSHAW (1954) showed that both *C. milnei* and *C. grahami* would ingest the microfilariae of *D. perstans* in approximately the same numbers as would be expected from the density in the donor's blood and the amount of blood meal taken by the flies. These observations by British workers in the Cameroons showed that *C. milnei* (= *austeni*) was the principal and most efficient intermediate host of *D. per-*

---

*The scientific name of the principal vector of *D. perstans* was referred to as *Culicoides austeni* Carter, Ingram et Macfie, 1920, by SHARP (1928) and later workers. However, NICHOLAS *et al.* (1955) re-examined the type specimens in the British Museum collection, and showed that *C. austeni* was a synonym of *Culicoides milnei* Austen, 1912.

stans in West and Central Africa, and that *C. grahami,* the principal vector of *D. streptocerca,* could only be a poor vector of *D. perstans.*

DUKE (1956), in British Cameroon, conducted a series of studies on the intake and development of microfilariae of *D. perstans* in *Culicoides grahami* and *C. inornatipennis.* The mean volume of blood ingested by *C. grahami* was estimated to be 0.044 mm³, and the volume ingested by *C. inornatipennis* was estimated to be 0.065 mm³. A volunteer, harboring the microfilariae of *D. perstans* at an average density of 2,357 per 50 mm³ and those of *L. loa* at 415 per 50 mm³, was fed upon by the two species of flies. In examinations of 120 *C. grahami* made immediately after the blood meal, the total number of microfilariae of *D. perstans* ingested was 300 (2.50 per fly) and that of *L. loa* was 4 (0.03 per fly); the number of the former was about 20% more than expected, while that of the latter was less than one-tenth of the number expected. In examinations of 100 *C. inornatipennis,* also made immediately after taking the blood, a total of 205 (2.05 per fly) microfilariae of *D. perstans* and 23 (0.23 per fly) of *L. loa* were found to be ingested. At dissection made seven to ten days later, 8 of 138 *C. grahami* contained a total of 18 infective larvae of *D. perstans,* and 7 of 17 *C. inornatipennis* contained a total of 8 infective larvae of *D. perstans.* It was concluded that both species of flies support the development of *D. perstans* microfilariae to the infective stage larvae, but not those of *L. loa;* moreover, it was concluded that *C. grahami* was only a poor or inefficient vector of *D. perstans.* In this small series of experiments, *C. inornatipennis* was apparently a more efficient vector of *D. perstans.*

Addendum:

Dipetalonema semiclarum Fain, 1974, was described as a new human parasite by the microfilariae found in the blood and skin samples from 52 persons in three villages in Equateur Province, Zaire. The microfilariae are unsheathed, resemble that of *D. perstans* and in many individuals both microfilariae were present together. The microfilariae of *D. semiclarum* are longer and broader (mean size of 198 × 5.2 μ in blood films) than those of *D. perstans,* and differ from them in the shape of the head, in having a shorter first nucleus, and in the presence of a characteristic clear band 25–40 μ long in the posterior half of the body. FAIN (1974), in his original report, described the structure of the microfilariae of *D. semiclarum* in comparison with other microfilariae reported from man and primates in Africa.

In connection with the problems of neurological disorders attributed to infection with *Dipetalonema pertans* reported in Africa (especially in Rhodesia), ORIHEL (1973) drew attention to the possible involvements of animal filariae as causes of such syndromes. The microfilariae recovered from two such cases of cerebral filariasis in Rhodesia and examined by him were similar to those of *D. perstans* in gross appearance, but were found to have inconspicuous sheaths and bore a striking resemblance to the microfilariae of *Meningonema peruzzii,* a filaria found in central nervous system of various African monkeys.

4B. *Dipetalonema streptocerca*
(Macfie et Corson, 1922)

This is a filarial parasite found in man in the tropical rainforest zone of western and central Africa. The microfilariae are found in the skin, and the adults were discovered only once from subcutaneous tissues of chimpanzee in Zaire. The parasite has been considered to cause little pathogenic effects on the hosts. *Culicoides grahami* and related biting midges have been incriminated as the vectors of *D. streptocerca*.

4B.1 Historical notes

This parasite was first discovered and described by MACFIE & CORSON (1922), who, while examining the skin of natives in Gold Coast (Ghana) for microfilariae of *Onchocerca volvulus*, found sheathless microfilariae of a previously unknown form, and named it *Agamofilaria streptocerca*. These authors found that the microfilariae of this new species could be distinguished easily from those of *O. volvulus* by the slender body and by the blunt, crook-shaped tail.

The same parasite was discovered later by SHARP (1927) from British Cameroon, by DUBOIS & VITALE (1938) from Zaire, by PHISTER (1952) from Upper Volta, by PHISTER (1954) from Ivory Coast, and by LANGUILLON (1957) from French Cameroon.

The adult form of *D. streptocerca* has not yet been demonstrated in human hosts, but PEEL & CHARDOME (1946) recovered and described females of *D. streptocerca* from the subcutaneous tissue of a chimpanzee, *Pan paniscus*, in Zaire.

4B.2 Geographic distribution

D. strentocerca is a parasite endemic in only the tropical rain forest zone of Africa, and has been recorded as to be occurring in the following countries: Ivory Coast, Upper Volta, Ghana, Cameroon, Zaire.

4B.3 The parasite

4B.3.1 Adults

The adults of *D. streptocerca* are known only by two females and a fragment of another recovered from the subcutaneous tissue of a chimpanzee, *Pan paniscus*, in Zaire, by PEEL & CHARDOME (1946).

4B.3.2 Microfilariae

The microfilariae of *D. streptocerca* are sheathless, taper at both ends, and in fixed specimens, the tail end is strongly bent like a fishhook or shepherd's crook. The tail has nuclei to the very end. They measure 180 to 240 μ in length and about 3 μ in diameter.

The positions of the fixed points as expressed in percentage distance from the anterior end are as follows: nerve ring, 26.9; excretory pore, 34.1; G-1 cell, 69.2; anal pore, 86.2 (after FAUST *et al.*, 1970).

The differential diagnosis of the microfilariae of *D. streptocerca* and *O. volvulus* can be easily made since the former are more slender, with crook-shaped and blunt-ended tails. The microfilariae of *D. streptocerca* have to be differentiated most carefully from those of *D. perstans*. In *D. perstans* the microfilariae are stouter, and the nerve ring, the G-1 cell, and the anal pore are situated farther forward than in *D. perstans*. The tail of *D. perstans* is not crook shaped as in *D. streptocerca*.

The microfilariae of *D. streptocerca* are found in the skin, but not in the blood. Their distribution in the skin at various body sites is quite different from those of *O. volvulus*, as pointed out by KERSHAW *et al.* (1954) and DUKE (1954). They are most numerous in the shoulder skin, less in the trunk, and very few, if any, are found in the skin of extremities. On the other hand, *O. volvulus* in Africa are most numerous in the calves and ankles, with few or none in the skin on the shoulders, trunk and arms.

4B.3.3 Larvae in the vectors

The microfilariae of *D. streptocerca* have been shown by CHARDOME & PEEL (1949) and DUKE (1954) to develop to the infective stage in a biting midge, *Culicoides grahami*, but no detailed study on the morphology of the developing stage larvae has yet been published.

4B.4 Pathogenesis

There have been no definite clinical signs attributed to the infection of *D. streptocerca*. MACFIE & CORSON (1922) found the microfilariae of *D. streptocerca* in the skin of 22 of 50 persons (44%) randomly selected in Ghana; all of them were apparently healthy. The occurrence of *D. strepto-cerca* has also been noted from the Cameroons, but there has been no report on its pathogenicity. However, DUBOIS *et al.* (1939), in Zaire, found the microfilariae of *D. perstans* at high rates among patients with elephantiasis of the legs or genital organs, and suspected that the parasite might be a cause of elephantiasis in this locale.

DUKE (1973) states, "The microfilariae, which are commonest in the skin over torso and mainly in the proximity of the adult worms, are usually asymptomatic, but they have been known to cause itchy rash which is clinically indistinguishable from onchocerciasis. There can be a positive Mazzotti-type reaction with this parasite, but it may not be elicited until higher doses of DEC are employed (i.e., over 200 mg). Both adult worms and microfilariae are susceptible to DEC, which can therefore produce a radical cure."

4B.5 Vectors

The vector of *D. streptocerca* was determined by CHARDOME & PEEL (1949), at Mbandaka, Zaire. They found that its microfilariae, ingested by a biting midge, *Culicoides grahami*, developed to mature stage in seven to eight days. HENRARD & PEEL (1949), in Zaire, further confirmed that 1.2% of 737 *C. grahami* caught at Gombe-Masaka village were naturally infected by the larvae.

DUKE (1954) observed that *C. grahami* fed on the legs below the knee (*streptocerca*-free area) was not infected, but the same species of fly fed on the shoulders and chest (*streptocerca* area) ingested the microfilariae; on dissection, made on the seventh or eighth day after the blood meal, 21 of 109 flies contained a total of 29 motile larvae measuring between 600 to 700 μ.

DUKE (1958) made a comparative study of the capacity of *Culicoides milnei* and *C. grahami* as vectors of *D. streptocerca*. A volunteer, heavily infected with the microfilariae of *D. streptocerca* and very lightly with those of *D. perstans*, was fed upon by the two species of biting midges at two locations: on the skin of the back and scapulae (the *streptocerca* area), and on the skin of the calves (the *streptocerca*-free area). None of 69 *C. grahami* fed on the *streptocerca*-free area contained microfilariae, and 5 of 222 *C. milnei* fed on the same area had the microfilariae of *D. perstans* but not of *D. streptocerca*. On the other hand, it was shown that out of 266 *C. grahami* fed on the *streptocerca* area, 40 flies (15.0%) contained a total of 65 microfilariae of *D. streptocerca*, while only one fly contained one microfilaria of *D. perstans*. Of 505 *C. milnei* fed on the same area, only 8(1.6%) contained the microfilariae of *D. streptocerca* (10 microfilariae, in total) and only 8 flies contained those of *D. perstans* (9 microfilariae in total). It was shown from these observations that *C. milnei* was a much less efficient vector of *D. streptocerca* than *C. grahami*, since the number of microfilariae of *D. streptocerca* ingested per fly was only 0.02 in *C. milnei*, in contrast to 0.24 in *C. grahami*. The question of whether the microfilariae of *D. streptocerca* ingested by *C. milnei* reach the mature stage could not be solved, because the host was also infected with the microfilariae of *D. perstans*. (One out of 167 *C. milnei* fed on the *streptocerca*-free area, as well as 5 out of 224 *C. milnei* fed on the *streptocerca* area were found to be harboring infective larvae when dissected between the seventh and tenth day. However, it was not clear whether these infective larvae were those of *D. streptocerca* or *D. perstans*.)

4C. *Mansonella ozzardi* (Manson, 1897)

Mansonella ozzardi is strictly a New World filaria, recorded from certain islands of the West Indies, Central America (Mexico to Panama), and South America (Colombia, Venezuela, the Guianas, Brazil, and Argentina). In contrast to the geographic distribution of *W. bancrofti* in these regions, which occurs mainly in the more urbanized areas along the coast, *M. ozzardi* is distributed almost exclusively among the aboriginal races (the American Indians) inhabiting the interior.

The adult worms have been recovered from visceral organs. The microfilariae appear in the circulating blood, and exhibit almost no periodicity. Extremely high microfilaria rates have been recorded in surveys conducted in Indian villages in the tropical zone, such as in the Guianas, and in Amazonas in Brazil. Though the microfilarial density in the blood of carriers in these regions often reaches surprisingly high levels, there are usually no manifest symptoms in the infected persons.

A biting midge, *Culicoides furens*, was incriminated as the vector in St. Vincent, West Indies. However, a black fly, *Simulium amazonicum*, was reported to be the vector in Brazil.

4C.1 Historical notes

M. ozzardi was recorded as a previously unknown filaria by MANSON (1897), who discovered the microfilariae in slides of blood smears, collected from residents of St. Vincent, West Indies, which had been sent to him in 1893 and 1895 by Hewsam. Manson stated, "In six of 152 St. Vincent slides I found numerous specimens of *Filaria nocturna* (*W. bancrofti*) and in ten of them an entirely new filaria which, at Blanchard' suggestion, I have named *Filaria demarquayi*." In the same paper, he also reported the discovery of two new forms of microfilariae in blood smears collected from aboriginal Indians in British Guiana by Ozzard, and sent to him the previous winter. One of them was sharp tailed, and closely resembled *Filaria demarquayi*; on the next page of this paper, he states, "I propose to call it provisionally *Filaria ozzardi*." The other species of microfilariae was blunt-tailed, and was judged probably identical with *Filaria perstans* described by MANSON (1891) from Africa. Thus, *F. demarquayi* and *F. ozzardi* were described in the same paper which appeared on 25 December 1897, in the

British Medical Journal, and the description of *F. ozzardi* was preceded by that of *F. demarquayi*. In this paper, Manson recognized six forms of human filariae: *F. nocturna* (= *W. bancrofti*) from Africa, India, the South Pacific, British Guiana, and the West Indies; *F. diurna* (= *Loa loa*) from West Africa; *F. demarquai* from the West Indies; *Filaria perstans* from West Africa; blunt-tailed *Filaria perstans* (?) from British Guiana; and sharp-tailed *Filaria ozzardi* from British Guiana. In this report, it was already recognized by Manson that *F. nocturna* was very common among people in coastal regions of British Guiana, but they were not infected with the unsheathed microfilariae, while aboriginal Indians were not infected by *F. nocturna* and highly infected by *F. perstans* and *F. ozzardi* microfilariae.

Low (1902) gave the following historical accounts:
Daniels in 1897 found that the sharp-tailed microfilariae were very common amongst the Indians in the interior of British Guiana, and Daniels (1898) found the adults form of the blunt-tailed microfilariae (*D. perstans*) at an necropsy of an Indian. In the following year, Daniels (1899) discovered the adults of the sharp-tailed form. Galgey, in St. Lucia, in 1899, found two adults of *Filaria demarquayi* at a necropsy of a native of this island. Manson compared these adults and found that those of the blunt-tailed form was identical with *Filaria perstans* of Africa, and those of *F. demarquayi* from St. Vincent and of *F. ozzardi* from British Guiana were also identical.

Low (1902) reported on the results of blood surveys conducted in various areas of the West Indies and British Guiana. Microfilariae of *F. demarquayi* (= *M. ozzardi*) were found in 23 (4.87%) of 472 persons in St. Lucia, 2 (1.3%) of 160 persons in Dominica, none of 600 persons in Barbados, 49 of 163 pure Indians in British Guiana (double infection of *demarquayi* and *perstans* in 38, *demarquayi* alone in 11, and *perstans* alone in 56), and 8 of 30 persons in St. Vincent were found to be infected with *F. demarquayi*.

As stated previously, microfilariae of this species were described by Manson (1897) by two names, *Filaria demarquayi* for the specimens sent from St. Vincent, and *Filaria ozzardi* for those sent from British Guiana; later they were recognized to be identical. However, the name *Filaria demarquayi* had been already used by Zurne (1891) for *W. bancrofti*, and thus Raillet (1908) proposed a new name *Filaria juncea*. In such a case, as pointed out by Leiper (1913), *Filaria ozzardi*, the second name proposed by Manson (1897), has priority over *Filaria juncea*.

The genus *Mansonella* was created by Faust in 1929, in honor of Sir Patrick Manson who described this species by the name of *Filaria ozzardi* (= *demarquayi*). However, the generic status of *ozzardi* is still uncertain, since the parasite is known only from the microfilariae (which are closely related to other *Dipetalonema*-microfilariae), and by the females.

As for the vector of *M. ozzardi*, Buckly (1934), in St. Vincent (West Indies), found that a biting midge, *Culicoides furens*, was naturally infected with the filarial larvae and that complete larval development took place in the fly in experimental infection studies.

4C.2 Geographic distribution

M. ozzardi is a parasite known only in man in the tropical Americas.
It has been recorded from the following countries and territories:
> Central America: Mexico (Yucatán Peninsula), Guatemala, Panama
> West Indies: Puerto Rico, Bahama Islands, St. Kitts, Guadeloupe,
> Dominica, St. Lucia, St. Vincent, Trinidad
> South America: Colombia, Venezuela, Guyana, Surinam, French
> Guiana, Brazil (mainly from Amazonas), Argentina (northern
> province), Bolivia

4C.3 The parasite

4C.3.1 Adults

According to Low (1902), the adult worms of *M. ozzardi* were recovered
on two occasions, once by DANIELS, in 1899, from an Indian in British Guiana, and again by GALGEY, in 1899, from an native of St. Lucia. These
worms were examined by Manson, who concluded that both were identical. These materials were studied further by RAILLET (1908) and LEIPER
(1913), but have been only poorly described.

The adult worm of *M. ozzardi* were recovered, on autopsy of the above
two cases, from the abdominal cavity, threaded into the mesenteries, or
embedded in the visceral adipose tissue. According to FAUST *et al.* (1970),
the male is known only from a posterior segment, 38 mm long and 0.2 mm
in maximum diameter. The caudal extremity has a sharp ventral curve
and a slightly bulbous termination. The females measure 65 to 81 mm in
length and 0.21 to 0.25 mm in diameter. The cuticula is smooth, the head is
unarmed, and at the caudal extremity, there is a pair of fleshy lappets.

4C.3.2 Microfilariae

The microfilariae of *M. ozzardi* have also been only poorly described.
They are sheathless, and appear in the circulating blood with almost no
periodicity. As stated previously, MANSON (1897), in his original report
on *Filaria demarquayi* from St. Vincent and *Filaria ozzardi* from Guyana,
differentiated them from *Filaria perstans* by the shape of the tail, the former
two being sharply pointed, and the latter being blunt.

The body length of the microfilariae of *M. ozzardi* is much shorter than
that of the microfilariae of *W. bancrofti*. RACHOU *et al.* (1954a) measured
each of 200 specimens of the microfilariae (all in blood smears) of *M. ozzardi*
from Amazonas, *W. bancrofti* from northern Brazil (Belém), and *W. ban-*

crofti from southern Brazil (Florianópolis), and obtained the maximum, minimum, and average lengths of 224, 150, and 191μ, respectively, for *M. ozzardi*, and 408, 224, and 292 μ, respectively, for *W. bancrofti*. FROS (1956) compared the microfilariae of *M. ozzardi* and *D. perstans* in alcohol-fixed blood smears collected from people in Surinam, and obtained the maximum, minimum, and average lengths of 232, 110, and 163μ, respectively, for *M. ozzardi*, and 207, 152, and 185μ, respectively, for *D. perstans*. He also pointed out that the microfilariae of *M. ozzardi* and *D. perstans* are differentiated by the structure of the tail end; the former being slender, tapering to a point at the end and devoid of nuclei; the latter containing nuclei to the very end, and usually thickened at the end like a drumstick around the last nucleus.

The microfilaria of *M. ozzardi* was illustrated by Faust (in FAUST *et al.*, 1970). According to this figure, the following percentages of the total body length were obtained by the present author for the fixed points:

BNC, 3.8; N, 21.0; EP, 34.8; EC, 39.2; G–1, 69.1; G–2, 76.2; G–3, 77.3; G–4, 78.5; AP, 80.1.

It has generally been admitted that the microfilariae of *M. ozzardi* appear in the circulating blood both day and night, and belong to a nonperiodic type. From statistical analysis of the data reported by RACHOU (1954), the microfilariae of *M. ozzardi* seem to show a weak diurnal periodicity (SASA & TANAKA, 1974; also see Section 11F.5). RESTREPO *et al.* (1962), in Colombia, also reported that the microfilariae of *M. ozzardi* exhibit a subperiodic appearance with a peak at 8 a.m. and the minimum density at 8 p.m.

4C.3.3 Larvae in the vectors

The full development of the larvae of *M. ozzardi* to the mature stage has been observed by BUCKLEY (1934) in *Culicoides furens*, but no detailed study on the morphology of the larval stages has yet been published.

4C.4 Pathogenesis

Most workers who have conducted epidemiological studies on *M. ozzardi* infection in South and Central America have recognized no specific symptoms, thus the parasite has been considered to be nonpathogenic, even when numerous microfilariae were present in the circulating blood. However, BIAGI & CASTREION (1957), in Mexico, reported that the parasite causes eosinophilia, especially in the early stage of infection. MARINKELLE & GERMAN (1970), in Colombia, reported that mansonellosis not only causes eosinophilia, but also severe articular pains, and thus is a major public health problem in the endemic area of Comisaria del Vaupes.

4C.5 Diagnosis

The diagnosis of *M. ozzardi* in man is usually made by demonstration of the microfilariae in the peripheral blood. Because the microfilariae show almost no periodicity (or a weak diurnal periodicity: see Section 4C.3.2), the blood examination may be made at any time of the day. The microfilariae should be differentiated from those of other filarial species by the morphological characteristics discussed in Section 4C.3.2.

At least in some endemic areas, there seem to exist many people showing microfilariae at extremely low levels. MARINKELLE & GERMAN (1970), in Colombia, found 96.1% of 332 adult Indians examined at Comisaria del Vaupes to be positive for the microfilariae; about 70% of the above positive cases, however, were so diagnosed only by the Knott's concentration method (see Section 10A.2.2.3), and those who showed microfilariae in 20 mm³ blood smears were only about 30% of the total positive cases.

BIAGI (1956) conducted a study of the immunodiagnosis of *M. ozzardi* infection in Mexico with skin tests and precipitin tests. The skin test antigen used was an extract of *Dirofilaria immitis* at a ratio of 1:8,000, and 0.1 ml was injected intradermally. Positive reaction (a wheal of 6 mm or greater) was seen in 13 of 17 cases carrying the microfilariae of *M. ozzardi*, but the test was considered of little diagnostic value because there were too many false positive reactions. The precipitin test was much less sensitive.

4C.6 Vectors

The vector of *M. ozzardi* was determined by BUCKLEY (1933, 1934) to be a biting midge, *Culicoides furens* (POEY, 1853), on St. Vincent Island, West Indies. In his experimental infection study, 27.5% of 200 midges fed on a *M. ozzardi* carrier were subsequently found to be infected with larvae in various developing stages, and the development to mature larvae was found to be completed in seven or eight days. Natural infection of *C. furens* was found in 5% of the midges caught at Calliaqua, St. Vincent.

The vector of *M. ozzardi* in other endemic areas in South and Central America and the West Indies has not yet been determined. In Brazil, however, CERQUEIRA (1959) conducted extensive studies on the transmission of *M. ozzardi* in the village of Codajás, on the Amazon, and incriminated the black fly, *Simulium amazonicum* Goeldi, 1905, as the vector. GARNHAM & WALLIKER (1965) reported that the only filarial parasite infecting man in this area was *M. ozzardi*, and there was no onchocerciasis among the inhabitants. *S. amazonicum* was shown to be anthropophilic; furthermore, developing filarial larvae, similar to those described by BUCKLEY (1934), were found in *S. amazonicum*; no other man-biting insects in this area, including *Culicoides* spp., were likely to be the vectors.

Garnham & Walliker (1965) visited the village of Codajaz in August 1964, and conducted epidemiological investigations on filariasis in this area. They examined 57 people between the ages of 2 and 68 years and found unsheathed microfilariae, indistinguishable from those of *M. ozzardi* described by Fülleborn (1929), in blood smears of 9 persons. None of the skin snips taken from the forearm of the people contained the microfilariae of *O. volvulus.* They also examined the blood of 52 wild animals, and found that 9 of 12 monkeys, 3 of 4 sloths, 5 of 11 rodents, 3 of 3 carnivores, 1 of 3 opossums, and 1 of 19 bats were carrying microfilariae in the blood, but none of the microfilariae were of *M. ozzardi* type.

4D. *Culicoides,* or the biting midge

Culicoides is a genus in the Family Ceratopogonidae, Suborder Nematocera, Order Diptera. They are small (1 to 4 mm) midges whose females are equipped with piercing and sucking mouthparts, hence, commonly called biting midges.

The Family Ceratopogonidae contains some 50 genera, among which four genera are medically important as bloodsuckers, namely, *Culicoides, Leptoconops, Forcipomyia,* and *Austroconops.* The genus *Culicoides* has a world-wide distribution, containing some 800 species, and many of them are severe pests of man and other vertebrates. Ceratopogonids, or biting midges, can be separated from other related insects, such as the nonbiting Chironomids, by the structure of mouthparts, peculiar wing venation, and the position of wings at rest (which are superimposed over the back). Most species of the Genus *Culicoides* have speckled wings.

The life cycle consists of egg, larval, pupal, and adult stages. The larvae are wormlike, slender, and smooth in shape, and are either aquatic or semi-aquatic. In water, they can be easily differentiated by their quick, eellike motion. Breeding places differ greatly according to species, and include swamps, river banks, wet soil with decaying plant materials, and rotting tree stumps and tree holes.

As stated before, *Culicoides furens* has been shown to be the vector of *Mansonia ozzardi* in St. Vincent, West Indies; *C. milnei* (= *C. austeni*) and *C. grahami* are vectors of *D. perstans* in Africa, and *C. grahami* and *C inornatipennis* are vectors of *D. streptocerca* in Africa.

5 # Filariasis due to *Onchocerca volvulus*

5.1 Historical notes

This parasite was described by the name of *Filaria volvulus* by LEUCKART (1893) from specimens obtained from nodules under the skin of a native on the Gold Coast (Ghana). This species was placed, by RAILLIET & HENRY (1910), into the genus *Onchocerca* Diesing, 1841, together with other species parasitic in animals. The genus *Onchocerca* was created by DIESING in 1841 with *O. reticulata* as the type species, which is a parasite of the horse, donkey, and mule in Europe. YAMAGUTI (1961) used an emended name, *Oncocerca* Creplin, 1846, for *Onchocerca* Diesing, 1841.

This parasite was eventually found to be widely distributed throughout the savanna and forest regions of Africa, affecting millions of people, and causing serious health hazards to large numbers of its victims in a number of countries. (See Chapter 7).

The occurrence of human onchocerciasis in the New World was noted first by ROBLES, in 1915, from Guatemala. Both PACHECO-LUNA (1918) and ROBLES (1919) described the eye lesions due to onchocercal infection. BRUMPT (1919) studied the material sent by Robles which consisted of one male and fragments of the extremities of two female worms. He named the parasite *Onchocerca caecutiens* because he considered that the specimens differed from the African form in the distribution of male papillae and in the larger size of spicules. However, subsequent studies carried out by FÜLLEBORN (1926) and SANDGROUND (1934), in which more material was examined, showed that while there was considerable variation among the specimens, there existed no consistent differences between the American and African forms, thus *O. caecutiens* was probably a synonym of *O. volvulus*.

The occurrence of eye lesions was once considered as pathognomostic to the American form of onchocerciasis, but since HISETTE (1932) reported onchocercal eye patients from the Congo, the common occurrence of eye disease associated with onchocercal infection has been noted in many African countries.

Based on these and other evidence, RUIZ REYES (1952) presented the view that onchocerciasis was brought to tropical America and became established when Negroes were imported from Africa to cultivate sugar cane and coffee. On the other hand, more recent studies by DE LEON & DUKE (1966) suggest that the Central American and African parasites are at least distinct physiological races in view of their compatibility with the *Simulium* intermediate hosts. Detailed clinical studies undertaken by WOODRUFF *et al.* (1966a, b), in Tanzania and Guatemala, also suggest that the African and American parasites differ in their pathogenicity. It has been further demonstrated by DUKE (1966a, 1967a) and DUKE *et al.* (1966, 1967b) that there are different physiological races of *O. volvulus* even in Africa itself; the savanna and forest forms in West Africa differ distinctly in the infectivity to the *Simulium* vectors, general epidemiology, and clinical manifestations (see Section 5.3.4).

The mode of transmission of *O. volvulus* was elucidated first by BLACK-LOCK (1926a, b), who demonstrated, in Sierra Leone, that the larval development takes place in a black fly, *Simulium damnosum*. In later studies by a number of workers, this species was found to be widely distributed in Africa, acting as the main vector of onchocerciasis in the majority of endemic areas in the savanna and forest regions. Another species, *Simulium neavei*, was shown to be the vector of onchocerciasis in certain regions of Zaire by HISSETTE (1932), and by MCMAHON (1940) in Kenya. The larvae and pupae of *S. neavei* and related species were found by MCMAHON (1951), in Kenya, to be living in streams in phoretic association with a crab species, *Potamonautes niloticus*. As for the vectors of *O. volvulus* in Guatemala, STRONG (1931, 1934) showed that the larval development takes place in three species of black flies, i.e., *Simulium ochraceum*, *S. metallicum*, and *S. callidum*, of which the first species is the most important vector.

The occurrence of onchocerciasis in other Central and South American countries has been noted rather recently, namely by HOFFMAN (1930) from Mexico, by ARENDS *et al.* (1954, quoted by ARENDS, 1966), and LEWIS & IBANEZ DE ALDECOA (1962) from Venezuela, by ASSIS-MASRI & LITTLE (1965) from Colombia, and by MORAES & DIAS (1972) from northern Brazil.

Control of *Simulium* vectors of onchocerciasis was begun in Kenya by GARNHAM & MCMAHON (1947) by the application of DDT into rivers. It was reported to have sucessfully eradicated the main vector, *S. neavei*, from certain endemic areas. The control of vectors in West Africa and America was apparently more difficult, but a large-scale control program of *S. damnosum* in the Volta River Basin area was initiated in 1973 under joint sponsorship of the International Bank for Reconstruction and Development and the World Health Organization.

5.2 Geographic distribution

Human onchocerciasis has been noted to be endemic mainly in the two regions: the tropical zone of Africa, and Central and South America. A small focus was found recently in Yemen, by FAWDRY (1957). Because the disease is transmitted by black flies of the genus *Simulium* whose larvae and pupae breed in swift-running waters, the endemic foci are usually located near rivers or streams in hilly or mountainous regions. Several species-groups of black flies with different biological characters are involved as the main vectors of onchocerciasis in different parts of the world, and the ecological features of the endemic areas sometimes differ greatly among the regions.

In Africa, onchocerciasis occurs throughout the greater part of the tropical rain forest regions and the savanna belt extending more than 6,500 km from the Atlantic coast of Senegal to the Indian Ocean coast of Tanzania, involving more than 30 million people. Here, the disease has the notorious name "river blindness," causing eye lesions in large numbers of people residing near rivers in the savanna and forest zones. Two black fly species act as the main vectors in Africa: *Simulium damnosum*, which breed in relatively large rivers and are found throughout the tropical regions of Africa; and *Simulium neavei*, which breed in small streams in the highlands of eastern Africa associated with certain fresh-water crabs.

In Central America, onchocerciasis has long been known to be endemic in the coffee-growing highland areas of Guatemala and Mexico. *Simulium ochraceum*, which breed in small streams in the mountainous region, have been noted to be the main vector. Onchocerciasis has been discovered rather recently in Venezuela, Colombia, and Brazil, where the endemic foci are located in the lowland hilly zones.

The countries from which human onchocerciasis has been reported to be endemic are as follows: (see Fig. 5-1 and 5-2)

Africa: Senegal, Sierra Leone, Liberia, Ivory Coast, Upper Volta, Ghana, Nigeria, Chad, Cameroon, Central African Republic, Zaire, Angola, Tanzania, Malawi, Kenya, Ethiopia, Sudan

Asia: southern Arabia (Yemen)

Americas: Mexico, Guatemala, Venezuela, Colombia, Brazil

5.3 The parasite

The adult worms of *Onchocerca volvulus* usually reside in the subcutaneous tissue of man. The microfilariae produced by the female worms are sheathless, and migrate to the skin of various body sites. The development from microfilariae to infective stage larvae takes place in the thoracic muscles of black flies of the genus *Simulium*.

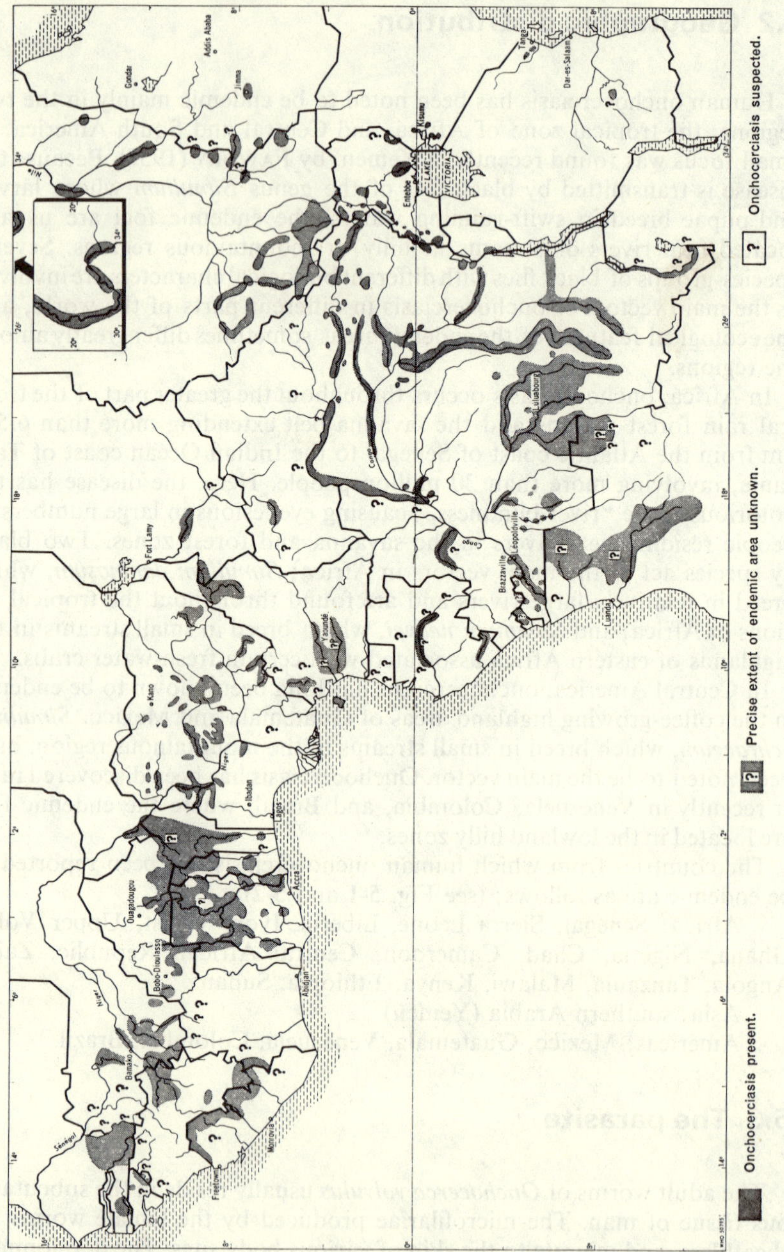

Fig. 5-1.   Geographic distribution of onchocerciasis in Africa (cited from WHO Expert Committee on Onchocerciasis, Second Report, 1966).

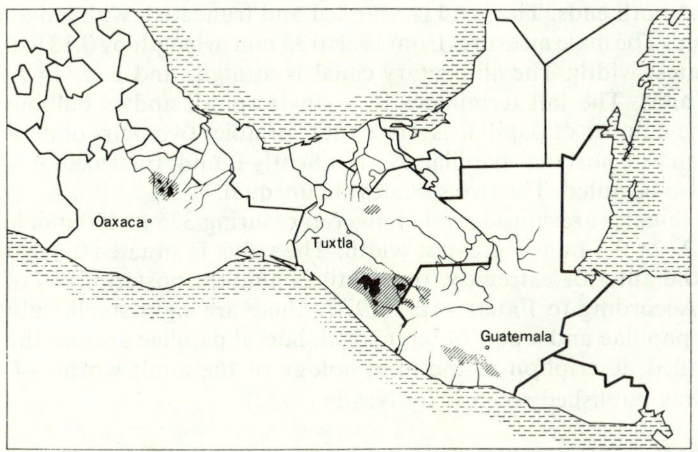

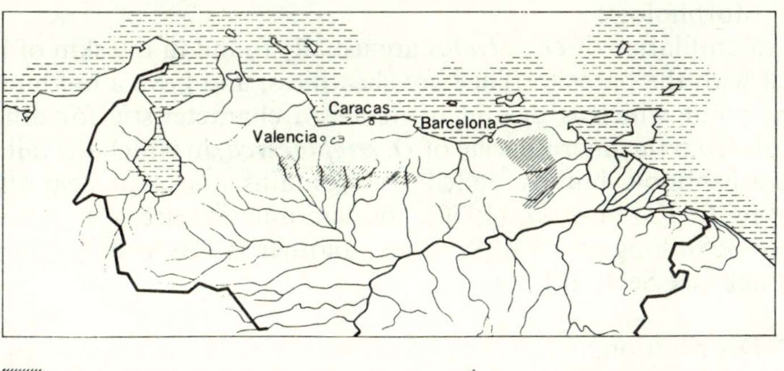

Fig. 5-2.   Geographic distribution of onchocerciasis in the Americas. (A) Mexico and Guatemala. (B) Venezuela (WHO Expert Committee on Onchocerciasis, Second Report, 1966).

5.3.1 Adults

The adult worms of *O. volvulus* have been collected, often in large numbers, from fibrous tumors (onchocercomas) in subcutaneous tissues, especially in areas where nodulectomy is a common practice in the treatment. They are creamy white, transparent nematodes, with conspicuous transverse annular thickenings of the cuticle which is reinforced externally by spiral thickenings. This cuticular structure is a peculiar characteristic of the genus *Onchocerca*.

According to STRONG (1934), the body of the adults are filiform and taper at both ends. The head is rounded and truncated, with a diameter of 0.04 mm. The male measures from 18.2 to 32 mm in length by 0.13 to 0.21 mm at greatest width. The alimentary canal is straight and ends in a subterminal anus. The tail terminates in a single spiral, and is bulbous at the tip. The number of papillae is somewhat variable; two pairs of preanal and two pairs of postanal papillae are frequently found. Intermediate papillae may also be noted. The two spicules are unequal.

The females are considerably longer, measuring 335 to 500 mm in length and 0.27 to 0.4 mm at greatest width. The vulva is situated 0.4 to 0.82 mm from the anterior extremity, or slightly behind the posterior end of esophagus. According to FAUST *et al.* (1970), there are eight small, submedian, sessile papillae and a pair of large, oval, lateral papillae around the mouth A detailed description of the morphology of the adult worms of *O. volvulus* was published recently by Neafie (1972).

5.3.2 Microfilariae

5.3.2.1 Morphology

The microfilariae of *O. volvulus* are usually found in the skin of humans infected with the parasite. They are sheathless, and have a tail tapering to a sharp point which is devoid of nuclei (a characteristic for differential diagnosis from the microfilariae of *D. streptocerca*, in which the tail is curved like a fishhook, bluntly ended and contains nuclei to near the end). According to FAUST *et al.* (1970), the microfilariae are of two sizes: one is 285 to 368μ long and 6 to 9μ thick, another is 150 to 287μ long and 5 to 7μ thick (see Section 1.3.3).

5.3.2.2 Distribution and density of microfilariae in the skin

It has been demonstrated that the microfilariae of *O. volvulus* are not evenly distributed in the skin of different parts of human body, and that probably the pattern of distribution differs according to the geographic race of the parasite. It is believed by most workers that the distribution of the density of microfilariae in the skin is correlated with the site of the adult worms, and KERSHAW *et al.* (1954a) showed, in West Africa, that the nodules are found mainly in the lower parts of the body (areas below the knee) where the density of the microfilariae is also the highest. The difference in the pattern of the distribution of the density of the microfilariae of *O. volvulus* and those of *D. streptocerca* in West Africa has also been clearly demonstrated by KERSHAW *et al.* (1954a, b) and DUKE (1954, 1956, 1962b).

On the other hand, the distribution pattern of the microfilariae of *O. volvulus* in East Africa is somewhat different, and NELSON (1958a) and WOODRUFF *et al.* (1966a) have shown that the main concentration of the microfilariae is around the buttocks and upper thigh. In Guatemala, DE LEON & DUKE (1966) estimated the distribution of the density of microfilariae of *O. vovulus* in different parts of the body from the numbers of microfilariae ingested by *Simulium ochraceum*, and found that the highest density was around the torso.

5.3.2.3 Microfilarial periodicity in the skin

It has been suggested by various workers that the density of microfilariae of *O. volvulus* in the skin might be dependent upon the time of day when the snips are taken or by other environmental conditions. WEGESA (1966, quoted by NELSON, 1970), in East Africa, showed that the density of microfilariae of *O. volvulus* in the skin is highest between 8 and 10 a.m. and around 6 p.m., coinciding with the peak activity of the local vector *Simulium woodi*. DUKE *et al.* (1967a), in the Cameroons, collected skin snips from 15 volunteers at intervals of one hour over a period of 24 hours and observed the microfilarial density per milligram of skin. When the carriers were considered in groups, an increase in microfilarial density occurred during the afternoon hours in both the forest and Sudan savanna forms; moreover, the 24-hour curves showed similarities to the curves for the temperature/saturation-deficiency and for the biting density of *Similium damnosum*. However, the fluctuations in the density of microfilariae were considered to be too small to affect the results of diagnosis. LARTIQUE (1967), in West Africa, also observed that the density in the skin was much higher at 4 p.m. than at 10 a.m. TADA & FIGUEROA MARROQUIN (1974) also conducted a study on the time changes in the microfilarial density in the skin of nine *O. volvulus* cases in Guatemala, by taking measured skin snips at four hour intervals over periods of 24 hours. The variation of the density was not consistent, and these authors considered that there was no circadian rhythm in the density of *O. volvulus* microfilariae in the skin.

5.3.3 Larvae in the vectors

A black fly species in Africa, *Simulium damnosum*, was demonstrated to be an efficient vector of *O. volvulus* by BLACKLOCK (1926a, b), in experimental infection studies with wild-caught flies. WANSON & PEEL (1945) and MUIRHEAD-THOMPSON (1957) successfully infected laboratory-bred *S. damnosum* with human *O. volvulus*. However, these authors did not describe the detailed morphology of the infective larvae. On the other hand, STEWARD (1937) showed that *Simulium ornatum* in Europe was a vector of *Onchocerca gutturosa* in cattle, and ANDERSON (1956) found that *Simulium venustum* was a vector of the bird filaria, *Ornithofilaria fallisensis* Anderson, 1954. It was further reported from Brazil by CERQUEIRA (1959) that larval development of *Mansonella ozzardi* took place in *Simulium amazonicum*.

It is, therefore, possible that wild black flies collected in endemic areas of human onchocerciasis may contain filarial larvae of animal origins, and methods are required, as in the examination of mosquitoes, to distinguish these different nematode species in order to confirm the natural infection with *O. volvulus*. In an endemic area of *O. volvulus* on the slope of Mount Elgon in Uganda, NELSON & PESTER (1962) observed that wild-caught

S. neavei were infected with three types of mature filarial larvae; out of 1,681 *S. damnosum* dissected, 18 had type A (more than 700 μ in length), 10 had type B (500 to 700 μ long), and 4 had type C (less than 500 μ long). Subsequent dissections of large numbers of Elgon *S. neavei* fed on patients with *O. volvulus* were made and compared with dissection of those fed on noninfected controls; they clearly demonstrated that the type B, medium-sized mature larva, was *O. volvulus*. Out of 132 *S. naevei* fed on an *O. volvulus* carrier and kept alive for seven or more days, 80 (60.6%) were found to contain mature larvae of *O. volvulus*, and the numbers found per fly varied from 1 to 42; of 198 flies of the same lot, 14 (7.1%) were found to be naturally infected with the type A larvae. Some of the wild flies were also infected by mermithids, which may be mistaken for "sausage stage" filarial larvae if examined carelessly. NELSON & PESTER (1962) gave illustrations and measurement data of the three types of filarial larvae found in *Simulium*, shown in Fig. 5-3 and Table 5-1.

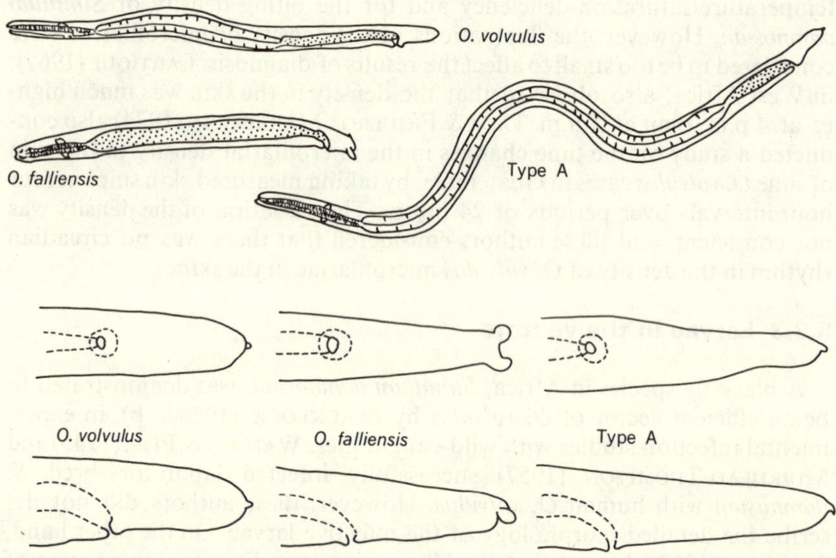

Fig. 5-3.   Three species of filaria larvae found in *Simulium* (after Nelson & Pester, 1962).

DUKE (1967) described three additional species of nematode larvae found in *Simulium damnosum* in West Africa, types D and E from savanna sites, and type F from forest sites. The measurement data and structure of these species are shown in Table 5-2 and Fig. 5-4. Type D and E are infective forms of filaria larvae, while it is not certain whether type E belongs to filaria or to other nematode groups.

Table 5-1.   Mean measurements (μ) of three types of mature filarial larvae found in *Simulium* (after NELSON & PESTER, 1962).

Species	*Onchocerca volvulus*	*Ornithofilaria fallisensis*	Type A
Head	9	9	11
Nerve ring	80	49	78
Anterior oesophagus	108	77	107
Posterior oesophagus	254	0	558
Maximum breadth	18.7	20.0	21.5
Intestine	163	322	90
Tail	31.2	33.0	48.2
Body length	566	432	803

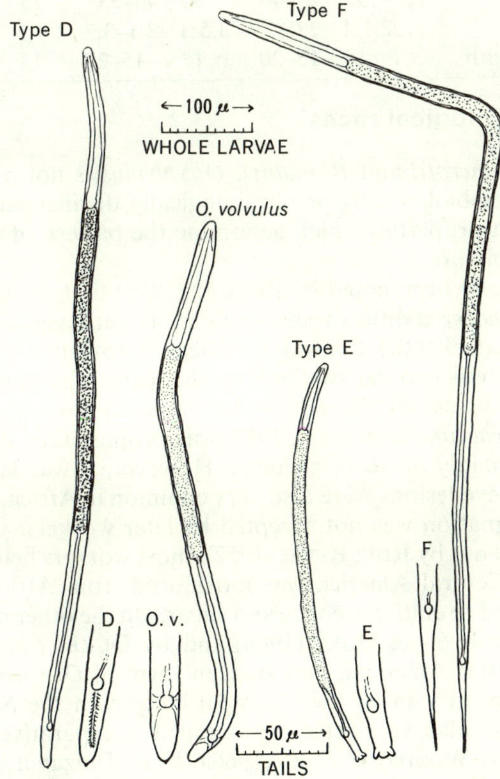

Fig. 5-4.   Semi-diagrammatic scale drawings from camera lucida projections of average-sized larvae of types D, E and F from wild *S. damnosum*, and a typical *O. volvulus* infective larvae. Some details of the ventral view of the tail end of each larva are given on a larger scale. (after Duke, 1967). *Ann. Trop. Med. Para.* 61:201

Table 5-2. Showing the mean and range of measurements (in microns) of 60 *O. volvulus* infective larvae, 15 larvae of type D, eight larvae of type E, and one larva of type F (after DUKE, 1967).

Structure measured	60 *O. volvulus* infective larvae		15 larvae of type D		8 larvae of type E		1 larva of type F
	Mean	Range	Mean	Range	Mean	Range	Mean
Total length	630	440–700	825	750–925	460	410–500	1,050
Head	8	8	10	10	5	5	10
Anterior oesophagus	127	90–140	165	140–200	65	55–85	150
Posterior oesophagus	270	190–320	370	270–475	305	240–345	435
Intestine...	190	130–220	230	190–320	60	50–85	350
Oesophago-intestinal ratio	2.1:1	2.0–2.6	2.3:1	2.1–2.4	6.1:1	3.6–7.3	1.7:1
Tail	35	25–40	50	45–55	25	20–30	115
Anal ratio	2.1:1	2.0–2.4	3.5:1	3.1–3.7	2.8:1	2.0–3.0	7.7:1
Maximum width ...	18	15–20	17	15–20	13	12–15	20

5.3.4 Physiological races

Like *W. bancrofti* and *B. malayi*, *O. volvulus* is not a uniform species, but comprises biologically or physiologically distinct races, each with its own inherent properties which determine the pattern of transmission and the clinical picture.

It has already been noted by BRUMPT (1919) that the Central American form of *Onchocerca* differs remarkably in its pathogenicity from the African form; namely, the Central American form mainly affects eyes and frequently causes nodular swellings on the scalp, whereas the African form is mainly a disease of the skin (other than on the scalp). A new name, *Onchocerca caecutiens* Brumpt, 1919, was proposed for the Central American form, mainly on these grounds. However, it was later realized that onchocercal eye lesions were also very common in Africa, so that Brumpt's specific designation was not accepted by later workers.

As pointed out by RUIZ REYES (1952), most workers believed that onchocerciasis in Central America was introduced from Africa when Negroes were imported to cultivate coffee and sugar. On the other hand, more recent studies by DE LEON & DUKE (1966) and by DUKE *et al.* (1967b) suggest that the Central American and African form of *O. volvulus* are, at least, different races in view of their compatibility with the *Simulium* vectors; this view was also supported by detailed comparative clinical studies undertaken by WOODRUFF *et al.* (1966a, b) in Tanzania and Guatemala.

DE LEON & DUKE (1966) conducted experimental studies on the transmission of Guatemalan and West African strains of *O. volvulus* by three species of Guatemalan black flies. Carriers of the Guatemalan strain of *O. volvulus* were exposed to bites of local black flies. *S. ochraceum* was shown to be the most efficient vector of *O. volvulus*, because it was markedly anthropophilic, ingested the highest numbers of the microfilariae, had the lowest mortality rate after infected, and allowed development of the largest numbers of infective larvae. The other two species, *S. metallicum* and *S. callidum*, were shown to be less efficient as vectors, but they also allowed the development of *O. volvulus* larvae to the infective stage. On the other hand, in the cases of carriers with African strains of *O. volvulus* (one with the forest strain and another with the Sudan savanna strain) exposed to the bites of Guatemalan black flies, the intake rates of the microfilariae by the three species of flies were of the same order as those recorded with *S. damnosum* feeding on the same volunteers in Africa. However, the numbers of microfilariae of the Guatemalan strain of *O. volvulus* taken by the three Guatemalan flies from human carriers harboring the microfilariae at similar densities were 20 to 25 times more than those of the African strains. It was further observed that the numbers of infective larvae of the West African forest strain developed in *S. ochraceum*, *S. metallicum*, and *S. callidum* were much smaller than those found in the forest strain of *S. damnosum*, the percentage being only 1.7%, 0.3%, and 7.3% of the ingested microfilariae, respectively, in contrast to 47% in *S. damnosum*. In the West African Sudan savanna strain of *O. volvulus*, the numbers of microfilariae ingested by the three Guatemalan black fly species were all of the same order as those in *S. damnosum*, but no development to the infective stage was observed in any of the Guatemalan flies. These results suggest that the Guatemalan strain of *O. volvulus* is physiologically quite distinct from either the forest or Sudan savanna strains of *O. volvulus* in West Africa.

DUKE *et al.* (1967 b) further conducted experimental studies on the intake and subsequent fate of microfilariae of a Central American strain of *O. volvulus* in West African *Simulium damnosum*. A group of over 1,000 *Simulium ochraceum* in Guatemala was infected with microfilariae from two Guatemalan *O. volvulus* carriers, transported by air across the Atlantic to Cameroon, and the infective larvae collected from them were inoculated to seven chimpanzees, 80 to 230 larvae per chimpanzee. *O. volvulus* microfilariae became detectable in skin snips after prepatent periods ranging from 9 to 19 months. Feeding experiments were carried out with the forest form and the Sudan savanna form of *S. damnosum*. For a known concentration of microfilariae in the skin, forest form of *S. damnosum* ingested 2 to 4.5 times as many microfilariae of the forest strain of *O. volvulus* as the Guatemalan strain. In both forms of *S. damnosum*, ingested parasites of the Guatemalan strain were rapidly eliminated as microfilariae, and very few developed to infective larvae. These results indicate that the Guatemalan strain and the West African forest strain of *O. volvulus* are physiologically different with respect to their compatibility with the West African *Simulium* vector.

DUKE *et al.* (1966) conducted experimental studies on the development of *O. volvulus* from forest areas of Cameroon (A), and that from the Sudan savanna area (B) in *S. damnosum* populations from the forest and Guinea savanna zones of West Africa (a) and those from sites in the Sudan savanna zone (b). It was demonstrated that (A) developed well in (a) but showed little or no development in (b); conversely, the larvae of (B) developed well in (b), but showed little or no development in (a). Hence, it was suggested that there were two strains of *O. volvulus* and two main physiological forms of *S. damnosum* in West Africa, and that these were coupled to form two distinct parasite-vector complexes, one extending over the forest and Guinea savanna zones, and the other confined to the Sudan savanna zones.

It has also been noted that the prevalence of eye lesions and blindness of onchocercal origin is greatest in the northern Sudan savanna zones. This situation is in contrast to that met in the forest and Guinea savanna zones where the forest type of parasite-vector complex prevails; here onchocerca infections may be widespread, numerous and very intense, but are associated with very little blindness (KERSHAW *et al.*, 1954; RODGER, 1959; BUDDEN, 1963a; QUERE *et al.*, 1963; and MONJUSIAU *et al.*, 1965). The relationship between the change from one complex to the other and the prevalence of blindness was seen most strikingly in the remote valleys of the mountain chain on the borders of Nigeria and Cameroon (DUKE *et al.*, 1966).

The borderlines dividing the forest, the Guinea savanna zone (the southern savanna area which is relatively humid), the Sudan savanna zone (the northern savanna area which is relatively dry), and the desert of the West Africa were studied by DUKE *et al.*, (1966). It was not clear whether the two forms of *S. damnosum* interbreed in nature, or constitute distinct biological species. Some morphological differences were pointed out between the two forms of *S. damnosum* by LEWIS & DUKE (1966), but it was not certain whether these differences were due to the influence of environment during the development, or to variation of a clinal nature.

5.4 Human onchocerciasis

5.4.1 Introduction

Because of its importance as a disabling disease and its wide distribution in Africa and the tropical Americas, large numbers of reports have been made on the pathology, symptomatology, diagnosis, and treatment of human onchocerciasis. Reviews on the problems of human onchocerciasis were published by a number of workers, including STRONG (1934), WANSON (1950), RODGER (1962), OOMEN (1969), NELSON (1970), DUKE (1972), BUCK (1974: editor), and the Pan American Health Organization (1974). Especially useful for practical purposes are the last two booklets published by the World Health Organization. In the first booklet edited by BUCK (1974a), presentations are made by various workers on the symptomatology, pathology, and diagnosis of onchocerciasis in general. In the second booklet, entitled "*Research and Control of Onchocerciasis in the Western Hemisphere*," reviews and discussions are made by some fifty invitees to a symposium on the various aspects of onchocerciasis research and control.

The pathological changes produced as a result of *O. volvulus* infection in man may roughly be classified into two categories: those caused mainly by the adult worms, and those caused by the microfilariae. The skin nodules, or onchocercomata (onchocercomas), are the main feature of the clinical manifestation caused by the adult worms. On the other hand, the microfilariae are apparently responsible for a variety of other often very serious pathological changes, especially in the skin and the eyes.

These clinical manifestations of onchocerciasis have been noted to differ by the geographic regions. As summarized by DUKE (1974b), the disease in the Western Hemisphere is characterized clinically by mild skin lesions, with the exception of the now rare erysipela de la costa, which usually affects the face of heavily infected children. In Guatemala and Mexico, the nodules and the skin microfilariae are predominantly distributed on the head and upper parts of the torso. This distribution is probably linked with the biting habit of the main vector, *S. ochraceum*, which mainly attacks the upper portion of the body. The risk of eye lesions and blindness here is particularly grave. In Venezuela and elsewhere in South America, where the main vectors are the less efficient and lower-biting *S. metallicum* and *S. exiguum*, infections tend to be less intense, and the distribution of nodules and microfilariae is not so much confined to the upper parts of the body. The risk of developing eye lesions here is less.

There also exist two forms of onchocerciasis in West Africa. In the forest zone, gross skin and gland lesions are seen, nodules are abundant, microfilarial concentrations are moderate, sclerosing keratitis is rare, and blindness rates seldom reach 3% in onchocerciasis patients. In the Sudan savanna zone, on the other hand, nodules are less numerous, gross skin and gland lesions are less frequent, but microfilarial concentrations are often very high, producing a high incidence of sclerosing keratitis; this is often associated with severe iridocyclitis, and these two regions are largely responsible for high blindness rates of up to 10%.

In central and eastern Africa, another clinical variant has been noted in areas where the parasite is transmitted by members of the *S. neavei* complex. For example, it has been noted in Zaire that the highest blindness rates and many head nodules are found in the southerly forests of the Kasai, where *S. neavei* is the vector. Further north on the forest savanna border in Uele, where *S. damnosum* transmits the parasite, there are few eye lesions, but gross skin lesions, hanging groins, and scrotal elephantiasis are common.

In the Yemen Republic, a form of *O. volvulus* is found which produces maximal concentrations of microfilariae in the lower legs and ankles, and the hypertrophic, blackened skin lesions called 'sowda' are commonly found.

5.4.2 Symptomatology

5.4.2.1 Reactions to the adult worms

The adult worms become lodged in the subcutaneous tissues, and gradual, fibrous encapsulations develop around them; however, in early stages
of the infection, especially in children and in lightly infected persons, the
adult worms of *O. volvulus* usually do not produce any detectable symptoms. NNOCHIRI (1964) found, in autopsy studies, that the adult worms in
the early stage of the infection live free in the subcutaneous tissues or
simply enclosed in loose fatty tissue. In later stages, however, chronic
inflammations, without acute symptoms, develop around the adult worms;
these eventually becomes nodules of various size. Calcification of adult
worms in the nodules was observed by KERSHAW *et al.* (1955).

As pointed out by STRONG (1938), in Guatemala and Mexico, the great
majority of the skin nodules are found on the scalp or near the eye, but in
Africa some 95% of the fibrous nodular encapsulations, or tumors, are
found in areas other than the head, i.e., on the chest, lower trunk, or near
joints.

The distribution of nodules among patients in Mexico recorded by RUIZ
REYES (1968, quoted by SALAZAR MALLÉN, 1974) was as follows: of a total
of 5,092 nodules, 1,917 (37.6%) were on the head, 993 (19.5%) were on the
crista iliaca, 630 (12.4%) were on the ribs, 564 (11.1%) were in the sacro-
coccygeal area, 244 (4.8%) were on the trochanter, 222 (4.4%) were on the
neck, 125 (2.45%) were on the shoulder and arm, 95 (1.9%) were in the
lumbar region, and 302 (5.9%) were on other parts.

The subcutaneous nodules, called onchocercomas, contain varying numbers of adult worms, and also numerous microfilariae. They are from a few
millimeters to several centimeters in diameter, and in Central America are
found most frequently on the head; in Africa, however, they are found on
the trunk and near joints, especially in sites where skin and bone are closely attached, such as on the trochanter, iliac crest, sacrum, ribs, elbow, and
knee joints. The nodules do not adhere to the skin, but sometimes attach
to the underlying periosteum. Cases of penetration of the skull leading to
epilepsy have been reported from Central America. Surgical extirpation of
the nodules and removal of adult worms has been shown to be an effective
measure in the treatment of onchocerciasis when the nodules are few, and
easily accessible, such as is often the case in the Central American form of
onchocerciasis. In Africa, the surgical removal is usually difficult to accomplish because the nodules are many, and widely spread over the body. The
nodules occasionally form abscesses which burst through the skin. They
disappear when effective doses of a macrofilaricide (e.g., suramin or trimelarsan) are administered.

5.4.2.2 Reactions to the microfilariae

The microfilariae are produced by female worms residing in the fibrous
tumors; they disperse into the subcutaneous and cutaneous lymphatics

over a wide range of the host's body. In many cases, the microfilariae migrate into the eye ball where they cause opacity of the eye and often damage the optic nerve. They cause various types of acute and chronic skin lesions, and lymphadenopathy of various body sites.

(a) Skin lesions

Various forms of skin lesions have been reported to be caused by onchocerciasis. The most common symptom is itching, which may be either confined to a certain area, such as the trunk in Africa, or may affect the whole body. The skin signs were classified by GOLDMAN & ORTIZ (1946) as licheniform, pigmentation, and eczematoid. OOMEN (1969) recognized two forms: eruption and diffuse changes.

As for the diffuse changes, there are hypertrophy and atrophy. Diffuse swelling of the skin without loss of the normal structure is a common sign, most often seen in the abdominal skin. Lichenification may follow, after a period of scratching caused by itching; the skin becomes dry, scaly, and inelastic, with coarse folds. This may lead to pachydermia, with true hypertrophy of the skin, and loss of fold pattern and follicles.

Atrophy of the skin is another common sign of long-standing onchocerciasis. Histologically, there is a marked loss of elastic fibers. On the lower legs, such atrophied skin is smooth and shiny, and the hair follicles and the normal pattern of skin folds are lost. On the thighs, the skin is loose and thin, as in the very aged. LAIGRET (1929), in Sudan, described the disease this way: "Onchocerciasis makes young people look like old and old people look like lizards."

Abnormal pigmentation appears in two forms: (1) depigmentation of irregular shape, sharply bounded, sometimes in large patches or in a mottled "leopard skin" pattern, most often in the pretibial region. The loss of pigment is nearly complete and the skin looks white or pinkish; (2) macular pigmentation, consisting of numerous, small spots, with a hypopigmented center and a hyperpigmented periphery (OOMEN, 1969).

The papular eruptions are rather acute symptoms associated with itching; they can appear within a few days and disappear spontaneously in a few weeks or months. In Africa, these usually affect the trunk and the proximal part of the limbs. Another type of onchocercal dermatitis was reported from southern Arabia, known by the name of "Soda," or "Sowda," in which rash is limited to a sharply bound area, most often located on the thighs (FAWDRY, 1957; GASPARINI, 1962).

CONNOR (1974) conducted histopathological studies of various forms of skin lesions and other changes encountered in onchocerciasis in different geographic regions. A large number of biopsy specimens collected from patients showing various macroscopical changes were examined histologically, and as a result, much new knowledge about the pathogenesis of onchocerciasis was revealed. The specimens studied and demonstrated in this paper included altered pigmentation, dermal swelling, scaling, papules, wrinking, lymphadenitis, 'sowda,' a macule that developed after treatment with DEC, an involvement of the aorta, and the kidney of a patient who died after DEC administration. A case report was described of a 61-year-old Zairian who was treated with DEC for two days, then became comatose and died five days later; the clinical diagnosis was pulmonary edema; autopsy uncovered large numbers of microfilariae in all organs studied, and many of the microfilariae were degenerating and had provoked an acute inflammatory response.

(b) Lymphadenopathy and other abnormalities

Lymphadenopathy is a common and typical sign of onchocerciasis. The glands are enlarged and firm but not painful. This symptom is found most commonly in the inguinal region in African cases, but in Central America, it may also be present in the axillae and the neck. In such cases, the microfilariae are often found in the glands, and hyperplasia of the lymphatic tissues, and later, diffuse fibrosis are recognized. In some parts of Africa, patients with "hanging groin", a saclike projection of loose atrophic skin containing a mass of large fibrotic glands, have been observed (NELSON, 1958b).

Scrotal involvements, such as "hydrocele," similar to those observed in bancroftian filariasis have been reported to be caused by *O. volvulus* in Zaire (RODHAIN 1952), and Uganda and Sudan (KIRK 1947, 1957, KIRK *et al.*, 1959). High rates of genital elephantiasis have been observed in endemic foci of onchocerciasis on the Uele River in northern Zaire, where bancroftian filariasis is absent (OUZILLEAU, 1913; DUBOIS, 1916; and DUBOIS & FORRO, 1939).

(c) Eye lesions

Ocular complications are the most serious and feared consequences of onchocerciasis; in some endemic areas in Africa and Central America, blindness due to *Onchocerca* infection affects from 5 to 20% of the adult population. The occurrence of ocular symptoms in onchocerciasis has also been noted in Guatemala, since the disease was discovered there by ROBLES (1915), and STRONG (1934) observed that ocular complications were present in 5% of onchocerciasis cases. In Africa, HISSETTE (1931, 1932) first called attention to the ocular complications of onchocerciasis in Zaire, and conducted extensive investigations. Detailed studies of the symptomatology and pathology of the eye lesions were made by RODGER (1957, 1959, 1960a, b, 1962), BODGER & BROWN (1957), BUDDEN (1958, 1962, 1963a, b), NEWMANN & GUNDERS (1963) CHOYCE (1958, 1966), and OOMEN (1969d).

The microfilariae of *O. volvulus* invade the cornea, causing vascular or interstitial, sclerotic keratitis, or congestion and edema of the conjunctiva. The microfilariae also migrate into the orbit, and using an opthalmoscope, they may be seen swimming in the anterior chamber of the eye. The microfilariae may cause inflammation of the iris, ciliary body, retina, and choroid, or they may invade the optic nerve, and result in partial or complete blindness. In Africa, this state is often called "river blindness." The eye lesions may be classified into the following categories:

(c–1) Anterior lesions: The cornea is frequently affected in onchocerciasis. The microfilariae in the cornea are considered to do little harm as long as they are alive; when they die, however, small infiltrations form around them, resulting in fluffy opacities similar to punctate keratitis due to other causes. In a later stage, these develop to dense infiltration, or "pannus," which usually starts in the lower half of the cornea and progresses.

The anterior chamber is also invaded by the microfilariae, and their death causes chronic iritis, which is one of the most consistent and pathognomonic signs of ocular onchocerciasis. The earliest sign is a loss of the lower part of the pupillary ruff. Later, the iris becomes blurred and loses its normal structure; pupillary reaction becomes sluggish. It finally becomes atrophic, often leading to synechia of the lens, or more rarely, the cornea; the pupil becomes narrow, fixed, and may be blocked by a white plug of secretions. The possibility of cataract formation due to penetration of the microfilariae into the lens was reported by RODGER (1957). SANGAGE (1967) described a chronic limbitis with brown pigmentation and multiple small nodules as typical of ocular onchocerciasis.

(c–2) Posterior lesions: Atrophy of the optic nerve and of the retina are also common ocular involvements of onchocerciasis. Chronic chorioretinitis with curious irregular pigmentations has also been reported. However, as pointed out by KERSHAW *et al.* (1954a), posterior eye lesions are not so common and typical as those lesions affecting the anterior parts of the eye; microfilariae are seldom found in the posterior parts, and there is no clear relationship between the intensity or duration of infection and the incidence of the posterior lesions. RODGER (1957) considered the possibility of involvement of vitamin D deficiency, and CHOYCE (1958) attributed these posterior lesions partly to hereditary factors.

5.4.3 Geographical variation of clinical manifestations

It has been noted by various workers that there exist great variations in the clinical manifestations among individuals in the same endemic areas, and also among patients in different endemic foci. For example, a status called "erisipela de la costa," an acute erisipelas-like eruption occurring most commonly on the face, accompanied by fever, headache, and photophobia, is seen only in Central America. WOODRUFF *et al.* (1966b) also pointed out the difference between the clinical pictures of onchocerciasis in Guatemala and in East Africa; they stated that the manifestation called "mal de morado," a raised, purplish eruption often in plaques, like "lichen planus," and affecting the upper body, is peculiar to the American form of onchocerciasis. It is a well-known fact that the majority of *Onchocerca* nodules in Central America are situated on the head, while those in Africa are mainly on the trunk.

The high incidence of eye lesions has been noted in Central America, and BUDDEN (1963a) observed that it is similarly frequent in the savanna part of Africa, but is much less common in the forest part of Africa.

Choyce (1966) compared the ocular complications of onchocerciasis in Central America, Africa, and the British Isles, and reported that the incidence of posterior lesions is more frequent in Africa, though the incidence of anterior lesions is nearly the same in Central America and in the African savanna.

The incidence of lymphadenopathy, represented by hanging groins, hydrocele, and scrotal elephantiasis, has been found to be common in the tropical forest areas of Africa in northern Zaire, Central African Republic, the West Nile province of Uganda, and the Bahr El Ghazar Province of Sudan, where eye lesions are relatively rare. On the other hand, such syndromes were reported to be rare in areas where the eye lesions are common, and the two types of endemic foci were found to be apparently isolated from each other in Zaire and Sudan (Kirk 1947, 1957; Fain & Halot, 1965).

5.4.4 Diagnosis

The diagnosis of onchocerciasis may be made by parasitological measures, by immunologic measures, or by clinical manifestations. As in other filarial infections, the only specific diagnosis that can be made is by demonstration of the parasite (either microfilariae in the skin or other tissues, or the adult in skin nodules). However, the detection of the parasite from infected persons is not always successful, especially in patients of the chronic stage. According to a review by Kagan (1963), various immunological methods have been proposed and tested for the diagnosis of onchocerciasis, but further studies are required before a reliable and practical method can be developed.

For practical purposes, the demonstration of microfilariae in skin snips or by scarification of the skin has been the most common practice. The examination of the skin must be made from those areas of the skin where microfilariae are most likely to be found, i.e., the hip or lower leg in African onchocerciasis, or the shoulder and head in the Central American onchocerciasis.

The phenomenon that persons infected with *O. volvulus* develop itching and a rash within a few hours after taking 2 mg per kg of diethylcarbamazine (DEC) has been used as an auxiliary measure for the diagnosis. This procedure is called the "Mazzotti test."

5.4.4.1 Methods for detection of microfilariae
(a) Examination of the skin
The microfilariae of *Onchocerca volvulus* can be demonstrated by examination of skin snips. The following methods were recommended by WHO Expert Committee on Onchocerciasis (1966):
In the prevalence survey, at least two skin snips should be taken from each person. The snips should be taken from the sites most likely to be heavily infected. For onchocerciasis in Africa and Venezuela, these are the

buttocks and the lower legs; in Mexico and Guatemala, they are the shoulders and buttocks. In *D. streptocerca*, the microfilariae are most numerous in the skin of the trunk and are absent or few in the extremities.

The skin snips are usually taken by insertion of a needle into the skin to elevate a cone of the skin, which is then cut off with a razor blade. The area snipped should be approximately 3 mm in diameter. For a quantitative examination, the snip is weighed rapidly on a torsion balance. The portion of tissue removed is placed on a microscope slide in a drop of water, teased with needle, and allowed to stand 10 to 15 minutes. The specimen is then examined under low-power magnification of a microscope, and the number and species of microfilariae are recorded. For detailed study of the morphology of the microfilariae, the specimen is dried, fixed in methanol for 30 seconds, and stained with Mayers hemalum or Giemsa's stain. For identification of the species, see Section 1.3.3.

TOUFIC (1969) introduced a simple instrument for taking skin snips for examination of the microfilariae. This is a modified scleral punch (la pince emporte-pièce) used by ophthalmologists for operation of glaucoma, and has been shown to enable rapid, almost painless and bloodless snipping of relatively uniform sizes. PICQ et al. (1971) conducted a quantitative observation on the numbers of the microfilariae of *O. volvulus* at various intervals from the time the skin snips were placed in distilled water. They found that about 50% of the total numbers being recovered in 120 minutes left the skin snips in 30 minutes period.

TADA et al. (1973) also conducted quantitative studies on the rate of recovery of the microfilariae of *O. volvulus* from skin snips. In a conclusion, these authors stated that maximum recovery of the microfilariae was obtained by incubating intact skin snips in a saline solution in a wet chamber for long periods, such as six hours or longer; the short incubation time recommended by previous workers, such as 20 or 30 minutes, yielded only about 50% recovery from the skin snips. It was also shown that the skin snips should not be teased as recommended by other workers because this caused loss of the microfilariae by mechanical injury. In one of their experiments, the cumulative percentages of the numbers of microfilariae recovered from skin snips were 36.2% after incubation of 20 minutes, 50.0% after 40 minutes, 60.1% after 60 minutes, 75.6% after 120 minutes, 86.9% after 240 minutes, and 93.4% after 360 minutes.

BRINKMANN (1973, 1974) also studied the recovery rates of microfilariae from skin snips after placed in physiological saline, and obtained two equations, one reflecting the fact that the weight and the area of the skin snips were related to its largest radius, and the other expressing the percentage of microfilariae emerging in relation to the time.

(b) Examination of the eyes

The detection of the microfilariae of *O. volvulus* in the anterior chamber of the eye can be made by direct examination, either with a slit-lamp, or with an ophthalmoscope, using a diopter lens of at least +20 magnification. This together with other ophthalmological examination methods, often constitutes an important measure for assessment of the ocular involvements.

(c) Examination of the urine and sputum

Occurrence of the microfilariae of *O. volvulus* in urine has been shown to be a relatively common manifestation of onchocerciasis, and it is suggested that urine examination should be included as a routine diagnostic procedure. Sporadic reports of the occurrence of the microfilariae in urine were made by SHARP (1926), PRICE (1961) and OOMEN (1969). Urinary onchocerciasis was studied systematically and reviewed by BUCK *et al.* (1969, 1971) and BUCK (1973). For example, they recovered the microfilariae in the urine of 11 % of the total population of a village in the Republic of Chad where onchocerciasis was hyperendemic. Microfilaruria was also shown to be common in Upper Volta and Ivory Coast by PICQ & ROUX (1972), in Cameroon by THOMAS *et al.* (1972) and ANDERSON & FUGLSANG (1973), in Ghana by ANTESON (1972), and in Mali by ROUGEMONT (1973). The recovery of *O. volvulus* microfilariae in urine was shown to be closely associated with the intensity of skin infection.

FUGLSANG & ANDERSON (1973, 1974) demonstrated that the microfilariae of *O. volvulus* in the blood and urine increased remarkably while the patients were treated with DEC. They treated 57 persons infected with *O. volvulus* in the United Cameroun Republic by oral administration of DEC. Twenty-four hours after the first dose the percentage of patients passing the microfilariae in the urine increased from 46% to 85%, and the mean number of microfilariae per specimen increased from 3 to more than 36. An early effect of DEC therapy seemed to be the mobilization of the microfilariae into the urine. In their second series of experiment, 20 patients heavily infected with *O. volvulus* and all with moderate to severe ocular infections were examined and treated with DEC. The patients were divided into two groups of ten heavily infected (more than 50 microfilariae per mg of skin snip) and ten less heavily infected (with less than 50 microfilariae per mg). The geometric mean numbers of microfilariae in the skin were 94 and 30 per mg, in the blood 3.0 and 1.0 per ml, and in the urine 1.0 and 0.2 per ml in the examinations conducted before the treatment. The patients were then treated with DEC for 14 days, during which time the mean numbers of microfilariae in the blood increased to 40 and 8 per ml on the 5–6th day and in the urine to 22 and 9 per ml on the 2nd–3rd day, after which they both diminished. At the end of the treatment the mean number of microfilariae in the skin had fallen to 7.2 and 2.9 per mg. Apparently microfilariae of *O. volvulus* are thus mobilized by DEC from some internal reservoir and liberated in the blood or discharged in urine.

ANDERSON (1974) found the microfilariae of *O. volvulus* in sputum of two patients who became collapsed after administration of DEC, and suggested that the microfilariae might be the cause of the respiratory distress.

5.4.4.2 Methods for immunodiagnosis

KAGAN (1963) reviewed various immunological methods which have been proposed for the diagnosis of *Onchocerca* infection in man, such as skin tests, complement fixation tests, hemagglutination tests, and fluorescent antibody tests. More recently, reports were made by BIGUET *et al.* (1964) on the precipitin test, by CIFERRI *et al.* (1965) on the skin tests with *Onchocerca* and *Dirofilaria* antigens, by LUCASSE (1962) and LUCASSE & HOEPPLI (1963), WOODRUFF & WISEMAN (1968) on the fluorescent antibody test, and by ROSE *et al.* (1966) on the hemagglutination test.

These immunological tests for diagnosis of *Onchocerca* infection in man are of little practical use because they were found to be unreliable either in specificity or sensitivity, or both. In his review, NELSON (1970) states:

> Some of these immunological tests may be of value in epidemiological studies and as a rapid check on control methods, but in preliminary surveys and for diagnosis of the infection in individual patients the only completely reliable method is to demonstrate microfilariae, either in the skin or eyes or in the material aspirated from nodules. If these procedures are negative then the Mazzotti test with a provocative dose of 50 mg of diethylcarbamazine is more reliable than the nonspecific immunological test. But even the Mazzotti test is not always positive. Occasionally patients with quite high densities of microfilariae in the skin show no obvious reaction and OOMEN (1967b) has found that the test is particularly unreliable in Ethiopia. Infections with *D. streptocerca* may mimic the early stage of onchocercal infection and the microfilaria which also occur in the skin can cause some confusion, but DUKE (1968d) maintains that the Mazzotti test is negative in cases of streptocerciasis except with doses of more than 200 mg. The test is negative in cases of *D. perstans* infection (RIVES & SERIE, 1967).

BUCK *et al.* (1973) studied serum immunogloblin levels in five villages in Chad, and in onchocerciasis patients with and without microfilaluria. IgG, IgA, IgM and IgD levels were determined by a quantitative immunodiffusion method with the plates commercially available. Immunoglobulin levels of persons with severe and mild onchocerciasis revealed different age patterns; the natural increase of IgG levels with age was not found in the group with severe infections, while IgD concentrations continued to rise from the youngest to the oldest age group. On the other hand, IgE levels were not affected by either infection intensity or clinical severity of onchocerciasis, but was highly correlated with *Schistosoma mansoni* infection.

5.4.5 Treatment

The treatment of onchocerciasis can be surgical (excision of nodules) or chemotherapeutic (administration of microfilaricidal or macrofilaricidal drugs).

5.4.5.1 Surgical treatment

Surgical removal of adult worms by denodulization has been practiced extensively in Guatemala and Mexico, where onchocercal nodules frequently occur on the head, thereby increasing the danger of ocular complications. In these countries nodulectomy is practiced not only in hospitals but also by teams of field workers as mass nodulectomy campaign in all endemic areas where the disease abounds. However, it can rarely be expected that all adult worms can be removed by the surgical method, and thus it is only a suppressive measure. In Africa, denodulization is rarely practiced because most adult worms are found scattered in subcutaneous tissues of various body parts.

5.4.5.2 Chemotherapy (also see Section 10E.1)

There have been many papers published on the chemotherapy of onchocerciasis, and reviews have been made by HAWKING (1955, 1958, 1973), WHO EXPERT COMMITTEE ON ONCHOCERCIASIS (1966), DUKE (1968a, b,c), and NELSON (1970). At least four groups of compounds have been shown to be chemotherapeutically effective against *O. volvulus*, namely DEC, suramin, and certain arsenicals and antimony compounds. DEC is effective against microfilariae of *O. volvulus*, and causes reduction or clearance of microfilariae from the skin or eyes at least for certain periods if sufficient doses are administered, and temporary cure of various skin or eye symptoms may be achieved by the drug. However, the adult worms survive even when large doses of DEC is repeatedly administered, and thus recurrence of the clinical symptoms is common when DEC treatment is suspended. Furthermore, DEC frequently causes severe side reactions, as will be discussed later.

Both suramin and some arsenical compounds have been shown to be effective against adult worms of *O. volvulus*, and thus can produce radical cure when adequate doses are accepted by patients. However, the arsenicals have sometimes caused serious side effects including fatal encephalopathy; therefore, they are no longer recommended in the treatment of any form of filariasis. Suramin is used only by intravenous injection; it also has certain side effects, though not so dangerous as the arsenicals. In any event, the control of onchocerciasis by mass administration of chemotherapeutic agents is considered by most workers to be impracticable at the present stage.

As a general method of drug treatment for complete cure of onchocerciasis, the WHO EXPERT COMMITTEE ON ONCHOCERCIASIS (1966) recommended a regimen consisting of a course of DEC, followed by a course of suramin, and eventually another course of DEC. The mass drug administration to people living in endemic areas of onchocerciasis has generally been discouraged unless measures to prevent the side effects of the drug and to control the vector are taken simultaneously. DEC alone does not cure the disease permanently. Suramin and other macrofilaricides are too dangerous for mass administration in the field. It should also be noted that where onchocerciasis coexists with *Wuchereria*, *Loa*, or *Dipetalonema* infections, mass administration of DEC for the control of these other filarial infections should be performed with great care in order to prevent the occurrence of severe side reactions.

(a) Diethylcarbamazine (DEC):

For individual patients with onchocercal infection without severe involvement of the eye, the dosage recommended by OOMEN (1969a) was 0.5 mg per kg of body weight (about 25 mg, or half a 50 mg tablet in adults), once on the first day, the same dose twice on the second day, and if the reactions are not too severe, 2 mg per kg three times daily for ten days. DEC destroys microfilariae in the skin within a few days, but has little effect on adult worms, and microfilariae reappear in the skin a few weeks after the end of treatment. Nevertheless, this destruction of microfilariae usually causes improvements in skin and eye conditions.

DEC frequently causes severe reactions in the skin, and also in the eyes when these are infected. The severity of the skin reaction is proportional to the density of microfilariae in the skin rather than to the dose, and is presumed to be caused by the liberation of antigens from the destroyed microfilariae. The infected skin parts become hot, swollen, and itch severely for several days; this is accompanied by a rise of body temperature, and swelling of the corresponding lymph nodes. The eyes, when infected, show conjunctivitis and photophobia. These symptoms usually subside after 3 to 5 days, and thereafter, large doses of DEC can be tolerated. Administration of cortisone (25 mg, four times daily for six days, beginning two days before administration of DEC) or of prednisone (5 mg, twice daily for five days, starting from one day before administration of DEC) was reported to be effective in diminishing the side reactions of DEC (MARKEL & TURNER 1957).

The microfilariae of *O. volvulus* may be cleared after sufficient doses of DEC are administered to the patients, but previous experiences by a number of workers have shown that they usually reappear in the skin of patients several months to a few years after the treatment is suspended. MAZZOTTI (1951b), for example, recorded in Central America the reappearance of numerous microfilariae from four to eight months after the treatment, whereas other patients remained free for 14 months. BURCH (1949) observed three out of nine patients to be free from microfilariae after seven to eight months, and BURCH (1950) found 3 of 20 patients free from microfilariae one year after receiving DEC in a dosage of 40 mg per kg. BURCH & ASHBURN (1951) recorded 14 of 46 patients remained free one year after treatment. In Zaire, WANSON (1952) observed the return of microfilariae between two and four months after treatment. HAWKING (1952) conducted a histological study of onchocerciasis treated with DEC.

A quantitative observation on the distribution and density of microfilariae in the skin by multiple skin snips, as well as their reappearance after DEC treatment, was conducted by DUKE (1957) in ten African volunteers in Cameroon. After examination of the multiple skin snips, each patient was given a three weeks' course of DEC starting on a low dosage of 50 mg per day of the citrate salt (which contains 50% of the base), working up to 450 mg per day by the end of the first week, and continuing at that level for two weeks, with the total dosage of 7.0 to 7.7 g of the citrate salt in each case. The dose was sufficient to destroy virtually all the microfilariae. At intervals from 3 to 13 months afterwards, further examinations of multiple skin snips were made to assess the rate of increase in the numbers and distribution of the microfilariae in the skin. It was estimated that the concentration of microfilariae returned to the pretreatment level within one to three years after cessation of the treatment, and the original pattern of microfilarial distribution was maintained during the posttreatment build-up.

DUKE (1968a, b, c) conducted a series of investigations on the effects of three groups of drugs on *O. volvulus*, i.e., DEC, the antimonial preparations (TWSb and MSbE), and three brands of suramine. In the first report (Duke, 1968a), quantitative studies were conducted on the effects of DEC on patients infected with the forest strain of *O. volvulus* and living in the Cameroon rain forest. Four weighed skin snip samples were collected from each patient, i.e., from the left and right calves and the left and right buttocks. In comparison of the microfilarial density (microfilarial count per mg in all snips) observed successively on 21 cases of the same untreated patients at intervals from 3 to 6 weeks, variations from 0.60 to 1.87 times were found to occur between the two examinations, with a mean of 1.03. In the experiments on the effects of DEC, a single course of treatment given at a total dosage of 7.7 g was again shown in 10 patients to clear almost all microfilariae in the skin and eye, but immediately after treatment the microfilarial concentration began to build up again, so that after one year they had reached from 30% to over 100% of their pre-treatment level, as reported in his previous paper (DUKE, 1957). In another series of experiments in which eight patients were treated with three courses of DEC (total dosage of each course was 7.0 g) given at six-month intervals, the results of examinations of eleven skin snips collected at each time from each patient showed that the rates of build-up were fairly constant each time and showed no reduction with succeeding courses. Thus, DEC was shown to have no significant lethal or sterilizing effect on adult *O. volvulus* worms, even when large doses were administered in three courses.

A detailed study on the effects of DEC in the treatment of onchocerciasis cases was made also by OOMEN (1969d). In general, the drug was shown to be very effective for the cure of clinical signs; "gale filarienne" (filarial scabies) often disappeared within a week, and improvements in pachydermia and skin atrophy became noticeable after one or two months; it seemed that nearly all signs of onchocerciasis were reversible. However, various grades of reactions, including death, were observed after the DEC administration. Of 327 onchocerciasis patients treated in the usual way with DEC, there was no reaction in only 72 cases (22.0%), 57 (17.4%) had late reactions (first signs more than 24 hours after the first dose of 50 mg), 184 (56.3%) had normal reactions (first signs of reaction within 24 hours from the first dose), and 14 (4.3%) had severe reactions (reaction within 24 hours, which subsequently became so severe that treatment with additional doses had to be stopped and sometimes corticosteroids were used). In other words, the Mazzotti test was negative in 40% of Oomen's patients.

In 184 patients who showed the normal reaction, itching, often accompanied by a papular or urticarial rash, developed and remained for several days. Fever was occasionally observed, and on rare occasions, there were joint pains and photophobia.

In the 14 cases with severe reactions, the itching was almost intolerable and often accompanied with urticarial rash: fever was nearly always present. Prednisone, in a dose of 30 mg per day, was very effective in controlling such reactions.

Of 327 onchocerciasis patients treated with DEC, seven died in circumstances suggestive of a fatal effect of the drug. These patients had the following features in common: (a) all were in poor general condition, (b) no clinical reaction occurred after administration of DEC, (c) all lapsed into an irreversible coma after a small amount of the drug (225 to 900 mg given in three to eight days), and (d) death ensued 4 to 12 days after the first dose.

ANDERSON (1974) described collapse which occurred during treatment of onchocerciasis with DEC. The trial took place in a Sudan-savanna village, where a small initial group of 15 patients was selected for out-patient treatment. Their infections were moderate to severe, with microfilarial concentrations per mg of skin at the buttock ranging from 40 to 245. Each was given a 50 mg tablet of DEC, a starting dose of a standard course adopted by DUKE & ANDERSON (1972) in the treatment of onchocerciasis. They all developed severe Mazzotti reactions, with early and pronounced tenderness and swelling of lymph nodes in the groin and axilla. Two to four hours after this initial dose most of them were so prostrated that it was difficult to persuade them to attend the further ocular examination. At this stage a man of about 30 years collapsed during slit-lamp examination and remained seemingly unconcious for about 10 minutes. His breathing was shallow and rapid, and pulse was weak at 135 per minute. After 2 hours of resting he was able to move around slowly, and within two days he was back to normal. Another patient, a 16 year-old male, who had received 50 mg Antistin with the first 50 mg dose of DEC, also developed severe general reactions with cough and shallow breathing. His condiction was unchanged at examination in his house the following morning (pulse 120 per minute, respiration 40 per minute), when he was given 100 mg Antistin and two APC tablets. By the evening he had improved sufficiently to receive 25 mg DEC together with 100 mg Antistin. He walked 500 m for examination the following morning. He was then given 50 mg DEC with 100 mg Antistin, and within 45 minutes he again collapsed during examination at the slit lamp. Sputum obtained at this stage contained several microfilariae of *O. volvulus*. Four other patients in the group were also observed to develop respiratory distress at some stage during the first five days of DEC therapy, usually soon after taking the drug. Subsequent groups were given steroid therapy (betamethasone 1 mg t.d.s.) as a routine for at least 24 hours prior to commencement of DEC treatment, and also during the first three to five days of treatment. Despite this one very heavily infected child developed acute respiratory distress within 30 minutes of taking the first 12.5 mg DEC, and again microfilariae of *O. volvulus* were recovered from his sputum.

LAZAR *et al.* (1968, 1970) considered that an ophthalmic preparation of diethylcarbamazine might be useful in treating ocular onchocerciasis, and studied its toxicity in animals. Two drops of 5% diethylcarbamazine dihydrogen citrate buffered to pH 7.0 with NaOH were placed in the eyes of 20 male and female rabbits three times daily, five days a week, for eight weeks. No abnormalities were observed at the end of eight weeks, both in ophthalmological examination with the slit-lamp, or in histological study. The compound showed good penetration into the anterior segment of the eye thus treated.

Duke (1968g) found that DEC was ineffective against adults of *O. volvulus* experimentally infected to chimpanzee, although the same drug was, according to Duke (1963), effective against *L. loa* in the same host.

(b) Suramin:

This is a drug known to be effective in the treatment of African trypanosomiasis, which has also been shown to be effective as a macrofilaricide in onchocerciasis (but not in other filarial infections). The drug has been used extensively by some workers in the treatment of human onchocerciasis, but there have been reports on the occurrence of severe reactions resulting from suramin treatment, including several fatalities due to exfoliative dermatitis and renal complications (VAN HOOF *et al.*, 1947; MASSEQUIN *et al.*, 1954; DUKE, 1968f; NELSON, 1955, 1970).

Suramin is given intravenously, at a dose of 0.5 g for an average adult, followed by 1 g at weekly intervals for a total dose of 4.5 to 5.5 g. The risk of serious side effects increases when this dose is exceeded. These side effects include fever, muscle pains, malaise, and sometimes generalized dermatitis; their occurrence is an indication to stop treatment. The most serious risk with this drug is kidney damage. When more than five erythrocytes per high power magnification field or protein is found in urine, treatment should be suspended until these signs disappear. The urine should be examined before each injection of suramin (OOMEN, 1969 d). For more detail, see Section 10 E.1.2.

(c) Arsenicals and other compounds:

Trimelarsan (pentylthiarsaphenyl-melamine, Melarsen W, Mel W) is a compound containing arsenic, introduced by FRIEDHEIM & JONGH (1959, 1960) in the treatment of *W. bancrofti* and *O. volvulus* infections in man. The compound was shown to be effective as a macrofilaricide of both *W. bancrofti* and *O. volvulus*, even after a single dose injection of 7.5 to 10 mg per kg of body weight, and there were, at one time, hopes that it would be of great value for mass treatment. Various dosage regimens, with a maximum total of 500 mg per adult given at one time, were tested; however, it eventually became clear that this compound may cause fatal arsenical encephalopathy, though in rare occasions (DUKE, 1966b; LAGRAULET *et al.*, 1966; BASSET & LACAN, 1967). Consequently, this compound is now not recommended for the treatment of any form of human filariasis.

A number of other drugs have been tested for the treatment of onchocerciasis, including niridazole, thiabandazole, and antimony compounds, but they were either ineffective or too toxic (DUKE & MOORE, 1967; DUKE & HAWKING, 1967; DUKE, 1968h).

(d) Metrifonate (trichlorfon):

SALAZAR MALLÉN *et al.* (1970) reported on a case of onchocercal dermatitis in a Mexican treated with metrifonate (trichlorfon; Bilarcil, Bayer). The drug was administered four times at two-week intervals in doses of 15 mg per kg. All manifestations of the disease receded or disappeared, and the number of microfilariae demonstrable in the skin by biopsy was reduced to less than half the original number. The drug was well tolerated (see Section 10E.2.3. trichlorfon).

SALAZAR MALLÉN & GONZALEZ BARRANCO (1971) further conducted trichlorfon treatment on 19 onchocerciasis cases in Mexico. The drug was administered orally after breakfast in single doses of 7.5 to 15 mg per kg of body weight, at two-week intervals, for a total of five to 16 doses. The treatment caused disappearance of two nodules after the second dose and had reduced the size of 25 out of the total of 65 nodules by the end of treatment. Nodules removed after four doses showed severe inflammatory reaction, and a majority of adult worms were nonmotile and showed damage to their reproductive organs. The rates of reduction of microfilariae in skin snips two weeks after administration of five or more doses were from 80% to 100%. The drug was well tolerated by all the patients. The side effects were seen in 12 of 19 patients; these were muscarine-like (colic in ten cases; nausea in nine cases; cough in six cases; vomiting in three cases; defecation in two cases), and were all mild and transitory.

According to a more recent report by SALAZAR MALLÉN (1974), onchocerciasis patients in Mexico under his control were being treated with daily doses of 10 mg per kg of trichlorfon for six days, with atropine sulphate to minimize the muscarinelike effects. The drug was shown to have definite though not uniform action against the larvae and adult worms, and produced a less severe therapeutic shock than DEC. (In Mexico, DEC is administered in the field in doses of 1 mg per kg daily for seven days; suramin is no longer used because of its toxicity; a trial with Mel W was promptly ended also because of its toxicity.)

In West Africa, DUKE (1972, 1974) conducted experimental treatments of onchocerciasis in human being and in chimpanzees, and showed that trichlorfon was a microfilaricide, but that even at doses as high as 22 mg per kg daily for six days, no action could be detected on the adult worms.

5.5 Vectors of *Onchocerca volvulus*

The mode of transmission of onchocerciasis was unknown until BLACKLOCK (1926a, b) demonstrated, in Sierra Leone, that the larval development of *O. volvulus* would take place efficiently in the black fly, *Simulium damnosum* Theobald, 1913. Later investigations by a number of workers in Africa have shown that this species is the most common man-biter and the principal vector of onchocerciasis in most of the endemic areas. Another black fly species, *Simulium neavei* Roubaud, 1915, was incriminated as an important vector in certain endemic areas of onchocerciasis in East Africa. In the endemic areas in the Americas, i.e., in Mexico, Guatemala, and Venezuela, *Simulium metallicum*, *Simulium ochraceum*, and *Simulium callidum* have been shown to act as vectors. A tremendous amount of literature is available on the bionomics of black flies in relation to the epidemiology of onchocerciasis in Africa and the Americas.

There have been large numbers of contributions made on the biology and ecology of the simuliid flies in relation to the transmission of human onchocerciasis in Africa and the Americas, and also in Canada, the United States, Europe and Japan where they are serious pests to man and animals. Comprehensive reviews were made by DeMeillon (1930), Hocking & Hocking (1962), Brown (1962), Lewis (1968), Nelson (1970) and Crosskey (1962, 1973) on the black flies in relation to the transmission of *O. volvulus*.

5.5.1 The black fly (Simuliidae)

The black fly, or Simuliidae, is one of the insect families of the suborder Orthorrhapha, order Diptera. The adults are usually small, dark flies with a stout body and a humpbacked appearance. The antennae are short, but consist of 11 segments. The wings are broad, without scales, hairs, or ornamentation; the anterior veins are stout, while the remaining veins are very weak. As in the case of mosquitoes, only the females are bloodsuckers.

The black flies usually breed in swift-flowing, well-aerated, clean water in hilly or mountainous regions. As a rule, it is necessary for a female fly to take a blood meal for the development of eggs. The eggs are deposited in a compact layer on the surface of rocks, leaves, and debris on swift-running streams. The egg cluster is usually covered with a yellowish creamy slime. This egg stage lasts about one week.

The larvae are soft skinned, creamy, somewhat cylindrical in shape, enlarged at both ends, and attenuated in the middle. The head bears two large fanlike organs for catching food. There is a leglike projection attached to the thorax. The larvae attach to rocks, leaves, and other matter (on crabs in the *S. neavei* group) in water by means of a disclike sucker at the caudal end of the body. They may be collected in enormous numbers from leaves or stones exposed to swift-running water. The larvae feed chiefly upon diatoms and algae. The larval stage lasts from two to three weeks in tropical areas.

At the end of the larval stage they spin boot-shaped cocoons from their cephalic glands. The cocoon is firmly attached to a leaf or rock in the stream. Pupation occurs in the cocoon. The pupa has a pair of long, branched respiratory tubes extending outside of the cocoon. The species may be identified in pupae by the shape of the cocoon and the respiratory tubes. The pupal stage lasts about two weeks, after which the adult emerges by breaking through the pupal skin and escaping from the water into the air.

5.5.2 The bionomics of the main vectors

(a) The main vectors of *O. volvulus* in Africa

Two black fly species-groups have been shown to act as the principal vectors of *O. volvulus* in the African region: the *Simulium damnosum* group, and the *Simulium neavei* group.

As for the vectors of onchocerciasis in Africa, DE MEILLON (1957) states:

> Two species of *Simulium*, namely *S. demnosum* and *S. neavei* are known vectors. A third, *S. renauxi* WANSON & LEBIED 1950, is said to be a vector in the western Belgian Congo but this is now regarded as a synonym of *neavei* by FREEMAN & DE MEILLON (1953). A few other species are known to attack man readily—namely *albivirgulatum* WANSON & HENRARD 1944, shown to be a nonvector, since microfilariae of *volvulus* do not develop beyond the thoracic stage; *merops* DE MEILLON 1950 bites man readily in Ngamiland but there is no onchocerciasis; similarly, the disease is absent in Madagascar, where *imerinae* ROUBAUD 1906 and *neireti* ROUBAUD 1905 bite. The absence of the disease may, of course, be due to the fact that it has not yet been introduced. In Angola *wellmani* ROUBAUD 1906 was originally caught biting viciously. Dr. Wellmann records that the flies were feared by the natives and on one occasion caused him to move camp; elsewhere in southern Africa and Ruanda Urundi it does not bite (FAIN, 1950). In the Dongola area of the northern Sudan, *griseicolle* BECKER 1903 occurs in vast swarms, and although only a small percentage bite man and the number of flies is so enormous that they constitute a definite nuisance, yet onchocerciasis is unknown in this region. *S. gariepensis* DE MEILLION 1953—a biting species very similar in behavior, and, for that matter, in morphology, to *griseicolle*—occurs in the southern Orange Free State, where onchocerciasis is unknown.

(a.1) The *Simulium damnosum* complex

Simulium damnosum Theobald, 1903, is a species complex widespread throughout tropical Africa. It is the most common human biter, and the main vector of onchocerciasis in most parts of the African region. Since BLACKLOCK (1926) first observed the development of *O. volvulus* larvae to the thoracic stage in this species in Sierra Leone, large numbers of reports were made on its bionomics and relation to the disease.

S. damnosum breeds on vegetation and rocks in various types of river systems. Its large-scale breeding has been noted in great rivers, such as the Congo and the Nile, and in their numerous tributaries flowing through thick forests and vast grasslands. It also breeds in seasonal streams on the edge of the desert in the northern savanna regions.

The adults of *S. damnosum* can be readily distinguished from other African simuliids by the greatly flattened front tarsi and the silvery pubescence of the front tibiae. Its pupae are very distinct from other species by the presence of a pupal gill consisting of short tubes resembling a bunch of bananas. The larvae have characteristic, paired, dorsolateral tubercles on the anterior abdominal segments.

A comprehensive review was made by DE MEILLON (1957) on the bionomics of *S. damnosum* in relation to the transmission of *O. volvulus* in the Ethiopian region. He cited as many as 45 references published before 1957. Especially important studies on *S. damnosum* were made by WANSON (1950) in Zaire, LEWIS (1948, 1953a, b, 1956, 1957, 1958a, b, 1960a, b) in the Sudan and West Africa, CROSSKEY (1954, 1955, 1956, 1957a, 1962) in northern Nigeria, DUKE (1962d, e, 1966a, 1967b, 1968b, c, i, j,), DUKE *et al.* (1966, 1967) in Cameroon, HOCKING & HOCKING (1962) in the Sudan, and DAVIES *et al.* (1962) in West Africa.

S. damnosum in Africa is not an uniform population. It is usually highly anthropophilic in its biting behavior, but zoophilic races have been found, especially outside of the endemic areas. Two distinct races have been identified by their compatibility with the respective onchocerca strain, *i.e.* the forest and Guinea savanna race and the Sudan savanna race (DUKE, 1966). DUNBAR (1966) differentiated four sibling species included in the *S. damnosum* complex from Uganda by studies on larval chromosomes. Dunbar (1969) further identified nine cytological segregrates in the *Simulium damnosum* complex.

DISNEY (1970b) investigated the variation within the *S. damnosum* complex in the forest zone of western Cameroon, and in addition to the Nile form, found a new cytotype in materials sent to Dunbar; two morphological forms differing in the shape of abdominal scales of their larvae were also recognized.

CROSSKEY (1955) made observations on the bionomics of adult *Simulium damnosum* in northern Nigeria, where the disease is intense and endemic foci are numerous. As for its feeding habits, *S. damnosum* is markedly anthropophilic, although it also attacks donkeys and dogs. The fly bites predominantly upon the legs below the knee; of 1,000 bites of *S. damnosum* studied by Crosskey, 946 were on legs below the knee, 29 on thighs, 24 on arms and hands, and 1 on the head. The legs were still the preferred site even when catchers lay down. Such a distribution of bites seems to be correlated with the quantitative distribution of the microfilariae of *O. volvulus* in the skin described by KERSHAW *et al.* (1954), who observed that the highest microfilarial density occurs in the legs, especially on the ankles. *S. damnosum* is a day-biting fly, and was observed to attack man from about 7 a.m. until 6.30 p.m. with a peak of activity at about noon. *S. damnosum* bites almost anywhere out-of-doors, with slightly shady places generally preferred; it rarely enters inside houses. As for the seasonal incidence, the adult population is extremely low in the dry season from

October to April, and rises rapidly during May and June when the rains begin.

As stated before, DUKE *et al.* (1966) carried out experimental studies utilizing *O. volvulus* from forest and savanna zones and *S. damnosum* from various bioclimatic zones of West Africa, and showed that there exist two strains of the parasite and two strains of vectors. The microfilariae of *O. volvulus* from forest areas of Cameroon developed well in *S. damnosum* from the forest and Guinea savanna zones of many parts of West Africa, but they showed little or no development in *S. damnosum* from Sudan savanna zones. Conversely, microfilariae of *O. volvulus* from the Sudan savanna area of Cameroon developed well in *S. damnosum* from Sudan savanna zones, but showed little or no development in flies from the Guinea savanna and forest zones. DUKE (1966 a) further observed that high intake of the Sudan savanna strain of *O. volvulus* microfilariae by the forest strain of *S. damnosum* increased the mortality of the flies only in the first 24 hours after ingesting the blood meal; furthermore parasites of the Sudan savanna strain of *O. volvulus* ingested by the forest form of *S. damnosum*, and those of the forest strain of *O. volvulus* ingested by the Sudan savanna form of *S. damnosus*, were eliminated mostly as microfilariae.

The biting activity and the longevity of *S. damnosum* in nature was studied in detail by LEWIS (1956. 1957, 1958a, b, 1960a, b, c, 1965). The parous and the nulliparous females could be differentiated by the presence or absence of relics in the ovarioles by the method described by DETINOVA (1962; see Section 10C.2.2); their physiological ages could be estimated from the rates of the parous females, or more precisely, by the frequency distribution of the numbers of the relics in the populations examined. It was demonstrated further that the peak of biting time of parous females came earlier than that of the nulliparous ones, and therefore, the size of the infection rate with *O. volvulus* and of the parous rate of the females differ greatly according to the time of day at which the flies are collected. A number of studies were made in reference to this important problem, and the results were reviewed by DISNEY (1970a).

(a.2) The *Simulium neavei* complex

Black flies of the members of the *S. neavei* complex are closely related in morphology and biology, and had been grouped into a single species, *S. neavei* Roubaud, 1915, until recently. They breed mainly in small streams in highland areas of East and Central Africa and nearly all species have an obligatory association with fresh-water crabs of the genus *Potamonautes*. This remarkable characteristic was first discovered by VAN SOMOREN & McMAHON (1950), in Kenya, and was confirmed in a number of other species in this group (i.e., *S. nyasalandicum*, *S. woodi*, *S. goinyi*, *S. hightoni*, and *S. ovazza*) by LEWIS & HANNEY (1965).

Black flies of the *S. neavei* complex has been incriminated as the main vectors of onchocerciasis in a number of endemic areas in East Africa. In

Amani, Tanzania, LEWIS (1960a, b; 1961a, b), as well as RAYBOULD (1967), showed that two species (unbanded and banded forms) of this complex inhabited this area, of which *S. woodi* De Meillon (banded form) was the only man-biting black fly and the vector of human onchocerciasis; another species, *S. nyasalandicum* De Meillon (Amani form, or unbanded form) was not a regular human biter.

Simulium neavei Roubaud, 1915 was reported to be the vector of onchocerciasis in Sankuru, Zaire (HISSETTE, 1932; STRONG, 1937), Kwango, Zaire (GEUKENS, 1950), and Nyanza Province, Kenya (McMAHON, 1940; BUCKLEY, 1949;). The occurrence of *S. neavei* has also been recorded from western Ankole and Kigura, Uganda (DE MEILLON, 1958), and several other localities in Zaire, Tanzania, and Kenya.

In Nyanza Province of Kenya, the endemic areas of onchocerciasis are restricted to the highlands (1,500 to 1,800 m above sea level) where the population density of *S. neavei* is highly concentrated. An overall infection rate of 10% was noted by McMAHON (1940) in this area. In western Zaire, GEUKENS (1950) found an infection rate of 100% in the local inhabitants, and WANSON (quoted by DE MEILLON, 1958) observed an infection rate of 50%, and an infective rate of 10% by dissection of 300 wild flies.

The eggs of *S. neavei* were observed in western Zaire to be deposited in clusters on vegetation near the cascades in which the crab, *Potamonautes*, lives. The larvae presumably migrate after hatching and seek out the crab host (WANSON, quoted by DE MEILLON, 1957). Larvae have only been found living in phoretic association with the crabs species *Potamonautes niloticus* in Kenya (McMAHON, 1951), and *P. lueboensis* and *P. lirrangensis* in western Zaire (WANSON & HOLEMANS, 1951). They are found attached around the eye stalks, mouth parts, bases of legs and dorsum of the carapace. The mature larvae spins its cocoon and also pupates on the crab host, especially around the sides of the carapace, rarely on mayfly pupae or on vegetation.

According to McMAHON (1951), at least three species of crabs are found in the rivers or streams of the breeding areas of *S. neavei* in Kenya, but only *P. niloticus* is used as the host. There are two black fly species closely related to *S. neavei*, whose larvae also develop commensally on the crab and are more widespread, but their adults do not bite man: *S. woodi*, known from Kenya, Uganda, Malawi, Zambia, and Ethiopia, whose larvae are found in the exhalant passage of the bronchial chamber of *P. niloticus*, and spins an unusually coarse cocoon (McMAHON, 1957a); and *S. nyasalandicum*, known from Malawi (Nyasaland), Kenya, and Uganda, found on *P. niloticus* both in the open country below 4000 ft and above the point where this crab is replaced by *P. granviki* in cooler upstream waters.

(b) Vectors of *O. volvulus* in America

Since BLACKLOCK (1926a, b) demonstrated for the first time in West Africa that the larvae of *O. volvulus* developed in *S. damnosum*, black flies have also been considered to be the vector of *O. volvulus* in Central

America. Robles (1919) considered, from epidemiological assumptions, that *Simulium* flies might be the vector of onchocerciasis in Guatemala. Hoffman (1930) reported on onchocerciasis in Mexico, and observed the development of microfilariae in *Eusimulium mooseri* (now a synonym of *S. callidum*). By later studies carried out in Guatemala and Mexico, the following three species were postulated to be the vectors of onchocerciasis in the Americas (Strong, 1931; Strong *et al.* 1934; Giaquinto, 1937: De Leon, 1957).

    Simulium ochraceum Walker, 1861

    Simulium metallicum Bellardi, 1859

    Simulium callidum (Dyar *et* Shannon, 1927).

Of the above three species, *S. ochraceum* was considered to be the principal vector because it was specifically anthropophilic, more numerous in the endemic areas than in the nonendemic areas, and tended to bite the upper half of the body where the microfilariae are most numerous. However, De Leon (1957), in Guatemala, dissected 3,561 black flies from September to December, and 1,143 black flies during December 1944, but found none of them to be infected with mature larvae of *O. volvulus*.

The first successful results in the experimental studies of the transmission of the American strain of *O. volvulus* by American blackflies were reported by De Leon & Duke (1966). Human carriers of the Guatemalan strain of *O. volvulus* were exposed to the bites of black flies at Finca El Amparo, in the department of Chimaltenango, situated in a heavily endemic area at a height of 4,500 ft above sea level. Full development of the filarial larvae to the infective stage was seen seven or eight days after ingestion of the microfilariae by *S. ochraceum*, *S. metallicum*, and *S. callidum*; however, their efficiencies as vectors of *O. volvulus* differed greatly. *S. ochraceum* was most numerous in the biting density, and ingested the largest numbers of microfilariae, highest survival rate after infected, and highest numbers of developed infective larvae; *S. callidum* was apparently more efficient than *S. metallicum* as an experimental vector, but neither species was likely to be of great importance because they are generally zoophilic, biting humans only in small numbers.

The vectors of onchocerciasis in the South American countries have not yet been confirmed. The endemic foci in Venezuela are located in a hilly region between 200 m and 1,300 m above sea level, mainly in sparsely wooded grasslands. Lewis & Aldecoa (1962), who conducted comprehensive studies on the bionomics of black flies in these regions, found 12 species, among which *Simulium metallicum* and *S. exiguum* were the common man-biting species.

The endemic area discovered from Colombia is also located on a relatively low plain, about 60 km inland from the coast, and only about 50 m above sea level. According to Barreto *et al.* (1970), almost the only man-biting black fly species was *Simulium exiguum*, and this species appeared to be the main vector of onchocerciasis in this region.

5.5.3 Control of *Simulium*-vectors of onchocerciasis

The use of DDT as a larvicide against *Simulium* was reported first by
FAIRCHILD & BARREDA (1945). The first successful trial for eradication of
the vector (*Simulium neavei*) from an onchocerciasis area was conducted
in Kenya by GARNHAM & McMAHON (1947).

Programs conducted by a number of workers in Africa have shown that
effective control and even eradication of the *Simulium* vectors of onchocerciasis is possible by systematic applications of larvicides to all the
streams and rivers where their larvae breed, for example, dripping DDT
at a concentration of 0.1 ppm for 30 minutes every ten days, for a period
of three months. Such larvicidal methods have already eradicated *S. neavei*
from western Kenya and *S. damnosum* from the Victoria Nile of Uganda,
and promising results have also been reported from certain endemic areas
of onchocerciasis in Zaire, and several West African countries, as described
by BROWN (1962) and McMAHON (1967). A standard method of DDT
treatment of rivers for eradication of simuliid flies was described by Mc-
MAHON (1957).

However, the extensive use of DDT and other chlorinated hydrocarbon
insecticides (BHC, dieldrin, chlordan, etc.) to control black flies poses
some serious problems; not only are such insecticides toxic to fishes and
other valuable animals and wild life, but also, they are biologically inde-
gradable and may cause future pollution of the environment, especially
when large amounts are applied for long periods. The use of insecticides
with lower toxicities to fish and other vertebrates, and those more easily
decomposed in nature, is recommended for this purpose. Insecticides,
such as "fenitrothion" used in Japan for the black fly control in rivers and
streams, or "Abate," (another organophosphorous compound) now used
in West Africa, are two examples of such larvicides.

(a) Methods for larvicidal operations

The control or eradication of black fly vectors of onchocerciasis has been
accomplished mainly by larviciding operations, although the control of
adult flies by the dusting of insecticides has been employed under special
circumstances with some success, such as reported from Leopoldville, in
Zaire (BROWN, 1962). DDT emulsifiable concentrate was recommended
by most workers as an effective and suitable formulation for this purpose.
Various equipment has been devised for insecticide application into rivers
and streams.

The dose of insecticides to be applied into water varies according to local
conditions, i.e., the length and speed of the flow, species of flies, the kind of
insecticide, and its formulation. The method most commonly adopted was
the application of 0.1 to 1.0 ppm DDT for 15 to 30 minutes of the river
flow. This usually results in complete kill of the larvae for length of 10 to
100 km downstream. The applications should be repeated several times at
10 to 14-day intervals. All the tributaries must be treated from the point
above which vector fly no longer develops. Several dosing points may be

necessary along the same river. Checking of the results by entomological surveys is essential for determining the dose, intervals, times of application, and the necessary dosing points.

In order to determine the dose of insecticide to be applied to a river, it is necessary to estimate the amount of river discharge. The unit "cusec" (cubic foot per second) has been used by most Western workers, but it is more convenient to measure the amount of river flow by "cubic meter per minute" as has been utilized in the black fly control program practiced in Japan (OGATA & SASA, 1955). The amount of river discharge in cubic meters per minute F is calculated from the formula: $F = W \times D \times V$, where W is the width of the river in meters, D is the mean depth of the river in meters, and V is the mean velocity of flow in meters per minute, all measured at one point. The dosage unit ppm (part per million) corresponds to a concentration of one gram per cubic meter, because the weight of one cubic meter of water is, roughly, one million grams. In measuring the amount of river flow, it is necessary to select a point where the diameter of the river is relatively straight for a certain length, and where the speed of flow is kept relatively constant for the entire width and for some length, otherwise, measurements of the mean depth and the mean velocity are difficult to obtain.

The flow speed can be estimated with either a current meter or float. Various types of current meters which measure the speed of water flow at one point are commercially available. Various types of floats have also been devised for measuring the water velocity. In small streams, the maximum surface velocity can be estimated simply by throwing rice husks or other small floating matter onto the surface of the water, and measuring the time required to pass two fixed points set 10 to 50 meters apart. The velocity V is then computed by dividing the fixed distance by the travel time. It should be noted that the velocity of water flow may vary greatly at different points of the river, and at different parts of the same section. In general, the water flows fastest on the surface and near the center of a stream; therefore, in order to estimate mean velocity, it is necessary to multiply by a correction factor, f, over the maximum velocity measured either with a velocity meter or with a float. The factor f varies, according to the depth of water and the structure of the river bed, from about 0.65 to 0.85 (MCMAHON, 1967).

(b) Progress of *Simulium* control programs

Kenya:

The first successful results of control or eradication of onchocerciasis vectors were achieved in Kenya, by systematic treatment of the breeding places of *S. neavei* with DDT. The first target area was an isolated focus of 65 square miles in the Kodera region called the Valley of Blindness, where onchocerciasis was found in some 70% of the inhabitants. The rivers in this area were treated in 1946 with 13 applications of DDT at 2 to 5 ppm for 30 minutes between January and June (GARNHAM & MCMAHON, 1947). The adult flies disappeared by March and never reappeared; new infections of onchocerciasis in children subsequently born in this region dropped to near zero (GARNHAM & MCMAHON, 1954; NELSON & GROUNDS, 1958).

A larger area of infestation (1,500 square miles) in the Kakamega-Kaimosi districts was treated, in a period from 1947 to 1948, with 11 applications of 1 to 2.5 ppm DDT for 30 minutes between November and April, but *S. neavei* reappeared in the northern half of the region in the following year. The Kisii and Kericho areas, together totalling 1,150 square miles, were also treated in a period from 1952 to 53 with ten applications of 0.5 to 1 ppm DDT for 30 minutes between October and January. By this time, the larvae were discovered to be breeding on a species of crab (VAN SOMOREN & MCMAHON, 1950; MCMAHON 1951, 1952), and the rivers previously treated were found to be only a part of the breeding ground. The Kakamega-Kaimosi sector was retreated in 1954 in order to cover 2,000 square miles, including all newly discovered breeding places. MCMAHON *et al.* (1958) reported that *S. neavei* had been eradicated from Kenya by these operations.

Uganda:

A large endemic area of onchocerciasis associated with the occurrence of *S. neavei* exists in eastern Uganda, on the western slope of Mt. Elgon, extending beyond the Kenya border. According to BARNLEY & PRENTICE (1958), this area was treated in 1957 with 12 applications of 0.5 ppm DDT for 30 minutes, at intervals of two weeks between January and April (the dry season). The operation in this area proved to be more difficult and extensive than initially thought because the topography was so complex, the breeding places were difficult to reach, and many new streams appeared during the rainy season; consequently, the operation never reduced the adult fly count to zero, and the numbers recovered to their normal level within a year, even though as many as 158 dosing spots were made in the Bulucheke area alone.

Much greater success was achieved with the Budongo forest located at the east end of Lake Albert (BARNLEY & PRENTICE, 1958). The prevalence of onchocerciasis was about 80% among the local population, and the infection rate of *S. damnosum* was about 20%. An area of 160 square miles was treated during a period between 1955 and 1956 with 0.5 ppm DDT for 30 minutes in 12 applications, at ten-day intervals. There were 20 dosing points on five streams in the forest. This resulted in the disappearance of *S. neavei* by the end of 1957.

In Uganda, there also existed endemic areas of onchocerciasis associated with *S. damnosum*. The most important among these was the region along the Victoria Nile from Victoria Lake to Kyoga Lake. According to BARNLEY (1958), the Victoria Nile, with a water flow of approximately 17,000 cusecs, was treated with 0.4 ppm DDT for 30 minutes, in 12 weekly applications during 1952. By the third application, adult *Simulium* had disappeared, and the number of flies remained low for three years. Onchocerciasis had afflicted 99% of the inhabitants on both sides of the river for a 45-mile stretch, but after the treatment this region became more densely populated. In 1956, the river was again treated with DDT at 0.2 ppm for 30 minutes, in ten weekly applications. No adult *S. damnosum* appeared in the four years after this treatment (BROWN, 1962). There still exist untreated endemic areas in Uganda because of the difficulties of transportation and inspection.

Nigeria:

As reported by BUDDEN (1956), onchocerciasis is highly prevalent among the people in Nigeria; he estimated that about 350,000 persons suffered from the disease, and of these, some 20,000 were blind. Over 50% of the reported endemic foci were observed in the Abuja and Pawa River areas south of Kaduna, in the Lokoja area around the confluence of the Niger and Benue rivers, and along Beli and Harwal rivers in the Adamawa region. CROSSKEY (1956) reported that *S. damnosum* bred in almost all rivers in northern Nigeria, except those in the dry north region above a latitute of 11° N. There are two distinct seasons in this region of Africa: a dry season from November to April, and a rainy season from May or June to October. Intensive breeding of black flies takes place during the rainy season.

As a result of these surveys, a pilot project for the control of *S. damnosum* by larvicidal treatments was organized by the Medical Department, and the first results were reported by CROSSKEY (1958). In contrast to the previous control projects which were applied to isolated endemic areas, such as in Zaire (WANSON *et al.*, 1949) and in Uganda (BARNLEY, 1953), Nigerian program was to be put into operation in an area where a network of nonisolated breeding rivers existed. For various reasons, the Abuja area of Niger Province was chosen; a preliminary survey was begun in late 1954, and treatments of the breeding rivers were begun early in 1956. In total, an area of some 1,200 square miles around Abuja Town was covered. Subsequent reports on the results were made by DAVIES *et al.* (1962) and DAVIES (1963, 1965, 1968).

For the first two years, technical DDT in diesel oil was used, then in 1956, a dose of 1.4 ppm DDT for 30 minutes, in 12 weekly applications at four points was applied at the end of the dry season from March to May. The treatment points were increased from four to seven in 1957. Beginning in 1958, DDT was used in miscible liquid form (25%); this was found to give equally good results, with the advantage of being easier to handle and apply. The dose was reduced to 0.5 ppm DDT for 30 minutes in 1958, and to 0.5 ppm DDT for 15 minutes in 1960. The density of black flies was reduced from 5.8 per fly-boy per hour to 0.15 per fly-boy per hour in 1956, and remained at this or higher levels thereafter, until 1960. Such a remarkable reduction, though not eradication, of the vector had reduced the incidence of onchocerciasis from the treated area. The operation will have to be repeated every year to keep the vector density as low as possible. The best results were obtained by application in the early wet season from May to July. The amount of *p,p'*-DDT consumed was 905.8 pounds in 1956,

1,489.6 pounds in 1957, 2,038.1 pounds in 1968, and 2,854.0 pounds in 1959.

Ghana:

Onchocerciasis is widespread in this country, especially in the northern region, where nearly 100% of inhabitants are affected, and some 20% of *S. damnosum* were found to be infected. Breeding of the black fly occurs in the Black, White, and Red Voltas, and their tributaries.

The first control experiment was performed in 1954, and tributaries of the White Volta were treated with DDT in oil at a concentration of 0.1 ppm for 15 minutes, applied seven times at four-day intervals in the rainy season (July and August). A reduction in the fly count of about 70% was observed in August only. The area was subsequently reinfested because some tributaries were left untreated (CRISP, 1956, quoted by BROWN, 1962).

Control experiments were later conducted on various rivers; for example, DDT applied in concentrations of 0.1 ppm for 30 minutes to the Black Volta in 1959 attained complete kill for 50 miles downstream. However, most of the treated areas were reinfested because the coverage of the tributaries was insufficient (BROWN, 1962).

The control of *S. damnosum* in the region of the Volta Dam, Ghana, was reported by KUZOE & HAGAN (1967). The construction of the Volta Dam was started in 1961, at Akosombo, and about 4,000 workers were engaged on the project. The prevalence of onchocerciasis was high in the lower Volta Valley; HUGHES & DALY (1951) reported an 82% infection rate among the people in Agbotia and 68.1% among the people in Atinpoku. In the present survey, *S. damnosum* was found to breed only in the perennial rivers in this region, and adult *Simulium* were most prevalent in the wet season, reaching a peak density in September and October.

DDT was used as a larvicide at dosage rates of 0.1, 0.3, and 0.4 ppm for 30 minutes, once every ten days for a period of three months, during three different treatment periods. The most effective time for treatment was found to be when the river was rising and when the discharge was above 8,000 cusecs. Successful elimination of the larvae was achieved for a distance of 30 miles downstream, and a remarkable reduction in adult *Simulium* density was achieved; however, reinfestation occurred rapidly. The practical difficulties of dosing a large river several hundred feet wide were overcome by using a motorized canoe on which the dosing gear was permanently mounted. The cost of the project was high mainly because of the large volume of larvicide needed to dose the Volta River; the total amount of larvicide used was 5,543 pounds for the period from July 1962 to March 1964. Dead fishes and crabs were observed only when the river was treated with a dose of 0.4 ppm.

Sierra Leone:

The entire country is infested by *S. damnosum*, with the exception of areas around the city of Freetown and the southern coastal plane; the prevalence of onchocerciasis is especially high in the hilly regions. The country is drained by nine rivers with a dry season discharge of 1,000 to 10,000 cusecs.

Systematic treatments were performed beginning 1957 on the Tonko-lili River, a tributary of the Seli River, where an iron mine was being developed. The onchocerciasis prevalence in the African population was as high as 85% (CONRAN & CONRAN, 1956). DDT was applied at doses of 1.0 to 0.5 ppm for 30 minutes, at two-week intervals, but it was necessary to repeat such treatments every year because of reinfestation of the fly from other untreated rivers (BROWN, 1962).

South of the Sahara:

The regions immediately south of the Sahara, between latitudes 9°N and 13°N, has been noted by the high prevalence of onchocerciasis. The first black fly control program was conducted in 1955, on Mayo Kebbi, in Chad; six successive applications of lindane at 1 to 2.5 ppm for 30 minutes were made at three points, during the dry season from February. The larvae and adults completely disappeared by March, but the flies returned in the next wet season (TAUFFLIEB 1955, quoted by BROWN, 1962).

A program for *Simulium* control was organized in 1956 by the Organisation Commune de Lutte Contre les Grandes Endémies, involving the governments of Dahomey, Togo, Ivory Coast, Upper Volta, Niger, and Guinea. Surveys were made, beginning 1956, of the epidemiology and vector biology. The Bougouri-Ba River, 400 km long, and flowing at about 70 cusecs in the dry season and 3,500 cusecs in the rainy season, was treated with DDT in kerosine at a concentration of 2.5 ppm for 30 minutes, in the dry season of 1957. This was effective for a length of 200 km, but not for 500 km long. Some fish were also killed (BLANC *et al.* 1958, quoted by BROWN, 1962).

WHO Onchocerciasis Control Program in the Volta River Basin area:

An international program for the control of onchocerciasis in the Volta River Basin is in preparation. The following are taken from a mimeographed report of the Mission for Preparatory Assistance to the governments of Dahomey, Ghana, Ivory Coast, Mali, Niger, Togo, and Upper Volta, represented by WHO and the International Bank for Reconstruction and Development (IBRD) as the executive agencies, and FAO and UNDP as associate agencies (August, 1973). The area to be covered under the program is one of the worst endemic onchocerciasis zones in the world extending over the seven countries, where it is estimated that over one million of the ten million inhabitants of the area (nearly 700,000 km) are infected, and that at least 70,000 are blind or have a serious impairment of sight. The main objective of the control program will be the destruction of the black fly larvae by application of insecticides into the rivers where they breed. The desiderata for a chemical compound lethal to the larvae are: (1) that it should not unduly affect nontarget fauna, especially fish; (2) that it should quickly decompose in the biological environment; and (3) that it should be effective as a black fly larvicide. Two compounds believed to best meet these requirements are Abate and methoxychlor. Although DDT is also effective against the *Simulium* larvae, its chemical stability and nonbiodegradability preclude its use.

Because of the inaccessibility by land of many of the breeding sites of *Simulium*, the only feasible method of applying the larvicide is from the air. In the case of large rivers that are sufficiently straight, light planes can be used, but narrow, twisting waterways, and those overhung with forest canopy require the use of helicopters. In the rainy season, when rivers flow swiftly, a single application may eliminate the *Simulium* larvae for up to 50 km downstream. In the dry season, relatively fast-flowing stretches of river may be interrupted by areas of still water, in which case, each of these stretches must be treated separately.

Because of the long life of the adult worm in the human host, sufferers from onchocerciasis may remain infective for as long as 15 years, even if not reinfected. The duration of a campaign must, therefore, not be less than this time.

The repopulation or settlement of the uninhabited fertile areas freed from the disease is another major objective of the Onchocerciasis Control Program. It is expected that major reclamation of deserted land will be possible some 18 months after the start of insecticide treatment in the zone concerned. It is planned to launch the program, which will last about 20 years, in 1974, after endorsement of the strategy proposed by all concerned. Funds in the neighborhood of US\$ 120 million will be required to finance the program, and a special fund for onchocerciasis is now being established. As an executive agency, WHO will assume technical responsibility, in conjunction with the governments involved. The executive organ will be the Steering Committee for Onchocerciasis Control in the Volta Basin area, representing the four sponsoring agencies (UNDP, FAO, IBRD, and WHO).

Zaire:

Black fly control programs have been undertaken in various endemic areas of onchocerciasis in the Congo River Basin. In the area around Leopoldville (Kinshasa), where nearly 100% of the native population was infected and some 16% of the adult *S. damnosum* were found to be harboring the larvae (WANSON *et al.*, 1949; WANSON, 1950), it was considered impossible to treat the river with insecticides, because the discharge of Congo was over 1,000,000 cusecs, even in low water. Adult control was attempted, first by dusting the infested vegetation with 10% DDT dust at 20 kg per hectare, but this proved ineffective. An Oxford aircraft was then engaged, and a DDT aerosol was produced by injecting a 20% DDT solution in three parts xylene and seven parts gas oil into the exhaust stack. Both sides of the river bank were treated with 20 kg of DDT per square mile between September and December 1948, and a virtually complete kill of adult flies and larvae in the river was obtained. In March and April 1949, the Ndjoue, Luwa, and Zumune rivers were treated, and this resulted in an apparently this area was kept free from *S. damnosum* only by continued annual applications (BROWN, 1962).

Control of *S. neavei* by river treatment in the onchocerciasis area around Bojuma, 60 miles west of Stanleyville, was reported by BROWNE (1960). A series of ten applications was made at ten-day intervals with 2 ppm DDT for 30 minutes. This treatment resulted in almost complete disappearance of the adult fly for an area of about 1,000 square miles, but it became reinfested six months later.

Simulium control in tropical America:

According to the report of the WHO Expert Committee (1966), the control of vector species of Simuliidae (*S. ochraceum, S. callidum*, and *S. metallicum*) was in progress in Mexico and Venezuela, but not in Guatemala or Colombia. As reviewed by CROSSKEY (1959), black fly control programs for the prevention of mass biting of man and livestock were also being conducted in Canada and the United States.

Onchocerciasis in Mexico and Guatemala is a disease associated with coffee-growing areas, and its boundaries are remarkably clear-cut. It occurs in mountainous terrain, which is generally well forested, at altitudes between 450 and 1,500 meters above sea level.

In Mexico, ground applications of larvicide (33% DDT in xylene and triton) was made to infested streams every 15 to 20 days throughout the year in the endemic areas in the states of Oaxaca and Chiapas, and marked reduction in the adult vector populations has been achieved. In Venezuela, a campaign was begun in 1958, and promising results were obtained during a pilot scheme, when DDT was applied to streams at points ten km apart at concentration of one ppm, which was reduced later to 0.5 ppm. (WHO EXPERT COMMITTEE, 1966).

Notes on *Simulium* control in Japan:

Black flies are serious pests of man and livestock in hilly and mountainous regions in Japan, and pilot studies and control programs have been conducted since 1952. The first pilot study for the control of black fly larvae was conducted at Seijo in Tokyo, and Myoko in Niigata. Based on the results of pilot experiments, an application of DDT emulsifiable paste, at the extremely small dose of one ppm per one minute flow volume, was recommended as a standard; this proved to be effective against black fly larvae for a distance of one to several km downstream. Later, DDT was replaced by certain organophosphorous insecticides, especially fenitrothion (Sumithion), which is less toxic to fish and biologically degradable. Results of the early studies were reviewed by OGATA & SASA (1955), and a comprehensive report was made by UEMOTO (1971) on the black fly control program in the city of Kyoto.

Part 2 | Geographic Medicine of Human Filariasis

6

Filariasis in the American region

The epidemiology of filariasis in the American Region is discussed in this text according to the three subregions, the North and Central Americas, the West Indies, and South America. Altogether four species of human filariae are known to be endemic in this region, namely *Wuchereria bancrofti*, *Dipetalonema perstans*, *Mansonella ozzardi*, and *Onchocerca volvulus*. A review was made on epidemiology of filariasis (excluding onchocerciasis) in the American region by Sasa (1974), and on that of onchocerciasis by Pan American Health Organization (1974).

6A. North and Central Americas

Filariasis due to *W. bancrofti* was once noted to be endemic in certain urban areas in the southern United States, particularly in and around the city of Charleston, South Carolina. Presumably, the parasite was introduced by immigrants from the West Indies and favored by the abundance of its vector, *C. fatigans*, in the Charleston area. The occurrence of clinical filariasis, such as chyluria, hydrocele, and elephantiasis of the legs, was reported to be common, and the microfilariae were demonstrated frequently during the period from the end of the last century until about 1920, but later, the disease gradually died out.

Sporadic reports have been made on the occurrence of *W. bancrofti*, *M. ozzardi*, and *O. volvulus* from various countries in Central America. The epidemiology of *W. bancrofti* infection in most Central American countries has not been investigated thoroughly, and it is still not clear whether the parasite has never become established or has not attracted the attention of medical workers. There are some old records from Mexico and Guatemala on the occurrence of *W. bancrofti*, but it is not known whether the transmission is still taking place. Relatively high microfilaremia rates were recorded from certain areas in Costa Rica, in 1947.

Table 6-1. The occurrence of clinical bancroftian filariasis (F), microfilaria carriers of *W. bancrofti* (W), *M. ozzardi* (M), *D. perstans* (P) and *O. volvulus* (V) in the countries or districts of the Americas as recorded in medical literature.

A. North and Central America

United States	F*	W*		
Mexico	F		M	V
Guatemala	F		M	V
Costa Rica	F	W		
Panama			M	

B. West Indies

Puerto Rico	F	W	M	
Dominican Republic	F	W		
Haiti				
Jamaica	F	W		
Cuba	F	W		
Bahama Islands			M	
Virgin Islands	F	W		
Anguilla				
St. Kitts	F	W	M	
Antigua				
Montserrat	F			
Guadeloupe	F	W	M	
Dominica	F		M	
Martinique	F	W		
St. Lucia	F		M	
St. Vincent			M	
Barbados	F	W		
Grenada				
Trinidad	F		M	P

C. South America

Colombia	F		M	V
Venezuela	F	W	M	V
Guyana	F	W	M	P
Surinam	F	W	M	P
French Guiana	F	W	M	
Brazil	F	W	M	V
Ecuador				
Peru				
Bolivia			M	
Paraguay				
Argentina			M	
Uruguay				
Chile				

*Once recorded but now absent or unknown.

Mansonella ozzardi infection is known from Mexico and Panama, and its possible role as the cause of some allergic conditions has been pointed out recently. *Onchocerca volvulus* infection is a serious problem in the hilly zones in Mexico and Guatemala. (See Fig. 6-1.)

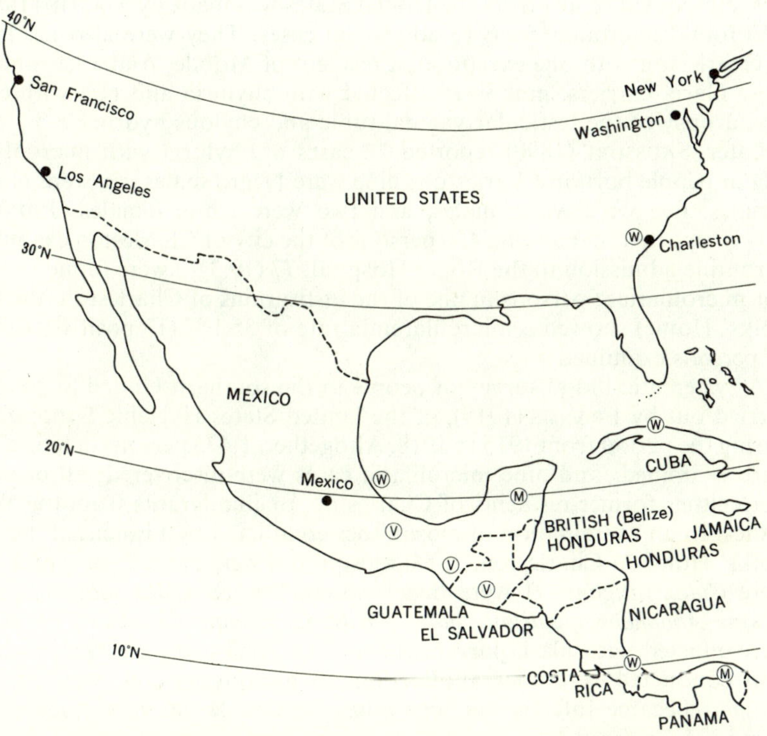

Fig. 6-1. Distribution of filariasis in North and Central Americas
W: *W. bancrofti,* M: *M. ozzardi,* V: *O. volvulus*

6A.1 The United States

Filariasis in the United States was recorded first by GUITERAS (1886), who was a resident of Key West, Florida. He found *Filaria sanguinis hominis* (*W. bancrofti*) in the blood of four Cuban immigrants to this island, who had apparently contracted the disease in their native country. Early in 1885, he moved to Charleston, where he found chyluria and elephantiasis to be common. In Charleston, he found microfilariae in the blood of a mulatto woman suffering from chyluria, and who had never been outside of the city except for five years that she spent in Augusta, Georgia. Later, he found another filaria carrier, a Negro suffering from hydrocele and elephantiasis of the scrotum. This patient was also a resident of Charleston and had never been outside of the city or its immediate neighborhood.

A subsequent report from the United States was made by MASTIN (1888), who found microfilariae in 13 additional cases. They were also residents of Charleston with one exception, a resident of Mobile, Alabama; among these filaria carriers, nine were affected with chyluria and two with chylous dropsy of the testicular vaginal tunic and chylous hydrocele.

Later, SAUSSURE (1890) reported 22 cases of chyluria with microfilaremia in people born in Charleston; nine were Negro males, six were Negro females, five were white males, and two were white females. JOHNSON (1915) reported that among 400 persons of the city of Charleston examined at routine admission to the Roper Hospital, 77 (19.3%) were found to harbor microfilariae; persons in one of the institutions of Charleston (the Old Folks' Home) showed a microfilaremia rate of 35.1% (13 positives out of 37 persons examined).

A systematic blood survey of people in the southern United States was carried out by FRANSIS (1919), of the United States Hygienic Laboratory, during the period from 1915 to 1918. Altogether, 1,475 persons in nine cities were examined, and nine microfilaria cases were discovered; all of them were either former residents of Charleston, or immigrants from the West Indies. In an examination of mosquitoes conducted by Francis, at the Old Folks' Home in Charleston, 1,000 mosquitoes were caught, of which 902 were *Culex fatigans*, 91 were *Aedes calops*, 5 were *Aedes solicitans*, and 2 were *Anopheles quadrimaculatus*. Of 65 *C. fatigans* dissected, 13 (20%) were infected with filaria larvae, and 4 (6.2%) had mature larvae. Francis also conducted experimental infections of mosquitoes and found that *C. fatigans* became infective at high rates, but no larval development was seen in *Ae. calopus*.

6A.2 Mexico

Mexico is located south of the United States and bounded on the southeast by Guatemala and Belize (British Honduras), between longitudes 15°N and 33°N. Mexico has an area of 1,966,500 km² and a population of 48,313,438 (1970).

Three species of human filariae have been reported to be endemic in Mexico, i.e., *W. bancrofti*, *M. ozzardi*, and *O. volvulus*. *Wuchereria bancrofti* was noted by Fülleborn (1929) and Mühlens (1932) to be spread along the Atlantic coast, but there have been no detailed studies or later reports on the epidemiology. Endemic foci of *M. ozzardi* have been found in the northwestern part of the Yucatán Peninsula. *Onchocerca volvulus* is a serious health problem in certain highland areas of southwestern Mexico.

Mansonellosis:

The occurrence of *M. ozzardi* in Mexico was recorded by FÜLLEBORN (1929), who found its microfilariae in materials sent to him by Hoffman. The endemic focus is located in the northwestern part of the Yucatán Peninsula, at about 20°N and 90°W. Epidemiological surveys were conducted by HOFFMAN (1930), MAZOTTI (1942), and BIAGI (1956a). BIAGI (1956a) obtained microfilaremia rates of 55.3% (973 positives out of 132 persons examined) in Tinun, 84.9% (62 of 73) in Nilchi, and 50.6% (46 of 91) in Tenabo, with the overall positive rate of 61.1% (181 of 296). Over 75% of adults above the age of 20 were found to be positive.

BIAGI (1956b) further reported on the results of clinical and immunological surveys using skin tests and precipitin tests with a *Dirofilaria immitis* antigen. No special clinical manifestations were observed, and no correlation was found between the immunological reactions and microfilaremia levels. However, the parasite was shown to cause eosinophilia, especially in the early stage of infection (BIAGI & CASTREION, 1957).

BIAGI (1957) made morphological studies and measurements of the length of microfilariae of *M. ozzardi* in Yucatán; their length was from 160 to 208 μ (mean: 183 μ) in specimens fixed in acetic acid solution, and from 192 to 232 μ (mean: 214 μ) in Formalin-fixed specimens.

Onchocerciasis:

Human onchocerciasis has been noted to be endemic in southwestern Mexico, and particularly in the states of Oaxaca, Chiapas and Guerrero (see Fig 5-2 and Fig 6-1). The situation is similar to that found in Guatemala, in that the infected areas are on highland slopes where coffee is grown, the clinical features are mainly represented by the development of tumors on the head and ocular lesions, and the same species of black flies act as the vectors.

According to a review by STRONG (1934), the occurrence of onchocerciasis in Mexico was noted by HARDWICK in 1928, who quoted a publication of LARUMBE from Oaxaca which noted the prevalence of a condition locally called "mal de la ceguera" (blinding sickness) and "mal morado" (purple sickness). HOFFMANN (1930) made detailed studies on its etiology and mode of transmission. Reports were made on onchocerciasis in Mexico by OCHOTERENA in 1930 and ARROY in 1931 on the histopathology of the skin, by DAMPF in 1931 on the transmission, TORROELLA in 1931 on ocular disturbances, DA SILVA in 1931 on the treatment, GUTIERREZ in 1931 on the complement fixation test, and MÜHLENS (1932) on epidemiology and clinical observations.

According to a recent review by Mallén (1974) on onchocerciasis in Mexico, there are three endemic areas in this country: one in the State of Oaxaca, which extends from 17°25' to 17°48' N and 96°12' to 96°48' W, and covers 1,400 km²; the other two are situated in the State of Chiapas, the northern one extending from 16°52′ to 17°7′ N and 92°29′ to 92°40′ W and covering 700 km², and the southern one extending from 15°4′ to 15°57′ N and 92°5′ to 93°7′ W and covering 6,800 km². This last focus includes a great part of the coffee plantations of Soconusco area and continues eastwards to the endemic area of Huehuetenango in Guatemala. The endemic areas are at altitudes from 600 m to 1,200 m above sea level. The rainy season in this area lasts from May to October, during which numerous small streams are formed to allow breeding of the *Simulium* vectors.

A national onchocerciasis control program was started in 1930. In 1940, a total of 160,837 persons from the Soconusco area were examined, and 24,384 onchocerciasis cases were discovered. An institute for the study of the disease was established in Huixtla in 1942. In 1965, the campaign was reorganized, and since then the operational functions have been undertaken by health authorities. In Chiapas, there are 13 teams to cover the two endemic areas, each team consists of five workers; in Oaxaca, where there are fewer patients, there is only one team of four workers. Under the supervision of physicians, these workers carry out most of the practical work, such as excision of nodules, administration of drug, and examination of skin biopsies. Entomologic work is supervised by one entomologist and two assistants, and working under them are 24 full-time workers and 124 other workers who apply 1 ppm of DDT emulsion in xylol, once a week at intervals of 250 m (Mallén, 1974).

6A.3 Guatemala

Guatemala is a republic situated south of Mexico, between latitudes 14°N and 18°N. It has an area of 108,900 km² with a population of 5,110,000 (1970). The regions on the Atlantic and Pacific coasts are not lowlands, while the interior is an extensive tableland some 600 to 1,500 m high, with several peaks exceeding 3,000 m in height.

Only *O. volvulus* is known to be endemic in Guatemala, and presents a serious health problem for the people in the endemic areas.

The occurrence of onchocerciasis was reported for the first time in the New World from the Pacific slope of Guatemala by ROBLES, in 1916, who described the disease in more detail in 1919 (ROBLES, 1919). In 1918 and 1921, PACHECO LUNA, and in 1917 and 1920, CALDERON confirmed these investigations, and further reports on the occurrence of the disease and its clinical features were made by ESTEVEZ in 1921, GUERRERO in 1921, MORA in 1922, SAENZ in 1922, MORALES in 1923, AZURDIA in 1924, and BARREDO in 1929.

According to STRONG (1934), the zone of infection constitutes a strip of territory within altitudes of about 2,000 to 4,500 feet above sea level, extending about 75 miles to the west of Yepocapa, and for nearly 75 miles to the southwest of it, reaching the southern part of the Department of Amatitlán. The eastern extension is somewhat less, touching only the northern part of the Department of Escuintla. The infected territory thus lies largely in the Departments of Chimaltenango and Solola, and in the northern part of Escuintla; the important municipal districts of Pochuta, Santa Barbara, and Chicacao are included in this endemic area. The territory in Amatitlán, nearly as far north as the town of Patin and extending south almost to the town of Guanagazapa in Escuintla, is probably also infected (see Fig. 5-2).

Onchocerciasis in Guatemala is almost exclusively associated with coffee plantations. The development of the coffee industry in this country has evidently had a marked influence upon the dissemination of the disease. Coffee is said to have been introduced to Guatemala in 1850, from Arabia, by a Spanish priest, and the coffee plantations on the Pacific slope were well established by the year 1880.

The vegetation in the coffee-growing area is semitropical, and the land is well irrigated by numerous, small, rapidly flowing streams of clear, cold water, all good breeding grounds for *Simulium*. The cultivation and preparation of coffee for export especially exposes the laborers to the bite of the black fly vectors. STRONG (1934) stated that it was not clear whether onchocerciasis in Guatemala was endemic among the Indians since old times, or whether they were infected while visiting countries where *Onchocerca*-carrying Africans had been imported as slaves. Strong also suggested that the infection in man in Mexico and Guatemala might have occurred from cattle infected with *Onchocerca gipsoni*, since no morphological differences could be found between this and human *O. volvulus*.

FIGUEROA MARROQUIN (1974) reviewed the status of onchocerciasis in Guatemala. The country is divided politically into 22 departments, among which the disease was found from seven, namely, Chimaltenango, Esquintla, Guatemala, Huehuetenango, Santa Rosa, Solola, and Suchitepéquez. The disease is distributed in four endemic foci, of which two are located in Huehuetenango in the northwest and are continuations of the infested zone in Mexico, especially the Soconusco focus of Chiapas; they have a total area of about 600 km². The third focus embraces the most infested municipalities in this country, such as Palin and San Vicente Pacaya in the Department of Escuintla, Chicacao in the Department of Suchitepéquez, Santiago Atitlán and San Lucas Tolimán in the Department of Solola, and Yapocapa, Pochuta, and Acatenango in the Department of Chimaltenango. Some coffee plantation populations in this focus have 100% infestation, 1% blindness, and 10% or more with ocular and skin lesions, even though fifty years have passed since the systematic denodulation campaign started. The fourth focus is situated in the rest of the infested departments, and the rates of infestation, as well as the disease manifestation, are much lower. These endemic foci are located in a zone 125 km long and 35 km wide, and the total area embraces some 4,500 km². The total number of people residing in the four endemic foci is estimated to be about 300,000, of whom 10% may be infected. Denodulization services by visiting the infested villages once every six months constituted the only control measure for the past fifty years, but there have been no signs of reduction in the infestation.

In a general examination of three districts in Guatemala in 1931, STRONG (1934) reported that about 54% of the inhabitants were found infected in Santa Emilia, about 40% in Moca, and about 58.6% in Santa Adelaida. The highest percentage, 66%, was found in the most populous portion of the district of Santa Adelaida near Santa Cristina.

STRONG (1934) also pointed out that the tumor found in Guatemala is, in the majority of the cases, situated upon the scalp, or in the region of the head; of 431 onchocerciasis cases with the tumor examined, only nine (2%) had nodules in regions other than the head. This coincides with the observation made by HOFFMANN (1930), in Mexico, who reported that the tumors were found upon the head in 92% of the cases examined, and constituted a great contrast to African onchocerciasis, in which the majority of the nodules are found on the trunk.

WOODRUFF et al. (1966) conducted a clinical and parasitological study comparing onchocerciasis in Guatemala and East Africa (Amani, Tanzania). In Guatemala, the percentage of people with microfilariae in skin snips, and the percentage with no demonstrable microfilariae in the skin snips but with a history of nodulectomy were, respectively: 67.65% and 23.53% of 102 persons examined at Moca, 86.96% and 4.35% of 46 examined at Olas de Moca, 33.33% and 38.89% of 18 at Panama, Ofelia los Andes and El Carmen Metzabal, 75.75% and 9.09% of 33 at Yepocapa, 100% and 0% of 24 at Panajabal, and 73.54% and 16.14% for the entire 223 persons examined. Some very large differences were encountered in the frequency of various clinical features of the disease in Guatemala and Tanzania. These differences included a greater frequency of iritis and keratitis, particularly severe sclerosing keratitis (but not of fundal lesions), and a lower frequency of skin lesions, especially those of the legs in Guatemala. Mal morado, erisipela de la costa, and leonine facies were encountered exclusively in Guatemala, occurring among the more heavily infected subjects. Differences were also encountered in the density and distribution of microfilariae in the bodies of Guatemalan and African subjects. Microfilarial densities in the legs were low in Guatemala, and those in the upper part of the body proportionally higher, but even the heaviest loads in Guatemala were smaller than those encountered in East Africa.

In a more recent survey of onchocerciasis in Guatemala, FIGUEROA MARROQUIN & GARCIA (1971, quoted by TADA et al., 1974) found 115 (73.2 %) microfilaria positives out of 157 inhabitants examined in Nimaya, and 122 (61.6%) positives out of 198 examined in Milan.

TADA et al. (1974) conducted epidemiological studies of onchocerciasis in Guatemala. In skin snip examinations, positive microfilaria cases were found in 58.5% of 31 persons examined in Monte de oro, 67.6% of 182 in Nimaya, and 46.1% of 245 in Milan. There was a definite difference in the microfilarial rate between males and females; the microfilarial rate of the females was lower than males in the age-group younger that 40 years. Onchocercomata were frequently found in younger persons, and half of the nodules found in Finca Nimaya were located in the iliac region. In the surveys of black fly vectors, four species were collected, i.e., *S. ochraceum*, *S. metallicum*, *S. callidum*, and *S. exiguum*, among which the first species was predominant.

Three species of black flies, *S. metallicum* (= *avidum*), *S. ochraceum*, and *S. callidum* (= *mooseri*) were incriminated as the vectors of onchocerciasis in Guatemala by STRONG (1931, 1934). DALMAT (1955) conducted an extensive study on the taxonomy, biology, and distribution of black flies in Guatemala with respect to the transmission of onchocerciasis. According to ROMEO DE LEON (1957), *S. ochraceum* is the main vector, because it is specifically anthropophilic, most numerous in the endemic areas of onchocerciasis, and tends to restrict its biting to the upper body, particularly the head. This species breeds in very small streams, and not in larger streams or rivers. *S. metallicum* is the second important vector with its bionomics similar to *S. ochraceum*; however, *S. metallicum* is less abundant in the endemic areas and more widely distributed over the country outside of the onchocerciasis areas, at altitudes ranging from just above sea level to 3,000 m. Furthermore, *S. metallicum* is less specifically anthropophilic. *S. callidum*, the third important vector, displays very little anthropophily, and is more numerous in onchocerciasis-free areas than in the endemic areas. Both *S. metallicum* and *S. callidum* breed in larger streams or rivers than *S. ochraceum*.

As of 1966, no insecticidal control of the vectors of onchocerciasis was being carried out in Guatemala (WHO Expert Committee, Second Report, 1966).

Note: As far as the published information collected by this author concerns, no human filariasis of any sort has been reported from the following Central American countries or territories:

Belize (British Honduras): Area, 23,000 km²; population, 119,645 (1970)
Honduras: Area, 112,000 km²; population, 2,582,000 (1970)
El Salvador: Area, 21,000 km²; population, 3,533,628 (1970)
Nicaragua: Area, 128,400 km²; population, 1,974,924 (1970)

6A.4 Costa Rica

A republic situated between latitudes 8°N and 11°N with an area of 50,900 km² and population of 1,710,083 (1970).

Filarial infection was investigated by BUTTS (1947), in Costa Rica, by house-to-house surveys of night blood in four sections of the Puerto Limón

area in early 1946. The microfilarial rates of the blood smears were 7.9%
of 706 persons examined at Cieneguita, 15.0% of 300 persons at Jamacia
Town, 3.0% of 100 persons at Bataan, 1.0% of 100 persons at Quepos, and
2.0% of 100 persons at Cahita. The microfilariae were nocturnally periodic, and were identified as those of *W. bancrofti*. Because of its abundance
in the areas surveyed, *C. quinquefasciatus* (= *fatigans*) was considered to
be the vector. Butts assumed that the infection was originally imported
from Jamaica and the West Indies, established in Limón, and was being
spread to other parts of Costa Rica from this focal point.

6A.5 Panama

A republic situated between latitudes 7°N and 10°N, Panama has an
area of 87,176 km² with a population of 1,425,343 (1970).

In Panama, the occurrence of endemic *M. ozzardi* was reported by Mc-
Coy (1933). The microfilariae were found in 53 (44.5%) of 119 Indians
examined in the Tuira River Basin, Darién Province. In addition to
Indians, Panamanian natives from five villages in Darién were examined,
and positive cases were found in all of five villages, though the rate was
usually low. However, in one of the villages where the natives were living
close to the Indians, 21.4% (6 of 24) were found infected, whereas the
Indians in the same area showed an incidence of 36%. A few cases of infection with *M. ozzardi* were found in the Chagres River Valley, but all of
them were recent arrivals from the Arato River Valley in Colombia. No
evidence was found that *M. ozzardi* was pathogenic to man.

6B. The West Indies

Two species of human filariae are known to be endemic in the West Indies: *W. bancrofti* and *M. ozzardi*. The latter is a parasite indigenous to
the native of these islands, and has been recorded from a few localities.
W. bancrofti, on the other hand, was probably introduced by slaves from
Africa, and later become established in the majority of the islands.

The West Indies are composed of a large number of islands lying
between the southeast coast of North America and northern coast of South
America, enclosing the Caribbean Sea. The islands are divided into three
groups, the Greater Antilles, the Bahama Islands, and the Lesser Antilles.
(See Fig. 6-2).

6B.1 Puerto Rico

Bancroftian filariasis has been known to be endemic in Puerto Rico at
medium to low grades as compared to other West Indies islands, and being

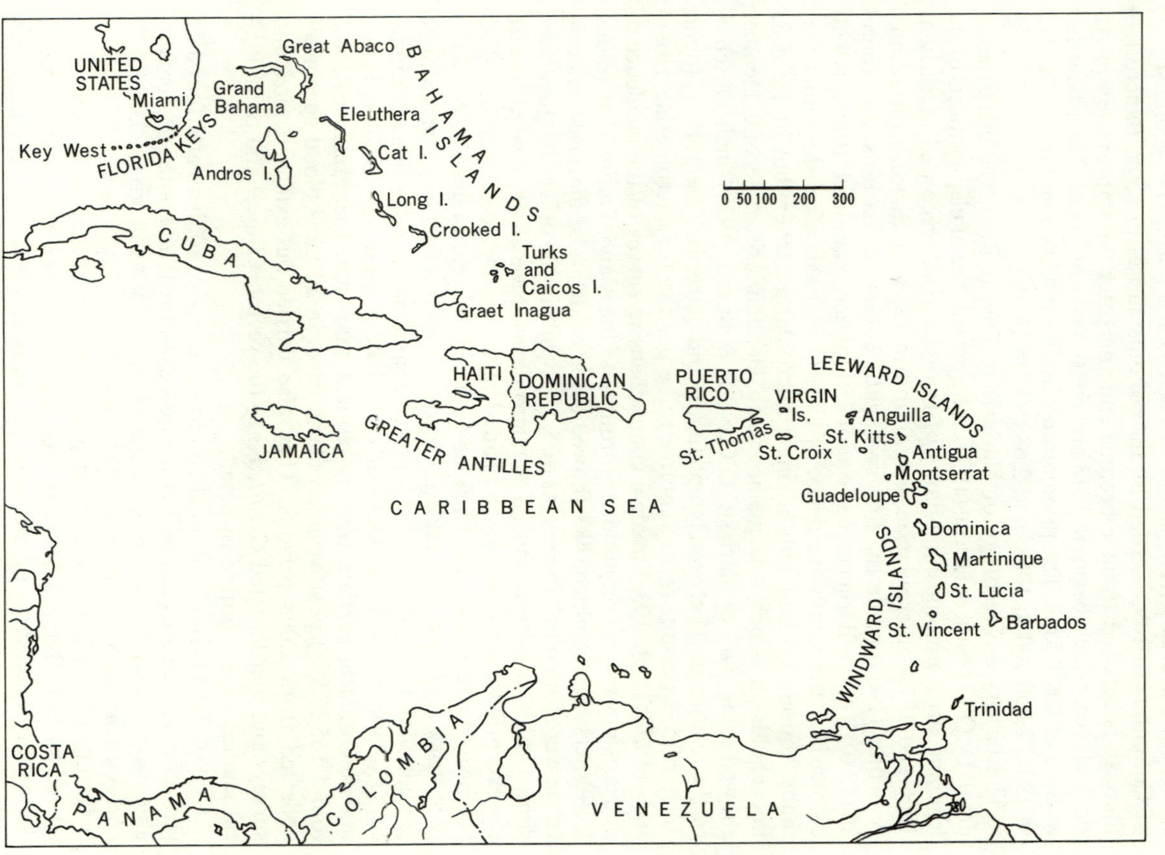

Fig. 6-2. A map of the West Indies (refer to Table 6-1).

a territory of the United States, a number of studies were made in the past by local, as well as by mainland U.S. workers, on the epidemology and control of the disease. The island was discovered during the second voyage of Colombus in 1493, settled by the conquistadores in 1505. Bancroftian filariasis is believed to have become endemic after the importation of African slaves, which began in 1513 and continued until 1820. The island has an area of 8,670 km². The population was about 45,000 in 1765, 1,543,000 in 1930, 2,350,000 in 1968, and 2,689,932 in 1970.

The history and ecology of filariasis in Puerto Rico was discussed in detail by O'CONNOR & HULSE (1935). The prevalence of elephantiasis of the legs and arms among inhabitants of the island was recorded as early as 1866 and 1875; microfilariae were found in 1893, by Spanish physicians. ASHFORD (1903) made the first systematic survey of filariasis, and found 30 (12.0%) microfilaria carriers out of 250 soldiers examined. BURKE (1928) emphasized the family incidence of clinical filariasis after she found that many households had only a single microfilaria carrier, but in 18 of 33 households in which one member had elephantiasis, a second member showed some signs of filariasis. O'CONNOR & BURKE (1928) further discussed the relationship between lymphangitis and filariasis. TAMPI (1931) found 7.7% of 518 persons from Santurce to be positive for microfilariae. HOFFMAN *et al.* (1928, 1932) made a comprehensive survey of the incidence of filariasis in various communities throughout the island, finding that among 4,590 persons examined, 483 showed some evidence of filariasis; microfilariae were found in 275 persons or 5.5%, while in the other 208 there were some clinical manifestations. The microfilariae were all *W. bancrofti*, with the exception of one person who had always lived in Vieques, an island off the eastern coast of Puerto Rico, and carried *M. ozzardi* filariae. ASHFORD & SNYDER (1933), while making a study of the treatment of filariasis with gentian violet, found 19 (3.75%) positive cases out of 480 soldiers examined. O'CONNOR & HULSE (1935) made an island-wide survey of clinical cases and microfilaria carriers (mostly clinical cases and their relatives), and found 165 (7.9%) positive microfilaria cases in 20 mm³ blood specimens collected from 2,098 persons. They also carried out extensive mosquito surveys and incriminated *C. fatigans* as the vector. Clinical and pathological studies were reported in detail.

OLIVER & OLIVER (1938) made a blood survey of soldiers and found 15 (1.9%) positive cases out of 749 persons examined; and noted the remarkable drops from the previous results obtained by ASHFORD (1903, 12.0%) and ASHFORD & SNYDER (1933, 3.75%).

Results of an island-wide blood survey of young Puerto Ricans were reported by BERCOVITZ & SCHWACHMAN (1946). The examination was made during the processing of male inductees for selective service. The inductees came from all regions of the island and represented those who were found to meet the minimum physical standards for military service. A total of 16,439 men between the ages of 18 and 38 years were examined. Examinations were conducted after 9:30 p.m. and a blood smear of approximately 20 mm³ was collected from each person. Altogether, 563 (4.42%) were found positive, and they were distributed practically all over the island. In the same year, HERNANDEZ MORALES & GONZALEZ BARIENTOS (1946) examined men in the Insular Penitentiary, and found 57 (4.5%) positive microfilaria cases out of 1,256 persons examined. The positive cases were distributed in thirty towns. A relatively high incidence of microfilaremia cases, 38 positives (7.2%) out of 529 examinees, was also observed in children in the government benefit institutions, in a survey reported by MALDONALDO et al. (1948).

HERNANDEZ MORALES & OLIVER GONZALEZ (1946) presented an interesting comment on the family incidence of filariasis, which had also been discussed by BURKE (1928). They examined clinical filariasis cases and their relatives who visited the hospital by a microfilaria concentration method from 10 ml of blood, using saponin as a hemolyser. Eight of 58 patients, as well as six (4.3%) of the relatives, were positive with this method. The authors commented that since the familial incidence of microfilariae in the blood of relatives was about the same as they encountered elsewhere in Puerto Rico, the spread of the disease due to close contact with the patients was minimal.

Observations on the effects of diethylcarbamazine (DEC) on the human microfilarial carriers, as well as on the vector mosquito infection, were carried out by MALDONALDO et al. (1950) in Puerto Rico. In a blood survey (20 mm³) of 269 boys (7 to 18 years of age) and 28 resident employees of an institution for boys, 29 boys (10.4%) and 2 employees were found to harbor microfilariae; 102 (14.7%) of 693 mosquitoes (all C. fatigans) collected at the institution were found infected with filarial larvae. DEC was administered to the positive cases in doses of 2 mg per kg, twice a day for 21 days, totaling 84 mg per kg. Blood examinations were repeated later, every month for 12 months, and most of them were found negative, though some cases occasionally showed low levels of microfilaremia. Remarkable drops in the rates of mosquito infection were also observed in monthly surveys conducted in the same institution. This study is considered to be an important contribution in the early stages of DEC use in the control of filariasis; not only did it demonstrate the long-term effects of the drug on microfilarial carriers under strict conditions, but it also showed, for the first time, the effects of DEC on the reduction in infectivity of the vector mosquitoes.

As for the clinical and pathological aspects of filariasis in Puerto Rico, LICHTERBERG & MEDINA (1957), JACHOWSKI et al. (1962), and GALINDO et al. (1962) emphasized the importance of W. bancrofti infection in the etiology of funiculoepididymitis, periorchitis, and hydrocele. Of 42 hydrocele cases histologically and serologically examined in Puerto Rico, 24 had positive or suggestive evidence of filarial origin, while filarial etiology could be eliminated in ten patients.

6B.2 Haiti

CHOISSIER (1923), in his report on the activities of the Hygienic Laboratory of the Republic of Haiti, stated, "Filariasis is quite common as evidenced by the many cases of elephantiasis seen among the native and the finding of *Microfilaria bancrofti* in the blood." This is apparently the only report on filariasis in Haiti.

6B.3 Dominican Republic

No information is available in the literature on filariasis in this country.

6B.4 Jamaica

STAFFORD *et al.* (1955) stated "Filariasis has not been reported from Jamaica and its dependencies."

6B.5 Cuba

The Republic of Cuba is situated just south of Florida and east of Mexico, with a total area of about 114,500 km², and a population of 8,523, 292 (1970). The main island lies between latitudes 20°N and 24°N.

The island was discovered by Columbus on his first voyage in 1492. After being conquered by Spain in 1519, many Negro slaves were introduced from Africa, presumably carrying with them *W. bancrofti*. The discovery of microfilariae of *W. bancrofti* was made by DEMARQUAY in 1863, in Paris, from hydrocele fluid of a patient from Cuba. GUITERAS (1886), in Key West, Florida, U.S.A., found the microfilariae of *Filaria sanguinis hominis* (= *W. bancrofti*) in the blood of four Cuban immigrants to this island, and assumed that they had contracted the parasite in their native country. Therefore, it appears highly probably that bancroftian filariasis was once endemic in Cuba. However, there have been no published report seen by the present author on filariasis in Cuba.

6B.6 The Bahama Islands

No information is yet available from the Bahama Islands, except for STAFFORD *et al.* (1955). They reported on the incidental finding of two cases of *M. ozzardi* microfilaria carriers who came from the Turks Islands and were admitted to the Hansen Home Leprosarium, in Jamaica.

6B.7 The Virgin Islands

The Virgin Islands are situated the farthest west of the Lesser Antilles, some 100 km east of Puerto Rico; they are composed of two groups: the British Virgin Islands and the United States Virgin Islands. The former has an area of 150 km² and a population of 8,650 (1967 estimate); no published report is available on filariasis. The U.S. Virgin Islands consist of St. Thomas, St. Croix, St. John, and about fifty other islands, with a total area of about 340 km², and a population of 63,200 (1970). Bancroftian filariasis has been reported to be prevalent in St. Croix but probably absent in St. Thomas.

St. Croix is an island 220 km² in area, with a population of about 12,000 (as of 1927), consisting principally of people of African blood. The two principal towns, Christiansted and Frederiksted, are situated 15 miles apart. There were some 60 plantations located in the rural areas of this island (HUGENS, 1927).

STENHOUSE (1925) reported on the prevalence of renal disease in St. Croix, and its relation to bancroftian filariasis He collected an unselected group of 100 case histories, and noted that 93 of them showed albuminuria, 30 were positive filaria blood cases with abnormal urine, and only one case was filaria positive and urine normal.

HUGHENS (1927) stated, "Upon arrival in the Virgin Islands the most impressive thing noticed in regard to the physical condition of the people is the large number having elephantiasis." He examined the records of 1,257 admissions to the Christiansted Municipal Hospital and found that 142 (110 males and 32 females) showed some clinical manifestations of filariasis; 76 males had hydrocele. In the Frederiksted Municipal Hospital, 260 males and 245 females were examined. There were 14 elephantiasis, 34 hydrocele, and 82 (31.5%) microfilaremia cases in the males; 11 elephantiasis and 79 (30.4%) microfilaremia cases in the female patients.

O'CONNOR & BEATTY (1938) made a study on the infection of mosquitoes with *W. bancrofti* larvae in St. Croix. Of 5,000 wild *C. fatigans* collected, 1,254 (25.1%) were infected and 115 (2.3%) harbored mature larvae. In 386 *Ae. aegypti* examined, 190 (49%) were found to be infected with microfilariae or young larvae, but no mature larvae were seen in this species. Likewise, no mature larvae were found in *Ae. taeniorhynchus. Anopheles albimanus* is limited in distribution in St. Croix, and mature larvae were found in one out of ten wild-caught females. *Culex habilitator* was also shown to be an excellent vector under experimental condition, but this species was never found in great numbers.

SAUNDERS (1941) reported on a comparison of the incidence of filariasis in the islands of St. Thomas and St. Croix. The disease had long been known to be prevalent in St. Croix, but there had been little reported from the neighboring island of St. Thomas. During April and May 1939, in St. Thomas, blood samples collected at random from 195 people visiting the hospital were examined by Knott's method (1 ml sample); only one individual, a 42-year-old Negro woman, who was born in St. Thomas and lived in Puerto Rico, was found to be harboring microfilariae. On the other hand, 50 of 200 persons examined at the Municipal Hospital in Christiansted, St. Croix, during the months from March to July 1939, had microfilariae in their 20 mm³ blood samples.

DONGLADE & FITZGERALD (1946) made a report about nine natives of St. Croix, serving in the U.S. Navy, who had asymptomatic microfilaremia.

A trial program for the control of filariasis in St. Croix by DDT residual house spraying was reported by KOHLER (1949) and BROWN & WILLIAMS (1949). The island had a population of 12,902 (in 1940) living in some 2,800 houses. DDT in 5% emulsion was sprayed on the walls of all houses in the amount of 200 mg of DDT per square foot; four rounds of spraying were conducted during the period from October 1946 to May 1948. Before this program was initiated, 13.3% of 1,311 children of school age had microfilariae of *W. bancrofti*, and 7.9% of 2,244 *C. fatigans* and 2.3% of 867 *Ae. aegypti* dissected were positive for filarial larvae. After the spray program had been conducted over a 21-month period, the following observations were made: the population of *C. fatigans* was reduced approximatly 50% in houses, the number of houses in which *C. fatigans* could be found was reduced by 57%, *Ae. aegypti* was completely eliminated from houses, there was a 50% reduction of *C. fatigans* containing *W. bancrofti* larvae, those containing mature larvae dropped from 0.40% to 0%, the microfilarial rate of school children dropped from 13.3% (1,311 children examined) to 10.6% (906 children examined), and the average microfilarial count in the children's 40 mm³ blood samples decreased from 74.1 to 45.8.

6B.8 Anguilla

No information is available on filariasis on this island.

6B.9 St. Kitts

LOW (1946, quoted by UTTLEY, 1959) reported *W. bancrofti* to be present in 32.8% of those examined in St. Kitts. ASHCROFT (1965) stated, "The microfilarial prevalence is also much lower than previously in St. Kitts (Lake, personal communication)."

BEYE *et al.* (1961), in a survey of helminthic infections among migratory workers from the British West Indies in the United States, found one of ten workers from St. Kitts harboring microfilariae of both *W. bancrofti* and *M. ozzardi*.

6B.10 Antigua

The prevalence of bancroftian filariasis on Antigua is probably greater than on any other island in the West Indies. O'CONNOR (1937) reviewed the literature referring to filariasis in Antigua, and also made comprehensive epidemiological studies. The first available reference to elephantiasis is by HENDY (1784). Hendy, considering the disease to be a monopoly of the Barbados, mentioned, as an exception, one case seen by him in Antigua. The disease had become a serious problem towards the end of last century, according to members of the meeting of the Leeward Islands Branch of British Medical Association in 1891 and 1892; MARSHALL, in 1915, and GRISWOLD, in 1918, referred to filariasis as one of the prevailing diseases in Antigua.

O'CONNOR (1937) made clinical and blood examinations of the general population of Antigua for evidence of bancroftian filariasis. In summary, a total of 2,526 persons (1,109 males and 1,417, females ranging from 3 to 87 years of age) were examined; microfilariae of *W. bancrofti* were found in 613 persons (24.3%), elephantiasis in 125 persons (4.9%), and hydrocele in 133 persons (12.0% of the males). The microfilaria rate was highest in the central clay area (26.3%), intermediate in the volcanic area (21.0%), and lowest in the limestone area (19.4%). *C. fatigans* was found to be a suitable vector. In this survey, two persons harboring microfilariae of *M. ozzardi* were discovered, both were born in Antigua and had never left the island.

UTTLEY (1959) reviewed the mortality and epidemiology of filariasis over the last hundred years in Antigua. The number of deaths from filariasis recorded in Antigua during the period from 1857 to 1956 was 357. The population was 36,000 a century ago and was about 55,000 in 1956. The average annual crude death rate by filariasis per 100,000 living was 24.2 from 1857 to 1866, but dropped to 0.4 in the period from 1947 to 1956. The number of deaths from filariasis during the past one hundred years was 147 males and 210 females, but the sex ratio of the population of this island was 754 males to 1,000 females at that time and thus the death rate was only slightly lower in males than in females (87.5:100). This paper also included a comprehensive review of filariasis in the West Indies.

6B.11 Montserrat

According to UTTLEY (1959), the annual reports of the Montserrat Medical Department state that filariasis is present, but there is no statement as to the species responsible.

6B.12 Guadeloupe

Both *W. bancrofti* and *M. ozzardi* are endemic in Guadeloupe, and elephantiasis, lymphangitis, chyluria, and other filarial diseases have been serious health problems. According to COURMES *et al.* (1968), some 30 reports were made on filariasis in Guadeloupe. CREVEAU, in 1870, discovered microfilariae in urine of a patient in Guadeloupe. STEVENEL (1913) found microfilariae in 4 (33.3%) of 12 night blood samples examined. LÉGER & LEGALLEN (1914) found microfilariae in 23 (15.2%) out of 150 persons examined at night. *M. ozzardi* was recorded for the first time from Guadeloupe by LE DANTEC in his textbook, *Précis de Pathologie Exotique*. Microfilariae of *M. ozzardi* were found in 6 of 210 persons examined in 1929 and 8 of 394 persons examined in 1930 by CLÉMENT. Previous surveys carried out by various workers have shown that the incidence of filariasis differs considerably by the locality; it is probably absent in Les Saintes and the French part of St. Martin, while Pointe-à-Pitre and Marie-Galante are the principal foci of *W. bancrofti*, and the population of Désirade is intensively infected by *M. ozzardi*. In Guadeloupe, indoor spraying of DDT or BHC was practiced periodically since 1950, as a measure against malaria and for *Ae. aegypti* control.

COURMES *et al.* (1968) conducted night blood examinations of 3,553 young men, conscripts from all over the islands. Microfilariae of *W. bancrofti* were found in 62 persons (1.73%) and those of *M. ozzardi* in 166 persons (5.79%); 40 persons showed a mixed infection of both species. *W. bancrofti* was found to be widespread over the archipelago of Guadeloupe, leaving free only certain tiny islands, such as Terre-de-Haut des Saintes, Désirade, St. Barthélemy, and French St. Martin. The incidence of *M. ozzardi* was higher, in general, than *W. bancrofti*, and apparently not affected by the insecticide spraying. Especially high rates were observed for Marie Galante (17.1%), Pointe-à-Pitre (13.5%), and Désirade (11.5%).

6B.13 Dominica

According to UTTLEY (1959), the annual reports from Dominica state that filariasis is present. ROBINSON (1958, personal communication) stated that the nematode has not been found, though an occasional case of elephantiasis occurs.

Low (1902) found two *M. ozzardi* carriers among 160 persons examined.

6B.14 Martinique

The occurrence of *W. bancrofti* in Martinique was recorded first by
NOC & STENEL (1913), who found its microfilariae in 4 (5.47%) out of 73
persons examined; lymphangitis and elephantiasis were also common. In
later examinations, microfilaremia was found in 2 (1.85%) of 108 persons
examined by MONTESTRUC & BERTRAND (1935), 8 (10.7%) of 70 persons
examined by FLOCH & LAJUDIE (1947), and 10 (9.52%) of 105 cases examined by MONTESTRUC (1949, quoted by MILLE *et al.*, 1961).

An extensive survey of filariasis in Martinique was conducted by MILLE
et al. (1961). In total, 243 (9.6%) out of 2,516 persons from various parts
of the island were positive for microfilariae of *W. bancrofti*. High rates were
observed in Le François (48 of 261, 18.4%) and Fort-de-France (58 of 398,
14.6%). The microfilariae were nocturnally periodic. *Culex fatigans* was
determined to be the vector.

6B.15 St. Lucia

UTTLEY (1959) reported that, "The annual reports state that filariasis is
present but do not specify the nematode."

Low (1902) found microfilariae of *M. ozzardi* in 23 (4.9%) of 472 persons examined.

6B.16 St. Vincent

UTTLEY (1959) stated, "No filaria present."

Low (1902) found microfilariae of *M. ozzardi* in 8 of 30 persons examined.

BUCKLEY (1933, 1934) conducted investigations on the transmission of
M. ozzardi in 1933, in Calliaqua, St. Vincent, and determined a biting
midge, *Culicoides furens* Poey as its vector. This was a common biting
midge in Calliaqua, where 37.7% of people were infected with *M. ozzardi*.
In his experimental infection study, of the 200 midges fed on *M. ozzardi* carriers, 27.5% were subsequently found to be infected with developing stages
of the parasite; the development to the infective stage was found to be completed in seven or eight days. Five percent of *C. furens* caught at Calliaqua
were found to be naturally infected with the developing larvae. The possibility that *Culicoides paraensis*, another species found in Calliaqua, might
act as a vector was not excluded.

6B.17 Barbados

ASHCROFT (1965) stated, "Filariasis in Barbados was once very notorious, and the term 'Barbados leg' was used as a synonym for elephantiasis. HUGHES (1750), HILLARY (1766), and HENDY (1784) all described typical cases of acute filarial fever and elephantiasis in Barbados. Elephantiasis is now rarely seen there, and in a recent survey (ADAMS & BYER, personal communication) the microfilaria rate was found to be very low."

UTTLEY (1959) stated, "BYER (1958), in a personal communication, informed the author that *W. bancrofti* is supposed to be the vector in Barbados, but that the pathologist has not been able to discover the microfilaria in the blood of any resident."

Low (1902) examined the blood of 600 persons in Barbados, but did not find microfilaria of *M. ozzardi*.

6B.18 Granada

UTTLEY (1959) stated, "No filariasis present (1930)."

6B.19 Trinidad

UTTLEY (1959) states, "Filariasis is not common as a cause of death (Annual reports)."

ASHCROFF (1965) also noted that filariasis was uncommon in Cuba or Trinidad, *M. ozzardi* was present on the north coast of Trinidad, as well as a small focus of *D. perstans* (SPENCE, personal communication).

6C. South America

Four species of human filariae are known to be endemic in South America: *W. bancrofti*, *M. ozzardi*, *D. perstans*, and *O. volvulus*, among which the first and the last species are pathogenic to man and of great public health importance in the endemic areas. Filariasis due to *W. bancrofti* is a serious health problem in the more urbanized parts of tropical South America; a number of reports have been issued from the Guianas and Brazil, but little published information is available from other countries. *M. ozzardi* is a human parasite indigenous to the Neotropical Region, and besides those cases reported from the West Indies, reports have been made about the infection among aboriginal Indians in the Guianas and

Brazil. *Dipetalomena perstans* has been found in the interior of the Guianas, on Trinidad, and in northern Argentina, again only among the aboriginal races. *Onchocera volvulus* has been noted from Colombia, Venezuela, and Brazil.

6C.1 Colombia

(1) *W. bancrofti*

MÜHLENS (1932) stated that *W. bancrofti* had been known in Colombia since 1917.

(2) *M. ozzardi*

Mansonella ozzardi was found to be endemic among the Indios in the eastern and the Amazonas regions of Colombia. According to RESTREPO *et al.* (1962), the first case was reported by OVALLE (1940); RENJIFO (1949) reported on 12 cases from eastern Colombia; BOTERO, in 1960, found 11 cases among Indios in the region of Turbo; the parasite was found also among Indios of Colombian Amazonas; and in 1961, 27 new cases were found among the Indios of Ticunas. A male patient with genital affections and showing microfilariae of *M. ozzardi* was reported by RESTREPO *et al.* (1962) from a region of Chocó. The microfilariae in the peripheral blood showed a subperiodic appearance with a peak at 8 a.m. and a minimum density at 8 p.m.

MARINKELLE & GERMAN (1970) reviewed the studies on mansonellosis in Colombia, and also the results of their epidemiological investigations carried out in Commisaria del Vaupés near the Brazilian border of Colombia. During 1967, clinical examinations and microfilarial surveys were made on 810 persons from the village of Mitú and environs. The area is surrounded by dense tropical rain forest inhabited by many dispersed Indian tribes. The authors collected 1 to 5 ml of blood from each person, and examined microfilariae by thick drop preparations, thin blood smears, and microfilaria concentration method with Knott's technique. It was demonstrated that 319 cases (200 females and 119 males) out of 332 adult Indians above the age of 12 years (208 females and 124 males) were positive for microfilariae of *M. ozzardi*, with an overall microfilaremia rate of 96.1 % (96.2 % in females and 96.0 % in males). On the other hand, only 3 out of 68 Indian children below the age of 12 years were positive. Of non-Indians in the Mitú area, 52 of 110 persons who had been in the jungle area over several months were also found infected. About 70 % of the above positive cases were diagnosed only by the Knott's concentration method, and those who showed microfilariae in 20 mm³ blood smears were only about 30 % among the total positive cases. The authors pointed out that mansonellosis would cause eosinophilia and severe articular pains, and thus the disease is one of the major public health hazards among the natives of Vaupés. No animal reservoirs of *M. ozzardi* were found among over 600 vertebrates of various species examined. Although black flies of the genus *Simulium* were abundant, none of them were found infected.

(3)   *O. volvulus*

The first confirmed case of onchocerciasis in Colombia was reported by ASSIS & LITTLE (1965). The patient was a 39-year-old Negro man from the Pacific port city of Buenaventura who had consulted an ophthalmologist at Cali because his vision was failing. Microfilariae were detected in the anterior chambers of both eyes. A skin snip was later taken from the same patient, and microfilariae of *Onchocerca* were found. The patient was admitted to the hospital for examination and treatment, and after a full course of DEC administration, the microfilariae disappeared from his eyes but not completely from his skin. The patient had lived in Buenaventura for only two years preceding the examination, having moved to that port city from a small settlement on the Rio San Juan de Micay, near the town of López, where he had been resident for first 37 years of his life.

Since it seemed likely that the patient had contracted onchocerciasis in an area near López, a team of scientists from various organizations in Cali was organized to make clinical, epidemiological, and entolological investigations of this area. The results were reported in two parts: by LITTLE & D'ALESSANDDRO (1970) on parasitological findings, and by BARRETO *et al.* (1970) on entomological findings.

López is an isolated town located in Department of Cauca, about 120 km south of Bucnaventura, on the Pacific coastal plain at the foot of the western Cordillera of the Andes (2° 56′ N, 77° 12′ W). It is about 60 km inland from the coast and has an altitude of about 50 meters above sea level. It was necessary for the research team to go first to Buenaventura, proceed by motor launch down the coast, and then up the Rio Micay (Micay River) to López.

In the Rio Micay area, each person was first examined by an ophthalmologist, and then by parasitologist who checked for skin nodules and microfilariae in skin snips. Of 292 persons (268 Negroes, 16 whites and 8 mestizos; 197 males and 125 females) examined, *Onchocerca* infections were detected in 44 (15.1 %; 43 Negroes; 22 males and 22 females). Most of the positive cases were from the settlement of San Antonio and other upstream areas, where 39 (29.5 %) of 132 persons examined were positive, while only 5 (3.1 %) out of 160 cases from López and the downstream areas were positive.

The ages of infected persons ranged from 7 to 60 years, the highest rate being in persons over 30 years of age. Microfilariae were found in the skin snips of 40 of the 44 positive cases; three cases were detected only by the discovery of nodules containing adult worms, and one was detected only by finding microfilariae in the eyes. Nodules were found on 20 cases, and it was possible to excise them from 17. Adult worms in nodules were detected from 10 of the 17 persons. The onchocercomata were located on the thorax in six cases, on the hip in three, and on the head in one. Two other locations in Columbia were examined for onchocerciasis by the team, but all of the 18 persons with ocular complaints at Puerto Melizalde and 109 persons from Caloto, a town about 60 km south of Cali, were negative.

As for the vector of onchocerciasis in this endemic focus, BARRETO *et al.* (1970) found on this expedition conducted in September that almost the only *Simulium* found biting on man was *S. exiguum*. Only small numbers of *S. mexicanum* and *S. ochraceum* also biting man or reared from pupae were collected. They concluded that *S. exiguum* appeared to be the principal vector of onchocerciasis in this region.

TRAPIDO *et al.* (1971) reviewed the historical and ecological evidence referring to the occurrence of an onchocerciasis focus at San Antonio on the Rio Micay in western Colombia. From a Spanish colonial document of the early eighteenth century, it could be established that some of the Negro slaves then working in gold mines on the Rio Micay had been brought there from West Africa. Although African Negro slaves, presumably infected with *O. volvulus*, were introduced at many places in Colombia (principally as labor in the explotiation of gold), the maintenance of *O. volvulus* transmission did not occur in most areas because of the presence of domestic livestock (equines and bocines), since *S. exiguum* and *S. metallicum* in these areas were fundamentally zoophilic. The Rio Micay focus was an exceptional situation where the absence of large numbers of such domestic animals resulted in "*Simulium*-man-*Simulium*-man" contact with a high enough frequency to maintain transmission.

GUTTMAN (1972) made studies on the biting activity of black flies in three types of habitats in western Colombia: the coffee-growing zone, the rain forest of the western coastal plain, and a focus of the 1967 episode of epizootic Venezuelan equine encephalitis (VEE), at San Antonio. Flies were collected simultaneously from horses, cows, and fly-boys exposed in these regions from 6 a.m. to 6 p.m., at bimonthly intervals in each area. About 29,500 simuliids were collected, consisting of *S. exiguum* (66%), *S. metallicum* (32%), *S. callidum* (2%), and a few specimens of *S. paynei* and *S. mexicanum*. Biting activity was greater in the VEE zone (58% of the total collection) than in the coffee-growing zone (28%) or the rain forest zone (14%). All simuliid species were highly zoophilic, although a larger proportion of *S. callidum* fed on man. Seasonal peaks of the biting activity of *S. exiguum* and *S. metallicum* usually coincided with periods of low rainfall. Diurnal fluctuations in biting activity with respect to hour, temperature, humidity, and wind velocity were recorded; it appeared that biting activity was inversely proportional to the wind velocity.

6C.2 Venezuela

(1) *W. bancrofti*

An endemic focus of bancroftian filariasis was reported by MÜHLENS (1927, quoted by MÜHLENS, 1932) from Puerto Cabello on the northwestern coast of Venezuela. The microfilariae were found in 14 (19%) of 74 laborers of the port. All the laborers were residents of the suburbs, and not of the town of Puerto Cabello. All Europeans residing in the town were negative, though some of them had stayed there for many years. MÜHLENS (1932) stated that he could not examine the night blood of the people in other areas, but it was highly possible that the disease was endemic in other coastal regions, especially in the area of Maracaibo, where many Negroes had immigrated from the West Indies.

(2) *M. ozzardi*

The occurrence of carriers of *M. ozzardi* was recorded from the high Orinoco region by BRICENO ROSI & MAYER (1949) and BAUMGARTNER (1953).

(3) *O. volvulus*

Onchocerciasis is endemic in two main areas, *i.e.*, the eastern area (east of Barcelona), and the western area (south of Valencia), and also in several localities in and near the State of Miranda (see Fig. 5-2). The infected areas are at altitudes between 200 and 1,300 meters above sea level, in a hilly region known as Cordillera de la Costa. In general, the vegetation consists of grass or sparce woodland, except for thick bush fringing the streams. The area is one of the drier parts of South America. Thus, the Venezuelan onchocerciasis area differs from other infected parts of Central America and Africa in that it is not high, and it has little or no thick forest (LEWIS & ALDECOA, 1962).

The occurrence of onchocerciasis in Venezuela has been noted by national workers since about 1950, and case reports were made by several workers in some local journals or in unpublished documents. According to ARENDS *et al.* (1954; quoted by ARENDS, 1966) two cases were found in central Venezuela; however, extensive investigations made subsequently have shown the prevalence of onchocerciasis in a wide zone surrounding the Lake Valencia (GARCIA OCAMPO *et al.*, 1957; PANALVER *et al.*, 1963; RIVAS *et al.*, 1964). Therefore, it is now considered that onchocerciasis is prevalent throughout the whole northern part of Venezuela.

LEWIS & ALDECOA (1962) also stated that the places they visited for entomological investigations into the transmission of onchocerciasis were all the known endemic areas which had been studied by various workers since 1948. These authors quoted three references: BRICENO IRAGORRY & ORTIZ (1957, *Bol. venez. Lab. clin.* 2:23), IBANEZ & CONVIT (1961, unpublished), and PENALVER (1961, unpublished).

Human onchocerciasis in Venezuela was also discussed by RIVAS *et al.* (1965).

LEWIS & ALDECOA (1962) conducted comprehensive studies on the bionomics of black flies in the onchocerciasis area in northern Venezuela. Among 12 species of *Simulium* encountered, special attention was paid to the two common, man-biting species: *S. exiguum*, which was abundant but of uncertain relation to onchocerciasis; and *S. metallicum*, which was regarded to be the main or only vector in the area studied.

According to CONVIT (1974), the studies done by the Department of Public Health Dermatology from 1958 delimited the extension of the disease to two main foci. One is in the eastern part of the country, namely, Anzoátegui, Monagas, and Sucre States, and the other in the central part including Aragua, Carabobo, Miranda, and Guárico States. Isolated cases were seen in the States of Cojedes, Falcón, and Yaracuy. The numbers and ratios of onchocerciasis patients found in these states during the period from 1959 to 1974 were as shown in Table 6-2. The numbers and ratios of

Table 6-2. Distribution of onchocerciasis in Venezuela and prevalence ratios per thousand persons examined per State (1959-June 1974); (After CONVIT, 1974).

State	Population in onchocerciasis areas	Examinations done*	Onchocerciasis patients found	Ratio $\frac{1}{1,000}$
Anzoátegui	201,336	118,410	2,748	23.20
Aragua	229,062	169,497	5,460	32.31
Carabobo	413,470	212,887	3,931	18.46
Cojedes	30,711	18,623	148	7.94
Falcón	8,732	1,885	5	2.65
Guárico	130,906	86,775	1,670	19.24
Miranda	165,777	204,028	4,450	21.81
Monagas	287,605	397,748	10,806	27.16
Sucre	301,686	340,306	10,636	31.25
Yaracuy	127,542	78,211	197	2.51
Total	1,896,827	1,628,370	40,051	24.59

*In the period covered by the investigation, several persons were examined more than once.

patients found every year from all Venezuela during the period from 1963 to 1974 were as seen in Table 6-3. The control of onchocerciasis in Venezuela consisted mainly of diagnosis by clinical signs, Mazzotti test, and skin biopsies, then treatment by administration of sodium suramin (Moranyl). Of 2,432 patients treated and observed, 21 had discrete albuminuria, and only three cases had severe complications; two had exfoliative erythrodermia lasting several months, and one had fever lasting a few weeks. A total of 33.8% of the patients treated presented some side effects (most frequently pruritus or palmoplantar edema). From 1961 to June 1974, 26,963 of 40,051 patients detected were treated with suramin. From the beginning of 1974, those who still showed microfilariae four weeks after finishing the treatment with suramin were further treated with DEC at a dose of 200 mg for three days.

Table 6-3. Onchocerciasis in Venezuela from January 1963 to June 1974; (after CONVIT, 1974).

Year	Persons examined	Cases detected	Prevalence ratios (per 1,000)
1963	113,353	3,098	27.330
1964	124,753	2,957	23.702
1965	96,920	2,442	25.196
1966	150,135	3,361	22.398
1967	223,937	5,054	22.568
1968	107,144	1,766	16.428
1969	138,612	2,683	19.356
1970	147,601	2,571	17.418
1971	124,636	1,787	14.337
1972	128,048	1,735	13.549
1973	100,272	1,615	16.606
1974	54,397	1,552	28.533

THE GUIANAS

The Guianas are situated on the northern coast of South America, north of the equator. They have been notorious for the prevalence of bancroftian filariasis, especially in the more urbanized coastal regions. This region is ecologically interesting because another two species of human filariae, *M. ozzardi* and *D. perstans*, are prevalent among the aboriginal Indians residing in the interior, where *W. bancrofti* is practically absent; furthermore, the distributions of the three species of human filariae among the races and according to the localities are quite different with respect to the breeding places of the vectors and the historical backgrounds of the individual human races.

The Guianas are divided into three regions: Guyana, or British Guiana; Surinam, or Dutch Guiana; and French Guiana. Although the ecological and epidemiological pattern of the filarial infections seems to be essentially the same throughout the Guianas, investigations of filariasis in each of the regions have been made rather independently by workers with different national backgrounds. It should be noted that certain important contributions to the knowledge of filariasis have been made from this region, and they will be discussed in the following sections.

6C.3 Guyana (British Guiana)

British Guiana, or the territory called Guyana since 1966, is located the furthest west of the Guianas, between latitudes 1° and 8° N. Guyana has an area of about 215,000 km² and a population of about 638,000 (as of 1964). The two principal towns, Georgetown and New Amsterdam, are located on the coast at the mouth of the Demerara and Berbice Rivers. It has long been recognized as a hyperendemic region of *W. bancrofti* infection. Recall that MANSON, in 1897, first described the microfilariae of *M. ozzardi* from the blood of an aboriginal Indian, collected by Ozzard in British Guiana. The adult worm of *D. perstans* was also first described by DANIELS, in 1898, from a specimen found in the mesentery of a native Indian from British Guiana.

According to GIGLIOLI & BEADNELL (1960), *W. bancrofti* infection is more prevalent in the urban and suburban population and in the larger villages, less so in smaller rural communities. It does not occur in the Indian populations of the sparcely inhabited interior, but asymptomatic infections with *D. perstans* and *M. ozzardi* are very common there.

(1)   *W. bancrofti*

Spot surveys for microfilaremia in urban areas were conducted by various workers in British Guiana. According to BEYE (1959, cited by BURTON, 1967), the following microfilaremia rates were obtained: DANIELS & CNYERS, 14.9% in 1896; WISE, 13.0%; ROSE, 20.8% in 1920; ANDERSON, 30.7% in 1921; and GRACE, 23.1% in 1927 to 1928.

Low (1908) found an incidence of 16.6% with microfilariae of *W. bancrofti* in 150 Guianese patients examined. ANDERSON (1924) and GRACE & GRACE (1931) conducted investigations of the incidence, epidemiology, and possible bacterial complications of bancroftian filariasis. GRACE *et al.* (1932) found a microfilaremia rate of 23.1% in 1,000 people. GIGLIOLI (1948) observed a 21.4% microfilaremia rate and a 5.3% elephantiasis rate near Georgetown. KENNEY & HEWITT (1949) reported that 255 of 1,241 (20.6%) people examined from Georgetown and New Amsterdam showed microfilariae in night blood.

RUMITI (1956) discussed the primary aspects of the disease syndrome of bancroftian filariasis in British Guiana, and concluded, "the conditions leading to the more commonly described states of bancroftian filariasis are: (1) the emigration of adult worms from their normal habitat, (2) death of the adult worm, (3) the blockage of the lymphatic system alone is not a sufficient cause to produce elephantiasis, and (4) bacterial complication itself is not the cause of a pathological manifestation of filariasis infection." He also made the interesting observation that microfilariae in the blood of patients disappeared or dropped significantly after removal of adult worms by operation for filarial varicolymphocele.

GIGLIOLI & BEADNELL (1960) reviewed the investigations on filariasis in British Guiana, and pointed out the very considerable reduction of the microfilaria rate in the city areas in recent years, presumably caused by installation of a modern sewer plant between 1926 and 1932. ANDERSON, in 1921, surveyed a centrally situated ward of Georgetown and obtained a general microfilaria rate of 30.5% out of 515 persons examined; the rate in children under 10 years of age was 19.5%. In 1947, 1,801 people in the same ward were examined by the same technique, and the rates were 12.1% for all people and 4.6% for children under 10 years of age. A total of 11,755 persons in various parts of British Guiana were examined in 1947; 2,005 were positive, with a microfilaremia rate of 17.1%.

In a more recent survey conducted from 1955 to 1961, 223,166 blood smears taken from people along the Guyana coastlands were examined, of which 17,698 (7.9%) were positive for *W. bancrofti* microfilariae. High rates were seen in some of the villages, for example, in Lodge Village, Georgetown, 503 out of 3,089 (16.3%) were positive in 1956; in Queenstown, 318 (20.0%) were positive out of 1,593 examined in 1957 (ADAMS, 1961, cited by BURTON, 1967).

Investigations of the mosquito vectors were conducted by GIGLIOLI (1948b) in Lodge Village. The species commonly found in houses were *C. fatigans*, *An. darlingi*, and *Ae. aegypti*. In *C. fatigans*, 37 (1.29%) of 2,852 females collected from infected households, as well as 46 (0.83%) of 5,501 collected at random were infected, and those with fully developed larvae numbered seven and three, respectively. In *An. darlingi*, 2 (2.74%) of 73 from the former group and 22 (4.27%) of 515 from the random group were infected, and 2 of the random group harbored mature larvae. None of *Aedes aegypti* was infected. It was also demonstrated that *An. darlingi* was as efficient as *C. fatigans* in the development of filaria larvae in experimental transmission studies.

The effects of DDT indoor spraying on the house-infesting mosquitoes were studied by GIGLIOLI (1948a). The insecticide used to cover the walls of houses was found to be excellent in the control of *Aedes aegypti* and *Anopheles darlingi* (the local vector of malaria), but had little effects on *C. fatigans*. The failure of DDT in the control of *C. fatigans* was also experienced by SYMES & HADAWAY (1947). CHARLES (1953) attempted control with DDT, chlordane, and BHC under various formulations, but appreciable reductions in the number of adult *C. fatigans* did not last longer than ten weeks with all the formulations tested.

BURTON (1964, 1967) made comprehensive studies on the habits and control of *C. fatigans* in Guyana. His investigations in Guyana from 1961 to 1963 under the Filariasis Research and Control Project have revealed that *W. bancrofti* is the only filarial parasite causing elephantiasis, and that *C. fatigans* is the primary vector; *M. titillans* and *An. aquasalis* are the secondary vectors. *C. fatigans* breeds primarily in pit latrines and secondarily in the clean, confined water of drums and barrels. Of 21,016 mosquitoes collected from houses, 39.9% were found on walls, 34.9% on clothing and other hanging objects, and 23.4% on or under furniture. Of 15,622 females caught, 9.6% contained *W. bancrofti* larvae and 0.5% contained its mature larvae. The flight range was found to be about 0.8 km. Control was achieved by a combination of antimosquito (spraying with gas-oil) and antiparasitic (chemotherapy with DEC) measures, which reduced the average microfilaremia rates in the Buxton control area from 17.7% to 2.2%. Over the same period, breeding in drums dropped from 14.25% to 4.7%, even though the drums were not treated or covered.

Pilot studies on the treatment of bancroftian filariasis cases with DEC

were conducted in large numbers of microfilarial carriers in British Guiana
for the first time by Kenney & Hewitt (1949) and Hewitt *et al.* (1950).
A total of 296 cases were treated with oral doses of from 0.2 to 2.0 mg
per kg, three times a day, and permanent cure of microfilaremia, as well as
acute symptoms, was observed in those treated with doses higher than
0.4 mg for 21 days or longer.

Edgehill (1961) conducted a filariasis survey and control program at
Port Mourant Sugar Estate, on the Courantyne coast of British Guiana.
The survey was begun in 1956 and continued for two and a half years. In
total, 3,539 persons were examined for microfilaremia, and of these, 2,815
were examined both parasitologically and medically. Microfilariae of *W.
bancrofti* were demonstrated in 399 persons (11.2%), and the highest rate
of 18.6% was observed among residents of Rose Hall Village. The racial
incidence was 24.4% in Negroes, 8% in East Indians, and 13.5% in other
races. Of 2,815 persons examined both parasitologically and medically,
234 (8.3%) had microfilaremia only, 80 (2.8%) had both microfilaremia
and clinical manifestations, 593 (21.0%) had only clinical signs, and 1,908
were negative for both signs. Elephantiasis was seen in 174 cases (6.5%),
48 in males and 126 in females, with 152 on the leg, 11 on the arm and one
case on the scrotum. DEC was administered in doses of 2 mg per kg, three
times a day, for ten days (180 cases) or for 21 days (312 cases); blood was
examined, in certain cases, at intervals of about one month. In average,
81.4% of those treated with the 21-day course and 67.9% of those treated
with the 10-day course were found negative at the subsequent blood examinations.

(2) *M. ozzardi* and *D. perstans*

The above two species of human filariae are known to be prevalent
among aboriginal Indians in Guyana, though both are apparently nonpathogenic. Manson (1897) described two species of microfilariae found
in blood smears collected from Indians in Guyana and sent to him by
Ozzard. One microfilaria had a blunt tail and was later determined to be
identical with *D. perstans*, already known from Africa; the other had a
sharp tail and was provisionally named *Filaria ozzardi*, but this was later
identified to be the same species as that found in the blood specimens sent
from St. Vincent and named, in the same paper, *Filaria demarquayi*.
Daniels (1897) found that the latter parasite was very common to the
Indians in the interior of Guyana. The adult worms of the blunt-tailed
microfilariae (*D. perstans*) were found by Daniels (1898), and those of the
sharp-tailed form (*M. ozzardi*) were found next year, also by Daniels
(1899), both at autopsy of Indians in Guyana.

Ozzard & Daniels (1897, cited from Low, 1902) showed that the two
species of microfilariae were found only in the people living in the interior
and not in those on the coast of the colony; moreover, as many as 58.3%
of the Indians in the interior were infected with one or the other, the blunt-
tailed form predominating over the sharp-tailed form. Low (1902) ex-

amined 163 pure-blooded Indians and found 105 (64.4%) to be infected with *D. perstans* or *M. ozzardi*; *D. perstans* alone was in 56, *M. ozzardi* alone was in 11, and 38 had double infections.

ORIHEL (1967) conducted an extensive survey of *D. perstans* and *M. ozzardi* infections among the aboriginal Indians of Guyana. A total of 9,506 persons, or approximately one-third of 30,000 Indians living in the interior were examined for evidence of filarial infection. The overall microfilaremia rate was 11.8% (1,121 positives) for both species, 10.3% (976 positives) for *D. perstans*, 0.5% (51 positives) for *M. ozzardi*, and 1.0% (94 positives) for the mixed infection. *M. ozzardi* was found to be distributed in only three of eight districts surveyed, whereas *D. perstans* infections were found in six districts. Where the two parasites were co-endemic, the mixed infection cases were found in significantly higher rates than expected from the random distribution. The results of the more recent surveys indicated that both *D. perstans* and *M. ozzardi* were not as prevalent among the Indians as reported by OZZARD (1897), DANIELS (1897, 1898), and LOW (1902), some seventy years before.

6C.4 Surinam (Dutch Guiana)

Filariasis due to *W. bancrofti* has also been noted to be prevalent in Surinam. The territory is located on the north coast of South America, between 2° and 6°N, and 54° and 58°W, covering an area of about 143,000 km². However, the inhabited area is estimated to be only 4,700 km². The total population, as of 1960, was estimated to be about 275,000, and the racial constitution of the population in the 1950 census was: black and mixed, 41%; East Indians, 35%; Indonesians, 30%; and others, 4%.

(1) *W. bancrofti*

The epidemiology of filariasis in Surinam was reviewed by BRUYNING (1961). In 1911, FLU reported on his investigations on the infection rate of different racial groups in the capital of Paramaribo. The highest rate was found in the low income class Creoles, with 50% in the males and 60% in the females. In the high income class Creoles, 23% were found infected. The rates in the other races were: 25% in Jews, 1.2% in Europeans, 6% in East Indians, and only 0.7% in Indonesians. In 1927, same author found a microfilarial rate of 25.9% in 244 persons examined.

WOLFF (1948) examined 4,851 persons of over five years of age and found that 22% harbored microfilariae. LAMPE (1950) demonstrated microfilariae in 24.8% of 1,214 individuals of the Creole group. FROS (1956) reported that 8,857 (17.4%) of 50,861 persons of all ages and races examined between 1949 and 1951 had microfilaremia, and the microfilarial rate and elephantiasis rate of the Creoles were 21.6% and 6.5%, respectively. The population of Paramaribo showed microfilaremia and/or clinical rates of as high as 24.2%. On the other hand, *W. bancrofti* was seldom encountered in rural areas with populations of East Indians, Indonesians, and Bush-negroes; in fact, in Surinam, elephantiasis is called "foto footoo" which mean "legs of the town."

According to BRUYNING (1961), *Culex pipiens fatigans* is the only vector of any importance in Surinam. *Aedes aegypti*, another common house mosquito, has never been found infected. In the northern outskirts of Paramaribo, *An. aquasalis*, *M. titillans*, and *Ae. taeniorhynchus* are acci-dental biters, but they are zoophilic in biting habits and are of no impor-tance as carriers of *W. bancrofti*. *Anopheles darlingi* is restricted in distribu-tion to the interior, and contrary to the situation in British Guiana, the species never has been of any importance as a vector of filariasis.

A detailed report on the results of a survey and control program of *W. bancrofti* infection in Surinam, which was conducted by the Division of Helminthology, Bureau of Public Health, was published by OOSTBURG (1974). From October 1969 to March 1971, a mass filaria survey covering all the districts was performed under this project, in which 120,745 persons or 31.4% of the whole Surinam population were examined.

In Paramaribo, for example, 79,613 persons, or 77.8% of the total inhabitants of the city, were examined; 1,637 (2.1%) were positive for microfilariae, 801 (1.0%) had elephantiasis, and 473 (0.6%) were found to have lymphangitis. The microfilaremia rate of 2.1% for this city was much lower than the 9.0% reported by VAN DER KUYP (1965) for the years 1959 to 1961, and 17.4% reported by FROS (1953) for the years 1949 to 1951. The elephantiasis rate of 1.0% observed in this survey was also lower than that of 1.1% found by VAN DER KUYP during 1959 to 1961 or 5.3% found by FROS during 1949 to 1951. The microfilaria rates and elephantiasis rates observed in other districts were much lower than those observed in Paramaribo.

The persons who were found to be carriers of microfilariae were request-ed to visit the filaria clinic of the Bureau of Public Health in order to receive a treatment with DEC. During 1969 to 1971 besides the people summoned for the mass blood survey, 712 patients were treated at the filaria clinic of their own will. Of these patients, 337 had elephantiasis, 101 had filaria attacks, but hydrocele was seen only in 11 and chyluria only in 3; 244 among them were positive for microfilariae, and 220 of them had no filarial symptoms.

(2) *M. ozzardi* and *D. perstans*

Filarial infections among the South American Indians residing in the rural areas of Surinam are quite different from those of Creoles and other races settled in coastal urban areas. *W. bancrofti* has been rarely found among these Indians, while the microfilariae of *M. ozzardi* and *D. perstans* are commonly found in their blood. FROS (1956) made a detailed study of filarial infection in various races of Surinam Indians. Unsheathed microfilariae (two species combined) were found in the blood of 28.7% of

881 lowland Indians and 1.9% of 208 Creoles, but *W. bancrofti* microfilariae were found in only 1 (0.48%) Indian and 5 (2.40%) Creoles. None of 200 upland Indians were positive for microfilariae. The lowland Indians living on the savanna belt were further classified into five groups, according to their residential areas, from east to west and the rate of infection of the two species were computed for each group. It was shown from these results that the incidence of *M. ozzardi* becomes higher, while that of *D. perstans* decreases, from east to west. Mixed infection of the two microfilariae were commonly encountered, especially in the western regions

6C.5 French Guiana

French Guiana is located east of Surinam and north of Brazil; it has an area of about 90,000 km² and a population of 51,000 (in 1970).

Filariasis due to *W. bancrofti* is also highly endemic in this region, and sporadic reports are available on the results of blood surveys, and on the relationship between filaria and lymphangitis or elephantiasis. For example, THÉSÉ (1916) examined 133 patients in a hospital and found 37 cases of *W. bancrofti* and 3 cases with *Filaria demarquayi* (*M. ozzardi*). BREMONT & LÉGER (1917) discovered 58 carriers of *W. bancrofti* out of 230 persons examined. LÉGER (1920) found 9 of 55 children to be positive. TISSEUIL (1936) observed microfilariae in 24% of 47 patients examined in 1934 and in 20% of 20 patients examined in 1935; furthermore, 18.6% of 241 cases examined at l'Institut d'Hygiène were positive.

FLOCH & LAJUDIE (1947) conducted parasitological and clinical surveys of people in French Guiana. Microfilariae of *W. bancrofti* were found in 59 (13.7%) of 430 Creoles, 8 (11.4%) of 70 people from Martinique, 4 (12.1%) of 33 people from Guadeloupe, 47 (14.4%) of 327 people originally from Guiana. However, since the microfilarial rates of persons with symptoms of endemic lymphangitis were practically the same as those without these symptoms, the authors could not believe that the disease was caused by *W. bancrofti*.

In a more recent review, MONTESTYUG *et al.* (1960) noted that most workers in French Guiana were more inclined to believe the streptococcal origin rather than a filarial origin for etiology of the endemic lymphangitis in this region, and apparently little effort had been made towards the control of *W. bancrofti* in French Guiana and the adjacent islands until then.

6C.6 Brazil

Brazil is a large country with an area of about 8,507,000 km² and a population of 93, 204, 379, as of 1970. The country is situated mostly in the tropical and subtropical regions, bordering on the north with the Guianas, a region known for the prevelence of *W. bancrofti*. Brazil is divided into 20 states, six territories, and a Federal District. The occurrence of filariasis (including imported cases) was reported from 16 of these areas, as shown in Table 6-5.

Besides *O. volvulus*, which was recently discoverd from near the Venezuelan border, two species of human filariae are known to be endemic in Brazil, i.e. *W. bancrofti* and *M. ozzardi*. The former is widely distributed in the more urbanized areas along the coast, and is an important public health problem, especially in the States of Para, Pernambuco, and Bahia. It has also been found sporadically in the inland of Amazonas, and along the southern coast, south to the States of Santa Catarina and Rio Grande de Sul. The actual number of persons infected or suffering from filariasis in Brazil is difficult to estimate, but RACHOU & FERREIRA (1958) considered that at least in the cities of Recife (population 750,000) and Belem (population 300,000) eighty thousand and forty thousand people, respectively, were affected with filariasis.

M. ozzardi in Brazil has been found exclusively among the people living in the rural, inland regions of Amazonas. The parasite is widely distributed among the aboriginal races, and its microfilariae are often found in high densities in the blood of people in the endemic areas. However, as elsewhere in the Neotropics, the parasite is apparently non-pathogenic to man.

Some important contributions were made in Brazil in the early history of filariasis research. While the etiologies of elephantiasis and chyluria were still unknown, the microfilariae were discovered for the first time in urine of patients suffering from hematochyluria, in August 1868 in Bahia, Brazil, by Wucherer. This was three years after Demarquay, in Paris, described the presence of the numerous tiny embryos in hydrocele fluid. Additional findings of microfilariae in thc urine of patients were reported in 1868 by DA SILVA LIMA in Brazil. He confirmed the presence of microfilariae in the peripheral blood of patients soon after it was reported by LEWIS, in 1872, in India. Contributions to the knowledge of bancroftian filariasis were also made in Brazil by SILVA ARAUJO (1820), PATTERSON (1878), MAGALHAES (1928), and others.

Since the national filariasis control program was established in Brazil in 1951, extensive surveys of filariasis and its vectors have been carried out throughout the country, and a tremendous number of reports have been made on its epidemiology and control. Some early contributions were made in Brazil on the use of diethylcarbamazine (DEC) in the treatment and prophylaxis of filariasis. In general, incidence of filariasis in Brazil was reported to be reduced considerably by the extensive blood surveys and intensive drug treatments of the carriers in most of the important endemic foci. However, being a large country in which the disease is widely distributed, filariasis still constitutes a serious public health problem in Brazil.

(1) *Wuchereria bancrofti*

So far as is known, *W. bancrofti* in Brazil is represented solely by the nocturnally periodic form, and is a type transmitted primarily by the domestic mosquito, *Culex pipiens fatigans*.

(1.1) The microfilarial periodicity

Observations on the periodicity of microfilariae were made by CAUSEY *et al.* (1945) in Belém. RACHOU *et al.* (1945b) and RACHOU (1954) compared the microfilarial periodicity in carriers residing in Belém (northern Brazil) and those in Florianópolis (southern Brazil) and its relation to the house-infesting activity of *C. fatigans*. Blood samples were collected once every hour during a 24-hour period in both cities. The distribution pattern of microfilarial density was essentially the same, although the variation in the times of sunset and sunrise by the season of year was remarkably different between the two localities, one situated in the tropics and another far south in the Temperate Zone. As for the relation of the microfilarial periodicity with the activity of the vectors, the authors took the numbers of *C. fatigans* found in houses as the indices of the activity, in place of the actual biting behavior of the mosquitoes, and thus only slight correlation could be demonstrated.

(1.2) Taxonomy of the parasite

There have been interesting reports made on the taxonomy of *W. bancrofti* based on purely morphological grounds. CARVALHO (1955) described three morphological variants for the microfilariae of *W. bancrofti* found in blood films collected from people in Recife, i.e., "typica,", "y," and "z." SCHACHER & GEDDAWI (1969) made detailed statistical analyses of the morphological structures of microfilariae collected from various localities in the world, and differentiated two groups from Brazil; one group had the same form as found elsewhere in the world, the other, corresponding to Carvalho's type "y," was significantly different. The 'latter was erected as a new species, *Wuchereria lewisi*, by SCHACHER (1969), with Recife (Pernambuco) as the type locality. No information is available on the differences in biological characters between the two groups (see Section 2B.4.2).

(1.3) Geographic distribution and incidence

Before the national filariasis control program in Brazil was initiated, several reports were made on the incidence of microfilaremia from various localities (see Table 6-4). In addition, a number of observations were made by various workers on the occurrence of clinical cases. These were reviewed by RACHOU & DEANE (1954).

The national filariasis control program was organized in 1951, as a project of "Departamento Nacional de Endemias Rurais" of the Brazilian Ministry of Education and Health. It was aimed at determining the endemic areas of filariasis in Brazil by a survey of microfilaremia and clinical cases, determining local vectors, controlling parasite carriers and vectors, and conducting the basic research necessary for epidemiological survey and control. By the blood surveys carried out from 1951 to 1953, microfilaria carriers were found in 16 of 58 localities surveyed. Until May 1953, carriers

Table 6-4. Microfilaremia rate of *W. bancrofti* reported from Brazil before 1950 (after RACHOU & DEANE, 1954).

States	Locality	Microfilaremia rate(%)	Author (year)
Amazonas	Manaus	2.0	Deane (1949)
Pará	Belém	10.8	Causey *et al.* (1945)
Bahia	Salvador	8.4	Patterson (1878)
Bahia	Salvador	9.5	Oliveira (1908)
Bahia	Salvador	12.0	Magalhaes (1928)
Bahia	Salvador	4.6	Pessoa & Andrade (1950)
Alagoas	Maceio	46.5	Coqueiro (1922)
Pernambuco	Recife	9.7	Azevedo & Dobbin (1952)
São Paulo	Caraguatatuba	0	Unti *et al.* (1953)

of microfilariae of *W*. bancrofti were found from four of five localities surveyed in Amapá, one of one in Guaporé, four of five in Pará, one of one in Alagoas, and 6 of 29 localities in Santa Catarina, but none from the States of Acre, Amazonas, Sergipe, and Paraná. Especially high rates were observed in Ponta Grossa (13.9%) of Santa Catarina, and Belém (9.8%), Vigia (5.2%), and Cameta (4.5%) of Pará. In all of the seven localities surveyed in Amazonas, high rates of infection of *M. ozzardi* were recorded.

A comprehensive report on the activity of the national filariasis control program was compiled later by RACHOU (1957a, b, 1960), and maps of the distribution of *W. bancrofti* and *M. ozzardi,* as well as detailed results of blood and entomological surveys conducted until then, were illustrated. From 1951 to 1958, 551 blood surveys were carried out in 21 states or territories, and a total of 477, 565 persons were examined. Microfilaria carriers were found in 89 of 538 localities surveyed (see Fig. 6-3). The endemic foci of *W. bancrofti* were mainly in urban or semiurban areas along the coast, but some inland towns in the States of Amazonas, Pará, and Bahia were also found to be infested.

A more recent report on the progress of the national filariasis control program in Brazil was made by FRANCO & DA SILVA LIMA (1967). Table 6-5 shows blood examinations conducted on 811, 361 persons in 852 localities in 24 states or territories; 4,310 persons were positive for microfilariae of *W. bancrofti* and 1,931 persons for those of *M. ozzardi*. Carriers of *W. bancrofti* were found in 16 states and territories, while those of *M. ozzardi* were almost exclusively found in Amazonas.

As for the epidemiology of filariasis in Brazil, the following reports are available for the respective states or territories:

General accounts: RACHOU & DEANE (1954), AZEVEDO (1955), RACHOU (1956), RACHOU (1957a, b), RACHOU (1960), FRANCO & DA SILVA LIMA (1967)

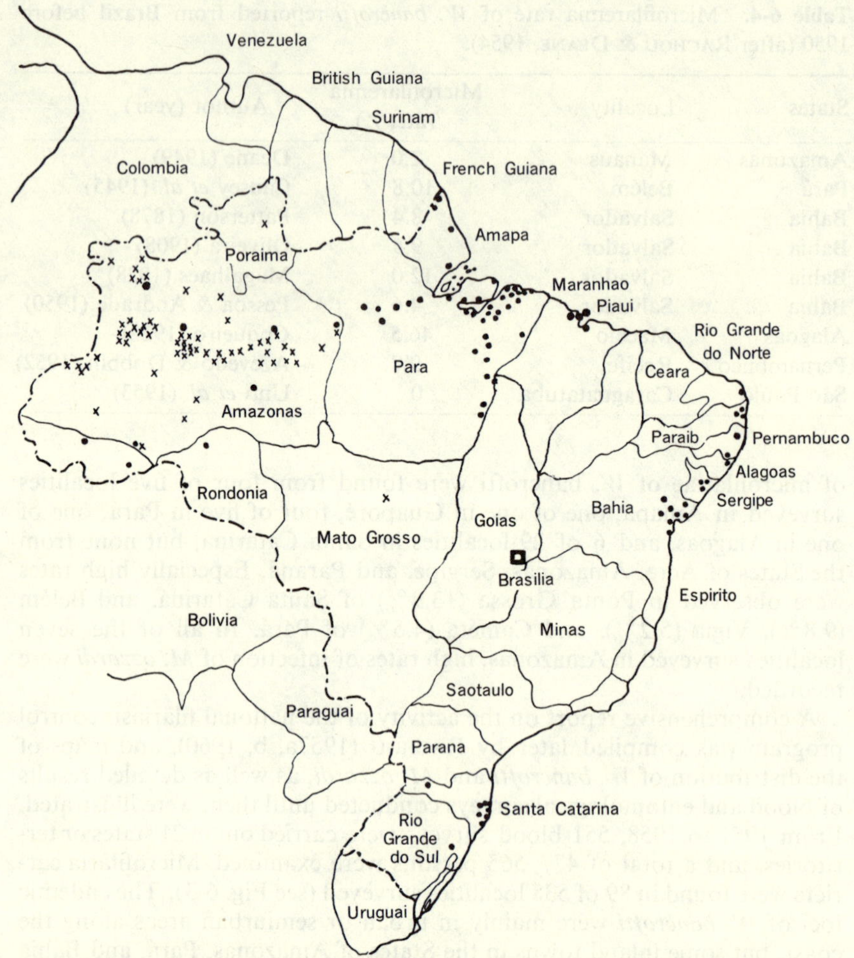

Fig. 6-3. Localities where microfilaria carriers of *Wuchereria bancrofti* (•) or *Mansonella ozzardi* (×) were discovered during the survey 1951–1958 (after Rachou, 1960; rearranged by the author).

Amazonas: Deane (1949), Rachou *et al.* (1955a), Rachou & Lacerda (1956a), Lacerda & Rachou (1956)

Amapa: Neves & Damasceno (1954)

Acre: Rachou *et al.* (1954d), Lacerda & Rachou (1956)

Rio Branco: Rachou *et al.* (1954d), Lacerda & Rachou (1956)

Guaporé: Lacerda & Rachou (1956)

Pará: Causey *et al.* (1945), Deane & Damasceno (1952), Athias & Gueiros (1963), Scaff & Gueiros (1967)

Maranhão: Rachou *et al.* (1958a)

Table 6-5. Results of microfilaria surveys carried out in Brazil under the national filariasis control program from 1951 to 1965 (after FRANCO & DA SILVA LIMA, 1967).

States or territories	No. of locali- ties	No. of persons examined	No. & % of persons with microfilaria			
			W. bancrofti		*M. ozzardi*	
Rondônia	13	6,833	8	0.11	0	0
Acre	15	6,438	2	0.03	0	0
Amazonas	104	43,583	40	0.09	1,921	4.41
Roraima	5	1,534	0	0	7	0.46
Pará	96	98,955	1,600	1.62	0	0
Amapá	24	44,686	190	0.43	0	0
Maranhão	25	22,910	55	0.24	0	0
Piaui	14	9,805	0	0	0	0
Ceará	2	16,504	0	0	0	0
Rio Grande do Norte	10	14,455	1	0.006	0	0
Paraiba	16	32,326	6	0.019	0	0
Pernambuco	36	66,280	1,763	2.06	0	0
Alagoas	10	15,809	19	0.12	0	0
Fernando de Noronha	1	809	0	0	0	0
Sergipe	35	26,003	3	0.012	1	0.004
Bahia	56	66,258	200	0.30	0	0
Espirito Santo	42	31,114	0	0	0	0
Guanabara	1	3	0	0	0	0
Paraná	28	13,289	0	0	0	0
Santa Catarina	178	167,310	391	0.23	0	0
Rio Grande do Sul	60	102,950	29	0.028	0	0
Mato Grosso	45	6,568	1	0.015	2	0.030
Goiás	35	15,662	0	0	0	0
Federal District	1	1,274	2	0.16	0	0
TOTAL	852	811,361	4,310	0.53	1,931	0.238

Pernambuco: RACHOU *et al.* (1956b), DOBBIN & CRUZ (1967, 1968)
Alagoas: DEANE *et al.* (1953)
Bahia: OLIVIERA (1908), MAGALHAES (1932), PESSOA & ANDRADE (1950), AGUIRRE *et al.* (1956), SHERLOCK & SERAFIN (1967)
Santa Catarina: FERREIRA & FERRAZ (1952a), RACHOU *et al.* (1954c), RACHOU *et al.* (1955b), FERREIRA *et al.* (1955)
Rio Grande do Sul: RACHOU *et al.* (1958b), FERRAZ *et al.* (1958)

(1.4) The parasite control

The national filariasis control program in Brazil has concentrated its efforts to only the control of *W. bancrofti* and not of *M. ozzardi*, since the latter is considered to be nonpathogenic to man (FRANCO & DA SILVA LIMA,

1967). After experiments and field experiences, it was judged that vector control was difficult and expensive, in view of the abundance of breeding places and development of insecticide resistance in *C. fatigans,* and that administration of DEC to microfilaria carriers was effective, and probably could achieve effective control of the disease by this method alone (RACHOU, 1957b).

In Ponta Grossa (Santa Catarina), where a high incidence of microfilaremia (14.5%) was observed in 1953 by RACHOU *et al.* (1955b), DEC treatment of the microfilarial carriers was begun in December 1953, at daily doses of 6 mg per kg for seven days. Repeated blood surveys were conducted thereafter from 1954 until 1957. In 1956, only 3 out of 118 persons examined had microfilariae. The authors considered that bancroftian filariasis could be controlled exclusively with the drug when it was given repeatedly to the microfilarial carriers. However, they also suggest that such a method, consisting of blood collection at night from everybody, and long-term treatment with the drug, cannot be practiced in big endemic centers such as Recife and Belém, where the total populations are 750 thousand and 300 thousand, respectively, and 80 thousand (Recife) and 40 thousand (Belém) filariasis cases exist (RACHOU & FERREIRA, 1958).

Various treatment schedules with DEC were tested on microfilaria carriers in the initial stages of the control program. RACHOU *et al.* (1955c) administered the drug at daily doses of 6 mg per kg for seven days to 43 carriers of *W. bancrofti* in Belém; by daily examination of the blood, they found out that a reduction of 82.8% in the number of microfilariae occurred after the first day of the treatment, and microfilariae disappeared from 46.6% of the treated cases. After the third day of treatment, these percentages increased to 93.1 and 63.1, respectively. Based on these results, the authors began to test a three-day schedule using the same daily doses, and a one-day schedule with a single dose of 10 or 12 mg per kg. On the other hand, NEVES & DAMASCENO (1954), in Belém, divided microfilaria carriers into four groups and compared the effects of daily administrations of 6 mg per kg over 7, 10, 15, and 21 days. The groups consisted of 183, 186, 158, and 171 persons, respectively, and blood examination were made before the treatment, after completion of the treatment, and thereafter, at monthly intervals for 12 to 18 months. When the blood examination was conducted 12 months after the treatment, for example, the microfilarial rates of the previously positive cases were 26.8% in the seven-day treatment group, 23.1% in the ten-day treatment group, 17.2% in the 15-day treatment group, and 9.8% in the 21-day treatment group. The average microfilarial count per person was reduced to 3.8% of the original level in the first group, 2.2% in the second group, 1.9% in the third group, and 0.3% in the fourth group.

RACHOU & SCAFF (1958) and RACHOU (1960) reported on the comparative efficacy of DEC administered at various total doses, i.e., 12 mg per kg given by single dose, or 6 mg per kg given daily for 3, 7, 10, 15, and 21 days; the microfilaremia rates and the relative densities of microfilariae per 20 mm^3 blood samples examined 12 months after completion of the treatment were highly correlated with the total dose administered to the microfilaria carriers.

Based on these experiments, the routine treatment of microfilaria carriers has been conducted as a rule, by the administration of 6 mg per kg of DEC for seven days. RACHOU (1960) reported that as of June 1959, in four major endemic areas of bancroftian filariasis in Brazil, i.e., Belém (Pará), Florianópolis (Santa Catarina), Castro Aves (Bahia), and Recife (Pernambuco), 902,532 persons, in total, were examined; of these, 63,423 persons were microfilariae positive, and 48,572 persons were treated with DEC. In Bara, Laguna Municipality of Santa Catarina, DEC was administered to the whole population of 12,000 in July 1957, and the microfilarial rate dropped from 9.4% in 1954 to 2.0% in 1958 and 0.8% in 1959; the average density of microfilariae per person also decreased from 0.9 to 0.1 and 0.03, respectively.

FRANCO & DA SILVA LIMA (1967) summarized the effects of the filariasis control activities since it began. Table 6-6 shows the considerable reductions in the microfilarial rates that were achieved in nine of the principal endemic areas.

Table 6-6. Comparison of microfilarial rates in nine endemic areas of bancroftian filariasis in Brazil before and after application of the control program (after FRANCO & DA SILVA LIMA, 1970).

Locality (State)	Year Started	Microfilarial rate Before Control	After Control
Belém (Pará)	1952	9.8	2.0
Cametá (Pará)	1952	4.5	0.4
Vigia (Pará)	1953	5.2	2.1
Soure (Pará)	1954	6.2	1.3
Recife (Pernambuco)	1954	6.2	1.8
Castro Alves (Bahia)	1957	5.9	1.0
Florianópolis (S. Catarina)	1967	1.4	0
Ponta Grossa (S. Catarina)	1953	13.9	0.5
Barra da Lague (S. Catarina)	1957	9.4	0

(1.5) The vector and its control

Wuchereria bancrofti in Brazil is endemic principally in urban or semi-urban areas and has been shown to be transmitted mainly by *C. p. fatigans*, although mosquitoes of the genera *Aedes* and *Anophleles* may occasionally act as secondary vectors in some rural areas. So far, *C. pipiens fatigans*, *Ae. scapularis*, *An. (N.) darlingi*, *An. (N.) tarsimaculatus* (= *aquasalis*), and *An. (K.) bellator* have been known to be naturally infected.

DAVIS (1935) conducted experimental infections of mosquitoes with *W.*

bancrofti in Belém and observed that development in the proboscis infection of mature larvae was obtained in *C. fatigans* Wiedeman, *M. (Rhynchotaenia) justamansonia* (Chagas), and *An. (Nyssorhynchus) tarsimaculatus* Goeldi. Advanced development of larvae occasionally took place in *An. (N.) bachmanni* Petrochi and *C. nigripalpus* Theobald, and retarded development was noted in one specimen of *An. (N.) tarsimaculatus* Goeldi. A slight degree of development, followed by degeneration, occurred in *Ae. aegypti* (Linnaeus) and in *Ae. fluviatilis* (Lutz). No metamorphosis was noted in *Ae. taeniorhynchus* (Wiedemann) or in *Ae. scapularis* (Rondani); and invasion of the thorax occurred only once in the former but never in the latter. For these and other epidemiological reasons, Davis considered that the chief vector in Bahia was, without doubt, *C. fatigans*.

CAUSEY *et al.* (1945) conducted parasitological and entomological surveys on the incidence and transmission of *W. bancrofti* in Belém. The examination of thick blood films from 5,000 persons from various sections of the city of Belém revealed that 541 (10.8%) of them harbored microfilariae of *W. bancrofti*. Elephantiasis was observed in 1.3% of the people examined. The youngest individual with microfilaremia was a 2-year-old boy, and the youngest person with elephantiasis was an 11-year-old boy. The principal vector was found to be *C. fatigans*. Among 1,014 *C. fatigans* dissected, 118 (11.6%) were positive for filaria larvae, and 8 (0.8%) of them harbored mature larvae. While making routine dissections for malaria infection in Belém, filaria larvae were found in three *An. darlingi* of 563 examined (one had mature larvae) and in two *An. aquasalis* of 332 examined (one also had mature larvae). Although the two anopheline species were shown to transmit filariae, these species were much fewer in numbers than *C. fatigans*. *Culex fatigans* were extremely abundant in the city of Belém. An average of 585 and 509 mosquitoes were collected per house during April and May, respectively, and 99% of them were *C. fatigans*. The microfilariae in the peripheral blood showed remarkable nocturnal periodicity.

In Belém, VIANA MARTINS, in 1944, also examined 81 specimens of *C. fatigans* caught in the Military Hospital and found 19 (23.5%) of them infected. PESSOA & ANDRADE, in 1950, observed an infection rate of 12.5% and an infective rate of 3.6% in 56 *C. fatigans* examined in a ward of Salvador, Bahia (cited from RACHOU, 1956).

After the national filariasis control program was organized in 1951, a country-wide survey of the vectors was begun in some 30 stations. RACHOU *et al.* (1955b), for example, observed in Ponta Grossa, a small village in the State of Santa Catarina, that out of 145 inhabitants examined (90.3% of the population), 14.5% had microfilaremia and 7.6% had elephantiasis; *C. fatigans* were collected in 77.8% of houses inspected with an average number of 4.7 per house, and out of 279 specimens dissected, 10.8% were infected with larvae of *W. bancrofti* and 0.7% had mature larvae. Among the mosquitoes caught outdoors with human bait, 3 of 39 *Aedes scapularis* were infected with larvae of *W. bancrofti*, and one of them had mature larvae.

In Manaus, the capital of the State of Amazonas, RACHOU & LACERDA (1956) made examinations of mosquitoes collected in houses, but none of 3,815 females of *C. fatigans* were infected. The microfilarial rate in this city was reported to be 2.0% for *W. bancrofti* and 0.6% for *M. ozzardi* by DEANE (1949), and 2.0% for the former and 0.4% for the latter by RACHOU *et al.* (1955a). However, in the district of the town São Raimundo, where most of the autochtonous carriers of *W. bancrofti* lived, 134 (1.37%) of 9,755 *C. fatigans* were infected, and 4 (0.04%) had infective larvae.

Detailed results of entomological surveys conducted by the members of the national filariasis control program were described for the years 1951 to 1955 by RACHOU (1956), for 1951 to 1958 by RACHOU (1960), and for 1951 to 1965 by FRANCO & DA SILVA LIMA (1967). From 1951 until 1955, 169,934 (99.6%) of the total of 170,691 mosquitoes examined were *C. fatigans*; these were collected in houses in 30 endemic areas of *W. bancrofti* distributed all over the country. Of a total of 90,171 *C. fatigans* dissected, 2,621 (2.91%) were infected and 241 (0.27%) had mature larvae. High infection rates were seen in Ponta Grossa (10.8%), Recife (7.3%), and Belém (6.5%). The correlation between the microfilarial rates of human populations and the infection or infective rates of the mosquito populations were shown by RACHOU (1960) for 11 localities surveyed from 1951 until 58.

In a more recent report by FRANCO & DA SILVA LIMA (1967), referring to the activities from 1951 to 1965, a total of 120,399 specimens of *C. fatigans*, collected in 12 states and territories, were examined; 2,720 (2.26%) were infected and 258 (0.21%) had mature larvae. High infection rates were again demonstrated in Pernambuco (7.32%) and Pará (4.02%).

As for the possibility of transmission of *W. bancrofti* by mosquito species other than *C. fatigans*, all previous workers in Brazil have agreed in that it is usually of minor significance. As stated previously, *Ae. scapularis* was once shown to be infected and harboring mature larvae by RACHOU *et al.* (1955b) in Santa Catarina. *Anopheles* (*N.*) *darlingi*, which was shown to be an important vector of *W. bancrofti* in British Guiana by GIGLIOLI (1948), was examined by DAVIS (1931) in Belém. He reported that 7.0% of 200 specimens examined were infected with filaria larvae. As stated previously, CAUSEY *et al.* (1945), in Belém, also found that 3 of 583 specimens dissected were infected and one of them had mature larvae. *Anopheles* (*N.*) *tarsimaculatus* (= *aquasalis*) was reported by the same authors in the same locality to be naturally infected, at rates of 0.60% (2 of 332) for all larvae and 0.30% (1 of 332) for mature larvae. As for *An.* (*Kerteszia*) *bellator*, RACHOU *et al.* (1955b) found that one of three specimens dissected in Ponta Grossa was infected with first stage larvae.

SHERLOCK & GUITTON (1967) made examination of *Culicoides paraensis* in Salvador (Bahia). This species of human-bloodsuckers was found to be quite abundant in this area. However, none of 1,019 specimens dissected were infected with larvae of *W. bancrofti*, while 34 of 1,112 specimens of

C. fatigans collected in the same area were found naturally infected.

Applications of DDT (2 g per m²) in houses as a measure of malaria control was reported by RACHOU *et al.* (1955b) to be an inefficient method to control *C. fatigans* in Ponta Grossa. Furthermore, possible manifestations of behavioral resistance in *C. fatigans* to dieldrin and in *An.* (*K.*) *cruzi cruzi* and *An.* (*N.*) *darlingi* to DDT was observed by RACHOU (1958). Development of insecticide resistance in *C. fatigans* in Belém was reported by MOURA LIMA & RACHOU (1959), who observed that only 2% mortality after exposure to 4% DDT and 3.3% mortality after exposure to 1.6% dieldrin was obtained after two hours with the WHO standard test kit.

In Belém, DDT house spraying had been conducted since 1946 for the purpose of malaria control. However, because of the development of resistance in *C. fatigans*, DDT was replaced with BHC in 1952, and was sprayed in houses at a rate of 300 mg of gamma isomer per m². Again, due to the development of resistance to this insecticide, dieldrin was used in 1955. This also became ineffective against *C. fatigans*, and contrary to what was expected, caused an increase in the density of the mosquitoes after its spraying (RACHOU, 1960).

The geographic distribution of mosquitoes in Brazil was reviewed by MATTOS & XAVIER (1965).

(2)   *Mansonella ozzardi*

The occurrence of *M. ozzardi* infection in Brazil was recorded first by DEANE (1949), who found its microfilariae in 12 out of 2,054 persons examined in Manaus, Amazonas. Later, country-wide blood surveys were carried out under the national filariasis control program, and RACHOU & DEANE (1954) reported that the carriers of *M. ozzardi* microfilariae were discovered from 1951 to 1953 in all of seven localities surveyed in the State of Amazonas, at rates varying from 4.6% to 28.6%. In a more recent review of the activities of the program published by FRANCO & DA SILVA LIMA (1967), a total of 1,921 positive cases (4.41%) were found among 43,583 persons examined at 104 localities in Amazonas (Table 6-5). According to RACHOU (1960), carriers of *M. ozzardi* were discovered in 66 of 538 localities in Brazil surveyed from 1951 to 1958. The localities where *M. ozzardi* carriers were recorded were all in the State of Amazonas, with the exception of two areas, one each in the States of Roraima and Mato Grosso. In Amazonas, the carriers were found in 64 out of 74 localities surveyed, and almost all the carriers were Indios. In this sense, the geographic and racial distribution of *M. ozzardi* is quite different from that of *W. bancrofti*, which occurs mainly in the coastal, more-or-less urbanized areas.

The microfilarial periodicity of *M. ozzardi* was observed by RACHOU & LACERDA (1954). They collected blood samples (20 mm²) every hour from 47 carriers and compared the percentages of positive persons for a 24-hour period. There was no periodicity recognized by this method. (Unfortunately, they did not show the microfilarial counts for each hour.)

The difference in the length of microfilariae of *M. ozzardi* and *W. bancro-*

fti was demonstrated clearly by RACHOU *et al.* (1954a). They measured 200 microfilariae each of *M. ozzardi, W. bancrofti* in a northern locality (Belém), and *W. bancrofti* in a southern locality (Florianópolis), in thick blood smears. The average, minimum, and maximum lengths observed were 191, 150, and 244 μ, respectively, in *M. ozzardi*, while those of *W. bancrofti* (excluding the sheath) were 292, 224, and 408 μ, respectively. There were no significant differences between the microfilariae of *W. bancrofti* from the north and south.

As for the vector of *M. ozzardi*, it was reported by BUCKLEY (1934) that a biting midge, *Culicoides furens*, on St. Vincent Island (West Indies) was naturally infected with the filarial larvae and that complete larval development took place in the fly in an experimental infection study (see Section 6B.3.10). In Brazil, however, CERQUEIRA (1959) made extensive studies on the transmission of *M. ozzardi* in the village of Codajás on the Amazon River, and incriminated the black fly, *S. amazonicum* Goeldi, 1905, as the vector. No onchocerciasis was found among the people he examined and although 70% of wild mammals and 17% of wild birds out of a total of 116 animals examined were found to harbor microfilariae, none of them were the *M. ozzardi* type. GARNHAM & WALLIKER (1965) made a survey of filariasis in the same village and found 9 of 57 people to be harboring the microfilariae of *M. ozzardi*, but none were infected with *O. volvulus*. They also found many of the wild mammals to be infected with various forms of microfilariae, but none of them were those of *M. ozzardi*.

(3)   *Onchocerca volvulus*

A focus of onchocerciasis was discovered recently in northern Brazil near the Venezuelan border. The first indigenous case was reported by BEARZOTI *et al.* (1967, quoted by MORAES *et al.*, 1973) from the far north Federal Territory of Roraima, but no further investigation has been made referring to this case. MORASES & DIAS (1972) reported finding two other cases in American women missionaries living on the Toototobi River, in the State of Amazonas, among Indians of the Waika Tribe. Both women had nodules in the sacral region that were several years old. Some months later, a third case was discovered by MORAES & CHAVES (quoted by MORAES *et al.*, 1973), also an American woman missionary living among the Waikas in the Surucucus Mountains of Roraima Territory, near the Venezuelan border.

MORAES *et al.* (1973) conducted an epidemiological survey of three Indian villages on the Toototobi River near where the missionaries established their post. The altitude of this area was about 180 m above sea level. A total of 91 Indians (49 men and 42 women among a total population of about 150) were examined. Biopsy of skin samples showed that 57 (30 men and 27 women) contained microfilariae of *O. volvulus*, with a rate of 62.6% (61.2% in men and 64.3% in women). Two of them were blind in one eye, and another complained of severe photophobia. Cutaneous manifestations were observed in a number of cases. The authors considered that the focus might be quite extensive covering both the territories of Brazil and Venezuela corresponding to the distribution of Yanomama Indian group to which the Waika tribe belongs.

Further studies on onchocerciasis in this region of Brazil were reported by RASSI (1974; quoted by MORAES, 1974), MORAES & CHAVES (1974), and MORAES (1974). In the Surucucus Mountains, a total of 57 Yanomama Indians were examined, and 47.3% among them were found infected. All the indians over 40 years of age were positive. In the Auaris River area, where the altitude is 670 m above sea level, a total of 102 indians were examined, and 25 (24.5%) had microfilariae in the skin. In these areas, nodules were found mostly on the scalp. Two indian men in the Surucucus Mountain region had unilateral blindness. Cutaneous manifestations were seen in all of the areas surveyed; the most frequent forms were slightly erythematous and highly pruritic papules on the buttocks and shoulder blades, and dry, shiny, and wrinkled patches of skin in the same regions. No elephantiasis or hanging groin case was seen in these areas.

According to RASSI (1974, quoted by MORAES, 1974), the predominant black fly species was *S. pintoi* (D'Andretta et D'Andretta, 1946) in the Auaris River area, *S. incrustatum* (Lutz, 1910) in the Surucucus Mountains, and *S. amazonicum* (Goeldi, 1905) (sensu lato) in the Toototobi River area. Only *S. amazonicum* in the Toototobi area was found naturally infected, with a rate of 0.72% (7 positives out of 972 specimens dissected). As stated previously, this was the species incriminated by CERQUEIRA (1959) as the vector of *M. ozzardi* in the Côdajas area of the State of Amazonas.

6C.7 Argentina

In northern Argentina, BIGLIERI & ARAOZ (1914, 1915)* discovered microfilaria in the blood of natives of Tucumán Province and named it *Microfilaria tucumana*. According to BIGLIERI (1923), this microfilaria has a sheath which is striated all along, like the body of a nematode. Its width measured by the Looss method is from 3.30 to 2.70 μ (mean 3 μ), and thus smaller than other known microfilariae. The microfilariae showed no periodicity, and apparently did not produce any trouble. In 1916, 150 cases were confirmed. Of 200 persons examined at this time, the microfilariae were found in 43 cases, and two of them were three years old.

MÜHLENS *et al.* (1925, quoted by FÜLLEBORN, 1929) and MÜHLENS (1926) made extensive blood surveys of this region, and found that the microfilariae were sheathless and of the type of *Microfilaria demarquayi*; they were found at high percentages among forest people, not only Tucumán Province, but also the Provinces of Salta and Jujuy in northern Argentina to the region around Yacuiba in Bolivia. VOGEL (1927, quoted by FÜLLE-

* *Prensa medica argentina*, 1914; *Anales dep. highiene*, August 1915; (quoted by BI-GLIERI, 1922)

BORN, 1929) studied these materials and confirmed that the microfilariae were identical with those of *M. ozzardi*. MÜHLENS (1932), in a review on filariasis in the Americas, stated that no microfilariae were found in other provinces (Chaco and Formosa) of Argentina or in Paraguay (Atyrá area), and also that, according to VINCENT & LOW, and BIGLIERI (1923), *Microfilaria tucumana* developed in *Stegomyia fasciata* (= *Aedes aegypti*) to the sausage stage.

DAVIS (1928) made a study on the experimental transmission of *M. ozzardi* (*Filaria tucumana*) in northern Argentina. Of 117 mosquitoes fed on a microfilaria carrier, two *An. tarsimaculatus*, one *An. albitarsis*, and one *Ae. aegypti* were found to be infected in the thoracic muscles, but the head and proboscis were not found invaded. In bedbugs (*Cimex lectularius*) and triatomas (*Triatoma infestans*) no larval development took place, but some of the microfilariae were found to remain alive in the gut contents for as long as two weeks.

7 | Filariasis in the African region

The epidemiology of human filariasis in Africa is more complicated than in any other region of the world because as many as five species of filariae are involved as causative agents, namely, *Wuchereria bancrofti*, *Loa loa*, *Dipetalonema perstans*, *Dipetalonema streptocerca*, and *Onchocerca volvulus*. The geographic distribution of each of these filariae is different, they take different blood sucking insects as intermediate hosts, and the features of the microfilariae are characteristic to each of the species. The microfilariae of the last two species are found in the skin and only rarely in the blood, while those of the first three species appear in the circulating blood. The periodicity is nocturnal in *W. bancrofti*, diurnal in *L. loa*, and nearly nonperiodic in *D. perstans*. The drug called diethylcarbamazine (DEC) has been proved to be more or less effective in the treatment of infections from all of these filariae, but the development of severe and often dangerous side reactions has been noted, especially in loiasis and onchocerciasis. To date, a large number of reports have been made on the epidemiology of filariasis in Africa, but there still exist large areas to be surveyed and treated by filariasis control programs.

Wuchereria bancrofti infection is widespread in Africa, and certainly constitutes a serious health hazard to people in the endemic areas, causing elephantiasis, hydrocele, lymphadenitis, and other clinical affections. Its distribution in Africa is rather patchy, and there exist large numbers of endemic foci isolated from each other by apparently *bancrofti*-free zones. The principal endemic foci are spread along the Indian Ocean coast, in some inland regions in eastern Africa, on Madagascar and some other Indian Ocean Islands, and along the southern coast of western Africa from Senegal to the western coast of central Africa. It is also endemic in certain inland regions of equatorial Africa, and in the Nile Delta. To date, the microfilariae are all known to be nocturnally periodic. The parasite indigenous to western and central Africa is a type more adapted for developing in anopheline vectors but less so in *Culex pipiens* s.l., while the parasite distributed in the Nile Delta, East African coast, and some Indian Ocean islands has been shown to be partly or fully adapted to development in *C. pipiens* s.l. STOLL (1747) estimated some 22 million people in Africa to be infected with *W. bancrofti*.

Loa loa is a human parasite indigenous to the tropical rain forest zones of western and central Africa, and so far as is known, the endemic area does not extend west of the Dahomey Gap nor east of the Congo River Basin and southern Sudan. Its microfilariae are diurnally periodic. The vectors are horse fly species of the genus *Chrysops*. The parasite causes various clinical symptoms, such as "Calabar swelling" of the skin, conjunctivitis due to migration of the adult worm, and various allergic reactions associated with high eosinophilia. The syndrome of meningoencephalitis and other severe reactions has been noted recently after administration of diethylcarbamazine (DEC) to loiasis cases harboring high levels of microfilariae.

Dipetalonema perstans is a parasite found in Africa and South America (the Guianas). In Africa, it is widespread and common over large areas of the tropical zone, covering western, central, and eastern Africa. In many endemic areas, the microfilarial rates approach almost 100% of the human adult population. The microfilariae are unsheathed and appear in the peripheral blood with almost no periodicity. The parasite has usually been regarded as nonpathogenic, but there have been recent reports, especially from eastern Africa, on its association with various allergic symptoms, such as transient swellings, joint pain, and pruritus associated with eosinophilia. Moreover, reports were made recently on cases in which the parasite apparently invaded the central nervous system causing symptoms of severe meningitis. In western Africa, *Culicoides austeni*, a night-biting midge, was incriminated as the vector.

D. streptocerca is a parasite also indigenous to tropical Africa. Its detailed geographic distribution is not yet well known, but it is apparently confined to the rain forest regions of western and central Africa. The parasite was first recorded in Ghana, and has been found to be very common in certain forest regions of Cameroon and Zaire. The microfilariae are sheathless, and found in the skin of infected people. Mixed infections of *D. streptocerca* and *O. volvulus* in the skin of people in the above regions are not uncommon, but they can be readily distinguished by that the tail part of *D. perstans* microfilariae is strongly bent like a fishing hook. Previous studies have shown that a day-biting midge, *Culicoides grahami*, is the principal vector.

O. volvulus is widely distributed in tropical Africa, especially in the hilly, mountainous regions. It has been reported to be endemic in most of the countries in western, central, and eastern Africa, south of the Sahara, including Senegal, Sierra Leone, Liberia, Ghana, Dahomey, Upper Volta, Chad, Central African Republic, Nigeria, Cameroon, Zaire, Angola, Malawi, Tanzania, Kenya, Ethiopia, and Sudan. Onchocerciasis is of great public health importance in these countries because the parasite causes serious skin lesions, and ocular complications which frequently lead to blindness. The microfilariae are sheathless; they are found in the skin but rarely in the circulating blood. Black flies, especially *Simulium damnosum* and *Simulium neavei*, are the vectors of *O. volvulus* in Africa.

In conducting epidemiological surveys of human filariasis in Africa, it is necessary to make examinations of microfilariae with at least three different methods in order to detect possible infections with the above five species, i.e., examinations of night blood for *W. bancrofti*, day blood for *L. loa*, and skin snips for *D. streptocerca* and *O. volvulus*.

As a matter of convenience, Africa is divided into five regions in this text, namely, (A) North, (B) West, (C) Central, (D) South and East Africa, and (E) Madagascar and other Indian Ocean Islands. The distribution of the five species of human filariae by the regions and the countries as recorded in medical literature is shown in Table 7-1 and Fig 7-1.

Table 7-1. Distribution of human filariae in Africa by the countries or territories.
W: *Wuchereria bancrofti*; L: *Loa loa*; P: *Dipetalonema perstans*; S: *Dipetalonema streptocerca*; V: *Onchocerca volvulus*

Country or Territory	Area (km^2)	Population (1970 est.)	Filarial Species Recorded
A. North Africa			
1 Egypt	1,001,684	33,239,000	W
2 Libya	1,758,857	2,010,000	
3 Tunisia	164,086	5,238,000	W P
4 Algeria	2,321,266	1,106,990	W P
5 Morocco	446,377	15,530,000	
6 Spanish Sahara	265,898	76,425	
7 Mauritania	1,030,305	1,160,000	
B. West Africa			
1 Senegal	197,083	3,930,000	W L P V
2 Gambia	11,133	374,770	W P
3 Guinea Bissau	36,111	530,000	W
4 Cape Verde Island	4,031	246,000	W
5 Guinea	245,761	3,920,000	W L P
6 Mali	1,239,230	5,031,500	W L P
7 Sierra Leone	71,713	2,627,000	W P V
8 Liberia	111,327	1,200,000	W P V
9 Ivory Coast	322,338	4,310,000	W P S V
10 Upper Volta	274,094	5,485,981	W P S V
11 Ghana	238,447	8,545,561	W S V
12 Togo	56,557	1,955,916	W V
13 Dahomey	112,577	2,718,000	W L P V

Country or Territory	Area (km²)	Population (1970 est.)	Filarial Species Recorded				
C. Central Africa							
1 Niger	1,188,540	4,020,000	W	L	P		
2 Chad	1,283,502	3,634,000	W	L	P		V
3 Nigeria	923,416	67,828,000	W	L	P		V
4 Cameroon	475,317	5,840,000	W	L	P	S	V
5 Ubangui-Shari	620,333	1,520,000		L	P		V
6 Equatorial Guinea	28,026	290,000					
7 São Tomé & Principe	963	61,000	W		P		
8 Gabon	264,900	500,000		L	P		
9 People's Republic of the Congo	341,870	1,089,300					
10 Zaire	2,343,208	16,585,944	W	L	P	S	V
11 Rwanda	26,338	3,736,000	W		P		V
12 Burundi	27,866	3,600,000	W		P		V
13 Angola	1,246,218	5,466,600	?	L	P		V
D. East Africa							
1 Mozambique	771,170	8,233,034	W				
2 Rhodesia	390,473	5,400,000	W		P		
3 Zambia	752,325	4,396,000	W	L	P		
4 Malawi	117,000	4,552,000	W				
5 Tanzania	944,837	13,273,000	W		P		V
6 Kenya	582,421	11,694,000	W		P		V
7 Uganda	235,946	10,461,500	W		P		
8 Somalia	637,538	3,000,000					
9 Ethiopia	1,221,374	24,315,000	W				V
10 Sudan	2,642,000	15,675,000	W	L	P		V
E. Indian Ocean Is.							
1 Madagascar	586,815	7,423,864	W				
2 Comoro Islands	2,234	267,000	W				
3 Mauritius	1,864	830,700	W				
4 Réunion	2,509	455,200	W				
5 Seychelle Islands	277	54,000	W				
6 Chagos Archipelago	197		W				

Note: The above figures are cited from "Webster's New Geographical Dictionary" 1972, G. & C. Merriam Co., Springfield, Mass. The areas given originally in square miles were converted to square km.

Reviews on the distribution and epidemiology of filariasis in Africa were made by HAWKING (1940a, for East Africa), HAWKING (1957), JORDAN (1960), HAMON *et al.* (1967), and HAWKING (1973).

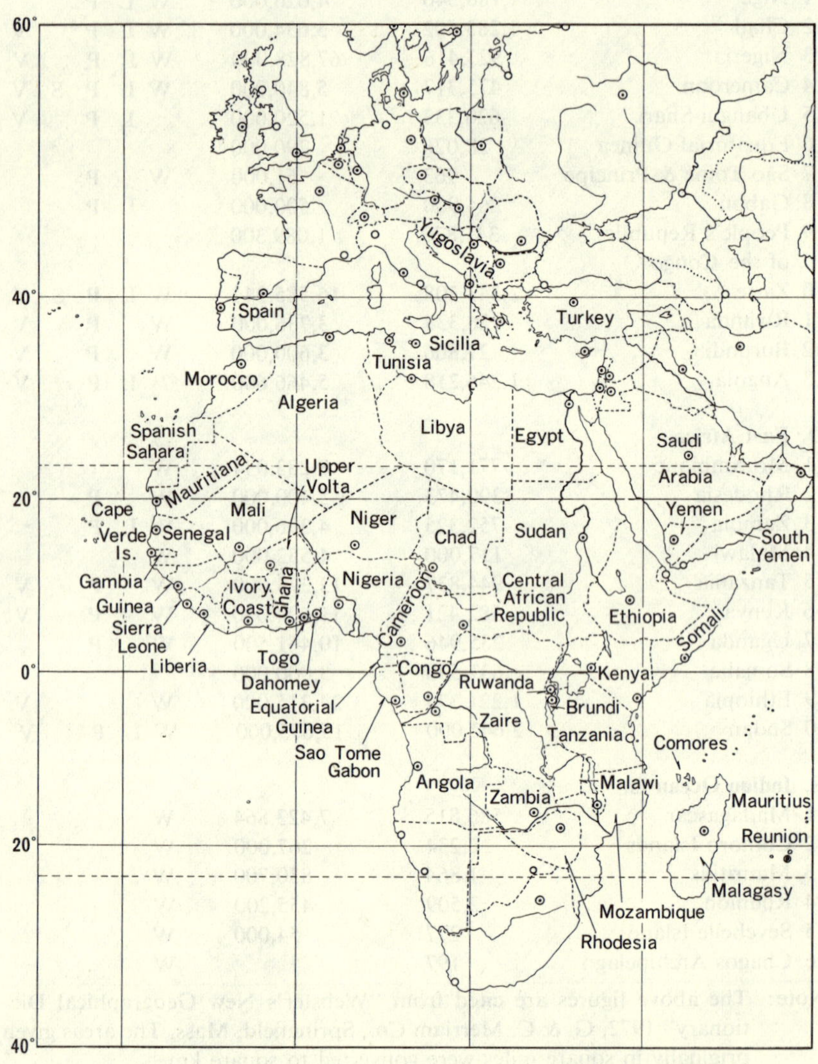

Fig. 7-1. Countries or districts of the African and European regions which involve endemic areas of filariasis.

7A. Northern Africa

The transmission of filariasis apparently does not occur in the vast desert region of the Sahara because of the scarcity of breeding places for the vectors and due to the dry climate. The sporadic occurrence of *W. bancrofti* infection has been noted on the Mediterranean coast, and especially on the Nile Delta. Case reports of *D. perstans* infection were made from Algeria and Tunisia.

BLATIN & JOYEUX (1908) reviewed the information on the distribution of *bancrofti*, *loa*, and *perstans* in Africa, and stated, "*Filaria bancrofti* is the only species that is endemic outside of the tropical zone, to the north in Egypt and probably in Algeria and Tunisia, and to the south in Natal and Transvaal." HAWKING (1973) stated, "Libya, Tunisia, Algeria, Spanish Sahara, and Mauritiana appear to be free from all kinds of filariasis. In Morocco and Tangier, bancroftian cases are said to have occurred but these seem to be rarities. The Canary Islands and Madeira appear to be free."

7A.1 Egypt

Egypt, or the territory of the Arab Republic of Egypt (formerly the United Arab Republic), is situated between 22° N and 32° N, and has an area of 1,002,000 km² and a population of 33,327,000 (1970 estimate). A large part of the land is desert, but areas along Nile River are well irrigated.

Filariasis due to *W. bancrofti* has been known to be endemic in certain areas in Egypt since ancient times, especially in the eastern part of the Nile Delta. MAHDI *et al.* (1963) state, "*Filariasis bancrofti* stands third in the list of endemic diseases in the U.A.R., the first is schistosomiasis and the second malaria. A spot survey among a population of about four million showed that the number of positives was estimated to be about a quarter of a million." The chief vector is said to be *C. pipiens*. A pilot control program was reported to have been launched in some limited endemic foci. The incidence in most endemic areas is considered to have decreased over the past 30 years, because of improvements in sanitary conditions.

In 1910, TODD & WHITE (quoted by BAZ, 1946) made a blood survey of several districts in Egypt, and obtained high percentages of infection (see Table 7-2). It was noted by BAZ (1946) that all of these villages had wells in the village and on the outskirts.

KHALIL (1935) made a survey of Kafr Ghatati Village, situated 14 km to the west of Cairo on the edge of the desert. Of the total number of inhabitants (1,038,985) examined at night, 26.5% were found to harbor microfilariae of *W. bancrofti*. The incidence was 28.6% among males and

Table 7-2. Distribution of filariasis in Egypt according to TODD & WHITE (1910, cited by BAZ, 1946).

District	No. of persons examined	No. of positive persons	Percent positive
Kafr El Ghataty	91	37	40.0
Abu Rowash	61	29	47.5
Bani Magdool	76	19	25.0
Kerdasah	79	23	28.0
Kafr Nassar	74	12	16.0
Nazlet El Simman	52	5	9.0

24.4% among females. The incidence of hydrocele was very striking, and out of 475 males examined, 122 (25.7%) had single or double hydrocele; 29 of 120 hydrocele cases had microfilariae in the blood, and this rate of 24.2% was slightly lower than the rate in the rest of the population (30.3%.)

KHALIL (1936) further reported on the results of a survey of Rosetta, an old port with a population of about 25,000 (in 1930) and famous as the location of the "Rosetta Stone." He stated, "Rosetta has been known for a very long time to be an endemic center of infection with filariasis and many cases of elephantiasis exist there. So much so that one of the vernacular names for elephantiasis of the leg in Arabic is 'Rosetta Leg'." Microfilariae of *W. bancrofti* were found in 12% of 250 persons in the center of the town, 10% of 150 persons in the south of the town, 8.8% of 250 persons in the south of the town, 6.2% of 250 persons in the west of the town, and 19% of 100 in a neighboring village, with an overall positive rate of 10.2% for this area. Among 1,000 persons examined, 18 (1.8%) had elephantiasis of one or both legs; of 107 males examined, 19 (17.8%) had hydrocele. Large numbers of *C. pipiens* larvae were found to be breeding in wells, and the incidence of filariasis was highly correlated with the number of wells in the areas.

As for the vector of bancroftian filariasis in Egypt, LOOSS (1914) stated that *C. fatigans* was the intermediate host; he described the metamorphosis of the larvae to the sausage-shaped stage and later to the fully formed, mature larvae.

KHALIL *et al.* (1932) conducted experimental infections of *C. pipiens* collected from a village near Cairo, and observed that the mosquito was a most efficient intermediate host of *W. bancrofti*; the females of *C. pipiens* fed on microfilaria carriers showed 100% infection of larval filariae, and the larvae of *W. bancrofti* completed their development in about 14 days at a temperature of 29° to 30°C, 15 days at 26°C, and 20 days at 23° to 24°C.

A general survey of filariasis in Egypt was reported by BAZ (1946). During the first six months of the year, officers working in antimalaria units were instructed to collect blood smears at night from people in their districts. As a result, a total of 9,115 persons in 25 districts of nine provinces were examined, and 121 cases (1.33%) in 13 districts were found to be harboring microfilariae of *W. bancrofti*. High incidences of microfilaria carriers were found mostly in districts where the people were still using wells. He also compared the microfilarial rates obtained by previous authors in Kafr El Ghataty (a small village near the Giza Pyramids) with those observed in 1954 and 1955; Baz attributed the reduction of filariasis to the filling up of the wells after the introduction of a perennial irrigation system in that district (Table 7-3). In this paper, the author stated that he found two races of *C. pipiens* in this country: one which breeds in wells and is anthropophilic and stenogamous, and another which has a wide range of breeding places and is zoophilic (see Section 2E.3).

Table 7-3. Incidence of filariasis in Kafr El Ghataty (after BAZ, 1946).

Year	Cases examined	positive Cases	Percentage positive	Author
1910	91	37	40.7	Todd & White
1934	1,100	291	26.5	Khalil Bey
1945	200	22	11.0	Baz
1946	200	10	5.0	Baz

Trial treatments of ambulant cases of bancroftian filariasis with DEC were reported by HALAWANI *et al.* (1949). The drug was administered three times a day, at doses varying from 0.9 to 2 mg per kg, for periods from 10 to 23 days, to 17 microfilaria carriers in Rosetta; microfilariae in three 20 mm^3 blood smears were counted before starting treatment and at varying intervals after treatment. Remarkable reductions in microfilaria density were observed in all cases, and cure from the attack of filarial fever was also noted.

SHAWABY *et al.* (1965) reported on the results of a country-wide blood survey, carried out by the Ministry of Public Health, to delimit the extent of the distribution of filariasis in Egypt. Blood samples were collected at night by house-to-house visits in 1,227 localities in 20 governorates, and a total of 504,276 blood films were examined. The incidence in 96 urban localities was about 0.3% out of 69,584 blood films. Filariasis appeared to be almost limited to the eastern part of the Nile Delta, and the infection there was widely spread. The microfilarial rate was 7.2% in Qalyubîya Governorate, 60.4% in Sharqîya, and 0.9% in Damietta. In the Canal Zone, the prevalence was only 0.1%, and the few cases detected were probably imported. Towards the west, the infection diminished, and in the center of the Delta, the incidence of positive films ranged from 0.005 to 0.08%. In the western part of the Delta, the rate was 0.1%, apart from Rosetta, where it was 1.2%. In urban Cairo, the rates ranged from 0.03% to 0.8%. In the Giza Governorate, the rate was 1.2%, and in two districts in Asyut the rates were 4.08% and 0.9%. Clinical filariasis cases were rare at the time of the survey and it seems probable that this change might have been due to the great reduction in the number of wells and other breeding places of *C. pipiens*.

A pilot program for the control of filariasis in Egypt was reported by MAHDI *et al.* (1963); the village of Marsafa, with a population of about 7,000, situated in the eastern part of the Delta, in Qalyubîya Governorate was selected as the program site. The preliminary phase extended throughout 1956, consisting of entomological, clinical, and parasitological surveys. In the preliminary blood survey, it was intended to cover the whole population, while during the rest of the year monthly collection of blood smears was restricted to a sample of 10% (about 700) of the population. In the control phase, which extended throughout 1957 and 1958, the following operations were conducted: a) destruction of mosquito larvae by weekly application of 0.5 to 1.0% lindane, and by elimination of artificial breeding places; b) destruction of mosquito adults by residual spraying of houses with 50% BHC water dispersible powder at a rate of 200 mg of gamma isomer per m², one cycle a year during March or April; c) treatment of microfilaria carriers and clinical cases with DEC.

Blood surveys of almost all the inhabitants were carried out four times during 1957 and three times during 1958. All positive cases detected in the surveys received DEC treatment at a dose of 6 mg per kg of body weight, administered as a single dose for ten successive days, totaling 60 mg per kg. The tablets were swallowed at nighttime in front of the field inspector. Moreover, patients showing any sign of filariasis were given the drug regardless of the results of their blood examination.

The phase of observation and maintenance extended throughout the years 1959 to 1962. In the 1956 survey of *C. pipiens*, adults were found to be present in premises all the year round, with an average of 5.1 per room; the density was highest in October and November, with an average of 11.7 and 9.7 per room, respectively. In 1957 and 1958, the same picture could be seen, but the density dropped remarkably, and the average number per room became 2.3 in October 1957 and 1.0 in October 1958. Remarkable reduction was seen also in the larval density in breeding places. The percentages of mosquitoes with all stages of filaria larvae and with mature larvae were 3.5% and 0.18% respectively, among 2,040 dissected in 1956; however, these percentages dropped to 0.95% and 0.7% among 733 dissected in 1957, and to 1.4% and 0.2% among 427 dissected in 1958. The microfilaria rate of the human population was 16.8% (1,085 positives of 6,457 examined), with an average microfilarial count per 20 mm³ blood smear per positive case of 9.5; this gradually dropped to 1.2% (81 positives of 6,636) and 1.0 per 20 mm³ blood smear in the third general blood survey in 1958. In the last four years (1959 to 1962), although the larviciding and residual spraying were stopped, the incidence of filariasis in Marsafa remained almost at the same level (1.2% to 0.8%).

ATA (1967) reported on the evaluation of the intradermal test in the diagnosis of bancroftian filariasis in Egypt. The antigen used was that prepared by Sawada and Takei from adult worms of *Dirofilaria immitis*. The ratio of the reaction wheal area to the control wheal area was suggested for evaluating the skin test, and a ratio of 1.25 was taken as a minimum for a positive diagnosis. The skin test could not differentiate between proven clinico-parasitological filarial patients and other inhabitants in an endemic area, but was negative in normal controls and in persons harboring intestinal nematodes in nonendemic areas. The positivity was independent of the presence of microfilariae in the blood of filarial cases. The frequency of positive reactions increased with the age.

7A.2 Algeria and Tunisia

SERGENT & FOLEY (1908) reported on the discovery of microfilariae of *Filaria perstans* in the blood of a 30-year-old man, who was born in Chellala (Hauts-Plateau oranais), Algeria, and who had never left the country.

The case of a *D. perstans* carrier was also reported from Tunisia by CONOR (1911). The patient had always resided in the Oasis of Gafsa, and was treated by 606 because of bilharziasis. Numerous microfilariae of *F. perstans* were demonstrated in urine on one occasion. Blood examinations were conducted a number of times, both day and night, but they were all negative.

7B. Western Africa

The belt of land in western Africa extending from Senegal to Nigeria, bordered by the Sahara Desert on the north and by the Atlantic coast on the south, is covered mostly by tropical rain forests and savanna. The region is highly populated. The amount of precipitation in this region is closely correlated with the latitude, i.e., smallest in the northern desert zone, increasing towards the south, and usually highest along the coastal belt. The vegetation, as well as the associated fauna, differs greatly with respect to the latitude and the rainfall.

Filariasis due to *W. bancrofti* and *D. perstans* is prevalent in many areas of this region. *Loa loa* infection has been noted, especially from the western part of this region; *O. volvulus* occurs in many areas along the rivers, and *D. streptocerca* has been found to be endemic in the forest areas of Ghana, Upper Volta, and Ivory Coast.

There have been two reports made on the results of general blood and skin surveys of people in the former French territories in West Africa. THIROUX (1912) conducted blood examinations of over 1,700 soldiers who came from various regions of French West Africa, and obtained the microfilarial rates of 29.0% for *D. perstans*, 23.8% for *W. bancrofti*, and 0.3% for *L. loa*, (Table 7-4). Both *D. perstans* and *W. bancrofti* were found to be widely distributed in these territories, with the exception of Mauritania. However, the distribution and incidence of the two parasites were rather independent, and an apparently negative correlation was seen between the two microfilarial rates.

Table 7-4. Microfilaria rates of soldiers of French West Africa by the regions (summarized from a report by THIROUX, 1912).

Region	No. examined	With *perstans*		With *bancrofti*		With *loa*	
		No.	%	No.	%	No.	%
Mauritania	7	0	0.	0	0.	0	0.
Senegal	287	22	7.7	135	47.0	2	0.7
Ivory Coast	114	60	52.6	9	7.9	0	0.
Dahomey	144	49	34.0	19	13.2	1	0.7
Haut-Senegal & Niger	718	203	28.3	163	22.7	2	0.3
French Guinea	498	180	36.1	94	18.9	1	0.2
Sierra Leone	9	1	11.1	3	33.3	0	0.
Total	1,777	515	29.0	423	23.8	6	0.3

PFISTER (1954) reported on the blood (daytime) and skin examinations of 10,169 adult Africans in various parts of French West Africa. In overall figures, 3,123 (30.7%) were positive for microfilariae of *D. perstans*, 388 (3.8%) for *W. bancrofti*, 581 (5.7%) for *O. volvulus*, and 10 (0.1%) for *D. streptocerca*. No carriers of *L. loa* were discovered. In the northern desert zone, only *W. bancrofti* was found. *D. perstans* was more prevalent in the savanna and wooded savanna (savane boisée) zones than in the desert or forest zones. *O. volvulus* was also widely distributed, but particularly prevalent along streams. The people in the forest had the lowest incidence of filarial infections. People in the savanna frequently harbored one or more filariae, but were generally healthy in appearance.

BRENGUES (1973) classified the land of western Africa into seven zones according to climatic features, and discussed their relationship to the epidemiology of bancroftian filariasis (Fig. 7-2).

Zone A is situated north of the region where *An. gambiae* and *An. funestus* coexist, and only *An. gambiae* (probably species B, according to Coz, 1973) is present. This species is quite localized and very rare because the annual rainfall is less than 300 mm. The daily temperature exceeds 30°C, which is over the range of normal development of filarial larvae in the vectors. In this region, bancroftian filariasis is practically absent.

Zone B is within the northern border of the region where *An. gambiae* s.l. and *An. funestus* coexist, but the annual precipitation is less than 500 mm and is restricted to the months of July, August, and September. The

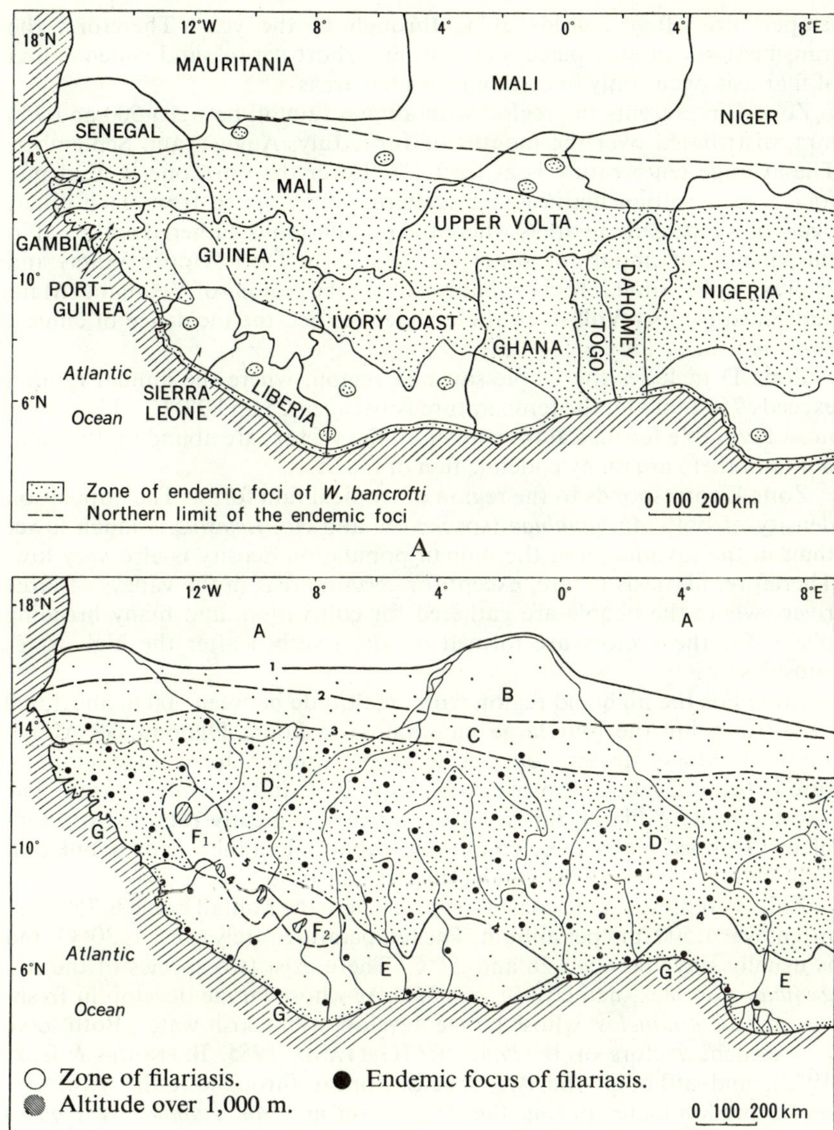

Fig 7-2.   Distribution of bancroftian filariasis in West Africa (after Brengues, 1973). A. Hypothetical distribution of bancroftian filariasis. B. Schematic illustration of zones (A,B,C,D,E,F, and G) with different prevalence of bancroftian filariasis. 1. Northern limit of area of coexistence of *An. gambiae* s.l. and *An. funestus*. 2. A line of 500 mm precipitation. 3. A line of 750 mm precipitation. 4. Northern limit of the forest. 5. The isothermal line of 25°C.

temperature often exceeds 30°C throughout the year. Therefore, the transmission can take place only during a short period, and endemic foci of filariasis occur only in certain restricted areas.

Zone C represents the region with annual rainfall between 500 and 750 mm, distributed over the months of June, July, August, and September. The average temperature is at least 1°C lower than in Zone B. Endemic foci of bancroftian filariasis are scattered and isolated from each other, occurring especially in areas where the population is gathered and fixed in the vicinity of important water sources, as in Dori (Upper Volta) and Niono (Mali). Similar foci probably exist in the regions of Yelimane (Mali) and Kaya (Upper Volta). In these endemic foci, the incidence of clinical cases is usually low.

Zone D includes the whole savanna region, where the annual rainfall exceeds 750 mm and the temperature is between 25 and 28°C. This zone is most favorable for filarial transmission, the vectors are abundant throughout, and there are many endemic foci of filariasis.

Zone E corresponds to the region of tropical rain forest. The population density of both *An. gambiae* (species A) and *An. funestus* is much lower than in the savanna, and the human population density is also very low. Therefore, filariasis is rare, except for certain areas in the valleys of large rivers where the people are gathered for cultivation, and many breeding places for the vectors are formed on the riverbed after the high water subsides.

Zone F is the highland region with an altitude between 500 m and 1,000 m surrounding the four large mountains: le Fouta Djaloon, les Monts Loma, le Massif de Seredou, and le Mont Nimba. The average temperature is below 25°C, and often goes below 20°C in the winter season. The development of filarial larvae in the vectors is greatly retarded or completely stopped under these conditions, even though the vector population may be high. Filariasis is almost nonexistent in this zone.

Zone G represents the coastal region, where the rainfall exceeds 750 mm, often over 1,500 mm per annum. The temperature rarely exceeds 30°C, and is usually stays between 26 and 27°C. There exist two species of the *An. gambiae* complex, namely *An. gambiae* A, whose larvae develop in freshwater, and *An. melas*, whose larvae develop in brackish water. Both serve as excellent vectors of *W. bancrofti* (GELFAND, 1955, BRENGUES & COZ, 1972), and although the two species appear throughout the year, *An. melas* predominates during the dry season and *An. gambiae* A does so during the rainy season. This zone is very favorable for the transmission of *W. bancrofti*, and there are many endemic foci of bancroftian filariasis.

The incidence of bancroftian filariasis varies greatly according to these zones and to the countries in western Africa. There are probably no endemice foci in Mauritania and very few, if any, in Niger. They do exist in Gambia, Guinea Bissau, in the southern regions of Senegal and Mali, in the western and the eastern parts of Guinea, in the northwest of Sierra Leone, in the center and south of Upper Volta, in the north of Ivory Coast, in the north, center, and southeast of Ghana, in Dahomey and Togo, and in the center of Nigeria. Foci possibly exist in certain coastal regions of these countries. In the forest zone of Sierra Leone, Liberia, Ivory Coast, and Nigeria, the foci may be also present, but they are probably rare and only localized.

7B.1 Senegal

Senegal is situated at the westmost point of Africa, on the North Atlantic coast between 12°N and 17°N. The territory is bounded on the north by the desert of Mauritania, and is mostly covered by rather dry grassland or savanna. Both *W. bancrofti* and *D. perstans* were found to be endemic in certain areas of this country.

It was observed by PELLETIER (1912) that elephantiasis of the scrotum was a relatively common affection in Senegal. He reported on cases of enormous swelling of the scrotum, in one case weighing 100 kg, other cases weighing 33 kg, 11 kg, 10 kg (two cases), and 7 kg. A high incidence of *W. bancrofti* infection (47.0%, 135 positives out of 287 soldiers examined) was reported by THIROUX (1912).

KARTMAN (1946) made an observation of the natural vectors of *W. bancrofti* in Dakar, Senegal. Natives suffering with elephantiasis were seen in some of the villages. In a routine check of native villages during a malaria survey, it was found that *An. gambiae* and *An. funestus* were predominant throughout the year, outnumbering all other mosquitoes, including *C. fatigans*. In the examinations conducted during 1944, 137 (36.6%) of 374 *An. gambiae* and 117 (15.6%) of 746 *An. funestus* were found to harbor filaria larvae.

DEJOU *et al.* (1950) made blood examinations (both at noon and midnight) of 152 male patients admitted to the Central African Hospital in Dakar. In all cases, 10 ml of blood were taken and hemolysed in 200 ml of water, or 1 ml of blood was added to 10 ml of 2% formalin solution, and the centrifuged sediment was examined for microfilariae. As a result, 14 cases (9%) were positive for microfilariae of *W. bancrofti*, and 22 (14%) were positive for those of *D. perstans*; 4 cases had mixed infection. These authors made a detailed study on the genital affections due to filariasis.

A high incidence of *W. bancrofti* infection in Casamance was reported by MCFADZEAN (1954) (see Section 7B.2.)

7B.2 Gambia

The Republic of the Gambia (a former British colony) is situated in western Africa at a latitude of about 13°N. It consists of a strip of land extending about 10 km on both sides of the Gambia River and about 350 km inland from the river mouth, with an area of about 11,000 km² and a population of 374,770 (1971).

MCFADZEAN (1854) reported on an investigation of filariasis in three villages of Gambia and a village in the Casamance region of Senegal. The incidence of *W. bancrofti* and *D. perstans*, respectively, was 38.3% and 10.2% in the coastal village of Kololi, 19.2% and 68.6% in the inland village of Jiboroh, 25.9% and 12.9% in the swamp village of Mandinari, and 39.5% and 9.5% in Elana in Casamance. A striking feature in the three Gambian villages was the small number of clinical filariasis cases as compared to the high morbidity in the village in Casamance, where 5.6% of the population had elephantiasis of the legs. The overall microfilaremia rates were almost the same in Kololi and Elana, but there was a higher rate in those under the age of ten years in Elana. The author considered that the early onset of microfilaremia and the high morbidity in the village in Casamance were both results of exposure to a more intense infection.

MCGREGOR & SMITH (1952) conducted a health, nutrition, and parasitological survey in a rural village of Kebena in West Kiang, Gambia. During the clinical survey, three cases of elephantiasis (two cases of the leg and one case of the arm) were found in 636 persons examined. About 20 mm³ blood samples were collected at night from 603 inhabitants; 220 (36.5 %) were found to harbor microfilariae of *W. bancrofti* and 203 (33.7%) had those of *D. perstans*; 102 among those infected had a mixed infection of the two parasites.

MCGREGOR *et al.* (1952) conducted a field trial of the control of filariasis with DEC in Kebena. The drug, in five daily doses of 5 mg base per kg of body weight, was administered to 181 *W. bancrofti* carriers. Of these, 69 had microfilariae of *D. perstans* as well as of *W. bancrofti*. Re-examination ten months after treatment showed that 64% of those treated were free of microfilariae of *W. bancrofti*, and the total number of microfilariae had been reduced by 94%. Microfilariae of *D. perstans* had been eliminated from the blood of 72% of those treated, with a 92% reduction of total load. The mode of occurrence of side effects was statistically studied. A conclusion was reached that, in spite of the very high therapeutic efficacy of DEC, its common toxic effects and high cost were disadvantages.

MINING & MCFADZEAN (1956) reported on the results of complement fixation tests of people in an endemic area of filariasis in Gambia due to *W. bancrofti* and *D. perstans*. The antigen used was an alcoholic extract of dried *Dirofilaria immitis*. The tests made on 55 sera from people in Hamburg were all negative, while in Gambia, 57% of 51 persons with the microfilariae of *W. bancrofti*, 25% of those with the microfilariae of *D. perstans*, and 23% of those with the mixed infection were positive; 33% of negative microfilaria persons in the endemic area were also CFT-positive.

7B.3 Guinea Bissau (fomerly Portuguese Guinea)

Located on the west coast of Africa between Senegal and Guinea at approximately 12°N, Guinea Bissau has an area of 36,000 km² and a population of 530,000 (1970).

In his review on filariasis in Portuguese overseas territories, FRAGA DE AZEVEDO (1964), stated that bancroftian filariasis was prevalent all over this territory because of its tropical climate, large precipitation throughout the year, and high population density. PINTO & ALMEIDA (1947) examined 986 persons of all ages in Castade Baixo and obtained a microfilaremia rate of 49.2%. ALMEIDA (1952) made a survey of the whole territory, and of 1,002 persons examined, 50.9% were positive for microfilariae of *W. bancrofti*. According to PINTO (1960), the microfilaremia rates in the coastal villages were 2.7% around Buba, 9.4% around Bissau, and 14.2% around Tpinto; however, those in the inland villages were 49.2% around Tpinto, 54.5%, 69.7%, and 11.7% around Mansoa, 41.6% in Bafata, and 18.9% in Farim. Elephantiasis and other clinical manifestations were extremely common. *An. gambiae* were found to be infected at a rate of 27.4 % among 336 specimens dissected. Pilot experiments on the control of filariasis with DEC were conducted in Bissau.

PINTO (1947, quoted by DEJOU *et al.*, 1950) made clinical and microfilarial surveys of *W. bancrofti* in Portuguese Guinea. Of 2,670 apparently healthy persons, microfilariae of *W. bancrofti* were found in 68%; of 1,523 persons with clinical signs of filariasis (adenolymphocele, epitrochlear adenitis, intrascrotal lesions), 47% were positive; of 469 elephantiasis cases, 20% were positive.

7B.4 Cape Verde Islands

A group of volcanic islands in the Atlantic Ocean situated in the west of Africa between 14°47′N to 17°13′N and 22°W to 26°W, these islands have a total land area of 4,033 km² and a population of 246,000 (1970).

FRANCO & MENEZES (1955) reported on a focus of Bancroftian filariasis verified in the region of Pedra Bajedo (São Tiago Maior) on the island of Santiago and its surroundings. Out of a total of 962 persons examined in 13 localities, 265 (27.5%) were found to harbor microfilariae of *W. bancrofti*. The localities where incidences of over 30% were observed were: Ponta da Achada (47.2%, 68 of 114), Achada Fazenda (43.1%, 22 of 51), Salina (40.3%, 48 of 119), Achada Igreje (39.4%, 13 of 33), and Cha da Silva (31.9%, 45 of 141).

Both males and females were similarly affected, while the rates were found to increase with age up to 40 years. Of 190 cases clinically studied. 20 had elephantiasis (9 were positive for microfilaremia), 88 were suspected of adenopathy (46 were positive), 8 had hydrocele (4 were positive), and 74 had no symptoms (20 were positive).

DE MEIRA (1961) reported on the results of control activities of various endemic diseases in Cape Verde. The endemic areas of *W. bancrofti* is rather limited to certain districts, and the vector is *Anopheles gambiae*. Anti-mosquito measure with DDT house spraying and mass administration of DEC (methods and dosages not described) were practiced. In November 1956, the infection and the infective rate of *An. gambide* obtained by dissection of 150 samples was 9.3% and 1.4% respectively, but these rates dropped gradually, and became to 1.33% and 0% respectively in December 1959. According to FRAGA DE AZAVEDE *et al.* (1969), the microfilaria rate for 1966 had fallen to 0.8% after 6 years of insecticide campaign.

7B.5 Guinea

Guinea (former French Guinea) is situated on the coastal region of West Africa between 13°N and 7°N. Area, 246,000 km²; population, 3,920,000 (1970).

THIROUX (1912) examined 498 soldiers from French Guinea, and obtained microfilaria rates of 18.9% for *W. bancrofti*, 36.1% for *D. perstans*, and 0.2% for *L. loa*.

PFISTER (1954) examined 352 persons in a savanna village, and found 146 (41.4%) persons to be positive for *D. perstans*, 14 (4.0%) for *W. bancrofti*, 44 (12.5%) for *O. volvulus*, and none for *D. streptocerca*; in another village in the forest, 380 persons were examined, of whom only 2 (0.5%) were positive for *D. perstans*, none for *W. bancrofti* and *D. streptocerca*, and 17 (4.5%) were positive for *O. volvulus*.

7B.6 Sierra Leone

A republic on the West African coast situated between 10°N and 7°N, Sierra Leone has an area of 71,740 km² and a population of 2,627,000 (1972). Its coastal belt is characterized by mangrove swamps; the country has rich agricultural fields and forests, as well as a high upland plateau in the northern region.

THIROUX (1912) detected three carriers of *W. bancrofti* and one carrier of *D. perstans* out of nine soldiers recruited from Sierra Leone.

BLACKLOCK (1922) conducted a study at Mabang, Sierra Leone, with an idea of detecting a relationship between the so-called signs of filarial disease and the occurrence of microfilaremia of *W. bancrofti*. Among 240 persons examined, 47 (18.8%) were positive for microfilariae of *W. bancrofti*, and the rate for those with some signs of filariasis was 21.0% (29 positives out of 138), in contrast to 17.6% (18 of 102) for those without signs of filariasis. The rate was 18.2% (2 of 11) in elephantiasis cases, 11.1% (1 of 9) in hydrocele cases, 22.6% (29 of 128) in those with enlarged glands, and 20.0% (3 of 15) in hernia cases. In this series, many of the "signs of filariasis" had no more of a correlation with the presence of microfilaria than did hernias, and some had even less. He concluded that to diagnose filarial disease from the discovery of enlarged glands, hydrocele, elephantiasis, and so on, might be just as misleading as diagnosing malaria simply from enlargement of the spleen.

GORDON *et al.* (1932) conducted a survey of the seasonal prevalence of house-hounting mosquitoes and their relation to the transmission of malaria and filariasis in the city of Freetown and in the adjacent native village of Kissy. Altogether, five species of anophelines and 14 species of culicines were collected, but there was a great predominance of anophelines over culicines (1,223:82 in Freetown and 3,763: 46 in Kissy). In Freetown, the only species of anophelines occurring in appreciable numbers was *An. funestus*, while in Kissy *An. costalis* and *An. funestus* appeared to be of equal importance. The densities of the two species were highly correlated with the rainfall; the rise in the *An. costalis* density started in May and reached a peak in July, about two months earlier than that of *An. funestus*. The infection of *An. costalis* with filarial larvae was seen in 14.6% for all forms and 2.7% for head and/or proboscis among 1,157 specimens dissected, while that of *An. funestus* was 8.0% and 1.2%, respectively, among 908 specimens dissected.

HICKS (1932) made observations on the transmission of *W. bancrofti* in Sierra Leone. The infection of *W. bancrofti* was common in Freetown, and according to the annual report of Connaught Hospital, microfilariac of *W. bancrofti* were found in 78 (9.1%) of 858 persons examined in 1913, 94 (9.7%) of 964 in 1914, and 7 (8.8%) of 80 examined in 1915 in the hospital. In prison, the rates were 11.8% (14 of 118) in 1914, 14.3% (29 of 203) in 1923, 19.0% (26 of 134) in 1930, and 20.6% (20 of 97) in 1931. Microfilariae of *D. perstans* were found in 13 of 2,454 persons examined in the hospital and in the prison. Among the mosquitoes studied, both *An. costalis* and *An. funestus* allowed complete development of larvae of *W. bancrofti*, and they were also found naturally infected. *Anopheles rhodesienses* and *An. squamosus* also allowed complete development, but they were not common human biters. No complete larval development was seen in *Ae. aegypti*, except for a single occasion when one out of 39 specimens dissected was found to have a proboscis infection.

THOMAS (1958) reported on the results of night blood examinations of prisoners in Freetown, and the civil population in Sierra Leone. The microfilariae of *D. perstans* were found in 4 of 897 native Africans in Freetown and also in 4 of 603 native Africans in Colony villages. In the examination of the adult male prisoners who had served less than three-month sentences, only 6 (3.37%) out of 178 native Africans were positive for the microfilariae of *D. perstans*, but 56 (31.5%) of them were positive for those of *W. bancrofti*. In the native African prisoners who had served longer than three-month sentences, 1 (0.19%) was positive for *D. perstans* and 104 (19.7%) were positive for *W. bancrofti*, out of 528 persons examined.

BLACKLOCK (1926a, b), while engaged in the study of onchocerciasis in the Konno district of Sierra Leone, discovered that a black fly was the vector of *O. volvulus*. He observed that the microfilarial rate of skin snips taken from adult males was as high as 42.3% (52 positives out of 123 persons examined). None of the persons examined in this district had the microfilariae of *D. streptocerca* in the skin. The black fly, *S. damnosum* Theobald, was also prevalent in this hilly country. By allowing wild flies to feed on restricted and heavily infected areas of the skin of human carriers, the gut infection was raised to 80% in one experiment, and the thorax infection to nearly 82% in another experiment. The developing forms of *O. volvulus* were found in the thorax after the infecting meal up to the seventh, eighth, and tenth days, after which no flies survived. In dissections of wild *S. damnosun*, 20 (2.6%) of 780 flies had microfilariae in the gut, and 15 (1.1%) of 1,320 flies had larvae in various developmental stages.

7B.7 Liberia

A republic in western Africa situated between 4°N and 9°N on the Atlantic coast; It has an area of 111,370 km² and a population of 1,200,000 (1970). Established as the Free and Independent Republic of Liberia in 1847, it was settled by freed American Negro slaves, and used to be under United States' protection. Investigations on tropical diseases, including filariasis, have been conducted by members of the Liberian Institute of Tropical Medicine in Marshall Territory, and other teams dispatched from the United States, and more recently by members of Tropeninstitut, Hamburg.

(1) *W. bancrofti* filariasis

STRONG (1930, quoted by DILLER, 1947) made a blood survey of 105 natives of Gbarnga, in central Liberia, and found one instance of *W. bancrofti* and one instance of *L. loa* infection. He also reported that elephantiasis was a common occurrence in Liberia. DILLER (1947) reported on the results of night blood surveys conducted by the Malaria Survey Unit of the U.S. Army in five villages in Liberia: Shangri-La, Paradise, Idlewylde, Village E, and Freetown; of a total of 955 persons examined, 84 (8.8%) showed microfilariae, and these were all *W. bancrofti* except for one case of *D. perstans*. In blood smears taken in the daytime, 14 cases of *W. bancrofti* infection and 2 cases of *D. perstans* infection were found out of 2,134 Liberian natives examined. No microfilaremia cases were found among

431 American soldiers who had been stationed in Liberia for a year or longer. Filaria larvae were found in 6 (0.92%) of 649 female *An. gambiae* dissected. Numerous cases of elephantiasis, notably scrotal enlargements, were observed among the Liberian natives.

Survey teams of the United States Public Health Service Mission to Liberia conducted sample studies of various endemic diseases from 1947 to 1950. The results referring to filariasis were reported by POINDEXTER (1950).

Blood smears were collected in three provinces and four of five counties of Liberia. Of 3,437 night blood smears examined, 342 (10.0%) were positive for microfilariae of *W. bancrofti*. The incidence differed greatly in each village, from the lowest of 0.8% (2 positives of 259) in Sanaquella district of Central Province, to the highest of 19.8% (16 of 81 adults) in Grand Bassa County; of 42,750 day blood smears collected in the same localities, 324 (0.76%) were positive for *W. bancrofti*. Hourly microfilarial counts were made on ten young adult microfilaria carriers, and remarkable nocturnal periodicity of *W. bancrofti* microfilariae was demonstrated in all cases. The distributions of malaria and filariasis were found to be not coincidental, and in the rural areas of the Vonjama-Massam Rolahun districts of Western Province, for example, over 80% of the children had enlarged spleens, 43% showed malaria parasites in blood smears, but microfilariae were found in only 1.0% of night blood smears.

YOUNG (1953) reported on microfilariae and trypanosomes found in a blood survey in Liberia. A total of 1,244 night blood smears (811 from adults) and 8,884 day blood smears (3,309 from adults) were collected in 18 localities covering various regions of Liberia; 4,34% (6.00% in adults) of night blood smears were positive for microfilariae of *W. bancrofti*. In the day blood smears, only 0.43% (30 of 8,884) were positive. All of the microfilariae found were identified as *W. bancrofti*. The incidence was highest in the coastal area (13.0%) and was much lower in other areas. The adults examined at Robertsport showed a positive rate of 23.9% (37 positives out of 155). Trypanosomes were found in five smears.

BURCH & GREENVILLE (1955) conducted a survey of microfilaria carriers in various localities of Liberia. In their previous blood surveys to determine the incidence of malaria, conducted during 1951 in two villages near Robertsfield, it was observed that as many as 7.3% of the individuals had demonstrable microfilariae in day blood smears. In the present survey, 53 (10.2%) of 520 night blood smears and 42 (3.0%) of 1,395 day blood smears contained microfilariae of *W. bancrofti*, No *L. loa* was observed, but six had *D. perstans*. The incidence of *W. bancrofti* was much higher along the coast than in the interior locations (6.1%, or 14 of 231 in the interior, 13.5% or 39 of 289 in coastal areas). Marshall Territory, near the Liberian Institute of Tropical Medicine, showed a positive rate of 16.4% (33 positives of 201) in night blood smears and 9.4% (34 of 362) in day blood smears. (Such high positive rates in the day blood samples were considered to be due to high microfilarial density of the population in these regions.) The observation of microfilarial periodicity in one case also showed remarkably consistent nocturnal appearance, though a few microfilariae were always detected during the daytime.

GELFAND (1955) conducted studies on the vectors of *W. bancrofti* in Liberia. Altogether, 15 species of wild-caught mosquitoes collected in Marshall Territory were dissected for examination for filaria infection; of these, 51 (19.5%) of 262 *An. gambiae*, 83 (27.1%) of 306 *An. melas*, and 132 (22.3%) of 592 *An. melas/gambiae* complex* were infected, and the percentages of those harboring mature larvae were 1.5, 3.6, and 1.9, repectively. All the other mosquito species (including 23 *C. fatigans*) were either uninfected, or did not have mature larvae. In addition, natural infections were found in *An. funestus* in a nearby locality.

Five species of indigenous, laboratory-reared mosquitoes were fed on a human donor who had microfilariae of *W. bancrofti*. *An, gambiae*, *An. melas*, and *C. thallasius* were readily infected and carried the infection to maturity within 13 to 14 days. *C. fatigans* and *Ae. aegypti* became infected at much lower percentages, and development of the larvae tended to be slower. In all three culicine species, many young, nondeveloping larvae were noted in the thoracic muscles. *An. melas*, which breeds in brackish water, was more heavily infected than *An. gambiae* in nature, and this was considered to be a reason that *W. bancrofti* was highly endemic in the coastal region.

GRATAMA (1969) made a study on the etiology of hydrocele in the southeastern territories of Liberia. Hydrocele was the most common surgical affections of male patients in this area, and in his previous survey reported in 1957, hydrocele accounted for 12% of all surgical cases. The materials for the present investigation were collected during routine work at the Firestone Cavalla Hospital; 176 hydrocele cases, admitted over the period from 1960 to 1964, were studied. Microfilariae were present in the hydrocele fluid of one-third of the patients; 14.5% among them had the microfilariae of *W. bancrofti*, 10.5% had those of *O. volvulus*, 0.6% had the mixed infection, and in 7%, identification was impossible. By applying the indications of JACHOWSKI *et al.* (1962) for the filarial etiology of hydroceles, they were, for the most part, filarial in origin. No difference could be established between hydroceles from the *W. bancrofti* group and the *O. volvulus* group on the basis of their clinical, surgical, and histopathological findings. Histopathological examination of removed testes failed to provide any indication that *O. volvulus* was a causative factor in the formation of hydroceles. The author made the conclusion that the majority of hydroceles in southeastern Liberia were caused by *W. bancrofti*, and although microfilariae of *O. volvulus* might be present in the hydrocele fluid by migration, they had no causal relationship to hydrocele formation.

BRINKMANN (1972) examined the night blood of 871 persons in 16 villages in Marshall Territory. The distribution of *W. bancrofti* infection was

---

* Dissected on the day of capture and therefore egg identification was not possible.

uneven over the different villages. The mean microfilarial rate was 12.7%. In the adult male, it was 26 to 32%, and in adult female, it was 8 to 12%. The rate was highest in the 40 to 49-year age-group. Villages close to the sea had higher rates than those inland. Hydrocele was found in 14.7% of all males and in almost half of the males in the 40 to 49-year age-group. Other filarial signs, including lymphadenitis, elephantiasis, and hemato-chyluria, were also commonly found. Malaria parasites were found in 26% of the blood smears, and onchocerciasis was found in 18.1% of the population.

MAASCH (1973) conducted quantitative studies on the transmission of *W. bancrofti* in urban, semiurban and rural areas in a coastal region of Liberia. Examination of over 20,000 (16 species) of mosquitoes indicated that *An. gambiae* and *An. melas* were the vectors, only single infections were found in *An. funestus* and *An. hancocki*, while the 3,000 *C. fatigans* were uninfected. It was calculated that in one rural area the residents would receive about 29,000 mosquito bites annually, of which 500 would be infective, conveying about 1,500 mature larvae. In another rural area the calculated mosquito bites were 10,000 per year, of which 200 would be infective conveying about 500 mature larvae. For the suburban area the figures were much lower, 5,500 bites per year yielding only 15 infective larvae. The transmission was not detectable in the city of Monrovia. Experimentally both *An. gambiae* and *An. melas* were highly susceptible to *W. bancrofti*, while *C. fatigans* was shown to be only 28% in the susceptibility of that of the anophelines. Due to this low susceptibility and the short life span, it was estimated that *C. fatigans* would require at least 30 times higher population density in order to be as effective a vector as the anophelines.

(2) *Onchocerciasis*

The occurrence of onchoceriasis in Liberia had been noted since 1926, when it was encountered by the Harvard African Expedition (STRONG, 1930). BURCH *et al.* (1955) made the first comprehensive survey of the disease in Liberia. Examinations were made on 2,423 male laborers from the Firestone Plantation at Harbel for the presence of palpable nodules; 469 (19.4%) of them were found to be positive. Approximately 90% of these nodules were located in the pelvic region. Microfilariae were found in 278 or 39.9% of 696 Africans examined by both skin biopsy and scarification smears. Nodules containing *O. volvulus* occurred in a significant number of cases in the absence of demonstrable microfilariae after skin biopsy and scarification smears; the highest percentage of onchocerciasis was demonstrated by combining the three methods of examination, *i.e.,* skin biopsies, scarification smears, and palpation for nodules. Small nebulae and other corneal opacities occurred more frequently among individuals with onchocerciasis than in those without this infection. In general, onchocerciasis was most common in the tribes from the interior of Liberia; the Kpelle, Gola, Mendi, and Gbandi tribes, especially, had high rates of infection; it was much lower among the Kru, Vai, and coastal Bassas. The microfilariae of *W. bancrofti* and *D. perstans* occasionally occurred in skin biopsies, especially in patients from the coast, where the prevalence of wuchereriasis was much greater.

FRENTZEL-BEYME (1973) conducted a detailed study on the prevalence of onchocerciasis and blindness in the population of the Bong Range, Liberia. Among a sample of 1,252 persons from a total population of about 15,000 people of the Kpelleh tribe in this area, 783 (63.2%) were carriers of microfilariae of *O. volvulus*. The infection was determined by a standard skin biopsy technique with Walser punch. The analysis of age-specific microfilarial rates revealed that at an age of 16–18 years more than 50% of the population became positive, and the number of "noninfected susceptibles" decreased annually by a rate of 0.92. The rate of blindness in the Bong Range was 1.18% and was more than twice as high as in onchocerciasis-free regions of Liberia. The average age of the complete blindness was 54 years, the onset of the blindness could be dated back to the average of 48 years. Among 1,131 subjects a bilaterally impaired vision was found in 8.3%.

GARMS (1973a) conducted an extensive survey of the distribution of *S. damnosum* in Liberia. Its breeding places were found to be distributed throughout the country, and the fly appeared to be most common in regions where the original tropical rain forest had been destroyed and replaced by farmland, rubber plantations, low bush or savanna. The larvae and pupae occurred in a surprizingly wide range of different habitats, and were observed not only in the rapids and waterfalls of all large rivers, but also in numerous smaller watercourses. This behavior may be due to the fact that at least four cytological categories of the *S. damnosum* complex differing in their breeding habits occur in Liberia. The 'Bandama' form was found in large rivers, while 'Yah' was inhabiting the smaller watercourses. 'Nile' and 'Soubre' were less common and seen only a few times in large rivers. Infections with *O. volvulus* were common in flies caught in the breeding areas of 'Bandana' and 'Yah'; the former form was considered more zoophilic, and contained larvae of animal filariae at high proportions.

GARMS (1973b) conducted quantitative studies on the transmission of *O. volvulus* by *S. damnosum* in the Bong Range, Liberia. The daily and annual cycles of biting densities, age compostion and infection rates of the *S. damnosum* population were studied for one or more years at seven catching stations. Dissections of 67,758 female *S. damnosum* revealed a mean annual parous rate of 10.9%; 17.2% of the parous flies carried filarial infections, 2.6% with mature larvae of *O. volvulus* and 3.0% with those of other filarial species. It was estimated that an average of 900 *O. volvulus* larvae were transmitted per man per year. This transmission rate was associated with a microfilarial rate of 63% in the human population.

7B.8 Mali

Mali (Sudanese Republic from 1958 to 1960, and French Sudan prior to 1958) is an inland country in western Africa, with an area of 1,240,000 km² and a population of 5,031,500 (1970). Its northern region is a part of the Sahara, while its southern part is crossed by the Upper Niger River and has large swampy areas.

THIROUX (1912) reported high incidences of *W. bancrofti* (27%) and *D. perstans* (46%) among soldiers from Bamako, the capital of Mali. LÉGER (1912) carried out blood surveys of people in the region of Bamako; in the examinations of night blood of 428 adults conducted during the rainy season, 61 (14.3%) were positive for *W. bancrofti* and 54 (12.4%) for *D. perstans*; in the examination of 525 persons conducted at about noon, 4 (0.75%) were positive for *L. loa* and 57 (10.8%) for *D. perstans*. In another survey, carried out during the dry season, 309 persons were examined at night and 35 (11.3%) were positive for *W. bancrofti* and 42 (13.6%) for *D. perstans*; out of 416 persons examined in daytime, 2 (0.48%) had *L. loa* and 39 (9.4%) had *D. perstans*.

BRENGUES *et al.* (1968, 1969), BRENGUES & COZ (1972, 1973), and BRENGUES (1973) reported detailed studies on the transmission of *W. bancrofti* in West Africa (Mali, Upper Volta, Niger, and Ivory Coast). In the Sahara zone of Hombori and Douentza, low microfilarial rates (less than 5%) were observed. More important foci of *W. bancrofti* infection were found from the regions of Niono, Markala, and Ségou, in the flooding zone of the Niger River. In the region of Ségou, the microfilaria rate was 26.5% in Boundo, 27.0% in Konodimini, and 11.9% in N'Gara.

In the region of Markala, the rate was 13.8% in Domgoma, 18.7% in Douabougou, 15.4% in Dougouba, and 2.6% in Sansanding. In the region of Niono, the rate was 8.3% in Kanabougou, 4.3% in Kourouma, 4.4% in Molodo-Banbara, and 2.0% in Niono "26."

According to BRENGUES & SALES (1971, quoted by BRENGUES, 1973), elephantiasis is rare in the region north of 14°N, but is rather common in the upper basin of the Senegal River (areas around Kayee and Yelimané), in the southern part of the flooded zone of Niger River, in the flooded zone of Bani River (areas of Djenné, San, and Tominian), in the south of the region of Bamako (areas around Bamako, Dioila, and Kangaba), in the upper valley of Sourou (area of Koro), and in the southern parts of Mali (areas around Sikasso, Bougouni, and Yorosso). In the hospital of "Point G" of Bamako, out of 5,518 surgical operations conducted from 1967 to 1970, 332 cases (6.0%) were hydrocele and 31 cases (0.56%) were elephantiasis. In Gabriel Touré Hospital in Bamako, there were 121 (13.1%) cases of hydrocele and 8 (0.88%) cases of elephantiasis, out of 922 operations conducted in 1971.

7B.9 Ivory Coast

Ivory Coast (Côte d'Ivoire) is a republic in western Africa situated between 11°N and 4°N on the Atlantic coast. It has an area of 322,463 km² and a population of 4,310,000 (1970). It was governed by France until it achieved independence in 1960.

THIROUX (1912) examined 114 soldiers from Ivory Coast and found 60 (52.6%) positive for *D. perstans*, 9 (7.9%) for *W. bancrofti*, and none for *L. loa*. PFISTER (1954) examined 633 persons from a village in the wooded savanna area, and observed 410 (64.8%) to be positive for *D. perstans*, 3 (0.5%) for *W. bancrofti*, 17 (2.6%) for *O. volvulus*, and none for *D. streptocerca*; among 893 persons from a forest village, 21 (2.4%) were positive for *D. perstans*, 1 (0.1%) for *W. bancrofti*, 37 (4.1%) for *O. volvulus*, and 3 (0.3%) for *D. streptocerca*.

In more recent reports by HAMON *et al.* (1967), BRENGUES *et al.* (1968), and BRENGUES (1973), it was also confirmed that *W. bancrofti* infection was rare in the forest zone, and microfilaremia was found in only one out of 502 persons examined in the region of Man, and in only 3 out of 1,789 persons examined in the region of Daloa. However, the infection seems to be common in the coastal villages, and in one of the surveys conducted in the region of Sassandra, 127 (10.0%) of 1,264 persons above the age of six years were positive.

In the hospital in Bouaké, 92 (3.13%) cases were hydrocele and 5 (0.17%) cases showed elephantiasis of the scrotum, out of a total of 2,938 patients surgically treated from May 1969 to June 1971. In the hospital in Abidjan, on the highland, 49 (1.89%) were hydrocele out of 2,529 surgical cases treated from June 1970 to November 1971 (BRENGUES, 1973).

7B.10 Upper Volta (Haute Volta, or the Voltaic Republic)

An inland country in West Africa situated north of Ghana between 9°N and 15°N, Upper Volta has an area of 274,000 km² and a population of 5,485,981 (1970). The territory consists mainly of plateau, with savanna in the northern part and a sparsely forested area in the south.

THIROUX (1912) examined 718 soldiers from the region of Haut-Senegal and Niger, and found high incidence of *W. bancrofti* (22.7%) and *D. perstans* (28.3%).

Pfister (1952) carried out blood and skin examinations for filariasis in various regions of Upper Volta. Daytime blood examinations were conducted in four regions located at different latitudes and with different amounts of annual rainfall. The incidences of both *D. perstans* and *W.*

bancrofti were found to be highly correlated with the latitude and the rainfall. In Bobo-Gaoua, located farthest south (10.5 to 11.5°N and having the greatest rainfall, some 1,200 mm per year), about 70% of the people examined during the daytime were positive for microfilariae of *D. perstans* and 5% for *W. bancrofti*. The rates decreased to 28% and 2.5%, respectively, in the area between 12° to 13°N where the average rainfall is 800 to 1,000 mm; the rates dropped to 12% and 2.1%, respectively, in areas between 13° to 14°N where the average rainfall is 600 to 800 mm, and to 4.7% and 0%, respectively, in the northernmost, dry area. In the northwestern region of Bobo-Dioulasso, 5,232 persons in 50 villages were examined for *D. perstans* infection; 85% of the old people, 67% of adult males, 58% of adult females, 25% of the boys, and 20% of the girls were found positive.

The blood examinations were conducted during the daytime for the purpose of detecting microfilariae of *D. perstans*; however, 44 (3.1%) carriers of *W. bancrofti* were discovered out of 1,440 persons examined. All of these *W. bancrofti* carriers were apparently healthy and free from clinical filariasis signs, such as elephantiasis and adenitis.

The distribution of onchocerciasis was also found to be higher, in general, in areas with larger rainfalls, but its incidence within the same region was quite uneven. In nine villages around Bobo-Dioulasso, 44 (10.2%) of 432 persons examined were positive for microfilariae and 22 (5.1%) had skin nodules. The overall microfilaria rate of the population surveyed was 6%, but villages near the valley of the Black Volta River (Volta Noire) were highly infected, and showed a microfilaremia rate of 20% in average. In some villages, the incidence was as high as 90%.

Four carriers of *D. streptocerca* were discovered. They were young men native of the Koudougou region, and visited Bobo-Dioulasso on their way back from a plantation in Ivory Coast; it was not certain whether they were infected in their native region, or while staying in Ivory Coast.

Results of blood surveys conducted recently by various workers in Upper Volta were reviewed by BRENGUES (1973). Carriers of *W. bancrofti* were found to be distributed in all the regions surveyed, though the incidence was quite variable by the localities. In general, the areas with high microfilarial rates were situated in the southern part where the annual precipitation is much higher than in the northern regions, and the incidence was highly correlated with the latitude. BRENGUES (1973) observed a high microfilarial rate of 38.7% (545 positives out of 1,407 persons examined) in Koupela, and also 39.9% (246 of 617) in Tingrela of the Banfora region. LAMONTELLERIE (1972) reported 7,812 positives (13.2%) out of 59,082 persons examined in 154 localities in the Banfore region.

BRENGUES *et al.* (1968) conducted comprehensive studies on the transmission of *W. bancrofti* in a savanna village of Tingrela. The main vector was shown to be *An. gambiae* s.l. and *An. funestus*. *Anopheles welcomei* was also found to be naturally infected. Observations were conducted during a period from August 1964 to November 1965 by night catches on human baits. The density of *An. gambiae* was high during the months from June to September, with a peak in August, while that of *An. funestus* increased later, being high during the months from November to February, with a peak in November. Mosquito specimens containing mature larvae of *W. bancrofti* were found only during the period from July to November in both species. Therefore, the transmission of *W. bancrofti* in this area seemed to take place not throughout the year but is concentrated to a season from July to November, with a peak in September. It was also estimated that the number of infective bites per man per year (from August 1964 to July 1965) was 20.7 by *An. gambiae* and 8.3 by *An. funestus* (a more quantitative discussion is made in Section 10A. 3).

Onchocerciasis has been found to be highly prevalent in the savanna area of the Volta Basin extending at least to the seven countries, i.e., Upper Volta, Dahomey, Niger, Togo, Ghana, Ivory Coast and Mali. An international program for onchocerciasis control in the Volta River basin area was launched in 1973 (see Section 5.5.3).

7B.11 Ghana

A republic formerly called Gold Coast, situated in West Africa between 5°N and 11°N, bounded on the south by the Gulf of Guinea, on the east by Togo, on the west by Ivory Coast, and on the north by Upper Volta. Ghana has an area of 239,000 km² and a population of 8,545,561 (1970).

As for *W. bancrofti* infection in Ghana, HAWKING (1957) stated, "Filariasis is moderately common and is widespread but it has not attracted much attention. It is said to be especially common at Navrongo in the northerly territories. During 1936 and 1937, out of 55,000 inhabitants admitted to hospital in the whole territory, there were 147 cases admitted for hydrocele and 134 cases admitted for elephantiasis; the true frequency of these conditions is probably higher than this." (from Gold Coast Medical Department Report, 1936, 1937, Accra)

MUIRHEAD-THOMPSON (1954) observed that in villages outside of Accra 9 out of 28 adults were carrying *W. bancrofti* microfilariae, and 4% of wild *An. gambiae* and 1.7% of wild *An. funestus* contained mature larvae.

Both *D. perstans* and *L. loa* are considered to occur in this country, but no definite information is available. However, important contributions have been made to the knowledge of *D. streptocerca* and *O. volvulus* by workers in this country.

MACFIE & CORSON (1922), when investigating the occurrence of larvae of *O. volvulus* in the skin of natives in Ghana, found sheathless larvae of a new filaria and named it *Agamofilaria streptocerca*. The microfilariae were found in the skin of 9 out of 24 cases selected for examination for *O. volvulus*, and also in one of 9 unselected autopsies. The larvae were sheathless, slender, tapering both anteriorly and posteriorly, and when fixed in

Ruge's solution, the body was shown to be almost straight, with the exception of the posterior extremity which was curved like the handle of a walking stick. The nuclei were large, two or three abreast in the middle of the larva, and completely filled the greater part of the body. The body length ranged from 180 to 240 μ and had a breadth of about 3 μ.

The larvae were found only in the skin, and none were found in the blood of the nine cases examined, though larvae of *D. perstans* were found in two cases. In sections of the skin, the larvae were lying in the tissue spaces of the *cutis vera* or *corium*, usually close to the *rete mucosum*. As for possible pathogenicity, lichenification of the skin was present in six of ten cases and there was a definite thickening in two others. In an examination of 50 men chosen at random in Accra, larvae of this species were found in 22 (44%) and those of *O. volvulus* in 17 (34%). No periodicity was observed with the larvae in the skin.

The authors pointed out that the larvae of this species may be distinguished at a glance from those of *O. volvulus* by their slender body, crook-shaped posterior extremity, and blunt tail. The larvae of *D. perstans*, from which larvae of this species have to be distinguished most carefully, are stouter, and the nerve ring, the G-1 cell, and the anal pore are situated further forward; when fixed in Ruge's solution, *D. perstans* larvae are straight and not crook-shaped at the posterior extremity.

The epidemiology of onchocerciasis, as well as the distribution and bionomics of its vector, *S. damnosum*, has been extensively investigated in Ghana by BERNER (1950, quoted by crisp, 1956b), HUGHES (1952), CRISP (1956 a, b), LEWIS *et al.* (1961) and SENKER *et al.* (1973). A map showing the distribution of *S. damnosum* and *O. volvulus* was compiled by CRISP (1956 b). It was based on the results of a three-year survey organized by the British Empire Society for Blindness, in 1952. The Gold Coast comprises three main regions: the lowlands of the coast, the basin of the Volta River, and the wide plateau in the north. Both *S. damnosum* and onchocerciasis were present along stretches of all the main rivers in the Northern Territories, and the fly was found in tributaries and in streamlets which flow for only a few weeks in the year. Outside the Northern Territories, the fly has a limited distribution; in Ashanti, for instance, it was found in a small area around Kintampo, while in the Gold Coast Colony, it was confined to a stretch of the Volta northeast of Accra.

7B.12 Togo

A republic in western Africa consisting of a strip of land about 100 km wide and extending about 550 km northward from the Gulf of Guinea, Togo was a German Protectorate prior to 1914, and later assigned to France, until it achieved independence in 1960. The coastal region is swampy, the northern region characterized by savanna, and the central region is mountainous. It has an area of 56,600 km² with a population of 1,955, 916 (1970).

Little is known about the epidemiology of filariasis in this country. HAWKING (1957) stated, "In the days of German administration, *W. bancrofti* was said to be present but not common."

BRENGUES *et al.* (1969) reported on the occurrence of endemic foci of bancroftian filariasis in southern Togo. In the region of Ancho, 452 persons were examined, and 8.0% of them had microfilariae, 5.7% had elephantiasis, and 3.2% had hydrocele. In the region of Porto-Seguro near Lake Togo, 505 persons were examined; 0.2% had microfilariae, 1.2% had elephantiasis, and 1.8% had hydrocele.

7B.13 Dahomey

A republic in western Africa occupying a strip of land extending from the coast of Gulf of Guinea to about 700 km north, Dahomey is situated between 6°N and 12.5°N. The territory consists of a hilly region in the northwest, plains in the east and north, and a marshy, coastal region in the south. It has an area of 113,000 km² with a population of 2,718,000 (1970).

THIROUX (1912) examined 144 soldiers from Dahomey, and found microfilariae of *W. bancrofti* in 19 (13.2%), those of *D. perstans* in 49 (34.0%), and those of *L. loa* in 1 (0.7%). PFISTER (1954) examined 62 persons from wooded savanna zone of northern Dahomey, and found 6 (9.7%) infected with *D. perstans*, 16 (25.8%) with *O. volvulus*, but none with *W. bancrofti* and *D. streptocerca*.

As pointed out by BRENGUES (1973), bancroftian filariasis is generally rare in the northern part of Dahomey but is very common in the south. According to THIROUX (1912), the microfilarial rate was 3.2% in soldiers from Nikki, Djougou, and Parakou in the north, but was 19.7% among those who came from Savalou and Abomey in the south. BRENGUES *et al.* (1969) found 20.3% to be positive among the people in the region of Athiéme on the lower valley of the Mono River, 8.1% in villages around Lake Aheme (Ouidah region), and 0.2% on the coast near Grand-Popo.

7C. Central Africa

7C.1 Niger

A republic in north central Africa, Niger is an inland country characterized by desert in its central and northern parts, and savanna in the southern part. The Niger River crosses it in the southwest, and the mountainous region of Air is located in the northern central part of this country. Niger has an area of 1,189,000 km^2 and a population of 4,020,000 (1970).

THIROUX (1912) found microfilariae of *W. bancrofti* in 6 out of 16 soldiers who came from Niamey. PFISTER (1954) examined 79 persons from the desert region of Say-Maradi and found microfilaria carriers of 5 (6.3%) with *W. bancrofti* and 1 (1.3%) with *D. perstans*, but none with *O. volvulus* or *D. streptocerca*.

BRENGUES *et al.* (1968) and BRENGUES (1973) observed that only 1 out of 205 persons examined at Tahoua, and 3 of 203 persons examined at Téra were positive microfilaria cases.

7C.2 Chad

Chad is an inland country in northern central Africa, situated between 24°N and 8°N; it has an area of 1,283,500 km^2 and a population of 3,634,000 (1970). The northern two-thirds of the territory is desert, while the southern part is well irrigated, and either forested or cultivated.

BOUILLIEZ (1916) made a survey of the distribution of various parasitic diseases in "Moyen Chari," in southern Chad, in an area near Fort-Archambault. As for filariasis, he found carriers of *Microfilaria nocturna* (= *W. bancrofti*) in 47 (21.7%) of 217 persons examined at night, *Microfilaria perstans* in 64 (35.4%) of 181 persons examined by day.

BUCK *et al.* (1969) reported on the results of the epidemiological study of onchocerciasis in two new endemic foci in the Republic of Chad: Ouli Bangala (7° 50′N and 15° 50′E) and Masidjanga (10° 10′N and 19° 20′E). In the first village, 398 persons of the total population of 401 were examined. Skin snips were collected from the back (about 2 cm above the iliac crest) of 373 persons with a corneal-scleral punch instrument (Holth; Lawton Co., 425 Fourth Avenue, New York), and microfilariae of *O. volvulus* were found in 316 (84.7%). Of 386 urine specimens examined, the microfilariae of *O. volvulus* were found in 44 (11.4%), and the eggs of *Schistosoma haematobium* were found in 26 (6.8%). Microfilariae in the urine were closely related to the intensity of skin infections (determined by microfilarial counts in skin snips) and to the distance of the residence from the Lim River, the only permanent habitat for *S. damnosum* in the area. BUCK *et al.* (1970, quoted by HAWKING, 1973) further conducted systemetic investigations of filarial infections among people in five contrasting villages in Chad.

SHABEL'NIK (1970) carried out examinations of school children and of hospital patients in the Prefecture of Guera for filarial infections. Of 4,253 day blood samples collected from schoolchildren, 8.37% were positive for microfilariae (species not determined). Of 1,000 hospital patients examined at Mongo, 15.7% were positive. Among these patients, 64 persons were infected with *D. perstans*, 50 with *W. bancrofti*, and 12 with both parasites.

BUCK *et al.* (1973) studied serum immunoglobulin levels of onchocerciasis patients in Chad (see Section 5.4.4.2).

VEDY & SIROL (1973) reported on results of a campaign against onchocerciasis in Chad carried out by the 'Services des Grandes Endémie.' The control operations included (a) clinical and parasitological surveys; (b) ophthalmological survey; (c) treatment by nodulectomy; (d) drug treatment with micro and macro filaricides; (e) antilarval measures in the streams; and (f) imagocidal measures. The *Simulium* vectors persisted in spite of these efforts in 1954/55 and 1956 to 1962. Finally, attempts to control onchocerciasis were abandoned in 1962. Surveys carried out under this program have revealed that the disease is prevalent in southern part of Chad where there are high rainfalls, large rivers and forests, and the infection rates in some areas such as Mayo Kebbi was nearly 100% with half of the people having impaired sight.

7C.3 Nigeria

The Federal Republic of Nigeria is bounded on the northwest and north by Niger, on the east by Cameroon, on the south by the Gulf of Guinea, and on west by Dahomey; it is situated between 4°N and 14°N. Nigeria has an area of 934,000 km² and a population of 67,828,000 (1971). The coastal plain varies in width from 16 km to 97 km; Jos Plateau is in the center with a maximum elevation of over 1830 m; there is a mountain range on its eastern boundary, while its extreme north is semidesert. The land was mostly under British administration until it achieved independence in 1960; a number of contributions to the study of filariasis referring to areas within the territory of Nigeria were made by British workers, in conjunction with those referring to the former British Cameroons.

The epidemiology of filariasis in Nigeria is complicated because of the diversity of the environmental conditions of the different regions. *W. bancrofti* has been noted to be highly endemic in some regions of northern Nigeria, but is apparently absent from the western plain and coastal areas of Ibadan and Lagos. On the other hand, *O. volvulus* is more extensively distributed and is a serious health hazard in many regions of Nigeria. Loiasis is also an important disease in this country, but *D. perstans* infection seems to be less common.

In Nigeria, ANNET *et al.* (1901, *Liverpool Sch. Trop. Med. Mem.* vol. IV, pp. 69–72, quoted by KARTMAN, 1946) found that 5.7% of 281 *An. gambiae* were infected with *W. bancrofti* larvae.

COURTNEY (1923) observed that microfilariae were among the most common parasites found in the blood of northern Nigerian natives, and also that microfilariae were frequently found in patients having certain common and trivial complaints, such as myalgia, chronic rheumatism, abscess, etc. In examinations of soldiers, prisoners, and other native people at Ilorin, Naraguta, and Ankpa, 73 (42.4%) of 172 persons examined had microfilariae. In infections of known pathological significance, microfilariae of *W. bancrofti* were found in 24 (13.9%) and those of *L. loa* in 8 (4.6%) of 172; these microfilariae were found in 16 (35.5%) and 6 (13.3%), respectively, of 45 patients examined for clinical reasons as being suspected of infection by either *bancrofti* or *loa*.

TAYLOR (1930) reported on the domestic mosquitoes of Gadau, northern Nigeria, and their relation to malaria and filariasis. Filariasis was found to be extremely common among the natives of northern Nigeria. The climate of this area is very dry, with an average annual rainfall of 28 inches, all of which falls between April and October. The river (Jemaari) flows about six months in the year, and during the dry season the only open water in the district is found to pools of varying size in the river bed. During this period, the inhabitants rely entirely on deep wells for their water supply. The breeding of mosquitoes was thus confined to the months from July to October.

During the period from June 1929 to March 1930, 2,134 anophelines (seven species) and 74 culicines (seven species) were collected from houses. The culicines constituted only 3.35% of the total collections; *C. nebulosus* made up nearly half of the total culicines, and no *C. fatigans* were collected. *Anopheles costalis* and *An. funestus* predominated over all other mosquito species and together formed 91.4% of the domestic anophelines. Dissections of 3,563 anophelines and 117 culicines collected from European and African dwellings were made, and it was observed that the infection rates with both malaria parasite and filaria were approximately the same. *Anopheles costalis* and *An. funestus* were the only species to be related to the transmission of malaria. Of 1,936 *An. costalis* dissected, 6.97% had immature filaria larvae and 1.65% had mature filaria larvae; also, of 1,260 *An. funestus*, 3.17% had immature larvae and 0.87% had mature larvae. *Anopheles costalis* was a little more than twice as heavily infected as *An. funestus*. Mature filarial infection was seen in one of 15 *Ae. ochraceus*, and immature infections in *An. pharoensis* and *An. squamosus*.

Onchocerciasis was first reported from northern Nigeria in 1908 by PARSONS. SHARP (1926) found microfilariae of *O. volvulus* in the skin of 55 out of 100 prisoners at Kaduna. Ocular onchocerciasis was reported to be an important cause of blindness in many parts of northern Nigeria by BUDDEN (1952). BUDDEN (1956) conducted an extensive survey of onchocerciasis, covering all the provinces, between November 1951 and August 1954. Two types of human investiagtion were carried out: the examination of persons with reduced vision and blindness, and total population surveys to determine the incidence of infection (by skin snips) and of reduced vision or blindness. In the vision examination, 5,170 patients were seen, of whom 1,789 were diagnosed to be blind (or unable to count fingers at distance greater than three meters). The total population surveys were conducted in 15 communities in the endemic areas and three communities in the arid, northern belt where there was no disease. In areas of heavy infection, 66.5% were found infected and 5.7% were blind due to onchocerciasis, out of 295 persons examined. In areas of moderate infection, 32.1% were infected and 1.0% were blind, out of 1,258 persons examined. In areas of light infection, 9.8% were infected and 0.1% were blind, out of 2,337 persons examined. Of the total population of 16,836,000 of this country at the time of the investigations, the numbers of people exposed to heavy, moderate, and light infection were estimated to be 158,000, 712,000, and 52,000, respectively; hence, about one-third of a million people were estimated to be suffering from the disease, and about 20,000 were blind due to onchocerciasis.

CROSSKEY (1954) made a sruvey of infection of *S. damnosum* with *O. volvulus* during the wet season in the Kudaru area of northern Nigeria; altogether, 1,680 wild specimens were dissected, of which 331 (19.7%) were found infected, 195 (11.6%) had developing forms, 108 (6.4%) had mature forms, and 28 (1.7%) had double infections. Some *S. damnosum* dissected were found to be infected with other parasites, including ciliates, hymenopterous larvae, mites, and nematodes other than *O. volvulus*. The bionomics of the adults of *S. damnosum* in northern Nigeria in relation to the transmission of *O. volvulus* were investigated by CROSSKEY (1955). CROSSKEY (1956) further conducted an extensive study on the distribution of *S. damnosum* in northern Nigeria. The fly was found to occur mainly between the southern border of the country (6°30 to 9°N) and 11°N. In the northwest, the range extends further than in the northeast, and reaches into the dry country, north of 12°N, in Sokoto Province. Within this range, the fly is not evenly distributed, but occurs only in particular areas. The fly is spread over about one-third of northern Nigeria, an area of some 90,000 square miles, but in this area there are numerous *damnosum*-free regions. The breeding distribution is linear along rivers, and limited in the far north by the absence of suitable perennial rivers and by the prolonged dry season. The *S. damnosum* foci tend to become more sporadic in the far north, and are of minor extent in the central plateau area, but some isolated foci may be heavily infested by the fly, giving rise to heavy infections with *O. volvulus*. In two particular areas, the northeast of Niger Province and southern Adamawa Province of Cameroon, numerous infected rivers form a network, giving the fly an almost continuous distribution over a very large area.

CROSSKEY (1957b) reported further on the infection of *S. damnosum* with *O. volvulus* in three areas in northern Nigeria: Abuja, Kudaru, and Loloja. It was unlikely that the transmission occurred in the dry season between November and April when the fly density was extremely low (usually between 0.01 and 0.2 flies per boy per hour); only 46 flies could be collected during this season, and none of them were found infected. On the other hand, the fly density showed two peaks during the wet season, one in early July and another in September. However, the infective rate of the flies was relatively low when the fly density was highest, and thus the rate of infective bites per person per day was found to be highest at Abuja in June (1.3) and in October (1.8).

Crosskey (1957a) reported that *S. bovis* De Meillon, 1930, which is a zoophilic species which usually bites cattle as the main host, bit man in localized areas in northern Nigeria when the fly density was high. At the dissection of 116 flies, 7 were found to be infected with filariae similar to those of *O. volvulus*; of these, 3 had infective larvae. The author suggested that *S. bovis* might act as a vector of human onchocerciasis in limited areas.

Cower & Woodward (1960) made a general survey of parasitic infections among employees of the Moor Plantation, Ibadan. As for filarial infections, 2 cases of *O. volvulus* carriers, 4 cases of *L. loa* carriers and 2 cases of *D. perstans* carriers were found among 100 males aged 15 to 48 years.

Cower & Woodward (1961) reported on parasitic infections recorded at University College Hospital, Ibadan, over a three-year period. Microfilariae of *L. loa* were diagnosed on 38 occasions in 5,150 blood films (0.7%). *Loa loa* is widespread in the eastern region of Liberia, Calabar, and Cameroon, and it is probable that there is some transmission occurring in the western region as well. *D. perstans* was identified only 15 times. As for *W. bancrofti*, there was no evidence of transmission in the Ibadan area, and its microfilariae were never found in night blood or hydrocele fluid. Although Cobban (1959) recorded 31 cases of bancroftian filariasis seen in the Outpatients Department from April 1957 to April 1958, the diagnoses were based on clinical observation alone and its microfilariae were never demonstrated. Cower & Woodward (1960), therefore, raised the possibility of clinical elephantiasis from non-filarial causes. The incidence of onchocerciasis was high enough to justify a special clinic in the hospital. Cower & Jackson (1964) reported on a case of onchocercal hydrocele without typical cutaneous manifestations of onchocerciasis, or infection with *W. bancrofti*. They reviewed the literature on elephantiasis, chylous hydrocele, and other abnormalities of the lymph system in Africa due to causes other than *W. bancrofti*, and particularly their association with *O. volvulus*.

Ngu & Konstam (1964) made clinical studies on chronic lymphoedema in western Nigeria. In 25 of the 65 patients studied, tuberculous adenitis was responsible for the lymphoedema. In 30 cases, the lymphoedema was due to chronic pyogenic infections, 26 arising in the lower leg and 4 in the scrotum. Seven patients had lymphoedema due to malignant or other infiltrations, and 3 were due to congenital anomalies. None of these cases could be confidently ascribed to filariasis.

Ngu & Folami (1965, quoted by Hawking, 1973) examined 1,340 night blood samples from 13 cities in western Nigeria, including Ibadan, Abeokuta, and Sapela. They found all of them negative for *W. bancrofti* aside from 2 (out of 93) from Benin City; however, the microfilariae of *L. loa* were found in 4.9% of night blood samples (*i.e.*, when the count is lowest).

A review was made by Cowper (1967) on helminthiasis in the western region of Nigeria, with special reference to the Ibadan area. *W. bancrofti* infection was very rare in this region. Its microfilariae were never seen in routine blood examinations at the University College Hospital during a three-year period (1957 to 60), and since then, it was seen only once. In a survey of the night blood of 1,340 hospital inpatients, microfilariae of *W. bancrofti* were found only in two cases, and they were both from Benin. In the same series, microfilariae of *L. loa* occurred in 4.9% and those of *D. perstans* in 2.0%.

On the other hand, Ibadan lies in the heart of the *Loa* belt of West Africa and its infection there is common. *D. perstans* is less common than *L. loa*, but GILLES (1961, quoted by COWPER 1967) found it at Akufo in 12 out of 828 blood films. Onchocerciasis is widespread in the western region, especially in the Ibadan area, as well as in the north and east of Nigeria. Epidemiological and pathological studies of onchocerciasis in western Nigeria were conducted by NNOCHERI (1964a, b).

OGUMBA (1971) made observations on the seasonal prevalence and filarial infection of house-infesting mosquitoes in Ibadan. Collections were made by the spray sheet method over a period of 15 months. *C. fatigans* was the predominant species, abundant throughout the year, with high population densities in the dry months (November to March). *Anopheles gambiae* and *An. funestus* showed higher densities in the wet season (April to October). Dissections were made of 2,128 wild female *C. fatigans* and 994 wild females of *An. gambiae* and *An. funestus*, but none contained developing filariae.

RODGER (1973) reviewed the *Simulium* control scheme at Abuja, North Nigeria, and its effect on the prevalence of ocular onchocerciasis.

7C.4 Cameroon

Cameroon (Federal Republic of Cameroon since 1960) is situated in central Africa between 2° to 13°N; it has an area of 475,317 km² and a population of 5,840,000 (1970 estimate). A German Protectorate was proclaimed in 1884, invaded by Anglo-French forces in 1914, and from 1919, it was divided into British and French administrative zones. In 1961, these were united and became independent.

The climate in the west is very humid and high in precipitation, with a short dry season and a long rainy season. In the south there are two dry and two wet seasons. The land can be roughly divided into four regions: the forest region in the south; the savanna region, extending from the edge of the dense forest to about 10° N; the steppe region which covers an area from southern Cameroon to the Chad border; and the mountain region in the west.

(A) Reports from the former British Cameroons
A series of extensive studies were made on the epidemiology of various

kinds of human filariasis in the area covering the former British Cameroons and Nigeria. Reports were made by Gordon *et al.* (1948, 1950), Kershaw (1950, 1951), Kershaw *et al.* (1953, 1954, 1955), and Nicholas *et al.* (1953, 1954, 1955). At least five kinds of human filariasis are known to be endemic in certain parts of this region, and especially important contributions to the knowledge of transmission and bionomics of the vectors of *L. loa, D. perstans, D. streptocerca*, and *O. volvulus* were made here by several workers. Kershaw *et al.* (1953) gave the following accounts of the general features of the distribution of various kinds of filariasis in the Nigeria and British Cameroon region.

> *Loa loa* is confined to the rain forest and its fringe and to the freshwater swamp, and is probably rare in the coastal mangrove swamps. The incidence of infection seems to be high in relatively undisturbed rain forests, higher in the artificial situation of rubber plantations, and lower in large towns. In the mountain grassland areas of the Cameroons, transmission does not occur, and the fall in incidence from the rain forest across the natural boundary to the grassland is very abrupt indeed.

> *Dipetalonema perstans* is widespread in Nigeria, with a high incidence in the rain forest in the Cameroons where the vectors are *Culicoides austeni* and possibly *C. grahami* and in the Bauchi Plateau. It occurs as far north as Kano, but is almost absent in a rubber plantation in the Niger Delta. These anomalies are, as yet, unexplained.

> *Wucheretia bancrofti* is probably widespread, though its incidence and intensity in the savanna country and the Bauchi Plateau is evidently high, since the microfilariae may be found quite commonly in blood films taken in the Cameroons.

> *Onchocerca volvulus* is widespread in Nigeria, and in very different types of country. It occurs in the rain forest, in the small coastal villages and in the more mountainous regions of the Cameroons, the more open country near the escarpment at Eungu, in eastern Nigeria, and on the escarpment of the Bauchi Plateau and the surrounding more gently sloping savanna country, and in the dry savanna near Sokoto. Eye changes are common in the Cameroons, though there are few complaints of blindness. Blindness is very common in the Bauchi Plateau, and the changes are most marked in the deeper structures of the eye. Skin changes are very obvious.

> *Dipetalonema streptocerca* occurs in the Kumba and Mamfe divisions of the Cameroons. Little additional information is available at present.

(1) *Dipetalonema perstans* and *D. streptocerca*

The vector of *D. perstans* was determined in a study by Sharp (1928) at Mamfe (5° N and 9° E). He stated, the prevalence of *D. perstans* infection in Mamfe division was recorded in 1925 to be 77% positives among over 1,000 persons from the whole area including the open grassland country. In June 1926, among 100 persons who were specially drawn from the dense forest area, no less then 92 showed microfilariae of *D. perstans* in blood. One of the garden boys, Peter, was selected as the bait. Sharp states "As a bait Peter had one drawback—namely the fact that his skin was infested with embryos of *O. volvulus* as well as with the little orphan, *D. streptocerca*." The bait was exposed to the bite of the fly in a tent put up on the back veranda of the Medical Officer's house. The tent had a small opening from which the flies entered. The opening was closed at 2 a.m., and the flies were collected next morning. The majority of flies thus collected were *Culicoides austeni* Carter *et al.*, 1920 (A synonym of *Culicoides milnei* Austen, according to NICHOLAS *et al.*, 1955). They were dissected to see day-to-day metamorphosis of the larva. Sharp states, "In the stomach of *C. austeni* only the microfilariae of *D. perstans* were found and none of those of *D. streptocerca* or *O. volvulus* was demonsrated." The development of the larvae was traced day to day, and by the end of eighth day, the fully developed larvae were found in the head, neck, and proboscis of the fly.

In the examination of wild-caught flies, 16 of 227 (5.8%) were found infected. *C. grahami*, which were far fewer in number, were found in the tent on only nine occasions. During the three days of life of two of these flies, development of the filarial larvae proceeded as in *C. austeni*.

The validity of the conclusions made by SHARP (1928) was later doubted by CHARDOME & PEEL (1949), HENRARD & PEEL (1949), and BERGHE & CHARDOME (1952). They observed in Zaire that *C. grahami*, and also probably *C. austeni*, very rarely took up the microfilariae of *D. perstans*, but showed a marked selectivity for the microfilariae of *D. streptocerca* (see Section 7C.10). On these grounds, they suggested that since one of Sharp's volunteers also had an infection with *D. streptocerca*, Sharp had observed the development of *D. streptocerca* and not of *D. perstans*.

However, the findings of the Belgian workers in Zaire concerning the inability of *C. grahami* to ingest the microfilariae of *D. perstans* were disproved by NICHOLAS *et al.* (1952). These workers demonstrated that the flies took up the microfilariae of both *D. perstans* and *L. loa*; the numbers found in the blood meals corresponded to the numbers expected from the density in the peripheral blood of the donors.

HOPKINS & NICHOLAS (1952) demonstrated conclusively that larvae of *D. perstans* would develop completely both in clean-bred *C. austeni* and in wild *C. grahami*. The numbers of mature larvae found in *C. austeni* were approximately what were expected from the estimated numbers of microfilariae ingested by the flies, but those found in *C. grahami* were much less than that expected, indicating that the parasite was less adapted for development in the latter species of *Culicoides*. Later, NICHOLAS & KERSHAW (1954) demonstrated that both *C. austeni* and *C. grahami* would ingest the microfilariae of *D. perstans* in approximately the same numbers as might be expected from the amount of blood taken up by the flies and from the microfilarial density in the donors' blood.

Interesting results were obtained by KERSHAW *et al.* (1954a, b) on the distribution of the microfilariae of *D. streptocerca* and *O. volvulus* in the skin of man. The microfilariae of *D. streptocerca* occurred most numerously in the skin of the shoulders, then on the trunk, but were few or absent in the extremities, especailly in the forearms and in legs below the knee. Those of

O. volvulus were found in large numbers in the skin of the extermities, but less in that of the trunk. These findings were further confirmed by DUKE (1954, 1956).

Later investigations in the British Cameroons were conducted on the intake of microfilariae and the larval development of *D. perstans* and *D. streptocerca* in various species of *Culicoides*. NICHOLAS & KERSHAW (1964) observed, under experimental conditions, that the microfilariae of *D. perstans* were ingested at much higher rates by *C. milnei* than by *C. grahami*, and that subsequent survival of the larvae was lower in *C. grahami* than in *C. milnei*.

DUKE (1954), in Kumba, observed the uptake of the microfilariae of *D. streptocerca* by *C. grahami* with a hope of interpreting more correctly the contradictory results obtained by CHARDOME & PEEL (1949) and HENRARD & PEEL (1949) in Zaire. The volunteer had been subjected to multiple skin snips and had a known distribution of the microfilariae of *D. streptocerca* in the skin (they were confined to the neck, shoulder, chest, upper arms, and torso, and were absent from the forearms and legs). He showed an average of 79 microfilariae of *D. perstans* and about 1,200 microfilariae of *L. loa* in 50 mm³ blood samples, but no microfilariae of *O. volvulus* in the skin. Wild *C. grahami* were allowed to feed on this volunteer, and those which fed on his shoulder and chest, as well as those which fed on his legs below the knee, were collected separately for further studies. None out of 500 wild *C. grahami* collected in the same place and dissected was found harboring filarial larvae. On the other hand, of 110 *C. grahami* fed on the shoulder and chest of the volunteer and dissected immediately after engorgement, the number and percentage of those harboring microfilariae were 90 (81.8 %) for *D. streptocerca*, 5 (4.5 %) for *D. perstans*, and 12 (10.9 %) for *L. loa*. Of 100 flies which had fed on the legs below the knee, none had microfilariae of *D. streptocerca*, 5 had those of *D. perstans*, and 20 had those of *L. loa*. Of 109 flies fed on the shoulder and chest and dissected on the seventh or eighth day, 88 were negative and 21 contained a total of 29 motile larvae. However, none of 143 flies fed on the legs below the knee (*streptocerca*-free area) found infected when examined on the seventh or eighth day. It appeared that *C. grahami* was an efficient vector of *D. streptocerca* but not of *D. perstans*.

DUKE (1956) in Kumba, also, conducted experimental studies on the intake of microfilariae of *D. perstans* by *C. grahami* and *C. inornatipennis*, and their subsequent development. By means of a gravimetric method, it was shown that the mean volume of blood taken by *C. grahami* was 0.044 mm³, and that by *C. inornatipennis* was 0.065 mm³ at one meal. The actual intake of the microfilariae of *D. perstans* was less than expected in both species. Both species took in fewer microfilariae of *L. loa* than was expected. No flies took in the microfilariae of *O. volvulus*, although the parasite was present in the skin on which they were fed. Full development of the larvae of *D. perstans* was shown to take place in both *C. grahami* and *C. inornatopennis*.

The intake of the microfilariae of *D. streptocerca* by *C. milnei* (= *aus-*

teni) was investigated further by DUKE (1958). A volunteer, heavily infected with *D. streptocerca* and only lightly infected with *D. perstans*, was selected and fed upon by both *C. milnei* and *C. grahami*. Of 497 *C. milnei* fed on the back and shoulders, 8 ingested the microfilariae of *D. perstans* and 8 ingested those of *D. streptocerca*. On the other hand, 40 (17.7%) of 226 *C. grahami* fed on the same body site were found to contain the microfilariae of *D. streptocerca* and only 1 out of 265 had those of *D. perstans*. Thus, the number of microfilariae of *D. streptocerca* ingested by 505 *C. milnei* was less than one-tenth of that ingested by 266 *C. grahami*.

HOPKINS (1952) carried out studies on the biology of *Culicoides* in the British Cameroons and their possible role as vectors of *D. perstans*. Collections were made mostly in villages in and around Kumba and in the forests. Near villages, 98% of the day biters were *C. grahami*. but away from the villages, *C. inornatipennis* were more common. Near villages, the majority of the night-biting midges were *C. austeni*, but at one site near Tiko, an unidentified night-biting species was very common. The breeding places of *C. grahami* and *C. austeni* were found to be mainly in decaying banana and plantain stems, and these habitats were closely associated with human dwellings. No developing filarial larvae were found in 1,500 *C. grahami* dissected. Developing filarial larvae were found in 3 out of 70 *C. austeni* taken near a village. Hopkins stated that GORDON & KERSHAW, in 1949, dissected 405 *C. grahami* collected in the Kumba area, and found 2 infected.

The bionomics of *C. austeni*, *C. grahami*, and other related species of the biting midges in the British Cameroons were studied further by NICHOLAS (1953a). *C. austeni* is a night-biting species, while *C. grahami* bites mainly in the morning and in the evening, but not at night. *C. austeni* readily enters buildings and passes through nets in search of a blood meal, but other species are only occasionally found indoors. *C. grahami*, *C. inornatipennis*, and *C. fulvithorax* are found biting in the forest canopy. The biting density of *C. austeni* falls to a low level with the onset of the dry season, but no such diminution was observed in the biting density of *C. grahami*. *C. austeni* must take a blood meal before the eggs can develop, and under laboratory conditions, wild flies oviposit on the third or fourth night after taking a blood meal. The eggs hatched on the third day after being laid, and the development from eggs to adults in material from rotting banana stems was completed in 25 to 28 days.

The distribution of various species of *Culicoides* in the British Cameroons was investigated by NICHOLAS *et al.* (1953) and KERSHAW *et al.* (1953).

   (a). In the rain forest zone, *C. grahami*, *C. milnei*, *C. inornatipennis*, and *C. fulvithorax* were caught biting man. *C. grahami* was common in the villages and in the forest reserves. *C. milnei* was common in the villages but were much less common in the reserves. *C. inornatipennis*

was common in the forest reserve and in small villages where the forest had not been extensively cleared. *C. distinctipennis* was caught only in the vicinity of mangrove swamps. *C. fulvithorax* was not a common man biter, and was found in the forest reserves.
(b). In the mountain grassland zone, *C. grahami* was always found in the vicinity of streams, and no other *Culicoides* were caught.
(c). In the savanna zone with relict forest, *C. grahami* and *C. inornatipennis* were the only species found.
In general, all of the above four species found biting man were observed to be breeding in the rotting stems of bananas and plantains, and the extensive cultivation of such nonindigenous plants had increased the biting density of *C. milnei* near the villages.

The dispersal of *C. grahami* and *C. milnei* in the clearings from their breeding sites was investigated by NICHOLAS (1953b). In the case of *C. grahami*, there appeared to be a linear regression between the logarithms of the biting density and the distance from the breeding site (rotting vegetation found in banana plantations), and the biting density fell to one-tenth of its initial value at a distance of 370 yards; the maximum distance at which *C. grahami* was observed to bite was 400 yards. On the other hand, the numbers of *C. milnei* collected in this experiment were much less because of the onset of the dry season, but the fly was found biting at least 400 yards from the nearest breeding site.

KERSHAW *et al.* (1953) made surveys of the incidence of infections with *L. loa* and *D. perstans* in human populations in various zones of the British Cameroons. The incidence of infection with *D. perstans* was high in the rain forest, where *C. grahami*, *C. inornatipennis*, *C. austeni*, and *C. fulvithorax* were present. On the abrupt forest fringe, where the population of *C. milnei* was apparently low, the incidence fell at the approach to the fringe, though not so rapidly as infection with *L. loa*. In the gradual transition zone, where both *C. grahami* and *C. inornatipennis* occurred, infection was present, though invididual infections might have been acquired elsewhere. In the grassland, where only *C. grahami* was found, the infection was absent. (The incidence of infection with *L. loa* was also high in the rain forest, where *Chrysops silacea* and *C. dimidiata* was present, but none was found in the grassland.)

NICHOLAS *et al.* (1965) reported on the distribution of *Culicoides* spp. in the British Cameroons. The authors pointed out that although it had been demonstrated by HOPKINS & NICHOLAS (1952), KERSHAW *et al.* (1953), and NICHOLAS & KERSHAW (1954) that *C. austeni* (= a synonym of *C. milnei*) was the principal vector of *D. perstans* and that *C. grahami* was the principal vector of *D. streptocerca* by DUKE (1954), the role played by other species of *Culicoides* in the transmission of *D. perstans* and *D. streptocerca* still remained to be investigated. Besides the above two species, *C. inornatipennis* and *C. nigerniae* were observed to feed on man, and altogether, eight species of *Culicoides* collected from breeding sites in the neighborhood of Kumba were reared from immature stages. By re-examination of the

British Museum collections, the authors pointed out that *C. austeni* Carter *et al.*, 1920 was a synonym of *C. milnei*.

(2) *Loa loa*

A series of extensive studies was conducted in the British Cameroons and neighboring areas on the epidemiology of *L. loa* infection and its transmission by *Chrysops* spp. The essential results were presented in a symposium arranged by GORDON (1955), and more recently by DUKE (1972 *Trans. Roy. Soc. Trop. Med. & Hyg.* Vol. 49, pp 97–157). As stated previously, the endemic areas of loiasis in this region are confined mainly to the rain forest zones, with *Chrysops silacea* as the principal vector, but the epidemiology of the disease has been shown to be more complex than previously thought since several other *Chrysops* species were found to be involved in the transmission of human and simian strains of *Loa*.

KERSHAW (1950) conducted some basic investigations on survey methods for infections with *L. loa* and *D. perstans*. The periodicity of microfilariae was investigated on nine microfilaria carriers (five cases with mixed infection, and four cases with *D. perstans* only) by recording the numbers of microfilariae found in 50 mm³ blood samples, taken at hourly intervals for 36 hours. Also, 64 prisoners in the Kumba Jail were examined once a day over a period of 13 days, and 194 Sapele villagers were examined every day for four days by Knott's method (KNOTT, 1939); the number of cases positive for microfilariae of *L. loa* and *D. perstnas* were 15 and 61, respectively, on the first day in the prisoners, but increased to 21 *L. loa* cases on the ninth day and to 64 *D. perstans* cases on the fifth day. In the villagers, the numbers diagnosed as positive on the first day were 42 for *L. loa* and 4 for *D. perstans*, but were 44 and 4, respectively, on the fourth day. The daily variation of the microfilaria counts was also recorded and statistically analyzed. Comparison was made among the microfilaria counts in blood samples obtained from right and left thumbs and from right and left veins; both in *L. loa* and *D. perstans*, significantly higher counts were observed in the thumbs blood samples than those taken from the vein.

KERSHAW *et al.* (1953) reported on the incidence of *L. loa* and *D. perstans* infections in relation to the ecological zones of human and vector habitats. The incidence of *L. loa* infection in man was found to be high in the rain forest zone where *Chrysops silacea* and *Ch. dimidiata* (both proven vectors) were present. In the abrupt forest fringe, where an additional species, *C. zahri* also occurred, the incidence was lower. In the gradual transition zone, and in the grassland where the breeding of *Chrysops* was unknown or absent, the infection was also absent.

DUKE & MOORE (1961) conducted a trial for controlling the transmission of loiasis in a rubber estate at Sapele, Nigeria, by the administration of DEC to the microfilaria carriers. In the pretreatment survey, 210 (12.9%) of 1,633 estate workers and 245 (12.9%) villagers examined showed microfilariae of *L. loa* in 50mm³ blood samples, with geometric mean numbers per positive film of 30 and 32, respectively. DEC treatment was given to

427 positive cases, at the dose of three tablets (each 200 mg) per day for 20 days, followed by a maintenance dose of one tablet per month administered on payday to only the estate workers. In the examinations made one month after completion of the original course, 15 out of 171 originally positive cases among the workers and 19 of 149 originally positive cases among the villagers were still positive, with geometric mean numbers of 8 and 15, respectively. In the later examinations made seven months after completion of the original course, the same positive figures were 20 of 109 in the workers and 38 of 118 in the villagers, with the geomctric means of 6 and 12, respectively. The drug was shown to be safely administered and to be efffective in reducing the infection potential to from 2 to 12% of the pretreatment level. However, about one-third of the population, when advised of the risk, refused to cooperate in the trial. Therefore, out of the total population of 5,120 in this area, 658 (11.1%) were estimated to show microfilariae before the treatment, 252 (4.9%) after one month, and 320 (6.3%) after seven months. The overall infection rate of *Chrysops silacea* in 1958, before the treatment, was 6.1% (798 infected out of 12,982 dissected), but in 1959, after the treatment, the rate dropped to 3.1% (379 of 12,315) or about one-half of the pretreatment level. In *C. dimidiata*, the infection rate was 2.0% (100 of 4,982) before the treatment and 2.2% (131 of 6,207) after; this suggests that *C. dimidiata* probably acquires infection from nonhuman reservoirs.

(3) *O. Volvulus*

ANDERSON *et al.* (1974a, b) reported on the results of detailed epidemiological and clinical surveys of onchocerciasis in Cameroon rain-forest and savanna villages. The total populations aged 5 years and over in 22 village groups were surveyed using standard techniques, and skin and eye lesions in 2,678 persons infected with *O. volvulus* were compared with those in 1,156 persons in whom the parasite was not detected. (a) Apart from itching and acute papular eruption, the signs in the skin and lymphatic system were (1) skin atrophy, (2) skin thickning due to lymphoedema, (3) skin depigmentation, (4) lymphoedema of external genitalia, (5) inguinal or femoral lymphadenopathy, and (6) hanging groin. (b) Apart from the presence of microfilariae in the cornea, anterior chamber, retrolental space and vitreous, the important ocular signs were (1) punctate keratitis (snow-flake, fluffy opacities), (2) sclerosing keratitis, (3) iritis with its sequelae, (4) post-neuritic and/or consecutive optic atrophy, and (5) choroidoretinitis. Blindness due to onchocerciasis was seen before the age of 20 years, and in persons aged 40 years and over it reached levels of 4.2% in the rain-forest and 14.4% in the savanna. In five selected hyperendemic savanna villages 34.1% of males aged 40 years and over were blind. These clinical signs were generally more severe in the savanna than in the rain-forest.

(B) Reports from the former French Cameroon

ROUSSEAU (1919) quoted some early records of filariasis in the German

Protectorate stage. In *Medizinische Berichte über deutschen Schutzgebiete 1909 to 1910*, ZIEMENN described, "*Filaria volvulus, F. bancrofti*, and *F. perstans* are highly prevalent in Douala; onchocerciasis is very common in Ebolowa; *F. diurna* and *F. perstans* are found in most adults in Dume." In the same series of reports for 1910 to 1911, WALDOW & PISTNER described filariasis in Douala, Kribi, and Edeah, with special reference to elephantiasis of the scrotum and legs. STECHEL discussed the differentiation of *perstans*, *loa*, and *volvulus*, and stated that elephantiasis also existed at various grades in Maka, Baia, and Kaka. HAUBOLD, in Moulundu, examined 215 recruited as railroad laborers, and found the infection of *F. perstans* in 80% and that of *F. diurna* (= *loa*) in 49%, including a mixed infection of 39%.

ROUSSEAU (1919) made examinations of blood in the hospital of Douala. Microfilariae of *L. loa* or *D. perstans* were found in the majority of people from the coastal region. Of 132 persons examined by day (from 9 a.m. to 5 p.m.), 48 had microfilariae. Elephantiasis was not common in Douala, but one or two cases were always found in the surrounding villages. *O. volvulus* was commonly found. He examined the blood of elephantiasis cases, but the only microfilariae he could find were those of *D. perstans*.

An extensive survey of the distribution of filariasis in Cameroon was reported by LANGUILLON (1957). The regions surveyed were: a) northern Cameroon, b) Adamaoua, the savanna region on the northern edge of the forest region in south, c) the mountain region in the west, and e) the forest region in the south. In total, 2,425 night blood samples (one thick smear), 7,271 day blood samples and 4,076 skin scarifications were examined for microfilariae. Altogether, five species were demonstrated, *W. bancrofti* mainly in the night blood, *D. perstans* and *L. loa* mainly in the day blood, and *O. volvulus* and *D. streptocerca* from the skin.

W. bancrofti: A large endemic area was discovered in northern Cameroon, where all of the five villages surveyed were positive; if Mokolo village, where the incidence was only 2.7% (4 positives out of 150) is excluded, the other four villages (Guider, Poli, Diamare, and Fort Foureau) show a gross positive rate of 18.2% (189 positives of 1,037 persons examined).

W. bancrofti was not found in the other three regions, with an exception in Douala Village in the forest region where 6 out of 88 persons (6.8%) were positive, and one *An. gambiae* was found to harbor filaria larvae. However, no cases of elephantiasis and adenitis were encountered in the north. The author considered that the presence of *W. bancrofti* was not a suffient factor in the etiology of elephantiasis, but the association with streptococci common in hot and wet countries was absolutely necessary, as demonstrated in the West Indies and in the Pacific.

D. perstans: This was found in all the regions, and an especially high incidence of 78% was seen in the southern forest region. In contrast to *W. bancrofti*, the incidence was lowest in the northern region, and a gradual decrease in incidence was observed as the locality proceeded towards the north, though an increase to 27% was seen in the western mountain range. Two forms of microfilariae were differenciated: the short, spiral form measuring about 110 μ, and the long, straight form about 200 μ long; the former was found in the forest region, and the latter in the savanna region.

L. loa: The incidence was generally lower than *D. perstans*, but exhibited a similar trend, in that the infection was highest in the forest region, becoming lower in the savanna region of Adamaoue, but slightly higher in the mountain region. Again, in contrast to *W. bancrofti*, no cases were found in northern Cameroon. The parasite is known to cause transitory edema, and eye complications when passing under the conjunctiva; these are frequent in Cameroon. In Europeans, it often causes prurigo on the skin of the shoulder, trunk, and hip.

O. volvulus: The incidence was found to be highest in the savanna region (19.6%), followed by the mountain region (11.0%), and the forest region (4.7%). Carriers of skin nodules were also very common, and of 1,722 persons examined, 19.6% had skin nodules and 20.0% had the microfilariae of *O. volvulus*.

D. streptocerca: This was shown to be endemic only in the forest region (8.7%), and no carriers were found in the mountain and savanna regions.

BECQUET *et al.* (1961) conducted a survey of malaria and filariasis in the region of Bahang (Bamileke, Cameroon), in the southern forest region. Of 412 day blood samples examined, 89 were positive for malaria parasites, of which 80 had *Plasmodium falciparum* and 14 had *Pl. malariae* (5 had mixed infection). Out of the same day blood samples, 53 harbored microfilariae of *D. perstans* and 11 had those of *L. loa*, with rates of 12.8% and 2.6%, respectively. Eight of them had mixed infections of the two filariae. No night blood examinations and skin scarifications were conducted.

7C.5 Central African Republic

Ubangi-Shari, or the Central African Republic, was the major part of the former French Equatorial Africa. It is situated between 3°N and 12° N, and, 14° E and 27° E, and has an area of 620,333 km² and a population of 1,520,000 (1970 estimate).

OUZILLEAU (1913) reported on filariasis in the region of the M'Bomou (Bomou) River in central Africa. The proportion of elephantiasis in this region varied from 0.3% to 3% according to the districts. Three human filariae had been known here: *D. perstans*, *L. loa*, and *O. volvulus*; *W. bancrofti* was absent in examinations of 1,500 blood samples collected by day and 400 blood samples collected at night. *D. perstans* was found in 64% of the native people over the age of 10 years. *O. volvulus* was found in

45% of the general population. *L. loa* was lower in incidence, and was found in only 16% of the people. Microfilariae of *L. loa* were found in 30% of persons with those of *D. perstans*, but only in 10% of those harboring *O. volvulus*. Adults of *L. loa* were frequently found in the subcutaneous tissue during surgial operations for hydrocele and hernia.

Because the distribution of elephantiasis was restricted to certain areas in this region, and *L. loa* and *D. perstans* were found almost all over central Africa, these two parasites were excluded from consideration as possible causes of elephantiasis. On the other hand, large numbers of microfilariae of *O. volvulus* were found by puncture of the inguinal lymph glands in all of the 79 elephantiasis cases examined. By the consistent presence of *O. volvulus* microfilariae in the local lymph glands of persons affected by genital elephantiasis, and by the coincidence of the distribution of elephantiasis and *O. volvulus* in this region, Ouzilleau concluded that *O. volvulus* was probably the causative agent of the local elephantiasis in M'Bomou.

7C.6 Equatorial Guinea

A republic (former Spanish Guinea) consisting of (1) Rio Muni Province, situated between Cameroon and Gabon, with an area of 25,994 km² and a population of 203,000 (1968 estimate), and (2) the island of Fernando Po with an area of 2,017 km² and a population of 61,197 (1960 census).

On Fernando Po, DENECKE (1941) reported that clinical filariasis was common among hospital patients in Santa Isabel, but microfilariae were only rarely found.

In Rio Muni, TOUMANOFF (1958) conducted a study on the transmission of filariasis in an area near the mouth of the Nunez River. Examination of the night blood of 250 persons in the coastal villages of Kamsar and Tassi-bili revealed 12 carriers (4.8%) of *W. bancrofti* and 5 carriers of *D. perstans*. Among mosquitoes collected in this area during December (dry season), *An. gambiae* var. *melas* and *Mansonia uniformis* were found infected with filaria larvae in the head and thorax. Also, *M. uniformis* collected in the northeast part of Rio Muni were infected. These two species were considered to be important vectors of *W. bancrofti* during the dry season.

7C.7 Sao Tomé and Principe

These islands in the Gulf of Guinea are a Portuguese overseas province. São Tomé is situated on the equator and Príncipe at about 1°N. Their combined area is 963 km² and combined population, 61,000 (1970).

FRAGA DE AZEVEDO *et al.* (1960) conducted surveys of filariasis on various groups of people in Príncipe. In their 1956 blood survey, a total of 4,014 persons were examined; 104 (2.6%) were found positive for microfilariae of *W. bancrofti* and 1,427 (35.6%) for those of *D. perstans*. The microfilaremia rates for *W. bancrofti* were by the order of people from Mozambique (7.7%), from São Tomé (3.1%), from Angola (1.9%), natives of Príncipe (1.7%), from Cape Verde (0.8%) and Europeans (0%). A high incidence of *D. perstans* infection was observed in all groups except Europeans, who were, however, infected at a rate of 7.4%.

Similar results were obtained in another survey conducted in 1958. Microfilariae of *D. perstans* were found at high rates among the natives of Príncipe and also among those from São Tomé. The incidence by the age groups was shown in a table. Microfilariae of *W. bancrofti* were found in the night blood samples of 15 (11.0%) of 136 adult natives of Príncipe, 13 (21.7%) of 60 persons from São Tomé, 35 (7.3%) of 482 from Cape Verde, 141 (41.8%) of 337 from Mozambique and 5 (50%) of 10 from Angola. Elephantiasis was fairly common among the infected people.

7C.8 Gabon

Gabon is situated on the western coast of central Africa between 2°N and 4°S. It has an area of 264,900 km² and a population of 500,000 (1970 estimate).

GALLIARD (1932) conducted a survey of filariasis in the southwestern part of Gabon during 1930. The area surveyed was between 1° S and 3° S, with the coast to the west, Ogooué River to the north, N'gounie River to the east, and Nyanga River to the south. The area was divided by two mountain ranges, and covered by forest or savanna. A total of 880 persons (137 adults males, 300 adult females and 443 children) were examined; 52.1% of them were found infected with *D. perstans*, and 10.4% with *L. loa*, including 6.3% with mixed infection. The microfilaremia rates for *D. perstans* were 41.5% in males, 53.5% in females, and 51% in children, those for *L. loa* were 22.6% in males, 8.2% in females, and 5.7% in children. *L. loa* was highest in the forest region, while *D. perstans* was highest in the savanna and the plain regions. No *W. bancrofti* carrier was found in this survey. VOYEL & RIOU (1939) reported that *W. bancrofti* cases were said to be abundant in the Adoumas region.

7C.9 People's Republic of the Congo

A republic in equatorial central Africa bounded by the Atlantic Ocean, Gabon, Cameroon, Central African Republic, Zaire, and Angola. The country is situated between 4°N and 5°S, has an area of 342,000 km², and a population of 1,089,300 (1970).

Information on filariasis in this country is scant. According to HAMON *et al.* (1967), the annual medical reports of 1955 to 1961 mention many cases of bancroftian filariasis. Hydrocele and elephantiasis are also known to occur in some parts.

7C.10 Zaire

Zaire (former Democratic Republic of the Congo, or Belgian Congo from 1908 to 1960) is a large, equatorial, African country situated between 5°N and 13°S. It has an area of 2,343,000 km² and a population of 16,585,944 (1970). The country occupies the greater part of the Congo River Basin, consisting mostly of low plateau, with marshes along the Congo in the northwest, mountain ranges in southeast with several peaks of about 6,000 feet, higher ranges along west shore of Lake Tanganyika, and high mountains on east

The country is divided into a Federal District and eight provinces: Bandundu, Bas-Zaïre, Équateur, Haute-Zaïre, Kasai-Occidental, Kasai-Oriental, Kivu, and Shaba. All of the five human filarial species are known to be endemic, and many important contributions have been made from Zaire on the epidemiology of these filarial infections.

An early record of a filariasis survey was reported by BRUMPT (1904), who made a long journey from Uele (Ouéllé), Ubangi (Oubangui), the upper, middle and lower Congo, as well as from upper to lower Kasai. A total of 1,225 persons were examined, and microfilariae of *Filaria diurna* (*L. loa*) were found in 224 (18.3%) and those of *D. perstans* in 597 (48.7%); 111 cases among them were mixed infections. *W. bancrofti* infection was not found in this survey, although night blood examinations were made on 15 persons, including six cases of elephantiasis.

(1) *Wuchereria bancrofti*:
According to VAN OYE & PIERQUIN (1961), who made a comprehensive review of the history of research on filariasis in Zaire (Congo), microfilariae of *Filaria nocturna* (= *W. bancrofti*) were discovered first in 1899 by VAN CAMPENHOUT, in the blood taken at 9 p.m. from a 14-year-old boy, a native of Bounda. VAN CAMPENHOUT & DREYPONDT also described, in the *First Report of 'Laboratoire Médical de Léopoldville'* (1899 to 1900), the presence of "microfilaires nocturnes" in Bas-Zaire. However, later blood surveys carried out at night by DUBOIS, in Pawa, and by CHESTERMANN, in Yakusu, did not show the presence of *W. bancrofti*. VAN DER BERGH (1941) stated that *W. bancrofti* was never confirmed, with precision, from Congo. It was also stated by AUGUSTINE (1951), "Contrary to apparent current belief, it (*W. bancrofti*) does not extend across tropical Africa, *i.e.*, it does not occur in the central Congo areas."

However, HENRARD *et al.* (1946, quoted by VAN OYE & PIERQUIN, 1961) recognized that *An. funestus* dissected at Matadi was frequently infected with filaria larvae; in an examination of specimens captured in the natives' hospital in Matadi and in the settlements near the Angolan border, 40 (4.9%) out of 820 mosquitoes dissected harbored mature larvae. They further conducted blood examinations of inpatients of the hospital in Matadi, and found microfilariae of *W. bancrofti* in 47 cases out of 1,500 persons examined.

In the meantime, two cases of *W. bancrofti* carriers were found out of 50 adult females examined by these authors at Ipamu, on the left bank of the Kasai River, in the Kwango region. They also found 14 cases of *W. bancrofti* carriers among 1,824 adult patients examined at the natives' hospital in Kinshasa (Léopoldville). They further confirmed that *An. funestus* was the most abundant mosquito species in the regions of Matadi and Songololo, and was the principal vector of *W. bancrofti*.

The results accumulated by medical workers in the Province of Léopoldville showed that the districts of Matadi, Thysville, Luozi, Idiofa, and Bandundu (Banningville) were infested by *W. bancrofti*. The same microfilariae were found also in Mbandaka (Coquilhatville).

FAIN (1947) reported on the results of filaria surveys conducted in the region of Bandundu (Banningville). All of the five human filaria species were detected in this region. *W. bancrofti* carriers were found in 169 (6.7%) of 2,510 persons examined. They were distributed along various tributaries of the Congo River, and the incidence by the river basin was 20% for the Kwango River, 3.4% for the Wamba River, 12% for the Kwilu River, 2.4% for the Inzia River, and 3.3% for the Kasai River. Among the villages along the Kwango River, the southern half showed a very high incidence of 30.9% (96 positives out of 311 examined), but the northern half had only one case (0.6%) out of 175 persons examined, and the endemic area seemed to be clearly separated from the nonendemic area by the river. In the southern and upper stream part, the incidence was 30% for *W. bancrofti*, 40% for *D. perstans*, 3% for *O. volvulus*, and 9% for *D. streptocerca*. Out of 277 persons (101 males and 176 females) examined in four villages in the endemic area, microfilariae of *W. bancrofti* were found in 87 (31.4%), lymphadenitis of the groin in 72 (26.0%), hydrocele in 13 (12.9% of the males), and elephantiasis of the legs in 11 (4.0%).

CHARDOME & PEEL (1949) examined 249 prisoners in Mbandaka (Coquilhatville). In the blood specimens collected at night the microfilariae of *W. bancrofti* were found in 4.81%, *D. streptocerca* in 44.98%, *D. perstans* in 55.02%, *O. volvulus* in 19.25%, and *L. loa* in 4.81% of those examined.

BELLEFONTAINE (1949) reported on the presence of a focus of *W. bancrofti* infection in the Territory of Yahuma, Basoko district. Examinations of night blood and skin scarification were conducted in 13 villages. Out of 54 adult males examined, 25 (46.3%) were positive for *W. bancrofti* in the night blood specimens, and 49 (90.7%) showed *O. volvulus* in the skin. These villages, along a road south of Yahuma, were thus recognized to be in a highly endemic area of both bancroftian filariasis and onchocerciasis.

LEJEUNE (1956, quoted by VAN OYE & PIERQUIN, 1961), in Kasongo-Lunda, observed that out of 188 cases of inguinal hernia operations, 12 cases had funiculitis with scrotal swelling typical to the lesion due to *W. bancrofti* infection. In 1957, a woman from the Territory of Bumba visited the Institute of Tropical Medicine in Léopoldville and was diagnosed to be a case of bancroftian filariasis. In a communication with the provincial doctor in Mbandaka (Coquilhatville, on the middle stream of the Congo River), he was informed that the presence of bancroftian filariasis is well known in Bumba, and the annual report for the province recorded 58 cases, 45 in Bumba, 2 in Banzyville, 5 in Gemena, and 6 in Ikela territories. In the eastern province, VAN OYE found the microfilariae in a patient of chyluria, in Yakasu, in 1947; BELLEFONTAINE (1949) reported on the presence of *W. bancrofti* infection in Yahuma, in the district of Basoko.

An endemic focus of bancroftian filariasis was reported by BROWNE (1960) from the Kasai-Oriental. The villages affected were all situated on the banks of the Congo River, to the east and west of Lomami, at about 1° N and 24°E., at an altitude of 410 m above sea level, and within the tropical rain forest. However, forest villages situated a few miles from the river were almost completely free from bancroftian filariasis, and the forest people who migrated to the river bank and established themselves there were found to have the same high incidence.

Nocturnal blood examinations by the three-drop method revealed a bancroftian microfilaremia rate of 63% in adult males, 67% in adult females, 9% in young people between 16 and 20, and 4% in children. Microfilariae of *W. bancrofti* were seen only on two occasions in the midday blood examinations of 294 adult persons. In an adult male population of 1,853, hydrocele was seen in 20%, inguinal lymphadenopathy in 27%, and chronic funiculitis in 68%. Elephantiasis had a low incidence and was of slight importance compared with hydrocele. *D. perstans* was present in the blood at a rate of 65% and *L. loa* at a rate of 8%. Onchocerciasis had a comparatively low incidence, and those with microscopic or clinical evidence totaled 12.1% of adult males living to the west of Lomami and 9.7% to the east of Lomami. *D. perstans* was seen only occasionally.

(2) *Dipetalonema perstans*:

According to the review by VAN OYE & PIERQUIN (1961), the presence of two varieties of microfilariae differing in size: one about 100 μ long and another about 180 μ long, were recognized by FIRKET in 1895 while investigating the microfilariae in the blood of sleeping sickness patients in Zaire (Congo). The microfilariae of *D. perstans* were confirmed by VAN CAMPENHOUT in 1899, in Boma, in a native prisoner from Banana. He also recognized the occurrence of small microfilariae usually associated with the typical form of *D. perstans*. The small form of microfilariae was also recorded by BRUMPT (1949), according to his textbook, in about one-tenth of the carriers of *D. perstans* in the Congo Basin. CHARDOME & PEEL (1951b, quoted by VAN OYE & PIERQUIN, 1961) reported that they found two different adult filariae corresponding to the short and the long form of the microfilariae.

FAIN (1947), in his report on the distribution of filariasis in the region around Bandundu, described that *D. perstans* was fairly evenly distributed in this region, with an overall incidence in about 60% of the adult natives. Of a total of 2,510 persons examined, 1,502 (59.8%) were found to be the carriers of microfilariae; the incidence was 68.6% (1,003 of 1,463) in male adults and 47.7% (499 of 1,047) in female adults. The incidence was 50% in the villages situated between the Wamba and Kwango Rivers, 67% in those between the Wamba and Inzia Rivers, and 67% in those between the Kwilu and Kasai Rivers. The infection was very high in certain villages on the banks of the Kasai River, and microfilaria carriers with over 1,000 per thick smear were not uncommon. However, no pathological manifestations were observed even in those harboring such high microfilarial loads.

(3) *Dipetalonema streptocerca*:

The human parasite, *D. streptocerca*, which was described first by MACFIE & CORSON (1922) in Gold Coast, was reported from Congo by DUBOIS & VITALE (1938) in the region of Bentngwe-Medjedje in Nepoko, Kasai-Oriental. Numerous microfilariae were discovered upon biopsy of the skin of leprosy patients. In the same region, DUBOIS *et al.* (1939) made skin biopsies and found *D. streptocerca* in 9 cases and *O. volvulus* in 6 cases out of 25 patients with genital elephantiasis; they also found 20 cases with *D. streptocerca*, and 3 or 4 cases with *O. volvulus* out of 20 cases with elephantiasis of the legs. In a control group of 16 apparently healthy persons, 16 had *D. streptocerca* and one had *O. volvulus*. The authors suspected that *D. streptocerca* might be a cause of elephantiasis of the legs, although no definite conclusion could be made from this study.

RODHAIN (1943) further reported on the presence of *D. streptocerca* in the regions of Lisala and Basankusu in the Province of Équateur. WANSON *et al.* found *D. streptocerca* in Léopoldville in 1945, and in Kibunzi in Bas-Zaïre, in 1946 (quoted by VAN OYE & PIERQUIN, 1961).

PEEL & CHARDOME (1946) conducted a study on filariae of chimpanzees, *Pan paniscus* and *Pan satyrus*, captured in the Province of Équateur, and discovered, for the first time, the adult worms of *D. streptocerca*. Two female worms were collected from the subcutaneous tissue of a chimpanzee, *Pan paniscus*. Microfilariae of *D. streptocerca* were also found in the skin of 6 out of 12 chimpanzees examined. Three new species were described from the chimpanzees: *Microfilaria rodhaini*, *Microfilaria binucleata*, and *Dipetalonema vanhoofi*.

FAIN (1947), in his extensive studies on the epidemiology of filariasis in the territory of Bandundu (Banningsville), found microfilariae of *D. streptocerca* in 308 (12.3%) cases out of a total of 2,510 persons examined. The incidence in males was 17% and was much higher than that of the 5% in females. The distribution of *D. streptocerca* was quite uneven; it was absent in areas along the Kasai River and the villages situated between this and the Kwili River, only two cases were found in areas along the Kwili River, and only five cases along its tributary, the Inzia River. However, the villages situated south of the territory between the Inzia and Wamba Rivers were highly infested. In the hinterland of Wamba-Kwango, about one-quarter of the adults were infected. In two villages on the bank of the Wamba, the incidence was as high as 75%. The author also pointed out that the incidence of goiter was high where *D. streptocerca* was prevalent; however, no special clinical manifestations were observed among the people infected with the parasite.

DUBOIS (1948) made a survey of blood and skin microfilariae in 13 localities around Pawa (Nepoko) in the northeastern province. Of a total of 266 persons examined, 197 (74.1%) were positive for *D. perstans*, 69 (25.9 %) for *D. streptocerca*, 61 (22.9%) for *L. loa*, and 21 (7.9%) for *O. volvulus*. With the exception of *O. volvulus*, which was found restricted to two localities, the other three filariae were positive in all the localities surveyed.

CHARDOME & PEEL (1949) conducted a survey of filariasis in the people of Avenue Boyera of Mbandaka (Coquilhatville). Of 290 persons (142 male adults, 126 female adults, and 22 children) examined, 79 (27.2%) had the microfilariae of *D. streptocerca*, 101 (34.8%) had those of *D. perstans*, 23 (7.9%) had those of *O. volvulus*, and 32 (11.0%) had those of *L. loa*. The microfilaria rates of 249 prisoners examined in the same city by day and by night, respectively, were 34.50% and 44.98% for *D. streptocerca*, 53.81% and 55.02% for *D. perstans*, 16.46% and 19.25% for *O. volvulus*, 8.00% and 4.81% for *L. loa*, and 0% and 4.81% for *W. bancrofti*. In examinations of children in three-quarters of this city, the microfilariae of *D. streptocerca* and *D. perstans*, respectively, were found in 204 (55.4%) and 218 (59.2%) of 368 persons in Bofidji-Ouest, 85 (46.4%) and 87 (47.5%) of 183 persons in Bofidji-Est, and 27 (19.9%) and 12 (8.8%) of 136 persons in Boluki.

These authors visited altogether 70 villages in the Coquilhatville region, and conducted over 8,000 skin scarification examinations. As a result, it was demonstrated that *D. streptocerca* was not present in villages on the bank of the Congo River, but became more prevalent towards the interior, as the distance from the river increased.

While staying in Coquilhatville, these authors carried out examinations of bloodsucking insects for infection with filaria larvae. The specimens included five species of mosquitoes, one species of *Phlebotomus*, one species of *Simulium*, and three species of *Culicoides*. In experimental infections, the microfilariae of *D. perstans* were frequently seen in *C. fatigans*, and although they survived up to four days in the stomach, no further development was observed.

Three species of *Culicoides* were found from this region: *C. austeni*, *C. grahami*, and *C. inornatipennis*. Their biting activity was highest in the morning from 6:30 to 9 a.m., and they could be easily collected while they were taking blood from microfilaria carriers. They were found to ingest microfilariae of *D. streptocerca*, but never those of *D. perstans* in the blood. This result was repeatedly confirmed by experimental feedings on carriers of either or both parasites. It was further observed that larvae of *D. streptocerca* completed their development in seven to eight days after being ingested by *C. grahami*, and reached a length of 574 μ and a width of 21 μ.

Further investigations were conducted by HENRARD & PEEL (1949) on the development of *D. streptocerca* in *C. grahami*. They selected Gombe-Masaka Village for the test station, where the microfilaremia rates of the adults (above the age of 20 years) were 55.2% (37 of 67 persons examined) for *D. streptocerca*, 31.3% (21/67) for *D. perstans*, 20.9% (14/67) for *L. loa* and 3.0% (2/67) for *O. volvulus*. Experimental feedings of *C. grahami* were conducted repeatedly on microfilaria carriers of either *D. streptocerca* or *D. perstans*, or those carrying both, and the results always showed that only those of *D. streptocerca* were ingested by the fly; none of the microfilariae of *D. perstans* were found in the stomach of the flies after they fed on the carriers. The development of *D. streptocerca* to mature larvae was found to be completed in the flies in about eight days. Also, by dissection of wild-caught *C. grahami*, the natural infection of larvae in the thorax or head was seen in 9 (1.2%) of 737 flies dissected.

From these results, they concluded that *Culicoides* was the vector of *D. streptocerca*, but not *D. perstans* as reported by SHARP (1928); by analysis of his work, these authors believed that the development of larvae seen by Sharp in *C. austeni* was probably that of *D. streptocerca* but not of *D. perstans*.

As for the investigation of the vector of *D. perstans*, HENRARD & PEEL (1949) observed a partial development of larvae in *Sarcopsylla penetrans*, but no development in *S. damnosum*. WANSON & PEEL (1949), in Kinshasa, reported that they did not see any *Culicoides* in this endemic area of *D. perstans*, and in examinations of the stomach content of large numbers of mosquitos, they could find its microfilariae in only two species of *Mansonioides* (*M. uniformis* and *M. africanus*) but not in *An. gambiae*, *An. moucheti*, or in other species. Also, no complete larval development was seen in experimental infections of *D. perstans* in various species of mosquitoes, including *An. gambiae*, *An. moucheti*, *Ae. aegypti*, and *C. fatigans*.

The occurrence of *D. streptocerca* in high densities in the region of Mbandaka (Coquilhatville) was noted by CHARDOME & PEEL (1949). VAN DEN BERGHE & CHARDOME (1952) reviewed the distribution and incidence of *D. streptocerca* infection in Zaire. The central area had by far the highest incidence, and it was estimated that practically 100% of adults south of Mbandaka and in the middle part of the Congo River harbored the parasite. The territories around Bandundu (Banningville) gave a microfilaria rate of 12% (Fain, 1947). In the lower Congo, the percentages ranged from 13.75 to 19.0%. More to the east, in the region of Idiofa, the incidence was reduced to 2.5%; it fell to 0% around Lusambo. No cases were found in the upper Katanga around Lubumbashi (Elisabethville), nor in the region along Lake Tanganyika. At Kindu, on the upper Congo

River, a very light incidence of 0.5% was observed. More to the north, in a region situated south of Kisangani (Stanleyville), the percentage rose to 31.0%, while to the east around Opienge, some 200 km from Kisangani, only 2.5% could be found. However, in the northeastern province of Uelé, the incidence was 24%. Since *D. streptocerca* was not discovered in Sudan (WOODMAN, 1949), Uelé seemed to constitute the northeastern limit of its distribution.

FAIN (1974) described a new species of filaria, *Dipetalonema semiclarum*, based on microfilariae found in the blood and skin of 52 people in three villages in Equateur Province, Zaire. (see Section 4B. Addendum).

(4) *Loa loa*:

According to VAN OYE & PIERQUIN (1961), microfilariae of *L. loa* was first described from Zaire by Van Campenhout in 1899, from the blood of a girl in Boma using name of *Filaria diurna*. Van Campenhout observed a number of cases affected by abrupt edematous swellings and attributed this to *Filaria loa*. The adults were also found in the eye. In 1906, BRODEN observed the microfilariae of *F. diurna* in the blood of a missionary who had stayed in Bamania and Baku, in the Province of Équateur. MOUCHET (1913) reported that microfilaria carriers were very common in Kinshasa. DUBOIS (1917) found *L. loa* at Amadi in Uele. SANDGROUND (1936) found it in Kama, in the district of Maniema.

In the review by VAN OYE & PIERQUIN (1961), *L. loa* was found to be widely distributed in Zaire, in the Provinces of Léopoldville, Coquilhatville, Stanleyville, Kasai, and Kivu. Although it was said that the parasite did not exist in Kantanga, Rwanda, or Burundi (Ruanda-Urundi), the Annual Reports of Medical Service of Congo and Ruanda-Urundi stated that numerous cases occur in all the provinces. In recent years, reports were made by a number of workers in Zaire on the nervous and psychiatric manifestations, including fatal cases of encephalitis, with the invasion of microfilariae of *L. loa* in the cerebrospinal fluid (BROWNE, 1954; DUBOIS *et al.*, 1955; JANSSENS, 1952; JANSSENS *et al.*, 1953; and KIVITS, 1952).

As for chemotherapy, LAGRANGE (1949) and WANSON (1949) reported that DEC was effective in clearing microfilariae of *L. loa* and *D. perstans* from the circulating blood, and in curing the skin swellings; however, its effects on adult worms remained unknown.

A more recent review on the distribution of loiasis and its vectors for the whole region of Zaire and Rwanda was made by FAIN (1969). In general, the endemic areas were confined mainly to the tropical forest zones and its edges, corresponding to the habitats of the principal vectors, *Chrysops silacea* and *Ch. dimidiata*. There were two important endemic foci with extremely high incidences: one in Uele near the northeastern border, and another in Mayumbe near the mouth of the Congo River. The disease was also spread in the surrounding regions at medium to low grades, for example, in most parts of the northeastern half of the country, as well as in the region of the lower Congo Basin.

The region of Mayumbe, in the lower Congo Basin, constitutes a part of the large equatorial forest zone of central Africa, and is close to the capital, Kinshasa (Léopoldville). Loiasis is hyperendemic in some of the villages, with positive rates of over 50%, or sometimes as high as 90% in the natives. In Kangu, KIVITS (1952) reported on four fatal cases of encephalitis with invasion of microfilariae of *L. loa* into the cerebrospinal fluid. FAIN (1969) also stated that such encephalitis cases are found in all the hospitals in this region, especially in chidren from 5 to 12 years of age. In most of these cases, the symptom appears soon after taking diethylcarbamazine (DEC), which is sold freely in the pharmacies and which people frequently use for various reasons. The two principal vectors breed abundantly and frequently attack man in the region from Boma to Kinshasa.

The distribution of loiasis, as well as its vectors, is interrupted by the vast dry plateau of Bateke, which extends from east and northeast of Kinshasa up to the border of Zambia and Tanzania. The absence of the two *Chrysops* species in Bandundu, situated 250 km east of Kinshasa, was confirmed by FAIN (1947a, c). Both the disease and the vectors are also unknown from Luluanbourg and Elisabethville (now Lumbashi) Provinces. In the Province of Coquilhatville (Équateur), FAIN *et al.* (1969) observed that the incidence of *L. loa* was low in villages about 300 km east of Mbandaka, right in the center of the vast flooded forest called "Cuvette Centrale."

In the Haut-Zaïre Province, loiasis is estimated to be highly endemic in the district of Uele, and also in the Kisangani (Stanleyville) and Kibali-Ituri districts. In Kivu Province, PEEL *et al.* (1952) found an incidence of 3.2% for *L. loa* among 1,682 native people examined in Bukavu.

FAIN *et al.* (1974) conducted microfilaria surveys (day and night blood examinations, skin snip examinations) of people in Mayumbe region. Altogether 2,476 persons in 32 villages were examined. The microfilariae of *D. perstans* were found in 39.8%, those of *L. loa* in 24.9%, and those of *D. streptocerca* in 49.3% of all the persons examined. On the other hand, the microfilariae of *O. volvulus* were detected in 38.5% of only 381 persons in six villages situated near Congo River in its narrow part, those of *W. bancrofti* were in the blood specimens of 32.1% of only 56 persons in one village situated in a swampy area close to Congo River. The microfilariae of *L. loa* were apparently nocturnally subperiodic; among 617 persons who showed the microfilariae in the blood, 16 (light infections) showed them only in night films and not in day films, and two had them more numerously in night blood than in day blood.

(5) *Onchocerca volvulus*:

O. volvulus has been found to be widely distributed in Zaire, and the endemic areas have been noted from all the provinces. According to VAN OYE & PIERQUIN (1961), the first record of onchocerciasis was made by BRUMPT (1904), who entered into Zaire in 1902 from the upper stream of Uele River, after staying in Ethiopia and the Upper Nile. The mission took a canoe and descended the river, finally reaching Léopoldville. Brumpt found 15 cases of onchocerciasis among the paddlers.

The occurrence of onchocerciasis in the district of Uele was reported by VEDY, in 1906, and by BRODEN & RODHAIN, in 1908, in Léopoldville. Later, extensive studies were conducted in Zaire by a number of workers. VAN OYE & PIERQUIN (1961) stated that 143 papers had been published about onchocerciasis, and its vectors in Zaire. A monograph on onchocerciasis in Zaire was compiled by VAN DEN BERGHE (1941). There have been six important endemic areas reported from Zaire: around Léopoldville (Kinshasa), in Lomani, Sankuru, Inzia, Uele, and Kivu (LEBRUN, 1954).

Since DUBOIS (1916) pointed out that elephantiasis patients in Uele were almost always infected with *O. volvulus* and the distribution of elephantiasis and onchocerciasis was nearly the same, a series of reports were made in Zaire incriminating *O. volvulus* as a cause of elephantiasis, especially the affection of genital organs (DUBOIS, 1917; DUBOIS & VITALE, 1938; DUBOIS & FORRO, 1939; and DUBOIS *et al.*, 1939). HISSETTE (1931, 1932) pointed out that in certain areas of the Kasai-Orientale, from the Sankuru-Lubilash River to the extreme northwest of Katanga, ocular affections due to *O. volvulus* were extremely serious, and some 20% of the population were blind and 50% had ocular complications.

Two species of black flies are responsible for the transmission of onchocerciasis in Zaire: *S. damnosum* in the endemic areas in Bas Lomani (SCHWETZ, 1930), Sankuru (HISSETTE, 1932), Uele (D'HOOGHE, 1934; VAN DEN BERGHE, 1941), Kinshasa (WANSON *et al.*, 1949); and *S. neavei* in Sankuru (HISSETTE, 1932, STRONG, 1937) and Kwango (GEUKENS, 1950). The larvae and pupae of the former species develop by attaching themselves to rocks, leaves, and other matter in the rivers, while those of the latter species are found almost always attached to freshwater crabs in streams, such as *Potamonautes lueboensis* and *P. lirrangensis* in the western Zaire (WANSON & HOLEMANS, 1951). The black fly vector in western Zaire was described under the name *renauxi* by WANSON & LEBIED (1950), but DE MEILLON (1957) regarded it to be a synonym of *neavei*.

Onchocerciasis transmitted by *S. damnosum* has been a serious problem in areas around Kinshasa, in the lower basin of the Congo River, and WANSON *et al.* (1949) observed that nearly 100% of the Africans here were infected, with 5% blind; 45% of the resident Europeans also had the disease. WANSON (1950) published a comprehensive study on the biology of the principal vector, *S. damnosum*, and the transmission, pathogenicity, prophylaxis, and therapy of onchocerciasis in this area. Investigations on onchocerciasis were made by FAIN (1947) and GEUKENS (1950) in Kwango, by PEEL *et al.* (1952) and DEMAEYER *et al.* (1955) in the Province of Kivu, by FAIN (1950) in Ruanda-Urundi (now Rwanda and Burundi), and by Van den DORPE (1958) in Kasai. From these and other studies, human onchocerciasis is now known to be endemic in all the provinces of Zaire, and future studies will probably show that the disease is spread across the whole region of the Congo Basin and most of central Africa.

More recent studies on the distribution of onchocerciasis and its vectors in Zaire were published by FAIN & HALLOT (1965). FAIN *et al.* (1969), in a study of filariasis in the region of Cuvette Centrale, examined 720 adults from ten villages, and found *O. volvulus* in 554 (76.9%), *W. bancrofti* in 4 (0.55%), *L. loa* in 16 (3.6%), *D. perstans* in 623 (86.5%), and *D. streptocerca* in 389 (54.0%); they pointed out that this region is an important and previously unknown focus of onchocerciasis.

7C.11.12 Rwanda and Burundi

Republics in eastern central Africa bounded on the east by Tanzania and on the west by Zaire; formerly the Belgian Trust Territory of Ruanda-Urundi, they achieved independence in 1962. Rwanda has an area of 26,340 km² with a population of 3,736,000 (1970). Burundi has an area of 27,870 km² and a population of 3,600,000 (1970). Most of the territories are at altitudes over 1,500 m, with high peaks of over 4,000 m.

Little is known about filariasis in this region. CORSON (1925) reported on the occurrence of *W. bancrofti* and *D. perstans* cases from Usumbara. FAIN (1969) stated that *L. loa* had never been seen in a systematic survey conducted in Rwanda, although *Chrysops distinctipennis* is present; he considers the altitude of 1,600 m to 2,300 m too cool for the development of the parasite in this vector. However, the occurrence of onchocerciasis in Ruanda-Urundi was reported by FAIN (1950).

7C.13 Angola

A former Portuguese overseas territory situated on the west coast of central Africa, south of Zaire, Angola is between 5°S and 18°S. It has an area of 1,246,000 km², and a population of 5,466,600 (1970).

As for bancroftian filariasis in Angola, FRAGA DE AZEVEDO (1964) stated in his review, "Although the widespread incidence of lymphatic filariasis throughout the province of Angola has been known for some decades, no detailed study of its distribution, incidence, and relative importance has been made. During my stay in Angola, a few years ago (1935), I was able to observe many cases of elephantiasis, lymph scrotum, hydrocele, lymphatic hypertrophy, and other symptoms which must certainly have been a result of infection with *W. bancrofti*."

MOURA PIRES *et al.* (1959) conducted a microfilaria survey in the Lunda district, in northeastern Angola bordering on Zaire. Fresh blood specimens collected by day from a total of 10,572 persons of all ages were examined, and microfilariae were found in 5,659. All microfilariae found in 400 blood smears, examined after staining with Giemsa, were those of *D. perstans*.

The distribution and incidence of infections due to *O. volvulus*, *L. loa*, and *D. perstans* in Angola were reviewed by CASACA (1967a). Among these, onchocerciasis was widely endemic in Angola and constituted an important health problem. The occurrence of *W. bancrofti* in Angola had not yet been confirmed, but CASACA (1967b) admitted the possibility of its existence, and stated that its probable distribution would be at the north of Angola only, namely, in the District of Cabinda and in the northern region of the District of Zaire.

Addendum: Southern Africa

The information on filariasis is scant or absent from southern Africa. HAWKING (1973) stated that *W. bancrofti* is probably rare or absent in Namibia and Botswana, and absent in South Africa, Swaziland, and Lesotho. *D. perstans* and other filariae are also absent from these countries.

7D. Eastern Africa

7D.1 Mozambique

A former Portuguese overseas province on east coast of Africa, situated south of Tanzania; between 10°S and 27°S, Mozambique has an area of 771,500 km² and a population of 8,233,032 (1970).

According to FRAGA DE AZEVEDO (1964), the prevalence of *W. bancrofti* in this province is considerable, but there are no detailed statistical data on its relative importance. In a survey of the adult population conducted in 1959 by FRAGA DE AZEVEDO & FARO, as well as that in 1960 by PINHAO (1961), the following incidences were recorded for *W. bancrofti* infection.

Zambezia: 5.4% of 185 day blood; 15.9% of 113 day blood.
Mozambique District: 5% of 200 day blood; 47.4% of 57 night blood
Cape Delgado: 6.7% of 105 day blood
Manica and Fofala: 10.9% of 350 day blood
Tete: 19.3% of 212 day blood

7D.2 Southern Rhodesia

A republic bounded on the northwest by Zambia (Northern Rhodesia); Rhodesia is an inland country situated between 15°S and 23°S and occupying a part of the Great South African Plateau with an average elevation of some 15,000 m. It has an area of 390,600 km² and a population of 5,400,000 (1970).

Information on filariasis is scanty. The occurrence of *W. bancrofti* has been recorded on a few occasions. *D. perstans* infection is widely distributed in the Zambesi River Basin and in the Burma Valley.

ALVES & VAN WYK (1960) reported on a focus of bancroftian filariasis in a village of the iron idol, "Chemombe," in the eastern Zambezi Valley, at 16°4'N and 29°47'E. A few adult males were seen with enlargements of the scrotum. Two ml of venous blood was drawn from 26 adults, put directly into 5 ml of a 2% glacial acetic acid and water solution; thick blood films were prepared from the sediment. Of 14 males, 5 were positive for *W. bancrofti*, 8 were positive for *D. perstans*, and two of them were positive for both. Of 12 females, 4 were positive for *W. bancrofti*, 4 for *D. perstans*, and one among the positives had a mixed infection. None of these cases showed any elephantoid reaction, but three of the cases suffered genitourinary pathology.

CONDY & HILL (1970) reviewed filarial infections in Rhodesian wild life, and discussed the possibility of human affections due to the animal filariae.

ROBERTS *et al.* (1971) examined the night blood of employees of the Game Department working in the Zambezi Valley, at the game camps in Mana Pools and Marangora. Of 109 persons (all adults) examined, 27 had microfilariae of *D. perstans*, 4 had those of *W. bancrofti*, and one had *Pl. falciparum*. One of the four subjects with *W. bancrofti* had small hydrocele.

According to HAWKING (1973), *D. perstans* infection in Southern Rhodesia is widespread, mainly in the Zambezi River Basin, and also in the Burma Valley. The distribution is patchy, with microfilaria rates of over 60% in some villages down to near zero in others. The endemic areas lie in a belt running from Kanyemba southwards through the Dande Tribal Trust Land and across the middle veld to the Silobela area west of Que Que, then westward through the Nkai and Lupane districts where the heaviest prevalence is found. There is a further belt extending southwards from Kariba along the Umniati River which joins the first belt in the Magondi Tribal Trust Land. There is a small focus to the east in the Bindura-Shamva district and another in the valley of the Gairezi River near the Mozambique border. There is an important focus in the Burma Valley immediately south of the Vumba near Umtali with a rate of 12%; from this area, several pathogenic infections have been reported (see below). A map of the distribution of *D. perstans* was given by CLARKE *et al.* (1971). In a village of the eastern Zambezi Valley, 50% of the people examined had *D. perstans* microfilariae (ALVES & VAN WYK, 1960). Transmission occurs mostly at altitudes between 800 and 1200 m above sea level. Above 1200 m, it paparently does not occur, and below 800 m, it occurs less frequently. It occurs in forest or semiforest areas but not in mopane forests. It is most frequent where surface water is plentiful.

Cases with clinical signs attributed to *D. perstans* infection have been especially noted from Southern Rhodesia. GELFAND & BERNBERG (1959) and BAKER *et al.* (1967) reported on cases with arthralgia, fever, and high blood eosinophilia. DUKE *et al.* (1968) described the case of a European with meningitis; microfilariae resembling *D. perstans* were found in the cerebrospinal fluid but not in the blood. They also described another similar case in an African patient. According to HAWKING (1973), the microfilariae were examined by ORIHEL (1973) who believed that these microfilariae were not those of *D. perstans* but from another filarial worm, *Meningonema*, which is a natural parasite of the talopin monkey and of *Cercopithecus aethiops*. In the monkeys, the adult worms are located in the central nervous system.

7D.3 Zambia

A republic, formerly called Northern Rhodesia, Zambia is an inland country bounded on north by Zaire and Tanzania, on the east by Malawi, on the southeast by Mozambique, on the south by Rhodesia and South-West Africa, and on the west by Angola. It covers an area of 752,600 km² and has a population of 4,396,000.

DANIELS (1901) stated, "The *Filaria nocturna* (= *bancrofti*) is found in many parts of British Central Africa, but its distribution is not uniform. Specimens of the blood of 687 natives were examined at night and this filaria embryo was found in 35 of them, or 5%. For convenience, I divided the districts from which the natives came as follows:

Highlands (Shire and Angoni)	137	No filaria
The Upper Shire River	120	Filaria in 1, or 0.8%
The Lower Shire River	52	Filaria in 13, or 25%
The Zambesi and Chinde Rivers	100	Filaria in 14, or 14%
Lake Nyassa (Southern half)	38	No filaria
Lake Nyassa (Northern half)	163	Filaria in 8, or 4.9%
Other districts	77	No filaria

The distribution of elephantiasis corresponds with that of filaria. It is well known to be present in the Lower Shire, the Zambezi, and at the north end of Nyassa Lake, and I have seen cases myself in each of these districts. *Filaria perstans* was found in one case only. This patient was a native of Mweneutambo, in British South Africa Territory" (abstracted).

BUCKLEY (1946) stated, "the first record of *W. bancrofti* in Northern Rhodesia (Zambia) appears to be from Mazabuka in 1938 (Medical Report) when three cases were reported by the medical officer. Three more cases were reported in the Medical Report for the year 1943. In a communication from the Health Department, evidence is to hand that *W. bancrofti* is present in natives of Feira District, near Luangwa-Zambezi confluence. However, there is some doubt whether the infections were contracted locally, or imported, and definite parasitological or clinical evidence of filariasis due to *W. bancrofti* endemic in N. Rhodesia is lacking. Likewise, *O. volvulus* has not been recorded from N. Rhodesia. *L. loa* was found by DE MEILLON (personal communication) from six natives in the Mankoya, Balovale, and Senanga districts in the Southern Province."

BUCKLEY (1946) made an extensive helminthological survey in Zambia. Blood films were examined for filariasis at the hospitals in Lusaka (172 individuals examined), Ndola (72), Fort Rosebery (20), Santa Maria Mission, Chilubi Island (40), Abercorn (69), Kasama (70), and Malole Mission (67). Of 459 night blood films, 25 (5.4%) showed microfilariae of *D. perstans*, and 3 (0.6%) those of *W. bancrofti*. The three carriers of *W. bancrofti* were found in Lusaka, Ndola, and Kasama, respectively. None of the *W. bancrofti* carriers were permanent residents of Northern Rhodesia; two of them were apparently imported cases, but one patient generally resided in Kashinga Village, near Malole Mission. Night blood specimens were subsequently taken from 67 individuals in the village but none of them were positive, and no elephantiasis cases were found in that area.

BARCLAY (1971), while working in routine outpatient clinics in various parts of Zambia, gained the impression that hydrocele was seen more commonly at the Zambia Flying Doctor Service clinics at East III and East IV in the Lukusashi and Lunsemfwa Valleys than at other clinics, and several villages in the neighbourhood of East IV clinic were visited. Night blood specimens were collected from 52 males and 25 females, and those of 10 males and 8 females were found to contain microfilariae of *D. perstans*. No microfilaria of *W. bancrofti* was demonstrated in this survey. Of 12 blood films obtained from adult males at East III, 4 contained microfilariae of *D. perstans*. It was also found that *D. perstans* infection existed in the neighborhood of Mpika. Although much of Zambia consists of a plateau of over 1200 m above sea level, these three areas are well below this altitude and are well wooded.

7D.4 Malawi (Nyasaland)

Malawi, formerly Nyasaland before 1964, is a long, narrow country situated inland of southeast Africa along the western shore of Lake Malawi (Lake Nyasa), between 9° and 17°S. It has an area of 117,000 km², and a population of 4,552,000 (1971).

(1) *W. bancrofti*:

Bancroftian filariasis has been known from two areas, the lower Shire in the southernmost part of the country, and the Songwe area at the northern end of Lake Malawi. The Songwe area is on the border between Malawi and Tanzania, and the Tanzania section of the northern Malawi Lake shore villages were investigated from 1950 by the East African Filariasis Research Unit (JORDAN, 1953).

ORAM (1958) reported on the results of epidemiological surveys conducted in the Malawi part of the north Malawi Lake shore. This area is about

250 km² in area and contains a population of about 15,000. It is about 1,500 feet high from the sea level but only a few feet above the lake level. Microfilairae of *W. bancrofti* were found in 6 (7.3%) of 82 persons examined in Karonga, 18 (19.6%) of 92 in Songwe, and 8 (30.8%) of 26 in Kyela. Among the populations of the three villages of 547, 616, and 497, those with clinical signs of filariasis numbered 5, 10 and 13, respectively; those with elephantiasis of the legs numbered 2, 2, and 1; those with elephantiasis of the scrotum numbered 2, 2, and 1; those with hydrocele numbered 8, 12, and 25; and those found with hernia numbered 0, 11, and 8.

ORAM (1960) further reported on the results of blood surveys conducted during August and September, 1957. Night blood was collected from about half of the villagers. The author stated, "All blood films were taken between 9.30 p.m. and 2. a.m. This caused a certain amount of difficulty and depended on the cooperation of the village headman. In the course of an evening quite a number of villagers would get bored and drift away before being examined. Fortunately, the author was well known by the people, otherwise it is unlikely that the survey would have been successful. In all, about half the total number of villagers were examined." Out of a total of 797 persons examined, 198 or 24.8% were positive for microfilariae of *W. bancrofti*. More males than females received the blood examination, and the microfilaremia rates were nearly the same for both sexes.

(2) *O. volvulus*:

Although it had been generally believed that onchocerciasis was prevalent in Malawi, apparently the first report on its distribution and prevalence was made only recently by BEN-SIRA *et al.* (1972). Onchocerciasis surveys were conducted during 1968 and 1969 in different districts of Malawi. In skin snip examinations of adult populations, only two out of 372 persons in eight places in the Northern Region and only two out of 821 persons in seven places in the Central Region were positive for *O. volvulus* microfilariae. In the Southern Region, 460 of 1,380 persons examined in Cholo District were positive, with a positive rate of 33.3%; of 909 persons examined in other nine places in the Southern Region, only three in three places were positive. Cholo District is situated at about 16°S in latitude and 35°E in longitude, and is part of Shire Highlands which form the eastern lip of the Great Rift Valley. The endemic area has an average altitude of over 3,000 feet, and it was estimated that at least 100,000 out of a total population of about 300,000 were infected.

7D.5 Tanzania

Tanzania is situated in eastern Africa, south of Kenya and Uganda. It was formerly divided into Zanzibar (a former British Protectorate consisting of Zanzibar Island, Penba Island, and adjacent small islands on the

Indian Ocean) and Tanganyika (formerly a republic of the British Commonwealth, and earlier, a greater part of German East Africa). In 1964, Zanzibar and Tanganyika were united as the independent United Republic of Tanzania. It has an area of 944,837km² with a population of 13,273,000 (1970).

The epidemiology of filariasis has been more extensively investigated in Tanzania than in any other region in East Africa. *W. bancrofti* infection has been known to occur mainly in five regions: 1) the offshore islands including Zanzibar; 2) the coastal region, including Dar es Salaam and other more urbanized areas, 3) the region south of Lake Victoria extending westwards to the shore of Lake Tanganyika, 4) the area around Tukuyu near the northern end of Lake Malawi; and 5) an inland area around Mahenge and Liwale in southern Tanzania. On the other hand, *D. perstans* infection has been recognized mainly from two areas, a) the area extending from western shore of Lake Victoria from southern Uganda to Lake Tanganyika, and b) the region around Liwale and the Mbemkuru River in southern Tanzania.

In the early years, when most parts of Tanzania were a German territory, the distribution of microfilaremia and clinical filariasis cases were recorded in the annual medical reports; these were reviewed by HAWKING (1940). FELDMANN (1905) reported the occurrence of *D. perstans* in the area around Bukoba, on the western shore of Lake Victoria. ENGELAND & MANTEUFEL (1911) found 9 (8.2%) *D. perstans* carriers and 13 (11.8%) *W. bancrofti* carriers among 110 prisoners examined in Mwanza, on the southern shore of Lake Victoria, and also reported on the occurrence of *W. bancrofti* and *D. perstans* carriers in Dar es Salaam and Tanga on the Indian Ocean coast in large numbers of routine blood examinations. ENGELAND (1920) examined blood specimens from 297 native soldiers both by day and at night in Dar es Salaam, and obtained 96 (32.3%) positives for *W. bancrofti* in the night blood, while only 6 (2.1%) were positive in the day blood; he thus concluded that the microfilariae of *W. bancrofti* on the East African coast was a nocturnally periodic form.

Spot surveys were made later by several workers in Tanzania; these will be described for each region. HAWKING (1940, 1943) reviewed previous records of filariasis in Tanzania, and described, in detail, the distribution of filariasis in East Africa. From 1950, the Filariasis Research Unit of the East African High Commission began extensive surveys of filariasis in Tanganyika, and the results were reported in a series of papers by JORDAN (1952, 1953, 1954, 1955a, 1956a,b, 1959, 1960a, 1962). JORDAN (1955b,c, 1960b) reviewed and discussed the economic importance and epidemiology of filariasis in Tanganyika.

KATAMINE *et al.* (1967) conducted blood examinations and skin tests with FPT antigen in a survey of filariasis. In Kilomboni on the eastern coast, 8 (7.3%) of 110 persons examined at night were positive for microfilariae of *W. bancrofti*; in Ilagala on the shore of Lake Tanganyika, 22

(7.4%) of 299 persons examined by day were positive for *D. perstans*, and 2 (5.3%) of 57 persons examined at night were positive for *W. bancrofti* microfilariae.

Studies on the transmission of *W. bancrofti* were conducted by McCarthy (1930) in Pemba, by Smith (1955) on Ukara Island of Lake Victoria, and by White (1971) in Northeast Tanzania.

7D.5.1 *W. bancrofti:*

7D.5.1.a Zanzibar and Pemba Islands

Howard (1918) reported on filariasis cases in Zanzibar, especially in reference to scrotal operations. He stated, "The most striking difference between the tropical diseases prevalent in the two regions (Zanzibar and Nyasaland) lies in the fact that filariasis does not occur in Nyasaland except in certain circumscribed localities, whereas it is exceptionally frequent throughout the island and town of Zanzibar." In examinations from 1911 to 1917 of the night blood of male patients entering the hospital (irrespective of the cause of their admission), 249 (31.6%) of 788 showed microfilariae of *W. bancrofti*. Howard further stated that hydroceles were common and large, hematoceles were fairly common, and so were lymphatic varix of cord, lymph scrotum, and elephantiasis; inguinal hernia was extremely common, and he believed that it was often due to filariasis.

Mansfield-Aders (1927) conducted investigations on malaria and filariasis in Zanzibar. Night blood was taken from 645 adult Africans from various parts of the island, and 169 (26.3%) of them were found to harbor microfilariae of *W. bancrofti*. *C. fatigans* was the most common mosquito in Zanzibar town. Engorged females were collected from houses in different parts of the town, kept in wide-mouthed test tubes and dissected on the twelfth day after capture; of 1,300 examined, 265 (20.3%) were positive for proboscis infection of mature larvae. Six species of *Anopheles* were found on the island, of which *An. costalis* (= *gambiae*) and *An. funestus* were most common; many of them were noted to harbor filaria larvae both in the thoracic muscle and the proboscis. Malaria was also found to be hyperendemic on this island.

Vasselo (1939) described acute funiculitis, which he stated was by no means uncommon in Zanzibar, but no reference was made to its relation to filarial infection.

Hawking (1943) reviewed the annual medical reports for Zanzibar (1912–38) and pointed out that filariasis was one of the major causes of hospitalization in this region; figures for the inpatients of the hospitals in Zanzibar town, Chake-Chake, Mkoani and Wete showed that these conditions were fairly evenly distributed throughout the Zanzibar Protectorate. In a total of 1,928 operations from 1929 to 1933, it was found that 29.7% were for hydrocele, 3.3% for elephantiasis of the scrotum, and 21.1% for inguinal hernia.

Filariasis has been noted also to be extremely common on Pemba Island,

and medical records from 1912 to 1927 all emphasized the importance and frequency of clinical filariasis on this island (HAWKING, 1943). DUNDERDALE (1921) found 20 (40%) of 50 people from Pemba harboring microfilariae of *W. bancrofti*. MCCARTHY (1930) made various medical examinations in Wete, Pemba, and in blood examinations conducted at night, found microfilariae (species not mentioned) in 35 (23.1%) of 156 adults, 9 (15.5%) of 58 children in the township, and 3 (16.7%) of 18 country children. As for the infection of mosquitoes, filaria larvae (stage not mentioned) were found in 8 of 96 *Culex*, 3 of 72 *Aedes*, and 1 of 58 *Anopheles* (species of mosquito not mentioned).

7D.5.1.b The East Coast Region

In Dar es Salaam, the capital of Tanzania, a large proportion of the inhabitants are immigrants from other parts of the country. ENGELAND & MANTEUFEL (1911) stated that 539 of 20,248 slides examined during the 1908–09 fiscal year and 325 of 19,604 slides examined during 1909–10 had microfilariae; of 50 slides containing microfilariae, 40 were those with sheath, and 10 were smaller and without sheath. In Tanga, a town on the coast in northern Tanzania, 303 of 13,704 slides examined contained microfilariae. The microfilariae were tentatively identified as those of *W. bancrofti* and *D. perstans*, respectively. ENGELAND (1920), in Dar es Salaam, examined the blood specimens of 297 soldiers at night, and found microfilariae of *W. bancrofti* in 96 (32.3%).

CORSON (1925), in Dar es Salaam, reported that out of 768 blood films collected mostly by day at the bacteriological laboratory, microfilariae were found in 6.7%. Also, of blood films collected between 10 and 11 a.m. from 140 school pupils, microfilariae of *W. bancrofti* were found in 8 (5.7%) and those of *D. perstans* in one (0.7%); of 140 blood films collected between 10 to 11 a.m. from prisoners, *W. bancrofti* was present in 7 (5.0%) and *D. perstans* in 5 (3.6%).

HAWKING (1940) conducted microfilarial and clinical surveys in Dar es Salaam and Mafia, and found carriers of microfilariae of *W. bancrofti* in 32.4% (60 out of 185 examined) of adult males and 18.2% (14 of 77) of adult females.

7D.5.1.c The Victoria Lake Region

JORDAN (1954b) examined microfilaremia among inpatients of the Mwanza Government Hospital, situated on the southern shore of Lake Victoria, where bancroftian filariasis is endemic. In the febrile cases, 52 (8.0%) of 651 males and 6 (5.3%) of 113 females were positive for microfilariae of *W. bancrofti*; in nonfebril cases (excluding hernia and filarial cases), 145 (20.6%) of 705 males and 48 (20.8%) of 231 females were positive. The positives among filarial cases were 8 (14.5%) of 55 with abscess and cellulitis, 6 (46.2%) of 13 with lymphadenitis, 8 (29.6%) of 27 with epididymo-orchitis and funiculitis, 13 (22.4%) of 58 with hydrocele, 1 of 1 with hematocele, 4 (12.9%) of 31 with elephantiasis of the serotum, 1

(3.4%) of 29 with elephantiasis of the legs, and 1 (5.6%) of 18 with scrotal abscess.

Results of filaria surveys conducted in the Lake Province was reported by JORDAN (1956c). This province has an area of 39,000 square miles and includes all the Tanganyika shores of Lake Victoria at an altitude of 3,720 feet. The area south and southeast of Lake Victoria is occupied mainly by Wasukuma, the largest tribe in Tanganyika, and most of this region is only a little above the level of the lake. A large area of the eastern part of the province is uninhabited with height near the northern province of over 5,000 feet.

Altogether, 33 villages in various districts were surveyed. The results showed that the province could be divided roughly into three areas: to the northeast and east, no filariasis was found; to the south and southeast of Lake Victoria, bancroftian filariasis is endemic; while to the southwest and west of the lake, infection with *D. perstans* was found. The latter focus of *D. perstans* infection extended over the northwest border into Uganda. Some islands in the lake also showed low to medium incidence of *W. bancrofti* infection.

In this survey, it was recognized that a relatively high incidence of elephantiasis occurred in areas where no microfilariae of *W. bancrofti* were found. For example, Runazi and Kaziramayaga Villages in the Biharamu-ro district, and Mabawa Village in the Ngara district had 9 cases altogether of elephantiasis out of 352 persons examined, while microfilariae of *W. bancrofti*, as well as those of *D. perstans*, were negative. In the Kibondo district of Western Province, adjacent to the above areas, elephantiasis was again found to be a common condition in persons who had never left the area; *W. bancrofti* infection was absent from this district. This focus of "nonbancroftian elephantiasis" was described by JORDAN *et al.* (1956a).

7D.5.1.d The Tukuyu Region

FISCHER (1932), in his comprehensive report on the pathology and epidemiology in East Africa, stated that he examined school pupils at Rwange, near the northern end of Lake Malawi, between 11 and 12 p.m. and found microfilariae of *W. bancrofti* in 32% of those from a district on the lake shore. HAWKING (1943) reviewed references of filariasis and elephantiasis in this area given in "*Medizinal-Berichte*" for years 1903 to 1910, and stated, a microfilarial rate in Tukuyu to be 17% of 42 persons examined."

JORDAN (1953) reported on the results of a filarial survey made in the southern highlands of Tanganyika during September and October, 1952 by the Filariasis Research Unit. Blood was examined at 14 villages in five districts, and approximately 30 mm³ of blood was collected from volunteers. For *W. bancrofti* infection, a high incidence was observed at Lusungo, with a population of about 3,000 and situated at the northern end of Lake Malawi; the microfilarial rate was 23% of 18 in children, 61% of 13 in adult males, and 54% of 13 in female adults. This endemic focus was considered to be confined to a small area with a radius of about 16 miles from the lake, among the natives in the villages situated on the lake shore Tukuyu and towns further north were negative for microfilariae of *W. bancrofti*.

7D.5.1.e The Southern Province

JORDAN (1954) reported on an extensive filarial survey of the Southern Province of Tanzania. This province is one of the least populated in this country because it consists of large tracts of waterless land and is infested by the tsetse fly; only the coastal belt and the Ruvumu River area in the south are well populated. Twenty-three villages in eight districts were surveyed, and the percentages of microfilaremia cases of *W. bancrofti* and *D. perstans*, as well as clinical cases, were presented in this paper. High microfilaremia rates of *W. bancrofti*, ranging from 73% to 13% in adult males, were observed in Kiwala, Lindi, Mikindani, Newala, and Masasi districts along the coast, and Liwale and Kilamarondo in the valley, but inland villages in the Songea and Tunduru districts were almost free from *W. bancrofti* infection. The distribution of *D. perstans* infection was more limited, but extremely high incidences were seen in some of the villages in the Kilawa and Tunduru districts. Microfilaremia of *W. bancrofti* and *D. perstans* was observed in several infants of ages from eight months to 18 months.

A second and previously unknown endemic focus of *W. bancrofti* in this province was discovered at Kimande, in the Iringa district, which has a population of about 1,500 and is situated in the valley of the Great Ruaha River. It is near an extensive swamp area and about 40 miles NNW of Iringa. Eighteen percent of 261 adult males and 6% of 250 adult females were positive for microfilariae, hydrocele was found in 7% of 281, and elephantiasis was found in 0.2% of 511 persons examined. A filaria incidence of 4% was also found at Rujewa (Mbeya district), situated at the southwest extremity of the Great Ruaha Valley; finding filariasis here suggested that the infection extended down the valley from Kimande. No indigenous cases of *D. perstans* infection were noticed in this survey. No evidence of nodule formation due to onchocerciasis was found among the several hundreds of persons examined in this region, although *S. damnosum, S. lepidum,* and *S. hargravesi* were present in the streams.

JORDAN (1955) reported further on the relationship between the infection rate and the microfilarial density of *W. bancrofti* and of *D. perstans* in the endemic areas in Southern Province of Tanganyika. It was shown by the analysis of surveys conducted in 1952 that the microfilaria rate of an area was related to the microfilarial density in both species. The incidence of infection with *W. bancrofti* and *D. perstans* increased with the age, but only in *D. perstans* infections was the increase accompanied by a consistent increase in the microfilarial density. The hydrocele rate of an area was also shown to be related to the microfilaria rate of *W. bancrofti*, and to increase with the age.

7D.5.1.f The Central Province

According to JORDAN (1955a), a filaria survey was carried out by the Filariasis Research Unit in ten villages in the Central Province; 2,623 night blood specimens were obtained, of these, 710 were from children under the age of 16, 905 were from adult males, and 1,018 were from adult females. Only 2 were found positive for microfilariae of *W. bancrofti*, and it seemed unlikely that these were indigenous infections. Only 7 hydrocele cases were seen, of these, 4 were from Shelui in Singida District, 2 at Makuru, and one at Mpapa. Also, 4 elephantiasis cases were seen during the survey. The Central Province has no coast line and no large lakes, most of the region has an altitude of 4,000 feet and over. The rainfall is between 30 to 40 inches; the mean maximum temperature is between 80°F and 85°F, the minimum temperature being between 60°F and 65°F. This climatic condition has probably not favored the transmission of *W. bancrofti*.

7D.5.1.g The Western Province

JORDAN (1956b) described the results of a filarial survey undertaken by the Filariasis Research Unit in nine villages of the Western Province. The microfilaremia rates in the adult males were from 0% to 6% for *W. bancrofti*, and from 0% to 37% for *D. perstans*. There were no extensive foci of either of the filariae in this province. The few villages in which cases of *W. bancrofti* were seen were generally on the edge of larger endemic areas in the Lake Province.

Note: As in other articles on filariasis by Jordan, the number of persons examined in each village and in total were not mentioned.

7D.5.1.h Transmission of *W. bancrofti* in Tanzania

As stated previously, three species of mosquitoes have been incriminated as the principal vectors of *W. bancrofti* in Tanzania: *C. fatigans, An. gambiae*, and *An. funestus*. The importance of these species differ according to the localities, namely, *C. fatigans* is the principal vector in urban areas, while the two anophelines are playing the major role in most of the urban areas.

In Zanzibar, MANSFIELD-ADERS (1927) found that 20.3% of 1,300 wild-caught *C. fatigans* become infected in the proboscis if kept until the 12th day before dissecting, and many *An. gambiae* and *An. funestus* were also infected. In Pemba, McCARTHY (1930) found infections in *Culex, Aedes*, and *Anopheles*. HAWKING (1940) reported that in Dar es Salaam, 81 (22.3%) of 362 *C. fatigans* were positive for filaria larvae, and 2 (0.6%) contained mature larvae; in Zanzibar, 9 (0.71%) of 1,265 *Culex* from houses were infected in the proboscis. MACKAY (1938) observed in Dar es Salaam during the routine examination of anopheline mosquitoes for malaria that 0.94% of *An. gambiae* and 1.21% of *An. funestus* contained filaria larvae.

SMITH (1955a,b,c,d) made a series of studies on the transmission of bancroftian filariasis on Ukara Island in Lake Victoria. The island is situated

3,750 feet above sea level, roughly square-shaped, with an area of 45 square miles and a population of some 17,000 Africans (called Bakara or Baregi). The temperature is fairly uniform throughout the year with minimum of 64°F recorded in July or August and maximum of 95°F in December. The rainfall is also fairly uniform, with the average for 1950–52 of 62 inches per annum. The mosquito fauna include 13 species of *Anopheles* and 29 culicines.

Of almost 6,000 night blood specimens obtained from the islanders by the East African Medical Survey Unit, 21% were positive for *W. bancrofti.* Infections occurred in all of 26 villages studied, but were high in some villages (30 to 40%) and low in others (6.6%). *D. perstans* and *L. loa* infections were absent from Ukara. Most of the villages with high incidences of *W. bancrofti* were situated near large rice-growing areas, where the density of *An. gambiae* and *An. funestus* was high.

The seasonal man-biting incidences by mosquitoes inside and outside the village huts were recorded. *An. gambiae* and *An. funestus* were by far the most common indoor biters, but they were also collected while biting outdoors in fair numbers. *Mansonia africanus* and *M. uniformis* were common outdoor biters in a village near a swamp. The inhabitants were bitten by *Ae. africanus* and *Ae. apicoargenteus* outdoors by day. Of 3,287 *An. gambiae* dissected, 65 (1.98%) were infected with filarial larvae and 19 (0.58%) had mature larvae. In *An. funestus,* 39 (3.18%) of 1,228 were infected and 13 (1.06%) of them had mature larvae. Of 93 *An. pharoensis,* 12 (12.9%) were infected, but not with mature larvae. No mature larvae were found in other mosquito species dissected. Results of precipitin tests showed that man and ox were the chief sources of blood to hut-resting mosquitoes. *An. gambiae* and *An. funestus* fed almost entirely on man, and *An. pharoensis* fed more on man than on ox. Culicines fed more on ox than on man. Hand-catches off on man, cow and goat in a hut confirmed the results of precipitin tests. From these results, *An. gambiae* and *An. funestus* were incriminated as almost entirely responsible for the transmission of *W. bancrofti* on Ukara Island, though some transmission may result from *An. pharoensis.*

WHITE (1971) carried out a quantitative study on the transmission of *W. bancrofti* in a coastal region of Tanzania, and elucidated some important aspects of the comparative importance of the three major vector species, *An. gambiae, An. funestus,* and *C. fatigans.* Three stations with contrasting environmental conditions were selected: Ubwari, a rural village near Muhenza town about 35 km inland from the coast; Maore village further inland in Gonja district; and an urban section of the sea port city Tanga. In each station, the numbers of mosquito bites per person were estimated on annual basis and the infectivity rates of each species were obtained by dissection.

In the urban parts of Tanga, the only significant filariasis vector was *C. fatigans.* This mosquito species was responsible for about 10,000 bites per person per annum, with an infectivity rate of about 0.23%. In the rural district of Ubwari, all three filariasis vectors were active, and their annual biting densities per person were 1,591 in *An. funestus*, 2,971 in *An. gambiae* A, and 3,058 in *C. fatigans*, with calculated infectivity rates of 6.1%, 2.4%, and 0.54%, respectively. The third locality, further inland at Maore, receives only about two-thirds as much rainfall annually as do Tanga and Muhensa. *Anopheles funestus* and *An. gambiae* (mainly species B) were found to be filariasis vectors here, with annual mean biting densities of 1,250 in *An. funestus* and 5,963 in *An. gambiae* per person per annum, and infectivity rates of 3.5% and 0.9%, respectively. Densities of *C. fatigans* at Maore averaged 3,603 bites per person per annum, but infective larvae were not observed in any of 360 specimens dissected.

From these data, it was calculated that during 1969, the mean personal exposure to the risk of infection with third stage larvae of *W. bancrofti* was due to the bites of 23 ± 15 infective mosquitoes at Tanga, to the bites of 185 ± 84 infective mosquitoes at Ubwari, and to the bites of 95 ± 66 infective mosquitoes at Gonja Maore. The apparent risks of filariasis transmission at Ubwari were due 52% to *An. funestus*, 40% to *An. gambiae* A, and 8% to *C. fatigans*. At Maore, the risks of transmission were due 46% to *An. funestus* and 54% to *An. gambiae*. From these results, it was indicated that *An. funestus* was a more efficient vector than *An. gambiae*. *C. fatigans* was least efficient and of little importance in the rural areas though it might be the most abundant mosquito.

CRANS (1973) conducted studies of experimental infection of *An. gambiae* (laboratory colony of species A, Kisumu strain) and *C. fatigans* (a colony from Tanga, Tanzania) with *W. bancrofti* in coastal East Africa (Tanzania). Uptake of microfilariae, survival of the vector after an infective blood meal, number of filarial larvae reaching the infective stage and percentage of mosquitoes harboring infective larvae after 14 days were compared in the laboratory. When the two species were fed simultaneously on the same carrier, *C. fatigans* ingested more than three times as many microfilariae, and 54% contained infective larvae after 14 days as compared to 9.0% of the *An. gambiae* colony. The mean number of infective larvae per positive mosquito was nearly twice as high in *C. fatigans*. The mortality rate over the 14 days after taking the infective meal was however about half in *An. gambiae* than in *C. fatigans*. The results of these studies suggest that in coastal East Africa *C. fatigans* is a far more efficient vector of *W. bancrofti* than *An. gambiae*, in contrast to the apparently reversed results obtained by some other workers in West and East Africa.

7D.5.2 *D. perstans*

Previous surveys have shown that *D. perstans* infection occurs in two regions in Tanzania, in the area from southern Uganda on the western side of Lake Victoria to the eastern shore of Lake Tanganyika, and the area around Liwale and the Mbemkuru River in the Southern Province. The occurrence of *D. perstans* in the Bukoba area on the western shore of Lake Victoria was noted already by FELDMANN (1904), who examined 6,000 persons in 12 localities, and found microfilariae of *D. perstans* in rates from 24 % to 86% of the people. FELDMANN (1905a) noted the frequent occurrence of *D. perstans* in banana-growing areas, and assumed that an argasid tick, which was found commonly infesting huts in banana gardens, to be the vector. He considered a form of worm found in the tick to be the developing larvae of *D. perstans*, but later FELDMANN (1905b) himself disproved this idea.

HAWKING (1940) reviewed the "*Medizinische Berichte*" in the German protectorate years and other records, and traced the above two endemic areas. JORDAN (1955b) reviewed the results of extensive blood surveys conducted by the Filariasis Research Unit, and found the parasite had a more extensive distribution in the Southern Province than had previously been recorded by Hawking. He also discussed the climatic conditions suitable for the transmission, and their relationship to banana growing.

7D.5.3 *O. volvulus:*

Man-biting Simuliids and human onchocerciasis have been reported from several parts of Tanzania by HAWKING (1940), GABATHULER & GA-BATHULER (1947), FREEMAN & DE MEILLON (1953), JORDAN (1956), WOODMAN (1958), and LEWIS (1960). One or more members of *S. neavei* complex were found at Amani, Kidodi, Njombe, and Ubena, and probably at Mahenge; *S. damnosum* was reported from Njombe, Tukuyu, and Ubena, and onchocerciasis exists in the Amani and Mahenge areas (LEWIS, 1960).

The endemic area at Amani in the Usumbara Mountains of northeastern Tanzania was surveyed by LEWIS (1960b). Single skin smears were taken from 30 persons, and microfilariae were found in 14 (46.7%); however, no symptoms were observed among the people. Of 359 flies dissected, 41.2% were found parous by the presence of follicular relics in the ovaries, and 12.8% of these were infected with nematodes (at least some of which were not *O. volvulus*).

Two members of the *S. neavei* complex were found in this region; they were designated the Amani unbanded and banded forms. (Scientific names were witheld until the taxonomy of the whole complex could be better understood). Larvae and pupae of both forms were found attached to the common local crab, *Potamon* (*Potamonautes*) *lirrangensis* Rathbun, but not on other two species of *Potamon*. The adults of the unbanded form were not seen biting man, while the banded form bit readily, but the density was relatively low at about five per man per hour, even in good catching places.

More detailed studies on the taxonomy, bionomics, and relation to onchocerciasis of the black flies in Amani area were reported by LEWIS (1961) and RAYBOULD (1967). *S. woodi* De Meillon, a member of the *S. neavei* complex, or the banded form of LEWIS (1960b), was shown to be the only black fly regularly biting man in this region, while another species of this complex, *S. nyasalandicum* DE MEILLON (Amani unbanded form) was shown to be nonanthropophilic.

LAING & WEGESA (1965) conducted a survey of onchocerciasis in the eastern Usambara Mountains of Amani and found 42% of the local inhabitants to be carriers of the microfilariae.

RAYBOULD (1967) conducted weekly 12-hour catches of man-biting *Simulium* for 13 months in a clearing near Amani. The biting cycle of *S. woodi* usually consisted of a morning and an afternoon peak and a midday lull. Parous flies had a rather different biting cycle from nulliparous flies. The morning and afternoon peaks of *S. adersi* were earlier and later, respectively, than those of *S. woodi*. *S. woodi* bit almost exclusively on the legs. Of 3,291 *S. woodi* dissected, 33.6% were parous, and 17.3% of these parous flies contained larvae at later stages of development.

GRANBACKA (1973) reported on the occurrence of an endemic area of onchocerciasis in southern Tanzania, on the shore of the northern end of Lake Malawi. The area is similar in general features to the onchocerciasis area reported from Malawi by BEN-SIRA *et al.* (1972), and on a plain on the western side of the Livingstone Mountains. In Lufilyo Village, 167 out of 260 (64.2%) had the microfilariae in skin snips. In Kambasegela Village near Mbaka River, 49 of 172 (28.5%) were positive. In Matema at the lake 5 of 70 (7.1%) were positive. Of 104 hospital patients examined, 46 (44.2%) were also positive. Skin nodules were common, and a lot of patients with big abscesses responded well to DEC without antibiotics. There were only a few patients with mild irritation of the eye.

7D.6 Kenya

Kenya is an East African country situated south of Ethiopia and Sudan, between latitude 5°N and 5°S, with an area of 582,421 km² and a population of 11,694,000 (1971). *W. bancrofti* is known to be highly prevalent in areas along the coast of the Indian Ocean and on adjacent islands. The inland region is apparently free from bancroftian filariasis, but some areas are infested by *D. perstans* and *O. volvulus*. *Brugia patei* was recorded from some animals of Pate Island and the coastal region, but no human infection has been noted.

7D.6.1 *W. bancrofti*

The prevalence of *W. bancrofti* infection along the coastal districts was noted by LOW (1903, quoted by HAWKING, 1943), who examined Swahili from the coast, working in Uganda. Low found that 26% among them were carrying microfilariae of *W. bancrofti*. DUNDERDALE (1921) stated that the annual report of the medical officer in Lamu for the years 1911 to 1912 gave a figure of 42 (35.6%) of 118 persons examined to be positive for filarial infection; in his own survey in the Tana River area (Lamu, Siyu,

Faza, Pemba, and other places), 132 (36.0%) of 367 persons examined in total were positive. According to HAWKING (1943), the following information was available:

Mombasa: In 1932, during the examinations of 5,410 routine blood films for malaria, microfilariae of *W. bancrofti* were seen 31 times, and those of *D. perstans* 17 times.

Digo District: In 1928, during a helminthic survey in which 15,112 men, 15,610 women and 11,246 children were examined, 44 cases of elephantiasis, 146 cases of hydrocele, and 113 cases of hernia were recorded.

Nairobi: During 1934, 1935, and 1937, 27,533 films from Africans were examined for malaria; microfilariae of *D. perstans* were seen in 138, and those of *W. bancrofti* in 12.

HEISCH *et al.* (1956, 1959) conducted epidemiological and entomological surveys of filariasis on Pate Island. In 1956, microfilariae of *W. bancrofti* were found in 52 (36.6%) of 142 males and 54 (28.4%) of 190 females examined, with the average counts per 20 mm^3 blood of 14.8 and 5.4, respectively. Of 142 males, 15 had elephantiasis and 22 had hydrocele; elephantiasis was also seen in 9 of 190 females. The youngest person with elephantiasis was ten years old. Of 46 persons with elephantiasis or hydrocele, only 11 (23.9%) showed microfilariae in their blood. DEC was given to all persons more than two years old who were living in Faza Village, and 1,200 out of a total population of 1,500 were treated by a daily doses of approximately 6 mg per kg for six days. Eight months later, the microfilarial rate decreased to 16% and the microfilarial density to 1.1 per 20 mm^3 blood.

Wild and domestic animals on this island were also examined, and seven species of filariae were identified; *Brugia patei* was found in dogs, cats, and genet cats. Three mosquitoes were found commonly in houses: *Ae. pembaensis* Theobald, *C. fatigans* Wiedemann, and *Ae. aegypti* (Linnaeus). Although high rates of infections with filarial larvae were seen in all these mosquitoes, the principal vector of *W. bancrofti* was determined to be *C. fatigans,* and the filarial larvae in other mosquito species were identified to be those of animal filariae.

NELSON (1959, 1960) made detailed studies on the morphology and identification of filarial larvae found in mosquitoes on Pate Island.

NELSON *et al.* (1962) conducted further investigations on filarial infections in man, animals, and mosquitoes on the Kenya coast. Ten districts along the coast were surveyed, and microfilarial rates of higher than 25% in the north to 10% in the south were observed. Adult males showed a higher rate than adult females. In Faza, for example, a microfilarial rate of 40.6%, elephantiasis rate of 16.8%, and hydrocele rate of 39.3% were observed among 89 males examined.

More than 1,500 animals representing 25 species were examined, and 18 species of filariae were found in 1,572 animals. *Brugia patei* was seen in dogs, cats, genet cats, and bush babies. Two distinct strains of *B. patei* were recognized: a nonperiodic form on Pate Island transmitted by *Ae. pembaensis,* and a nocturnally periodic form on the continent transmitted by *M. uniformis* and *M. africanus.* No *Brugia* infections were seen in man. More than 4,000 mosquitoes were dissected, and mature larvae of *W. bancrofti* were found in *An. gambiae, An. funestus,* and *C. fatigans.* No other mosquito species contained mature larvae of *W. bancrofti,* though often infected with animal filariae. In coastal towns and villages, *C. fatigans* was predominant and acted as the main vector of *W. bancrofti* throughout the year. In inland villages, *An. gambiae* and *An. funestus* were more important as the vectors, but in most areas they failed to maintain a high transmission level because of the short rainy season.

In a review by HAWKING (1943, 1957), he noted that most of the inland districts of Kenya has not been thoroughly surveyed, but are believed to be free from *W. bancrofti.* COHEN (1960) found cases of elephantiasis in Ethiopia and inland Kenya, but regarded them as "idiopathic lymphoedema."

SOMEREN *et al.* (1955) studied the taxonomy, distribution, and behavior of mosquitoes of the Kenya coast. A total of 121 species were listed, and their localities of collection, biting habits, larval breeding places, and morphological variations were discussed.

7D.6.2 *D. perstans*

D. perstans is probably not endemic in the coastal and the inland region around Nairobi. According to HAWKING (1943), the microfilariae of *D. perstans* were noted in Nairobi only twice in 7,984 blood films from Europeans examined for malaria during the years 1932 to 1937 but were seen in 138 of 27,533 films from Africans during the same period. (The Africans included many immigrants.) *D. perstans* is known to be endemic on the northern and western shores of Lake Victoria, in the territories of Uganda and Tanzania, but apparently does not extend to the eastern shore of the Kenya territory. All of 130 examinations at Kisumu and 150 at Wasemi, near Kisumu, were negative.

7D.6.3 *O. volvulus*

Onchocerciasis in Kenya is confined to Nyanza Province in the west, and its principal vector is *S. neavei* ROUBAUD, 1915. Results of extensive surveys of the disease and the vector were reported by McMAHON (1940–1957) and BUCKLEY (1949, 1950). Experiments for the eradication of *S. neavei* were initiated by GARNHAM & McMAHON (1947, 1954) using DDT dripped into the rivers. A comprehensive report on the epidemiology of onchocerciasis and the eradication of *S. neavei* was made by McMAHON *et al.* (1958) and BROWN (1962).

Nyanza is the most westerly province of Kenya, approximately 40,000 km² in area; its altitude varies from 1135 m at the level of Lake Victoria to 4270 m at the summit of Mount Elgon. Onchocerciasis exists in three main foci. The first and most recently discovered is mainly in Uganda, on the western slope of Mount Elgon, with small extension to Kenya. The second, and by far the largest, is in northern Nyanza and involves parts of Kakamega and Kaimosi districts. The third, which is really a collection of four foci, is in southern Nyanza, and includes the large Kipsonoi and Kuja River areas, as well as two small foci at Kodera and Riana.

In the surveys conducted by BUCKLEY (1949) in Nyanza Province, before application of the control program, high microfilaria and ocular complication rates were reported.

Extensive epidemiological surveys were carried out in these endemic areas, and according to MCMAHON *et al.* (1958), the percentages of people positive for the microfilariae of *O. volvulus* and those with ocular complications were, respectively, 49% and 10% at Kodera (near Kisii), southern Nyanza, 21% and 1.6% at Riana (near Kisii), 29% and 1.8% at Ngoina (near Kericho), southern Nyanza, and 72% and 10.5% at Kaimosi, northern Nyanza.

Surveys of adults and immature stages of *S. neavei* were conducted extensively convering most of the endemic areas. Since the larvae and pupae are found attached to the freshwater crab, *Potamonautes niloticus,* the breeding places were sought by trapping the crabs using various methods, especially bait traps and box traps, designed for this purpose.

The campaign for the eradication of the vectors of onchocerciasis in Kenya began in 1939 by intensive surveys of onchocerciasis and its vectors. GARNHAM & MCMAHON (1946) reported on the successful eradication of *S. neavei* from Kodera district with the aid of DDT dripped into rivers at rates of 0.5 to 1.0 ppm for 30 minutes. In 1950, the immature stages of *S. neavei* were discovered to be breeding in phoretic association with a freshwater crab (*P. niloticus*) by MCMAHON (1951, 1952) in the Kipsonoi River near Kericho; as a result, a more complete survey of the breeding places was carried out. It was demonstrated in the Kakamega and Kaimosi areas that large numbers of tributaries and small streams in forested areas where adult *S. neavei* were captured in abundance did not harbour the earlier stages of this fly, and that the rivers outside of the forests which were not included in the original insecticide treatment in 1947 contained large numbers of *S. neavei* larvae.

Larviciding with DDT at a rate of 0.5 ppm for 30 minutes was begun in September 1954 and continued for a period of three months, covering all rivers and streams of northern Nyanza. As a result, adult catches and searches for immature stages of *S. neavei* remained negative for nearly a year. In December 1955, the upper reaches of Yala River were found to be infested, and these were treated for three months beginning February 1956; *S. neavei* was eradicated from this area also. MCMAHON *et al.* (1958) stated that the eradication program in Nyanza Province of Kenya was successful for most of the endemic areas of onchocerciasis, involving about 40,000 km^2.

7D.7 Uganda

Uganda is an inland country north and west of Lake Victoria, with an area of 235,946 km² and a population of 10,461,500 (1972 estimate).

7D.7.1 *W. bancrofti*

In a review by HAWKING (1940, 1943), he stated that endemic areas of *W. bancrofti* are considered to be widespread throughout Uganda according to estimates from medical and hospital records of elephantiasis and hydrocele, but systematic surveys on the distribution of parasite carriers and vectors have not yet been made in this country. The incidence of clinical filariasis cases has been reported to be especially high in areas north of Lake Victoria, in the Teso, Lango, West Nile, Tororo, and Ankole districts.

BURKITT (1951) stated, "In the district of Lago, hydrocele is very common. The incidence over large areas exceeds 25% of the adult male population, varying geographically from 30% in the east to 1% in the west. The size of the hydrocele sack is immense, the average content of one sack being a little over a pint. In examining just over 300 cases, I found bilateral hydroceles in 43%. The largest was a bilateral hydrocele with ten pints in one sack and 34 fluid ounces in the other." Microfilariae were found in the fluid in 17 out of 130 cases examined.

SPENCER (1962), in Lira District Hospital, Lago, also reported on clinical aspects of bancroftian filariasis in the Lago district. Some 25 % of the male patients in Lira Hospital were admitted because of lesions believed to be filarial. These patients were drawn from every county, and almost every village in the district. As for the clinical signs, episodic adenolymphangitis, genital filariasis, hydrocele, elephantiasis, synovitis, arthritis, and Fournier's disease (widespread gangrene of the scrotal skin) have been especially noted.

7D.7.2 *D. perstans*

Dipetalonema perstans is densely distributed over most of the region between Lake Victoria and Lake Kioga; the percentage of adults found infected ranged from 50 to 60% round Kampala and Entebbe to 91% in the Sese Islands (HAWKING, 1943).

7D.7.3 *L. loa*

According to POLTERA (1973), the occurrence of loiasis in Uganda was denied by WOODMAN (1958; loc. cit.). However, NNOCHIRI (1971; loc. cit.) found *Loa* microfilariae in Ugandan Africans who had never left the country. POLTERA (1973) conducted a retrospective study of 40 conjunctival biopsy materials at the Department of Pathology, Makerere University, Kampala, from 1967 to 1972, and found portions of nematode in 18 cases. Two among them were gravid females bearing sheathed microfilariae of *Loa*. In 22 biopsies worm granulomata or a worm track were observed. The patients were not only from the southern region, but also from eastern and western regions of Uganda.

7D.7.4 *O. volvulus*

Uganda has several large endemic foci of onchocerciasis. These are further classified into two types: those transmitted by *S. neavei,* and those transmitted by *S. damnosum*. Extensive programs for the control of Simuliid vectors have been in progress since 1955, and BROWN (1962) gave a detailed review on the distribution of the vectors and on the results of the control operations (Fig. 7-3).

S. neavei infested areas: (1) on the western slope of Mount Elgon in eastern Uganda, extending partly into Kenya, (2) in the foothills of the Ruwenzori Mountains in Kigezi Province, (3) the Bogama-Budongo region along the escarpment of Lake Albert, and (4) in the highlands of West Nile Province, extending partly into Zaire.

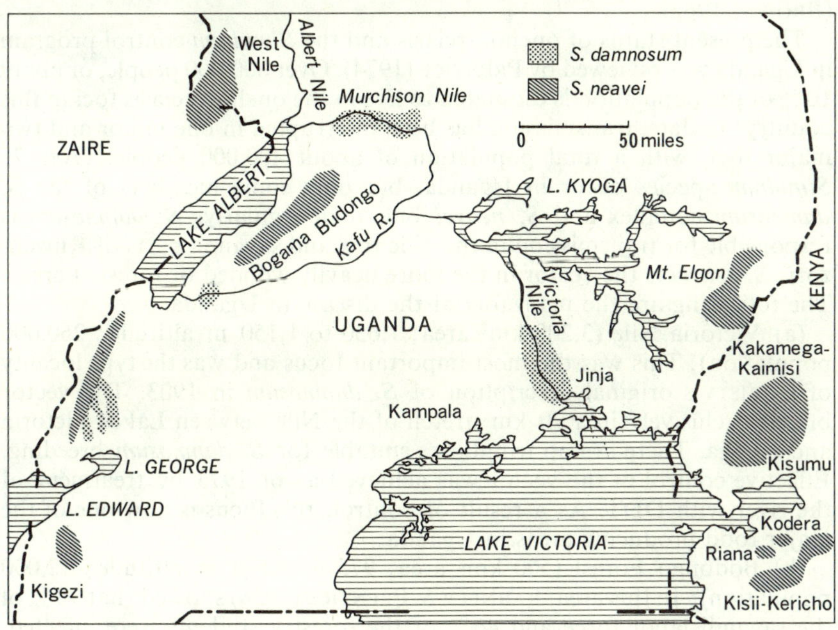

Fig. 7-3. Distribution of *S. neavei* and *S. damnosum* in eastern Africa (Uganda and Kenya). (After Brown, 1962).

S. damnosum is known to breed in (1) the Victoria Nile River connecting Lake Victoria and Lake Kyoga, (2) the Murchison Nile River from Atura to Lake Albert, and (3) the lower reaches of the rivers draining the Ruwenzori Mountains. There are several other rivers where the fly species are suspected of breeding.

According to BARNLEY (1958), the Victorial Nile, with approximately a 17,000 cusec flow, was treated in 1952 with DDT at 0.4 ppm for 30 minutes in 12 weekly operations. By the third application, *S. damnosum* had disappeared, and remained low for three years thereafter. The river was again treated in 1956 with DDT at 0.2 ppm for 30 minutes in weekly applications, and no *S. damnosum* appeared in the four years after treatment. Onchocerciasis had afflicted 99% of the inhabitants, on both sides of the 45-mile stretch of the rapids, but after the treatment this area became more densely settled because of the eradication of the black fly vector.

The Murchison Nile, with a flow of approximately 20,000 cusecs, was also treated in 1959 with DDT at 0.2 ppm for 30 minutes applied in 11 weekly treatments from January to April. The fly count fell to zero after the second application, but the fly reappeared by July, and large numbers of larvae were found in the Nile and its tributaries by October. In this case, the results were unsatisfactory because of the presence of tributaries in the Murchison game areas which were inaccessible to the control operation (BROWN, 1962).

The present status of onchocerciasis and the *Simulium* control program in Uganda was reviewed by PRENTICE (1974). Over 800,000 people, or about 10% of the population is estimated to live in the onchocerciasis foci in this country; to date, transmission has been interrupted in one minor and two major foci, with a total population of about 400,000 people. Over 75 *Simulium* species occur in Uganda, but only some members of the *S. damnosum* complex and *S. neavei* bite man regularly. *S. damnosum* is responsible for transmission in the Nile foci and savanna parts of Ruwenzori; *S. neavei* is the vector in the more heavily wooded or forested areas. The following are the main foci of the disease in Uganda.

(a) Victoria Nile (3,200 km² area; 1,030 to 1,150 m altitude; 260,000 population): This was the most important focus and was the type locality of CHRISTY'S original description of *S. damnosum* in 1903. The vector breeds exclusively in a 70 km stretch of the Nile between Lakes Victoria and Kyoga. There are no tributaries suitable for *S. damnosum* breeding. Effective control of the vector was achieved as of 1973 by treatment of the river with DDT. As a result of control, this focus is now one of the major food producing areas in Uganda.

(b) Bodongo Forest (500 km² area; 975 to 1,190 m altitude; 12,000 population): In this area, BARNLEY & PRENTICE (1958) showed that 78% of the sawmill labor force and 46% of the forestry students were infected. Trial control of *S. neavei* by application of DDT started in 1955, with ten applications per year at a dose of 0.5 ppm for 30 minutes, at ten-day intervals. The treatments were effective, and nearly complete eradication of *S. neavei* was achieved by 1962. The operation cost was approximately £500 per year, including monitoring costs.

(c) Masaba (Mt. Elgon): (1,000 km² area; 1,050 to 2,130 m altitude; 160,000 population): Onchocerciasis transmitted by *S. neavei* occurs on the densely populated southern and western slopes, with prevalence rate reaching 80% noted among adults. A *Simulium* control operation was initiated in 1957 by application of DDT at 140 dosing points, at a dose of 1 ppm. A resurvey of one of the focus in 1972 revealed that the prevalence dropped to between 5 and 10%, which may in part be accounted for by deforestation.

(d) Kabalega (Murchison) Nile (1,500 km² area; 760 to 950 m altitude; 15,000 population): A trial control of *S. damnosum* was attempted in 1959 to protect the work force during the construction of a hydroelectric power station.

(e) West Nile district (5,000 km² area; 900 to 1,500 m altitude; 120,000 population): NELSON (1958) reported a 56% prevalence rate in four villages. The vector is *S. neavei*. A pilot control scheme was initiated in 1955 by 12 weekly applications of DDT at a dose of 0.5 ppm for 30 minutes, on eight points of the six major streams. No further work was undertaken.

(f) Kigezi (1,500 km² area; 1,065 to 2,436 m altitude; 50,000 population): This focus is mountainous and extends into Zaire. Barnley (1949) reported prevalence rates of up to 80%. The vector is *S. neavei*. No control action has yet been taken.

(g) Ruwenzori (1,6000 km² area; 910 to 2,130 m altitude; 130,000 population): This focus is on the foothills of the 5,100 m high Ruwenzori Mountains, and extends into neighboring Zaire. High prevalence of onchocerciasis was noted, and trial control of the vector, *S. damnosum*, was initiated in 1971.

A new focus of onchocerciasis was reported by VAN DE WERD (1973) east and south-east of Lake George. Small rivers flow into the lake and a large part of the population in this small area was found to be suffering from the disease. The microfilariae were found in the skin snips of 68 out of 149 persons examined, nodules were seen in 20, and the eyes were affected in 32. *S. damnosum* was identified in some catches.

7D.8 Somalia

Somalia, or Somali Democratic Republic, is a country situated on the coast of the Gulf of Aden and the Indian Ocean, with a population of about 3,000,000 (1970 estimate) and an area of 638,000 km². Much of the country is semidesert and hilly or mountainous. No published information on filariasis is available. HAWKING (1973) stated, "Probably *W. bancrofti* is rare and the other filariae absent."

7D.9 Ethiopia

Ethiopia is a mountainous country lying between 3°N and 18°N, with an area of 1,221,000 km² and a population of 24,315,400 (1970).

7D.9.1 *W. bancrofti* and elephantiasis

The only record of *W. bancrofti* infection in Ethiopia was a correspondence by LUDERS (1937), a mission doctor, who stated, "In Bedelle, I have newly found *Filaria bancrofti* in centrifuged sediment of urine of a patient, who visited me because of hematuria."

The occurrence of *W. bancrofti* filariasis was reported also recently by McCONNEL & SCHMIDT (1973) from Gambela, Illubador province. The microfilariae were detected by filtering one ml of diurnal blood in 20 (24%) of 82 adult Anuak residents. Six of 2,531 *An. gambiae* and eight of 2,286 *An. funestus* contained third stage larvae of *W. bancrofti*. Filaria larvae were absent in 1,227 *Mansonia africana* and 2,001 *M. uniformis*.

OOMEN (1969c) reported that elephantiasis was common and widely distributed in Ethiopia, and in market counts*, 2.72% (6,770 cases) out of 247,908 persons inspected in 56 market places in various regions of this country were found to have elephantiasis. OOMEN (1969b) also discussed the etiology of elephantiasis, and concluded that although its cause in Ethiopia remained unclear, its association with filariasis could be excluded because "*W. bancrofti* is absent from Ethiopia," and the geographic distribution of elephantiasis is essentially different from that of onchocerciasis.

7D.9.2 *O. volvulus*

Onchocerciasis has been noted to be widespread, especially in southwest Ethiopia. BRYANT (1935) stated in the first report on onchocerciasis in Sudan that "it is possible that it exists also in Gambela, in Abyssinia," without mentioning the background for this suspicion. According to OOMEN (1969), an Italian scientific mission of JACONO, GIAQUINTO & BUCCO, in 1939, reported the discovery of onchocerciasis cases in Bonga. While they were staying in Ethiopia, 169 cases with positive skin snips were detected in this area; of these, 76 had photophobia, 34 had diminished vision, 7 were blind, and 33 had pruritus. In 1944 to 1945, a general medical survey was conducted in Ethiopia by the United States Technical Project, and "numerous positive cases were seen in Shebe (40 km from Bonga). COSSAR in 1948

*A method for epidemiological survey of disease manifestations formerly used for determination of incidence of goiter; one person counts the number of persons above the age of 16 who came into the market place, and another person counts the number of patients.

reported on 4 cases diagnosed in Gore and in 1951 on 50 cases in Jima. AKLILU LEMA reported high rates of infection in villages along Gojeb River near Bonga at the First African Conference on Onchocerciasis held in Brazzaville, in 1954. GRENIER & OVAZZA (1956) conducted a survey of *Simulium* in Ethiopia, and mentioned the common occurrence of onchocerciasis around Jima and Gore. TORYE (1966, quoted by OOMEN, 1969) carried out a medical survey of the Say Say people in the Blue Nile Gorge and reported a high incidence of onchocerciasis.

An extensive study on the clinical and epidemiological aspects of onchocerciasis, as well as on elephantiasis of the legs in Ethiopia was reported by OOMEN (1969). Out of 1,087 in-patients (765 males and 322 females) of all ages examined at the provincial hospital in Jima, the capital of Kefa Province, 230 (215 males and 15 females) were positive for microfilariae of *O. volvulus* in skin snips, with positive rates of 28.1% in males and 4.7% in females. The rates of persons above the age of 15 years were 29.7% (207 of 698) in males and 5.2% (15 of 286) in females. In 513 patients with positive skin snips, the most common signs were gale filarienne, macular dispigmentation, lichenification of the skin, and inguinal adenopathy; 25% among them suffered severely from itching; onchocercomata occurred in 12.8%, and suspect eye lesions only in six cases.

A survey of onchocerciasis based on the prevalence of the microfilariae in skin snips were conducted covering 38 locations and 3,854 persons in southwest Ethiopia. Of these places, seven were practically negative; the age and sex distribution of the positive rates of the people in 31 endemic areas were studied. The male rate (32.6%) was almost double that of the female rate (15.7%).

The present survey showed that the endemic area was spread over southwest Ethiopia covering some 132,000 km², with a population of 2.5 million of the provinces of Kefa, Ilubabor and Welega, and roughly 500,000 were estimated to be infected. Tentative boundaries of the endemic area beyond which the disease was considered to be practically absent because of high altitude and other reasons could be located as a result of this study. Of 38 places surveyed, 4 places showed high endemic levels of over 60% positive skin snips among the males over 15 years of age, 14 showed medium levels of 31 to 60%, and 13 places showed low levels of positive rates between 6 and 30%.

In general, the disease was more endemic to rural areas than to urban areas. Eye lesions were rare in all of the places visited, though slightly more common in the lowlands. The clinical appearances differed considerably between places above and below 1,000 m in altitude. Gale filarienne and its sequel, macular dyspigmentation, were common in the highlands and absent in the lowlands, while skin hypertrophy and onchocercomata were about five times more common in the lowlands than in the highlands with identical endemic levels.

Large numbers of *S. damnosum* and *S. woodi* were caught in a number of highland locations and Oomen considerd that both transmitted the disease here. No *Simulium* could be caught in this survey in the lowlands. It was estimated that the transmission in the highlands is perennial and not very intensive, while that in the lowlands is seasonal and intensive.

IWAMOTO *et al.* (1973) conducted an epidemiological and clinical survey of onchocerciasis in Ilubabor Province in southwestern Ethiopia. In examinations of skin snips, the microfilariae of *O. volvulus* were found in 70 (51.4%) of 136 persons examined at Abdella and 36 (66.7%) of 54 persons examined at Didessa; the positive rate in adult males was 80.7% (41 of 51) in Abdella and 71.4% (20 of 28) in Didessa. Various types of skin lesions due to onchocerciasis were observed among the villagers. Elephantiasis of the legs was also common, although it was not sure whether it was of onchocercal origin. Onchocercomata were found mostly around the iliac crest, ribs, and shoulder girdle. In four patients who were treated with DEC, severe pruritus occurred in three, and remarkable reductions in the microfilarial density in the skin snips were observed in all the cases.

7D.10 Sudan

Sudan is situated south of Egypt and on both sides of the middle stream of the Nile River. It has an area of 2,505,000 km² and a population of 15,675,000 (1971 estimate). The northern part of the country is an extention of the Libian Desert and is very dry though irrigated by the Nile River, while the southern half is hilly and mountainous and has larger precipitation.

Four species of human filariae are known to be endemic in the southern and more humid parts of Sudan, namely, *W. bancrofti*, *L. loa*, *D. perstans*, and *O. volvulus*. Dracontiasis used to be prevalent in the dry, northern areas.

The known endemic areas of *W. bancrofti* are confined to near the southern edge of Sudan (Equatoria and Bahr-al-Ghazal) and to the region near Nuba Mountain. *L. loa* has been found to be common among people in southern Sudan, near the edge of the tropical rain forest region, bordering the Central African Republic and Zaire (Congo). *D. perstans* has a wider distribution than *L. loa*. *O. volvulus* is prevalent in the Bahr-al-Ghazar area between latitudes 6° and 7° N, where "Jur," or "Sudan endemic blindness" is common.

CRUICKSHANK (1936) in a review of tropical diseases in southern Sudan, states, "The three known filaria in southern Sudan are *D. perstans*, *L. loa*, and *O. volvulus*, So far, *W. bancrofti* infection has not been identified. *D. perstans* is almost universal. At Wau, in a series of examinations of 642 persons of the general population I found 64% harbored *D. perstans*, The known distribution of *L. loa* is limited to the territory adjoining the Belgian Congo and French Equatorial Africa, chiefly the country of the Zande tribe. Last year's figures for Li-Rangu Hospital show that 38% of all male admissions (691) and 20% of all female (396) harbored this parasite. *O. volvulus* is found in all the *L. loa* areas and extends north to the limits of the fly belt. Its distribution east of the Nile has not been worked out but it is known to occur on the Abyssinian border. Dracontiasis has a patchy distribution over most of the areas except in the Zande country and in the western extremity. In the Nile Valley, all the country east of the Nile, and the cattle areas west of the river it is endemic. In the Yei District bordering Uganda, it was estimated that ten years ago, 60% of the population had guinea worm." He also pointed out that *L. loa* might be a factor in the causation of elephantiasis and hydroceles, and *O. volvulus* to be another cause of elephantiasis of the genitalia, and hydroceles.

7D.10.1 *W. bancrofti*

The occurrence of *W. bancrofti* infection in Sudan was reported by WOODMAN & BOKHARI (1941), who demonstrated the first clear instance of its microfilariae after examination of more than 1,500 films of day and night blood of cases showing sheathed microfilariae (these were mostly *L. loa*). Some dozen cases were subsequently found between 1937 and 1938. The areas surveyed were in Bahr-al-Ghazal Province near the border of Zaire, between latitudes 4° and 6° N and longitudes 27° and 31° E. The main features are open savanna forest, a rainfall of approximately 51 inches, an altitude of 2,000 feet, and temperature range between 54°F to 100°F. No actual cases of elephantiasis and hydrocele revealed either the microfilariae or the adults.

WOODMAN & BOKHARI (1941), in the same paper, also referred to the common occurrence of hydrocele in certain areas in Sudan. In the hospital of Meride, 80% of all operations performed were for hydrocele, and 240 were radically treated in one year. However, neither microfilariae nor adults of *W. bancrofti* was found in these materials, and microfilariae of *O. volvulus* were found on only one occasion. In other papers, WOODMAN (1948, 1949) reviewed the problems of filariasis in Sudan, and stressed the failure to find *W. bancrofti* in association with elephantiasis and hydrocele. He drew attention to the possible association between *L. loa* and these clinical symptoms.

KIRK (1957, 1960) reviewed the distribution of filariasis in Sudan, and reported on another endemic focus of *W. bancrofti*, which was discovered in 1944 by Mohi Din Mahdi, in the area round Kadugli, in the Nuba Mountains, southwest of Khartoum. The occurrence of elephantiasis in the Nuba Mountains had been known for years, but this was the first identification of the causal filaria. The microfilariae were nocturnally periodic. The author stressed the need for similar surveys in other areas where clinical filariasis existed, particularly the country along the Ethiopian border, where cases of hydrocele and elephantiasis were frequently reported by administrative officers.

KIRK (1957) stated that no study had been made to determine the vectors of *W. bancrofti* in the Sudan.

According to KIRK (1960), no instances of *W. bancrofti* infection were noted in central and northern Sudan in the thousands of blood films examined annually in local hospitals and dispensaries, although suitable vectors, such as *An. gambiae*, breed abundantly in these well-irrigated areas.

ABDALLA (1974) found the microfilariae of *W. bancrofti* in the blood of five cases of elephantiasis and hydrocele. The patients were from two regions of Sudan other than the Nuba Mountains, *i.e.*, a village near Yabus River in southern Blue Nile Province near the Ethiopian border, and another in Dafur province near Zalingi. Four of the above five cases were from the former village, and of 20 persons examined in this village, six were positive for *W. bancrofti* and ten for *O. volvulus*. This author suspected that *W. bancrofti* might be more widely distributed in this country than previously admitted.

7D.10.2 Other filariae

Loa loa was reported by CRUICKSHANK (1936) to occur mainly in the Zande country, on the northern edge of the tropical rain forest region. WOODMAN (1949) found the distribution of *L. loa* to be between 4° and 6°N, extending westwards into French Equatorial Africa and southwards into Zaire. ABBOT (1950) also reported that loiasis was very common in the Zande area. KIRK (1957) stated that about 20% of the native population and 23% of the European and Syrian officials were infected. *D. perstans* has a wider distribution than *L. loa*, but is less precisely known. In the Bahr-al-Ghazal Province, it occurs throughout the areas of distribution of *L. loa* and *O. volvulus* (WOODMAN. 1949).

O. volvulus was recorded by LAIGRET (1929), and was reported by KIRK (1947) to be prevalent in the Bahr-al-Ghazal Province; *S. damnosum* was found to be the principal and possibly the only vector. MORGAN (1958) reported on onchocerciasis in northern Sudan. A study on *Simulium* in Sudan was conducted by HOCKING & HOCKING (1962).

7E. Madagascar and other Indian Ocean Islands

Filariasis due to *W. bancrofti* has been shown to be endemic in certain parts of Madagascar, and some adjacent islands in the Indian Ocean, such as the Comoro Islands, Reúnion, Mauritius, the Seychelle Islands, and the Chagos Archipelago. The incidence in some areas has been reported to be extremely high. There seems to exist two different epidemiological types of bancroftian filariasis in this subregion: the African type transmitted by the *An. gambiae-funestus* complex and endemic in Madagascar, and the Indian type transmitted by *C. fatigans* on other smaller Indian Ocean islands. Other filariae have not been reported from this subregion.

Reviews on the epidemiology of filariasis referring to this subregion were made by Hawking (1957, 1973), Brygoo (1958), Hamon *et al.* (1967), and Brunhes (1973).

7E.1 Malagasy (Madagascar)

Malagasy Republic occupying the island of Madagascar, is situated in the Indian Ocean east of the African continent, between 12°S and 26°S. It has an area of 587,000 km² with a population of 7,423,864 (1970). The island is almost entirely covered by plateau and mountains. Its eastern coast has high precipitation and is covered mostly by tropical rain forest, while its central region and western coast are dry consisting of savanna or semidesert.

W. bancrofti is the only human filaria presently known to be endemic in Madagascar. Although the island has many rivers and streams, and *Simulium* flies are abundant, especially on the east coast, *O. volvulus* has never been found to be endemic. Bancroftian filariasis is endemic throughout the lower zones of Madagascar and is particularly prevalent in the eastern coastal zone.

(a) Distribution

The occurrence of filariasis in Madagascar has been noted since old times. According to Brygoo (1958), Vivie, in 1903, described the frequent occurrence of lymphangitis and elephantiasis in the northwestern region of the island. Fontoynont & Leopold Robert in 1909 reported to "la Société des Sciences Médicales de Madagascar" that microfilariae were found in 38 out of 50 patients examined at the hospital of Tananarive, the capital of Madagascar. However, later workers have never confirmed the occurrence of filariasis in this high plateau region. On the other hand, the occurrence of a number of clinical filariasis cases were noted by Sicé (1927), Cloitre (1928), Sanner *et al.* (1936). and Radaody-Ralarosy & Guidoni (1940).

As for the epidemiology of bancroftian filariasis in Madagascar, Randriambelo (1950) conducted the first blood survey in the region of Farafangana and found about 40% of the people to be infected. After this report was published, mobile teams for health inspection examined this region in more detail, and a preliminary report was compiled by Beytout (1952). Doucet (1950) made a study of the mosquito fauna of this region, and found that *An. funestus* in Vangaindrano was infected by various stages of filarial larvae.

In 1955, the Director of Sanitary and Medical Services of Madagascar decided to make a general survey of filariasis covering the whole island. Thick blood smears were collected by mobile teams at night, after 8 p.m., and were then sent to the Pasteur Institute of Madagascar for staining and examination. By the end of August 1957, a total of 18,384 persons were examined; blood specimens were collected from 60 out of 83 districts on the island and from 272 out of 475 villages. A summary of the results of these investigations were reported by BRYGOO (1958).

It has been demonstrated from this survey that bancroftian filariasis is widely distributed in Madagascar, especially in the regions along the east coast; especially high incidences were noted in the districts on the southeast coast and the coastal districts of Fianarantsoa Province. The rates in this region varied from 20.35% in the Vohipeno district to 36.64% in the Ifanadiana District. The microfilarial rates were also high in some districts of the Tamatave Province, such as 24.19% in Fénérive, 15.87% in Brickaville, and 15.24% in Tamatave. Endemic foci were also found from northern parts of the east coast, such as the Vohémar district of Diégo-Suarez Province, and several districts in Majunga Province.

(b) Taxonomy

In the course of these blood surveys carried out in the southeast coastal region, GALLIARD & BRYGOO (1955) recognized that the microfilariae found in the thick blood smears of people in Manakara, Fort Carnot, Lahorano, and Ifaho showed an appearance similar to those of *B. malayi*; they were twisted and irregular in shape accompanied by secondary undulations in addition to the principal waves, and were different from the regular, graceful appearance of those of *W. bancrofti*. Their length was between 180 and 275 μ, close to the length (165 to 265 μ) of the microfilariae of *B. malayi*, but shorter than those of *W. bancrofti* (over 300 μ). The nuclei of the Madagascar microfilariae were overlapping and difficult to differentiate as in the case of *B. malayi*; they were different in arrangement from *W. bancrofti*, which are separated and easily countable. On the other hand, these microfilariae differed from those of *B. malayi* in the absence of caudal nuclei, in the position and size of the anal or excretory pores, etc. From this evidence, a new name, *Wuchereria bancrofti* var. *vauceli*, was proposed for this type of microfilariae. These descriptions were also given by GALLIARD *et al.* (1955). This variety was later raised to a full species, *Wuchereria vauceli*, by GALLIARD (1959). SOUVEINE *et al.* (1955) demonstrated that the microfilariae on the eastern coast of Madagascar were a nocturnally periodic form.

BRYGOO (1958), in his paper on the review of filariasis in Madagascar, stated that *W. vauceli* was not the sole cause, but was usually mixed with the typical *W. bancrofti*; on the east coast, the former represented about 95% of the positive cases, while in Ankazoabo, *W. bancrofti* was apparently the sole agent. On the other hand, CHABAUD & CHOQUET (1958) stated that the microfilariae of *W. vauceli* were apparently indistinguishable from those of *Dipetalonema petteri* Chabaud et Choquet, 1955, described from lemurs from Madagascar, and suggested the possible occurrence of animal reservoirs for *W. vauceli*. However, as stated previously (Section 2B. 4.2), SCHACHER & GEDDAWI (1969), as well as SCHACHER (1969), made nuclear count studies of the microfilariae of *W. bancrofti* collected from various localities in the world and those collected from the type locality of *W. vauceli*; they concluded that there was no structural characteristics for separating *W. vauceli* from *W. bancrofti*, and also that the secondary, kinked attitude described as one of the attributes of *W. vauceli* microfilariae was possibly caused by shrinking upon protracted drying of the blood films, or delay in dehemoglobinization. These authors concluded that *W. vauceli* was a synonym of *W. bancrofti*.

BRUNHES *et al.* (1972) made extensive studies on the epidemiology of human filariasis in Madagascar, and in the observations on the characteristics of the microfilariae and mature larvae also concluded that there were no significant differences between those of Madagascar and those of typical *W. bancrofti* from the Comoro Islands, and that *W. bancrofti* was the only filarial worm infecting man in Malagasy. In this report, high incidences of microfilaremia cases was observed in Fort Carnot (57.6%, or 19 of 33 hospital patients), Ifanadiana (38.9%, or 7 of 18 hospital patients), and rural communities of Haute-Mananano (19% of 46 young people from various villages).

(c) Transmission

The distribution of bancroftian filariasis in Malagasy is in essentially rural areas and especially high incidence has been noted in villages along the eastern coast, while the disease is practically absent from urban areas and central high plateau regions. In contrast to bancroftian filariasis on the Comoro Islands which is mainly transmitted by the urban mosquito, *C. fatigans*, the disease in Malagasy has been noted to be transmitted by anopheline mosquitoes, especially by *An. gambiae* and *An. funestus*.

DOUCET (1951) made a study of mosquito vectors of filariasis for the first time in Malagasy, and found 8.3% (10 of 120) of *An. funestus* collected at Vangaindrano to be infected with filaria larvae. BRUNHES (1969) examined mosquitoes in the region of Manakara, and found 7 with mature larvae and 6 others with immature larvae, out of 214 *An. funestus* examined; in the east coast, 3 of 239 *An. gambiae* were infected, and 2 of them had mature larvae of *W. bancrofti*. Natural infections with third stage larvae of *W. bancrofti* were also shown in an endemic area in Ifaho (Haute-Mananano) in 69 out of 21,537 *An. funestus*, 25 out of 8,374 *An. gambiae*, and 1 out of 127 *An. pauliani*; in the same study series, third stage larvae of *Setaria* were found in 2 of 21,537 *An. funestus*, 1 of 675 *An. coustani*, and 42 of 4,685 *M. uniformis*.

Under experimental conditions, MOREAU (1965) studied the development of *W. bancrofti* in *C. fatigans* in Majunga (northeastern Madagascar); out of 72 female mosquitoes which were fed on a *W. bancrofti* carrier with moderate microfilaremia density, and kept under natural conditions for 12 days, 33% were found to be infected. BRUNHES (1969) also conducted laboratory experiments with various mosquito species, and the parasite was shown to develop to the mature stage in *An. gambiae* A, *An. gambiae* B, *An. coustani*, *An. mascarensis*, *C. fatigans*, and *C. antennatus*.

When *An. gambiae* B were raised at different temperatures in the laboratory, larvae of *W. bancrofti* reached the mature stage after 27 days at 20°C, after 14 days at 25°C, after 11 days at 30°C, but the development was slower at 35°C. The percentage of the females carrying mature larvae was 81% among those kept at 20°C, 91% at 25°C, and 69% at 30°C. In *C. fatigans* (Tananarive strain) raised under the same conditions, the percentages of females carrying mature larvae were much lower, namely, 3% at 20°C, 10% at 25°C, and 36% at 30°C.

In a more recent study on the experimental infection of Madagascar mosquitoes with *W. bancrofti* by BRUNHES *et al.* (1972), development to mature larvae was seen in 2 of 4 *An. fuscicolor*, 1 of 1 *An. squamosus*, 1 of 2 *An. pauliani*, 1 of 1 *An. mascarensis*, 1 of 2 *An. coustani*, 2 of 2 *An. gambiae*, and 8 of 9 *C. antennatus*, but none of 26 *M. uniformis* and other Culicine specimens tested were found to harbor mature larvae.

A comprehensive study and review on the transmission of bancroftian filariasis in Madagascar was presented by BRUNHES (1973). In the study of filaria transmission in a rural environment, four villages on southeast coast along Mananano River were selected, where BRUNHES *et al.* (1972) conducted parasitological and epidemiological investigations. The result of 60 collections of man-biting mosquitoes both indoors and outdoors was that 19 species (10 *Anopheles*, 4 *Culex*, 3 *Aedes*, and 2 *Mansonia*) were found to attack man. In Ifaho and Mahavelona, the number of total catches by order were: 6160 *An. gambiae*, 3685 *M. uniformis*, 584 *An. coustani*, and 163 *An. funestus* (163); in Stephaville and Manaville, the numbers by order were 17393 *An. funestus*, 3183 *An. gambiae*, 1715 *M. uniformis*, and 153 *An. coustani*. *An. gambiae* was collected more from outdoors than indoors (4952 versus 4352), while in *An. funestus*, the number collected indoors slightly exceeded those collected outdoors (10280 versus 7276); *M. uniformis* was shown to be a markedly exophilic mosquito (indoors, 1131 versus outdoors, 4296). Natural infection with mature larvae of *W. bancrofti* was seen only in *An. gambiae*, *An. funestus*, and *An. pauliani*; *M. uniformis* was found to harbor only the larvae of animal filariae (*Setaria* and *Dirofilaria*). The transmission of *W. bancrofti* was found to occur mainly during the season from November to April when the mean temperature is high enough for the larval development; little transmission occurs during the winter season from April to September. The density of the vectors is also dependent upon the rainfall; on the eastern coast, they are abundant except for a short, dry season from August to October. Therefore, the transmission was found to be most intensive during the wet and warm season from December to March. The rate of development to mature larvae was shown to be higher in *An. gambiae* than in *An. funestus*, but since the latter has a longer life span, the natural infection rate with mature larvae was higher in *An. funestus* than in *An. gambiae*.

In the urban environment around the city of Tananarive, both *An. gambiae* and *C. fatigans* coexisted with the latter found to breed throughout the year, but bancroftian filariasis was apparently absent from this region.

During the year 1971, 52 night catches were conducted, and altogether, 4236 *C. fatigans* and 120 *An. gambiae* were captured; none of them were found to be harboring third stage larvae. In experimental transmission studies, the percentage of infective female mosquitoes which had fed on a carrier from the Comoro Islands harboring 100 microfilariae per 20 mm³ blood 14.5 days before was 87.4% of 103 *C. fatigans* and 75.5% of 49 *An. gambiae*, with the average number of infective larvae per mosquito of 8.9 and 5.1, respectively. The percentages of mosquitoes containing mature larvae 14.5 days after feeding on a carrier in Madagascar harboring 95 microfilariae per 20 mm³ blood were 41.7% in *C. fatigans* from Tananarive, 45% in *C. fatigans* from Majunga, and 92% in *An. gambiae*, with the average number of mature larvae per mosquito of 3.8, 2.4, and 8.1, respectively. These results indicate that *W. bancrofti* in Madagascar is more adapted for development in *An. gambiae* than in *C. fatigans*, while the relationship is probably reversed in the *W. bancrofti* strain in the Comoro Islands.

Other observations on the transmission of *W. bancrofti* were conducted in two urban areas: in the town of Majunga situated on the west coast where it is generally hot and dry, and in the town of Tanatave on the east coast where it is cooler and more humid. In the Province of Majunga, 6.5% out of 1,514 persons examined were microfilaria positive, but clinical filariasis was extremely rare, and only one out of 43 *C. fatigans* dissected was found to contain second stage filaria larvae. The extensive house-spraying program with DDT as a measure of malaria control was considered to be at least partly responsible for such a poor transmission data for filariasis. In the province of Tamatave, BRYGOO (1958) observed a microfilaria rate of 9.6% out of 5,027 persons examined at night, and because of the abundant breeding of *C. fatigans* in the urban area, the future spread of *W. bancrofti* into the towns was also feared.

7E.2 The Comoro Islands

A group of volcanic islands in northern Mozambique Channel between the continental Africa and Madagascar, at about 12°S; it includes four main islands; Great Comoro (1,148 km² and 118,924 inhabitants), Mohéli (290 km² and 9,545 inhabitants), Anjouan (424 km² and 83,829 inhabitants), and Mayotte (374 km² and 32,609 inhabitants) (BRUNHES, 1973). The total area is 2,235 km²; the total population is 267,000 (1970).

LAFONT, in 1905 (quoted by BRYGOO & ESCOLIVET, 1955), reported on the frequent occurrence of elephantiasis in the Comoros and stressed the need for control of the vectors and for further research on filariasis in these islands.

ROUFFIANDIS (1910) reported that 90% of the population of Mohéli, 80% of Mayotte, 30% of Anjouan, and 5% of Great Comoro were affected by filariasis. Among the various races in the Comoro Islands, the "Mahore," or the autochthonous people on Mayotte and Mohéli, and the "Makoi" imported as slaves from East Africa, were the most severely affected, while those from Madagascar, as well as Arabs and Europeans mainly residing on Great Comoro, were much less affected. Of the male population of 3,000 on Mayotte, 80% had filarial manifestations; 59% had elephantiasis of the scrotum associated with adenolymphocele and chylous hydrocele, 12% had lymphoscrotum accompanied by elephantiasis of the legs, 5% had adenolymphocele only, 3% had elephantiasis of one or both legs, and 1% had various forms of hematochyluria, chylous ascites, and lymphatic abscesses.

SULDEY (1918), in a communication on leprosy and endemic diseases on Mohéli, stated that among 261 filariasis patients examined, 61 cases (37%) had elephantiasis (left leg, 24; right leg 12; both legs 15; and scrotum 10), 13 cases had adenolymphocele, and 26 cases had hydrocele.

BRYGOO & ESCOLIVET (1955) conducted a comprehensive survey of filariasis on Mayotte and Mohéli Islands. On Mayotte, a total of 1,442 persons, or 14.4% of the adult population, were examined, and microfilariae were found in 536 (37.2%); of 706 males, 339 (48.0%) were positive, and of 736 females, 197 (26.8%) were positive. The rates by the villages varied from 20.5% to 55.5%. On Mohéli, 1,996 persons were examined, and 873 (43.7%) were positive, with rates of 48.8% (517 of 1,060) in males and 38.0% (356 of 936) in females. The rates varied from 24.7% to 48.7% by the villages. The microfilariae were all those of the classical type of *W. bancrofti*, and the variety *vauceli* described by GALLIARD & BRYGOO (1955) from Madagascar were not found among them. Out of 6,636 persons examined in Mayotte and 5,736 persons examined in Mohéli, elephantiasis was seen in 55 (0.8%) and 98 (1.7%), respectively. Four species of anophelines and four species of culicines were found on Mayotte, and six species of anophelines and eight species of culicines were found on Mohéli. Among the known vectors of *W. bancrofti*, *An. gambiae* and *An. funestus* were found on both islands, and *C. fatigans* was found on Mohéli.

A survey of filariasis in the island of Anjouan was reported by Prod'hon (1972). The total population of the island was 83,829 in 1966, of which 52,897 (25,772 males and 27,125 females) were above the age of ten years. Thick blood smears were collected at night after 9 p.m. from 1,607 persons in nine villages (1,565 were above the age of ten years), of whom 347 (45.4%) out of 764 males and 316 (37.5%) out of 843 females were positive for the microfilariae of typical *W. bancrofti*. Each of the nine villages surveyed showed a high incidence of filariasis, with the gross microfilarial rate varying from 26.5% to 56.7%.

A comprehensive study on the epidemiology of filariasis on the island of Mayotte was conducted by BRUNHES (1973). In the village of Sada, of 668 males and 758 females examined, 228 (34.1%) males and 275 (36.3%) females were positive; the rates among the persons above the age of ten years were 46.3% (184 of 397) in males and 44.0% (214 of 486) in females.

The median microfilarial density (MfD-50) per 20 mm^3 blood samples among the positive cases was 17.2. Out of 668 males and 758 females examined clinically, 17 males and 18 females had elephantiasis; hydrocele was found in 19% (75 of 397) of the males above the age of ten and 35% of 77 males above the age of 50.

In the village of Chiconi, 33.4% (162 of 485) of the males and 17.1% (83 of 485) of the females above the age of ten were examined; 34.5% among the males and 21.7% among the females examined had microfilariae in 20 mm^3 blood samples. The value of MfD-50 was 18 for the male carriers and 8 for the female carriers. Of 162 males above the age of ten, 11 had hydrocele but none had elephantiasis of the leg; of 83 females examined, 2 had elephantiasis of the leg.

In the village of Bandele, where clinical signs of filariasis among the inhabitants were most conspicuous, 23 (38.3%) of 60 males above the age of ten showed microfilaremia, and 10 (16.7%) of them had hydrocele or elephantiasis; among 24 females above the age of ten examined, 10 (41.6%) had microfilaremia and 1 (4.2%) had elephantiasis. In this village, the MfD-50 was 37 among the male carriers and 14 among the female carriers.

Blood examinations were also conducted on 209 persons admitted to the hospital of Mamutsu and Dzaoudzi on Mayotte Island; 83 or 39.7% among them were positive for microfilariae. Of 94 patients who showed some clinical signs of filariasis, 17 had elephantiasis of the legs, 64 had hydrocele or elephantiasis of the scrotum, and 12 had both elephantiasis of the legs and pathological deformation of the scrotum; the microfilaremia rate among the 94 cases was 21.5%. Out of 304 persons who underwent surgery from 1969 to 1971, 105 (34.5%) were hydrocele cases.

As for the mosquito fauna of Comoro, BRUNHES (1973) confirmed the Occurrence of 34 species: 6 *Anopheles*, 8 *Aedes*, 2 *Eretmapodides*, 1 *Mansonia*, 1 *Ficalbia*, 1 *Orthopodomyia*, 12 *Culex*, and 3 *Uranotaenia*. On Great Comoro, 199 *C. fatigans* were examined, of which 12 (6.0%) were infected with filaria larvae and 3 (1.5%) had mature larvae of *W. bancrofti*; 77 *An. gambiae* were also examined, of which 3 were infected, but none had mature larvae. In Mohéli, 1,199 *C. fatigans* were dissected, of which 5.2% were infected and 0.5% were infective; none of 12 *An. gambiae* were infected. In Mayotte, 75 (1.9%) out of 4,026 *C. fatigans* and 18 (0.6%) of 2,844 *An. gambiae* dissected had mature larvae of *W. bancrofti*. From this and other evidence, the author considers *C. fatigans* to be the principal vector of *W. bancrofti* in the Comoro Islands, and *An. gambiae* to be a secondary vector in some parts of the islands.

7E.3 Mauritius

Mauritius is an island situated in the Indian Ocean at a latitude of about 20°S and about 720 km east of Madagascar; it has an area of 1,900 km^2 and a population of 830,700 (1970). It has been independent since 1968.

The incidence of filariasis in Port Louis, the capital of Mauritius, was reported by KIRK (1928). In 1925, he examined approximately 20 mm³ of blood at night collected from 51 hospital patients, and found microfilariae of *W. bancrofti* in 16 (31.4%). In another examination of night blood of the general population of Port Louis conducted in 1927, microfilariae of *W. bancrofti* were found in 74 persons, with a microfilaremia rate of 11.2%. The rate for adult males above the age of 16 was 15.4% (36 of 234) and that for adult females was 9.0 % (20 of 221). Microfilariae of species other than *W. bancrofti* were not found in these surveys. Clinical filariasis was common among the hospital patients. The common mosquito species were *C. fatigans* (very common), *Ae. albopictus* (very common), *An. costalis* (relatively common), and *Ae. argenteus* (relatively rare).

According to HUEHNS (1953), a blood survey was conducted in 1928 by Pilot, in the Flacq district, and 17% were found showing microfilariae. In the same year, 25% of the inmates of the mental hospital and 9.6% of patients admitted to the Port Louis Civil Hospital showed microfilariae in the blood.

GEBERT (1937) reported that bancroftian filariasis occurred throughout the island. In blood examinations of hospital patients, 9.1% of the males and 3.0% of the females from Port Louis, as well as 11.6% of the males and 3.1% of the females from other districts were positive for microfilariae of *W. bancrofti*. He also showed that *C. fatigans, An. costalis, An. funestus*, and *An. maculipalpis* were all capable of acting as vectors.

HUEHNS (1953) conducted a blood survey in 17 villages covering the whole island of Mauritius and including the two main towns, Port Louis on the coast and Curepipe, in the center of the island. Of 1,930 civilians examined, 213 (11.0%) were positive; of 700 Mauritian recruits, 58 (8.3%) were found infected. Positive cases were distributed all over the island, and the highest incidence was 38% of Campe Creoles (Albion). The periodicity of the microfilariae was definitely nocturnal. Elephantiasis and other clinical manifestations of filarial infection occurred on the island, but were relatively infrequent.

7E.4 Réunion

An island of the Mascarene Islands in the Indian Ocean, 684 km east of Madagascar, on about 21°S; Réunion is 2,510 km² in area, with a population of 455,200 (1971). It has been an overseas territory of France since 1946.

According to BRYGOO & BRUNHES (1973) and BRUNHES (1973), bancroftian filariasis has been noted to be prevalent in Réunion; THERON, in 1897, reported that 81 (1.4%) of 5,743 young men examined for medical service were exempted because of hydrocele, and 20 (0.35%) others were also exempted because of elephantiasis. HEIM & CALLOT (1969) conducted night blood examinations on 908 patients (222 males and 686 females) admitted to the hospital, and found microfilariae in 11.67% (12.16% in males and 11.51% in females).

Studies on mosquitoes in Réunion were reported by HAMON & DUFOUR (1954), and HAMON (1956) in connection with the control of malaria. BRUNHES (1973) collected six species of mosquitoes by six night collections: *An. gambiae* s.l., *C. p. fatigans*, *C. tritaeniorhynchus*, *Ae. albopictus*, and *Ae. fowleri*. In this study, none of the mosquitoes collected were found infected with mature filaria larvae; it was also estimated that bancroftian filariasis on this island was taking a course of spontaneous disappearance, possibly due to the extensive application of insecticides as malaria control measures. Under experimental conditions, *C. fatigans* was shown to be highly adapted for the development of *W. bancrofti* larvae.

7E.5 The Seychelles Islands

The Seychelles are a British colony consisting of about 90 islands scattered in four groups over a wide area of the western Indian Ocean, east of Northeast Tanzania, on about 4°S and 56°E. They have a total area of 277 km^2 with a total population of 54,000 (1972).

The distribution and epidemiology of filariasis in the Seychelles and the Chagos Islands were reported by LAMBRECHT (1971b). The Seychelles were not populated until the first French colonists from Mauritius settled on Mahe Island along with African laborers in 1756. The present population comprises of a mixture of descendents of the first European and African settlers and of later immigrants from Africa, India, and China. The occurrence of elephantiasis and other signs of bancroftian filariasis were recorded in the *Annual Reports of the Medical Department* for 1926 and 1931. FRÖLICH (1968, quoted by LAMBRECHT, 1971b) made a preliminary night blood survey and found the microfilariae of *W. bancrofti* in 20% in one area of Mahe, and in several areas of Praslin. In this survey, 2 ml of venous blood was drawn from each person, hemolysed in 10 ml of 2% formalin and centrifuged; the sediment was examined. As a result, microfilariae were found in 63 (3.5%) of 1,780 persons examined in Mahe, 100 (17.1%) of 586 examined in Praslin, 16 (7.4%) of 216 examined in La Digue, and 9 (4.5%) of 200 examined in Silhouette. In an examination of 20 mm^3 blood samples collected from 25 persons on Denis Island by LAMBRECHT (1971b), 4 (16.0%) were positive.

As for the mosquito fauna of the Seychelles, MATTINGLY & BROWN (1955) recorded 14 species (5 *Culex*, 5 *Aedes*, 1 *Mansonia*, and 3 *Uranotaenia*). *Ae. aegypti*, *Ae. albopictus*, and *C. fatigans* were the most common mosquitoes; *Anopheles* species were absent from the islands. According to LAMBRECHT (1971b), the infection rate of *C. fatigans* with all stages of larvae and with mature larvae of *W. bancrofti* were 1.6% and 0.23% respectively, out of 434 specimens collected at Port Glaud (Mahe). In experimental infection studies, three groups of *C. fatigans* fed on microfilaria carriers became infected with mature larvae at the rates of 60%, 45%, and 50%, but none of *Ae. albopictus* experimentally infected contained mature larvae in examinations conducted 11 to 14 days after taking the blood containing microfilariae. In the Seychelles, *C. fatigans* was regarded as to be the only vector of *W. bancrofti* from these observations. A comprehensive report on the ecology of the Seychelles mosquitoes was published by LAMBRECHT (1971a).

7E.6 The Chagos Archipelago

The Chagos Archipelago consists of numerous islands and coral reefs lying in the Indian Ocean between 4°S and 8°S, and between 70°E and 73°E south of the Maldive Islands and east of the Seychelles Islands. Diego Garcia, Peros Banhos, and Salomon, the three main atolls, have been inhabited since the latter part of the 18th century. Area, 197 km². The archipelago is part of the British Indian Ocean Territory, which was created in 1965.

LAMBRECHT (1971b) conducted night blood examination of 20 mm³ samples collected from people in the three main atolls, and found the microfilariae of *W. bancrofti* in 14 (15.6%) of 90 persons examined on Diego Garcia (population, 319), 3 (15.0%) of 20 on Salomon (population, 182), and 20 (24.1%) of 83 on Peros Banhos (population, 151). LAMBRECHT & VAN SOMOREN (1971) reported on the occurrence of three species of mosquitoes in the Chagos Archipelago: *Ae. aegypti*, *Ae. albopictus*, and *C. fatigans*. Of 120 *C. fatigans* collected on Diego Garcia, three were infected with various stages of filarial larvae, and one had mature larvae of *W. bancrofti*.

7F. Filariasis in Europe and Near East

Sporadic records of the occurrence of clinical or microfilaremia cases of bancroftian filariasis were made from Yugoslavia (Macedonia), Italy (Sicily), Greece, Spain, and Portugal, but for many years no fresh cases have appeared in these countries (HAWKING, 1973). In Israel, WITTENBERG (1968) recorded that *W. bancrofti* infection was recognized among immigrants from India, but no new cases have since appeared. Two endemic foci of bancroftian filariasis have been found from Turkey. No published records on the occurrence of indigenous filariasis cases are available from the Middle East countries, i.e., from Iraq, Syrian Arab Republic, Jordan, Iran, Bahrain, Oman, Democratic Yemen, Kuwait, Qatar, and Saudi

Arabia, although imported cases have been found in some of these countries.

In Yemen, *O. volvulus* was found among patients suffering from a skin disease locally called "soda."

7F.1 Europe

CASTELLANI (1917) stated, "on August 15, in Skoplje (capital of Macedonia in southern Yugoslavia), and in 1916 near Monastir (a seaport town in Tunisia, North Africa), I have seen two cases of acute lymphadenitis with erythematous rash and great enlargement of the left leg in both cases. In the Skoplje case, the blood taken at night was seen to contain *Microfilaria bancrofti* on two occasions. I have seen also in Macedonia three cases of typical elephantiasis of the leg, and one in Naples." He had also seen a typical case of endemic funiculitis in Macedonia, in 1915.

FAMULARI (1915) reported on a case of filariasis in a woman, 52 years of age, who had never been out of Sicily. She spent most of the time in Messina, but when the town was devasted by an earthquake a few years ago, she was forced to reside at a place named San Stefano Soprano for two years, after which, she returned to Messina. She then began to suffer from the illness. The urine was found to exhibit the characteristics of filarial infection, and microfilariae were found in it. More microfilariae were found in the blood taken at night. The author considered that filariasis had become endemic in Sicily having probably been introduced in recent years.

7F.2 Turkey

Turkey is situated between the Black Sea and the Mediterranean Sea, between 36°N and 42°N. It has an area of 780,576 km² and a population of 35,666,549 (1970).

Two isolated endemic foci of bancroftian filariasis have been found in this country. One was reported by YUCEL & DESCHIENS (1960) and DESCHIENS *et al.* (1961) from the region of Elazig, eastern Turkey, at about 38°E and 40°N. It is in a mountainous region with an average height of about 1,000 m above sea level, comprising a high valley of the Euphrates River. Among some 50,000 inhabitants of this area in the village of Elazig and the vicinity, 13 cases of filariasis were detected, of which 9 were thoroughly investigated. They showed lymphangitis, lymphadenitis, and some had elephantiasis of the leg. Microfilariae typical of *W. bancrofti* were demonstrated from the night blood of one out of three cases examined. Unpublished observations conducted by SCHACHER & THORSON in 1965 (quoted by HAWKING, 1973) suggest that this focus has died out.

The second focus was reported from the town Alanya in Antalya Province, southern Turkey, facing the Mediterranean Sea. According to SIPA-HIOGLU (1959, 1966), microfilariae were found in 243 (2.72%) of 8,920 persons examined. The parasite was believed to have been imported from Alexandria and Rosetta in Egypt, with which Alanya has long had close ties through frequent boat crossings.

7F.3 Onchocerciasis in South Arabia

Indigenous cases of onchocerciasis were reported by FAWDRY (1957) from Yemen, South Arabia, which constitutes, so far as is known, the only endemic area of the disease outside of Africa and Central America. A peculiar skin disease called "soda" (from *sawad* meaning black) had long been noted by local people, and had also been frequently seen by physicians in Aden. The natural course of the disease, as deduced from detailed histories of 50 sufferers is as follows:

> An itching is noticed in the leg below the kneee, and during the next few weeks it spreads gradually upwards and downwards to cover the whole of the skin of the lower leg except for the sole of the foot. There is slight swelling of the leg and, as a result of the scratching, small pimples and boils form, which burst and leave circular scars of 0.5 to 1 cm across; gross secondary infection may produce an impetiginous rash over the whole area and painful inflammation. It does not give rise to the large tropical ulcers which are common among other Yemenis from the same area.
>
> The area of itching slowly spreads up beyond the knee and usually reaches to the sacroiliac region behind, the iliac crest at the side, and the inguinal ligament in front.
>
> The skin becomes coarse in texture, thickened, and inelastic, so that round the knee, especially, there may be thick folds; generally edema is slight. The change in color which gives the disease its name is not noticeable in the very dark, but in light or medium-skinned Arabs, the color of the limb contrasts oddly with that of the remainder of the body. The lymph node enlargement is quite considerable and roughly related to the area of skin involved at the height of the disease. The individual nodes may be up to 2 to 3 cm long and 1 to 2 cm broad, usually being a cluster of three or four. They have a rubbery consistency and are very different from the harder, smaller glands of chronic inflammation.

Of 50 patients with "soda," only 5 had subcutaneous nodules; adult worms of *O. volvulus* (identified by Buckley) were recovered from all of the three nodules biopsied. The microfilariae of *O. volvulus* were also found from skin of 3 of 10 "soda" dermatitis cases, but not from the skin of the remaining 7 cases. No macroscopic eye lesions were found in any of the 50 cases.

Fawdry (1957) considers that the skin disease of South Arabia called "soda" is somewhat different from the typical skin lesions described for onchocerciasis, but since adults and microfilariae of *O. volvulus* have been found in some of the cases, it is probable that the worm is the cause of the dermatitis.

FAWDRY (1957) also stated, "Elephantiasis of the bancroftian type is occasionally seen here (Aden); during the current investigation, four males have come with gross firm edema of the leg, distinguished at once from *soda* by the absence of itching, the normal color of the skin, and normal femoral glands. No other signs of filariasis, such as transient swellings, nocturnal fever, or microfilariae in the blood, have been discovered."

ANDERSON *et al.*(1973) reported on results of further studies on onchocerciasis in Yemen. The occurrence of larvae and pupae of *Simulium damnosum* was reported from the endemic area by MERIGHI *et al.* in 1969 (Ann. Inst. Super. Sanita 5:197). In a survey of 110 males in July 1972 in the village of Al Barh, 59 cases (53.6%) were onchocerciasis and 14 of them were 'sowda' patients. Blindness due to onchocerciasis was not seen, but the microfilariae were present in the anterior chamber in 14%, and in the cornea in 30% of the positive cases.

8 | Filariasis in the Asian region

South and East Asia represents the largest and most highly populated area in the world where filariasis is endemic; the population infected was estimated by STOLL (1947) to be as many as 200 million. Two species of human filariae are endemic in this region; *Wuchereria bancrofti* (the nocturnally periodic race) and *Brugia malayi* (both the nocturnally periodic and nocturnally subperiodic races).

Wuchereria bancrofti is widely distributed throughout the tropical and subtropical zones of Asia, with the exception of the desert areas in the southwest. Its distribution however, is, patchy and uneven. For example, it is highly endemic almost all over India, though the incidence varies a great deal among various districts. In Sri Lanka, the endemic foci are found restricted mainly to the southwestern coastal belt. Thailand is nearly completely free from endemic *W. bancrofti,* except for small foci in certain jungle villages. The disease used to be widely distributed in southern China, but the island of Taiwan is practically free from indigenous *W. bancrofti.*

Brugia malayi is a human parasite indigenous to only the Asian region. Its distribution is apparently interrupted towards the west beyond Pakistan and Iran by the desert, towards the north by he Himalayas and the Mongolian desert, and towards the southeast by the zoogeographic line (Weber line) separating New Guinea from the Moluccas Islands (see Fig. 2-4). The endemic foci of *B. malayi* are usually more restricted and patchy than those of *W. bancrofti,* but both parasites are frequently coendemic, and mixed infections in the same individual are not uncommon.

Two physiological races have been noted within the species-complex of *B. malayi*: the nocturnally periodic race and the nocturnally subperiodic race. The latter has been recorded from forest areas in Malaysia, Indonesia, and the Philippines, while the former has a wider geographic distribution. These races are further subclassified into epidemiological types according to the ecological characteristics of the main vectors. (For details of the epidemiology of *B. malayi,* see Section 2C.)

National filariasis control programs are in progress in some countries, such as India, Sri Lanka, Malaysia, China, and Japan. Pilot control programs have been organized in several other countries. However, so far, successful and satisfactory results have been obtained only from certain limited areas. The methods and procedures adopted for the control of the disease have varied a great deal among the different countries.

8A. South Asia

8A.1 Pakistan

The Islamic Republic of Pakistan (former West Pakistan) is bounded on the west by Iran and Afganistan, on the east by India, and on the south by the Arabian Sea. It has an area of 818,000 km², and a population of 53,990,173 (1969).

As pointed out by KORKE (1933) and NAPIER (1946), filariasis was considered to be nonendemic in areas of the Indian Subcontinent, north and west of a line drawn from Karachi to Delhi, because of the dry climate. WOLFE & ASLAMKHAN (1969) conducted night blood examinations of 160 persons in Karachi whose nighttime occupation might predispose them to infection, and also, 103 native-born children and adults from the congested center of the city; none of them were found to be carrying microfilariae. On the other hand, 4 carriers of *W. bancrofti* were found among 209 persons who had migrated from known endemic areas: two from Patna, one from Kerala, and one from the Chittagong district of Bangladesh. Because large numbers of people had migrated from India and Bangladesh into Pakistan during the last twenty years, and because *C. p. fatigans* is abundant in Karachi and other areas, the authors pointed out the need for more large scale surveys in order to investigate the possibility of transmission of filariasis in this country.

8A.2 India

The Republic of India has an area of 3,184,000 km² and a population of 546,955,945, as of 1971. It is composed of a continental part, situated between 8°N and 37°N, and certain Indian Ocean islands (the Andaman and Nicobar Islands, the Laccadive, Minicoy, and Amindivi Islands). The continental area may be divided by physical features into the three well-defined regions: the Himalayan region in the north, the Indo-Gangetic plain between the foothills of the Himalayas and the Vindhya Mountains, and the plateau region in the southern and central part. The land is divided into 21 states and nine Union Territories.

Filariasis is widespread in India, and is known to occur in all states except Punjab, Himachal Pradesh, Jammu Kashmir, and Rajasthan, all of which lie in the northwestern part of the country. The population exposed to the risk of infection is estimated to be as large as 136 million, as of 1971, thus, the number of persons infected and/or suffering from the disease is by far the largest among the countries where filariasis is endemic. However, the epidemiology of filariasis in view of the parasite species concerned is rather simple, since only two forms are involved: the nocturnally periodic *W. bancrofti* (mainly the *urban type* transmitted by *C. fatigans*) and the nocturnally periodic *B. malayi* (mainly the swampy area type transmitted by *Mansonia* mosquitoes).

8A.2.1 Historical notes

According to RAGHAVAN (1957), filarial infections were recorded in India as early as the sixth century B.C., by the famous physician SUSRUTA, in Chapter 12 of the *Susruta Samhita;* the description of the signs and symptoms of this disease by MADHAVAKARA (seventh century A.D.) in his treatise *Madhava Nidhana* (Chapter 39), holds good even today. More recently, CLARKE, in 1709, called elephantiasis of the legs in Cochin, South India, "Malabar legs."

The discovery of microfilariae in the peripheral blood of infected human hosts was made first by LEWIS (1872), in Calcutta, nine years after these microfilariae were recorded from hydrocele fluid of a patient from Cuba, by Demarquay, in Paris. Lewis proposed a name "Filaria sanguinis hominis" for this parasite, and in 1877 gave a detailed description of the adult parasite recovered from a patient in Calcutta.

Spot surveys of filariasis were conducted in India before World War II by a number of workers, such as CRUICKSHANK & WRIGHT (1914) in Cochin, ROY & BOSE (1922) in Orissa, CRUICKSHANK *et al.* (1923) in a village near Madras, and KORKE (1927, 1928, 1929a) in Bihar and Orissa. KORKE (1929b) recognized in Orissa the occurrence of an atypical form of microfilariae beside those of typical *bancrofti,* and reported that these were morphologically closely related to those described by BRUG (1927) from Indonesia by the name of *Filaria malayi.* IYENGAR (1932, 1933, 1938) conducted detailed epidemiological studies on filariasis in Travancore (Kerala), and confirmed the occurrence of *B. malayi* in these regions. SUNDAR RAO (1736) also demonstrated, in two towns in Orissa, that the infection consisted entirely of *B. malayi.* The adult worms of *Filaria malayi* of BRUG (1927) were first discovered and described by RAO & MAPLESTONE (1940) from a patient in Kerala.

As for the vectors of filariasis in India, *C. fatigans* was demonstrated to be the main vector of *W. bancrofti* when CRUICKSHANK & WRIGHT (1914) observed its complete larval development in this mosquito in Cochin,

Kerala. However, IYENGAR (1941) found natural infections with *W. bancrofti* larvae in *An. philippinensis,* in a rural area of Bengal. The main vectors of *B. malayi* were demonstrated to be *Mansonia (Mansonioides)* spp. by IYENGAR (1932, 1933, 1938), in Kerala.

8A.2.2 Geographic distribution

As stated before, *W. bancrofti* is widely distributed in India, and has been recorded from at least 12 states, i.e., Andhra Pradesh, Assam, Bihar, Gujarat, Kerala, Madhya Pradesh, Maharashtra, Mysore, Orissa, Tamil Nadu, Uttar Pradesh, and West Bengal, and also from some centrally administered territories, such as the Andaman and Nicobar Islands, the Laccadive, Minicoy, and Aminidivi Islands, Goa, and Pondicherry. The disease is represented mainly by the type transmitted by the house mosquito, *C. fatigans,* and is usually more prevalent in urban areas than in the rural. However, the occurrence of a rural *type* of filariasis bancrofti transmitted by anopheline mosquitoes has also been noted from India.

B. malayi in India is more localized in its distribution, and has been recorded from the states of Kerala, Andhra Pradesh, Assam, Madhya Pradesh, Orissa, and West Bengal. So far as is known, the microfilariae are all nocturnally periodic, and the main vectors are the swamp-breeding mosquitoes of the subgenus *Mansonioides.*

Being a large country with high population density, the determination of the distribution and the extent of prevalence of filariasis in India has been a difficult problem. MEGAW & GUPTA (1927) first published a filaria map of India based on information collected from various states. More recently, JASWANT SINGH & RAGHAVAN (1953) brought out the salient points of filariasis in India, and compiled a filaria map based on reports received from states and reports previously published by various authors. The map has been revised several times in connection with the progress of country-wide filariasis survey activities. The National Filaria Control Program (NFCP) was initiated under the direction of the central government in 1955, and since then, a tremendous amount of information has been accumulated on the epidemiology and control of filariasis in India. Reports of the Assessment Committee on the NFCP were published in 1961, 1967, and 1971. Reviews on the epidemiology of filariasis in India were also made by RAGHAVAN (1957) and RAMAKRISHNAN *et al.* (1960).

The occurrence of *W. bancrofti* infection in a rural area of India was reported by IYENGAR (1941). In general, the distribution of bancroftian filariasis in India had been considered to be characteristically urban, and its absence from rural areas was attributed to the fact that *C. fatigans,* the chief transmitter of the infection, occurred mainly in urban areas. It was also noted that malaria and *W. bancrofti* infection did not ordinarily occur together, not because of any antagonism between the two infections, but

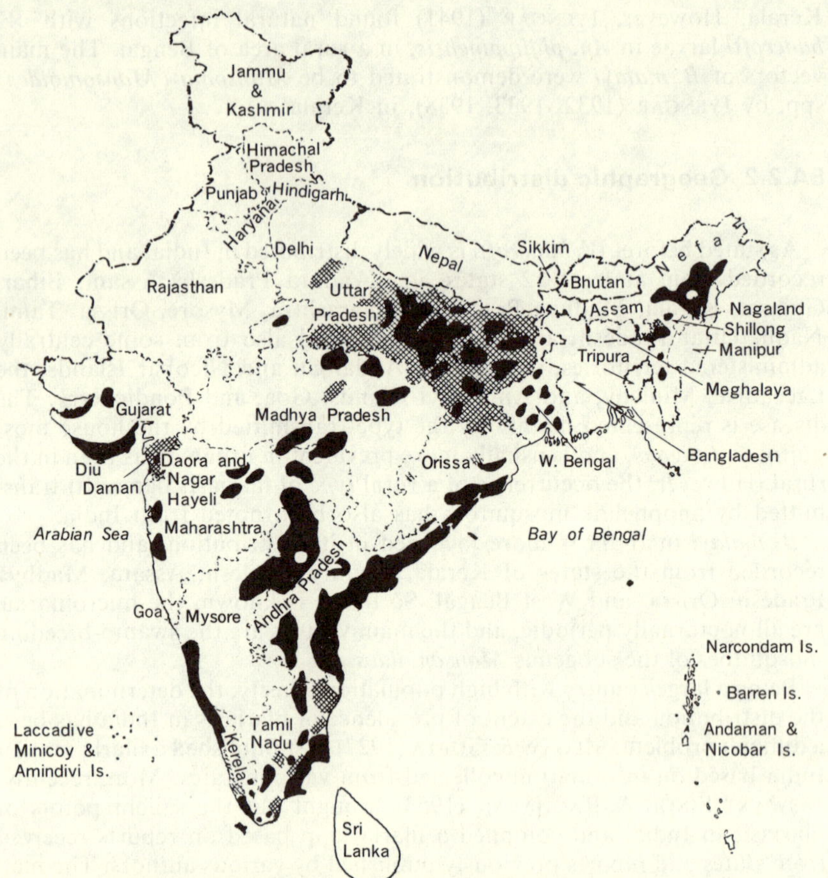

Fig. 8-1. Filaria map of India (1958) (*Indian Council of Medical Research,* 1971).

AREA SURVEYED: *W. bancrofti*
AREA SURVEYED: *B. malayi*
AREA KNOWN TO BE FILARIOUS

because of the difference in breeding habits of the major vectors. However, during a malaria investigation in Illambazar-thana in the Birbhum district of Bengal, cases of endemic filariasis were observed in several typically rural villages. In Bharatpur Village, 9 (17.6%) of 51 persons examined had microfilariae, and in Nabagram, 10 (16.7%) of 60 examined were also positive; the microfilariae were all those of *W. bancrofti*. Six persons out of 111 showed elephantiasis of the legs, and one of them had elephantiasis of the scrotum as well. These cases were all negative for microfilariae in the peripheral blood. In all the villages with cases of filariasis, a high incidence of malaria was also noticed, and the spleen rates among children

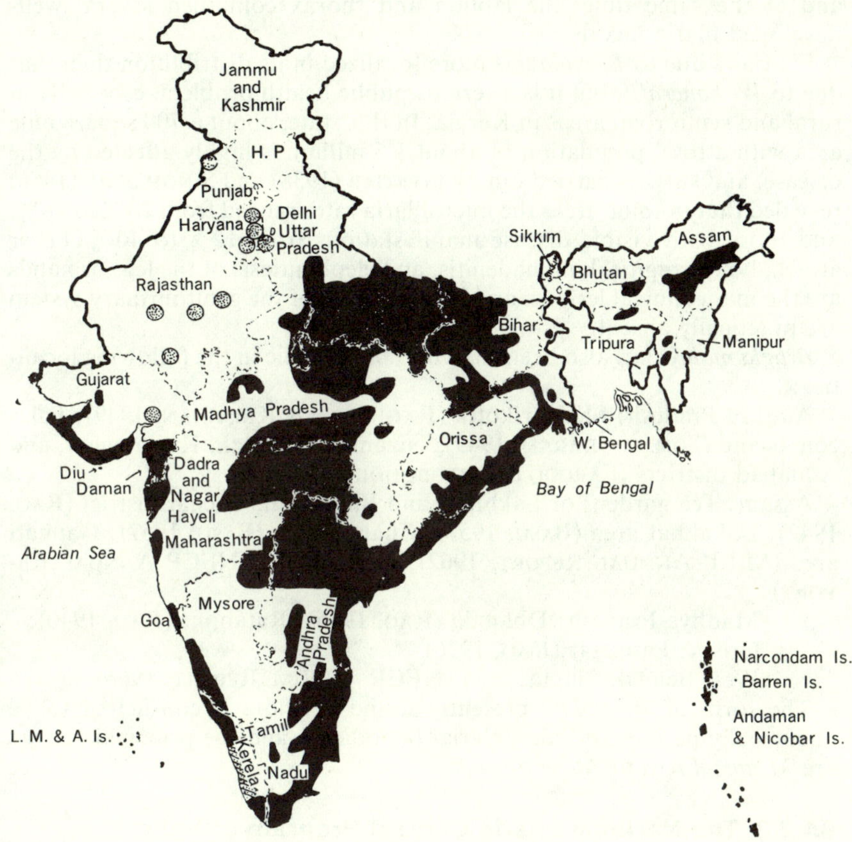

Fig. 8-2. Filaria map of India (1969) (*Indian Council of Medical Research,*
1971).
W. bancrofti AREA:
B. malayi AREA:
W. bancrofti infection detected during recent surveys:

in the above two villages were 50.0% and 84.2%, respectively. The vector
of malaria in these areas was *An. philippinensis,* and its natural infection
rate with malaria parasite was 7.2%. Also, 2 out of 13 *An. philippinensis*
caught in these villages, as well as 6 out of 104 specimens of the same
species caught in the neighboring village of Baruipur, contained well-
developed larvae of *W. bancrofti.* One of the specimens of this species
collected from the village of Nabagram showed both filarial and malarial
infections; the salivary glands were packed with innumerable sporozoites,

and at the same time, the labium and thorax contained several well-developed filaria larvae.

Filariasis due to *B. malayi* is more localized in its distribution than that due to *W. bancrofti*, but it is a serious public health problem, especially in rural and semiurban areas in Kerala. In this state, about a 700 square mile area with a total population of about 1.5 million is highly affected by the disease, and surveys carried out by IYENGAR (1938) and SINGH *et al.* (1956) revealed that in some areas the microfilaria rates ranged from 20% to 38%, and those with visible disease manifestations from 12% to 40%. Fever attack, lymphangitis, lymphadenitis, and elephantiasis of the legs or hands are the main clinical lesions, and involvements of the genitourinary system are practically absent.

Brugia malayi has also been shown to be endemic in the following localities:

Andhra Pradesh: Sri Harikotta (RAGHAVAN & KRISHNAN, 1949); Palacole Island (SOMASUNDARAM, 1949); Nizambad, Medak, Karimnagar, and Adilabad districts (FAROOQ & QUTUBUDDIN, 1946).

Assam: Tea gardens of Lakhipur and Binakandi, Cachar district (RAO, 1942); Bokakhat area (BASU, 1957); Chabua area (BASU, 1957); Gauhati area (M.I.I. ANNUAL REPORT, 1962); Tezpur area (NFCP ANNUAL REPORT)

Madhya Pradesh: Dhamda (RAO, 1945); Ratanpur (RAO, 1940);
Orissa: Patnagar (RAO, 1936)
West Bengal: Siliguri area (NFCP ANNUAL REPORT, 1966)

The form of *B. malayi* presently found in India is considered to be nocturnally periodic in microfilarial periodicity, and the principal vectors are *M. annulifera* or *M. uniformis*.

8A.2.3 The National Filaria Control Program of India

8A.2.3.a Organization and planning

Filariasis as a public health problem in India and the need for its control were discussed in detail by JASWANT SINGH & RAGHAVAN (1953); the National Filaria Control Program (NFCP) was organized based on the suggestions of these authors. A pilot experiment for the control of filariasis was initiated in Orissa, jointly sponsored by the state government, the Indian Council of Medical Research, and the Malaria Institute of India (now, the National Institute of Communicable Diseases). The objectives and the plan of work were as follows:

1. To determine the dose schedule that would be suitable for mass administration of DEC; 2. To evaluate the suitability of each of the following methods, viz: (a) Mass drug administration on the basis of the selected dose schedule, (b) recurrent antilarval measures, and (c) recurrent antiadult measures by indoor residual spray of DDT in doses of 100 and 200 mg per square foot; 3. To assess the results of the above measures by (a) vector density, (b) infection rate in the vector, (c) infectivity rate in the

vector (all weekly), (d) the prevalence and the number of attacks of fever, lymphadenitis, lymphoedema, etc., per person at monthly intervals, and (e) microfilarial rate in the community determined by annual surveys.

The project terminated in 1955, and a detailed report of this experimental study was published in the *Technical Report of the Scientific Advisory Board of the Indian Council of Medical Research* (1954, pp. 371–6). The results showed that all three methods of control were effective in some measure or the other, though each of them also had its drawbacks. It seemed that a multiple approach using all the three methods was essential. Based on the results of this experiment, the Indian government decided to initiate a country-wide control program.

The NFCP, since its launching in 1955, has been gradually expanded and has continued activities in epidemiological surveys, drug treatment of the infected populations, and control of vector mosquitoes. In principle, filariasis control is carried out by each state, and the central government provides assistance in training, coordination, planning, etc. The central coordination is carried out by the headquarters at the National Institute of Communicable Diseases (NICD, formerly the Malaria Institute of India) in Delhi. Reviews on its activity were made by RAMAKRISHNAN *et al.* (1960), INDIAN COUNCIL OF MEDICAL RESEARCH (ICMR) (1961, 1967, 1971), and EDESON (1973). Annual reports have been issued since 1965 from the Institute describing the activities during the current year.

When started in 1955, the NFCP had as its objectives: (a) to carry out filariasis surveys throughout the country in order to determine the extent of prevalence, the type of infection, and the vectors concerned; (b) to undertake large scale pilot studies to evaluate the known methods of filariasis control; and (c) to train the personnel necessary for the program. Filaria survey and control units were established in the states participating in the scheme; 22 such units were allotted to nine states (Andhra Pradesh, Bihar, Bombay, Madras, Madhya Pradesh, Kerala, and West Bengal) from 1955 to 1956, and 47 units were allotted to participating states from 1958 to 1959.

The activities of a control unit under the program were directed to: (a) preliminary surveys covering 3 to 10% of the total population to be protected, (b) control operations (drug administration and mosquito control), and (c) assessment of the results. The mass treatment was carried out over a period of five successive days with the daily doses of about 4 mg of DEC per kg of body weight (200 mg daily to adults, 150 mg to adolescents between the ages of 12 to 18 years, 100 mg to children between 6 to 12 years old, 50 mg to children between 2 to 6 years old). The mosquito control operations consisted of both antiadult measures (indoor residual spraying with dieldrin at 50 mg per square foot was recommended) and antilarval measures (water soluble BHC powder, 6.5% gamma, was recommended).

As a result of epidemiological surveys conducted by the units during this period, it was estimated that at least 64 million people (24 million in urban areas and 40 million in rural areas) resided in filarious areas in 12 states of India, as compared to the original estimate of 25 million at the start of this program.

As a result of the five years of activity of the NFCP, the committee (1961) stated that 1.(a) the filariasis problem in the country is far greater than envisioned previously, (b) bancroftian filariasis spreads centrifugally from urban to rural areas, (c) there is a large risk of filarial transmission being established in new areas, (d) no area, therefore, can be considered free from the risk of transmission before a study is made on the spot; 2. that (a) none of the synthetic imagocides available so far is capable of significantly intercepting filariasis transmission, (b) mass drug administration with DEC has limitations and restricted value in a control program in the country, and (c) antilarval measures wherever adequately adopted have proved useful. The committee therefore recommended that the program be modified so that control be based solely on measures against larvae of the vector, *C. fatigans*, directed only to urban endemic areas, and that mass administration of DEC be abandoned as a control measure.

As stated before, the program as modified on the recommendation of the Indian Council of Medical Research Assessment Committee in 1961 has dealt entirely with the use of larvicidal oil to control *C. fatigans* in endemic urban areas only, i.e., those with a population of 20,000 and

Table 8-1. Statewise distribution of areas surveyed, and estimated population at risk of filaria infection (ICMR, 1971).

State	Population (million)	Total number of districts	Districts surveyed	Population at risk (million)
Andhra Pradesh	36	20	12	14.44
Assam	11.9	11	5	1.00
Bihar	46.4	17	9	21.20
Gujarat	20.6	19	10	4.57
Kerala	16.9	9	9	4.00
Madhya Pradesh	32.4	43	30	6.20
Maharashtra	39.6	26	6	4.50
Mysore	23.6	19	3	1.73
Orissa	17.5	13	8	7.83
Tamil Nadu	33.7	13	12	13.00
Uttar Pradesh	73.7	54	28	47.00
West Bengal	34.92	16	13	10.00
Andaman Island	—	—	—	0.01
Laccadive Islands	—	—	—	0.02
Pondicherry	0.4	—	—	0.37
Goa	0.6	—	—	0.31
Total	388.2	260	150	136.28

above. The control measures suggested were: 1. recurrent antilarval measures throughout the year with the use of a mosquito larvicidal oil, 2. reorganization of the units, 3. establishment of new units, 4. prevention of filariogenic conditions in town expansions and in new townships, and 5. adequate disposal of sewage.

The Second Assessment Report on the National Filaria Control Program, published in 1971, reviews its activities during the period from 1961 to 1970. As a result of surveys conducted during this period, it became evident that the problem was far more extensive than previously estimated, and over 136 million people are now considered to be living in the endemic areas of filariasis. The statewise distribution of areas surveyed, and the estimated populations at risk are shown in Table 8-1.

In the Second Assessment Report (1971) the committee suggested a standard staffing pattern of the NFCP units by eight grades from A to H, for different sizes of population, and recommended reorganization of the existing units in each state; they also recommended the establishment of new units to deal with the 60 million population at risk, as against the original estimate of 25 million. The committee further recommended the allotment of 70 units altogether (from grades A to F) in 13 states or territories, and in future, to distribute 94 units (from grades A to H) in various states. Reinforcement of the organization at the state level by the establishment of a special bureau for filariasis, and also at the headquarters at the National Institute of Communicable Diseases was also recommended.

8A.2.3.b Control measures and method for their evaluation

Previous blood surveys in India have shown that nocturnally periodic *W. bancrofti* transmitted by *C. fatigans* is the predominant filarial parasite in India. It is widespread along the coastal regions, extending inland into Tamil Nadu, Andhra Pradesh, Madhya Pradesh, Uttar Pradesh, and Bihar, where it exists mainly along the great rivers, spreading into Assam.

It has been emphasized in India that bancroftian filariasis is mainly a disease of urban areas, from where it spreads centrifugally. Accordingly, emphasis has been placed on the control of filariasis in urban areas, and any program for the control of filariasis in rural areas was considered a research project. However, the Second Assessment Report (1971) pointed out the importance of filariasis in rural areas, and estimated that out of the total population at risk of about 136 million, some 85 million would be living in rural areas. Thus, a special project was initiated in Maharashtra State for studying the problem of rural filariasis.

When the NFCP was started, three methods were applied for the control of *W. bancrofti* infection: (1) mass drug administration, (2) residual house spraying against adult mosquitoes, and (3) larviciding. However, the First Assessment Committee recommended that the first two methods be discontinued because of operational difficulties or unsatisfactory results; only the larviciding in urban areas with populations over 20,000 has been practiced since then.

The First Assessment Committee of ICMR (1961) recommended the collection of the following indices for evaluation of the control measures: (1) vector density, (ten man-hour density of *C. fatigans*), (2) vector infection rate, (3) vector infectivity rate, and (4) microfilaria rate in children of the age-group 5 to 15 years. The data accumulated from the states concerned have been published by NICD members under the group title of *"Filariasis in India—Facts and Figures"* Part 1, Andhra Pradesh, by SINGH *et al.*, 1967a; Part 2, Assam, by BASU *et al.*, 1967a; Part 3, Bihar, by RAGHAVAN *et al.*, 1967a; Part 4, Gujarat, by SINGH *et al.*, 1967b; Part 5, Kerala, by BASU *et al.*, 1967b; Part 6, Madhya Pradesh, by RAGHAVAN *et al.*, 1967b; Part 7, Maharashtra, by BASU *et al.*, 1968; Part 8, Mysore, by SINGH *et al.*, 1968. Summaries of the above results are given also in the Assessment Report of ICMR (1971).

Generally speaking, some reductions in microfilaria rates were observed in areas where mass drug administration was carried out with good or fair coverage, but the rates of reduction have usually been much lower than those observed in similar antifilariasis programs in other regions of the world. Some decreases in vector density, vector infection rates and infectivity rates, and microfilaria rates of human populations have also been observed in survey results reported after the mass drug administration program was abandoned and only larvicidal operations were continued as the sole control measure. However, EDESON (1973) points out that the true value of survey results accumulated so far in India is difficult to assess because of the varying standards in the performance of parasitological and entomological techniques, due to the shortage of supervisory staff. The blood examinations, for example, were conducted by collecting unmeasured blood samples from a finger prick, and the smears have been stained with J.S.B., which is a poor stain for studying the structure of microfilariae but which has been traditionally used because it is inexpensive. Therefore, although tremendous amounts of facts and figures have been presented annually as survey results, they lack reliability as criteria for the comparison of rates and densities, and for differentiating the microfilariae of *B. malayi* from *W. bancrofti*.

8A.2.3.c Control of *Brugia malayi* infection

A pilot scheme for control of *B. malayi* was proposed for Kerala, by the ICMR (1961) in its First Assessment Report on the NFCP. The largest single endemic tract of *B. malayi* in India is located along the coast of Kerala, in the districts of Quilon, Allepy, Kottayam, Ernakulam, and Trichur, and on many islands in Vembaned Lake. The population is about 1.5 million in an area of about 650 square miles. The project was actually started in January 1966 by NICD and four localities (Arror, Turavoor North, Thuravoor South, and Vayalar West) were selected as experimental control zones, using BHC as a residual insecticide against the vector mosquitoes. Another five localities were kept unsprayed for comparison purposes.

Field trials instituted by the Malaria Institute of India from 1954 to 1955 showed that the adults of *Mansonioides* species, unlike *C. p. fatigans*, are highly susceptible to DDT and BHC; furthermore, BHC, at a dose of 40 mg gamma isomer per square foot was observed to have a residual effect lasting over 20 weeks after a single spray. When the operation was carried out on a larger scale in 1966, the vector density in the sprayed areas showed a remarkable decline when compared to the unsprayed areas. Data on the age determination of the vectors showed the absence of parous mosquitoes during some months in the sprayed areas. The microfilaria rate in the sprayed areas showed a decline from 20.67% in 1966 to 7.5% in 1970, while the rates in the unsprayed area were 8.83% in 1966–67 and 6.95% in 1970. However, the transmission of *B. malayi* infection was found to be continuing even in the sprayed areas, and rather reluctant results have been accumulated in the mosquito infectivity rates. The coverage of the house spraying has been steadily declining due to public resistance, which is partly due to the increases in the bed-bug problem.

Chemotherapy with DEC has not been attempted as a routine method of control because of its side effects, which are generally more severe than in the treatment of *W. bancrofti* carriers. However, the Assessment Committee (1971) suggested the necessity to undertake studies on the feasibility, acceptability, and other factors associated with administration of DEC. The committee also discussed the problem of *Pistia* control for the prevention of breeding of the vector mosquitoes.

8A.2.3.d Problems of DEC administration in India

India was one of the first countries to introduce diethylcarbamazine (DEC) for the treatment and control of filariasis. The drug was previously used in the mass treatment of people in the endemic areas of filariasis in the experimental control project initiated in Orissa in 1949. When the National Filariasis Control Program was started in 1955, mass treatment with DEC was adopted as one of the main control measures. The dosage scheme suggested was a daily administration of about 4 mg per kg of body weight (200 mg for adults, 150 mg for adolescents of 12 to 18 years, 100 mg for 6 to 12 year-olds, 50 mg for 2 to 6 year-olds) over a period of five consecutive days, with the total dose of about 20 mg per kg.

The results of the mass drug administration conducted in various states with the above standard method were evaluated by a number of workers: by PATEL & PARANJPEY (1958) in Bombay State, by NANDA *et al.* (1960) and DIWAN CHAND *et al.* (1961) in Uttar Pradesh, by RAMAKRISHNAN *et al.* (1960) for all India, by GONSALVES (1960) in Mysore, by VARMA *et al.* (1961, 1964) and BOSE & SINHA (1965) in Bihar, and by NAIDU (1962) in Andhra Pradesh. NAIR (1968, 1971) conducted special studies on the side reactions caused by DEC in asymptomatic *B. malayi* and *W. bancrofti* carriers.

According to the Assessment Report of 1961, some 5.62 million persons out of 14.1 million population under the 47 units were treated with mass drug administration up until December 1960; the proportion which took the full five-day course ranged, with different units, between 38.3% and

97.6%. However, many unpleasant reactions were observed following the drug administration, and an average of 16.5% of 3,650,902 persons complained of some adverse reactions from the drug. The mass drug administration produced varying degrees of reduction in the microfilaria rate, as well as the mean microfilarial density in the community, and there appeared to be a general direct correlation between the percentages of population treated and the reduction in the microfilaria rate among the different units. However, the decline in the mean microfilarial density in the community did not show any such correlation. The reduction in the mean microfilarial density at the end of one year following drug administration ranged from 10.9% to 84.6%.

DIWAN CHAND *et al.* (1961) conducted a special study for the evaluation of mass therapy with DEC in Faizabad, Uttar Pradesh. In a precontrol survey of a study area, 12.5% of 4,550 persons examined were positive for microfilaria, with an average count per 20 mm³ of blood of 16. The microfilariae were all those of *W. bancrofti*, and 68 (2.83%) out of 2,402 *C. fatigans* dissected were infected, among which 21 (0.87%) had infective stage larvae. Mass drug administration was conducted; 61.1% of the population took the drug for all five days, and 66.3% took the drug for varying number of days. At the posttreatment blood survey conducted on 2,936 persons, the microfilaria rate dropped to 6.3%, and the average count in 20 mm³ blood dropped to 6.

SINGH *et al.* (1962) made observations on the effect of DEC on the microfilarial density during the course of treatment scheduled under the National Filaria Control Program of India. The dose schedule adopted was 4 mg per kg of DEC administered daily, in a single dose for a period of five days, 20 mg per kg in total dose. Forty-four microfilaria positive cases, all *W. bancrofti* infection, were selected, and a measured quantity of 20 mm³ blood smears were prepared every night, between 9:30 p.m. and 11:30 p.m., every day for six days beginning just before the start of the treatment. At the blood examinations made before the drug was administered, all of 44 cases were positive, and the total number of microfilariae in all cases was 1,743. At the second examination made one day after the initial dose was administered, the total microfilaria count decreased to 288, and 8 persons became negative. The total count and the number of negative cases, respectively, were 189 and 15, at the third examination, 74 and 24 at the fourth, 46 and 27 at the fifth, and 62 and 27 at the sixth examination. At the seventh examination, made one day after completion of the five-day treatment, the total count was 59, and 25 of 44 previously positive cases became negative, with a so-called cure rate of 56.9%; the remaining 19 cases, or 43.1%, were still positive, with counts varying from 1 to 7.

In general, the results of the mass drug administration operations conducted from 1957 to 1969 in India were far from satisfactory when compared with those obtained in other countries, such as Ceylon, Japan, and some Pacific islands. The following factors are pointed out as the main causes of such failure: (a) the dosage scheme adopted in this program, i.e., five daily doses of 4 mg per kg, 20 mg per kg in total, was not sufficient to clear the microfilariae or to eradicate adult worms in most filaria carriers, (b) the rates of coverage of the populations under control were much lower than levels sufficient for interruption of transmission, and (c) there were too many refusals or objections to the drug treatment because of the unpleasant side reactions. It was most unfortunate that the dose recommended by the Indian authorities was sufficient to cause the side effects but was insufficient to cure the disease.

As stated before, the mass drug administration program was abandoned by recommendation of the First Assessment Committee in 1960 because: (a) there was poor coverage in most of the areas and unpleasant reactions following administration, (b) administration of the drug failed to clear the microfilariae in some individuals, and in certain areas, the reduction in the levels of microfilaremia did not persist, and (c) decline in the infectivity rate of mosquitoes after drug administration was not appreciable in most areas.

The use of DEC in the control of filariasis in India was re-evaluated in the 1971 Assessment Report. Although its mass administration in daily doses had been abandoned since 1960, the committee suggested that the selective treatment of microfilaria positive cases may be practiced in some rural areas, or the mass drug administration program with spaced doses (administration at weekly or monthly intervals) could also be applied in India, since both techniques were reported to be effective and successful in a number of other countries. Pilot studies on the mass treatment by supplying DEC-medicated salt are also in progress with promising results. The committee concluded that in the planning of any measure for the control of filariasis in India, a uniform pattern of approach in all areas of the country is not feasible, as had been adopted in the National Malaria Eradication Program. The committee also suggested that the function of filaria clinics already established in a number of localities in India be directed not only as centers for treatment, but also for the promotion of health education in various facets of the filariasis problem.

NAIR (1968) carried out an analytical study on the clinical reactions in asymptomatic *B. malayi* carriers caused by DEC therapy. A temporary clinic was opened at Thuravoor, Kerala State, a place highly endemic for *B. malayi*. Three blood smears, each 20 mm^3 in volume, were taken during the night from people who voluntarily came to the clinic. After determining the density of microfilariae, DEC citrate, containing approximately 51% of the base, was administered orally between 8 p.m. and midnight, at various dosage regimens; careful observation of the volunteers was made until any reactions that developed had subsided completely. The pulse rate and oral temperature were recorded three times a day, and other clinical signs or symptoms were also recorded. As criteria for the assessment of the results, the severity of reactions was classified into one of four degrees in the case of fever (I: up to 99 °F, II: 99 to 101°F, III: 101 to 103°F, and IV:

above 103°F), and into one of three degrees in the case of headache or body pain (slight, moderate, and severe). The microfilaria carriers were classified by density into five groups: below 1, 1 to 10, 11 to 30, 31 to 50, 51 to 100, and over 101 per 20 mm³ blood.

In general, the reactions in the asymptomatic *B. malayi* microfilaria carriers were very severe. Many of them were completely prostrated and had to rest in bed during the reaction period. Common symptoms were very high fever accompanied by chill, rigors, severe headache, and bodyache. These reactions occurred within 6 to 12 hours and reached a maximum in 24 to 36 hours after the drug administration. There was delirium in one case and convulsion in another. But these severe reactions subsided in two to four days, and nothing untoward occurred. However, general malaise and weakness persisted for varying periods even after the reaction had subsided. Anorexia was common, and nausea or vomiting occurred in a large number of the patients.

There was a significant correlation between the microfilarial density and the intensity of reaction among 77 carriers who received a single dose of 6 mg per kg of body weight; 41.5% of them had fever between 99°F and 101°F, and 32.5% between 101°F and 103°F. The correlation coefficient between the microfilarial count and the degree of fever was 0.434, with the standard error of correlation being 0.092, which was significant.

The duration of reaction was found to be correlated also with the microfilarial density of the carriers treated with a single dose of DEC at the rate of 6 mg per kg. The average duration according to the microfilarial density was 0 hour (no reaction) in the group with counts below 1, 40.24 hours in those with counts from 1 to 10, 40.8 hours in those with counts from 11 to 30, 42.9 hours in the group with counts from 31 to 50, 45.5 hours in those with counts from 51 to 100, and 55.1 hours in those with counts of over 101.

Observations were also made on the relationship between the dosage and the intensity of reaction. From the results, the author considered that the intensity of the reaction appeared to increase up to a dosage of about 4 to 6 mg per kg, and there was no further notable increase in the intensity when the dosage was increased up to 16 mg per kg. Both the intensity and duration of the reaction appeared slightly more in those who received treatment for three to five days than in those who were treated for only one or two days. The reactions, such as headache, and body pain, were less in children of 11 years and below than in the older age-groups, but the intensity of the fever did not differ between the two age-groups.

NAIR *et al.* (1971) studied the relationship between the intensity of reaction and the microfilaremia load at the time of DEC administration to asymptomatic *W. bancrofti* carriers in Fort Cochin, Kerala. They classified the microfilaria carriers into three groups: (1) those showing up to ten microfilariae per 20 mm³ of blood examined, (2) those with 11 to 50, and (3) those with above 50 microfilariae. Four common reactions, i.e., fever, headache, body pain, and abdominal pain, were taken as the criteria, and the grade of each reaction was classified further into mild, moderate, and severe reactions. It was concluded that the incidence of reaction was higher in persons with a high microfilaria load than in persons with a low load, but that this observation was true only up to a particular level, beyond which no proportional increase in the incidence was evident; they also concluded that there was no statistical evidence to indicate that there was any correlation between the microfilaria load and the intensity of reaction, and that the type of reaction, namely, fever, body pain, headache, and abdominal pain were independent of the initial microfilaria count.

8A.2.4 Epidemiology of filariasis in different states and territories of India

8A.2.4.a Andhra Pradesh

Andhra Pradesh is a state in southeast India with a population of some 43 million (1971). According to HAWKING (1973), filariasis occurs mainly in two regions: one along the eastern coastal region of the Bay of Bengal, and another in an inland northwestern area, around Kamareddi.

According to SINGH et al. (1967a) and ICMR (1971), filaria surveys were carried out by the units in Mandapetta, Guntur, and Hyderabad during 1955, 1956, 1958, and 1964. Out of 20 districts, 12 districts were covered by the surveys. Of the total population of 36 million (29.7 million in rural areas and 6.3 million in urban areas), 14.4 million were estimated to be exposed to the risk of infection. The microfilaria rates varied from 13.8% in Karimnagar to 0.6% in Guntur. Two control units (Mandapetta and Kamareddi) were reorganized, and in addition, two modified units were set up at Visakhapatnam and Hyderabad mainly to help with the urban malaria problem. Only 0.6 million people were being protected by antilarval measures as of 1967.

DHAR et al. (1968) conducted studies on the seasonal prevalence, resting habits, host preference, and filarial infection of C. fatigans in Rajamundry, Andhra Pradesh.

FAROOQ & QUTUBUDDIN (1946) carried out an epidemiological study of filariasis in Hyderabad state. A preliminary survey carried out from 1940 to 1942 showed that the disease was endemic in a roughly kidney-shaped area of 4,800 square miles covering adjacent portions of the Nizamabad, Medak, Karimnagar, and Adilabad districts, with an average altitude of almost 1,500 feet. The present study was undertaken in 24 villages around Kamareddi, covering a population of 43,593. House-to-house visits were made in search of persons showing filarial signs; thick blood smears approximately measuring 20 mm³ were taken at night from diseased and healthy persons selected at random. As a result, 692 filarial disease cases were recorded, of whom 615 had elephantiasis of the leg (88%), 15 had elephantiasis of the hand alone, elephantiasis of the hand and leg in 35, elephantiasis of the scrotum alone in 20, and elephantiasis of the scrotum and leg in 7. Of 722 persons whose blood was examined, microfilariae were found in 92 persons, giving an average microfilaria rate of 12.7%.

Naidu (1962) reviewed the progress of the filariasis control program in Andhra Pradesh. The state has about 36 million people living in 20 districts; eleven of these districts constitute the Andhra component, which was formerly part of the composite Madras State, while the remaining nine districts constitute the Telengana component, which formed a part of Hyderabad State prior to reorganization in 1956. In the Andhra component, filariasis was known to be prevalent for a long time in most of the coastal districts, while in the Telengana component, a survey conducted in 1940 showed that the districts of Karimnagar, Medak, and Nizamabad had filariasis.

In Andhra, the regional malaria organizations at Visakhapatnam and Bellary undertook filaria surveys in certain districts, upon which were based the first antifilaria measures in 1950. In Telengana, some malaria and filariasis control activities, night blood surveys, mass chemotherapy, and antilarval measures were initiated from about 1953. The new Andhra State participated in the National Filaria Control Program in 1954. In Andhra, two survey units were established in 1955–56 and surveys covering a total population of 156,000 were conducted. Based on the results, a control unit was established in 1956, in the district of East Godavari. In Telengana, one control unit and one survey unit were allotted during 1955; mass therapy covering nine villages was started in April 1957, and completed by August 1958.

In the Andhra region, the mass therapy by the Mandapetta unit was initiated from March 1956 to January 1957, and was completed within a period of ten months. The standard dose of DEC was administered to 212,843 persons out of the total population of 277,802 in 117 villages, and 1,389,207 tablets of DEC were consumed. As a result, 61.6% of the population was covered, but the net coverage for the full five-day treatment came to only 41.1%. Side reactions to DEC were seen in 33,489 persons, and 2,241 persons passed the round worm (Ascaris) during the course of treatment.

In Telengana region, the Kamareddi unit undertook mass therapy from May 1959, and completed it in March 1960. The total number of persons who took the drug was 201,947, and the unit covered 66.6% of the population under control, but the coverage for the full five-day treatment was only about 23% of the whole population.

The results of blood surveys in samples taken before and after the mass therapy are shown in Table 8-2. Although the microfilaria rates were lower in the posttreatment surveys than in the pretreatment ones, the rates still remained considerably high, even after the drug treatment. In a conclusion, the author stated, "Evidently, the effect of the one-round mass therapy on the reservoir of infection was unsatisfactory. There were difficulties in the way of adequate coverage by mass therapy, and if measures had been conducted as thoroughly as originally envisaged, the effect would have been more encouraging. However, the difficulties for conducting the mass therapy were considerable." The author also concluded that the ideal set of operations for the present appears to be: (1) mos-

Table 8-2. Results of blood surveys before and after mass therapy with DEC in Andhra Pradesh (after NAIDU, 1962).

Place	Pretreatment survey			Posttherapy survey Treated people		
	No. exam.	No. positive	% positive	No. exam.	No. positive	% positive
Mandapetta	3,124	559	17.8	123	17	13.8
Puram	3,609	605	16.7	327	25	7.6
Yeditha	1,915	252	13.2	234	13	5.5
Akkapur	255	38	14.8	139	8	5.7

quito control by intense antilarval measures, supplemented by (2) imagociding with pyrethrum or BHC, (3) provision of drainage as a permanent measure, and (4) parasite control by instituting a more systematic mass chemotherapy with a regular follow-up.

8A.2.4.b Assam

Assam is a state in northeast India with an area of 181,000 km^2 and a population of 14,857,314 (1971).

Both *W. bancrofti* and *B. malayi* are endemic; the former mainly in the center of the state and the latter in two large areas in the center and south. Apparently, filariasis occurs particularly in villages of the major tea plantations, having been brought there by immigrant laborers (HAWKING, 1973).

According to the Assessment Report of ICMR (1971) and NICD Report by BASU *et al.* (1967), there has been only one unit established in Gauhati since 1965, and out of 11 districts in the state, only five have been covered by surveys. The population exposed to the risk of filariasis was estimated to be 1.0 million out of a total population of 11.9 million (10.9 million in rural areas and 1.0 million in urban areas). Only 0.1 million people among them are protected by antilarval measures.

SUNDAR RAO (1942) reported on filariasis endemic in the tea gardens in the southeast of the Cachar district in lower Assam. The tea gardens of Lakhipur and Binakandy were surveyed, and filariasis due mainly to *B. malayi* was found to be endemic in seven out of nine villages investigated. Out of a total of 2,445 persons examined, 115 (4.7%) had microfilariae in the peripheral night blood. Of these carriers, 5 had *W. bancrofti* infection, and they were found only in the village of Lakhipur. *B. malayi* carriers were found in seven villages, and microfilarial rates of as high as 28.2% (37 of 131) and 18.9% (10 of 53) were found in Naidar and Robipur, respectively. Signs of filarial disease were seen in 110 (4.5%) persons, including 89 cases of elephantiasis of the leg, 16 cases of elephantiasis of the arm, 4 cases of elephantiasis of both the leg and arm, and one case of hydrocele. The villages situated in the midst of extensively cultivated land were practically free from filariasis, while the villages situated in the midst of swampy areas showed a high incidence.

BASU (1957) conducted filariasis surveys of two areas of Assam, one in the Sibsagar and another in the Lakhipur district. Six tea gardens and 19 villages were included in Sibsagar, and 2 tea gardens and 12 villages in Lakhipur. The total populations in both areas was about 27,843, of whom 3,952 were examined. In the Bokakhat area of Sibsagar, 2,213 persons were examined; 73 (3.3%) had filarial disease manifestations and 100 (4.5%) showed microfilaremia. Both *W. bancrofti* and *B. malayi* infections were noted, the former in 26% and the latter in 74% of the carriers. In the Chabua area, 1,739 persons were examined; 32 had disease manifestations, and 138 showed microfilaremia. *W. bancrofti* was in 81.3%, and *B. malayi* in 18.7% of the positive cases. Both *C. fatigans* and *M. uniformis* were found to be abundant in these areas, and infective larvae were found in *C. fatigans*.

8A.2.4.c Bihar

A state in northeast India, Bihar has an area of 174,000 km² and a population of 56,387,296 (1971).

Filariasis due to *W. bancrofti* is apparently spread almost all over the state, especially in the urban areas in and around the towns of Patna, Muzaffarpur, Gaya, Ranchi, Monghyr, Bhagarpur, and Darbhanga (HAWKING, 1973).

According to the NICD Report by RAGHAVAN *et al.* (1967) and the Assessment Report of ICMR (1971), surveys were carried out by Filaria Survey Units of Gaya and Patna from 1955 to 1956, and eight filaria control units were allotted to the state. Out of 17 districts in the state, nine have been covered by the surveys, and the population exposed to the risk of filariasis was estimated to be 21.3 million in 1969 out of a total population of 46.4 million. Only 1.1 million people are presently being protected by antilarval measures. In the "filariometric data" regarding the eight control units from 1960 to 1969, the mosquito density was shown to fluctuate and was not reduced significantly, but steady decreases have been observed in the vector infection rates, infectivity rates, and the microfilaria rates. The percentages of positive microfilaria cases in the 5 to 15 year age-group in 1963 to 1964, and in 1969, were, respectively, 7.2 and 2.0 in Monghyr, 4.5 and 1.9 in Patna, 2.7 and 1.1 in Ranchi 8.9 and 1.3 in Bhagarpur, 10.5 and 4.1 in Darbhanga, and 12.9 and 3.2 in Gaya.

In Bihar, KORKE (1927) carried out blood surveys on prisoners in jails in Bhagarpur and Gaya, and obtained 32 positive cases (19.3%) out of 166 persons examined. The microfilariae were nocturnally periodic, and were identified as *W. bancrofti*.

KORKE (1928) further reported that filariasis was endemic in some areas in Bihar and Orissa, such as Barachatti, Madanpur, Wazirganj, Barun, Aurangabad, Daudhagar, Hasua, Jehanabad, Gaya Town, Bihar, Giryak, and Puri. Out of a total of 1,254 persons examined in these areas, 150 (12.0%) were microfilaria positive, and 203 showed some clinical signs. There were 50 positive microfilaria cases out of 203 (24.6%) persons with clinical signs and in 100 of 1,051 (9.5%) persons without clinical signs. The microfilariae were identified as *bancrofti*, and morphological studies were carried out both on the microfilariae and the developing stages in *C. fatigans*. The microfilariae in one of the cases studied showed nocturnal periodicity.

KORKE (1929a) reported on the results of filarial surveys conducted at 24 different places in the Gaya, Patna, Purnea, and Balasore districts in Bihar and Orissa. Out of a total of 2,321 persons examined in all the areas, 328 were positive for microfilariae and 285 had some clinical signs, with the gross microfilaria rate of 14.1% and the disease rate of 12.3%; 50 (17.5%) of 285 cases with clinical signs and 278 (13.7%) of 2,036 persons without clinical signs were positive for microfilaria. The author stated that the predominant species was *W. bancrofti* (occurrence of other filarial species was not mentioned). The incidence of filariasis was found to be highest in a cultivated area situated at sea level, and lowest or nothing in the sub-mountain and plateau area. A notable clinical feature was the affection of the genitals in the area above sea level and affection of the lower extremities in the areas at sea level.

KORKE (1927, 28, 29a), during the survey of filariasis in Bihar and Orissa, recognized the occurrence of an atypical form of microfilariae which was morphologically different from the typical *bancrofti*. KORKE (1929 b) further investigated the problem, and confirmed that the atypical form was observed in the Balasore district of Orissa, and possessed morphological characters closely resembling the *Filaria malayi* reported by BRUG (1927). KORKE also noted that elephantiasis of the lower extremities was more prevalent in the areas where the atypical form was found in numbers, while hydrocele was more prevalent in the areas where the typical form of *bancrofti* was predominant.

KANT *et al.* (1956) made observations on the incidence of filariasis in Patna, Bihar. Blood and clinical surveys were conducted in 16 wards of the city with a total population of 114,568, and 9,485 or 8.3% of the people covering all ages and sexes were examined; 2,869, or 30.1%, were found to have some clinical signs and 1,780, or 18.7%, were positive for microfilaria. They showed age and sex distribution of the disease and microfilaria rates.

The results of extensive activities on epidemiological survey and control of filariasis in Bihar were reported by VARMA *et al.* (1960–64), and by RAGHAVAN *et al.* (1967). In Bharalpur, for example, VARMA *et al.* (1961a) found a microfilaria rate of 21.4% and a disease rate of 35.1% out of 6,625 people examined. In the rural populations around the town of Bhagarpur, VARMA *et al.* (1961b) recorded an average microfilaria rate of 12.8% and a disease rate of 23.8% in surveys of ten villages. In another eight villages, VARMA *et al.* (1961c) examined 1,324 persons (15.2% of the population) and observed an average microfilarial rate of 4.1% and a disease rate of 25.2%. In the Monghyr area, VARMA *et al.* (1962) obtained a microfilarial rate of 11.9% and a disease rate of 17.1% for the urban population, and the corresponding figures of 4.3% and 7.9% for the rural population.

The effectiveness of the mass drug treatments according to the standard course of DEC administration (4 mg per kg, once a day for five days, 20 mg per kg in total) was evaluated by VARMA *et al.* (1964) in the special study area, as well as in the other areas in Bhagarpur, Bihar. In the study area, the microfilaria rate and disease rate in the pretreatment survey were 21.4% and 35.1%, respectively. Out of the total population of 30,700, 71.8% took the drug, and 65.3% took the full dose of 20 mg per kg. The microfilaria rate and the disease rate in the posttreatment examination was 11.5% and 27.3%, respectively, so that the effect of the drug treatment was obviously unsatisfactory. The mosquito infection rate was 10.1% before the treatment and 12.2% after the treatment.

BOSE & SINHA (1965) reviewed the progress of the filaria control program in Bihar from 1956 through 1963. Filariasis is endemic in the urban and peripheral areas in Bihar; *W. bancrofti*, transmitted by *C. fatigans*, is the main form causing the disease in this state. The population at risk to filariasis in Bihar was estimated to be 5.0 million in 1960. Two survey units were established in 1955–56, one at Patna and the other at Gaya, and eight filaria control units were started in 1956. Mass therapy with DEC was launched from September 15, 1958 to February 14, 1959 for a period of five months. Filariasis in Patna was also reported by SEN & PURI (1965).

8A.2.4.d Gujarat

Gujarat is a state in West India with an area of 187,100 km² and a population of 26,660,929 (1971).

Filariasis occurs in almost all the coastal districts, especially around Bulsar, Surat, Junagadh, and Jamnagar. According to the NICD Report by SINGH *et al.* (1967b) and the Assessment Report of ICMR (1971), filaria surveys were carried out by the Filaria Survey Unit of Rajkot from 1956 to 1959. Four control units were allotted to the states. Out of 19 districts in the state, 10 have been covered by the surveys, and population exposed to the risk of infection was estimated to be 6.3 million of a total population of 20.6 million. Only 0.5 million people were being protected by antilarval measures (1964 figures).

RAGHAVAN (1951) conducted a survey of filariasis in Porbandar, Saurashtra (Gujarat), and obtained a microfilaria rate of 10.1% among 2,999 persons examined; clinical signs were seen in 205 (6.8%) among them, of whom 17 were positive for microfilaria. The microfilariae were all those of *W. bancrofti*.

PAWAR & MITTAL (1968) observed, in Jamnagar, a microfilaria rate of 2.5% and disease rate of 1.2%, mostly elephantiasis of the legs and various lesions of the genitalia.

8A.2.4.e Kerala

A state in southwest India bordering on the Arabian Sea, Kerala has an area of 38,900 km² and a population of 21,210,397 (1971). Filariasis is prevalent among people in this state, especially among those residing in the lowland coastal belt. Both *W. bancrofti* and *B. malayi* are present, and the latter is more prevalent here than in any other state of India. The state may be divided into three zones: (a) a low coastal belt, with many inland waterways and lagoons (which is the zone with most of the filariasis), (b) an undulating middle zone with some foci, and (c) a mountainous zone (the Ghats) to the east, which is apparently free from infection (HAWKING, 1973).

Filariasis in Kerala has been intensively investigated by a number of workers during the past sixty years. Under the NFCP, filaria surveys were carried out by two units during the period from 1955 to 1960. Until 1969, 20 control units were functioning in the state, but all of these units were reorganized according to the pattern recommended by the NFCP Assessment Committee, and six of them were disbanded. All nine districts in the state have been covered by the surveys, and the population exposed to the risk of filariasis as estimated in 1964 was 4.0 million out of a total population of 16.9 million. Only 1.25 million people are being protected by antilarval measures (BASU *et al.*, 1967).

The distribution of filariasis in the coastal belt of Kerala was reviewed by JOSEPH & PRASAD (1967). The climate of this region is generally hot, temperatures ranging between 79°F and 90°F, with a high degree of relative humidity, reaching up to 90%; the rainy season extends from June to November, and annual rainfall sometimes exceeds 200 inches. The surveys conducted under the National Filaria Control Program covered the entire coastal belt in the period from 1956 to 1961. Both *W. bancrofti* and *B. malayi* are found, often coexisting in the same areas, but the former is usually more prevalent in urban areas while the latter is mainly a rural infection. High microfilaria rates, above 10%, were observed in Pachathiri (12.2%, both *W. bancrofti* and *B. malayi*), Parathur (*B. malayi* only), Quilandi Town (14.85%, *W. bancrofti* only), Feroke (11.86%, *W. bancrofti* only) and Allepy Town (13.6%, both *W. bancrofti* and *B. malayi*).

CRUICKSHANK & WRIGHT (1914) made a detailed study on filariasis in Cochin, a city situated on the southwestern coast of Kerala. A total of 1,000 persons (761 males and 239 females) were examined by house-to-house visit; microfilariae were found in 15 mm³ measured smears of 209 cases (175 males and 34 females). They showed frequency distribution of the microfilarial counts and the positive rates according to the age-groups.

The clinical signs observed by the authors were: 112 cases of elephantiasis of the legs, 12 cases of elephantiasis of the arms, 30 cases of elephantiasis of the scrotum or vulva, 5 cases of thickened lymphatic trunks, 6 cases of chyluria, 9 cases of orchitis, 77 cases of hydrocele, 514 cases of enlarged groin glands, 368 cases of enlarged axillary glands, and 294 cases of filarial fever. The observations on adult worms were made in 23 specimens surgically removed from patients known to be suffering from filariasis. Morphological descriptions of the adult worms were presented. The examination of day and night blood of 31 cases showed that the microfilariae were nocturnally periodic. The morphological study of the microfilariae indicated that they were all those of *Filaria bancrofti*. *C. fatigans* in Cochin was found to serve as an efficient vector of the local filaria.

IYENGAR (1932) reported that the type of filarial infection occurring in two adjacent coastal areas in North Travancore, namely, Shertalai and Ambalapuzha, was different from the infection observed in other parts of India; firstly, the microfilariae found in the human carriers in this area were different from those of *W. bancrofti*, and secondly, the chief transmitter of the infection was *M.* (*Mansonioides*) *annulifera*, and consistently negative results were obtained with *C. fatigans*, both in natural and experimental infections. The microfilariae exhibited a definite nocturnal periodicity, but their morphological characters were quite similar, in many ways, to those of *Filaria malayi* described by BRUG (1927) from the Malay Archipelago. In Travancore, both types of filarial infections were found to occur, those due to *W. bancrofti* in urban areas, and those due to the other type in rural, coastal, sandy areas in the north. In the urban area, *C. fatigans* was a common species and acted as an efficient vector both in nature and under conditions of experimental infection. In the latter areas, *C. fatigans* was sparse and had not been found infected, experimentally or in nature, while *M. annulifera* was common; 26% of over 900 *M. annulifera* specimens dissected were infected, and reached the mature stage in 11 days when experimentally infected.

IYENGAR (1933) reported on the results of surveys of filariasis in Trivandrum, the capital city of Travancore, situated on the southwestern seacoast of India. All microfilariae observed in man in this city were those of *W. bancrofti*. Blood and clinical examinations were carried out in 24 sections of this city; a total of 3,268 persons (10.5%) of 31,005 examined were positive for microfilariae, and 1,025 (3.31%) had filarial symptoms. High degrees of positive correlation were seen among the population density, the microfilarial rate, the average number of microfilariae per positive film, the disease rate, and the infection rate of *C. fatigans* observed in the 24 sections. In general, the flat, lowland area in the center of the city had a heavier infection, with microfilaria rates of 15 to 20%, while the outskirts of the city had lower infection rates.

LYENGAR (1938) compiled a detailed report on the epidemiology of filariasis in Travancore. The state was divided into 30 'taluks,' or districts, and had a population of 5,096,000 according to the 1931 census. Two types of filarial infection were found to occur in Travancore, namely, those due to *B. malayi* and *W. bancrofti*. Two urban districts, Quilon and Trivandrum, were endemic areas of only *W. bancrofti*, while *B. malayi* was endemic in all of the remaining 11 districts, and mixed endemicity of the two species was seen in six districts. The author classified the districts into the three types: the districts with extensive filarial incidence (Shertalai, Amalapula, Karthigapalli, Karunagapalli, Vaikam and Paroor), the districts with localized endemic foci (Pathanapuram, Kottarakara, Neduman-gad, Vilevencode, Kalkulam, Quilon, and Trivandrum), and districts with little or no endemic filariasis (Kunnathnad, Todupula, Pathanamthitta, Shencotta, Neyyattinkara, Agasthiswaram, and Tovala).The author presented various interesting results accumulated in this extensive survey.

Detailed studies were also made by IYENGAR (1938) for the first time on *B. malayi* infection in India. Naturally caught mosquitoes from an endemic area in Pattanacaud were examined. Eight out of 17 mosquito species examined were found infected. Comparatively high infection rates were observed in *M. annulifera* (438 of 1,928; 22.7%), *M. uniformis* (9 of 174; 5.2%), and *M. indiana* (4 of 80; 5.0%); 3 of 205 (1.5%) of *An. barbirostris*, 2 of 3,978 *C. gelidus*, 3 of 3,237 *C. vishnui*, 2 of 172 *Culiciomyia pallidothorax*, and 1 of 1,118 *An. subpictus* were also found infected. *Culex fatigans* was rare in the area, and only two were examined; neither was infected. About 400 laboratory-reared *C. fatigans* were fed on *B. malayi* carriers and examined 5 to 15 days after the feed; all the mosquitoes failed to develop the infection except for a solitary specimen which showed a few young larvae in the thoracic muscle. Control experiments with *M. annulifera* showed normal development of the worms. Bionomics of *Mansonioides* mosquitoes, including the egg-laying habits, larval development, host plants, seasonal incidence of larvae and adults, and feeding habits were investigated in detail. The periodicity of microfilariae observed in five cases were definitely nocturnal. The author proposed a modified method of estimating the periodicity (periodicity index: average counts between 9 a.m. and 4 p.m. divided by average counts between 9 p.m. and 4 a.m.) in place of the method employed by Brug (ratio of number of microfilariae at noon divided by number of microfilariae at midnight).

Schemes for the control of filariasis were started in three areas in Travancore: (1) a rural area in Shertalai with *B. malayi* infection, (2) the urban area of Trivandrum with *W. bancrofti* infection, and (3) the town of Eraniel where both *W. bancrofti* and *B. malayi* infection occurred. In Shertalai, the main measure for *B. malayi* control in the selected area of about 25 square miles consisted of the removal of *Pistia* (the host plant of *Mansonioides* larvae) by hand, started in October 1934 by special workers. Considerable reduction in *Mansonioides* mosquitoes was observed as compared with the number of catches in an untreated area. At the blood examinations conducted in April 1937, no new infection was seen in 71 children, two years old and under, examined in the treated area, whereas 11 of 56 children of the same age-group in the untreated area were found infected. In Trivandrum, the control measures were directed against *C. fatigans*, and periodic treatment with larvicides of all the breeding places was started in October 1932. Within two months after starting this work, the incidence of *C. fatigans* was brought down by more than 85% as shown by test catches. In Eraniel, where both *B. malayi* and *W. bancrofti* were endemic, the above two measures were applied, i.e., the treatment of breeding places of *C. fatigans* with larvicides, and the clearance of *Pistia* from tanks and pools. These control measures effected a striking reduction in the incidence of mosquitoes, and test catches showed a reduction of 92 to 94% after four months and of 98% after seven months.

JASWANT SINGH *et al.* (1956a) conducted surveys of Ernakulam and Mattancherri, Travancore-Cochin state. In Ernakulam, 7,328 persons were examined, and 519 *W. bancrofti* cases and 47 *B. malayi* cases, including 9 mixed infection cases, were found. In Mattancherri, 5,017 persons were examined, and 681 *W. bancrofti* cases and 71 *B. malayi* cases were discovered, among which 15 cases had the mixed infection. *B. malayi* was encountered in the peripheral wards, especially towards the southern end of the town.

JASWANT SINGH *et al.* (1956b) carried out field studies on the effects of residual insecticides on the vectors of *W. bancrofti* and *B. malayi* in the Ernakulam area of Travancore-Cochin, and observed that DDT, dieldrin, and BHC applied at dosages of 200 mg, 50 mg, and 44 mg, respectively, per square foot, were effective against *C. fatigans* for 13 to 14 weeks, and were also effective in reducing the population of *Mansonioides* mosquitoes for at least 20 weeks after the spraying. In general, *Mansonioides* was considered to be more susceptible to these insecticides than *C. fatigans*.

JASWANT SINGH *et al.* (1956c) conducted epidemiological and entomological surveys of filarial infections in Shertalai Taluk, Travancore-Cochin State. The area was surveyed by IYENGAR (1938) and high endemicity rates ranging from 31.2% to 65.2% were recorded. The average microfilarial rate was 29% and exclusively due to *B. malayi* infection. In the present survey carried out during the period from March to May 1955, 8,463 persons, covering 3.3% of the population, were examined for microfilariae and disease signs; 1,776 persons (20.9%) showed microfilariae in their night blood, while external manifestations of filariasis were found in 2,011 (23.8%). Sixteen cases (all from Shertalai) among the microfilaria positive persons had the microfilariae of *W. bancrofti*, and seven of them had these microfilariae in association with those of *B. malayi*. The authors noted that *W. bancrofti* had begun to establish itself in this town with the advancing urbanization. The disease manifestations were elephantiasis of the legs in 1,298 cases, elephantiasis of the hands in 44 cases, elephantiasis of the legs and hands in 142 cases, fever and lymphangitis in 516 cases, and filarial scrotum in 11 cases. The youngest age at which microfilariae were detected was in a girl one year old, and elephantoid swelling of both legs was recorded in a boy three years old. As for entomological observations, a total of 13 species of mosquitoes were collected from Shertalai Taluk (five species of *Culex*, including *C. fatigans*, two species of *Mansonia*, one species of *Armigeres*, and four species of *Anopheles*); developing filarial larvae were found in only *M. annulifera* (92 positives of 1,830 dissected, or 5.0%) and in *M. uniformis* (1 positive of 62, or 1.6%).

RAGHAVAN *et al.* (1958) conducted a filaria survey of hill-tribe settlements in Quilon and Trivandrum Districts. In this region IYER (1901) recorded 27 cases of filariasis from Pathanaparum, and IYENGAR (1938) recorded high rates of microfilaremia and disease cases in association with hyperendemic malaria. In the present survey, 471 persons comprising 42% of the total population in the five settlements were examined, and the microfilaria, disease and endemicity (both combined) rates were 25.9, 28.9, and 46.3 percent, respectively. The microfilariae were all those of *B. malayi*. Only two among them had enlarged spleen, and none of them was positive for malaria prasites. Of 11 species of *Anopheles*, one species of *Mansonia*, and four species of *Culex* collected and dissected, infection with advanced stages of filarial larvae was found only in 3 of 32 *M. uniformis* examined in February 1957; none of 312 *C. fatigans* examined were infected.

NAIR & ROY (1958) conducted a filaria survey of Eriyad Panchayat, Granganore Taluk, in the Trichur district of Kerala. Night blood smears of about 20 mm³ were prepared from 1,787 persons (9.4% of the total population), and 197 (11.0%) were found to be positive for the microfilariae of *B. malayi*; no *W. bancrofti* microfilariae were found among those examined. The number with filariasis manifestations were 201 (11.2%), of whom 20 (10.0%) were microfilaria positive. No genitourinary affections were observed, and only lymphoedema or elephantiasis of the limbs were encountered (112 cases on one leg, 46 cases on both legs, 21 cases on one hand, 5 cases on both hands, and 17 cases on both leg and hand). Of 292 female mosquitoes from 16 species dissected, filarial infection was found in only 2 of 77 *M. annulifera* and 1 of 16 *M. uniformis*.

NAIR *et al.* (1959) reported on a filaria survey of Edapally Panchayat, in the Ernakulam district of Kerala. In the previous survey reported by IYENGAR (1938), a microfilaria rate of 15.7% and a disease rate of 11.04% were recorded from the same area. In the present survey conducted from January to February 1957, 631 persons (5.1% of the total population) were examined at night, and 74 (11.7%) were microfilaria positive in approximately 20 mm³ blood smears, and 66 (10.5%) showed disease manifestations. The microfilariae were all those of *B. malayi*, except for one case who also had those of *W. bancrofti*. The disease manifestations were all elephantoid condition of the legs and/or hands.

JOSEPH *et al.* (1960) carried out pilot studies on the control of filariasis due to *B. malayi* in Kerala. The following four measures were tried: (a) *Mansonioides* control by indoor residual spraying of dieldrin at 50 mg per square foot, from May to June 1958 and January 1959; (b) *Mansonioides* control as above, accompanied by mass therapy with DEC, 200 mg for adults per day for five days; (c) *Mansonioides* control through *Pistia* clearance by manual removal; and (d) *Pistia* clearance as above, combined with DEC mass therapy.

The indoor application of dieldrin reduced the density of *M. annulifera*, the main vector of *B. malayi*, to practically zero for at least six months, but its effect on *M. uniformis* was much shorter and lasted only for two months; it had led to a remarkable increase in the prevalence of dieldrin-resistant *C. fatigans*. *Pistia* clearance was a lengthy process which had to be carried out continuously throughout the year; it was found impracticable over large areas. Mass therapy with DEC was not a feasible preventive measure against *B. malayi* in Kerala, because with the best efforts, it had not been found possible to cover more than 50% of the experimental populations, due to refusals to take the drug for fear of the adverse reactions.

NAIR *et al.* (1960) carried out a filaria survey of Fort Cochin, Kerala, from August to September 1957. Of 8,581 persons examined, covering 28.7% of the population, the microfilaria rate, the disease rate, and the endemicity rate observed were 11.3%, 6.1%, and 17.2%, respectively. Of 969 microfilaria positive cases, 931 (96.1%) had only the microfilariae of *W. bancrofti,* 33 (3.4%) had only those of *B. malayi*, and 5 (0.5%) had those of both species. Of 520 persons with filarial disease signs, 2.1% showed microfilariae, while 11.9% of 8,061 apparently healthy persons were microfilaria positive. Of 548 mosquitoes collected and dissected, 48 (13.7%) of 443 *C. fatigans* were found infected with filaria larvae and 12 (3.4%) had infective stage larvae.

NAIR (1962) conducted a survey of Ponani, a coastal town in Panchayat, in the Palghat district of Kerala. In a previous survey carried out in 1953 in Panchayat, a microfilaria rate of 13.7%, a disease rate of 19.7%, and an endemicity rate of 33.4% were recorded. In the present survey, 1,555 (5.5% of the population) were examined, and a microfilaria rate of 14.4%, a disease rate of 15.0%, and an endemicity rate of 28.0% were obtained. The microfilariae were all those of *W. bancrofti,* except for two persons who had those of *B. malayi*. The microfilarial periodicity in four *W. bancrofti* carriers, observed by recording counts in 20 mm³ blood samples collected at one-hour intervals, was typically nocturnal.

JOSEPH & PEETAMBARAN (1963) conducted a filaria survey of the Trichur Town area of Kerala, between December 1960 and October 1961. Out of 8,386 persons examined, 226 (2.7%) were positive for microfilariae; all the microfilariae were those of *W. bancrofti*. Disease manifestations were found in 35 persons, and these were all elephantiasis of the legs; no case of genital or urinary involvements was observed. Out of 2,506 mosquitoes collected, 2,431 were *C. fatigans*, and 9 of 1,808 *C. fatigans* dissected were infected with filaria larvae.

JOSEPH *et al.* (1963) made observations on the comparative hospitability of the water plants *Salvinia auriculata* and *Pistia stratiotes* to *M. annulifera*, the main vector of *B. malayi* in Kerala. The former was a recently introduced plant, while the latter was the normal host plant. It was found both in laboratory and field experiments that where the plants grew together, the mosquito preferred *Pistia* to *Salvinia* for oviposition by a ratio of about 4:1, with nearly 70% of the larvae attached to the Pistia. The larval mortality was about twice as much in pure *Salvinia* ponds as in the pure *Pistia* ponds. It was concluded that *Salvinia* is not a favorable host for *M. annulifera*.

NAIR & BHATNAGAR (1968) reported on the results of a filaria survey of Trichur Town, which was formerly believed to be free from filariasis. However, at examination of 1,578 persons in 18 wards, a gross microfilarial rate of 4.4%, and a disease rate of 1.3% were obtained. The microfilarial density of the positive cases was relatively low in general; of a total of 70 positive cases, 27 persons had counts of 1 to 5, 11 with counts of 6 to 10, 10 with counts of 11 to 20, 5 with counts of 21 to 30, 9 with counts of 31 to 50, 3 with counts of 51 to 100, and 3 with counts of over 100. Of 21 clinical cases, 17 had elephantiasis of the leg, 3 had hydrocele, and one had both elephantiasis of the leg and hydrocele. *Culex fatigans* was found to be breeding in numerous polluted water collectors, and the adult density was 24.6 per man-hour. Two of 227 *C. fatigans* examined were positive for mature larvae. Infection was not seen in *An. subpictus*, *C. vishnui*, or *C. gelidus*.

8A.2.4.f Madhya Pradesh

A state in central India, Madhya Pradesh was formerly called Central Provinces and Berar; it has an area of 1,844,650 km² and a population of 41,449,729 (1971).

Filariasis due to *W. bancrofti* is widespread, but generally at relatively low rates. *Brugia malayi* has been found in Ratanpur, in the Bilaspur district, and constitutes the only human filaria in this region. According to the NICD Report by RAGHAVAN *et al.* (1967) and the Assessment Report of ICMR (1971), filaria surveys were carried out by two survey units, Raipur and Satna, from 1956 to 1965. Out of 43 districts in the state, 30 have been covered by the surveys, and the population exposed to the risk of filariasis was estimated to be 5.9 million (1964) out of a total population of 32.4 million (1961 figures). Three A-type control units were established at Chhatarpur, Tikamgarh, and Satna.

PARK (1961, 1962a, 1962b) reported on the results of a series of filariasis surveys conducted in the Rewa Division, Satna District, and Chhatarpur District of Madhya Pradesh.

SUNDAR RAO (1940) reported that filariasis was endemic in Ratanpur, in the Bilaspur district of the Central Provinces, and that the infection consisted entirely of *B. malayi*. The town is situated at an elevation of about 1,000 feet above sea level, and had a population of 4,950. Night blood was taken from 191 persons representing all the wards of Ratanpur, and microfilariae were found in 31 cases (16.2%). A house-to-house survey showed that out of a population of 2,000 examined, 78 had elephantiasis of the legs or arms, with the filarial disease rate of 3.9%; 49 of them were males and 29 were females; 35 cases had elephantiasis of one leg, 42 had that of both legs, and one had elephantiasis of the arm. Elephantiasis of the genitals, hydrocele, and chyluria were entirely absent. *M. annulifera* was the most common mosquito species, and its breeding places were mainly the large water tanks densely covered with *Pistia*. The author also referred to the fact that *B. malayi* had been found to be endemic also in Shertalai in North Travancore, Balasore and Patnagarh in Orissa, Comilla in East Bengal, and Sylhet in Assam.

SUNDAR RAO (1945) observed that Dhamda village of the Durg district of Central Provinces also had endemic filariasis due entirely to *B. malayi*. Of 120 persons examined, 16 (13.3%) were found to show microfilariae in the night blood. A house-to-house survey for filarial disease showed that in the whole population of 3,628, 80 persons had elephantiasis of the legs or hands, and no cases of hydrocele, chyluria, or genital involvements were observed in this area. *M. annulifera* was the most common mosquito, and was the only species that was found infected. The towns reported as the endemic foci of *B. malayi* by the author, i.e., Patnagarh in Orissa, and Ratanpur and Dhamha in Central Provinces, were all at one time the important trade centers of the ancient Hindu kings, and so still had relics of a large number of tanks covered with *Pistia stratiotes*, the favorite host plant of *Mansonoides* mosquitoes.

8A.2.4.g Maharashtra

A state in western and central India, Maharashtra comprises the southeastern portion of the former Bombay State. It has an area of 307,270 km^2 and a population of 50,295,081 (1971).

Filariasis due to *W. bancrofti* occurs in the western coastal zone, and in various inland areas towards the northeast, especially around Nagpur; the infection is intense in many areas. According to the NICD Report by BASU *et al.* (1968), and Assessment Report of ICMR (1971), filaria surveys were carried out by the survey unit of Nagpur during the years 1955–56. Out of 26 districts in the state, six have been covered by the surveys, and the population exposed to the risk of filariasis was estimated to be 4.5 million out of a total population of 39.6 million (1961 census). The state has 4.5 control units distributed in the Nagpur district, Nagpur Municipal Corporation, Chanda, Bhandara, and Bassein. None of the units were reorganized and thus, have both rural and urban components. Data referring to vector density, vector infection, infectivity rates, and microfilaria rates in the 5 to 15-year age-group were reported for the years from 1962 to 1969. The mosquito density in all units except Bassein has been showing an upward trend. The microfilaria rates have been rather stable in Nagpur (7.0% in 1962–63 and 7.3% in 1968), increasing in Chanda (2.8% in 1962–63, 6.7% in 1968) and in Bhandara (1.8% in 1962–63, 3.5% in 1968), and slightly decreasing in Nagpur Corporation (4.6% in 1963–64 and 2.8% in 1968) and in Bassein (4.5% in 1962–63 and 2.9% in 1968).

Filariasis surveys were also conducted by BASU *et al.* (1967) in Greater Bombay. PATEL & PARAHJPEY (1958) conducted observations on mass therapy with DEC for filariasis control in Bombay State. KALRA *et al.*

(1967) reported on the occurrence of a larvivorous fish *Lebistes reticulatus* (Peters) breeding in sewage water at Nagpur (see Section 10D.3.2.3).

8A.2.4.h Mysore

A state in southern India, Mysore occupies a plateau region of southern Deccan, with hills in the west. Its area is 191,760 km², with a population of 29,224,046 (1971).

Filariasis due to *W. bancrofti* occurs along the coastal belt to the west (continuing into Kerala) and in the northeast corner (joining Andhra Pradesh). Filaria surveys under the NFCP were carried out during the years 1957 to 1962 and from 1966 to 1967; out of 19 districts, three have been covered by the surveys. The population exposed to the risk of filariasis was estimated to be 1.8 million in 1964 out of a total population of 23.6 million (1961 figures). Only 0.2 million people are being protected by antilarval measures (NICD Report by SINGH *et al.*, 1968).

KRISHNASWAMI (1955) reported on filariasis in the municipality of Mangalore, a town on the west coast of Mysore State, at about 13°N and 75°E. Altogether, 7,402 persons in 25 wards, or 6.3% of the total population of 117,095 (1951 census) were examined; 1,112 (15.0%) were positive for microfilariae of *W. bancrofti* in their night blood, and 704 (9.5%) had disease manifestations of filariasis (elephantiasis of the legs, hydrocele, and chyluria). The age distribution of microfilaria and disease rates were recorded. Filarial infection was seen only in *C. fatigans* and not in other culicine or anopheline mosquitoes; the infection rate of *C. fatigans* was 12.1% of 1,784 dissected in March 1954, 15.1% of 1,064 dissected in April, and 17.6% of 539 dissected in May.

SUBRAMANIAM & TAMPI (1958) conducted observations on the seasonal prevalence and filarial infection of *C. fatigans* in Mangalore Town. The average density per man-hour of female *C. fatigans* varied from a low of 11.2 in July to a high of 39.7 in November, while the infection rate was highest in June (23.2%) and lowest in January (3.2%). They showed the relationship between the monthly precipitation, mosquito density, and filarial infection rate.

GONSALVES (1960) made an evaluation of the results of mass therapy with DEC carried out in Mangalore Town under the NFCP. NANJUNDIAR & JEEVANDHARA KUMAR (1961) reported on a filaria survey in the Gulbarga district of Mysore.

8A.2.4.i Orissa

Orissa is a state on the east coast of India, with an area of 155,860 km² and a population of 21,934,827 (1971).

Both *W. bancrofti* and *B. malayi* occur in the state. The former is widely distributed, and particularly prevalent in the coastal zone around Chatrapur, Rampur, Puri, and Cuttack. The latter has been recorded from two inland areas, from the Balasore district by KORKE (1929, see Bihar), and from Patnagarh by RAO (1936).

Filaria surveys under the NFCP were carried out in Orissa by four survey units (two at Khurda and two at Raipur) from 1955 until 1957. Five control units were allotted to the state: at Khurda, Ranpur (transferred subsequently to Bhubaneswar), Chatrapur, Puri, and Cuttack. Out of 13 districts in the state, eight have been surveyed, and the population exposed to the risk of filariasis was estimated to be 7.8 million out of a total population of 17.5 million (1961 figures, from the ICMR-1971 Report). Relatively high microfilaria rates have been observed in the 5 to 15-year age-group, for example, 13.3% in Khurda, 9.2% in Bhubaneswar, 6.0% in Chatrapur, 11.0% in Cuttack, and 13.1% in Puri (1960 to 1961 surveys).

Roy & Rose (1922) reported on filariasis at Puri, where they found the disease was prevalent. Of 571 unselected persons examined at Puri Jail and Sadar Hospital, 156 or 27.3% showed microfilariae in blood, and 160 showed clinical manifestations of filariasis; 75 with fever and lymphangitis, 10 with filarial abscess, 9 with elephantiasis of the scrotum, 44 with elephantiasis of the leg, 3 with elephantiasis of the arm, 4 with that of the vulva, 3 with that of the penis, 2 with orchitis and funiculitis, 2 with synovitis, 2 with chyluria, and 6 with hydrocele. The total number with elephantiasis was 63, or 11% of the persons examined. Microfilariae were found in 120 (29%) of 411 apparently healthy persons, 17 (22.6%) of 75 cases with lymphangitis and filarial fever, 6 of 63 cases with elephantiasis, 6 of 10 with filarial abscess, and 2 of 2 with chyluria. The microfilariae showed nocturnal periodicity, and various developmental stages of the larvae were seen in *C. fatigans*. Among various drugs tested, sodium antimony tartrate was found to be effective in reducing the microfilariae when injected daily, beginning with 2 cc of 2% solution and rising to 5 cc.

Sundar Rao (1936) reported that filariasis was endemic in the town of Patnagarh in Orissa, where the infection consisted entirely of *B. malayi*. The town was the capital of Orissa until 1899; it is situated at an elevation of about 500 feet above sea level, and is the second biggest town in the state. The blood survey of people in this town revealed that 186 (17.8%) of 1,047 persons examined were positive for microfilariae of *B. malayi*. The microfilarial rate varied from a high of 40.0% (22 of 55) to a low of 3.2% (4 of 125), according to the wards surveyed. The microfilarial rates according to the age-groups were fairly uniform, and a rate of as high as 21.0% was seen in the youngest age-group of 1 to 5 years. The youngest child showing microfilaremia was four years old. A remarkable difference of the age distribution of the microfilarial rates from that of *W. bancrofti* was noted by the author. The clinical signs were found in 127 of 3,887 persons examined, with a gross filarial disease rate of 3.3%. Of those showing clinical signs, 65 (51.2%) had elephantiasis of the legs, 9 had elephantiasis of the forearm and hand, 4 had elephantiasis of both leg and arm, and 49 had filarial lymphangitis of the leg or arm. Elephantiasis of the genitals, hydrocele, and chyluria were entirely absent. All the microfilariae were identified as those of *B. malayi*. Of 110 *M. annulifera* examined, 23 were found infected, and one out of 23 *M. uniformis* was also positive for filarial larvae. *C. fatigans* were rather rare, and none of 28 was infected.

MAHAPATRA (1961) gave figures for the 1956–57 filariasis surveys in Orissa.

8A.2.4.j Tamil Nadu

A state in South India, Tamil Nadu was formerly called Madras State. It has an area of 130,000 km² and a population of 41,103,125 (1971).

Filariasis due to *W. bancrofti* occurs along the eastern coastal zone and in some inland areas. Relatively high microfilaria rates were observed in the 1955–59 surveys under the NFCP from several districts, such as 11.20% in Chingleput, 9.63% in North Arcot, 9.56% in Tanjore, and 8.38% in South Arcot (RAMAKRISHNAN *et al.* 1960a). Four control units were established in the state from 1956 to 1958. Out of 13 districts in the state, 12 have been covered by the surveys, and the population exposed to the risk of filariasis was estimated to be 13.0 million out of a total population of 33.7 million (1961 figures).

CRUICKSHANK *et al.* (1923) carried out a filarial survey of the whole village of Saidapet near Madras, and obtained a microfilarial rate of 20.05% (152 of 758 examined) in those with signs of filarial disease, and that of 25.5% (192 of 752) in those without signs of filarial disease. The authors pointed out that in their experiences, microfilariae were less commonly found in those with the recognized signs of filarial disease than in those without these signs, and that their results were quite different from those observed by MANSON-BAHR (1912) in Fiji and Ceylon, where this relationship was reversed.

SOMASUNDARAM (1949) carried out a filariasis survey of Palacole, a municipal town in the deltaic taluk of Narsapur in the West Godavari District of the Madras Presidency. The town had a population of 19,829 at the 1941 census. Night blood was taken at random from about 50 people in each ward. Out of 556 slides examined, 83 (14.9%) were positive for microfilariae, which were all identified as those of *W. bancrofti*. A survey of clinical filariasis was made on 5,957 persons, of whom 474 (7.5%) showed some clinical signs; of these, 363 (76.6%) had elephantiasis of the leg, and 134 of them were males and 229 were females. Elephantiasis of the scrotum was seen in 88, that of the arm in 14 cases. Chyluria was found only in one case. One peculiar aspect observed by the author was that *Mansonioides* seemed to be the chief vector of bancroftian filariasis in this town, and *C. fatigans* seemed to play only a minor role. *Mansonioides* larvae were found breeding abundantly in tanks associated with *Pistia*, and represented the most abundant mosquito. The infection with filaria larvae was seen in 31 of 250 *Mansonioides*, 1 of 48 *C. fatigans*, none of 185 *An. subpictus*, and none of 24 other species dissected.

RAGHAVAN & KRISHNAN (1949a) carried out an epidemiological study of malaria and filariasis in Sri Harikotta Island, Nellore, Madras Presidency. The island had a population of 5,492 at the 1941 census, but it had dwindled down to about 3,900 at the time of the survey because of the ravages of malaria, filariasis, and malnutrition. About 20 mm^3 of peripheral blood was drawn at night, and both thick smears and thin films were made for examination of microfilaria and malaria parasite. Of 709 persons examined, "microfilariae similar to *B. malayi*" were found in 175 (22.1%), and clinical signs of filariasis were seen in 102 (14.4%). The clinical cases observed were: 56 persons with elephantiasis of either of the lower extremities, 21 persons with that of both lower extremities, 11 persons with that of either of the upper extremities, 7 cases with involvements of both upper extremities, 5 cases with involvement of both lower and upper extremities, one with hydrocele, and one with chyluria. None of the 102 cases with clinical manifestations showed microfilariae in the peripheral blood, and at least two cases with hydrocele or chyluria were those who had come from a *W. bancrofti* endemic area. Malaria parasites were found in 29 persons, 11 with *Plasmodium falciparum*, 14 with *Pl. vivax* and 4 with *Pl. malariae*. Both microfilariae and malaria parasites were coexisting in 7 cases (2 *Pl. falciparcum* and 5 *Pl. vivax*). The periodicity of microfilariae observed in three cases was definitely nocturnal, and the values of the periodicity index proposed by IYENGAR (1938), calculated by the following formula: "Average counts between 9 a.m. and 4 p.m. divided by the average counts between 9 p.m. and 4 a.m., multiplied by 100," turned out to be 0.100 in all of the three cases. Altogether, 19 species of mosquitoes were collected on the island, among which 42 (including 21 specimens of head/proboscis infection) of 169 *M. annulifera* and 3 (including one head/proboscis infection) of 18 *M. uniformis* were infected with filaria larvae, and one of 54 *An. culicifacies* had oocysts. Larvae of the above *Mansonia* species were found breeding abundantly in ponds covered by *Pistia* and contaminated with organic matter.

RAGHAVAN & KRISHNAN (1949b) further observed that microfilariae of *B. malayi* in a carrier of Sri Harikotta Island did not develop when experimentally fed by *C. fatigans* and *An. stephensi*, but underwent normal development to the infective stage in *M. annulifera*, and confirmed the evidence reported by LICHTENSTEIN (1927) from Indonesia and by IYENGAR (1932) from North Travancore, that *C. fatigans* was refractory to *B. malayi*.

8A.2.4.k Uttar Pradesh

Uttar Pradesh is a state in North India at the foot of the Himalayas, comprising mostly of the valleys of the Ganges and Yamuna Rivers. It has an area of 294,370 km^2 and a population of 88,299,453 (1971 figures).

Filariasis due to *W. bancrofti* is widespread in the state, especially in its eastern part. According to the Assessment Report of the Indian Council of Medical Research (1971), filaria surveys in Uttar Pradesh were carried out by the filaria survey units of Basti, Jaunpur, Ghazipur, Kanpur, and Lucknow during the period from 1955 to 1962. At present, ten control units are functioning in the state; out of 54 districts in the state, 28 have been covered by the surveys and the population exposed to the risk of filariasis was estimated to be 32.9 million out of the total population of 73.7 million (1961 figures).

Reports on the results of filariasis surveys were made by a number of workers: RAGHAVAN *et al.* (1957) for Basti Town, RAHMAN *et al.* (1957a) for Ballia Town, RAHMAN *et al.* (1957b) for Basti Town, GUJRAL (1958) for urban, semiurban, and rural filariasis in Ballia District, RAHMAN *et al.* (1959a) for Bahraich Town, RAHMAN *et al.* (1959b) for Barabanki, NANDA *et al.* (1960) for Barabanki (including observation on mass therapy), DIWAN CHAND *et al.* (1961a) for Ghazipur, DIWAN CHAND *et al.* (1961b) for Deoria, DIWAN CHAND *et al.* (1961c) for Gonda, DIWAN CHAND *et al.* (1961d) for Bahraich, DIWAN CHAND *et al.* (1961e) for Faizabad (including observation on mass therapy), DIWAN CHAND *et al.* (1962) for Gorakhpur, SINGH *et al.* (1963d) for rural Sitapur District, SINGH *et al.* (1963e) for Sitapur Town, SINGH *et al.* (1964) for urban filariasis in Lucknow, and by PUTATUNDA & SINGH (1967) for Gaur, Varanasi District.

GUJRAL (1958) conducted a comparative study of the endemicity of filariasis in urban, semiurban, and rural areas of Ballia District, Uttar Pradesh. The microfilaria rates were 12.0% (383 positives out of 3,179 persons examined) in the urban area, 10.9% (193 of 1,764) in the semiurban area, and 9.7% (273 of 2,813) in the rural area. The percentages of persons with disease signs were 34.5% in the urban, 27.1% in the semiurban, and 19.9% in the rural area. The number of filariasis cases attending dispensaries were also highest in the urban area, and had increased 11.84 times in the urban, 7.68 times in the semiurban, and 2.55 times in the rural areas during the previous five years. The infection was exclusively due to *W. bancrofti* in urban, as well in the rural areas, and the vector responsible for its transmission was *C. fatigans.*

SINGH (1960) reviewed the geographical distribution of filariasis in Uttar Pradesh. Filariasis surveys had been carried out in three out of five natural divisions of the state: the east plain, the central plain, and the hill-plateau; the Himalayan, as well as the west plain division, was still left unsurveyed. In general, the endemicity rates were highest in the districts in the east plain division, moderate in the central plain division, and lowest in the hill-plateau division.

Filariasis in the city of Lucknow, the capital of Uttar Pradesh, was investigated by SINGH *et al.* (1964). During the survey, conducted over a period of two years (1960 to 1962), 436 (5.44%) of 8,011 persons examined were found harboring microfilariae of *W. bancrofti*, and the average count per 20 mm³ blood was 6.80. Disease manifestations were seen in 185 (2.30 %) of the people examined, of whom 121 had hydrocele, 10 females had some genital involvements, 53 had elephantiasis of the leg, 7 had elephantiasis of the arm, and 8 had chyluria. Of 1,512 *C. fatigans* dissected, 82 (5.4%) were infected and 4 (0.26%) harbored mature larvae; none of 80 *Anopheles* were positive for infection.

8A.2.4.1 West Bengal

West Bengal is a state in northeast India, comprising the delta of the Ganges around Calcutta. Its area is 87,680 km² with a population of 44,440,095 (1971).

According to the ICMR Assessment Report (1971), filariasis surveys in West Bengal were carried out by the filaria control unit at Contai, during the period from November 1959 to October 1960. Out of 16 districts in the state, 13 have been covered by the surveys. The microfilaria rates observed were: 11.7% in Midnapore; 7% in Bankura, Birbuhum, and Murshidabad; and 5% in Nadia, Hooghly, Howrah, Calcutta, 24-Parganas, Maldah, Darjeeling, Jalpaiguri, and Cooch Behar (sample sizes are unknown for all of these districts). The total population covered by the surveys was 0.72 million. The population exposed to the risk of filariasis was estimated to be 10.0 million out of a total population of 34.91 million.

In a survey of parasitic infections in a rural community of the Bandipur Union in West Bengal, about forty miles north of Calcutta, CHOWDHURY & SCHILLER (1968) found only 2 microfilaria cases (*W. bancrofti*) out of 875 blood specimens collected at night (between 10 p.m. and 1 a.m.). Hookworm eggs were found in 78% of the fecal specimens examined.

ROZEBOOM *et al.* (1968) conducted seasonal observations on the transmission of filariasis in urban Calcutta. In the days when KNOWLES & BASU (1934) made observations on mosquitoes and mosquito-borne diseases in Calcutta, it was reported that filariasis was only slightly endemic, and that transmission could occur throughout most of the year without showing epidemic waves. ACTON & RAO (1930), on the other hand, stated that in Calcutta the favorable period for transmission did not synchronize with the breeding of *C. fatigans* as was seen in other localities, and consequently, the microfilaria rate was low. There have been, however, many changes in Calcutta since the completion of earlier studies, and many refugees and other immigrants carrying filariasis are believed to have settled in and around the city. The breeding sites of *C. fatigans* are more stabilized and no longer affected by rainfall to the extent they were in former years. As a result, the mosquito density in 1966–67 was found to be highest during the cold, dry months of February and March, at low levels during the hot, dry months (April to June), and again relatively high throughout the rainy season from July to November. The natural infection rate with mature larvae of *W. bancrofti* ranged from 0 to 1.0% during the cold months, and from 1.8 to 4.3% during the warm months. From biting rates, infective larva rates, and intensities of infections, it was estimated that anyone living in this area would have the risk of being bitten about 50 times during the year by infective mosquitoes carrying a total of at least 180 third stage larvae. There are two transmission seasons: late February to early April, and during the warm rainy weather from July to November. An important factor inhibiting higher transmission rates is the high daily mortality rates of the mosquito, which ranged from around 20 to 30% through most of the rainy, warm season.

8A.2.4.m Goa

Goa is a former Portuguese territory on the west coast of India, about 250 miles south of Bombay, and is composed of Goa, Daman, and Diu. It was annexed to India in 1962. It has an area of 3,636 km² and a population of 626,978 (1970).

The occurrence of filariasis in Goa was first reported by DESSAI (1952). However, according to MESQUITA (1959), the disease was already widely spread over the territory. Following a case-finding campaign begun in 1953, it was found that 5.3% of 9,708 persons examined were infected; among them, 7,456 were natives of Goa, with an infection rate of 5.4%. The highest incidence was recognized between the ages of 10 and 20 years; the percentages were 6% in males and 4.7% in females. The incidence by races were: 8.4% of 273 Mohammedans, 8.3% of 2,495 Hindus, 4% of 4,206 Christians, 0.7% of 1,656 Africans, and 0.2% of 405 Europeans. Trial administration of DEC was carried out on 371 persons.

In Diu, VAGA (1959) made a report on filariasis and its control. Of 1,995 persons examined from the total population of some 4,000 in this town, 10% were found to be infected. Elephantiasis was found in 61 cases (3%).

According to the Assessment Report of ICMR (1971), filaria surveys were carried out in Goa from 1960 to 1964. Out of a total population of 0.6 million persons in Goa, about 2.5 lakhs were covered by the surveys. The surveys were confined to urban areas only. The population exposed to the risk of infection was estimated to be 1.5 lakhs out of the total population of 6 lakhs. Three A-type units were allotted to the Union Territory in 1965–66, and these units are required to send only vector density data. The vector density in Panaji registered a decline from 121.1 (10 man-hour density of *C. fatigans*) in 1966 to 61.6 in 1969, in Margao from 69.7 in 1967 to 37.2 in 1969, and in Mapusa and Vasco from 96.8 in 1967 to 37.2 in 1969. The microfilaria rate in Panaji came down from 3.1% in 1960 to 0.7% in 1964 and remained more or less so from 1965 to 1969; in Mapusa, the rate declined from 4.2% in 1961 to 1.3% in 1969; in Margao, the rate was 1.7% in 1961 and 1.1% in 1969.

8A.2.4.n Pondicherry

A centrally administered territory of India and a former French coastal settlement, Pondicherry is situated south of Madras at about 12°N. It has an area of 474 km² and a population of 471,347 (1971).

A filaria survey in Pondicherry Settlement was reported by NAIR (1960).

In Pondicherry Town, 742 (10.3%) of 7,184 persons examined were positive for *W. bancrofti* microfilariae. In Pondicherry communes, 464 (3.9%) of 11,940 persons were positive. Analysis was made on the age and sex incidence of microfilaria carriers and clinical cases.

According to the Assessment Report of ICMR (1971), one filaria control unit was allotted to Pondicherry settlement in 1961, and the microfilaria rate among the age-group of 5 to 15 years was 8.9% in 1962–63, 8.6% in 1963–64, 6.8% in 1964–65, 3.0% in 1967, and 3.0% in 1968.

8A.2.4.o The Laccadive, Minicoy, and Amindivi Islands

A centrally administered territory of India, these island groups comprise about 20 islands in the Arabian Sea west of Kerala State, situated between 8°N and 12°N. They have an area of about 30 km² and a population of 31,798 (1971).

A survey of filariasis was carried out by SUBRAMANIAM *et al.* (1958) during the period from December 1954 to February 1955. Of ten inhabited islands of the Laccadive Archipelago, with a total population of about 20,000 as of 1955, nine were surveyed, with the exception of Bitra. The islands of Kalpeni, Androth, Agathi, Kiltan, Chetlat, and Kadamath were found to be endemic for *W. bancrofti*, while Minicoy, Kavarathi, and Ameni were free from filariasis. Of a total population of 11,846 (1951 census) on the six islands where filariasis was shown to be endemic, 10 to 37% were examined, and microfilaria rates ranging from 4.2 to 18.2% and disease rates from 0.80 to 29.7% were recorded. *Wuchereria bancrofti* was the only parasite; *B. malayi* infection, *Mansonia* mosquitoes, and the *Pistia* plant were not encountered. *Culex fatigans* was the only vector proved by the dissections.

A second survey of the Laccadive Archipelago was carried out by NAIR (1961) in April 1958. Altogether, 4,855 persons, comprising 23.3% of total population, were surveyed, and *W. bancrofti* was found to be endemic in six of ten inhabited islands, with microfilaria rates ranging from 11.8 to 21.7% according to the islands. *W. bancrofti* was the only parasite detected, and the periodicity of the microfilariae was strictly nocturnal.

8A.2.4.p The Andaman and Nicobar Islands

These island-groups are a centrally administered territory of India, comprising two groups of islands in the Bay of Bengal, about 650 km west of lower Burma, situated between 7°N and 15°N. They have a population of 115,090 (1970 census) and an area of 8,293 km².

BASU (1958) reported on malaria and filariasis in Andaman and Nicobar. The local filaria control unit surveyed about 9,000 people in 1956–57 on Car Nicobar, Nancowry, Kamotra, and the Trinket Islands, about 15% of the population; they found an infection rate of 4% and disease rate of 0.9%. The parasite was *W. bancrofti* only. During this period, 1,134 *C. fatigans* were dissected, and infection was noted in 15 mosquitoes. In 1958, the unit conducted a blood survey of people in the Nicobar group, and found 3 (2.8 %) of 106 night blood samples and 28 (8.9 %) of 316 day blood samples to be positive for the microfilariae of *W. bancrofti*. In the present survey, 85 persons in Champin and Malacca in Nancowry group of the Nicobars were examined at night, and 6 (7.1 %) among them were found to be positive for *W. bancrofti*; two among them had elephantiasis of legs. Since the microfilaria rate of day blood samples was higher than that of night blood samples, it was suggested that *W. bancrofti* in this region might be a subperiodic form. Altogether, eight species of *Anopheles* were record-ed by CHRISTOPHERS in 1911; he concluded that among these, *An. ludlowi* (= *An. sundaicus*) was the only important malaria carrier. The local filaria control unit recorded seven species of mosquitoes from Nicobar, and noted the development of filarial larvae, including the infective stage, in *C. fatigans*.

According to the Assessment Report of ICMR (1971), a modified malaria cum filaria control unit was allotted to the islands located in the Car Nicobar group in 1955. Another unit located at Port Blair, has been functioning since December 1967.

RUSSEL *et al.* (1975) carried out filaria surveys and field experiments in the Andaman and Nicobar Islands during January and February, 1974. There were two distinct forms of *W. bancrofti* infection, i.e. a nocturnally periodic form in Port Blair, and a subperiodic form in Nancowry, Chowra and Carnicobar of Nicobar group of islands. The microfilaria rates in Ter-ressa and Chowra (Nicobar) were more than 13 %, but the disease rate was low (2.9 % or less). The microfilaria rate and the mean microfilarial den-sity were highest in the afternoon as compared to forenoon and night. *C. p. fatigans* was shown to be an efficient vector of the nocturnally periodic form in Port Blair, but the subperiodic form in Nancowry and Chowra developed only in about nine percent of *C. p. fatigans* experimentally fed on microfilaria carriers.

8A.3 Nepal

A kingdom on the northeastern border of India, Nepal is bounded on the north by Tibet, China, on the east by Sikkim and India, and on the south and west by India; it is situated between latitudes 26°N and 31°N. Nepal has an area of 140,743 km^2 and a population of 11,237,616 (1971). The southern portion, Terai, is subtropical in climate, rather flat, and cul-tivated or forested; the central part is hilly or mountainous, temperate in climate, and mostly level cultivated, with high population density; the northern part is occupied by the high mountain range of the Himalayas.

Filariasis due to *W. bancrofti* is probably endemic in this country, at least in areas around the capital city of Katmandu, since chyluria is one of the common diseases seen by the physicians (personal communication at the All Nepal Medical Conference held in Katmandu, in February

1971). JONES *et al.* (1970) also reported on hematuria and chyluria cases in Nepal. Mosquito fauna of Nepal were recorded by PETERS & DEWAR (1956).

JUNG (1973) conducted a preliminary survey of the prevalence of filariasis in Nepal. Examinations of night blood films and clinical signs were conducted on about 5,000 persons in nine areas (three urban, two semi-urban and four rural areas). Elephantiasis was found in 1.2 to 17.8% and microfilariae were found in 0.8 to 17.7% of the people examined in different areas. Active transmission was shown to be occurring both in rural and urban areas, and infection occurred as high as 1,900 m above sea level.

(No information is available concerning filariasis in Sikkim and Bhutan.)

8A.4 Sri Lanka (Ceylon)

Sri Lanka is an island in the Indian Ocean, south of India, with which it is connected by a chain of shoals called the Adam's Bridge; it has an area of 65,610 km² with a population of 12,514,00 (1970 estimate). Sri Lanka is situated between 5°55′ and 9°51′N, and 79°43′ and 81°53′E. It achieved independence from Britain in 1948. The island is composed of a central hilly region and the surrounding plain, which divides itself into the northern, the southwestern, and the southeastern plains. The southwestern portion receives rainfall during both monsoons: the northeast moonsoon which lasts from October to April, and the southwest monsoon from May to September. The rest of the country is more or less dry, and receives rainfall during either of the monsoon seasons.

Filariasis due to *W. bancrofti* is endemic mainly on the southwestern coastal belt, which is highly populated and rich in rainfall. *Culex fatigans* has been incriminated as the principal vector. A well-organized antifilariasis campaign has been in operation since 1947. Endemic foci of *B. malayi* were reported from several rural areas, but results of recent surveys indicate that the infection has terminated in most of the previously known endemic areas.

8A.4.1 Historical notes

The earliest scientific record referring to filariasis is found in the Ceylon Administration Report of 1879 wherein ONDAATJE reported a case of elephantiasis in Kandy Hospital and two cases in Matale Hospital. In the Administration Report for 1892, KYNSEY recorded one case of *Filaria sanguinis hominis* at the Matara Hospital (quoted by ABDULCADER, 1961).

BAHR (1914) carried out a filariasis survey of the island, and reported the occurrence of bancroftian filariasis in Ambalantota, Hambantota, Tangalla, Illekumulla, Matara, Galle, and Induruwa in Southern Province,

Kurunegala, Hiripitiya, and Puttalam in Northwestern Province, and Mutur and Toppur in Eastern Province. He examined 1,824 blood samples from 1,308 persons and found microfilariae of *W. bancrofti* in 43 samples (2.4%). The highest rate was 26.6% in Toppur. Clinical manifestations were detected in 57 persons: 47 cases of elephantiasis, 7 cases of hydrocele, 1 case of lymph scrotum, and 2 cases of chyluria. Enlargement of the epitrochlear or inguinal glands without obvious filariasis signs was noticed, and 7.5% of these cases showed microfilariae in their blood.

SWEET & DIRCKZE (1934) carried out a survey of filariasis in Southern Province, in 1925. In Galle Town, 605 persons were examined, 35 (5.8%) had microfilariae in night blood specimens and 7 (1.2%) had elephantiasis. In Galle District, 1,193 persons were examined, 19 (1.6%) were microfilaria positive and 10 (0.8%) had elephantiasis. In Matara District, 566 persons were examined, 8 (1.4%) had microfilariae and 3 (0.5%) had elephantiasis. In Hambantota District, 1,007 persons were examined, 101 (10.0%) had microfilariae and 22 (2.2%) had elephantiasis. Species identification was not done by these workers.

CARTER (1933) conducted an epidemiological survey of filariasis in Toppur, northeastern Ceylon, and found microfilariae of *B. malayi* in night blood samples of 34.4% (44 of 128) of the adults and 25.0% (11 of 44) of the children examined. He found 29 cases of elephantiasis of the extremities, but there was no case of genital involvement. Altogether, 1,313 mosquitoes collected in this area were dissected; 77% were *Mansonioides*, and infection with filarial larvae was seen in 37 (17 *M. annulifera* and 20 *M. indiana* or *M. uniformis*). This report is the first record of *B. malayi* in Ceylon.

A more detailed study on the epidemiology and clinical manifestations of *B. malayi* filariasis in Ceylon was reported by DASSANAYAKE (1938, 1939).

ABDULCADER (1961) referred to the results of an extensive filariasis survey conducted from 1937 to 1939 by Dassanayake and his associates, covering almost the whole island. A total of 10,989 persons in four provinces were examined; 1,684 (18.1%) were positive for the microfilariae of *B. malayi* and 32 (0.3%) were positive for those of *W. bancrofti*. The latter was confined to Galle and Matara Towns in the southwestern coastal belt, while *B. malayi* was found in Southern Province (6.8%, or 405 positives out of 5,922), Northwestern Province (29.8%, or 1,153 of 3,871), Eastern Province (10.4%, or 111 of 1,063) and North-Central Province (11.3%, or 15 of 133). The results indicated that at least at this time in Ceylon, *B. malayi* was much more prevalent and widely distributed than *W. bancrofti*. By this time it was established that *B. malayi* in Ceylon was transmitted by *M. annulifera, M. uniformis*, and *M. indiana,* which breed in large irrigation tanks and channels, in association with the water plant *Pistia strationes*.

After the termination of World War II, many cases of clinical filariasis were reported from the southwestern coastal belt of Sri Lanka, and an antifilariasis campaign was inaugurated on 24 October 1947, by the government of Ceylon and assisted by WHO. Reviews of progress of the project were made by IYENGAR (1949), KERSHAW (1961), ABDULCADER (1961, 1962, 1965a, b). ABDULCADER & PADLEY (1960), EDESON (1963), ABDULCADER & RAJAKONE (1965), ABDULCADER & SASA (1966), DISSANAIKE (1969), and HAWKING (1973).

According to ABDULCADER & SASA (1966), the Antifilariasis campaign consists of the headquarters (with a central laboratory) located in Colombo, and 17 peripheral units (as of 1966) distributed along the coastal belt and supervised by medical officers of the respective health districts. The activities are directed mainly to: 1) night blood examination of people under the control areas by house-to-house visits by local technicians to collect unmeasured blood samples (one drop from finger prick, or about 20 mm^3), and microscopical examination of the thick blood smears by some thirty microscopists at the central laboratory; 2) distribution of DEC to the microfilaria cases by house-to-house visits of local health inspectors, at a standard dosage of 6 mg per kg of body weight once a day, 18 doses in total; 3) treatment with DEC of clinical filariasis cases who visit filariasis clinics set up in the health districts concerned; 4) entomological investigations of the vector (dissection of mosquitoes and search for the breeding places), and control of the vectors, mainly by larviciding with applications of malathion in diesel oil, on a weekly cycle.

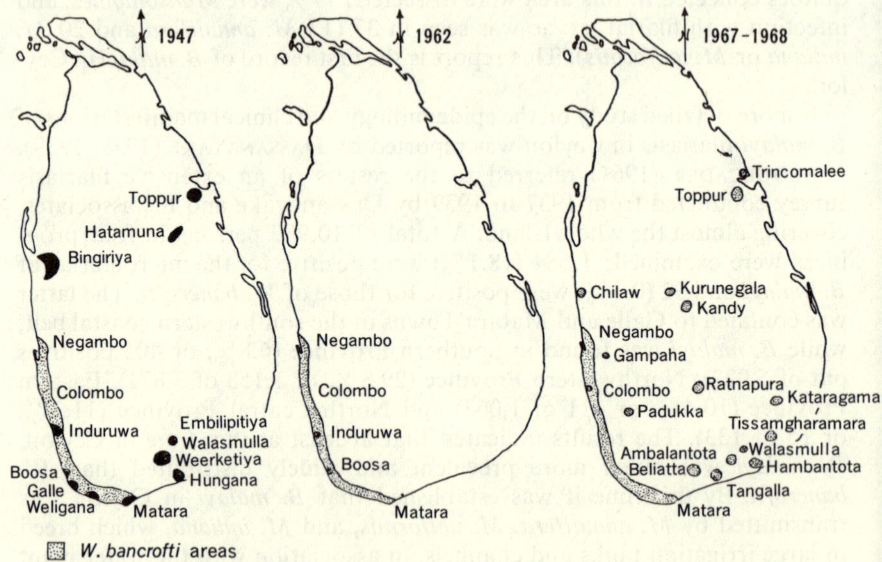

Fig. 8-3. Distribution of endemic areas of *W. bancrofti* and *B. malayi* as observed in the microfilaria surveys conducted in 1947, 1962, and 1967–68. (cited by DISSANAIKE, 1968).

8A.4.2 Distribution of Infection

The results of blood examinations shown in the annual reports of the Antifilariasis campaign are shown in Table 8-3. It is noteworthy that *W. bancrofti* infection is widely distributed in all the areas along the south-western coastal belt from Negombo to Matara at relatively low density levels (from 1.2 to 4.9% in 1963–64), and that the transmission is still going on in most of the areas despite tremendous efforts made for control. (Table 8-4). The areas being surveyed have been expanded each year, and new endemic foci have been detected in every year; therefore, the gross microfilaria rates shown in the table are only slowly decreasing, though some 85 to 90% of the individual positive microfilaria cases have turned out to be negative in the posttreatment blood examinations.

According to HAWKING (1973), the microfilaria rates of the districts in the coastal belt from Negombo to Matara in 1966 to 1967 ranged from 0.4 to 3.9%, with a mean rate of 1.3%. It was later recognized that the endemic belt extends more widely from Kataragama to Chilaw, covering an area of some 1300 km². In 1970–71, the microfilaria rate in this belt ranged from 0.03 to 3.7%, with a mean rate of 0.6%. Furthermore, probe surveys since 1966 have shown infection in many other areas, for example, Yeyangoda (4.9%), Gampoha (5.3%), Beliatta (3.6%), Chilaw (3.5%), Tangalla (3.4 %), Ambalantota (3.2%), Tissamagharamara (2.85%), Hambantota (1.9 %), Ganemulla (1.75%), Walasmulla (1.6%), Anuradhapura (1.2%), Kurunegala (0.75%), Weliweriya (0.7%), Ratnapura (0.55%), Matale (0.3%), Batticaloa (0.25%), and Badulla (0.2%). WIJETUNGE (1967) reported that transmission of filariasis was also taking place on the university campus at Peradeniya, in central Ceylon.

The microfilariae detected in the blood examinations by the antifilariasis campaign since 1959 have been all those of *W. bancrofti*, with the exception of two *B. malayi* carriers discovered in 1967 and 1970 from near Colombo and from Nattandiya, respectively. The colombo case was a six-month-old baby and the latter case was nine months old.

8A.4.3 Clinical cases

In Table 8-3, it is noteworthy that some 2,500 new cases with clinical manifestations were detected every year from the endemic belt, although the general microfilaria rate in this area is relatively low. The attack rates per 1,000 ranged from 0.59 (Ja-ela) to 4.73 (Ambalangoda), and were found to be highly correlated with the microfilaria rates of the respective districts (Table 8-4). In Dehiwala Clinic, for example, 3,480 cases altogether were examined before 1965; 2,075 (59.6%) were females and 1,405 (40.4%) were males. Lymphoedema and elephantiasis of the limbs were the most common symptoms and represented 98.5% (2,043 cases) among the female patients and 66.9% (940 cases) among the male patients. Genital

Table 8-3. A summary of achievements of the Antifilariasis Campaign, Sri Lanka (after ABDULCADER & SASA, 1966).

	1959	1960	1961	1961/62	1962/63	1963/64	1964/65
No. of blood films examined	81,809	132,161	114,260	126,892	219,539	396,774	405,274
No. of blood films positive	2,323	4,832	3,871	4,378	7,995	11,460	7,347
Rate positive (%)	2.84	3.66	3.39	3.45	3.64	2.89	1.81
No. of post-treatment films examined	584	3,369	5,164	8,074	12,773	22,194	24,864
No. positive	106	691	810	1,268	2,374	3,978	2,720
Rate positive	18.2	20.5	15.7	14.6	18.6	17.9	10.9
No. of *C. p. fatigans*							
Collected	9,119	15,505	11,735	16,586	15,677	24,985	24,465
Dissected	5,991	10,091	9,032	10,269	8,761	14,727	15,687
% with all larvae	2.2	2.3	1.6	1.6	2.0	1.7	1.3
% with mature larvae	*	*	*	0.6	1.1	0.7	0.5
No. of breeding places sprayed	73,254	77,349	86,413	84,911	106,770	105,477	103,775
No. filled with earth	423	248	732	1,630	1,431	645	641
No. of catch-pit latrines converted to water-seal type	1,105	2,855	1,734	1,032	1,197	1,642	762
No. of clinical cases treated	5,706	9,308	7,319	9,959	9,525	5,495	4,830
No. of new cases detected	2,215	1,949	2,553	2,718	2,889	2,754	2,520
Per capita cost (Rupees)	0.74	0.84	0.81	0.87	0.90	1.78	2.11

*Not available.

Table 8-4. Results of microfilarial, clinical, and vector surveys conducted under the Antifilariasis Campaign, Sri Lanka, 1963/64 (ABDULCADER & SASA, 1966).

District	Estimated popu-lation	Microfilaria survey					Average Mf. per		Clinical cases		Mosquito infection	Percentage	
		No. examin.	% examin.	No. posi-tive	% posi-tive	Total Mf. count	posi-tive	total exam.	No. obs.	Attack rate per 1,000	No. dis-sected	All larvae	Mature larvae
Negombo	45,262	36,013	79.9	580	1.61	8,040	15.83	0.223	85	1.88	853	1.18	0.58
Ja-ela	5,060	5,673	112.1	65	1.15	1,033	15.89	0.182	3	0.59	149	0.00	0.00
Wattala	12,666	4,710	37.2	145	3.08	2,659	18.34	0.565	38	3.00	802	1.74	0.99
Peliyagoda	23,110	14,184	61.4	653	4.60	11,182	17.52	0.788	96	4.15	1,675	3.22	1.13
Kolonnawa	29,182	21,287	72.9	801	3.76	8,504	10.62	0.399	59	2.02	1,864	2.20	0.53
Kotte	66,794	30,820	46.1	954	3.10	17,928	18.79	0.582	314	4.25	636	1.25	0.47
Dehiwela	100,000	77,002	77.0	2,015	2.62	20,132	9.99	0.261	271	2.46	832	1.80	0.72
Moratuwa	77,543	50,215	64.8	780	1.55	7,534	9.67	0.150	106	1.42	197	1.12	0.00
Panadura	20,868	20,302	97.3	367	1.81	3,067	8.16	0.151	50	2.47	387	0.52	0.52
Kalutara	22,868	18,221	79.7	237	1.30	2,441	10.30	0.134	20	0.87	1,575	0.51	0.31
Beruwela	15,361	7,551	49.2	281	3.72	2,762	9.83	0.366	49	3.19	250	0.80	0.80
Alutgama	17,951	5,161	28.8	227	4.40	3,201	14.10	0.620	34	1.89	123	0.81	0.00
Ambalangoda	28,900	18,479	63.9	874	4.73	17,313	19.81	0.937	108	4.73	466	0.44	0.00
Galle	74,505	38,770	52.0	1,902	4.91	28,830	15.16	0.744	248	3.33	215	1.86	0.93
Unawatuna	9,038	6,815	75.4	266	3.88	2,207	8.30	0.324	27	2.99	313	0.96	0.32
Weligama	15,545	10,679	68.7	277	2.59	2,716	9.81	0.254	15	1.04	340	2.94	2.06
Matara	33,000	24,004	72.7	815	3.40	13,531	16.60	0.564	43	1.27	1,111	1.98	0.99
Total	597,653	389,886	65.3	11,239	2.88	153,080	13.62	0.393	1566	2.62	11,788	1.70	0.708

involvements were seen in 30.0% (422 cases) of the male patients. Chyluria was seen only in two cases (after ABDULCADER & SASA, 1966).

8A.4.4 Vector

Previous entomological investigations conducted in Sri Lanka have shown that the only major vector of *W. bancrofti* in the endemic belt is *C. fatigans*, which breed in various water collection devices around houses. CHOW & THEVASAGAYAN (1957) made detailed observations on the bionomics and the effects of various insecticidal measures against this mosquito. Large numbers of mosquitoes were collected and dissected every year for examination of filarial infection (see Table 8-3). A study of the age composition of natural populations of *C. p. fatigans* in relation to the transmission of *W. bancrofti* was conducted by SAMARAWICKREMA (1967).

ABDULCADER (1965) reported on the results of entomological surveys carried out in the *W. bancrofti* endemic belt in Ceylon by workers of the entomological unit of the Antifilariasis Campaign. Collections of adult mosquitoes were conducted from human dwellings and cattle sheds during the period from 1949 to 1962. A total of 318,887 female mosquitoes were collected and identified from both controlled and uncontrolled areas. *Culex fatigans* was the predominant species among those collected from the dwellings in all the areas, and constituted 70.8 to 86.1% of the total collections. The second most numerous species was *M. uniformis,* which ranged from 4.1 to 13.9%; the third was *C. tritaeniorhynchus.* In cattle sheds, on the other hand, the prevalence of mosquitoes was (by order): *M. uniformis, C. tritaeniorhynchus, C. gelidus,* and *C. p. fatigans.* The specimens from dwellings involved 24 mosquito species, and those from cattle sheds contained 25 species. The infection with *W. bancrofti* larvae was seen only in *C. fatigans,* at a rate of 5.9% (6,924 of 115.529) among those collected from dwellings, and of 4.1% (245 of 6,015) among those collected in cattle sheds. Infections with some animal filariae were seen in *M. uniformis, M. annulifera, C. tritaeniorhynchus, Armigeres obturbans,* and *An. barbirostris.*

8A.4.5 Control measures

The work undertaken by the antifilariasis Campaign of Sri Lanka, assisted by WHO, represents one of the best organized programs of this sort, and has achieved remarkable results in the prevention of the disease, which otherwise must have expanded intensively. The measures have been directed to both parasite and vector control.

For parasite control, extensive blood surveys have been in progress since 1959. In house-to-house visits of health inspectors, usually over 50% of the population in target areas have been examined at least once a year. Persons found to be positive, as well as their immediate contacts, are treated with DEC, 6 mg per kg of body weight daily, totaling 18 doses, as a rule. The drug is also distributed by house-to-house visits. Follow-up blood examinations of the previously positive cases have shown that over 80% among them become negative, as shown in Table 8-3.

The vector control is undertaken by the staff of the district units, and emphasis has been placed on larval control with insecticide application. Malathion in diesel oil was formerly used, but fenthion in water is now utilized. It was intended that every potential breeding place of *C. fatigans* be treated once a week by the insecticide. Guppies (*Poecilia reticulata*) have been released into some permanent water collection tanks, such as coconut husk pits and abandoned wells, since 1965, with successful results. Much public health education has been also undertaken by the profession-al staff.

8A.5 Maldives

The Maldives is a republic consisting of 19 clusters of coral islands (at-olls) scattered over a long and narrow belt in the Indian Ocean, southwest of Ceylon, between latitudes 7°N and 1°N and longitudes 72°E and 74°E. It has a total land area of approximately 298 km² and a population of 114, 469, as of 1970 (census). The archipelago consists of over 2,000 islands, of which approximately 200 are inhabited. All the islands are essentially flat, mostly just a few feet above the high tide level; they are covered by dense vegetation consisting mainly of coconut palms. The only mammals ex-isting, except for man, are the rat (*Rattus rattus* var. *wroughtoni*), a large frugivorous bat (*Pteropus medius*), and a common shrew (*Crocidura muri-nus*); no domestic animals, such as cows, horses, sheep, dogs, pigs, or cats are present.

IYENGAR (1952) reported on the results of a filariasis survey conducted by a WHO team from January to March 1951. Filariasis was known to be endemic in the three southern atolls of the Maldives, namely, Haddumatti, Suvadiva, and Addu. Surveys were made by the team in three villages of Haddumatti, where a total of 3,646 persons were examined; a filarial dis-ease rate of 13.1%, microfilaria rate of 26.1% and a filarial endemicity rate (both combined) of 36.0% were obtained. These same rates were 24.3%, 18.9%, and 40.1%, respectively, for 9,767 persons in 16 villages of Su-vadiva, and 8.8%, 14.1%, and 21.5%, respectively, for 5,423 persons in six villages of Addu Atoll. The microfilariae were all those of *W. bancrofti*. High incidence of cases with elephantiasis of the legs and with hydrocele or elephantiasis of the scrotum was noted especially in Suvadiva and Addu. Altogether, 13 species of mosquitoes were recorded during the investiga-tion, of which *C. p. fatigans* constituted 92% of the total number of mos-quitoes caught inside dwellings. The main breeding place of *C. p. fatigans* were the step-wells, where the water was generally heavily polluted with organic matter. Infection with filarial larvae was found in 429 of 1,729 *C.*

p. fatigans, 4 of 22 *An. tesselatus*, 2 of 45 *C. sitiens*, 4 of 12 *C. tritaeniorhynchus*, 1 of 41 *Ae. albopictus*, 1 of 6 *Ae. aegypti*, but none of 18 *C. stylifurcatus*, 3 *C. parainfantulus*, or 5 *Armigeres obturbans*.

8A.6 Bangladesh

Bangladesh, or formerly East Pakistan, includes the former East Bengal area and the Sylhet portion of Assam of pre-partition British India. It is surrounded by the states of West Bengal and Assam of India, Burma, and the Bay of Bengal. It has an area of 142,780 km^2 and a population of 59,330,000 (1969). The land is largely the delta of the Great Ganges and Brahmaputra River systems and over 85% of the country is an alluvial plain with yearly flooding. More than 90% of the people live in a rural environment.

A review on the epidemiology of filariasis in Bangladesh was made by WOLFE & ASLAMKHAN (1971). Hydrocele was recognized as being prevalent in lower Bengal by CHEVERS in 1886. SUNDAR RAO, in an unpublished report (quoted by MEGAW & GUPTA, 1927), first worked out the distribution of filariasis in India, in which two places now in Bangladesh are covered; microfilariae were found in 13 of 100 persons examined in Dinajpur Town, and in 2 of 35 persons examined in Pabna Town. The occurrence of *W. bancrofti* was reported by CHAKRAVARTTY (1927) in Noakhali District, and by RAO (1930) from neighboring Sandwip Island. RAO (1940) described *B. malayi* from Comilla and Sylhet.

SANDOSHAM *et al.* (1962) reported on the discovery of a nocturnally periodic form of *B. malayi* microfilariae in the blood of one out of 13 rhesus monkeys (*Macaca mulatta*) captured in the Chittagong area of Bangladesh. Of 71 *M. uniformis* experimentally fed on the monkey when the parasite density was 8 to 9 per 60 mm^2, 30 mature larvae were found 11 days after taking the blood meal. Another monkey was infected with a *Dirofilaria* microfilariae.

WOLFE & ASLAMKHAN (1968, 1971) conducted blood examinations (20 mm^3 samples collected between 8 p.m. and midnight) in 39 institutions (27 hospitals and 12 student hostels) in various districts of Bangladesh. Altogether, 4,190 persons were examined, and 118 (2.8%) were positive. The microfilariae were all those of *W. bancrofti*, except for those of *B. malayi* in two cases from the Chittagong area. Positive cases were found in all of the 17 districts surveyed. The highest prevalence of filariasis was found in Dinajpur District in the northwestern corner of the country, where almost 14% of those examined from all parts of the district were positive. The neighboring districts of Rangpur and Pabna, as well as Barisal District in the south, also had relatively high prevalence rates. Positive cases were also found throughout the Chittagong Hill Tracts. Only 2 cases out of 215 persons examined in the Dacca City were positive. In general, the microfilaria rate was more than double in males (3.5%, 95 positives of 2,749 examined) than that in females (1.6%, 23 of 1,441)

BARRY *et al.* (1971) carried out a survey to determine the prevalence and distribution of filariasis in Thakurgaon, an area of 645 km² in the Dinajpur District of Bangladesh. A multistage, stratified sampling scheme was employed. The area was divided into 106 designated sample units on the basis of population and jurisdictional delineation. After distribution into three strata, 35 sample units were selected for survey from a table of random numbers. With the stipulation that the total sample be 5.0% of the population, or 9,500 examinations, it was determined that 54 households per sample unit would yield the required sample size. Census data reporting an average of five persons per household indicated an expected number of 270 examinations per sample unit. Clusters of about 54 houses were delineated on maps prepared by the Malaria Eradication Program Office. One cluster per sample unit was randomly selected for a complete house-to-house survey.

The survey was carried out between July 1969 and January 1970. A single sample of peripheral blood, 20 mm³ measured by calibrated pipette, was taken from the finger, and thick smears of 15 mm² were prepared. The smears were stained with 2% Giemsa and the entire film was examined to count the microfilariae. The blood samples were collected between 8 p.m. and midnight. Physical examinations were performed to detect the clinical manifestations of filariasis.

As a result, 9,624 persons (5,201 males and 4,423 females) were examined from 2,032 households. Microfilariae were detected in 1,618 (16.8%), or in 946 (18.2%) of the males and 651 (14.7%) of the females. Clinical manifestations were observed in 973 persons (946 males and 27 females). A total of 2,330 (24.2%) were detected to be either microfilaria carriers or afflicted with objective clinical manifestations. The median microfilaria density per 20mm³ blood of the positive cases was 14.0. The microfilariae were all *W. bancrofti*, and periodicity studies conducted on three microfilaria carriers demonstrated a strictly nocturnal occurrence.

WOLFE & ASLAMKHAN (1972a, b) conducted epidemiological and entomological investigations on bancroftian filariasis in two villages in Dinajpur District, Akcha, and Madarganj. The microfilarial rates of the two villages (all ages) were 15.6% (95 of 602) and 16.4% (138 of 841), with male disease rates of 21.7% and 20.6%, respectively. Disease manifestations were almost exclusively hydrocele, with only a rare case of scrotal or limb elephantiasis. Only one female was found to have elephantiasis, and over one-third of the adult males had hydrocele. In these two villages of a nonurban focus of nocturnally periodic bancroftian filariasis, ten species of *Anopheles*, one species of *Tripteroides*, three species of *Mansonia*, eight species of *Aedes*, two species of *Armigeres*, and 11 species of *Culex* were identified among a total of 20,642 mosquito specimens collected in houses and on human and cattle bait. Of 3,545 *C.p. fatigans* dissected, 373 (10.5%) were found infected with all stages of filaria larvae, and 40 (1.1%)

had mature larvae of *W. bancrofti*. Infective *C. p. fatigans* were found only during the rainy season from March to August. This species was never found biting cattle. The only other mosquitoes found infected with mature larvae of *W. bancrofti* were those of the *C. vishnui* complex (*C. annulus, C. pseudovishnui*, and possibly *C. tritaeniorhynchus*), in which 12 specimens were infected and 2 had mature larvae of *W. bancrofti* out of 5,569 dissected. The periodicity of microfilariae in three bancroftian filariasis cases from Akcha, Thakurgaon, and Dinajpur, as observed from the microfilarial counts in 20 mm^3 blood samples taken at two-hour intervals, was all strictly nocturnal.

8A.7 Burma

The Union of Burma is a republic in Southeast Asia, bounded on the west by India and Bangladesh, on the northeast by China, on the east by Laos, and on the southeast by Thailand. It extends from 10°N to 28°30′ N. It has an area of 678,034 km^2, with a population of 26,980,000 (1969).

Fillariasis due to *W. bancrofti* and *B. malayi* has been noted to be endemic in Burma, but published information is scant. *Brugia malayi* was reported by SIMMONS (1944, quoted by HAWKING, 1973) but no further information is available. *Wuchereria bancrofti* is considered to be widely distributed, and the survey team appointed by the Directorate of Health Services obtained the figures shown in Table 8-5, by blood examinations carried out from 1960 to 1965 in 14 districts of Burma.

Table 8-5. Results of blood examinations undertaken by survey teams appointed by the Directorate of Health Services, Burma, from 1960 to 1965 (quoted by HAWKING, 1973).

District	Population	Blood films examined	Microfilaria rate
Rangoon	670,203	185,093	4.7%
Bassein	526,000	31,524	3.5%
Hmawbi	191,000	36,803	2.4%
Mergui	165,000	31,147	4.2%
Tavoy	160,000	24,932	2.8%
Hanthawaddy	314,000	54,223	1.4%
Kyaukpyu	188,000	21,479	4.5%
Akyab	562,000	65,864	2.6%
Toungoo	283,000	44,449	1.6%
Thaton	229,000	55,270	1.2%
Moulmein	357,000	101,043	3.0%
Pegu	471,000	117,034	0.8%
Prome	299,000	82,064	1.9%
Sandoway	102,000	29,333	0.6%

According to a review prepared by ABDULCADER (1971), filariasis in Burma was apparently introduced from India rather recently, especially during the British administration when there was no restriction on immigration into Burma from India. By 1931, some 7% of the Burmese population consisted of Indian immigrants, mostly concentrated in the Rangoon and Akyab districts. Blood surveys for the detection of microfilariae were started in Rangoon in 1925, and the first case was reported in 1932. In the 1930's, only a few clinical cases of filariasis were reported, and they were mostly among Indians. In 1957, however, a blood survey of 1,892 patients and staff of the Rangoon General Hospital revealed the presence of *W. bancrofti* microfilariae in 144 cases (7.6%), and 14% of *C. p. fatigans* captured in the hospital were infected.

A Filariasis Research Unit (FRU) was set up in Rangoon by WHO in 1962, with the agreement and support of the Burmese Government; Dr. De Meillon was appointed as the first project leader. Its first three years activity was devoted to the study of the insect vector. A tremendous amount of information on the bionomic and epidemiological aspects of *C. fatigans* was accumulated by the staff and collaborators. These results were published in a series of papers by DE MEILLON and associates in 1967 (*Bull. Wld Hlth Org.*, Vol 26, No.1). Reviews on later activities of the FRU were made by WILLIAMS (1968), ABDULCADER (1971), and GRAHAM *et al.* (1972).

DE MEILLON *et al.* (1967a) carried out laboratory experiments to determine the duration of immature stages of *C. p. fatigans*. At a temperature of $28.1 \pm 0.7°C$, the mean incubation period of eggs was 27.11 ± 0.57 hours. Females spent a longer time in the larval stage (135.3 ± 4.4 hours) and in the pupal stage (34.16 ± 0.74 hours) than did the males in the larval stage (118.4 ± 2.4 hours) and in the pupal stage (32.95 ± 0.75 hours). There was no 24-hour pupating and emerging rhythm.

DE MEILLON *et al.* (1967b) conducted further observations on the oviposition of *C. p. fatigans*. There were two peaks in the arrival of gravid females at a breeding site (sewage ditch): one just after sunset, and the other at sunrise. The oviposition cycle was biphasic, the two peaks coinciding, in calm weather, with the two arrival peaks; wind and rain caused a marked disturbance in the oviposition cycle. The mean duration of the gonotrophic cycle depended on the time of feeding. Roughly speaking, two-thirds of the mosquitoes that had their blood meal before midnight oviposited after two days (the third night) and the remaining one-third after three days, whereas practically all of the mosquitoes that had their blood meal after midnight oviposited after three days (the fourth night).

DE MEILLON & KHAN (1967) reported on observations on the flight activities and resting habits of *C. p. fatigans* in Rangoon.

LINDQUIST *et al.* (1967) carried out experimental studies on the flight range and dispersion of *C. p. fatigans* tagged with radioactive ^{32}P in Rangoon. In the first field experiment, larvae were reared in water in vats containing radioactive phosphoric acid at a concentration of 0.05μ Ci/ml, and were released at the station where they were originally collected. About

583,000 tagged mosquitoes were released from the vats from January 15 th to the 27th. Later, collection of adult mosquitoes was done by hand in houses; of a total of 46,275 *C. p. fatigans* of both sexes caught over the 23-day period, 31 males and 36 females were radioactive. Mosquitoes of both sexes were found to disperse fairly evenly in all directions, and could be collected on the outermost "circle No. 15" (i.e., 46 m × 15 = 690 m from the release point). Two males and one female were caught at a station across the Rangoon River, 880 m distant from the release point. In the second experiment, approximately 280,000 adult *C. p. fatigans*, one to three-days-old were released on a street at twilight. A total of 117 (34 males and 83 females) radioactive mosquitoes were contained among 64,695 *C. p. fatigans* captured during a period of ten days after the release. The distribution of radioactive specimens according to the five concentric circles [at distances of 200 yd (183 m)] was 40 (34%) in circle No.1, 36 (31%) in circle No.2, 19 (16%) in circle No.3, 16 (14%) in circle No.4, and 6 (5%) in circle No.5. Assuming that 70% of the released mosquitoes stayed in the survey area, the total number of *C. p. fatigans* occurring in this circle was estimated to be 43.7 million.

DE MEILLON *et al.* (1967d) found, in Rangoon, that *C. p. fatigans* not only feeds and rests indoors, but also rests outside, in a variety of shelters, such as underground drains, unoccupied shelters, vegetation, etc. The lower parous rate and higher 'green mosquito rate' in outside catches as compared with indoor catches led the authors to assume that newly emerged *C. p. fatigans* (showing green color) rest for some time out-of-doors before setting off to feed. On the other hand, the mosquitoes biting outside were similar in parous rate and infective rate to those biting inside and resting inside, and thus the authors pointed out the chance of acquiring infection out-of-doors should also be seriously considered in a filariasis control campaign.

DE MEILLON *et al.* (1967e), in Rangoon, conducted experimental studies on the infection and reinfection of *C. p. fatigans* with *W. bancrofti*, and the loss of mature larvae in blood feeding. The rate of growth and development of *W. bancrofti* larvae in mosquitoes already infected from a blood meal ten days before was nearly the same as that in the control (uninfected) group, and there seemed to exist no immunity in mosquitoes against the infection with filaria larvae. In the second experiment, a volunteer harboring microfilariae of *W. bancrofti* at average densities per 20 mm^3 of 64.3 at 9:10 p.m, 118.0 at midnight and 111.7 at 5:20 a.m. was exposed to the mosquito bites from 9:20 p.m. until the next morning. These mosquitoes were kept in cages, and a part of them were allowed to feed on chicken 12 days after the infective meal. The mosquitoes were dissected after the second blood meal and the results were compared with those dissected on the same day without providing the opportunity of taking the second blood meal. Of 60 mosquitoes dissected immediately before the second blood meal, 54 (90.0%) were infected, and a total of 329 third stage larvae were recovered, with the average of 6.1 per infective mosquito. On the other hand, the number of infective larvae found in seven infective mosquitoes dissected immediately after the second meal was 25 (3.6 per mosquito), and that found in 65 infective mosquitoes dissected one-half day after the second blood meal was 223 (3.4 per mosquito). Thus, 41 % of the infective larvae were estimated to be lost from the mosquitoes at the time of the infecting feeds.

DE MEILLON & SEBASTIAN (1967) reported on qualitative and quantitative characteristics of adult *C. p. fatigans* populations according to time, site, and place of capture in Rangoon. In Kemmendine, where pit latrines are very rare, the heavy monsoon rains have a cleansing effect and adult mosquito populations drop sharply during the rainy season. In Okkalapa, however, pit latrines form the only sanitary measure and the rainwater-diluted pit latrines become sites for widespread breeding of *C. p. fatigans*. In observations on adult *C. p. fatigans* at nine stations in Kemmendine, the average density per man-hour was 22.0, the proportion parous was 0.48, and of a total of 21,921 females dissected, 1,050 (4.8%) were infected with all stages of filaria larvae, and 79 (0.36%) had infective stage larvae.

DE MEILLON *et al.* (1967f) conducted an evaluation of *W. bancrofti* infection in *C. p. fatigans* in Rangoon. A "risk of infection" index was introduced, which is directly proportional to the three principal parameters that determine the extent of transmission, namely, the biting density of the vector, the proportion parous to the total number biting, and the proportion infective to the total number parous. The intensity of transmission of *W, bancrofti* by *C. p. fatigans* in Rangoon was studied analytically by Hairston & De Meillon (1968—see Section 10A.3).

8B. Southeast Asia

8B.1 Thailand

Thailand has an area of approximately 514,000 km² and a population of 34,152,000, as of 1970. The land may be dividied roughly into five geographic regions: 1) the hilly region in the northwest, with a rainy season from May to October, and a dry season from November to April: 2) the central, alluvial region which is low and flat, with extensive flooding during the rainy season; 3) the dry plateau region in the northeast, traversed by tributaries of the Mekon River; 4) the densely forested area in the southeast at the head of the Gulf of Siam; and 5) the southern peninsular region consisting of a narrow strip of land situated between the Indian Ocean and the South China Sea.

Both malayan and bancroftian filariasis are present in Thailand (Fig 8-4). The former is endemic in swampy areas along the eastern coast of the peninsular region, and is a serious health problem for the people in several provinces; the parasite is mostly the nocturnally periodic form, but the occurrence of a subperiodic form of *B. malayi* has also been recorded recently from this region. A nocturnally subperiodic form of *W. bancrofti* was recently discovered to be endemic among people in the deep forest areas in West Thailand near the Burmese border. No indigenous case of the urban type of *W. bancrofti* has been observed in Thailand, although its potential vector, *C. fatigans*, is abundant in cities and towns.

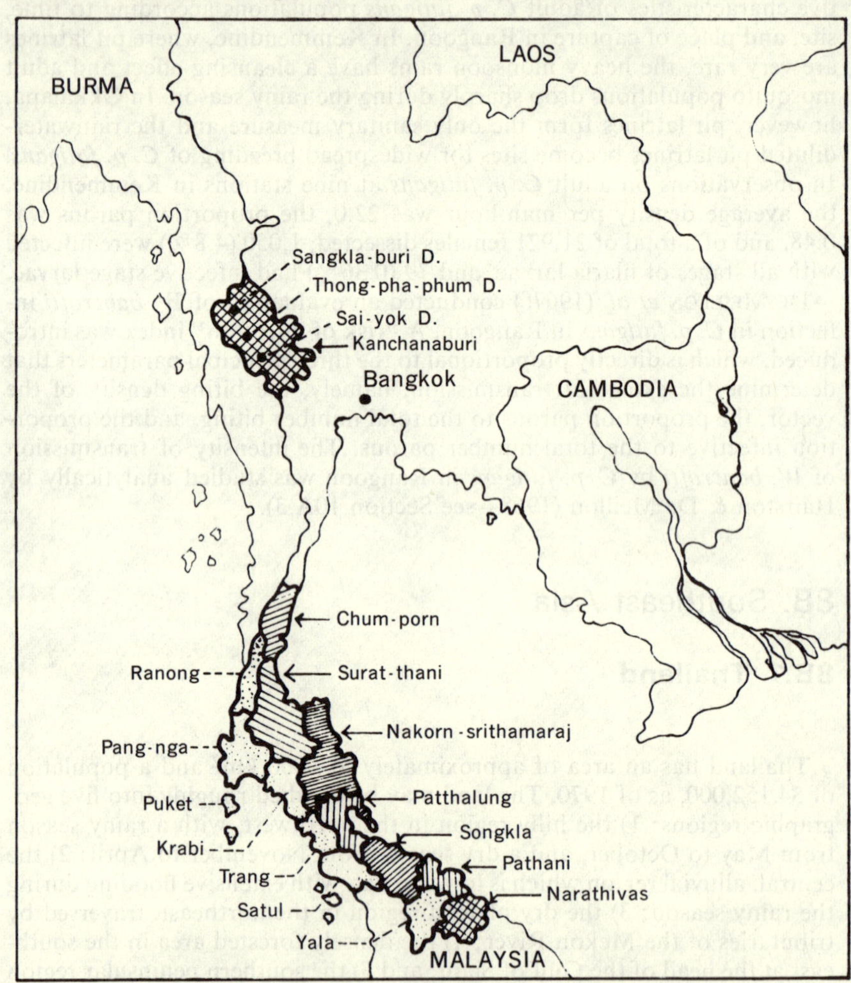

Fig. 8-4.   Map of Thailand, Showing the known or suspected endemic areas of filariasis and the areas of unknown infections (after RAMACHANDRAN, 1969).

Area of bancroftian filariasis (known and suspected).
Area of malayan filariasis (known or suspected).
Area of unknown infections.

8B.1.1 Malayan filariasis in Thailand

According to IYENGAR (1953), the Public Health Department of Thailand noted the frequent occurrence of elephantiasis in the peninsular part, and called for the reporting of the disease by the headmen of the villages in this region. As a result, elephantiasis cases were reported from 10 of 15 provinces of the peninsular region, namely, Pattani, Narathiwat, Phathalung, Nakhon-Srithamrat, Suratthani, Chumphon, Yala, Krabi, Trang, and Ranong. The province of Nakhon-Srithamrat headed the list with 1,246 cases, followed by Pattani with 603 cases. As for the four provinces of Yala, Trang, Krabi, and Ranong, which are not in the eastern coastal area, only a small number of cases were reported, and it seemed likely that they were mostly imported from endemic foci outside these provinces

An epidemiological survey of four provinces in this area was reported by IYENGAR (1953). The collection of thick blood smears and examination of clinical filariasis was conducted by house-to-house visits (between 8 p.m. and midnight) of some 15 to 30% of the houses in villages under the investigation. The microfilaria rate and elephantiasis rate observed were 29.7% and 4.2% for the total of 13 villages in Pattani Province, 11.5% and 7.5% for two villages in Phathalung Province, 15.4% and 6.5% for 11 villages in Nakhon-Srithamrat Province, and 16.9% and 5.2% for six villages in Suratthani Province, respectively, with an overall microfilaria rate of 21.0% (863 positives out of 4,112 cases examined) and elephantiasis rate of 5.2% (215 cases). All the microfilariae were those of *B. malayi*, with an exception of those of *W. bancrofti* from a Chinese boy who was born on Hainan Island, South China, and had lived there until the age of 11 years. Of 215 cases with clinical filariasis, 109 had elephantiasis of one leg, 95 had that of both legs, 7 had that of both legs and one arm, 1 had that of one leg and both arms, 1 had that of both legs and both arms, and 2 had hydrocele. Genital affections commonly seen in *W. bancrofti* cases, such as elephantiasis of the scrotum, hydrocele, epididymitis, and funiculitis, were absent, with the exception of two hydrocele cases (both had travelled extensively outside southern Thailand and had lived previously in India or elsewhere).

Investigations of mosquito vectors were carried out extensively in the endemic areas in southern Thailand. Altogether, 64 species of mosquitoes were collected and identified, and 2,499 specimens belonging to 40 different species were examined for the presence of filarial larvae. Natural infection of *B. malayi* larvae (various stages) was found in 17.3% (9 of 52) of *M. annulifera*, 11.4% (5 of 44) of *M. uniformia*, 8.8% (28 of 317) of *M. indiana*, 6.9% (9 of 131) of *M. longipalpis*, 11.7% (42 of 358) of *An. barbirostris*, 3.7% (3 of 81) of *An. nigerrimus*, 3.6% (3 of 83) of *An. sinensis*, 4.0% (1 of 25) of *An. albotaeniatus*, 3.3% (1 of 30) of *An. umbrosus*, and 1,2% (1 of 83) of *C. sitiens*. None of 299 *C. fatigans*, 52 *C. tritaeniorhynchus*, 71 *C. vishnui*, and 134 *Ae. aegypti* was found infected.

NAIR & CHAYABEJARA (1961) conducted a study on the periodicity of microfilariae of *B. malayi* in three human carriers in southern Thailand, one from Nakhon-Srithamrat Province and another two from Pattani Province. Three 20 mm³ blood smears were prepared from each carrier at two-hour intervals, and the average counts per 20 mm³ smear were recorded. The microfilariae were noted to be strictly nocturnal in periodicity. It was also noted that in the Giemsa-stained blood smears, many of the microfilariae were ex-sheathed, with their sheaths lying separately.

HARINASUTA *et al.* (1970a) reported on epidemiological studies of malayan filariasis in Chumporn Province, southern Thailand. A total of 20,115 persons in 165 villages were examined, of whom 470 (2.3%) were positive for the microfilariae of *B. malayi*. The microfilaria rates varied from 0.4% to 10.8% according to the villages. Elephantiasis was found in 259 cases (1.3%). The true endemic focus appeared to be at Bangluke Canton of Muang District, where the microfilaria rate was 10.8% and the elephantiasis rate was 3.3%.

The microfilarial periodicity studied in 18 positive cases was found to be all nocturnal, with the observed peak varying from 10 p.m. to 6 a.m. Blood samples of 110 cats, 98 dogs, and 5 monkeys were examined, and *B. malayi*-like microfilariae were found in two of the cats. An extensive survey of mosquitoes in this area was conducted, and *Mansonia* was found in 71.6% of a total of 37,908 specimens collected at Bangluke Canton. Of a total of 36,201 mosquito specimens dissected, the infection with mature larvae of *B. malayi* was found only in four species of *Mansonia*, with rates of 0.28% (25 positives out of 8,823 specimens dissected) in *M. indiana*, 0.22% (22 of 10,159) in *M. uniformis*, 0.16% (4 of 2,474) in *M. bonneae*, and 0.04% (1 of 2,790) in *M. annulata*.

A pilot project for the control of malayan filariasis in Thailand was started in 1963 in a village in Kanjanadit District of Suratthani Province, southern Thailand, and the results were reported by HARINASUTA *et al.* (1964, 1970c). In 1963, 977 persons (99.5% of the total population of 1,023 of the village) were examined, and microfilariae of *B. malayi* were positive in 21.1% of the blood samples (two thick smears of 20 mm³ each) collected from each villager. Elephantiasis was found in 5.3% of the population. Microfilarial periodicity studied in 25 cases was all nocturnal. Of 4,136 mosquitoes of various species identified and dissected, *B. malayi* larvae were found only in 2 of 338 *M. uniformis*, one with second stage larvae and another with mature larvae.

Two methods were employed for the control of filariasis: parasite control by mass administration of DEC to as many of the villagers as possible, and the vector control by DDT spraying to all houses once or twice a year. DEC was administered at a dose of 5 mg per kg of body weight, once a week, for six weeks; in 1963, 888 persons (86.8% of the population) received the drug, and although considerable side effects were observed in nearly all microfilaria carriers, the microfilaria rate dropped from the pretreatment level of 21.1% to 2.2% after one month, to 2.2% after one year, 0.4% after two years, 0.4% after three years, 0.9% after five years, and 0.5 % after six years. No infection in the mosquitoes was observed after the drug administration was practiced in 1963, except for second stage larvae found in two *M. uniformis* in 1965.

The occurrence of a nocturnally subperiodic form of *B. malayi* was reported by GUPTAVANIJ *et al.* (1971) from Banduat Canton, in Chumporn Province of southern Thailand. Blood examinations were made of 443 persons (about 40 % of the total population), and 22 (4.97 %) were positive for the microfilariae of *B. malayi*. There were also 16 cases of elephantiasis of the leg, who were all negative for the microfilariae. Results of a microfilarial periodicity study on three cases, by collecting 20 mm³ blood samples at two-hour intervals for a period of 24 hours, showed that they were a subperiodic form which peaked at night. On dissections of 24,626 mosquitoes, mature larvae of *B. malayi* were found in 10 of 5,036 *M. bonneae* and 3 of 7,045 *M. uniformis*. Blood examinations were also made on 66 cats, 98 dogs, 16 rats, and 11 other rodents; *B. malayi*-like microfilariae were found in only one cat. As stated previously, nocturnally periodic *B. malayi* infections were reported to be widely distributed in southern Thailand, involving at least seven provinces, including Bangluke Canton of Chumporn Province near Banduat Canton, but the authors could not find any difference between this subperiodic *B. malayi* and the previously known periodic *B. malayi* as far as infection rate, clinical signs, or mosquito vectors were concerned.

8B.1.2 Bancroftian filariasis in Thailand

The occurrence of a subperiodic form of *W. bancrofti* was reported by HARINASUTA *et al.* (1970b,d) from Sangkla-buri District, Kanchanaburi Province of West Thailand. The Faculty of Tropical Medicine was informed in December 1964 of many cases of hydrocele occurring among the villagers, and survey teams visited the area from 1965 to 1968. A study of microfilarial periodicity of three cases revealed that the parasite was a nocturnally subperiodic form of *W. bancrofti* (HARINASUTA *et al.*, 1970b). Results of more comprehensive studies were compiled by HARINASUTA *et al.* (1970d). The filariasis cases were discovered from all of ten villages surveyed along the Kwai-Noi, with an overall microfilaria rate of 13.1 % and a clinical filariasis rate of 8.7 % among 1,549 persons examined. The disease was also endemic along the Maenam Mae Klong River, where out of 524 persons examined in ten villages, 2.3 % had microfilaremia and 1.9 % had hydrocele. Results of the study of microfilarial periodicity by collecting 40 mm³ blood samples from 17 positive cases at two-hour intervals revealed that the parasite was a nocturnally subperiodic form (the periodicity index calculated from the original data by SASA & TANAKA, 1972, was 53, being intermediate between the values of the previously known periodic and subperiodic forms of *W. bancrofti* and *B. malayi*; see Section 11F.5). A total of 9,079 mosquito specimens belonging to 47 species were dissected; mature larvae were found only in 6 of 2,750 specimens of the *Ae. niveus* group. No *W. bancrofti* microfilariae were found in the blood of 31 cats and 12 dogs examined.

In contrast to the neighbouring countries like Burma, India, and South Vietnam, where the nocturnally periodic *W. bancrofti* transmitted by *C. fatigans* is highly endemic in certain urban districts, the occurrence of this type of *W. bancrofti* infection has never been observed to be endemic in large cities in Thailand, although the vector breeds abundantly in most urban areas. SASA *et al.* (1965a,b,c) conducted a series of studies on *C. fatigans* and its natural enemies in Bangkok. Its biting cycle was shown to be a nocturnal type with a single peak at about midnight, similar to the pattern of the periodicity of microfilariae of the nocturnally periodic *W. bancrofti*. An average of 753.2 *C. fatigans* per man per night were observed to be biting from January to August in the garden or a room of the Faculty of Tropical Medicine in Bangkok. The guppy, *Poecilia* (*Lebistes*) *reticulata*, which had been introduced from South America as a pet fish, was found to be breeding in some polluted sewage water pools in Bangkok; it was shown to be highly effective as a biological control measure of *C. p. fatigans* when introduced to such breeding places. Comparative studies were made on the toxicity of insecticides to the fish, larvae of *C. p. fatigans*, and *Ae. aegypti*; it was demonstrated that chlorinated hydrocarbon compounds, such as DDT, BHC, and dieldrin, were more toxic to the fish than to the mosquito larvae, while some organophosphorous insecticides, including fenitrothion, fenthion, and ronnel, were toxic to the fish only at concentrations several hundred times higher than that effective in killing all the mosquito larvae.

8B.2 Laos

Laos is bounded on the north by China and North Vietnam, on the east by North Vietnam and South Vietnam, on the south by Khmer, and on the west by Thailand and Burma. It lies between 14°N and 24°N, and 100°E and 108°E. Its area is 236,707 km², with a population of 3,033,000 (1971).

Although filariasis due to *W. bancrofti* and *B. malayi* is known to be endemic in neighboring countries, such as Thailand and North Vietnam, little is known about filariasis in Laos. BEDIER (1925), in a report on the function of the laboratory in Vientiane, described a single case of filariasis due to *W. bancrofti* from Vientiane.

8B.3 Khmer (Cambodia)

Khmer Republic, or Cambodia (Cambodge), is in the southern part of Indochina, bounded on the north by Thailand and Laos, on the east by

South Vietnam, and on the south by the Gulf of Siam. It lies between 10°N and 15°N, and 102°E and 108°E. Its area is 180,966 km² and its population, 6,818,200 (1970).

Little is known about the status of filariasis in Khmer. CANET (1950) stated that there had been no evidence of the occurrence of filariasis in Cambodia. CANET (1952) conducted an extensive blood survey of people in southern Indochina, and although he found a number of *W. bancrofti* infections among the people in South Vietnam, all of the blood samples collected from Cambodians in three localities, i.e., 100 persons in Chup, 138 in Kompong-Cham and Phnom-Penh, and 149 in Soctrang, were negative.

8B.4 North Vietnam

North Vietnam, or the Democratic Republic of Vietnam, is bounded on the north by China, on the east by the Gulf of Tonkin, on the south by South Vietnam and Laos, and on the west by Laos. It lies between 17°N and 23°N, and 102°E and 107°E. It has an area of 164,040 km², with a population of 19,900,000 (1970).

North Vietnam includes the territories called Tonkin in the north and the northern part of Annam in the south. Tonkin consists roughly of the three regions: the delta of the Red River, a middle hilly region, and a high mountainous region. Much of the work on filariasis was done during the time of French occupation, i.e., prior to 1955. Both *B. malayi* and *W. bancrofti* was known to be endemic. The former has a patchy distribution in some swampy areas in the delta, where *Mansonioides* mosquitoes act as the main vector. The latter is more widely distributed covering all three regions of Tonkin, though the incidence is usually not very high.

In 1951, there was an outbreak of *B. malayi* filariasis among French and North African servicemen after returning home from North Vietnam. The main syndrome was eosinophilia, enlargement of lymph glands, and asthmalike attacks, and was quite different from that seen among the autochthonous people in endemic areas of malayan filariasis.

In Tonkin (North Vietnam), MATHIS (1909) reported on three cases infected by *Microfilaria nocturna*, observed at the Military Hospital of Hanoi. The first case was a 21-year-old male, born in the province of Ha Dong, and admitted to the hospital because of hydrocele and inguinal lymphadenitis. The second case was a 29-year-old male, also born in Ha Dong Province, and admitted because of hydrocele. The third case was a 23-year-old man, born in Kien An Province, and suffering from epididymitis. Microfilariae were demonstrated from their blood, and also from the fluid of the hydrocele. The author stated that filariasis was never a rare disease in Indochina as believed by previous workers, but was common, especially in Tonkin.

MATHIS & LEGER (1910) carried out blood surveys of a total of 3,010 natives from the provinces of North Indochina, except for two provinces of Tonkin and three provinces of Annan. Most of those examined were prisoners, but some soldiers and hospital patients were also included. As a result, microfilaria carriers were found in all the provinces of the delta region of Tonkin, with a gross positive rate of 4.96%; high incidence was recorded from Hanoi (27 of 300, or 9.00%), Haiduong (10 of 118, 8.67%), Nam Dinh (10 of 136, 7.35%), and Kien An (5 of 77, 6.49%). Positive cases were also found in two of the four provinces in the middle region of Tonkin, namely, Vinh Yen and Phuto, where 5 of 352 (1.46%) persons examined were positive. In the high region of Tonkin, 10 positive cases were found out of 604 persons examined in four of nine provinces, namely, Tuyenquang, Moncay, Langson, and Caobang. No microfilaria carriers were found among 280 prisoners from three provinces of North Annan.

(In this report, the author did not recognize the occurrence of the two species of filariae in this region.)

GALLIARD (1936a,b: 1937) published a series of papers on filariasis in Tonkin, and discovered for the first time in Indochina the occurrence of *B. malayi* in the Hanoi area. It was noted that in a hospital in Haiduong, a town about 40 km from Hanoi, 156 cases of elephantiasis had been seen during the past five years, but there were no cases showing chyluria or hydrocele. By examination of 170 blood specimens taken from patients of this hospital, he found microfilariae of *B. malayi* in 23 cases. Later, he carried out blood surveys of people in three regions of Tonkin, and recognized the coexistence of *B. malayi* and *W. bancrofti*. It was demonstrated that *malayi* was more prevalent in the low delta region than in the middle and high regions, and that the indicence was about twice higher than *bancrofti* in areas near the mouth of the Red River, such as in Nam Dinh and Thai Binh. However, this relation was reversed in the high or mountainous region, where *W. bancrofti* was predominant, and the only positive case of *B. malayi* discovered here was an immigrant from Ha Giang.

GALLIARD & PHIEM (1939) conducted a study of periodicity on a *B. malayi* carrier from the province of Ha Dong. The patient had insufficience of aorta, and had been admitted to a hospital in Hanoi. The microfilarial counts in 2 mm^3 of the cutaneous blood showed nocturnal periodicity and became almost zero during the day, but the time of the peak count varied greatly according to the day of observation, and at one time showed two peaks at 10 p.m. and 4 a.m. with a remarkable reduction at midnight. The authors considered that there was no particularity in periodicity of *B. malayi* as was reported by some Dutch workers in the Malay Islands, and that the irregularity of the appearance of the peak was probably due to the unusual health condition of the patient.

DESTOMBES (1952) reported on the results of blood examinations carried out in Tonkin; of 730 persons examined, 9.7% were positive, among which 8.3% were the *malayi* cases.

Sery *et al.* (1961) at the Czechoslovakian Hospital in Haiphong carried out filarial surveys in North Vietnam. From 1958 to 1959, 21 cases suspected of filariasis were examined at the hospital; 12 had elephantiasis of the leg and 9 had elephantiasis of the genital organs, hydrocele, or chyluria. Microfilariae of *W. bancrofti* were found in thick blood smears of two cases with elephantiasis of the scrotum. Most of those suffering from elephantiasis of the leg were from the province of Haiduong. Blood surveys were made on 808 persons in nine provinces of North Vietnam; microfilariae were found in 15 (1.9%) persons, of whom 9 were *B. malayi* cases, 4 were *W. bancrofti* cases, and 2 were undetermined. Seven clinical cases were found among them, five with elephantiasis of the leg and two with that of the scrotum. *Wuchereria bancrofti* cases were found in the provinces of Thai Binh and Hai Ninh, while *B. malayi* cases were in Thai Binh, Haiduong, Laocay, Thai Nguyen, Laocay and Hai Ninh provinces.

Since most of the patients with elephantiasis of the leg who visited the hospital were from a village in the province of Haiduong, a special survey was conducted here. Thick smears were taken from 256 persons from 9 to 68 years old; 27 (10.5%) showed microfilariae of *B. malayi*. Microfilariae were also detected by utilizing a concentration method from 4 of 24 persons who were negative in the thick smears. Clinical manifestations were seen in 102 persons (49 females and 52 males), or 39.5% of the people examined in this village.

Do-duong Thai (1964) gave general accounts on the parasitic diseases in North Vietnam, in which he presented a review of the information on filariasis in this country.

Galliard (1957) reviewed a series of reports on an outbreak of filariasis due to *B. malayi* among French and North African servicemen after they returned from North Vietnam to Algeria. Altogether, about 150 cases were diagnosed for filariasis in 1951. As a result of war conditions, most of the patients had been operating in the bush and swamps in contact with *Mansonioides* mosquitoes while they were staying in Tonkin. Some cases were repatriated after having spent between six months and two years at the front. In others, the symptom appeared from six to eight months after their return home.

The typical syndrome occurring among the servicemen was quite different from that seen among the native people. The three main associated symptoms were eosinophilia, enlargement of the lymph glands, and bronchitis with attacks of asthma. The blood was free from microfilariae, but microfilariae were found from the lymph glands by puncture, or by putting sections of lymph glands in saline for a few hours. Of 100 cases examined by Carillon, 69 cases were North African and 31 were French. The number admitted to hospitals and the reason for admission were as follows: adenopathy, 25; asthma, 13; edema and lymphangitis, 11; bronchitis, 7; eosinophilia, 7; routine pulmonary radiological examination, 10; other reasons, 10. In all cases, administration of DEC was dramatically effective.

These unusual syndromes associated with *B. malayi* infection among the soldiers probably represented an early phase of the evolution of the disease. The reason that such syndromes had never been recognized among the native people is either that only advanced stages of the disease attracted the attention of the workers, or perhaps, the disease itself takes a different course when people are continuously exposed to the infection from a young age.

8B.5 South Vietnam

South Vietnam is bounded on the north by North Vietnam, on the east and south by the South China Sea, and on the west by Khmer and Laos; it lies between 8°N and 17°N, and 103°E and 109°E. Its area is 173,740 km², with a population of 18,332,000 (1970).

South Vietnam includes the area called the southern part of Annam in the north, and Cochinchina in the south. The former is generally hilly except for a narrow coastal belt, while the latter is represented largely by the Mekong Delta. Much of the work on filariasis in South Vietnam was done during the time of French occupation, prior to 1955; little information is available about its present status.

In contrast to North Vietnam where *B. malayi* infection is a serious health problem in the Red River Delta area, no endemic area of this species of filaria has been noted from South Vietnam. On the other hand, *W. bancrofti* infection seems to be widely distributed, even in the city of Saigon. Except for the classical form of *W. bancrofti* which is nocturnally periodic and transmitted by *C.p. fatigans*, the form found among natives of the hilly region in the north is possibly a nocturnally subperiodic race of *W. bancrofti*, such as that discovered from West Thailand by HARINASUTA *et al.* (1970b).

The first report on filariasis from Cochinchina was made by NOC (1908), who found microfilariae of *Filaria bancrofti* in a European in Saigon. The patient was a 17-year-old male, born in France, but living in Saigon since he was two-and-half-years old. He spent five years in a school in Basse-Cochinchina. The patient had suffered from febrile attacks since 1905, and was admitted because of lymphadenitis.

BAUCHE & BERNARD (1912) stated that human filariasis was very rare in the central Annam area south of Tonkin.

In South Annam, CADET (1916) reported on three cases of filariasis from Phantiet; one case was a European. KOUN (1923) observed a case of chyluria in a European in Annam.

In Cochinchina, NOC (1908) reported on a case of filariasis in a European in Saigon. BROQUET & MONTEL (1909) also observed a case of filariasis in a native of Annam. GUERIN & LE CHUITTON (1923), as well as GUE-

RAN (1924) and LE CHUITON (1923, 1924), conducted blood surveys in Saigon and found microfilariae of *bancrofti* in 9 of 200 (4.5%) prostitutes, 13 of 83 (15.5%) fishermen, and 2 of 16 (12.5%) Tonkinese residents of Cochinchina. The development of the larvae in *C. p. fatigans* was also confirmed. According to the 1953 report of Pasteur Institute of Saigon, only one positive case was found out of 3,296 persons examined in South Vietnam (after SERY *et al.*, 1961).

CANET (1950) carried out epidemiological studies on filariasis among different races in southern Indochina. One of his studies was carried out from 1947 to 1948 in the region of Honquan and Bassin du Song Be, situated near the northern extremity of the province of Thudaumot, about 120 km north of Saigon. Three different races were residing in this mountainous region: the "Tonkinois" from the delta of the Red River and the "Cochinchinois" from southern Vietnam (both laborers of the agricultural plantation); and the "Mois-Stiengs" living in the forest. In the "Tonkinois" immigrants, night blood samples were taken from 397 males and 25 females; 51 *W. bancrofti* cases and one *B. malayi* case were found among the males, while the females were all negative. Examination of the day blood of the same population yielded only one positive case. In the examination of 2,000 Vietnamese who came from lower Cochinchina, only two cases with *bancrofti* were discovered. No positive cases were found among 500 Cambodians from the region of Chup (Kompong-Cham); however, of 267 "Cochinchinois" who had stayed in Quanloi plantation for more than two years, 3 cases were found positive for *bancrofti*. On the other hand, the results of examinations of the people of the Stieng villages showed a very high prevalence of *W. bancrofti*. Of 3,743 persons in 43 villages examined during the daytime between 4 p.m. and 5 p.m., 300 (8.01 %) were positive; the microfilaremia rate was 12.5% (170 of 1.355) in male adults, 6.9% (85 of 1,226) in female adults, and 3.8% (44 of 1,162) in children of both sexes. In one of the villages examined both day 5 p.m.–6 p.m. and night 11 p.m. to midnight, the positive rates were 30.9% (30 of 97) and 40.9% (47 of 115), respectively.

The above result is surprising not only because of the unusually high incidence of microfilaremia in an endemic area of *W. bancrofti*, but also by the unusually high positive rates obtained by daytime examination as compared with those of the nighttime. It is possible that bancroftian filariasis among the mountain people in southern Indochina represents the same subperiodic form as that found from the mountainous regions of western Thailand.

It was also recognized, in two series of studies in the Stieng villages of this region, that the microfilarial rates were considerably higher among those who were living in huts and not engaged in systematic labor (56 positives out of 706 persons examined; 7.93%), than among those who were employed as laborers of the agricultural farms (23 positives out of 802 examined; 2.86%).

Another fact which was unusual was the absence of clinical filariasis among the Stiengs. Some 7,000 people were examined, with at least 500 microfilaria carriers included, but not a single case of elephantiasis, hydrocele, or chyluria was encountered; eosinophilia, though, was relatively high with 9% in the average and often exceeding 20%. Canet considered that *C. p. fatigans* was probably the vector of *W. bancrofti* among the Stieng, because 6% of the mosquitoes collected in the villages were infected.

CANET (1952) reported on the results of his second series of filariasis surveys in southern Indochina in the year from 1950 to 1951. The surveys convered areas of the southeastern part of Cambodia, lower Cochinchina and the plateau of southern Annam. A total of 2,422 persons of the three major races residing in 13 localities were examined. All the people of the Cambodian race examined at three localities (Nos. 6, 8 and 11) were free from the microfilariae. On the other hand, high prevalence of bancroftian microfilaremia were seen among the populations of Moi race (Stiengs and Rhades), which are of Malay-Polynesian origin, residing in the regions of medium altitudes (from 80 to 1,000 m high) in the western and southwestern parts of Annam Mountains. The hyperendemic zones extended to the hilly areas in the north of Saigon around Locninh and Budop, and to the east of Saigon at Courtenay. The prevalence was much lower among the Rhade race at Ban Me Thuot, where the altitude is about 500 m, and almost no infection was seen in the low plain area of Cambodia. In all of these hyperendemic zones, the incidence in the males was higher than in the females, and that clinical manifestations were almost absent despite the presence of high microfilaria rates (Table 8-6).

CANET & JAHAN (1949) reported on the results of the treatment of filariasis with DEC at the hospital of Quanloi. The drug was given to ten *W. bancrofti* carriers, of whom nine were symptomless, and one had hydrocele. The patients received three or four tablets per day, each containing 0.1g of the active base, for four to ten consecutive days, as the initial treatment. The patients received the second treatment ten days to one month later, and all the patients took in total at least 3g (maximum 8g) of the drug. At the blood examination conducted after completion of the treatment, all of ten patients became free from microfilariae, but two became positive again when re-examined three months later. The author concluded that DEC was a promising drug in the treatment of filariasis.

COLWELL *et al.* (1970) conducted epidemiological and serological investigations of filariasis in native populations and American soldiers in South Vietnam. In 1967, the microfilariae of *W. bancrofti* were incidentally observed in 15% of thick blood films taken for examination of malaria from 121 Montagnard residents of Song Be district. Song Be is located only a few kilometers northwest of Hon Quan, where CANET (1950) reported a presumably subperiodic type of *W. bancrofti*. In this connection, several localities in South Vietnam were selected and blood surveys with Knott's concentration method were conducted on different ethnic groups, as well as on U.S. soldiers stationed in the vicinity of the endemic areas. The

Table 8-6. Results of blood examination of people in southern Indochina (after CANET, 1952).

	Race	Locality	Male adults			Female adults			Children		
			No. exam.	No. pos.	% pos.	No. exam.	No. pos.	% pos.	No. exam.	No. pos.	% pos.
1	Moi-children	Honquan	—	—	—	—	—	—	74	1	1.35
2	Moi-Stiengs	Xacat	41	1	2.4	44	0	0	52	0	0
3	Tamon	Minh-Thanh	39	2	5.1	41	1	2.4	51	0	0
4	Moi-Stiengs	Locninh	51	11	18.6	52	7	13.5	19	0	0
5	Moi-Stiengs	Budop	225	32	14.2	231	27	11.7	182	7	3.8
6	Cambodian	Chup	66	0	0	34	0	0	—	—	—
7	Cham	Kompong-Cham	75	0	0	25	0	0	—	—	—
8	Cambodian (Khmère)	Kompong-Cham and Phnom-Penh	138	0	0	—	—	—	—	—	—
9	Cochinchinois	Soai-Rieng	57	2	3.5	20	0	0	—	—	—
10	//	South Cochinchina	240	3	1.3	112	1	0.9	78	0	0
11	Cambodian	Soctrang	149	0	0	—	—	—	4	0	0
12	Mountain Stiengs	Courtenay	74	24	32.4	54	9	16.7	42	6	14.3
13	Moi-Rhadè	Ban-mé-Thuôt	50	2	4.0	25	1	4.0	—	—	—

microfilariae of *W. bancrofti* were found among 13 of 60 Montagnards and 2 of 27 Cambodians at Bu Dop, 6 of 72 Montagnards at Song Be, 3 of 37 Montagnards at Hon Quan, and 1 of 20 Montagnards at Minh Thanh. None of the Vietnamese or U.S. soldiers in the same localities or in Saigon were found infected. In contrast to the observation by CANET (1950), clinical cases with obstructive filariasis were frequently seen among the Montagnards, and the results of periodicity studies in 16 Montagnards infected with *W. bancrofti* showed that the microfilariae were a nocturnally periodic (not subperiodic) type. Tests of filarial antibodies with the soluble-antigen fluorescent antibody (SAFA) were conducted; SAFA yielded much higher positive results than the demonstration of microfilariae with Knott's method, and the results of the two methods for diagnosis of filarial infection were found to be highly correlated.

8B.6 Philippines

The Republic of the Philippines is situated on an archipelago consisting of about 7,100 islands; it lies approximately 805 km off the southeast coast of the Asian continent, between latitudes 5°N and 19°N. It has a total area of 299,420 km² and a population of 37,008,419 (1970).

Two species and two forms of human filariae are known to be endemic in the Republic of the Philippines: the nocturnally periodic *W. bancrofti*, and the nocturnally subperiodic *B. malayi*.

The endemic areas of *W. bancrofti* are scattered widely in many islands, and are located mostly in rural environments. The large cities are practically free from filariasis. The most peculiar feature of the epidemiology of bancroftian filariasis in this country is that its distribution is highly associated with the industry of abaca (hemp) growing. In these endemic areas, *Ae. poecilus*, a mosquito species which breeds in the leaf axils of the abaca plant, acts as the principal vector. Bancroftian filariasis transmitted by *An. minimus flavirostris*, also the main vector of malaria in this country, has been recorded to be endemic in rural areas. The urban type of bancroftian filariasis transmitted by *C. p. fatigans* has also been recorded from southern Luzon.

The occurrence of endemic foci of *B. malayi* has been recorded recently from four regions: Palawan, southern Sulu Islands, Agusan Province of Mindanao, and Samar. So far as is known, the microfilariae are all nocturnally subperiodic, and a swamp-breeding mosquito, *M. bonneae*, is the vector in all of these endemic areas. A review was published recently by Cabrera & Arambulo (1973) on human filariasis in the Philippines.

8B.6.1 *W. bancrofti* infections

The occurrence of filariasis in the Philippines was first recorded in a circular issued in 1901 from the Office of the Chief Surgeon, Philippines Division, which noted the discovery, by STRONG, of the microfilariae of *Filaria nocturna* in the blood of a European resident of Iloilo (PHALEN & NICHOLS 1908). CALVERT (1902) discovered an adult filaria in sections of the iliac lymphatics on autopsy of a Filipino plague victim; he also found two microfilaria cases out of 426 prisoners examined. The species of filaria was not given, but it had a nocturnal periodicity. WHERRY & McDILL (1905) reported a case of hematochyluria in a Japanese woman, in whose blood was found microfilariae having a nocturnal periodicity, and which were considered to be *Microfilaria bancrofti.*

ASHBURN & CRAIG (1906) found a microfilaria in a Visayan prisoner in Bilibid Prison, in Manila, and described it as a new species, *Filaria philippinensis.* ASHBURN & CRAIG (1907) found the infection of the same microfilaria in four persons, who were all natives of the province of Ambos Camarines, Luzon Island, and gave a detailed morphological description and a description of its development in *C. fatigans.* The authors believed that the microfilariae they found in the Philippine natives differed from *Filaria nocturna* Manson (namely, *W. bancrofti* of present workers) in the absence of nocturnal periodicity, in the lack of pathogenicity in man, and in some morphological characters. In these papers, the authors recorded the finding of small numbers of microfilariae in blood smears taken day and night; all five cases they examined had no symptoms, and in a table for differentiation of microfilariae, it was pointed out that *Filaria philippinensis* had a serrated retractile band and spicule on the head, while *F. nocturna* had six lips. Complete development of the parasite was observed in *C. fatigans.*

However, PHALEN & NICHOLS (1908a) reported on cases with microfilariae morphologically identical with *Filaria philippinensis* but having a nocturnal periodicity; they also reported the occurrence of a number of clinical cases with hydrocele or elephantiasis from various localities in the Philippines, including Luzon. These authors carried out a field survey in the southern parts of Luzon, covering the provinces of Ambos Camarines, Albay, and Sorsogon. Thirty-four cases with well-marked elephantiasis were observed, and microfilariae with nocturnal periodicity were seen in 11 of 80 persons of the general population and 9 of 37 prisoners examined in Albay. The microfilariae were identified as those of *W. bancrofti.* It was stated in this paper that this malady was well known among the natives by the name of "titibac," and that the entire labor class of this section worked with hemp (abaca). These authors attributed the disease to the effect of that plant: some believed that elephantiasis was due to the direct effect of the sap of the abaca upon the skin, but a more prevalent idea connected the disease with the strain upon the legs incident to hemp stripping, followed by getting the feet wet.

PHALEN & NICHOLS (1908b) further gave notes on the distribution of *Filaria nocturna* in the Philippine Islands. Beside the prevalence of the disease in southern Luzon discussed in their previous paper, unpublished reports led them to believe that the same might be true of Davao, Mindanao, and the east coast of Samar. The authors carried out blood examinations of people in Parang, Cotabato, Cudarangan, Duluan, Overton, Cebu, and Manila, and obtained positive cases from all of these areas except for Duluan; in total, 29 of 1,178 persons examined were positive. PHALEN & NICHOLS (1909) further discussed the distribution of filaria in the Philippines based on results of blood examinations carried out in areas covering nearly the whole of Luzon, the principal islands of the Visayan group, the northern end of Mindoro, and the scattered sections near the coast of Mindanao. A total of 6,384 persons were examined, including 4,883 enlisted personnel of the Philippine Scouts, and 127 cases were found positive. High infection rates of over 5% were seen in southeastern Luzon, and the islands of Leyte, Samar, and Bohol, while the rate was less than 1% in the greater part of Luzon and the populous islands of Panay, Negros, and Cebu. The authors pointed out that the distribution of the disease in the Philippines was probably very wide but rather irregular and uneven; they could not give an adequate explanation of the cause of such a patchy distribution.

Later workers, such as LOPEZ-LIZAL & PADUA (1926), GUZMAN (1933), and AFRICA et al. (1935) also noted that the microfilariae exhibited a distinct nocturnal periodicity. AFRICA et al. (1935) stated, "Our results seem to point out definitely to the existence of a periodic type of human microfilaria in the Philippines, contrary to the current belief expressed in textbooks and in the general literature. Of course, this finding does not necessarily discount the possible presence in this country of the nonperiodic type known to occur in Samoa, Fiji, Tokelau, Wallis, the Ellice Islands, and Tahiti, which the results of the investigation of Ashburn and Craig seem to indicate." The authors also considered that the periodic form might have been introduced from China, while the nonperiodic form accompanied Malays in their early colonization of the Philippines.

In the study of the microfilarial periodicity by AFRICA, et al. (1935), a male Philippine patient suffering from scrotal elephantiasis was examined, and blood samples, each 2 mm³, were taken at two-hour intervals over a period of 24 hours, nine times during August through January. Contrary to the currently prevailing belief expressed in textbooks and general literature, the microfilariae showed a definite nocturnal periodicity. On one occasion, 1 cc of venous blood was examined at 4 a.m. and 12 noon; the nocturnal blood yielded 17,340 microfilariae, whereas not a single microfilaria could be demonstrated in 1 cc of the day blood.

RECIO (1940), in a review on surgical aspects of helminthiasis in the Philippines, pointed out that one engaged in the practice of medicine for some time invariably meets cases of filariasis, usually in the form of hydrocele of varying sizes; he noted also that his own observations and those with whom he corresponded showed the disease to be quite frequent in Bicol Province, Samar, Leyte, Romblon, Masbate, Surigao, and certain parts of Mindanao.

Avery (1946) reported on the results of blood surveys of native populations of the San Pedro Bay (Leyte Gulf) area conducted during March and April 1945. All microfilariae found in this survey were identified as *W. bancrofti*. The number of natives examined, percentage of positives, and the number of microfilariae per positive slide (thick smear, volume unmeasured) obtained at night surveys were, respectively: 353, 2.8%, and 8.4 at Tolosa, Leyte; 300, 1.3%, and 3.5 at Salcedo, Samar; and 436, 9.6%, and 27.7 at Mercedes, Samar. The figures obtained at day blood surveys of the same population at Mercedes, Samar, were 353, 3.4%, and 8.6, respectively; the percentage and the count were considerably lower at day than at the night. Thus, the author referred to the strain he encountered as exhibiting a modified nocturnal periodicity.

Tubangui & Cabrera (1948) conducted a survey for filariasis in Irosin and Juban, two island towns in the province of Sorsogon; they also examined some of the inmates of the New Bilibid Prison at Muntinlupa, Rizal. Thick blood smears were taken at night between 9 and 10 p.m., and measured smears (usually 20 mm^3) were prepared from some of the positive cases at four-hour intervals to study the periodicity. In Irosin, 35 cases (26 males and 9 females) of 242 persons (157 males and 85 females) examined were positive, while in Juban, 6 of 30 males and 1 of 9 females were positive. In the New Bilibid Prison, a total of 823 male prisoners representing 45 provinces were examined, and 37, or 4.5%, showed microfilariae. Those prisoners who were positive were: 2 of 10 from Albay, 1 of 16 from Bohol, 1 of 6 from Camarines Sur, 1 of 31 from Capiz, 2 of 10 from Davao, 6 of 105 from Leyte, 3 of 26 from Oriental Misamis, 2 of 12 from Romblon, 13 of 78 from Samar, 4 of 15 from Surigao, and 2 of 16 from Zamboanga. The results also suggested the spotty and uneven distribution of filariasis in the Philippine Islands. Microfilarial counts in 20 mm^3 blood smears taken at four-hour intervals from 12 cases from various provinces all showed a remarkable nocturnal periodicity.

An important contribution to the epidemiology of filariasis in the Philippines was made by Cabrera & Tubangui (1951), who conducted a study on mosquito vectors in Sorsogon. Prior to this study, Ashburn & Craig (1907) and Tubangui (1927) observed complete larval development of the parasite in *C. fatigans* under experimental conditions, but no natural vectors had yet been determined in the Philippines. Two towns in Sorsogon were selected: Irosin (Poblacion) and Casiguran (Barrio Mabini). The former is an island town where 35 of 242 (14.5%) persons examined were positive, and in the latter, 18% of 68 persons were positive. In experimental infections with laboratory-reared mosquitoes, complete larval development was seen in *C. quinquefasciatus* (= *fatigans*) and in *C. annulirostris* within 13 to 14 days, but the development did not go beyond the sausage stage in *Ae. aegypti*. In the town of Irosin, 513 naturally caught mosquitoes were dissected; 441 were *C. quinquefasciatus* and 56 (12.7%) were infected only with immature larvae; and all the other five species were negative. In

Barrio Mabini, a total of 635 mosquitoes representing five species were dissected; 43 of 309 (14.0%) *C. quinquefasciatus*, 49 of 140 *Ae. poecilus* and 2 of 56 (3.6%) *M. uniformis* were infected; it was noted that more than half of the infected mosquitoes of *Ae. poecilus* harbored the infective stage larvae, while nearly all of the larvae found in the other two species were immature. These authors recognized, for the first time, the importance of *Ae. poecilus* as the vector of *W. bancrofti* in the Philippines; since the larvae breed in the water contained in the leaf axils of plants, the close correlation between the prevalence of the disease and the abaca plantations in the Philippines was ascribed to the peculiar breeding habits of this mosquito species.

The distribution of filariasis in the Philippines was further investigated by ROZEBOOM & CABRERA (1956). There were 30 malaria control field units (part of the six-year malaria control program) distributed throughout the malarious areas of the Philippines. Taking advantage of these units, about 50 night blood samples were collected from a rural community within each unit. It was also noted whether abaca was present in the locality where the blood samples were collected. In addition, night blood samples were collected by the authors from rural communities in Albay, Leyte, and Palawan. As a result, a total of 1,970 blood films from 36 localities were examined, and 94 persons (4.8%) from 13 localities were found positive. The microfilaria rate among the 706 persons examined in these positive localities was 13.3%. Of 13 microfilaria positive localities, abaca was grown in ten localities (76.9%), while microfilaria carriers were found only in two out of other 23 non-abaca growing areas; thus, there was a strong correlation between filariasis and abaca growing. Blood examination was also conducted on 184 prisoners at the New Bilibid Prison who came from the previously known endemic areas of filariasis, and 24 (13.1%) were positive for microfilariae. Laboratory colonies of *C. p. fatigans* from Sorsogon and Manila were found to support full development of *W. bancrofti* larvae when experimentally fed on one of the prisoners.

In some communities of Sorsogon (southeastern province of Luzon) in the Bicol Peninsula, BAISAS (1958) demonstrated that *C. p. fatigans* was playing its classic role as a vector of *W. bancrofti* in a tropical urban environment.

An isolated focus of *W. bancrofti* infection was reported by ROZEBOOM & CABRERA (1963, 1964) from Mountain Province of Luzon. A series of 69 night blood films taken at Bontoc by the Malaria Eradication Unit at Tabuk were examined, and the microfilariae of *W. bancrofti* were found in 20, or 29%. In a later blood survey conducted at Barrio Calaccad, 30 (10.7%) of 280 persons examined were positive. A total of 70 species and subspecies of mosquitoes were collected and identified from this area, including 16 *Anopheles*, 20 *Aedes*, and 16 *Culex* species. The species most frequently collected were *C. whitmorei*, *Ae. vexans nocturnus*, and *Ae. albopictus*. Natural infections of *W. bancrofti* were found in 5 of 321 *An.*

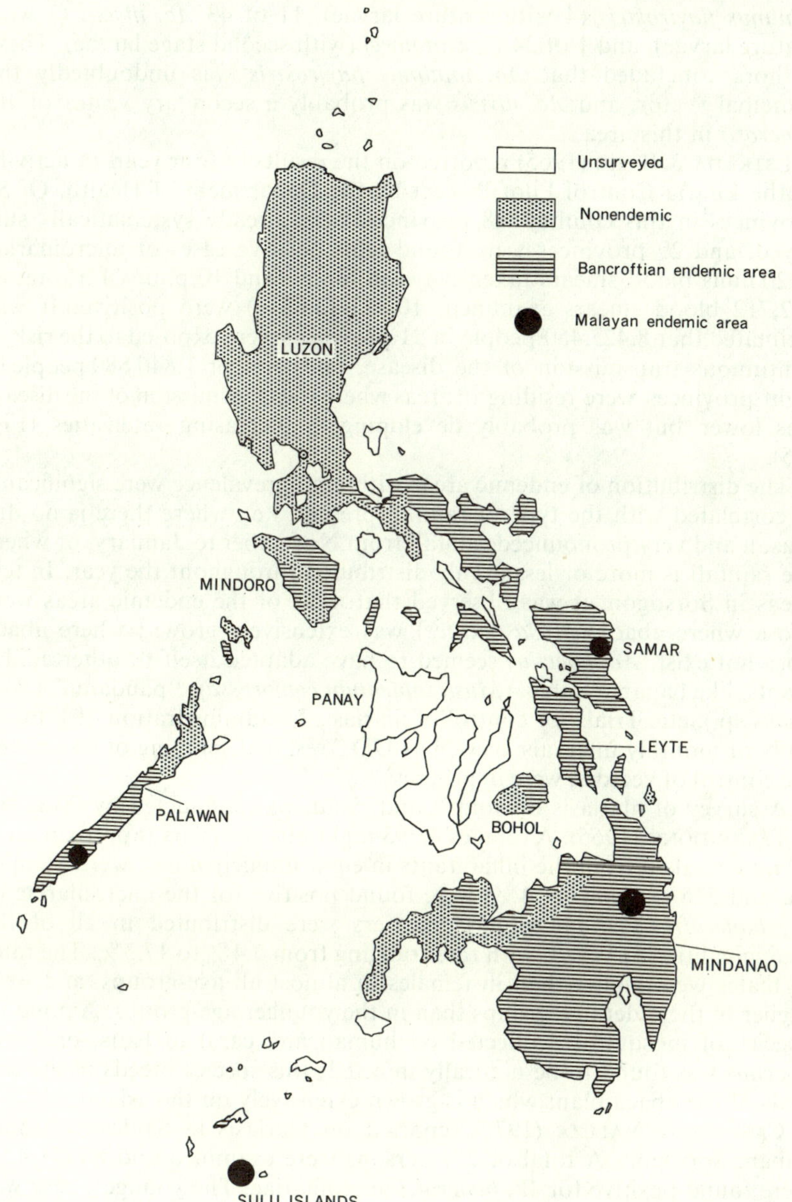

Fig. 8-5. Distribution of filariasis in the Philippines (adapted from map in Estrada & Basio, 1965, *J. Philipinne Med. Assoc.* Vol. 41, pp. 100–153).

minimus flavirostris (4 with mature larvae), 11 of 43 *Ae. niveus* (2 with mature larvae), and 1 of 34 *C. whitmorei* (with second stage larvae). These authors concluded that *An. minimus flavirostris* was undoubtedly the principal vector, and *Ae. niveus* was probably a secondary vector of *W. bancrofti* in this area.

ESTRADA & BASIO (1965) reported on the results of four years of activity of the Filaria Control Pilot Project by the Department of Health. Of 56 provinces in this country, 48 provinces were already systematically surveyed, and 29 provinces were found with positive cases of microfilariae in 20 mm³ blood smears taken between 6 p.m. and 10 p.m. Of a total of 282,712 blood smears examined, 10,823 (3.83%) were positive. It was estimated that 8,423,450 people in 21 provinces were exposed to the risk of continuous transmission of the disease, and another 1,846,880 people in eight provinces were residing in areas where the transmission of the disease was lower but was probably developing in increasing intensities (Fig. 8-5).

The distribution of endemic areas with high prevalence were significantly correlated with the type of rainfall present, i.e., where there is no dry season and very pronounced rainfall from November to January, or where the rainfall is more or less evenly distributed throughout the year. In test areas in Sorsogon, it was observed that most of the endemic areas were those where abaca (*Musa textiles*) was extensively grown; where abaca does not exist, *Ae. poecilus* seemed to have adapted itself to other axillar plants, like banana "saba" (*Musa sapientum compressa*), "pandanu" (*Pandanus* sp.), etc. Trials for control of filariasis by administration of DEC at daily or monthly intervals, as well as DDT residual spraying of houses for the control of vectors, were in progress.

A survey of filariasis on Jolo Island, Sulu, was conducted by CABRERA & TAMONDONG (1966). A total of 4,593 night blood smears (approximately 20 mm³), taken from the inhabitants in eight municipalities, were examined, and 526 persons (11.4%) were found positive for the microfilariae of *W. bancrofti*. The microfilaria carriers were distributed in all of the municipalities surveyed, with rates ranging from 3.4% to 17.3%. The rates in males were higher than in females in almost all age-groups, and were higher in the older age-groups than in the younger age-groups. Among 16 species of mosquitoes collected on human and carabao baits, only *Ae. poecilus* was found to be naturally infected; this species breeds in the leaf axils of the abaca plant which is grown extensively on this island.

CABRERA & VALEZA (1972) reported on filariasis in Sablayan Island, Juban, Sorsogon. A total of 757 persons were examined and 86 (11.4%) were found positive for *W. bancrofti* microfilariae. The youngest case was a four-year-old boy. The prevalence rate was higher in males than in females. A total of 1,551 mosquitoes belonging to five genera and 22 species were collected; 16 *Ae. poecilus* were found harboring larvae of *W. bancrofti*, and one had *D. immitis* larvae.

8B.6.2 *B. malayi* infections

The occurrence of *B. malayi* infections in the native people in the Philippines was first reported by CABRERA & ROZEBOOM (1964) from Palawan. Of a total of 314 natives from nine villages in Barrio Panitian, on the southwestern coast, 104, or 33.1 %, were positive for microfilariae; furthermore, of 58 positive films which were properly stained, 51 had the microfilariae of *B. malayi* and 15 had those of *W. bancrofti*, including 8 cases of mixed infections. One of 2 domestic cats examined at Gungnan showed microfilariae similar to that of *B. malayi*. *Mansonia dives*, a swamp-breeding mosquito, was most abundant, and 5 of 922 specimens dissected were found infected with the filarial larvae, including mature stage larvae of *B. malayi*. None of 525 specimens of 22 other mosquito species were positive. A more detailed study on *B. malayi* infections in Palawan was reported by ROZEBOOM & CABRERA (1965 a). In contrast to the endemic areas of *B. malayi* in Palawan, which are restricted to the swamp forest zone, *W. bancrofti* was found more scattered in rural areas of this island. ROZEBOOM & CABRERA (1965b) showed that *An. minimus flavirostris* acted as the major vector of *W. bancrofti* in one of the villages.

CABRERA & ROZEBOOM (1965) demonstrated that *B. malayi* in Palawan was a nocturnally subperiodic form, while *W. bancrofti* in Palawan and in Mountain Province of northern Luzon was a nocturnally periodic form; each parasite retained its own characteristic periodicity in the blood of mixed infection cases (see Section 11F.5; Table 11-19).

CABRERA & TAMONDONG (1966) conducted a more extensive survey of the people in the province of Palawan, in order to determine the extent and distribution of *B. malayi* and *W. bancrofti* infections. Of a total of 3,726 persons (2,088 males and 1,638 females) examined, 204 (139 males and 65 females) were positive for the microfilariae of *W. bancrofti*, with a microfilaria rate of 5.5 % (6.5 % in males and 4.0 % in females); those positive for *B. malayi* numbered 184 (132 males and 52 females), with a rate of 4.9 % (6.3 % in males and 3.2 % in females). The endemic areas were found to be restricted to the swamp forest areas in Quezon, along the southwestern coast of Palawan Island, and no additional focus was detected; *W. bancrofti* cases were distributed in nearly all regions of the island. The microfilaria rates among males exceeded the females in almost all ages for both species of filaria, and those of *B. malayi* in children were higher than those of the adults, while this relationship was reversed in *W. bancrofti* infection. The microfilaria densities among cases of *W. bancrofti* were higher than those of *B. malayi* in both sexes.

CABRERA (1966a) conducted trail treatments of *B. malayi* cases in Palawan with DEC. The drug was administered to 44 microfilaria carriers at daily doses of 12 mg per kg for 12 days, and all of them, with the exception of one case who had a high microfilarial count, became negative after the treatment. Approximately 95 % of them had the fever reaction (for details, see Section 2C.5.).

CABRERA (1966b) reported on the results of an experimental infection study of three common mosquito species with *B. malayi* in Palawan. *Mansonia bonneae*, the known natural vector of malayan filariasis in Palawan, showed high infection rates, up to 83%, and it took 11 days after feeding for the development of mature larvae. On the other hand, no complete larvae development was observed in *C. p. fatigans* or *Ae. albopictus* from Manila when fed on the same *B. malayi* carriers.

The second endemic focus of *B. malayi* in the Philippines was reported by CABRERA & CRUZ (1968) from the southern Sulu Islands. Altogether, 120 cases out of 3,695 persons examined were positive for microfilariae; those of *W. bancrofti* were found in 91 persons and those of *B. malayi* in 29 persons. The average microfilaria count of *W. bancrofti* was eight times higher than that of *B. malayi* in males and four times higher in females. The microfilarial periodicity was nocturnally periodic in *W. bancrofti* and nocturnally subperiodic in *B. malayi*. The cases infected with *B. malayi* were found in 11 municipalities on three islands, Siasi, Tandu'Bas, and Bongao, but the incidence was low and clinical cases were rare. The prevalence of *W. bancrofti* cases was highly correlated with the extent of abaca growing of the communities.

A third endemic area of malayan filariasis in the Philippines was discovered by CABRERA & TAMONDONG (1970) from Agusan Province, Mindanao. Night blood smears (two thick smears of approximately 20 mm^3 each) were collected from individuals residing close to freshwater swamps on this island, and out of a total of 5,446 persons covering nine provinces examined, 106 (1.95%) were found positive for *W. bancrofti* microfilariae, 25 (0.46%) for *B. malayi* microfilariae, and 4 with mixed infections. Most of the *B. malayi* cases were found from Agusan Province, where 2,034 persons were examined, and 25 (1.23%) were positive for *B. malayi*, and 32 (1.57%) were positive for *W. bancrofti* in towns near swampy areas. Four *B. malayi* cases were found scattered in North Davao Province, but they were considered to have contracted the parasite in the swampy area in Agusan, or elsewhere. Based on the average microfilarial count in relation to the age composition of the subjects, it appeared that malayan filariasis was introduced in Agusan and Sulu much more recently than in Palawan. The incidence and distribution of *W. bancrofti* cases in Mindanao were found to be closely correlated with the extent of abaca growing.

WESCESLAO *et al.* (1972) found the fourth endemic focus of *B. malayi* in eastern Samar. A total of 14,543 persons in 22 barrios and 17 sitios were examined; 700 (4.81%) were positive for *W. bancrofti* microfilariae, 47 (0.32%) were positive for *B. malayi* microfilariae, and 4 of the carriers had a mixed infection. *W. bancrofti* carriers were found in all of the 39 places, with the highest microfilaria rate of 16.6% (60 poritives out of 361 persons examined) in the sitio of Sta. Cruz. *Brugia malayi* carriers were discovered in six places, and the highest rate was also 4.4% (16 of 361) in Sta. Cruz. A study of the microfilarial periodicity of *B. malayi* in 13 carriers indicated that the parasite is a nocturnally periodic type, with the average percentage at noon being 5.7% of the peak at midnight. The authors stated that this type of microfilarial periodicity of *B. malayi* had not been found in the Philippines.

8B.7 Malaysia

Malaysia is a federation consisting of 11 states in West Malaysia (Malaya) on the Malay Peninsula, and two states (Sabah and Sarawak) on the island of Borneo. Its total area is 33,274 km², with a population of 10,424, 325 (1970). The land lies between latitudes 1°N and 8°N, and the climate is mostly tropical-oceanic.

Both *W. bancrofti* and *B. malayi* are endemic in many areas in Malaysia. *W. bancrofti* known from Malaysia is mostly a rural type, adapted for development in anophelines rather than in *C. p. fatigans*. Two races of *B. malayi* have been discovered from West Malaysia: a nocturnally periodic race endemic mainly in rice paddy areas, and a nocturnally subperiodic race endemic mainly in swamp forest areas. A large number of important contributions to the knowledge of filariasis have been made by post-World War II workers in West Malaysia.

8B.7A Filariasis in West Malaysia (Malaya)

8B.7A.1 Historical notes

The first record of filariasis in Malaya, or west Malaysia, was published by DANIELS, (1908), who found microfilariae of *Filaria bancrofti* in the blood of 3 cases of 100 examined at the Kuala Lumpur General Hospital. Of these, two were Tamils, and one was Chinese. The infections were thought to have been imported. He stated also, "Dr. McClosky informs me that the case of elephantiasis admitted at the District Hospital in the last four years is only three, though the total admissions for all cases amount to 17,804 in that period," and "*Culex p. fatigans* was shown to be here, as elsewhere, an efficient intermediate host."

The first investigation on endemic filariasis was made by STRAHAN & NORRIS (1934) in Wellesley North, while serving as medical officers of this province. They recognized that elephantiasis was fairly common in the northwest corner, and carried out blood surveys and clinical examinations of a rice paddy area along the coast, south of the Muda River. In one of the villages, they obtained blood films from 34 male adults, and found microfilariae in 8 (23.5%); twelve of them had elephantiasis. The doctors tried to examine women and children also, but they refused, so that no blood films were obtained from women or children. In this article, it was stated that the microfilariae were identified by Dr. Sandosham, in Singapore, to be *Microfilaria malayi*. The authors considered that filariasis in this area was not a recent introduction, because cases as old as 75 years of age had been affected for over thirty years. The occurrence of filariasis in Kedah was recorded by VICKERS & STRAHAN (1937).

A special investigation on filariasis by the Institute of Medical Research was begun in 1936, and the results were described in its annual reports from the year 1936 to 1940; results were also reported by POYNTON & HODGKIN (1938). As a result, filariasis due to *B. malayi* was shown to be endemic in certain rural areas, epsecially on the lower reaches of the Pahang, Perak, and Bernam Rivers. A considerable number of elephantiasis and lymphangitis cases was recorded from these areas. It was estimated that about 1,500 individuals in these areas were suffering from some clinical manifestations, and of 983 elephantiasis cases recorded from these areas, 819 were Malays, 159 were Tamils, and 5 were Chinese. In four of the estates in the endemic areas on which the whole population was examined, the elephantiasis and microfilaria rates were 18.2% and 10.8% in 662 males over 10 years of age, 2.9% and 4.5% in 375 females over 10 years of age, and 0.3% and 3.3% in 361 children under 10 years. Natural infections with mature larvae were found in *M. longipalpis* (now known to be composed of two species: *M. dives* and *M. bonneae*) and *M. uniformis*. POYNTON & HODGKIN (1939) further reported on a discovery of two kinds of microfilariae in the blood of the monkey, *Macaca irus*, trapped in one of the endemic areas on the Perak River; one of them was identical with that of *B. malayi*.

In these surveys, the infection with *W. bancrofti* was found only sporadically from hospital patients and on some estates. Of 13 cases harboring the microfilariae of *W. bancrofti*, 10 were Tamils from India, 1 was Chinese from China, and 2 were Straits-born Tamils.

The investigations on filariasis in Malaya were resumed after World War II, chiefly by workers in the Institute for Medical Research, Kuala Lumpur; remarkable contributions to the knowledge of filariasis were made, especially during the fifteen-year period from 1950. Comprehensive reviews on the achievements made during this period were published by LAING (1960), WILSON (1961), Edeson (1962), and RAMACHANDRAN (1969). A filariasis research unit was established in 1953 at Kuantan, in Pahang, and since then, tremendous amounts of information regarding filariasis in Malaya have been accumulated. A separate division for filariasis research was established in 1968 within the Institute for Medical Research at Kuala Lumpur, and work on basic and applied research in filariasis has been further reinforced. Some contributions have also been made by other organizations, including the University of Malaya Medical School and other government institutions.

Results of previous surveys have shown that *B. malayi* is the predominant species as the cause of human filariasis in Malaya, and *W. bancrofti* is known only from certain small endemic foci in rural areas, or among immigrants from India, China, and other filarious regions. It should be noted that two races of *B. malayi* have been found in Malaya: a nocturnally periodic and a nocturnally subperiodic one. The two races are not only isolated from each other in geographic distribution and ecological zones, but they also differ in some other physiological characters and in their affinity for the vectors and for the final hosts.

8B.7A.2 *Wuchereria bancrofti* infections

Wuchereria bancrofti infection in Malaya was recognized by DANIELS (1908) in two Tamils and one Chinese among 100 patients of Kuala Lumpur General Hospital. It was also found sporadically among the Tamils and Chinese from hospital patients and estate laborers in surveys carried out by POYNTON & Hodgkin (1938). WILSON & REIN (1951), therefore, considered that *W. bancrofti* infections in Malaya were rather rare and usually imported cases. The occurrence of an urban form of *W. bancrofti* infection was reported later by WILSON (1954) from Penang, and by DANARAJ *et al.* (1958) from Singapore, where *C. p. fatigans* was considered to be responsible for transmission. However, recent studies have shown that *W. bancrofti* is more widely distributed than originally considered, especially in rural areas, and is endemic among the Malays and aborigines.

REID & EDESON (1957) reported on the occurrence of infection of *W. bancrofti* among native Malays in a rural area in Pahang. WHARTON (1960) carried out a detailed study on the mosquito vectors. The site chosen for the investigation was Singgora, a scattered kampong of some 500 people living in narrow valleys in the upper reaches of the Pahang Rivers, about 40 miles from the coastal areas where *B. malayi* is highly endemic. There was a mixed infection of the two filarial species, and a blood survey by Edeson revealed microfilaria rates of 10% (20 of 193) for *W. bancrofti* and 11% (22 of 193) for *B. malayi*. Mosquitoes were caught, mainly by human-bait net-trap (130 nights) and by bare-leg catches (188 nights), and a total of 4,406 and 4,796 specimens were collected by the respective methods. These specimens represented five species of *Mansonia (Mansonioides)*, three species of *Mansonia (Coquillettidia)*, 14 species of *Anopheles*, 16 species of *Culex,* seven species of *Aedes*, three species of *Ficalbia,* and one or more species of the genera *Armigeres, Aedomyia, Harpagomyia, Tripteroides*, and *Uranotaenia*. A total of 6,083 mosquitoe were dissected, but infective larvae of *W. bancrofti* were found from only one of 502 *An. letifer*, and those of *B. malayi* from 2 of 602 *M. longipalpis*. The number of *C. p. fatigans* was only 8 out of over 9,000 mosquitoes collected on human bait during this period. *Anopheles letifer* (now *An. whartoni* REID, 1963) was suspected to be the main vector for various reasons. In an experimental infection study with this species, 9 of 16 mosquitoes that fed on a carrier who had 0.8 microfilariae per 1 mm³ blood, and survived for 11 or more days were infected, all with fully mature larvae of *W. bancrofti*. In *C. p. fatigans*, only 13 were infected and 5 harbored mature larvae out of 529 dissected after ten days; the development of this rural strain of *W. bancrofti* was found to be very poor in this species. On the other hand, the same *C.p. fatigans* colony fed on two *W. bancrofti* carriers from Singapore was found to serve as an excellent intermediate host, and the larval development was approximately 20 times more efficient than in the rural strain. A quantitative study was made with the urban strain of *W. bancrofti* with regard to the development in *C. p. fatigans*.

LAING & WHARTON (1960) reported a 16% microfilaria rate among aborigines living in Bukit Lanjan, a small village 10 to 12 miles from the city of Kuala Lumpur. Nine of 43 persons examined were positive for microfilariae, and of these, 6 showed both *B. malayi* and *W. bancrofti*, 2 with *B. malayi*, and 1 with *W. bancrofti* only. A more detailed investigation of this area was carried out by RAMACHANDRAN *et al.* (1964). There were 230 aborigines and 148 Malays living in this area, and microfilariae were found in 29 (17.3%; 15 with *B. malayi* only, 10 with *W. bancrofti* only, and 4 mixed infection cases) of 167 aborigines and 2 (*B. malayi* only) of 110 Malays examined. Both *B. malayi* and *W. bancrofti* were shown to be the periodic type by blood examinations carried out on six cases (including two mixed infection) at two-hour intervals. Mosquito trapping with human bait was conducted for 70 nights, but no infective larvae of *Brugia* or *Wuchereria* was found in over 1,000 mosquitoes dissected. The dominant mosquitoes caught were *An. maculatus*, *M. dives*, *C. annulus*, and *Ae. albopictus*. Experimental feedings of various colonies of *C. p. fatigans* from Malaya on a *W. bancrofti* carrier showed that all the colonies were capable of supporting the development to the infective stage, though the infective rates were different according to the colonies.

WHARTON *et al.* (1963) carried out extensive surveys of filariasis and malaria among the aborigines in Selangor and Pahang. *W. bancrofti* was found to be endemic throughout the coastal regions, lowlands, and inland hills, especially in the lowlands on both sides of the central mountain range, with microfilaria rates varying from 2% to 18% according to the villages. Subperiodic *B. malayi* was present in the coastal and lowland areas, whereas aborigines living in the inland hills were infected with periodic *B. malayi*. Malaria parasite rates were low (2 to 6%) in coastal areas, moderate (7 to 31%) in most lowland areas, and high (37 to 86%) in the inland hills. Dissections of wild-caught mosquitoes and experimental infections showed *An. letifer* was the vector of malaria and periodic *W. bancrofti* in one lowland settlement of Selangor, while in an inland hill settlement in Selangor, the malaria vector was *An. maculatus* and the vectors of periodic *B. malayi* were *M. dives* and *An. donaldi*.

The distribution of filarial infections among aborigines of various tribes from various states of Malaya was studied by ONYAH (1967), who carried out blood examinations at Gombak Hospital on patients and their accompanying relatives. A total of 1,964 aborigines from the states of Selangor, Negri Sembilan, Johore, Perak, Kelantan, and Pahang were examined, and those who carried *W. bancrofti* or *B. malayi* were found in all the states, with overall positive rates of 2.8% (56 cases) and 8.5% (168 cases), respectively.

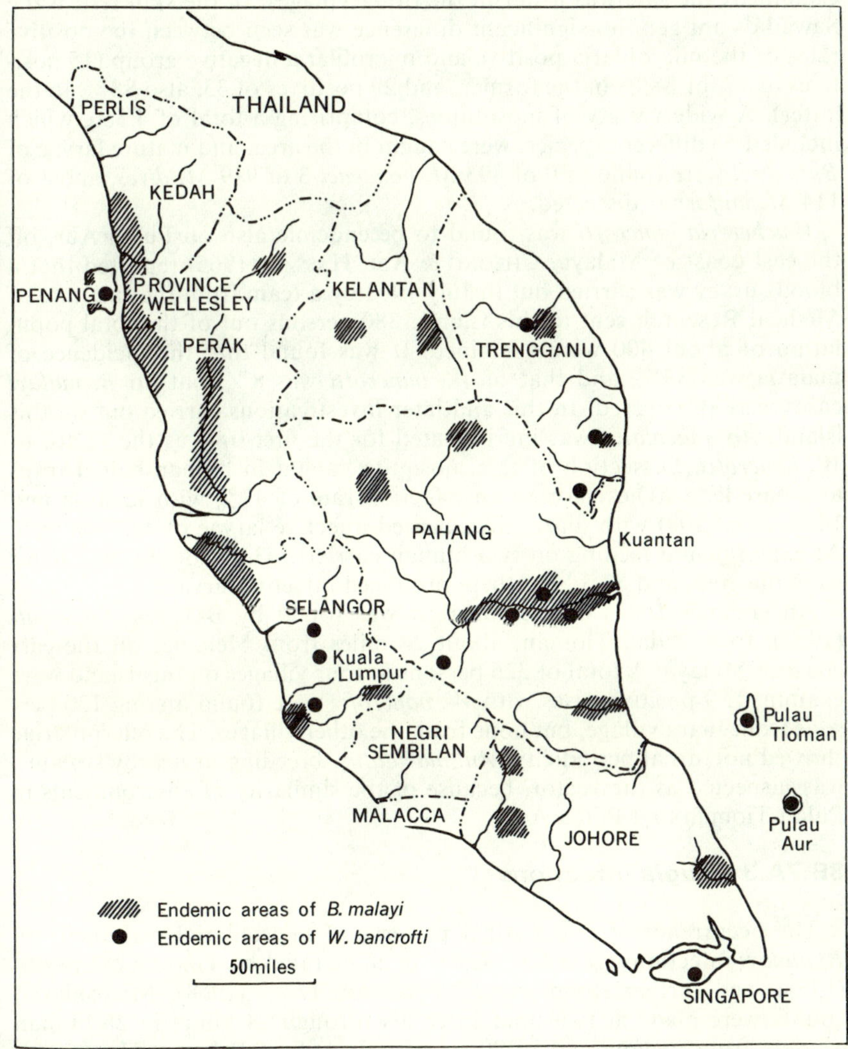

Fig. 8-6. Main endemic areas of filariasis, West Malaysia, 1968 (after Ramachandran, 1969).

Ramachandran *et al.* (1970) reported on the results of a filariasis survey in Ulu Treganu, near the east coast and north of Pahang. Of 591 persons examined from four villages, 13 (2.20%) were positive with *W. bancrofti* and 25 (4.23%) with subperiodic *B. malayi*. Two of the positive cases had mixed infection. One of the villages (Bukit Tadok) showed a relatively high prevalence rate, and 16 *B. malayi* carriers and 9 *W. bancrofti* carriers (including 2 mixed infection cases) were found out of 137 persons examined; the rate was lower in the other villages. In the skin test, using Sawada's antigen, no significant difference was seen between the positive rates of the microfilaria positive and microfilaria negative group (15 positives of 17, or 88%, in the former, and 29 positives of 33, also 88%, in the latter). A wide variety of mosquitoes, comprising a total of 4,550, which included 53 different species, were caught in the area, and mature larvae of *B. malayi* were found in 9 of 893 *M. bonneae*, 3 of 919 *M. dives*, and 1 of 114 *M. uniformis* dissected.

Wuchereria bancrofti was found to be endemic also on Pulau Aur, off the east coast of Malaya. Cheong & Abu Hassan (1965) reported that a blood survey was carried out in July 1963 by a team from the Institute of Medical Research sent to this island; 380 persons out of the total population of about 400 were examined. It was found that the incidence of malaria was 35%, and that of *W. bancrofti* was 8%, but no *B. malayi* cases were discovered. In this and later investigations carried out on this island, *An. maculatus* was incriminated for the first time as the vector of *W. bancrofti*. Dissection of this mosquito caught in human-baited traps and bare-leg catches showed an infection rate of 43% with malaria and 14% (30 of 208) with filaria; five carried infective larvae of *W. bancrofti*. At experimental feeding on two human carriers, 63.9% of *An. maculatus* were infected, and 82.3% of them produced infective larvae.

An endemic focus of *W. bancrofti* was found by Balasingam *et al.* (1967), from Pulau Tioman, about 24 miles from Mersing, off the east coast of Malaya. A total of 326 persons in four villages on this island were examined; 9 positive cases with *W. bancrofti* were found among 130 persons from Juara village, but none from the other villages. The microfilariae showed nocturnal periodicity. *An. maculatus*, breeding in nearby streams, was suspected as the vector, because of the similarity of environments in Pulau Tioman and Pulau Aur.

8B.7A.3 *Brugia* infections

The occurrence of two distinct patterns of microfilarial periodicity in *B. malayi* infections were first clearly demonstrated by Turner & Edeson (1957), and further summarized by Wilson *et al.* (1958). Microfilarial counts were made at two-hour intervals through 24 hours in 26 human carriers from Penang and in 20 carriers from East Pahang. The former showed a marked nocturnal periodicity; only 8 of 26 persons showed small numbers of microfilariae at 11 a.m., but all were positive at examinations from 9 p.m. to 5 a.m. In the latter, microfilariae were found in the peripheral blood even during the day in all cases, and the nocturnal rise in counts was much less marked. It was also pointed out that the periodicity observed by WILSON (1950) in two cases from Kedah was markedly nocturnal, but those observed by NEVIN, in 1938, in aborigines at Pinta, Perak, by POYNTON & HODGKIN (1938), in two cases from the lower reaches of Perak River, and by POLUNIN (1951), in aborigines in the upper reaches of Perak River were the type with less noticeable nocturnal periodicity.

The differences between the two forms of *B. malayi* in man in Malaya were summarized by WILSON *et al.* (1958) (see Section 2C.4.2). The two forms differ remarkably in their microfilarial periodicity, their efficiency in the development in different mosquito species, and their development and reproductivity in animal hosts, such as cats. They also differ from each other in microfilarial appearance, i.e., whether empty sheaths are common or rare, the mean length; however, no other morphological characters for the distinction of the two forms has ever been recognized in microfilariae, nor in adult or larval stages in the mosquito vectors. In Malaya, the periodic form occurs in Kedah and Penang in the northwest, and the subperiodic form is common in the eastern state of Pahang, but recent surveys suggest that the two forms may occasionally occur together at the same place, depending presumably on the presence of their main vectors.

The investigations in the past by various workers have shown that a large number of filarial species are parasitic in animals in Malaya, among which the species belonging to the genus *Brugia* are considered of special medical importance. The finding of a microfilaria indistinguishable from that of *Filaria malayi* in the common Kra monkey, *Macaca irus*, was reported by POYNTON & HODGKIN (1939). Soon after the establishment of the filariasis research unit in Pahang, EDESON *et al.* (1955) reported that sheathed microfilariae, apparently indistinguishable from human *B. malayi*, were found in some wild and domestic animals, for example, from 3 of 55 Kra monkeys, 3 of 20 slow loris (*Nycticebus coucang*), 1 of 1 banded leafmonkey. (*Presbytis melalophos*), 4 of 5 domestic dogs, and 12 of 31 domestic cats. Upon examination of the adult worms recovered from the lymphatic systems of the infected animals, they recognized two different species; one was closely related to *B. malayi* in man and was found in the Kra monkeys and cats, and another was distinct from it and found in dogs and cats. The microfilariae of the former type developed efficiently in *M. longipalpis*, *M. uniformis*, and *M. annulata*, the same as those of *B. malayi* in man, but those of the latter type were inefficient in *M. longipalpis* and developed efficiently only in *M. annulata*. BUCKLEY & EDESON (1956) made a detailed study on the morphology of the adults, and named the former as a new species, *Wuchereria pahangi*, while the latter was treated as *Wuchereria* sp. (? *malayi*). The authors point out that the most remarkable differences between the two species are seen in the terminal portion of the males; the tail length (the distance from the anus to the end) is shorter, the ratio of two spicules is smaller in *B. pahangi* than in *B. malayi*, and the distal part of left spicule of *B. pahangi* is much shorter and thinner and lacks the spatulate termination so characteristic of the latter species. Also, *B. pahangi* is shorter in body length (both males and females) and devoid of the minute cuticular bosses which occur in the adults of *W. bancrofti* and *B. malayi*.

In the meantime, EDESON & WHARTON (1957) reported on the successful transmission of subperiodic *B. malayi* in man to the domestic cat by direct inoculation of infective larvae obtained after feeding laboratory-reared *M. uniformis* on a human carrier. The prepatent periods of the five infected cats were 80, 81, 82, and 96 days. The microfilariae were indistinguishable from those of the human donors which developed normally in the vector mosquitoes, and the adult worms recovered from those cats corresponded to the description of *B. malayi* by RAO & MAPLESTONE (1940), as well as that by BONNE *et al.* (1941) from Indonesia. EDESON & WHARTON (1958) further succeeded in transmitting human *B. malayi* to the long-tailed macaque monkey (*Macaca irus*), the Rhesus monkey (*M. rhesus*), the slow loris (*Nycticebus coucang*), the civet cat (*Virerra tangalunga*), and the domestic cat. The strains from man were passed successively through different animal species, and thus it was established that the subperiodic *B. malayi* in man and various animals is the same species.

The success of the experimental transmission of *B. malayi* in man to various animals in Malaya made it possible to recover and study the anatomies of many adult worms, and BUCKLEY (1960) erected a new genus, *Brugia*, with *malayi* as the genotype. *Wuchereria pahangi* BUCKLEY et EDESON, 1956, as well as *W. patei* BUCKLEY, NELSON et HEISCH, 1958, were included in this new genus. It was pointed out that the members of *Brugia* differ from *Wuchereria* s. str. (*bancrofti* is the only member left in this genus) not only in the structure of microfilariae, but also in the structure of the spicules and caudal papillae. This idea has been accepted by later workers, and filariae of the *malayi* group, formerly called *Filaria* spp. or *Wuchereria* spp., have become known as *Brugia* spp.

The studies on *Brugia* species in Malaya were further extended by surveys of animal infections by LAING *et al.* (1960). The people in East Pahang were found to be showing microfilaria rates of about 40%, as of 1953. *B. malayi* was found occurring naturally in 19 of 25 dusky leaf-monkey (*Presbytis obscurus*), 9 of 88 domestic cats, 1 of 44 common palm civet, 4 of 116 macaque monkeys, 1 of 7 wild cats, and 2 of 11 pangolin (*Manis javanica*). *B. pahangi*, on the other hand, was found in 18 of 88 domestic cats, 5 of 25 dogs, 8 of 25 slow loris, 12 of 44 palm civets, as well as in a wild cat, tiger, pangolin, moon rat, and giant squirrel. The periodic *B. malayi* was considered to be rare or absent in animals other than man. At this stage of the blood survey, the authors differentiated *B. pahangi* from *B. malayi* mostly by microfilariae, since it was found that microfilariae of *B. pahangi* were significantly longer (215 to 270 μ in Giesma-stained thick smears) than those of *B. malayi* (170 to 230 μ).

Attempts were made by EDESON *et al.* (1960a) to infect *B. malayi* and *B. pahangi* in animals to man. A strain of *B. malayi* originally obtained from man and transmitted through a macaque monkey to a cat was inoculated into two volunteers who had infective larvae that had developed in *M. longipalpis* (now *dives*), but neither of them subsequently developed microfilariae. However, one of the two other volunteers inoculated with infective larvae of *B. pahangi* obtained from *Armigeres obturbans*, which had fed on a cat, developed microfilariae 84 days later, and these persisted in small numbers for 56 more days. All the four volunteers suffered from episodes of lymphangitis, lymphadenitis, edema in the inoculated limb beginning one month after the inoculation, eosinophilia ranging from 18 to 32% after 12 or 13 weeks, and all showed positive complement fixation and skin tests at about 12 weeks. One volunteer from each pair developed subcutaneous modules in the inoculated arm about four months afterwards. (Unfortunately, there is no statement in this paper referring to the numbers of infective larvae inoculated to the volunteers, nor to the volunteers' previous history. It is stated that one of the volunteers infected with *B. malayi* had two microfilariae of *B. malayi* at a blood examination made on the day of the inoculation, and that he might have had some immunity already developed before the inoculation.)

The results of experimental transmission of *B. pahangi* were reported by EDESON *et al.* (1960b). Among various mosquito species tested, *M. annulata*, *An. barbirostris*, and *Armigeres obturbans* were found to be the efficient vectors, but *M. longipalpis* was less efficient and *M. uniformis* was a poor vector. The parasite was successfully infected by direct inoculation of infective larvae to domestic cats, slow loris, and civet cats, but no monkeys became infected. The prepatent period in cats was from 59 to 83 days, and microfilariae were maintained for more than two and a half years.

8B.7A.4 Mosquito vectors

Many valuable contributions have been made by various workers concerning the mosquito vectors of filariasis in Malaya, and reviews were made by LAING (1960), WILSON (1961), WHARTON (1960), SANDOSHAM (1964), and RAMALINGAM *et al.* (1968).

8B.7A.4.1 Vectors of *W. bancrofti*

Wuchereria bancrofti infections in Malaya have been fairly well defined into the two types, an *urban type* found from the cities like Penang and Singapore, and a *rural type* which is widely distributed, affecting mainly the Malays and the aborigines residing in rural areas. The two types are differentiated not only by the terrains where the disease is endemic, but also by the species of the mosquito vectors. The *urban type* is considered essentially the same as that endemic in most other Southeast Asian countries, such as India and Sri Lanka, and is transmitted mainly by the common tropical house mosquito, *C. fatigans*. DANIELS (1908) already recognized that *C. fatigans* in Kuala Lumpur was an efficient vector.

As for the vectors of the *rural type* of *W. bancrofti*, WHARTON (1960) carried out an extensive mosquito study in an area in inland Pahang, where *W. bancrofti* and periodic *B. malayi* were coendemic; he incriminated *An. letifer* (now *An. whartoni*) as the major vector of *W. bancrofti*. He also found that *C. p. fatigans* was approximately 20 times less efficient as the vector of this *rural type* of *W. bancrofti* than in the *urban type* of *W. bancrofti* tested at the same time. This is an important evidence suggesting the existence of physiological and genetic differences between the two types of *W. bancrofti*. WHARTON *et al.* (1963) further observed at Bukit Mandul, Selangor, that 5 of 2,867 *An. letifer* were naturally infected with mature larvae of *W. bancrofti*, and both *An. letifer* and *An. maculatus* served as efficient experimental vectors of local *W. bancrofti* in the aborigines. Natural infections of *An. maculatus* with mature larvae of *W. bancrofti* were reported by CHEONG & ABU HASSAN (1965) from Pulau Aur. This species is considered to be the main vector of *W. bancrofti* in the other offshore islands, including Pulau Tioman (BALA-SINGAM *et al.*, 1967).

8B.7A.4.2 Vectors of subperiodic *B. malayi* and *B. pahangi*

The investigation on the mosquito vectors of *B. malayi* in Malaya was carried out first by POYNTON & HODGKIN (1938), who examined the mosquitoes caught in human-bait traps in the endemic areas on the Bernam and the Pahang Rivers. They found natural infections with mature larvae in *M. longipalpis* and *M. uniformis* in both areas.

The investigations were succeeded and extended by WHARTON (1957 a, b), who carried out detailed experimental studies on the mode of development of *B. malayi* in *M. longipalpis* at a field laboratory in Kuantan. This species was found to be very receptive to the microfilariae of subperiodic *B. malayi*, ingesting more microfilariae than expected from the density in the donor's blood and the amount of blood fed by the mosquito; mature larvae appeared as early as the tenth day after the infection. The relationship between the density of microfilariae in the donor's blood and the rate of infection, as well as the number of infective larvae that developed in the mosquitoes, was quantitatively studied, and a method was developed to calculate the "index of experimental infection," representing an estimate of the number of mature larvae produced in each mosquito. The index rose as the density of microfilariae in the donor increased, reached a peak in the 3 to 11 microfilariae per mm^3 range, and fell away when the density was higher (see Section 10A. 3; Fig. 10-1).

WHARTON (1962) published the results of comprehensive studies on the biology of *Mansonia* mosquitoes in relation to the transmission of *B. malayi* in Malaya, with special reference to the subperiodic form in the endemic area in Pahang. Six species of the subgenus *Mansonioides*, namely, *M. annulata*, *M. annulifera*, *M. bonneae*, *M. dives* (= *longipalpis*), *M.*

indiana, M. uniformis, and three species of the subgenus *Coquillettidia,* i.e., *M. crassipes M. nigrosignata, M. ochracea,* had been known prior to this study. *Mansonia (C.) aureosquammata* was added as a new record for Malaya and *M. (C.) hodgkini* was described as a new species. The morphological description, illustrations, and keys for identification were presented, and the methods for collection of the immature forms and adults were described in detail. The basic types of breeding places are (1) the open swamp for *M. uniformis* and *M. crassipes,* (2) the forest edge where open swamp and forest meet (all species are found but this was the typical breeding place for *M. annulata*), and (3) the swamp forest for *M. dives, M. bonneae,* and *M. nigrosignata. Mansonia ochracea* is found in all three locales. In a study of seasonal prevalence carried out over four years, all species were present throughout the year, though the population density was remarkably influenced by the rainfall. Precipitin tests of the blood in adults caught resting in the vicinity of houses showed that 10% of *M. dives/bonneae* and 2% of *M. uniformis* had fed on man. All species of *Mansonia* preferred to attack in the open rather than inside houses, and the biting activity was highest shortly after dusk.

In laboratory studies on the development of various filariae in the mosquitoes, it was shown that: (1) subperiodic *B. malayi* developed excellently in all the swamp forest species, i.e., *M. dives, M. bonneae, M. annulata,* and *M. uniformis;* however, (2) for periodic *B. malayi,* only *M. uniformis* was a good host, and only a few larvae developed in *M. dives* and *M. annulata* but none developed in *M. bonneae;* and (3) *M. annulata* was the only good host for *B. pahangi,* while *Armigeres subalbatus* was an excellent experimental host for *B. pahangi* but a poor host for both subperiodic and periodic *B. malayi.* The differences between the standards of host efficiency were measured by an index of experimental infection which related the survival rate, infective rate, and the numbers of mature larvae, with the microfilarial count at the time of feeding. In the swamp forest area studies, *M. dives, M. bonneae, M. annulata,* and to a lesser degree *M. uniformis* were the only mosquitoes regularly found infected with *Brugia* larvae; the infection rate of *M. dives/bonneae* was 1.1 to 1.4% around houses compared with 0.7% in the swamp forest two miles from human settlements. It was estimated that man would receive approximately 30 infective bites per year at night inside houses, and about 0.08 infective bites per hour in the period immediately after dark.

8B.7A.4.3 Vectors of periodic *B. malayi*

When WILSON *et al.* (1958) reported on the occurrence of two forms of *B. malayi* in Malaya, it was already recognized that the major vectors of each form were different, and they listed *M. longipalpis, M. annulata,* and *M. uniformis* as natural vectors of the subperiodic form, while those of the periodic form were considered at that time to be *An. barbirostris,* the *An. hyrcanus* group, *M. indiana, M. uniformis,* and *M. annulifera.* In a later survey carried out by REID *et al.* (1962) in the endemic foci of periodic

B. malayi in northwest Malaya, including Penang Island, *An. campestris* (formerly known as the dark-winged form of *An. barbirostris*), *M. indiana*, *M. uniformis*, and possibly *M. annulifera* were incriminated as the major vectors. Some 23,600 mosquitoes caught in the Kedah, Krian, and Penang areas were dissected from 1947 to 1958, among which natural infections with mature larvae were demonstrated in 19 of 3,573 *An. campestris*, 2 of 4, 424 *M. indiana*, and 1 of 4,316 *M. uniformis*, but not from any other anopheline or culicine mosquitoes. None of the *An. hyrcanus* group were naturally infective, though over 10,000 specimens were dissected and some immature filarial larvae were demonstrated. However, the development of periodic *B. malayi* in the above four mosquitoes after being experimentally fed on local donors was equally efficient.

Both periodic *B. malayi* and *W. bancrofti* were found to be endemic in the inland hill regions of Selangor by WHARTON *et al.* (1963), as noted before. The vectors of periodic *B. malayi* in these regions were determined to be *M. dives* and *An. donaldi*. Malaria and periodic *B. malayi* infections were also common among aborigines living in the isolated forest areas of Kelantan at altitudes of 500 to 1,200 feet; *An. maculatus* was identified as the vector of malaria, but the vector of *B. malayi* remained unknown.

8B.7A.5 Treatment and control

As discussed before, previous surveys carried out by various workers have shown that three kinds of filariasis are distributed in Malaya: the nocturnally periodic *W. bancrofti*, the nocturnally periodic *B. malayi*, and the nocturnally subperiodic *B. malayi*. The endemic foci of each type of filariasis are distributed in a complicated pattern, largely depending upon the prevalence of the mosquitoes that act as efficient vectors of each type of parasite. In general, the two forms of *B. malayi* occur more or less isolated from each other, though there are some areas in which the two forms are suspected to be coendemic. The *rural type* of *W. bancrofti* has been found often to be coendemic with either of the two *B. malayi* forms, but it also is known to occur singly on some offshore islands, as stated before.

The basic studies and pilot experiments for the control of filariasis in Malaya were started in 1953 by workers of the Institute for Medical Research in Kuala Lumpur and its field laboratory in Pahang, where sub-periodic *B. malayi* is highly prevalent; a tremendous amount of important information has been accumulated by these groups. Field studies were also started in northwest Malaya, or the Penang-Kedah area, in 1950; a national filariasis campaign was organized, and a nation-wide control activity initiated from about 1960.

8B.7A.5.1 Pilot studies on filariasis control

WILSON (1950) conducted a preliminary experiment of the use of DEC in the treatment of *B. malayi* carriers at the hospital of Sungei Patani, in the state of Kedah. Diethylcarbamazine dihydrogen citrate, manufactured by Lederle Laboratories Division, American Cyanamide Co. was used, and 20 persons with symptomless blood infections of *B. malayi*, 8 with clinical filariasis and no microfilariae, and one with both, were treated in varying doses and for varying periods. The compound was administered orally, at single doses of approximately 2 mg per kg of body weight, three times a day, as a rule. In the microfilarial carriers, the drug, in doses of 0.28 mg per kg three times a day and over, quickly cleared microfilariae from the blood of 18 patients, and only 5 showed recurrences out of 11 re-examined 10 to 13 months later. However, most of them developed severe reactions within 6 to 12 hours after the first dose, with temperatures of 103°F or more, headache, and nausea or vomiting. These symptoms disappeared by the third day even when drug administration was continued. The reactions were less severe in patients with clinical filariasis without microfilaremia. Although the drug had little immediate effect on clinical symptoms, some cases later reported a considerable degree of freedom from filarial fever, or the reduction of swelling.

TURNER (1959) reported on the results of the treatment of *B. malayi* cases with DEC in single daily doses. Seventy cases from endemic areas of the periodic form on Penang Island were hospitalized, and different dosages of the drug were administered every day, once per day. Although as little as 0.25 mg per kg per day reduced the microfilaria count by 63%, the effect was considered too slow, and larger doses were recommended. Febrile reactions occurred in 54 of 55 microfilaria carriers when the dosage was high enough to remove microfilariae, but did not occur in patients with negative blood films. Also, after the febrile reaction had subsided, large increases in dosage never provoked a recurrence of the febrile symptoms. TURNER & SODHY (1959) further reported on the trial mass treatment of *B. malayi* filariasis in a community on Penang Island with the single, daily dose regime. The initial dosage was determined by the patient's blood survey result, for example, 0.5 mg per kg to those with 30 or more counts per 20 mg of blood, 1.0 mg per kg to those with less than 30 microfilariae per 20 mg of blood, and 2.0 mg to those who were microfilaria negative. The initial dosage was repeated if a febrile reaction occurred, and in other cases, or when the reaction waned, the dose was increased by the order of 1.0, 2.0, 4.0, 8.0, 10.0, and 12.0 mg per kg. In a preliminary night blood survey, in which 92% (144 of 156) of the people in the village were examined, 27%, (39 of 144) were positive with 20 mm³ blood samples. The treatment policy was to give everybody at least 100 mg per kg body weight of Banocide (DEC citrate) in an uninterrupted course of single, daily doses. However, various difficulties were encountered, and only 30% of them received uninterrupted doses totaling more than 60 mg per kg; when the trials ended after 48 days, 86% had received total dosages of more than 40 mg per kg. At the blood resurvey carried out five weeks later, only 2 of 31 previously positive cases remained positive, and all of them became negative at the second resurvey conducted 42 weeks later.

However, the author concluded that mass treatment of *B. malayi* filariasis involves many difficulties and needs to be supervised because of the high incidence of febrile reactions, and that simpler schedules were preferable.

The above information obtained by WILSON (1950) and TURNER (1959) suggested that DEC would be very efficient in the control of the parasite carriers and in the treatment of acute filarial cases, but at the same time they warned of the danger of unsupervised mass treatment with the drug because of the occurence of the marked clinical reactions in the microfilarial carriers, which would be much more severe than those reported in the treatment of *W. bancrofti* infection. In the meantime, KESSEL *et al.* (1953) and KESSEL (1957), in Tahiti, reported on the successful control of nonperiodic *W. bancrofti* infection by administration of DEC in monthly doses. EDESON & WHARTON (1958) conducted a pilot experiment for the control of microfilaria carriers with monthly or weekly doses of DEC at a hospital in East Pahang, and also obtained promising results. Various dosage schemes were tested, ranging from 0.5 mg per kg to 6 mg per kg, given either once a week or once a month, six times, as a rule. At the end of treatment, all dosage regimes had reduced the microfilarial counts by at least 93%, and doses of 4 to 6 mg per kg had reduced the counts by 99%. Almost every microfilarial carrier suffered a sharp febrile reaction after the initial dose, and the reduction of the initial dose could not eliminiate the reaction completely. However, very few patients suffered any such reaction after the second or subsequent doses, despite the occasional persistence of numbers of microfilariae.

The control of the vectors of *B. malayi*, as well as the rural form of *W. bancrofti* in Malaya, has been considered difficult in most instances, because of the existence of extensive and inaccessible vector breeding places, and also because of the outdoor biting habit of most *Mansonioides* species. WHARTON & SANTA MARIA (1958) conducted experiments on the effects of DDT, dieldrin, and gamma BHC on the behavior and mortality in human-baited window-trap huts of *Mansonioides* mosquitoes in East Pahang. *Mansonia longipalpis* represented the majority of mosquitoes trapped in the huts. Dieldrin at 100 mg per square foot was clearly superior to the other insecticides, killing 100% of the *M. longipalpis* for two months, and maintaining a kill (24 hour) of over 50% for about six months.

Following hospital trials with monthly and weekly doses of DEC conducted by EDESON & WHARTON (1958), and the observations in window huts with residual insecticides for the control of vector mosquitoes by WHARTON & SANTA MARIA (1958), a field study for the eradication of *B. malayi* infection was carried out by WHARTON *et al.* (1958) in three Malay settlements in East Pahang. In the first settlement, Sawah, DEC was given to the whole population once a week; the first dose was 0.5 mg per kg, the second dose was 1 mg per kg, and the six final doses were each 5 mg per kg. In the second settlement, Tanah Puteh, DEC was given in monthly doses of 5 mg per kg for six months. In the third settlement, Ubai, dieldrin was sprayed in the houses at 100 mg per square foot at six-month intervals. Weekly administration at Sawah reduced the microfilaria rate from 49% (38 of 78 persons) to 10% (8 of 78) and the mean number of microfilariae per 20 mm³ blood from 19.7 to 0.26 at re-examination one month after end of the treatment. Monthly drug administration at Tanah Puteh reduced the microfilaria rate from 35% (42 of 119) to 6% (7 of 119) and the mean count from 11.2 to 0.16 also one month after end of treatment. In both areas, the microfilaria rates and counts had risen slightly one year later. Spraying with dieldrin at Ubai over a period of two years had no effect on the microfilaria rates and densities (35% of 215 and 12.6 before the spraying, 45% and 15.2 one year after spraying, and 41% and 12.6 two years after the spraying). In all three areas, there was no observable difference in the intensity of transmission, as measured by the biting and infection rates of *M. longipalpis*, although observations in houses showed that dieldrin killed large numbers of the mosquito and the drug treatment was shown to effect a tenfold reduction in the infectivity of the population of mosquitoes. It was believed that the lack of observable effect on transmission was partly due to the small areas under control and partly to the presence of untreated reservoirs of *B. malayi* infection in domestic and wild animals.

The experiences of pilot experiments of mass treatment with various dosage regimes indicated, as stated by WILSON (1961), that weekly doses were the easiest to organize; the regime of 5 mg DEC citrate per kg of body weight, once a week for six doses was, therefore, adopted for general use.

The results of observations on the effect of DEC on *B. malayi* and *B. pabangi* infection in cats reported by EDESON & LAING (1959) were surprisingly different from those experienced in man. In spite of large doses (up to 100 mg per kg of body weight) given orally or intraperitoneally, microfilaria counts fell relatively slowly, and microfilariae continued to circulate for six to ten months after the course of treatment. However, at least some of the adult worms of both species were shown to be killed by the drug and death was followed by calcification.

Results of a long-term epidemiological survey of an endemic area of the subperiodic *B. malayi* in East Pahang was reported by WILSON & RAMACHANDRAN (1971). The village selected was Kampong Ubai, where a pilot control experiment of residual house spraying with dieldrin was conducted every months (WHARTON *et al.*, 1958; WILSON, 1961). Blood surveys were conducted every year from 1953 to 1960. The microfilaria rate of the villagers was about 40% from 1953 to 1956, and later gradually dropped to about 20% in 1960. The mean microfilaria count per 20 mm³ blood dropped from 17.5 (per all films) and 43.4 (per positive film) to 4.5 and 23.6, respectively. The results suggested that the vector control experiment with house spraying of residual insecticide was only slightly effective as a measure for the control of *B. malayi* filariasis (see Section 10A.3).

8B.7A.5.2 Epidemiological surveys

As in other areas, information on the occurrence of elephantiasis is regarded as suggesting the presence of endemic foci, and blood examinations of the whole or sampled population have been the measure for determining the prevalence of infection in the communities in Malaya. POYNTON & HODGKIN (1938) emphasized the enlargement of inguinal lymph nodes as indicative of filarial infection, but WILSON & REID (1959) noted that several patients with high microfilaria counts had no perceptible enlargement of any lymph node, and EDESON (1955) showed that enlargement of the nodes in Malay children in nonfilarious areas was as common as in the highly infected kampongs of Pahang.

In Malaya, examination of measured blood samples (20 mm^3) with Sinton's capillary tube technique has been adopted as a standard for microfilarial surveys since it was used by FIELD (1948). WILSON (1956) recommended the staining of the thick blood smear with a 1:50 dilution of Giemsa stain in phosphate buffer solution (pH 7.2) for one hour. This technique was found to produce a color contrast between the microfilariae of *W. bancrofti* and *B. malayi* which facilitated identification. (Before this report appeared, most workers recommended Brug's original method of staining with hematoxyline and examination of the detailed structure, such as the presence or absence of caudal nuclei, but WILSON presented a much simpler criterion useful in mass diagnosis.)

Data referring to the results of microfilarial and clinical surveys on fairly large populations in Malaya were reported by POYNTON & HODGKIN (1938), HASSAN (1957), WILSON (1961), and SANDOSHAM (1964).

The microfilaria rates by age and sex in the Penang-Kedah area and in the Pahang area were discussed by WILSON (1961). In Pahang, the infection rates reached higher levels and rose somewhat more steeply. In the Penang-Kedah area, the total infection rate in females was little different, at all ages, from that in males. In Pahang, however, there was a well-marked tendency to lower rates in females from 10 to 55 years old. In the Kedah-Penang area, the youngest infected child was 13 months, and the microfilaria rate rose to a peak of 56% in males at age 9 to 10. In Pahang, the youngest infected child was age three months; the microfilaria rate in both sexes increased rapidly to reach 57% at age 4 to 5 years, and the tendency to a consistently lower rate in females first became apparent from about 10 years and up. (See Section 11A.2.)

The relation between total infection rate and microfilaria density was also discussed by WILSON (1961). In area KG, with a high total infection rate of 57% in 687 persons, microfilaria density in males was almost at its maximum in the earliest age-group and varied little thereafter; in females, it showed the same peculiar fall and later rose as did the curve of the total infection rate. In area LJB with lower total infection rate of 33% in 622 persons, mean microfilaria densities both in males and females rose steadily with increasing age. In these areas, there was no direct relationship between infection rate and microfilaria density.

A detailed account of the clinical features of *B. malayi* filariasis was published by TURNER (1959a). The early stages of a natural infection seem to be symptomless, even when large numbers of microfilariae appear in the blood; many have no detectable enlargement of lymph nodes. The first initiation of the disease is an attack of adenolymphangitis, usually accompanied by fever. These recur at irregular intervals. In Pahang, WILSON (1961) observed that children from six years upwards suffer from such attacks, but in the Kedah-Penang area, the symptom appears much later. The episode may be accompanied by some swelling of the affected limb. This is at first temporary, but later becomes permanent elephantiasis. The swellings and elephantiasis almost always affect the leg, frequently both legs, and seldom extend beyond the knee. The arms are rarely affected, and scrotal elephantiasis was seen only once.

According to WILSON (1961), the microfilaria rate of those who are suffering from elephantiasis is considerably lower than that of persons without elephantiasis in the same areas, both in the Kedah-Penang area (the periodic form) and in the Pahang area (the subperiodic form), as shown in Table 8-7.

Table 8-7. Microfilaria rate of persons with and without elephantiasis in two endemic areas in Malaya (after WILSON, 1961).

Area	Without elephantiasis		With elephantiasis	
	No. of persons examined	Mf. rate	No. of persons examined	Mf. rate
Kedah-Penang	1,563	37%	108	2%
Pahang	3,828	43%	279	10%

8B.7A.5.3 Filariasis control campaign

The outline of activity and status of the filariasis control campaign in Malaya was reviewed by HASSAN (1959), WILSON (1961,1969), SANDOSHAM (1964), and RAMACHANDRAN (1969). Control in Kedah has been carried out as a public health measure by the State Health Department since 1956. For some years before, houses had been sprayed with residual insecticides at six-month intervals as an antimalaria measure, at first with DDT (200 mg per square foot), and later with dieldrin. Mass treatment with DEC was started in 1956, at doses of 5 mg per kg of body weight given once a week for six weeks. WILSON (1961) reported that the microfilaria rate of 26% in 3,135 persons dropped to 1.5% at re-examination 7 to 12 months later, and the mean microfilaria count per 20 mm³ blood from 2.6 to 0.2. Most positives were re-treated, and in 815 persons re-examined two years after their first course of treatment, the microfilaria rate had been reduced from 23% to 0.5%, and the mean count from 3.36 to 0.02. It was also reported by SANDOSHAM (1964) that in Bukit Meriam, Kedah, the microfilaria rate of 26% and the mean count of 2.59 in 3,227 persons examined before the treatment dropped to 1.5% and 0.18, respectively, at examination of 3,135 persons 7 to 12 months later; at the survey of whole area in 1962, the rate and count remained as low as 0.9% and 0.1, respectively, in 2,972 persons, or only 0.51% positives in 2,741, excluding immigrants from untreated areas.

In East Pahang, the pilot experiment conducted by WHARTON *et al.* (1958) was intended to cover larger areas. SANDOSHAM (1964) reported that in the Pahang Tua Irrigation Area, where the microfilarial rate was 36% and mean count per 20mm³ blood was 17.5 in 1,519 persons at the survey in 1953, the rate and count were 31% and 7.1, respectively, in 1,632 persons in 1957 at the start of mass treatment; the figures dropped to 5% and 0.5, respectively, in 1,712 persons in 1958. However, while only the previously positive microfilaria cases were re-examined and treated during the subsequent years, the rate rose to 12.4% and the mean count to 0.6 in 729 persons at the survey carried out in 1962. This result suggested that in such areas where animal reservoirs play an important role as a source of infection, re-treatment of all positive cases every two years would not be sufficient, and mass treatment of the whole population should be resorted to every few years in order to achieve effective control of the disease.

8B.7B Filariasis in East Malaysia

Although little is known about the status of filariasis in this region, a few reports made in the past indicate that at least two species of filariae are endemic: the nocturnally subperiodic *B. malayi* in freshwater swamp areas, and the nocturnally periodic *W. bancrofti* in the inland hilly areas of primary forest.

ZULUETA (1957), while engaged in a malaria survey project in Sarawak and Brunei from 1952 to 1953, reported on the results of detection of microfilariae in the blood films collected for the purpose of malaria survey. In this project, nearly 10,000 people were examined for spleen enlargement by five teams, covering a large part of the two regions; blood films were taken during the daytime, from every alternate person, as the rule. The localities where microfilaria positive cases were detected reached over 30 villages. These were mostly *B. malayi*, and the endemic areas were usually in the flat coastal land along the large rivers of Sarawak. *W. bancrofti* infections were also found at special surveys directed to the mountain regions, especially in upper Tinjar, where the villages were in the Tinjar Valley about 150 m above sea level, and surrounded by abrupt mountains covered by dense jungle. At examinations of mosquitoes carried out in an endemic area of *W. bancrofti* in this valley, 44 of 5,492 *An. leucosphyrus* and 4 of 263 *An. barbirostris* were found to be infected with filaria larvae (stages and species not indicated).

In the state of Sabah, the northeastern part of Borneo closest to the Philippine Islands, BARCLAY (1965, 1969) carried out detailed surveys on filariasis. Prior to these investigations, CLARKE, in 1951, reported tha the saw two cases of elephantiasis while investigating the health of the Muruts. REGESTER (1956), while studying the primitive communities of Muruts and Dusuns, found 3 to 10% were microfilaria cases of *W. bancrofti* according to night blood films examined from several parts of the interior. BARCLAY (1965) carried out a survey of three villages in the Brunei Bay area, and found microfilariae of *B. malayi* in 11 of 48 at Sinapokan, 1 of 32 at Milikai, and 1 of 65 at Labidan. Results of blood examinations of some domestic and wild animals were all negative for *Brugia*.

Extensive surveys of filariasis in various areas of Sabah were carried out by BARCLAY (1969). Microfilaria cases were detected from eight areas surveyed; *B. malayi* was in five areas in the southwest and northeast, and *W. bancrofti* cases were in six areas (three areas had mixed infection). The *Brugia* cases were mostly in freshwater swamp areas, while the *Wuchereria* cases were found in hilly areas of primary forest. Infective larvae of *Brugia* species were detected from 3 of 1,465 *M. dives/bonneae* examined, and all the other 13 mosquito species were not infected. Of animals examined, microfilariae of a *Brugia* species thought to be *B. pahangi* were found in cats. Most people found infected were asymptomatic. In areas where *B. malayi* was endemic, the most common clinical manifestation seen was elephantiasis of a mild degree affecting the legs below the knee. In areas where *W. bancrofti* was endemic, the most common lesion seen was hydrocele. A summary of results of this survey is shown in Table 8-8.

8B.8 Singapore

Singapore is an island situated close to the southern extremity of the Malay Peninsula, at about 2°N and 104°E. It is a republic with a population of 2,110,400 (1971) and an area of 583 km². As in Hong Kong, the majority of the people reside in highly urbanized areas.

Filariasis has apparently not attracted the attention of public health workers in Singapore until recently. WHARTON (1960), in a report on experimental study of the vector of a rural strain of *W. bancrofti* in Pahang, Malaya, stated that *C. fatigans* fed on two *W. bancrofti* carriers from Singapore proved to be an efficient vector, while the same mosquito was only a poor vector for the rural strain of *W. bancrofti*.

DANARAJ *et al.* (1958) conducted a survey of 902 persons in the city of Singapore, and found microfilariae (all *W. bancrofti*) in 5.5%. The infections were mostly in adult Indian and Chinese immigrants who had lived in Singapore for from 1 to 30 years. It was calculated that local infections accounted for about 30% of the cases seen among Indians and about 80% of those among Chinese and Malays. The chief clinical manifestation was elephantiasis of the legs, followed by hydrocele and chyluria. *Culex fatigans* was found to be the vector.

Table 8-8.   The distribution and prevalence of filariasis in Sabah (rearranged from data reported by BARCLAY, 1969).

| | | | | Microfilaria carriers | | | | Clinical | |
| | | | | B. malayi | | W. bancrofti | | cases | |
Area	Estimated population	No. & % examined		No.	%	No.	%	No.	%
1. Brunei Bay	32,000	3,227	10.1	181	5.61	0	0.	19	0.59
2. West coast	250,000	6,530	2.6	4	0.06	0	0.	0	0.
3. Benkoka	10,000	1,159	11.6*	206	17.77	*51	4.40	9	0.78
4. Sugut-Labuk-Kinabatangan	21,000	3,117	14.8	297	9.53	17	0.55	22	0.71
5. South-east	86,000	4,961	5.8	7	0.14	0	0.	0	0.
6. The Interior	81,000	6,243	7.7	0	0.	8	0.13	0	0.
7. Upper Kinabatangan & Upper Menggalong	11,000	2,402	21.8	0	0.	114	4.75	17	0.71
8. Banggi Island	5,000	273	5.5	0	0.	3	1.10	0	0.

*Includes 24 cases of mixed infection

COLBOURNE & NG (1972) made an assessment of filariasis transmission in Singapore. During the previous five years, 129 cases were diagnosed as filariasis in two general hospitals in Singapore, and the rate among Indians was highest (53 cases, 41 per 100,000), followed by Malays (20 cases, 8.6 per 100,000) and Chinese (55 cases, 3.6 per 100,000). Three districts in Singapore were found where the number of cases were three times higher than expected. (Anson, Geylang and Joo Chiat). Investigations for infected mosquitoes were then conducted in six districts, including the above three districts. A total of 2,895 *C. fatigans* were dissected, 49 (1.7%) were found to be infected, and 2 (0.07%) had larvae in the head. Of 259 patients examined in two general hospitals, 5 (1.9%) had *W. bancrofti* microfilariae in their night blood smears.

8B.9 Indonesia

The Republic of Indonesia is situated on an archipelago extending from longitudes 95°E to 141°E and latitudes 7°N to 11°S. It has a total area of 2,018,600 km² and a population of 121,089,000 (1970).

Being a large country composed of several thousand islands scattered over the southwest Pacific Ocean, the epidemiology of filariasis is extremely complicated in this country. The nocturnally periodic race of *W. bancrofti* is widely distributed from the westmost island of Sumatra to the eastmost territory of West Irian, and a variety of mosquito species indigenous to each area are participating in its transmission. *Brugia malayi* is also widely endemic and is usually more prevalent than *W. bancrofti* in Sumatra, Kalimantan, Sulawesi, and the adjacent small islands, but its distribution is apparently limited by the Weber line which separates Irian from the Ceram-Ambon Islands. Both nocturnally periodic and subperiodic forms of *B. malayi* are known from this country. Because West Irian belongs zoogeographically to the Papuan zone, and the ecology of filariasis and its vectors is quite different from other areas of Indonesia, filariasis in this region is discussed in Section 9C.

8B.9.1 Historical notes

Filariasis in Indonesia was first reported by HAGA & VAN EECKE (1889), who gave descriptions of several cases of elephantiasis of the scrotum and penis, and found embryos of *Filaria sanguinis* in the tissues. Later, filarial infections were reported from Java by FLU (1918) and GOMPERTS (1926), from Sumatra by OOSTINGH (1923), MILITAIR GENEESKUNDIGE DIENST (1923), and LICHTENSTEIN (1927), from Kalimantan (Borneo) by FLU (1918), from Sulawesi (Celebes) by FLU (1918), GOMPERTS (1926), and ERBER (1927), from Maluku (the Molucca Islands) by GOMPERTS (1926), SCHIJVESCHUURDER (1927), and COOL (1927), from the Sunda Islands

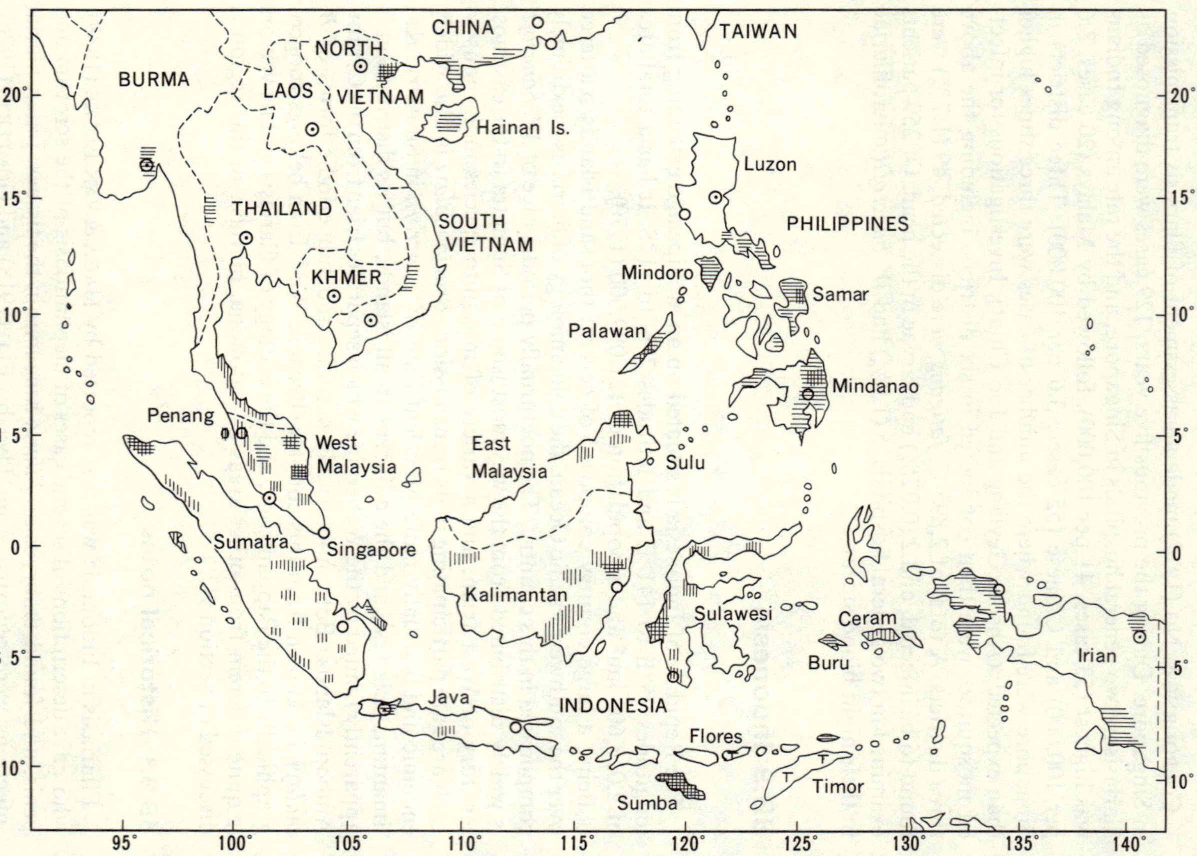

Fig. 8-7. Distribution of endemic areas of *B. malayi, W. bancrofti* and Timor-filaria in Southeast Asia (adapted from various authors' reports).

(Soemba, Savoe, Timor, and Flores) by KUYER (1922), RODENWALDT & ESSED (1923), and GOMPERTS (1926), and from New Guinea by LEIMENA (cited by COOL, 1927). BRUG (1928, 1931) presented comprehensive reviews on the distribution of filariasis in Indonesia.

LICHTENSTEIN (1927), while conducting experimental studies on the transmission of a filaria in Bireuen, on the north coast of Sumatra, found out that the microfilariae ingested by *C. fatigans* did not develop in this mosquito, such as demonstrated by BRUG (1920) for the filaria in Batavia (Djakarta). He recognized the Bireuen filaria to be different from the previously known *Filaria bancrofti*. The blood specimen was sent to Brug for identification of the microfilariae. BRUG (1927) made comparative studies on the morphology of the microfilariae with those of *Filaria bancrofti*, and identified the Bireuen filaria as a new and distinct species. There were differences in the structure of the tail and other parts of the microfilariae, in the efficiency of *C. fatigans* as the carrier, and in the absence of symptoms other than elephantiasis. The species was named *Filaria malayi*. BRUG (1928, 1931b) further made comprehensive studies on the microfilariae of both species, and pointed out various morphological characters that differentiated *malayi* from *bancrofti* (see Section 2A.2.3).

The principal vector of this new species of human filaria was determined by BRUG & DE ROOK (1930) in a study carried out at Dermajoe (Benkoelen, Sumatra). In this area, 47.5% of the inhabitants were found to be showing microfilariae of *B. malayi*, and *W. bancrofti* as well as *C. fatigans* was totally absent. Two species of mosquitoes, *Taeniorhynchus (Mansonioides) annulipes* and *T. (M) annulatus* were extremely abundant. The results of experimental infections with these mosquitoes showed that 101 of 109 (93%) of the former and 148 of 178 (83%) of the latter species dissected at varying intervals from one-half to 17 days after engorgement with the infected blood were found to be positive for filarial larvae. The authors also made morphological studies on various stages of the larvae developing in the mosquitoes. Natural infections were seen in 6 of 323 *annulatus* and 4 of 339 *annulipes*, but not in other mosquito species. The proboscis infection was found both in naturally and experimentally infected mosquitoes.

In determining the natural vectors of filariasis in the particular endemic area, BRUG & DE ROOK (1930) utilized a unique and efficient method. A microfilaria carrier was exposed to mosquito bites for a certain period of a day, and as soon as a mosquito had inserted its proboscis in the skin, a test tube was carefully put over it and held in position until the gnat was fully engorged and flew into the test tube. In this way, about five catchers were occupied with a donor, in order to catch all the mosquitoes. The mosquitoes in the test tubes were kept in a humid condition as long as they survived, and were identified and dissected as soon as they were found dead. With this method, they could obtain the biting rhythm and preva-

Taeniorhynchus is a synonym of *Mansonia*

lence of man-biting mosquitoes, as well as the mode of development of the filarial larvae in each species of the mosquitoes. This method was later used by the Dutch and Indonesian workers in determining the vectors of different localities.

This report by BRUG & DE ROOK (1930) is historically important not only as the first paper dealing with the vector of malayan filariasis, but also in that the authors incriminated, for the first time, the mosquitoes of the genus *Mansonia* as the carriers of human disease. Apparently, the biology of this group of mosquitoes was still unfamiliar to the workers at that time. BRUG (1931b) stated,

> "I regret that I cannot give you particulars regarding the biology of the *Mansonioides* species with which we dealt. They are fierce man-biters. The bite may be felt as a sting, unlike that of *Stegomyia fasciata*. The subsequent itching is moderate, at least for a tropical "old hand." These mosquitoes enter at 7 o'clock in the evening. Their attacks begin at about 8 o'clock and become unbearable at 10 o'clock. They enter the house by preference when it rains; even heavy rain does not check them. We could not explain how they managed to fly through the rain. After sunny days there were few mosquitoes. This is quite different from our experience in Batavia, where a rainy afternoon means a mosquito-free evening.
>
> In spite of the tremendous number of *Mansonioides* imagos, a fourteen-day search failed to reveal us a single breeding place; SENIOR WHITE (1927) had the same experience with *T. (M.) uniformis* in Ceylon. There was a large swamp near our village with virgin forest within it. In this forest we could find very many adult *Mansonioides* throughout the day, but no larvae were detected. We failed also to obtain adults with mosquito nets suspended on the water."

(The present author had the same experience with *M. uniformis* in Okayama, Japan, in 1946. It took two weeks before I could find their breeding place in a nearby swamp, in which no mosquito larvae were collected previously by using a dipper. Since the larvae are firmly attached to the roots of water plants by inserting the tip of siphon, it is necessary to collect the larvae by shaking the host plant vigorously in a water tub.)

The adults of this new filaria, as well as its taxonomic status, remained unknown, until RAO & MAPLESTONE (1940) discovered both males and females in man in India. They described the morphological characters, and placed this species into the genus *Wuchereria* Seurat, 1921, with *bancrofti* as the type species. The adult worms were also found and described by BONNE *et al.* (1941), in Batavia, from a male Malay who had suffered from leukemia and died after an operation for calcus vesicae. Later, several new species related to *malayi* were discovered from animals, and BUCKELY (1960) created a new genus, *Brugia,* with *malayi* as the type species, as explained in Section 2C.1.

As for the geographic distribution of the two filarial species, BRUG (1931a) collected the information by sending a circular of inquiry to all medical men in Indonesia and compiled a map from their responses. As a result, he stated that both species were found in Sumatra, Java, Borneo, and Celebes, though generally *malayi* was more frequent. In Java, however, where filariasis was relatively rare, *bancrofti* seemed to be predominant. In New Guinea and on the small island of Kabaena, south of Celebes, only *bancrofti* was found and was highly prevalent. In villages where both species occurred, the number of mixed infections was significantly greater than might be expected according to the laws of probability. In villages where *malayi* only was found, elephantiasis and lymphagitis of the limbs were the predominant symptoms, and others were rare or absent; in pure *bancrofti* regions, however, affections of the genitalia largely outnumbered elephantiasis of the limbs. *Microfilaria malayi* showed nocturnal periodicity, but less strictly so than *bancrofti* of nocturnal form, and the ratio between the number present in the blood during daytime and that at midnight was about 1:15, with extremes of 1:3 to 1:50 in *malayi*, but less than 1:100 in *bancrofti*.

Additional information concerning the distribution of the two species of filariae in Indonesia was collected by a number of later workers; LIE & REES (1958) and LIE (1971) published revised maps. A third species of human parasite, which is now tentatively called the "Timor filaria," was described recently by DAVID & EDESON (1965) from Portugese Timor, and was reported by OEMIJATI & LIEM (1966) to occur also in the Indonesian part of the island.

A number of noteworthy contributions have been made from this region on the mosquito vectors of filariasis. As for *W. bancrofti, C. p. fatigans* was incriminated as the principle vector of the urban form, such as is endemic in Jakarta, by BRUG (1920), FLU (1929), SOEWADJI (1939), LIE *et al.* (1958), and CHOW *et al.* (1959). The rural form of *W. bancrofti* infection in New Guinea (West Irian) was found to be transmitted mainly by the local anopheline mosquitoes according to observations made by ELSBACH (1937b), DE ROOK (1955, 1957a, 1957b, 1959), TOFFALETI & KING (1947), and VAN DIJK (1959), though other mosquito species, including *C. p. fatigans, Ae. kochi, M. uniformis*, etc., might also be involved. On the other hand, *B. malayi* was shown to be transmitted mainly by species of *Mansonia*, with some involvement by *Anopheles*, by BRUG & DE ROOK (1930) and REES *et al.* (1958) from Sumatra, by JURGENS (1932) and BRUG (1937) from Celebes, by KARIADI (1941, '42) OEY (1942), and KLOKKE (1961) from Kalimantan, and by LIE *et al.* (1960) from Java.

8B.9.2 Epidemiology

As stated before, both *B. malayi* and *W. bancrofti* are widely distributed in the islands of Indonesia. The occurrence of both species was reported from Sumatra, Java, Kalimantan, Sulawesi, and the adjacent islands, while only *W. bancrofti* has been found in West Irian and Kabaena. The distribution of *B. malayi* seems to be confined towards the east up to the island of Ceram and to the islands of Sumba, but not further. Both periodic and subperiodic forms of *B. malayi* were reported to be found by LIE *et al.* (1960) from Sumatra.

The islands that belong to Indonesia are divided into the two major zoogeographical regions: the southwestern Asiatic region and the Melanesian (or Papuan) region. The distribution of filarial parasites, as well as the vectors, is also clearly defined according to the regions. For example, *B. malayi* is a parasite confined to the Asiatic region, while some Melanesian anopheline mosquitoes are higly adapted as vectors of *W. bancrofti.*

8B.9.2.a Filariasis in Sumatra

Filariasis, especially that due to *B. malayi*, has been recognized to be widely distributed throughout Sumatra. In a review on the distribution of filariasis in Indonesia, BRUG (1928) pointed out that filariasis was widely endemic in Sumatra from the northern region of Atje (Acheh) along the east coast to Djambi and Palembang. As mentioned previously, *B. malayi* was described first by BRUG (1927) by the name of *Filaria malayi* from a blood specimen collected from a carrier in Bireuen (Acheh, Sumatra), and thus North Sumatra represents the type locality of this parasite. The mosquito vector of this parasite was also determined first on this island, at Dermajoe (Benkoelen, Sumatra), in a study carried out by BRUG & DE ROOK (1930), where they found *M. (Mansonioides) annulipes* and *M. (M.) annulata* were by far the most prevalent man-biting mosquitoes, both being efficient vectors of *B. malayi.*

In the review on the distribution of *B. malayi* and *W. bancrofti* in Indonesia compiled by BRUG (1931a), more than 30 localities were recorded from Sumatra as the endemic foci of *B. malayi*, scattered along both the northern and southern coasts of the island. Heavy infection has been found in many localities, such as the microfilarial rate of 54% (71 of 131) in Dermajoe, 43% (19 of 23) in Idi, 40% (35 of 88) in Sipang Kiri, and 33% (22 of 62) in Meulaboh. On the other hand, *W. bancrofti* was recorded only from a few localities near the northern extremity of Sumatra and from Sarolangoen, inland of southern Sumatra, and always coendemic with *malayi.*

There have been only a few contributions made on the epidemiology of filariasis in Sumatra after the survey made by BRUG (1931a). SCHEEPE (1935) carried out an extensive survey of villages in the highlands of Indragiri, examined a total of 5,519 persons out of some 50,000 population, and found an overall positive rate of 29.0% (471 of 1,625) in male adults, 14.5% (245 of 1,689) in female adults, 12.7% (274 of 2,155) in children, and 17.9% (990 of 5,519) for the whole population. The number of patients with microfilariae and with manifest elephantiasis were 60 in males and 20 in females, and those with the periodic appearance of pre-elephantiasis signs numbered 42 in males and 10 in females. Several villages in this region showed microfilarial rates above 30%, such as 37.6% (38 of 101) in Kelampean, 36.7% (110 of 300) in Polakpisang, and 36.1% (73 of 202) Pasirbongkal. The microfilariae detected were all those of *B. malayi*, and neither hydrocele nor elephantiasis of the scrotum was observed. The mosquitoes most abundant were *M. annulipes*, followed by *M. uniformis*.

LIE & REES (1958) carried out a survey in Bengkulen, South Sumatra, and found that 39.3% of 6,608 persons examined were carrying microfilariae of *B. malayi*. LIE *et al.* (1960b) reported both periodic and subperiodic *B. malayi* to be endemic in this swamp forest area. REES (1958, unpublished, cited by LIE, 1970) obtained an infection rate of 1.4% and an infective rate of 0.4% in 699 naturally caught *M. annulata*.

A survey of filariasis at Bireuen (the type locality of *B. malayi*) was carried out by a joint team of the Indonesian and Japanese workers in August 1973, in order to determine which of the two physiological races (or subspecies) of *B. malayi* was first dealt with by the original authors (Lichtenstein, 1927; Brug, 1927). The survey team revealed that both *B. malayi* and *W. bancrofti* were still endemic among the people in this area. A study of the periodicity of the microfilariae of *B. malayi* in five cases and that of *W. bancrofti* in one case was conducted by taking 60 mm^3 blood samples at two-hour intervals over a period of 24 hours. Both were found to be the nocturnally periodic race, with the periodicity index of 89.44% in *B. malayi* and 107.35% in *W. bancrofti* (SASA *et al.*, in press).

8B.9.2.b Filariasis in Kalimantan (South Borneo)

The information referring to the endemicity of filariasis in southern Borneo is very meager, as it is for northern Borneo. The common occurrence of elephantiasis in the Bandjermasin area was recorded by HELFRICH in 1860. KNOCH, in 1898, described the case of man in Muara Teweh (central Borneo) with hematochylothorax, whose thoracic fluid contained numerous microfilariae. FLU (1918), in Batavia, examined nine persons from Borneo and found one microfilaria carrier. The above records were the only information when BRUG (1928) made a review on filariasis in the then Nederlandsch Indië.

In a review on the distribution of filariasis prepared by BRUG (1931) and based on questionnaires sent to all the medical workers, two endemic areas were traced in South Borneo. One of them was around Balikpapan, the oil center of East Borneo, and another was in the Hulu Sungei, the fertile, hilly district to the northeast of Bandjermasin. In the latter area, the existence of *B. malayi* infection had already been demonstrated by HAGA (1929) based on nine cases observed in the villages of Rantau, Kandangan, and Barabai. A heavy infection of both *B. malayi* and *W. bancrofti* was estimated to exist in the former area, as KOTTER found 7 *malayi* and 9 *bancrofti* positives (including 4 mixed infections) out of 21 persons examined at Djenparing.

KARIADI (1938) carried out epidemiological and entomological surveys of malayan filariasis prevalent around Martapura, in the Hulu Sungei in southeastern Borneo. The overall microfilarial rates in the inhabitants of nine villages were 32.3% (196 of 606) in adult males, 27.1% (26 of 96) in adult females, and 11.8% (11 of 93) in children. Mosquitoes, especially *M. (Mansonioides) uniformis, M. (M.) annulifera,* and *An. barbirostris typicus* were very abundant in this area, and high natural and experimental infection rates were observed with the above three species. KARIADI (1941) further reported that in Martapura, *An. hyrcanus X* breeds very abundantly in the wet season of the year, and is capable of carrying *Filaria malayi,* though the susceptibility was lower than *M. uniformis* and *An. barbirostris.*

OEY DJOEN HOAT (1942) carried out observations on the vectors of *B. malayi* in Boven Mahakam,Kalimantan, where the villagers showed a microfilarial rate of about 50% (39 of 77 examined were positive). In an artificial infection experiment with mosquitoes that attacked a microfilaria carrier, four species of the genus *Mansonia* were collected and examined at varying intervals after engorgement. The overall infection rate was 76% (35 of 46) in *M. (Mansonioides) longipalpis,* 70% (24 of 74) in *M. (M.) annulata,* 74% (74 of 99) in *M. (M.) indiana,* and 26% (21 of 80) in *M. (Coquillettidia) crassipes.* Proboscis infection of the mature larvae was also observed in the last species, and thus, aside from the already known vectors which belong to the subgenus *Mansonioides,* a species of the subgenus *Coquillettidia* was added as a vector of *B. malayi.* The author also conducted a study on the host plants of these *Mansonia* larvae.

In the endemic area of *B. malayi* west of Bandjermasin, KLOKKE (1961) carried out a systematic epidemiological survey. The area investigated was near the mouth of one of the Great Dayak Rivers (Kahaian), rich in swamps, canals, and pools. In the villages of Pankoh and Badirih, nearly 80% of the population was examined; the microfilarial rates were 38.4% (130 of 338) in the males and 22.7% (90 of 396) in the females; elephantiasis was seen in 28 males and 9 females. Night catches of mosquitoes inside the houses by one man for two hours yielded 133 specimens which contained 61 (45.9%) *M. longipalpis,* 37 (27.8%) *M. annulata,* 14 (10.5%) *M. ochracea,* 6 (4.5%) *M. novochracea,* 6 *C. vishnui* group, and 6 *An. barbumbrosus.* At the dissection of a part of the mosquitoes, 1 of 5 *M. ochracea,* 1 of 18 *M. longipalpis,* and 3 of 14 *M. annulata* harbored the infective larvae. Besides the predominant occurrence of the known vectors of filariasis that belong to the subgenus *Mansonioides* of *Mansonia,* the relative abundance of the big yellow mosquitoes of the two species of the subgenus *Coquillettidia,* i.e., *ochracea* and *novochracea,* and the natural infection of the latter, was specially noted by the author.

8B.9.2.c Filariasis in Java

The occurrence of filariasis due to *W. bancrofti* in Jakarta (Batavia) has been known for many years. FLU (1918, 1921) carried out microfilaria surveys in Jakarta, and found 3 positive cases out of 160 (1.9%) in 1918, and 91 positives out of 895 (10.6%) in 1921. BRUG (1920) examined the suitability of *C. fatigans* in Jakarta as the intermediate host of bancroftian filariasis; he observed that 13 of 33 mosquitoes fed on a microfilaria carrier were infected, including those with the mature larvae after 14 days. FLU (1929) observed the natural infection of *C. fatigans* in an area where 9 of 73 people were microfilaria positive. KEUKENSCHRIJVER (1929), at Catharina Hospital, found that 68 of 1,482 (4.6%) male and 19 of 701 (2.7%) female Javanese were microfilaria positive. However, GOMPERTS (1926) found no positive cases among 619 persons in Bandung and 120 persons in Madura. BRUG (1931) stated that filariasis was relatively rare in Java, and *bancrofti* was apparently the predominant species.

SOEWADJI PRAWIROHARDJO (1939) carried out an experimental infection study in Jakarta on the development of *W. bancrofti* larvae in 19 mosquito species. The donor was a woman of about 80 years, carrying large numbers of microfilariae in night blood. The infection with the filarial larvae was observed in all the mosquito species tested, but the development to the infective stage was seen only in four species of *Culex* and in all of the six species of *Anopheles*; the larval developments remained more or less incomplete in the other four species of *Culex*, two species of *Aedes* (*Stegomyia*), one species of *Arimigeres*, and two species of *Mansonia*.

The first systematic survey of filariasis in Jakarta was carried out by LIE *et al.* (1958). Night blood samples were collected from people in three sections (two urban and one semirural) of the Rawasari district. Microfilariae of *W. bancrofti* were found in 547 of 7,048 (7.8%) of the blood smears. The rate was higher in females than in males in the young age-group (from 6 to 30 years), while the relation became reversed in older age-groups (over 31 years). The microfilarial periodicity studies in 14 cases showed a remarkably nocturnal pattern. Although no elephantiasis was found, 14 of 92 males examined showed hydrocele, and lymphnode swelling was frequently found in both men and women.

CHOW *et al.* (1959) made a comprehensive study on the vectors of filariasis in the Rawasari district of Jakarta from 1956 to 1757. *C. p. fatigans* was the only species found to harbor the larvae of *W. bancrofti* in this area, and the infection rate among 24,271 *C. p. fatigans* dissected was 1.8% for all stages of larvae and 0.3% for mature larvae. It was established that transmission occurred throughout the year, with a maximum in September. The density of larvae of all stages per dissected mosquito was 0.12 and that of the infective stage larvae was 0.014. The "potential transmission index" *was calculated to be 0.26. As for the bionomics of *C. p. fatigans* in this area, the study revealed that the density was highest in July and August,

---

*The potential transmission index was calculated by multiplying (A), the "average number of mosquitoes caught per minute" by (B), the "density of average number of all stages (first to third stages) of filarial larvae per dissected mosquito" (KESSEL, 1957). (A) was 2.2 and (B) was 0.12 in this study in Jakarta.

that mosquito nets, clothes, hanging objects, and furniture were the preferred resting places, and that feeding took place mostly after midnight.

The information on the epidemiology of filariasis in the same area of Jakarta was studied further by LIE *et al.* (1960). The inhabitants of the study area showed a microfilarial rate of 16.3 % (32 of 196 examined), with an average microfilarial count per 20 mm³ blood per positive case of 33.6. A total of 17,247 *C. p. fatigans*, the only vector in the area, were dissected; 7% harbored ex-sheathed larvae, 3.5% harbored *Wuchereria* larvae of all stages including the infective, while only 0.1 % harbored infective stage larvae. Analysis of the results according to the positive and negative houses showed that the positive rates with the early larval stages were significantly higher in houses with microfilarial carriers, but no significant differences were seen in those with the second stage and older. The transmission rate in this area was low, because *C. p. fatigans* in Jakarta was short-lived. At the dissection of 2,025 mosquitoes for examination of the follicular relics, 1,724 (86.0%) were found nulliparous, 268 (13.2%) had one relic, 32 (1.6%) had two, and only 1 had three relics. Out of 17 mosquitoes harboring second stage larvae, 7 had one relic and 10 had no relic. Out of 3 mosquitoes with infective stage larvae, 1 had two relics, 1 had one relic, and 1 had no relic. The authors concluded that, with such a short-lived vector, transmission of *W. bancrofti* in Jakarta was possible only because of the high density of the mosquito, and that filariasis was mainly a domestic infection here, though not a family infection.

An endemic area of *B. malayi* in the delta of Serajoe, on the southern coast of middle Java, was investigated by RODENWALDT (1933a); this represented the only epidemiological study carried out in Java outside of Jakarta. The author carried out a sampling examination of 50 male adults, 50 female adults, and 50 children from people of five villages in the delta and six villages near this region and outside of the delta. All the microfilariae found in these areas were of *B. malayi*. The overall microfilaria rates in the delta region were 32.0 % (80 of 250) in male adults and 31.6 % (79 of 250) in female adults; the overall microfilaria rates of people outside of the delta, however, were lower, with 4.7 % (14 of 300) in male adults and 1.3 % 4 of 300) in female adults. The elephantiasis rate in adults was 19.6 % in the delta region and 4.5 % in the region outside of the delta. RODENWALDT (1934) further carried out investigations on the transmission of *B. malayi* by local mosquitoes, and obtained experimental infection rates of 66.6 % in 12 *M. uniformis*, 71.4 % in 7 *M. indiana*, and 88.9 % in 18 of the *An. hyrcanus* group. RODENWALDT (1933b) also gave a detailed morphological description of the microfilariae of *B. malayi*.

8B.9.2.d Filariasis in Sulawesi

As in Sumatra and Borneo, filariasis due to both *B. malayi* and *W. bancrofti* has been recognized to be endemic in many areas in Sulawesi (Celebes), and generally, *B. malayi* was found more frequently than *W. bancrofti*. In the review compiled by BRUG (1931), more than 20 localities were already listed as endemic foci of *B. malayi* from the mainland of Celebes, but *W. bancrofti* was recognized only in a few areas, generally coendemic with *B. malayi*.

The occurrence of endemic filariasis in Celebes had already been noted by FLU (1918), GOMPERTS (1926), and ERBER (1927), before BRUG (1927) differentiated *malayi* from *bancrofti*. ERBER (1927) carried out a blood survey of 15 districts in Mamoedjoe, on the west coast of Celebes, and found 276 positives out of 1,027 (24.9%) in total. Although he described it as *Filaria bancrofti*, this was probably all or mostly the *malayi* infection. He gave comparative figures of the microfilarial counts in 20 mm^3 of blood taken at 11 p.m. and that of 1cc (1,000 mm^3) taken at 11 a.m. from 30 positive persons, and obtained a total count of 275 microfilariae in the former and 1,284 in the latter; hence, the night blood contained 10.7 times more microfilariae than the day blood.

VAN SLEE (1930) reported on the results of blood surveys also carried out in Mamoedjoe. A total of 1,024 villagers (about 90% were males) were examined, and 261 *malayi* carriers and 12 *bancrofti* carriers (including 8 mixed infections) were detected. *W. bancrofti* was found from only two districts. In the comparative study of the microfilarial counts between 20 mm^3 night blood and 1 cc day blood samples on 50 *malayi* carriers, the total count came out to be 607 in day samples and 1,970 in night samples, with the night day ratio being 15.1 : 1. Elephantiasis and swelling of the lymph nodules were the major clinical signs, and no chyluria cases were observed.

JURGENS (1932) conducted a study on mosquito vectors in the Mamoedjoe area. The mosquitoes most abundant were *An. barbirostris*, followed by *M. annulipes*, and natural infection rates of 8.9% (19 of 214), and 2.7% (2 of 75) were obtained for the respective species in a village with a microfilarial rate of 37%. An experimental infection study was also carried out according to the method of BRUG & DE ROOK (1930). A total of 15 mosquito species were collected on a microfilaria carrier. The overall infection rate was 83% (90 of 108) in *An. barbirostris* and 64% (28 of 44) in *M. annulipes*, and mature larvae were obtained in both species. An unidentified species of *Aedes* was most abundant, but only 8 of 175 were infected, and one of them, dissected after ten days, contained one nearly mature larva. Based on these observations, the author regarded *An. barbirostris* as the primary and *M. annulipes* as the secondary vector of *B. malayi* in this area.

TESCH (1937) carried out a study on filariasis in the Paloe, Donggala, and Parigi divisions, in the northern arm of Celebes Island. The species of parasite found in this region was *B. malayi*, and elephantiasis and lymphangitis were the major clinical signs. In the lowland region in Paloe Valley, 32 of 691 (4.6%) had elephantiasis, and 415 of 668 (62.1%) were microfilaria positive in nine villages of southern Paloevlakte. In northern Paloevlakte, 266 persons in five villages were examined; there were no elephantiasis cases, but microfilariae were detected in 34 (12.7%). In the coastal region, 10 of 337 (2.9%) had elephantiasis and 74 of 305 (24.2%) had microfilaremia in nine villages of Donggala, while in 18 villages in Parigi, 13 of 723 (1.8%) had elephantiasis and 95 of 457 (20.9%) were microfilariae positive. In the mountain region, the elephantiasis rate and the microfilarial rate were 0% (0 of 180) and 11.8% (19 of 160), respectively, in four villages of Pekawastreek, and 0.2% (1 of 702) and 10.8% (59 of 545), respectively, in 15 villages of Koelawistreek. The rates in the mountain region were generally lower than in the valley or coastal regions, but the filarial carriers were found in areas up to almost 1,000 m above sea level. The microfilaria rate and the elephantiasis rate found in these villages were highly correlated. The periodicity of the microfilariae in the blood was studied by comparison of the microfilarial counts in 1 mm³ blood samples taken with Sahli pipettes from 30 microfilarial carriers, four times a day, at noon, 4 p.m., 8 p.m., and midnight. The results suggest that the parasite in this region is a nocturnally periodic type. In a survey of immigrants from central Java who resided in a colony in Kalawara, near Paloe, the infection rate and the elephantiasis rate were found generally lower than in the natives in the surrounding villages, and both rates were correlated with the length of period spent in this colony.

BRUG (1937) reported on interesting results concerning the mosquito vector of *B. malayi* in Kalawara (Paloe Division, Celebes), where epidemiological studies were carried out by TESCH (1937). In an artificial infection experiment using a carrier of *B. malayi*, a total of 143 mosquitoes classified into nine species were collected; 96 were *An. barbirostris typicus*, and 95 (99%) of them were found infected at later dissections. The development of larvae in this mosquito was excellent; mature larvae were detected as early as 6.5 days after the infection, and not a single immature larva was seen at dissections made 9.5 and 10.5 days after the infection. The species was also most commonly found in human dwellings, and represented 89.1% of a total of 304 mosquitoes collected in houses. Of 271 *An. barbirostris* caught in houses and dissected, 22 (8.1%) were infected, some with mature larvae. Other mosquito species were rather rare, and none was infected except for a single *An. bancrofti*. *Mansonia* species were considered to be of no practical importance. Although *An. barbirostris* in other parts of the Malay Archipelago was known to attack man only rarely, the species readily sucked the blood of man in Kalawara, while *An. bancrofti*, which is generally recorded as very anthropophilic, was found in fair numbers in cow sheds but did not seem to attack man in Kalawara.

PARTONO *et al.* (1972) conducted a survey of endemic foci of *B. malayi* in Margolembo, southern Sulawesi. Three villages were selected for the study; village I (Kalaena) with a population of approximately 250 consisted of Javanese transimmigrants who settled in the area in 1939; village II (Sindu Binangun) was inhabited by about 200 people who came to the area from central Java eight months prior to the survey; and village III (Margolembo), an old, established village consisting of a mixed population of 1939 Javanese transimmigrants and native Sulawesians with a population of approximately 500. Quantitative night blood samples of 20 mm³ were collected between 8 p.m. and 2 a.m., and skin tests were done with a Sawada type filarial antigen prepared from adult *Dirofilaria immitis*.

As a result, 215 persons of all ages were examined in village I, and *B. malayi* microfilariae were found in the blood of 71 (33.0%) and symptoms of filariasis in 44 (16 with elephantiasis, 28 with lymphangitis, lymphadenitis, etc.), with an overall filariasis rate of 44.1%. In village II, only one case out of 150 persons had microfilariae and another with recurrent fever. In village III, 270 persons of all ages were examined, and 32.5% had microfilariae and 14.8% had symptoms, with an overall filariasis rate of 41.4%. In the skin test, 46% of persons of all areas without microfilaremia or symptoms were positive, while only 29% of those with microfilaremia or symptoms were positive.

A study of microfilarial periodicity in 12 cases of *B. malayi* carriers in Margolembo revealed that the parasite was a nocturnally periodic race. (SASA & TANAKA, in 1972, obtained the periodicity index of 86.87 and the best estimate of the peak hour was 23.5 from their result). Of a total of eight species of mosquitoes collected and dissected, only *An. barbirostris* were found to be naturally infected, with a rate of 11.7% (13 of 112) for all stages of larvae and of 3.5% for mature larvae. It was also demonstrated that of a total of 135 *An. barbirostris* kept alive after feeding upon a microfilaria carrier, 43.4% were found to carry larvae, and the development to the third stage larvae was completed within six to eight days.

8B.9.2.e Filariasis on other smaller islands of Indonesia

The occurrence of *Wuchereria* infection on Boeton (Butung) and Kabaena Islands situated close to and south of the southeastern arm of Celebes was recorded by BRUG (1931). In Kabaena, REELING KNAP (1930) carried out a blood survey of the inhabitants, and found only *W. bancrofti* in 28 of 96 (29%) of the persons examined. A total of 32 cases with hydrocele and other scrotal involvements were recorded from all of the eight villages. BRUG (1938) carried out a study of mosquito vectors in a coastal village on Kabaena. About 20% of the adults in the village harbored microfilariae of *W. bancrofti*. A total of 902 mosquitoes belonging to ten species of *Anopheles* and six species of *Culex* collected in houses were dissected, but natural infection was seen only in 3 of 171 *An. aconitus*, 1 of 37 *An. leucosphyrus* var. *hackeri*, 1 of 201 *C. p. fatigans*, and 3 of 200 *C. alis-vishnui* mixture; none of the larvae were mature, and none of 201 *An. barbirostris typicus* were infected. In an artificial infection experiment, nine species of *Anopheles* and seven species of *Culex* ingested the infected blood, and complete development to mature larvae was seen in *An. barbirostris*, *An. aconitus*, *C. fuscocephalus*, *C.whitmorei*, *C. p. fatigans*, *C. alis-vishnui*, and *C. annulirostris*. The development was completed in 10.5 to 14.5 days. In *C. alis-vishnui*, *C. tritaeniorhynchus*, *C. bitaeniorhynchus* and *Ae. albopictus*, the ingested filarial larvae often survived as long as 10.5 to 14.5 days, but failed to complete the development. Therefore, the author calculated two artificial infection indices, a "crude" and a "corrected" index. The mosquitoes containing only larvae of retarded stages were considered as negative in the determination of the "corrected" index.

In the Molucca Islands, the occurrence of filariasis was recorded from Ceram by GOMPERTS (1926), WIRTH (1927), and SCHIJVESCHUURDER (1927), as shown in the list compiled by BRUG (1928). Also BRUG (1931) cited the results obtained by Lodder, who found 6 *B. malayi* carriers out of 44 persons in Hatenoeroe, Ceram. On Buru Island, west of Ceram, SOETRISNO (1940) carried out detailed epidemiological studies. As on the island of Kabaena, only *W. bancrofti* was found from inhabitants of this island, and the overall microfilarial rate in 832 persons examined was as high as 51.8% (431 positives). The rates were 63.8% (186 of 298) in adult males, 49.0% (98 of 200) in adult females, 45.5% (89 of 195) in children above six years of age, and 40.1% (58 of 139) in those under six years. (These rates are unusually high for an endemic area of *W. bancrofti*.) Forty persons among 832 people examined had elephantiasis. Microfilarial counts were made in 18 persons at intervals of three hours, and the periodicity was shown to be a nocturnal type, with a peak at 3 a.m. (It is also unusual that the counts at 6 p.m. and 6 a.m. were nearly as high as the peak counts.) No mosquito vectors were determined by the author.

Only a few records are available referring to filariasis in the Lesser Sunda Islands. BRUG (1931) cited the results of blood surveys conducted by other medical workers; in Sumba, 12 of 70 (17.1%) examined were positive (7 with *malayi*, 7 with *bancrofti*, including 2 mixed infection). On Flores Island, four areas were surveyed by Bloemsma, and 128 (27.5%) of 465 persons were positive (68 with *malayi* and 87 with *bancrofti*, including 27 mixed infection). Also, the presence of unidentified-microfilaria carriers and elephantiasis cases was also recorded from Alor Island, Timor Island, Roti Island, and Savoe Island. One of 56 persons in Atamboea, Timor, was recorded to be a carrier of *malayi* in the table by BRUG (1931).

The occurrence of an endemic area of the nocturnally periodic form of *B. malayi* was confirmed recently from Ceram Island, Maluku, Indonesia. A team composed of Dr. Ch. E. Pupella and his associates from the Health Department of Maluku, and two Japanese scientists (M. Sasa and T. Kurihara) visited a small village (Rumalurung) in the Taniwel district on the northern coast, in March 1972. Of a total population of about 104 in this village, elephantiasis of the legs of the advanced stage was found in five persons and the microfilariae of *B. malayi* in eight cases. The periodicity, as studied from microfilarial counts in six 10 mm^3 blood samples collected from five cases at two-hour intervals, was a typical nocturnally periodic form (SASA & TANAKA, 1972).

The occurrence of the new type of microfilariae of 'Timor-filaria' described by DAVID & EDESON (1965) from Portuguese Timor was also reported from the Indonesian part of Timor by OEMIJATI & TJOEN (1966) and OEMIJATI & PARTONO (1971). The following results were obtained by their surveys: 1) In Kupang, the capital of East Nusa Tenggara, 63 hospital patients were examined and one had the microfilariae of *W. bancrofti* and another had those of the Timor filaria; of 85 student nurses, 1 had *W. bancrofti* and another 2 had the Timor filaria. 2) Of 199 prisoners in Atambua, 2 showed *W. bancrofti* microfilariae and 7 showed the Timor microfilariae; of 86 prisoners in Kafamenanu, 2 had *W. bancrofti* and 1 had the Timor microfilariae. 3) In the survey of villages, the Timor microfilaria was found in 1 of 196 examined at Oepura, 1 of 119 examined at Oemanu, and 2 of 101 examined at Mananas, while the microfilariae of *W. bancrofti* were found in 25 of 200 examined at Fatumetan and 1 of 101 examined at Mananas. 4) In Wini, a small seaport in the north, 29 of 74 persons examined had microfilariae; 14 had those of *W. bancrofti* only, 1 had those of the Timor filaria only, and 14 had mixed infections. Patients showing elephantiasis, lymphoscrotum, and recurrent lymphadenitis with fever were common. 5) On the island of Rote, west of Timor, 22 of 90 persons examined had only the Timor microfilariae.

The periodicity of the Timor microfilariae examined in four carriers was shown to be a nocturnally periodic type with the peak at midnight or 4 a.m. The microfilariae showed a marked resemblance to those of *B. malayi*; the curves of the body are mostly angular, and the nuclei are densely packed. But the overall length was much longer (258 to 302 μ) than those of *B. malayi,* and the cephalic space was very long (length: width is 3 : 1).

KURIHARA & OEMIJATI (1975) reported on the occurrence of the Timor type of microfilaria in man on Flores Island. Blood samples (30 mm³) were collected on 20 December 1973, from 105 persons (47 males and 58 females) ranging in age from 10 to 88 years; 12 (8 males and 4 females) were positive for microfilariae (all the Timor type), with a positive rate of 11.4% (17.0% in males and 6.9% in females). Elephantiasis was seen in 14 cases (13.3%) and only 1 of these were positive for the microfilariae. The sheath of the microfilariae was not stained with Giemsa's solution, the cephalic space was longer than wide (2.5 to 3.3 : 1), the threadlike tail contained two nuclei, and the body lengths of 38 microfilariae were 279.93 μ in average (range, 261 to 314 μ; standard deviation, 14.5 μ).

8B.10 Timor

Portuguese Timor (as of 1974) occupies the eastern half of Timor Island in the Indonesian Archipelago, situated about 9°S and 125° to 128°E. Its area is 14,920 km² and its population is 610,541 (1970).

A study of filariasis in Portuguese Timor was carried out by FRAGA DE AZEVEDO *et al.* (1958). The occurrence of elephantiasis was reported in 1955, from 7 out of 23 districts, 73 cases in total, and especially high incidences were recognized in Manatuto (44 cases out of the whole population of 4,124), and Baucau (14 cases out of 13,700). Altogether, 3,350 persons in 29 localities were examined by looking for microfilariae in fresh blood collected by day, and 2% were found to be infected with *B. malayi*. Tests at night on 48 males showed 10.4% to be infected. The microfilaria carriers did not show any clinical signs. On the other hand, 103 cases of elephantiasis were found in three localities, with rates of 3.4% at Laleia, 1.9% at Manatuto, and 0.3% at Vemasse. However, it was not possible to attribute these cases to filarial infection.

DAVID & EDESON (1964, 1965) reported the occurrence of two types of microfilariae in the blood of the native people in Portuguese Timor. One was identified as *W. bancrofti*, while the other resembled the microfilariae of *B. malayi* but had constant differences; this was named "Timor microfilaria." A group of healthy young males aged 18 to 22 years, who were recruited from all over Portuguese Timor, were examined during the period from 1962 to 1964 by taking approximately 20 mm³ blood from 7 p.m. to 9 p.m.; of a total of 982 persons examined, Timor-microfilariae were found in 3.5%. In a later survey carried out during 1964, attempts were made to examine whole households. Of a total of 1,462 persons examined in ten areas, 108 (7.4%) had Timor-microfilaria only, 38 (2.6%) had *W. bancrofti* microfilaria only, and 25 (1.7%) had both; the former was found in all of the areas surveyed, with a highest rate of 15.3% (39 of 255) at Manatuto, while the latter was found in five of ten areas surveyed with a high rate of 18.7% (29 of 155) at Batugade, on the coast near the border with Indonesian Timor. Clinical filariasis cases were very rare, and only 17 elephantiasis cases were found in the whole area surveyed in 1964.

It was noted that the sheaths of some of the microfilariae of *W. bancrofti* stained a pale pink with Giemsa; this finding was in contrast to these authors' previous experiences with *W. bancrofti* from Malaya and Ceylon, where the staining of *W. bancrofti* sheaths was rare. The *W. bancrofti* appeared to be of the nocturnally periodic form.

The Timor-microfilariae in air-dried, Giemsa-stained films measured 287.0 μ in average (range of 265 to 323 μ), and are thus considerably longer than those of *B. malayi* (234.1 μ in average in the periodic form and 199.0 μ in the subperiodic form of Malaya. The tail ends in a threadlike process containing two caudal nuclei, resembling the tail nuclei of *Brugia* spp. microfilariae. Besides the difference in overall length, the Timor microfilariae differed from those of *B. malayi* in the ratio of length to width of the cephalic space (3 : 1 in the former and 2 : 1 in the latter), and in the failure of the sheath to stain with Giemsa. (For a detailed description of the microfilariae, see Section 2D.) The Timor-microfilariae are nocturnally periodic (see Section 11F.5). The Timor-microfilariae were found to be very susceptible to DEC treatment, and administrations at daily doses of 400 mg for seven days cleared the microfilariae from the circulating blood in all of 7 cases and that at 200 mg daily for seven days cleared the microfilariae in 9 of 12 cases. The febrile reaction was much less severe than that which occurred when carriers of *B. malayi* were treated.

8C. East Asia

8C.1 People's Republic of China

The area governed by the People's Republic of China includes eastern and central parts of the continent of Asia and a number of offshore islands, between latitudes 17°N to 58°N, and longitudes 74°E to 135°E. Its area is 10,256,330 km², with a population of 773,654,000 (1970). It is administratively divided into two municipalities, 21 provinces, and five autonomous regions.

8C.1.1 General epidemiology

Filariasis due to *W. bancrofti* and *B. malayi* was widely endemic in southern and central China, and the number of infected persons was probably the largest in the world except for India. Some historically important contributions about human filariasis, such as the discovery of microfilarial periodicity and of the transmission by mosquitoes, were made by the pioneering studies of MANSON, in 1878, in Amoy (Section 2B.1).

The occurrence of *B. malayi* infection in China was discovered by FENG (1933a), and the parasite was later found to be widely distributed. Extensive surveys and control activities were begun by the People's Government in 1953, and detailed information on the distribution and incidence of filariasis in China was later accumulated.

According to LI HUEI-HAN (1959b) and KUNG CHIEN-CHANG (1959), about 20 to 30 million Chinese people were affected by filariasis due to *Wuchereria bancrofti* and *Brugia malayi*. The former was widespread in the provinces of Shantung, Anhwei, Kiangsu, Chekiang, Fukien, Kwantung (including Hainan Island), Hunan, Hupeh, Honan, Kwangsi, Kweichow, and Szechuan. Provinces where *B. malayi* infection have been recorded are Kiangsu, Anhwei, Chekiang, Fukien, Kiangsi, Hunan, Hupeh, Honan, Kwangsi, Kweichow and Szechuan. In other words, both species are coendemic in at least 11 provinces, while only *W. bancrofti* occurs in the additional provinces, namely, Taiwan, Kwantung, and Shantung. The endemic areas extend from 18°N to 37.5°N in latitude.

In general, the endemic areas of filariasis are distributed along the coastal belt of southern and central China, and also along both banks of the Yangtse River. The incidence is usually higher in the rural areas than in the urban areas. Only the nocturnally periodic race has been found both in *W. bancrofti* and *B. malayi*. Besides the mosquitoes of the *Culex pipiens* complex, which are the most common vectors of *W. bancrofti* throughout South and East Asia, members of the *Anopheles sinensis* group have been shown to be the more important vectors of *W. bancrofti* in rice paddy areas.

The same group of anopheline mosquitoes have also been incriminated as the main vector of *B. malayi* in rural areas. In some coastal areas, *Aedes togoi* was found to act as the vector of *B. malayi* like in the coastal endemic areas in Japan and Korea.

8C.1.2 Historical notes

Some important contributions to the knowledge of human filariasis were made from China in the early stages of filariasis studies, especially noteworthy are those made by MANSON while staying in Taiwan from 1865 to 1870 and in Amoy from 1871 to 1883. In Taiwan and Amoy, Manson began to accumulate notes on enlarged groin glands, elephantiasis, and chyluria, with special reference to their interrelationships. Following the discovery of microfilariae in the blood of patients by LEWIS, in 1875, in Calcutta, MANSON made detailed studies on the mode of appearance of the microfilariae in a number of cases, and discovered their nocturnal periodicity in 1877. The next year, Manson published a note on the development of filarial larvae in the mosquito, *Culex fatigans*, which he called the "nurse." He further discovered in 1880 the adult filaria in a lymph scrotum in a Chinese patient, and confirmed the finding of BANCROFT in Australia. In 1881, he succeeded in reversing the nocturnal periodicity of the microfilariae by inducing his patient to sleep in the day and keep awake at night. These early contributions by MANSON were described in detail in the *China Maritime Customs Reports* (1872 to 1882) published from Shanghai (See Section 2B.1).

As for the epidemiology and distribution of filariasis in China, MANSON (1877) examined the blood of 670 persons at Amoy, and found microfilariae in 62, or 9.25%. Those who were examined were mostly the hospital patients randomly selected. Only ten of the filarial carriers were the residents of Amoy, and the rest were mainly from various parts of southern Fukien.

RENNIE (1881) examined the blood of 182 inpatients of a hospital in Foochow and found microfilariae in 25 (13.7%). Of these positive cases, 14 were from Futzing, 6 from Hinghwa, and 5 from Foochow.

WHYTE & CAMB (1909) conducted a detailed study in South China (Kwantung Province) on the relationship between the microfilarial periodicity and eosinophilia in six microfilaria carriers, and observed that the hour at which the maximum number of microfilariae in the blood was not, as had been often stated, always midnight, but that the number was often less at that hour than both earlier and later; furthermore, the degree of eosinophilia often corresponded with the number of microfilariae in the circulating blood.

JEFFERY & MAXWELL (1911), in their general accounts on the diseases of China, referred to the distribution and common occurrence of elephantiasis in southern China.

MAXWELL (1921) gave detailed accounts on the clinical aspects of filariasis in China based on 20 years of study carried out in Fukien Province while he was engaged in a medical mission. According to the author, the distribution of filariasis throughout China was somewhat peculiar, and roughly speaking, the infection did not spread north of the Yangtse Valley. Following the line of the Yangtse River west, the disease was found sporadically along both banks and also in Kweichow and southern Szechwan, getting less and less frequent as one ascended the river. Coming back to the coast from the mouth of the Yangtse down to the Tonkin border, there was a belt some 25 to 40 km broad, and the major portion of the disease was found in this coast belt; most of the islands off the coast were also infected, but not heavily. When one passed inland beyond this belt, the infection was practically lost, although occasionally a small patch of infection was found on the higher reaches of a river, for it tended to spread upward along the banks of all the rivers between the mouth of the Yangtse and the Tonkin border, but not to any considerable distance. Kiangsu was entirely free from the disease, and Fukien, away from the coast belt, was also uninfected.

The case incidence, according to MAXWELL (1921), varied with the region, and broadly speaking, increased towards the south. Taking a large hospital at about the middle of the coast belt (Changpu, Fukien), he found a percentage of 2.4 of filarial cases who came to the hospital for some diseases connected with the infection; but this did not represent the incidence of filarial infection in this region, and his figures gave a percentage of 24.8 of the general population infected with the parasite. Besides these figures, 3.39% of the general population showed no embryos in the blood but presented signs of old filarial disease, while 16.1% of another series were found, on microfilarial examination, to be infected, but presented no signs and no history.

The nature of the disease Maxwell saw in 260 hospital patients were: 48 cases of elephantiasis of the scrotum, 44 cases of lymph scrotum, 91 cases of elephantiasis of the leg, 33 cases of filarial abscess, 8 cases of filarial gangrene of the scrotum, 6 cases of lymphatic fistula, 4 cases of chyluria, and 26 cases of other filarial diseases. Of the 260 cases he examined, only 5 were women.

LEE (1926), in Peking Union Medical College, received information from a physician that a microfilaria carrier of *W. bancrofti* was seen in a native of Hsuchofu, Kiangsu Province, and that elephantiasis was occasionally seen in this region. He conducted a survey in Kiangsu, the province on the lower basin of the Yangtse. At a preliminary investigation of the distribution of elephantiasis in the Chinkiang area, it was noted that the disease had a patchy distribution and was more prevalent in regions north of the Yangtse River than on the southern side. A total of 363 persons were examined in Chinkiang for the presence of microfilariae in the blood, of whom 7 of 119 (5.9%) from Hsuchofu and 31 of 195 (15.9%) from the Tsing Kiang Pu district were found infected. Two of 33 immigrants from other provinces were also found positive, and one of them was a native of Shantung Province. He found only 4 cases of clinical filariasis in Hsuchofu, but discovered 17 cases of elephantiasis in Tsing Kiang Pu in a survey of the general population. He further found some microfilaria carriers and clinical cases in Suining and Szeyang, in the district between Hsuchofu and Tsing Kiang Pu, and assumed that filariasis was widely distributed in the whole part of Kiangsu Province lying north of Yangtse River. He also found 15 of 25 *C. pipiens* collected at a house in Tsing Kiang Pu to be infected, and noted that the microfilariae had nocturnal periodicity in two cases examined in this area.

FENG (1931a, b) conducted investigations on mosquito vectors of filariasis in the areas around Woosung, a small town on the southern side of the Yangtse River where the author found a high prevalence of bancroftian filariasis. The area was a lowland, surrounded by ditches and rice paddies, and was an ideal habitat for the breeding of *An. hyrcanus sinensis* and *C. tritaeniorhynchus*. *C. p. pallens* was rare in the rural areas, where elephantiasis of the legs was very common, whereas the town of Woosung had much less elephantiasis and more *C. p. pallens*. On examination of mosquitoes caught in houses, 9% of the houses in Woosung Town and 33% of the houses in the country villages had infected mosquitoes. Natural infection with filarial larvae was seen in 16% of *An. hyrcanus sinensis*, and 16% of the infected specimens contained mature larvae of *W. bancrofti*. About 13% of *C. p. pallens* caught in nature also harbored filarial larvae, but none of these were in the infective stage. Filarial larvae of only the early developmental stages were found in wild *C. tritaeniorhynchus*, *Armigeres obturbans* (= *Ar. subalbatus*), and *Ae. albopictus*. From these results, he concluded that *An. hyrcanus sinensis* was the principal vector of bancroftian filariasis in Woosung and probably along the whole Yangtse River Valley.

FENG (1933a) conducted a blood survey of prisoners in a prison in Amoy; of 161 persons examined, 22 (13.6%) were found positive for *W. bancrofti*, and a *B. malayi* carrier was also found among them, for the first time in China. The *malayi* carrier was from Wenchow, Chekiang. Of 22 *bancrofti* carriers, 13 were from the mainland of Fukien Province, 5 were from other provinces, and 4 were natives of Amoy. However, no elephantiasis cases were seen in the city of Amoy for the two months that Feng stayed there. On return to Peking, FENG examined old slides kept in his laboratory, and discovered a collection of 94 slides, all containing microfilariae of *malayi* only. These slides had been sent from Huchow, Chekiang Province, in 1929 for teaching purposes.

In Amoy and the nearby villages, FENG (1933a) found five species of mosquitoes to be common in houses: *C. p. fatigans*, *Ar. obturbans*, *Ae aegypti*, *Ae. albopictus*, and *An. minimus*. Natural infection with *bancrofti* larvae was found only in *C. fatigans*, with a rate of 9% (16 of 169) in the city and 15% (7 of 46) in the villages. He also found 5 of 205 *An. minimus* infected with filarial larvae of an undetermined species.

FENG (1933b) made comprehensive studies on the comparative anatomy of the microfilariae of *malayi* and *bancrofti* in China, and discovered a number of new characteristics useful in differentiating the two species. In this report, the author stated that *Microfilaria malayi* had been found very frequently in cases of filariasis in Huchow, Chekiang Province. FENG (1934) found that *An. hyrcanus sinensis* and *M. uniformis* in this district were the suitable intermediate hosts of *B. malayi*.

FENG & YAO (1935) reported on the results of blood examinations of 2,112 patients admitted to Huchow General Hospital. The microfilariae of *B. malayi* were found in 42 cases and those of *W. bancrofti* in 6 cases, of whom 4 cases were the mixed infections. Among them, those infected with *W. bancrofti*, including the 4 mixed infection cases, were all from the northern part of the district, namely Changhsing and Nanshun. The cases from all the other parts of the district situated south of Lake Taihu were infected with *B. malayi* only. The microfilarial periodicity observed six times in four *B. malayi* carriers in good physical condition was markedly nocturnal, but one tuberculous case, who was very much debilitated and whose sleeping habit was irregular, showed microfilariae in peripheral blood all through the day.

FENG (1936) conducted experimental infections of *An. hyrcanus sinensis* with *B. malayi*, and gave detailed accounts on the morphology of the larvae developing in the mosquito.

HU (1934) made an examination of blood smears of 146 prisoners at Paoshan, Kiangsu Province, and found microfilariae of *W. bancrofti* in 24 of 140 males and 3 of 6 females, with a positive rate of 18.5% (27 of 146 examined). Of 27 positives, 17 were the natives of Paoshan, and the other 10 were from eight other areas.

HU *et al.* (1937) conducted surveys of filariasis in the Foochow and Futsing regions. During the period from June to November 1936, 500 persons were examined for microfilariae at Foochow Christian Hospital. The thick smears were prepared from 10 p.m. to midnight. Of 367 inpatients examined, 23 (6.3%) were found with microfilariae in their blood, and 4 of 102 hospital staff, as well as 1 of 31 hospital servants, were also positive, with the total number of positives being 28 (5.6%) out of 500. Of these positive cases, 4 were *malayi* and the remaining 24 were *bancrofti* infections. Those who were infected with *malayi* were from Nanping, Fuan, Kienow, and Yuki, while those with *bancrofti* were 9 cases from Foochow, 6 from Futsing, 4 from Diongloh, and one each from Saipu, Mintsing, Yungtai, Pingtan, and Nanping.

The authors made a trip to the Futsing region for a survey of filariasis. In Futsing City, 151 persons were examined at a hospital and 12 (7.9%) were positive for *bancrofti*. Another 115 persons in the prison of this city were examined; 26 (22.6%) were found positive for *bancrofti*.

A survey was also made in the town of Lungtien, where they were informed that elephantiasis was common. Of 40 hospital patients examined, 3 (7.5%) were positive for *bancrofti*. The authors saw many cases of elephantiasis in the town and surrounding rural areas.

LIU (1937) reported on the results of a survey conducted in Changsha, an inland city and the capital of Hunan Province. Of 79 inpatients of Hsiang Ya Hospital examined, 2 cases (2.5%) were found positive for *B. malayi*. The author also reported that he had seen the infection of *B. malayi* in a patient suffering from marked elephantiasis of the scrotum who was a native of southern Hunan.

Such is an outline of the pre-World War II studies on human filariasis in China (excluding Taiwan). After World War II and especially since the communist government established control over mainland China in 1950, filariasis was taken up as one of the main targets of public health activities, and systematic studies on the epidemiology and control were begun. The outline of the achievements were published in 1959–1960 in the *Chinese Medical Journal* and other periodicals, but unfortunately no detailed reports are available about later contributions.

8C.1.3 Distribution and Incidence of Filariasis by the Provinces

8C.1.3.1 Shantung

According to Li Huen-Han (1959a), the Antifilariasis Bureau was established in Shantung Province in 1955, and surveys and control programs for filariasis were initiated. Among 123,121 persons in 52 counties, 8,787 (7.1%) were positive for the microfilariae of *W. bancrofti*. Cases with clinical signs, such as hydrocele and elephantiasis, were not uncommon. Over 6,000 cases in different endemic areas were treated with DEC by various dosage schemes. *Culex pipiens pallens* was incriminated as the main, or the only vector. In some experimental areas, antilarval measures (elimination of breeding places, spraying with BHC) and house spraying with DDT and BHC were also performed.

The distribution of filariasis in the southeastern coast region of Shantung was investigated by Ma *et al.* (1958). Provincial Antifilariasis Station, Shantung (1959) reported that 52 of 67 hsiens under survey were positive for filarial infection, and all the heavily infected ones were in the southern part. The microfilaria rates varied from 0.03% to 26.0%. All the microfilariae were those of *W. bancrofti*, except three cases who came from known endemic areas of *B. malayi*. In mosquito surveys conducted during 1956–57, 22 species were collected, among which 94% of adult collections were *C. p. pallens*. Of 5,873 adult mosquitoes belonging to six species dissected, only *C. p. pallens* was positive for infective larvae, and immature larvae were found in *An. sinensis*.

Yu Yuan *et al.* (1959) conducted mosquito surveys in 16 selected localities in Shantung Province; 25 species belonging to four genera were found, and of 1,924 mosquitoes dissected, only *C. p. pallens* was found to be infected with filaria larvae. The highest infection rate was 13.5% of Ssushui, Southern Shantung, and the lowest was 0.75% of Tsingtao.

8C.1.3.2 Anhwei

Both *W. bancrofti* and *B. malayi* are endemic (Li, 1959b). In a village in northern Anhwei, in 1958, 209 out of 1,009 blood specimens examined after administration of 25 to 100 mg of DEC contained microfilariae of *B. malayi* (KUNG & WANG, 1959).

8C.1.3.3 Kiangsu

The occurrence of elephantiasis and the relatively high incidence of microfilaria carriers in Chinkiang were noted by LEE (1926). HU (1934) examined the blood of prisoners in Paoshan, a town located about 12 miles north of Shanghai, and recorded 24 positives (17.1%) out of 140 males and 3 (50%) of 6 females. According to LI (1959b), the microfilaria rate varied from 5.8% to 17.8%. KUNG *et al.* (1959a), in a survey of Chentse Hsien, found that both *W. bancrofti* and *B. malayi* were prevalent in this region. Out of 2,377 villagers surveyed, 318 (13.4%) were found positive for microfilariae. Those with *bancrofti* only, *malayi* only, and mixed infections were 39.3%, 43.4%, and 17.3%, respectively. Malayan filariasis was more prevalent in the southern region of the peninsula, whereas the bancroftian type was endemic chiefly in the northeastern villages near Soochow.

HSU WEI-NAN (1958) conducted an investigation into filariasis in 6,736 persons at the Da Ma Dun Cooperative Farm in Kiangning, Kiangsu. The infection rate in the total number of persons was 5.9%, and 7.8% in males and 4.0% in females. Persons above 16 years of age showed the highest infection rate. After the age of 40 the incidence was the same in both sexes. *Culex pipiens pallens* had a wide distribution over the whole area, and the percentages of infected mosquitoes in three villages on the cooperative farm were 18.4, 12.23, and 8.53, respectively.

At Nanking Army Hospital, LI HUEI-HAN (1959b) stated that 2,049 patients were treated with DEC in 1955. CH'EN TZU-TA *et al.* (1959a, b) conducted a series of investigations on the treatment of filariasis with various dosage schedules using DEC, and stated that of 372 cases treated with intensive dosages, 330 were *W. bancrofti* carriers, 31 were *B. malayi* carriers, and 5 had a mixed infection.

8C.1.3.4 Hupeh

Both *W. bancrofti* and *B. malayi* are endemic, and apparently the latter is predominant. According to LI HUEI-HAN (1959b), the report in 1956 from Wuchang, Hupeh Province, stated that of 1,230 cases of malayan infection, 861 (70.5%) had simple, acute, inflammatory attacks and 363 (29.5%) had both inflammatory attacks and elephantiasis. WU (1959) conducted a survey of filariasis and its vectors from May to November 1957 at Tutitong, a village 30 km south of Wuchang. The infection rates, including cases of lymphangitis and elephantiasis, in two agricultural cooperatives with a total population of 1,074 were 49.00% and 34.18%. All the worms found were of the malayan type. Of 285 *An. sinensis*, 92 *C. tritaeniorhynchus*, and 144 *C. fatigans* dissected, the infection with filaria larvae was seen in 25.61%, 4.3%, and 2.1%, respectively; infective larvae were found only in *An. sinensis*, with a rate of 3.5%.

8C.1.3.5 Chekiang and Shanghai

The occurrence of many elephantiasis cases in Ningpo was noted by MEADOWS (1871). FENG & YAO (1935) examined 2,112 hospital patients in Huchow, and found 44 cases (22.1%) to be positive for microfilariae; 38 had the microfilariae of *B. malayi* only, 2 had those of *W. bancrofti* only, and 4 had both microfilariae.

MOMMA (1942a, b) conducted a series of blood surveys in order to find out the distribution of *B. malayi* and *W. bancrofti* infections in Chekiang and Kiangsu Provinces. At Tinghai on Chow-Shan Island, and at Huchow, south of Lake Taihu, *W. bancrofti* and *B. malayi* were found to be coendemic. In five towns of Chekiang located south of the Tsian-Tung River, i.e., at Ningpo, Chiangko, Chen, Shaohsing, Shiaoshang and Hsihsing Chen, all the microfilariae found were those of *B. malayi*. On the other hand, all the microfilariae found among the people examined at three towns in Kiangsu Province, i.e., Ihing, Nant'ung and Kunshan were those of *W. bancrofti*. The results are summarized in Table 8-9.

Table 8-9. A summary of the results of blood survey reported by MOMMA (1942a, b).

Province	Locality	No. examined	No. positive	Percent positive	Species of Mf.		
					W. banc.	*B. mal.*	Both
Chekiang	a. Ningpo	146	11	7.5	0	11	0
	b. Chiangko Chen	54	13	24.1	0	13	0
	c. Shaohsing	265	5	1.9	0	5	0
	d. Shiaoshang & e. Hsihsing Chen	310	10	3.2	0	10	0
	f. Tinghai	168	19	11.3	12	4	3
	g. Huchow	195	25	12.8	16	9	0
Kiangsu	h. Nant'ung	318	4	1.3	4	0	0
	i. Ihing	478	41	8.6	41	0	0
	j. Kunshan	196	7	3.6	7	0	0

CHANG *et al.* (1955, quoted by FAN *et al.*, 1957), in Chiashan, examined 2,631 hospital inpatients and staff members, and found microfilariae in 204 (7.8%); 161 had the microfilariae of *W. bancrofti*, 38 had those of *B. malayi*, and 5 had both microfilariae.

Both *W. bancrofti* and *B. malayi* were found to be endemic in the Ta-Chen Archipelago, offshore islands of Chekiang Province. The people on these islands were evacuated in February 1955, and some 18,000 refugees came to settle in Taiwan. Members of the Taiwan Antimalaria Research Institute in Chaochow examined 239 blood slides of the refugees and found 30 (12.5%) to be positive for *B. malayi*. Based on these findings, extensive blood surveys were conducted in Taiwan and the results from 58 scattered camps in southern Taiwan of the evacuees from Ta-chen were published by Wu & Huang (1955), and those referring to 49 refugee settlements in northern Taiwan were reported by Fan *et al.* (1957). In the former report, it was stated that a total of 8,848 persons were examined and 831 (9.4%) were positive for microfilariae, of whom those of *W. bancrofti* were found in 43, and those of *B. malayi* were found in 793 (both including 5 cases of mixed infection). The refugees were from 13 islands of Ta-chen, and the microfilaria rate according to the districts varied from 2.38% to 11.40%.

In the Pao-shan district of Shanghai, Hsieh *et al.* (1960) found 1,630 (1.3%) of 122,252 persons examined were positive for the microfilariae of *W. bancrofti*. In four villages in Chingpu, 4.1% of 7,379 persons were positive for the microfilariae of *B. malayi*. The Shanghai Antischistosomiasis Bureau (1959) reported the incidence of filariasis in the suburbs of Shanghai was 2 to 5%, and about 20% in some places. With the help of over 1,000 students, blood-smear examinations of 320,000 persons were conducted, in the eastern and northern suburbs and in Paoshan Hsien, and also mass blood examinations of 300,000 persons were carried out in Chianting Hsien. About 10,000 cases of filariasis were discovered in these two suburbs and two hsiens, and were treated accordingly, i.e., with a single dose of DEC on one night. Filariasis (and also malaria and ancylostomiasis) was said to be practically eliminated from these areas after two months of hard work.

8C.1.3.6 Hunan

Filariasis due to both *W. bancrofti* and *B. malayi* is endemic (Li Huei-han, 1959b). Fan & Hsu (1958) stated that 80 patients were examined at Changsha in 1937, and 2 were infected with *B. malayi*.

8C.1.3.7 Kweichow

Chin Ta-husiung *et al.* (1959) summarized the results of filariasis surveys in Kweichow Province. The disease was distributed in the eastern part of the province, where 27 hsiens were involved. The occurrence in the western part with high altitudes was not demonstrated. Endemic areas of filariasis could be divided into two sections with latitude 27°N as the boundary. In the northern section, filariasis due to *W. bancrofti* was prevalent, with the incidence varying from 10% to 20%. This area and some adjacent hsiens in Szechuan Province formed big endemic zone of bancroftian filariasis. The chief vector was *C. fatigans*, while *An. sinensis* and *C. tritaeniorhynchus* might play a secondary role, though no infective larva has ever been found in them. The southern part formed, with the neighboring hsiens of Kwangsi and Hunan Provinces, a large endemic zone of malayan filariasis, where *An. sinensis* was the chief vector. More than 10% of the population was infected, and the incidence might be as high as 30% to 50% in some villages. Mixed infection with *W. bancrofti* was occasional.

8C.1.3.8 Kiangsi

WANG CHIAO-PIAO *et al.* (1959) conducted a survey of two small villages in Tiehlu Hsiang of Fengch'eng Hsien, situated in a narrow valley surrounded by high mountains. There were ponds and irrigation ditches, and all the land was under rice cultivation. Of 614 persons in the two villages examined, microfilariae were found in 82 (13.4%), and clinical manifestations in an additional 52 persons, with a total of 134 cases (21.8%). The youngest filarial case was 13 months old. Of 82 cases with microfilariae, 69 contained those of *B. malayi* only, 8 with *W. bancrofti* only, and 5 had mixed infections. Investigation of those with microfilariae of *W. bancrofti* suggested they contracted the infection elsewhere. During this investigation, 13 species of mosquitoes were encountered, among which *An. sinensis* was the most common species occurring in human dwellings. Of 210 *An. sinensis* dissected, 9 (4.3%) were infected, and 2 (0.95%) contained infective larvae of *B. malayi. C. p. fatigans, C. tritaeniorhynchus,* and *Ar. obturbans* were negative for filarial infection.

8C.1.3.9 Szechuan

According to LI HUEN-HAN (1959b), both bancroftian and malayan filariasis were present, and the rate of infection was between 21.8% to 27.8%.

8C.1.3.10 Fukien

The historical studies by MANSON (1876–82) on bancroftian filariasis, including the discovery of the mosquito intermediate host and the microfilarial periodicity, were conducted in Amoy, where Manson found a high prevalence of the disease.

As previously stated, FENG (1933a) examined 161 prisoners in Amoy, and found 22 among them to be positive for microfilariae of *W. bancrofti*, and one for *B. malayi.* He also found *C. fatigans* and *An. minimus* infected with filarial larvae.

HU *et al.* (1937) examined 500 persons in a hospital in Foochow, and found 24 (4.8%) to be positive for *W. bancrofti* and 5 (1.0%) for *B. malayi.* In Futsing City, 12 (7.9%) of 151 hospital patients and 26 (22.6%) of 115 prisoners were positive for *W. bancrofti.* In Lungtien Town, 3 (7.5%) of 40 hospital patients showed microfilariae of *W. bancrofti.*

CHEN (1948) conducted blood surveys of the general population, hospital patients, and prisoners in several districts of Fukien, and demonstrated that both *W. bancrofti* and *B. malayi* were widely endemic.

LIN & CH'EN (1958) conducted epidemiological surveys of filariasis in and around the city of Foochow. The microfilariae of *W. bancrofti* were found in 9.11% (582 positives out of 6,391 persons examined) in the urban area, 7.40% (160 of 2,160) in the rural areas, and 5.24% (26 of 494) in the mountainous areas. As for the mosquito vectors, 74 (4.88%) of 1,514 *C. fatigans* dissected were found to be infected, and 9 (0.59%) among them had mature larvae, while none of the specimens of other mosquito species were infected. There was no correlation between the fluoride content of the drinking water or the incidence of mottled teeth and the incidence of filariasis among the villages surveyed. The absence of correlation between fluoridation and filariasis in areas around Foochow was further confirmed by LIN *et al.* (1959). This contradicted the report from India (SUBRAMANIAM, 1953) that filariasis was absent in areas with a high fluoride content in water, and that sodium fluoride was effective in the treatment of filariasis.

8C.1.3.11 Kwantung

According to LI HUEI-HAN (1959b), the microfilaria rate in Kwantung was 1 to 30%, and both *W. bancrofti* and *B. malayi* were present. CHU SHIH-HUEI *et al.* (1959a) conducted a detailed filariasis survey of Ts'unghua Town, about 56 km northeast of Canton, from 1956 to 1967. Altogether, 5,599 persons from six localities were examined, of whom the microfilariae of *W. bancrofti* were found in 666 (11.9%). Of 2,229 *C. fatigans* dissected, 10.5% were found to harbor filaria larvae of various stages.

CHU SHIH-HUEI *et al.* (1959b) reported on filariasis in Chung Hua Hsien, Kwantung. Altogether, 1,459 farmers were examined, and 415 (28.6%) were found to be positive for the microfilariae of *W. bancrofti*. The rate in the town of Tse Kao rose with the increase in age, and the highest microfilarial rate of 54.49% was found in the age-group 41 to 50 years. Among 1,134 *C. fatigans* dissected, 7.4% were found to be infected. As for the clinical signs, chyluria and involvements of the external genitalia were the chief signs; 58 cases had a history of chyluria, and only 2 cases had elephantiasis of the legs.

8C.1.3.12 Hainan Island

WANG YUNG-HSIANG (1959) carried out a survey of eight small villages of the Li Nationals in Paisha Hsien in the central part of Hainan Island. Of 580 persons examined, 129 (22.2%) had microfilariae of *W. bancrofti* in the blood. The positive rates of the various villages ranged from 13.3 to 47.4%. Though the microfilarial rates were not too low, there seemed to be no cases of elephantiasis or chyluria, and the local people did not know about these conditions. Eight species of *Anopheles*, one species of *Culex*, and one species of *Armigeres* were collected from human dwellings. Upon dissection, only *An. minimus*, *An. jeyporiensis candinensis*, and *An. leucosphyrus* were found to be infected, and infective larvae were encountered in all of these three mosquito species. *An. minimus* constituted about 90% of all mosquitoes found inside houses.

8C.1.3.13 Kwangsi

According to HAWKING (1973), both *W. bancrofti* and *B.malayi* apparently occur here. In Paochiangtun and neighboring villages of Lungsheng, the filarial index (microfilaria rate plus disease) was 38.6%.

8C.1.4 Vectors of filariasis in China

In the transmission of *W. bancrofti*, *Culex pipiens* s.l. is considered to be the most common and important vector throughout China. In certain rice paddy areas, mosquitoes of the *An. sinensis* group have also been shown to be an important vector. In South China, some tropical anopheline species were found to be involved in the transmission. The transmission of *B. malayi* in rural areas in China is accomplished mainly by *An. sinensis*, while *Ae. togoi* was incriminated as the principal vector in some coastal villages.

(a) *Culex pipiens* Linnaeus, s.l.

As in Japan, three ill-defined races of the *C. pipiens* complex are considered to be occurring in China: *C. p. fatigans*, a tropical and anautogenous race in southern China; *C. p. pallens*, an anautogenous race in the Temperate Zone; and *C. p. molestus*, an autogenous race. The first two races were shown to act as excellent vectors of *W. bancrofti* in various regions of China.

The development of filarial larvae in this species was first shown by MANSON (1878), in Amoy, South China. Natural infections of filaria larvae were observed by LEE (1926) in Kiangsu, by FENG (1933a) in Amoy, and by JACKSON (1936) in Hong Kong. As reviewed by LI (1959b), extensive entomological surveys were conducted from 1953 under the national filariasis control program of China; natural infection rates of *W. bancrofti* were found in 16.2% of *C. p. pallens* in the Choushan Islands from 1953 to 1954, 12% at Chentse in Kiangsu in 1957, 43.6% at Hsin Village in Hsueh-ch'chen, 49.9% at Chia Village, and 31.9% at Wu Village in Tsouhsuen in Shantung Province. In 1957, a further survey of 14 hsiens in Shantung showed a natural infection rate of 16.9%. In an artificial infection experiment, more efficient development of the larvae of *W. bancrofti* was seen in *C. p. pallens* than in *An. sinensis*.

As for *C. p. fatigans* which occur in South China, LI (1959b) recorded natural infections in 4.88% examined in Fukien Province, and 12.4% in Kwangtung Province. The infection rate by artificial infection was 94.5%.

Both *C. p. pallens* in the Choushan Islands and *C. p. fatigans* in Kwangsi were shown to be inhospitable for the development of *B. malayi* (LI 1959b).

(b) *Anopheles sinensis* Wiedemann, 1828

FENG (1931) observed at Woosung, a rural village on the southern side of the Yangtse River surrounded by rice paddies, that *An. sinensis* was the most common mosquito found in houses; 16% of them were naturally infected with larvae of *W. bancrofti,* and 16% among the infected mosquitoes had mature larvae. FENG (1934) further found that this species was the principal vector of *B. malayi* in Huchow of Chekiang Province. LI (1959b) recorded natural infection rates with *W. bancrofti* of 14.3% in the Chou-shan Islands from 1953 to 1954, 9.22% at Chentse in 1957, and 8.5% in 14 hsiens in Shantung Province in 1957. The natural infections with the *B. malayi* larvae in this species was 67.7% of 130 specimens collected in the Choushan Islands from 1953 to 1954, and 43.9% of 41 specimens collected at Lungsheng, Kwangsi Province. Positive findings with infective stage larvae were also obtained in Hunan Province and Kweichow Province.

Two races (or species) differing in the morphology of eggs were recognized within the *An. sinensis* group in China; one with a wide-decked egg (wide form, *An. sineisis* Wiedemann) and another with the narrow-decked egg (narrow form, or *An. lesteri* Baisas & Hu). Both races were hospitable for the development of *B. malayi* larvae (KUNG, 1959). At Hangchow, Chekiang Province, natural infections with *B. malayi* larvae were seen in 41 % of the former and 61 % of the latter race (Li, 1959b).

(c) Other anophelines

Mosquitoes of the genus *Anopheles* other than the *sinensis* group are probably important vectors of filariasis in South China. For example, WANG (1959), KUNG (1959), and LI (1959b) found *An. minimus* and *An. jeyporiensis candinensis* naturally infected in a survey conducted at Paisha, Hainan Island, in 1957.

(d) *Aedes (Finlaya) togoi* (THEOBALD, 1907)

LI (1959b) and GUN (1960) reported that *Ae. togoi* in the Choushan Islands were naturally infected with both *B. malayi* and *W. bancrofti,* and also that it was an excellent intermediate host of both filariae under experimental conditions. This mosquito breeds in brackish water and is found only within 3 to 5 km along the seacoast.

(e) *Mansonia uniformis* (THEOBALD, 1901)

This is an important vector of *B. malayi* in South Asia. In China, FENG (1934) demonstrated that both *M. uniformis* and *An. sinensis* were suitable vectors of *B. malayi* in Chekiang. LI (1959b) reported that 11 of 632 specimens dissected in the Choushan Islands were found infected, but none of them had mature larvae. Because of its restricted distribution in China, he concluded that *M. uniformis* is a minor vector.

8C.1.5 Control

According to LI (1959b), the People's Government has made a resolute attack on diseases since liberation, and the Institute of Parasitic Diseases of the Chinese Academy of Medical Sciences was charged with the duty of training large numbers of physicians and health workers to specialize in the control of parasitic diseases. Since 1953, numerous control and research institutions for parasitic diseases and filariasis have been established in Shantung, Kiangsu, Anhwei, Kwangsi, Hupeh, Fukien, and many other provinces.

According to LI (1959b), a course of 7 to 10 days of treatment with 200 mg of DEC has been utilized as a standard in endemic areas in Kiangsu, Chekiang, Hunan, Hupeh, Kiangsi, Anhwei, and Shantung Provinces. With this treatment schedule, it was observed by the Nanking Army Hospital that clearance of bancroftian microfilariae occurred in 87.1 % of the cases studied, and the cure rate after 11 to 17 months was 92.9 %. The action of DEC on *B. malayi* carriers was even more pronounced. In Shantung Provincial Institute for the Control of Filariasis, 85.3% of 153 *W. bancrofti* carriers treated with the above schedule (200 mg, three times a day for seven days) became negative by the end of treatment, and a cure rate of 70.2% was obtained in examinations of 151 patients. About half of the patients treated with DEC developed reactions, such as chills and headache, but none of the reactions were important enough to confine the patients to bed.

Especially noteworthy are the extensive studies by Chinese workers on the use of DEC in the treatment and control of filariasis. (LI, 1959b; KUNG & WANG, 1959; CH'EN *et al.*, 1959a, b; LI *et al.*, 1959; CH'EN, 1964). Among various dose regimens tested, a method of administration of DEC in a large single dose was recommended by some workers. For example, the EPIDEMIC PREVENTION DEPARTMENT OF FUKIEN (1959) tested a method of administration of DEC by a single dose of 1 g, or a total dose of 1.5 g divided into two doses. In the single dose treatment at night, the microfilariae disappeared in 92% of 15,914 cases in Nanp'ing region. As to the remote result of the treatment, observations in Minch'ing showed that the microfilariae disappeared from the blood in 93.4% immediately after the treatment, and in 96.6% of 90 cases re-examined three months later. HSIEH *et al.* (1960), in Shanghai, also gave 1 g of DEC in a single dose to adult patients, and obtained a clearance rate of 82.8% in 154 *B. malayi* cases and that of 60.4% in 708 *W. bancrofti* cases.

LI (1959b), in a conclusion, stated:

> Through the investigations and numerous surveys on filariasis carried out since liberation in many provinces throughout China, we have obtained a good knowledge of the degree of endemicity, the main mosquito vectors, and the epidemiology of the disease. The achievements during the past nine years in the treatment and prevention of the disease have laid a firm foundation for the eradication of filariasis. Many provinces have already trained large numbers of personnel to fight the disease. Extensive work on filariasis case surveys and extermination of mosquito carriers has been carried out, and up to the present filariasis has been basically eradicated in 38 *hsiens*. Under the leadership of the Chinese Communist Party and through the efforts of the great masses of the people, we have full faith that the disease can be practically eradicated throughout the country before the end of 1959.

An important report on the mode of action of DEC, antimony, and arsenic compounds as macrofilaricides was published by CH'EN (1964). In trial experiments for the treatment of filariasis with DEC and some antimony and arsenic compounds, it was demonstrated that these drugs could kill adult filaria worms when sufficient doses were administered under appropriate dosage regimens. Special nodules were found to be formed after treatment with the drugs, from which dead adult worms of *W. bancrofti* and *B. malayi* were demonstrated many times by surgical removal and dissection. In 1954, it was also shown that a short intensive administration of DEC was effective in the treatment of filariasis (see 2B.5.2), and beginning this year, DEC was produced on a large scale in this country.

There were "only 16 deaths" among several millions of cases given mass therapy since 1953. The causes of death were pulmonary edema, pharyngeal edema, bronchopneumonia, and a cerebral type of subtertian malaria in two cases each; high fever with collapse in four cases; and toxic hepatitis, heart failure, acute colitis, and unknown in one case each.

8C.2 Taiwan and Adjacent Islands

Taiwan (Formosa) is an island off Fukien Province, situated between latitudes 21.8°N to 25.4°N, and longitudes 120°E to 122°E. It has an area of 35,970 km² with a population of 14,810,929 (1971). Taiwan (including the Pescadores and some adjacent islands) was ceded from China to Japan in 1895, returned to China after World War II, and became the seat of the Chinese Nationalist Government in 1949. Besides the mainland of Taiwan, the Pescadores, the Kinmen Islands (Quemoy Islands), and the Matsu Archipelago situated in the Taiwan Strait are also under administration of the Chinese Nationalist Government.

It is rather strange that the mainland of Taiwan is practically free from indigenous filariasis, though a small focus was discovered recently from near Tainan City. However, the problem of imported filariasis among large numbers of evacuees from the mainland China is a great concern to the health workers. Indigenous filariasis due to *W. bancrofti* in the Pescadores has been noted since the islands were under Japanese control. Filariasis in the Quemoy and Matsu Islands is also discussed in this section, because these were surveyed by workers under the Nationalist Government.

8C.2.1 Main Island of Taiwan

The main island of Taiwan was considered to be free from indigenous filariasis until FAN & HSU (1955) reported on endemic foci of *W. bancrofti* in southern Taiwan, especially at Hsinhua, about 8 km east of Tainan City, where 134 (1.63%) of 8,210 persons examined were positive for the microfilariae, and 27 (0.33%) had clinical filariasis symptoms.

In connection with the Civil War between the communist and the nationalist regimes, large numbers of soldiers and civilians from various regions of mainland China moved and settled in Taiwan from 1949 to 1955, many of them carrying *W. bancrofti* and/or *B. malayi*. For example, 24,780 military personnel in Taiwan, Kinmen, and Penghu were examined from 1951 to 1954, and 1,151 (4.64%) among them were found to be carrying microfilariae, 740 with *W. bancrofti,* 369 with *B. malayi,* and 42 with both species. (FAN & HSU, 1963). In the examination of evacuees from the

Ta-Chen Islands of Fukien, WU & HUANG (1955) found 38 carriers of *W. bancrofti* microfilariae, 788 carriers of *B. malayi* microfilariae, and 5 carriers of both species out of a total of 8,848 persons examined in 58 refugee camps in southern Taiwan, with the overall positive rate of 9.4%. FAN *et al.* (1957) examined the evacuees from Ta-Chen in 49 refugee settlements in northern Taiwan, and found 13 carriers of *W. bancrofti* microfilariae and 347 carriers of *B. malayi* microfilariae out of 5,335 persons.

8C.2.2 Pescadores

The Pescadores (Penghu Islands) are an archipelago consisting of about 48 islands, situated between Taiwan and mainland China, at about 23°N. They have a total area of about 127 km² and a population of 82,785 (1954).

The occurrence of filariasis in the Pescadores was reported by GOTO & HARAYO (1919). TANAKA (1937) examined 229 Chinese dockyard laborers at Makung Navy Base, and found 27 (16.2%) to be positive for the microfilariae of *W. bancrofti*. YOKOGAWA *et al.* (1939) conducted a survey of filariasis in four villages, and found 126 positive cases (7.8%) out of a total of 1,608 persons examined; the positive rates according to the villages were 10.8% in Huhsi, 11.5% in Kongti, 7.4% in Watung, and 2.3% in Hokaito.

After World War II, FAN & HSU (1953) conducted epidemiological surveys of 13 villages on Makung, Peihsa, and Hsiyu Islands, and found 218 (14.3%) to be positive for the microfilariae of *W. bancrofti* out of a total of 1,529 persons examined. The microfilaria carriers were distributed to all the villages surveyed. Results of statistical analysis of the data were reported further by FAN & HSU (1957a). DEMOS *et al.* (1954) conducted a survey of Huhsi Village, and found 17 (17.7%) of 96 persons examined to be positive for the microfilariae of *W. bancrofti*.

8C.2.3 Kinmen Islands

Kinmen (or Quemoy) Islands are located close to Amoy Island and to the shore of Fukien. They consist of Kinmen Proper, Little Kinmen, and two other islets. Kinmen Proper lies at about 25.26°N and 118.04°E, has an area of 160 km².

A survey of filariasis in five villages in Kinmen Proper (Ta-Kinmen) and two villages in Little Kinmen (Shiao-Kinmen) was conducted in 1952 by FAN & HSU (1954, 1957b). In the five villages of Kinmen Proper, 1,163 out of the total population of 2,203 were examined, and 238 (20.5%) were found to be positive for the microfilariae of *W. bancrofti*. In the two villages of Little Kinmen, 260 of the total population of 417 were examined, and 34 (14.0%) were positive for the microfilariae of *W. bancrofti*.

A more detailed epidemiological survey was reported by FAN *et al.* (1972, 1973) and WANG & FAN (1973). Bancroftian filariasis was shown to be prevalent among the Kinmen Chinese, with a microfilarial rate of 10% in average, an average microfilarial density of 17 per 20 mm³ blood, a clinical rate of 12%, a mosquito infection rate of 10%, and an average of 5.6 larvae per infected mosquito. It was thus estimated that about 7,000 out of the total population of 60,000 would have clinical manifestations in different degrees.

Based on these data, a five-year filariasis control project was organized in 1972 to cover the Kinmen Islands, and a detailed report was published by FAN *et al.* (1974a). In the present survey, a total of 20,018 persons in 55 villages of four townships were examined, and microfilariae were found in 1,764 (8.8%); clinical manifestations were found in 282 (19.2%) of 1,470 persons examined. The microfilarial rates according to the townships were 10.9% (1,038 positives out of 9,522 persons examined) in Kinnin, 7.5% (104 of 1,385) in Kincheng, 6.1% (482 of 7,843) in Kinhu, and 11.0% (140 of 1,268) in Liehyu. The age and sex distribution of the microfilarial rates and the densities per 20 mm³ blood were also demonstrated. The microfilarial rate, the average density, and the clinical filariasis rate in 9,522 civilians in 21 villages were 10.9%, 17.7, and 21.5%, respectively, while those in 2,428 soldiers stationed in nearby camps were 0.1%, 26.3, and 0%, respectively. In the latter, microfilaria carriers numbered only three, two were Kinmen Chinese and one was from the mainland; all of 1,832 Taiwanese soldiers were negative.

Entomological surveys were conducted in 43 villages in the Kinmen Islands during the period from August 1972 to April 1973. In the collection of mosquitoes resting inside houses, a total of 4,717 specimens were identified, among which the most abundant was *C. p. fatigans* (3,893, or 81.4%). Of 330 *C. p. fatigans* collected during the warmer season from August to December and dissected 5 to 16 days after capture, 35 (10.6%) were found infected, and 27 (8.1%) contained mature larvae of *W. bancrofti*. Of 614 *C. p. fatigans* collected during the winter season from February to April and dissected 3 to 22 days later, 43 (7.0%) were infected and only 11 (1.8%) among them had mature larvae. Extensive surveys of breeding places of *C. p. fatigans* and other mosquito larvae were conducted, and fenitrothion (Sumithion) was sprayed as a mosquito larvicide at a rate of 0.2 g per m². In the unsprayed area, 9.5% (337 of 3,548) of the potential breeding sites were positive for mosquito larvae and pupae, while in the sprayed area, only 0.7% (59 of 8,166) of the similar possible breeding sites contained mosquito larvae (they were all immature larvae and none contained fourth instar larvae or pupae).

A drug treatment program was implemented on microfilaria carriers detected in the blood surveys conducted on the Kinmen people. Two different dosage regimens were tested: a ten-day treatment course (200 mg on the first day, 300 mg on the second day, 400 mg on the third day, 500 mg on the fourth day, 600 mg on the fifth to the tenth days, for 5 g in total), and a twelve-day treatment course (100 mg on the first day, 200 mg on the second day, 300 mg on the third day, 400 mg on the fourth day, and 500 mg each on the fifth to twelfth days, also 5 g in total). There were no significant differences in the efficacy between the two schedules, since the cure rate was 82.3% in the former and 80.3% in the latter, and the microfilaria reduction rate was 94.9% in the former and 97.3% in the latter. However, the rate of persons with some side reactions was 63.9% in the latter, significantly lower than the 85.5% of the former. The number and percent of *C. p. fatigans* containing all stages of larvae and mature stage larvae were 52 (11.9%) and 46 (10.5%) of 438, respectively, in a survey conducted before the drug administration; both fell to 15 (2.2%) and 6 (0.1%), respectively, of 680 female *C. p. fatigans* collected and dissected after the microfilaria carriers were treated with DEC.

Fan *et al.* (1974b) reported on the results of clinical investigations of filariasis on the Kinmen Islands. Physical examinations combined with blood examinations at night were carried out on a group of 1,708 villagers in September 1971. Clinical manifestations were seen in 205 (12.0%), microfilariae of *W. bancrofti* were found in 291 (17.0%), and 423 persons (24.7%) had either clinical manifestations or microfilaremia, or both.

8C.2.4 Matsu Archipelago

The Matsu Archipelago is situated about 17 km off southeast coast of Fukien at about 120°E and 26°N. The total land area is 34 km² and the population is 10,358 (1954 census). The people are living in 39 villages on five islands.

A survey of filariasis was conducted by Fan & Hsu (1957c) during December 1953 and January 1954 in eight villages on three islands. In the four villages on Nankan Island, 347 persons out of the total population of 2,488 were examined, and 32 (9.2%) were positive for the microfilariae. In the two villages on Peikan Island, 200 persons of the total population of 846 were examined, and 24 (12.0%) were positive. In the two villages on Paikan Island, 64 of 987 were examined, and 15 (23.4%) were positive. All the microfilariae were those of *W. bancrofti*. The overall microfilaria rate was 11.6% (71 positives out of 611 persons examined).

8C.3 Hong Kong

Hong Kong is a British Crown Colony situated at about 22.5°N and 114°E, 145 km south of Canton. It has an area of 1,030 km² with a population of 3,950,000 (1971). It is a commercial and industrial center in Southeast Asia, highly urbanized, with most of the people living in high-story buildings.

Because Hong Kong is surrounded by filariasis endemic areas, it is presumed that the infection occurs at least among the large numbers of immigrants from China, but no recent information is available. The only record on filariasis in Hong Kong is as follows.

Jackson (1936) reported on filarial infection in man and mosquitoes in

Hong Kong. The author, while engaged in the investigation of malaria in Hong Kong as the Government Malaria Officer, encountered microfilariae in a number of specimens taken for examination for malaria. In one survey a total of 3,733 thick blood smears were taken at about 10 a.m. during the period from 1933 to 1935 from prisoners admitted to Victoria Goal; 45 (1.21%) were positive for *W. bancrofti* and 63 (1.69%) were positive for malaria. Also, in June 1932, the author examined thick blood smears taken at night from 106 inhabitants of Little Hong Kong, and found 13 (12.3%) to be positive for *W. bancrofti* microfilariae. However, clinical cases seemed to be rather rare in Hong Kong, and the number of filarial cases reported from all of the government hospitals in Hong Kong was 2 in 1932, none in 1933, 4 in 1934, and 7 in 1935. Natural infections with filarial larvae were seen in 59 of 2,432 *An. minimus,* 5 of 165 *An. jeyporiensis candinensis,* and 6 of 442 *C. fatigans* dissected during 1932. In experimental infections, full development of the larvae was seen in *C. fatigans, An. hyrcanus sinensis, An. minimus, An. maculatus,* and *Ae. togoi.*

8C.4 Korea

Korea consists of a peninsula on the east coast of Asia and a number of adjacent islands. It is divided at present, by the 38°N parallel into South Korea (the Republic of Korea), which has an area of 98,440 km² and a population of 29,207,856 (1966), and North Korea (Democratic People's Republic of Korea), which has an area of 120,670 km² and a population of 14,000,000 (1970).

Human filariasis has been recorded only from South Korea. Endemic areas of *B. malayi* are found mainly in three regions, i.e., Cheju Island and some nearby islands in the southern coastal district, Nonsan and some other localities along the Keum-gang River, and the Yongju area of Kyongsang-buk-Do Province. Although there were some pre-World War II records on the occurrence of *W. bancrofti* filariasis from Korea, these were probably misdiagnoses of *B. malayi* filariasis, and all the microfilariae found in man in various endemic areas in Korea by recent workers have been identified as those of *B. malayi.* The main vector on Cheju Island is *Ae. togoi,* while that in the peninsular regions is probably *An. sinensis,* the same as in the continental regions of China.

8C.4.1 Historical notes on pre-War studies

The first record of the occurrence of filariasis in Korea is probably a case report prepared by YUN (1927), who described the pathology of an autopsy case of a 29-year-old male patient with elephantiasis of both legs, who contracted the disease in Chung Cheong Nam-Do and died at Kyoto University Hospital in Japan. The author gave detailed accounts on the pathological changes of various organs, and stated that he found a male worm of *W. bancrofti* in an inguinal gland.

OH (1929) reported on finding filariasis in Korea. The author had observed microfilariae in the blood of 24 cases, all natives of Korea; of these, 20 were carriers of *Filaria bancrofti*, and the other 4 cases were, according to the author, those of *Filaria perstans*, because the microfilariae of the latter cases had no sheath and showed no periodicity. Twelve of the 24 cases were apparently healthy, and the rest had filarial disease manifestations. One male and three female adult filariae were recovered from a cyst on the left arm of a patient. The cases were from 12 different localities of southwestern regions of the Korean Peninsula.

MOON (1939a) conducted an epidemiological survey of endemic elephantiasis which he found to be prevalent among people in areas around Nonsan Gun and Buyeo Gun of Chung Cheong Nam-Do, The disease is called "Shunchuntari" or "pittun," by the local people, and the frequent attack of fever associated with inflammation is called "pinarim" or "tari-shungsung." A total of 161 cases (137 males and 24 females) were examined by the author, and detailed accounts on the clinical histories and disease manifestations are described. Age distribution of the onset of the disease was shown in the table. More males than females were affected, and 159 (98.9%) of 161 cases were farmers working in rice paddies. The seasonal distribution of the onset, as well as the recurrence of the fever attack, was highly associated with the labor for rice cultivation, highest in October at the time of harvest, next in August at the time of weeding, and then in June at the time of rice planting. Blood examinations of the people were not conducted. In a conclusion, the author pointed out that endemic elephantiasis in South Korea was different from that associated with filariasis known from Japan and China, since it was confined to only the lower legs or forearms, and no cases with involvements of the genital or urinary systems were seen in this area.

MOON (1939b) further conducted clinical and epidemiological studies on endemic elephantiasis on Cheju Island after he was informed of the occurrence of a disease similar to that found in South Korea by a health worker stationed on this island. While staying on the island in January 1939, he collected general information about the disease, and examined 26 elephantiasis cases from various villages. He found them to be clinically identical with those found in South Korea. It was noted that the disease was prevalent in villages along the southeast coast of the island, involving some 5 to 10% of all the villagers, rather rare in other coastal villages, and absent from the inland areas. He postulated various factors as possible causes of the disease, but could not come to a definitive conclusion. He pointed out that the disease in South Korea was associated with rice cultivation, but since there were no rice paddies on this island, it was difficult to discover a common factor causing the same disease. This report is probably the first record of endemic elephantiasis on Cheju Island, but this group of workers did not make blood surveys.

The occurrence of *Microfilaria malayi* Brug in Korea was reported first by SENOO (1943), and detailed descriptions of the results of blood surveys conducted by Senoo from 1942 to 1944 in southern Korea were published by SENOO & LINCICOME (1951). Thirteen villages in southwestern Korea, eight villages in southeastern Korea, and four villages on Cheju Island were randomly selected without regard for the endemicity of the disease. Of a total of 5,001 persons examined, 604 (12.1 %) were found to be positive for microfilariae of *B. malayi*, and none of them were found to be carrying the microfilariae of *W. bancrofti*. *B. malayi* carriers were found in all of the four villages on the Island, where the overall microfilaria rate was 26.6% (268 positives out of 971 persons examined; 26.5%, or 155 of 585 males, and 26.7%, or 103 of 386 females). In southwestern Korea, four villages in South Ch'ungchong Do, five villages in North Cholla Do, and four villages in South Cholla Do were surveyed, and microfilaria carriers were found in all the villages; the overall microfilaria rate was 11.2% (285 positives of 2,548), or 11.8% (160 of 1,352) in males and 10.5% (125 of 1,196) in females. In southeastern Korea, five villages in North Kyongsang Do and three villages in South Kyongsang Do were surveyed; significant numbers of microfilaria carriers were found only in Togyedong Village where 27.0% (55 of 204) were positive. The other villages in this survey were completely or nearly free from the infection; the overall positive rate in the southeastern region was 4.1% (61 positives of 1,428 persons examined). From these results, malayan filariasis was found to be prevalent on Cheju Island and in the southwestern region of Korea.

8C.4.2 Filariasis on Cheju Island

Cheju (Quelpart) is an island located south of the Korean Peninsula at about 33.5°N and 127°E. It has an area of 1,792 km² and a population of 281,662 (1960 census). The island is mostly rocky and mountainous and has only small plain areas. There are numerous rock pools along the coast and in the river and stream beds, which serve as ideal breeding places for *Ae. togoi*, the main local vector of *B. malayi*. The island is notorious for the high incidence of elephantiasis due to *B. malayi*, and reports have been made on its epidemiology by MOON (1939b), HUNTER *et al.* (1949), SENOO & LINCICOME (1951), LEE (1961), SONG *et al.* (1964), LEE *et al.* (1964, 1965), SOH (1965), SEO *et al.* (1965, 1966), MOON (1968), KOH *et al.* (1971), KATA-MINE *et al.* (1971), KOH (1972), SEO *et al.* (1973), and SEO & KANG (1973).

HUNTER *et al.* (1949) carried out epidemiological surveys of parasitic infections in southern Korea, and reported that 2 of 35 blood specimens examined on Cheju Do Island were positive for *B. malayi*, but 23 examinations for filariasis on the mainland of Korea were negative.

LEE (1961) examined 229 children under 15 years old (132 boys and 97 girls) from six villages on Cheju Island and found microfilariae of *B. mala-yi* in 26 (11.4%) of both sexes, 11 (8.3%) boys, and 15 (15.5%) girls. Positive cases were found from 5 of 6 villages surveyed. The rates according to age-groups and sex was 4.2% (3 positives out of 71 examined) in boys and 2.6% (1 of 39) in girls for the age-group 0 to 4 years, 12.2% (5 of 41) in boys and 20.5% (9 of 44) in girls for the age-group 5 to 9 years, and 15.0% (3 of 20) in boys and 35.7% (5 of 14) in girls for the age-group 10 to 14 years. The girls showed significantly higher rates than the boys except for the age-group 0 to 4 years.

LEE *et al.* (1964), in 1960, surveyed Wimi-Ri Village, Nam-Cheju-Kun, on the southern coast of Cheju Island. Of a total population of 1,776, 356 persons (200 males and 156 females) were examined, and the microfilariae of *B. malayi* were found in 22.2% of the total persons examined, and in 20.5% of the males and 24.4% of the females. Elephantiasis was seen in 53 cases, or 2.98% of the whole population of 1,776, and in 1.96% (16 cases) of 815 males and 3.89% (37 cases) of 951 females.

According to SOH (1965), the same village was surveyed again in 1965, after five years. Among a total of 73 persons examined both times, 11 among the previously negative cases became microfilaria positive at the second examination, and 2 among the previously positive cases developed elephantiasis and became negative for the microfilariae. The other 15 previously positive cases remained microfilaria positive at the second examination.

KATAMINE *et al.* (1971) presented a summary of a joint study between Korean and Japanese workers on the epidemiology of filariasis on Cheju Island. A village (Wimi) situated near the coast with a population of 1,700 was selected for the study. Blood examinations were conducted on 1,059 persons, of whom 221 (20.9%) were found to be positive for *B. malayi* microfilariae, and 78.9% were skin test positive. The villagers residing in the zone within 300 m from the coast showed higher microfilaria and skin test rates than those residing inland of the zone (26.0%:23.0% in the microfilaria rate, 30:10 in the median microfilaria density, and 85%:75% in skin test). The percentage ratios (coastal:inland) of patients showing clinical signs were 30.4%:20.6% for the fever attack, 17.0%:7.2% for lymphangitis, and 4.4%:1.6% for elephantiasis. Altogether, 12 species of mosquitoes were collected and examined, among which 4 species, *C. p. pallens* (72.9% of the total), *Ae. togoi* (24.4%), *Ae. albopictus*, and *Ar. subalbatus* were found inside houses. The infection with filaria larvae was seen in 27 (8.8%) of 308 *Ae. togoi* dissected, among which 5 mosquitoes contained mature larvae, while only 2 of 504 *C. p. pallens* were infected with first stage larvae. In conclusion, malayan filariasis in this area is transmitted mainly by *Ae. togoi*, which breeds in tide pools on the beach, and the incidence is highest among people residing in areas closest to the beach.

SEO *et al.* (1973; abstract only) made an observation on the periodicity of *B. malayi* microfilariae in nine carriers on Cheju by counting the numbers of microfilariae found in 30 mm^3 blood samples collected at two-hour intervals over a period of 24 hours. In average, the peak count was seen at 1:30 a.m. and the ratio between the maximum and the minimum count was 8.07. It was concluded that *B. malayi* on Cheju is a nocturnally periodic strain similar to that reported from Penang by TURNER & EDESON (1957).

SEO & KANG (1973; abstract only) made a mathematical approach for the epidemiological analysis of malayan filariasis in Wimi-Ri Village of Cheju Island. For the age distribution of the skin test positive rate, the simple catalytic model $y = 0.864 \, (1 - e^{-0.157t})$ could be applied. For the age distribution of the microfilaria rate, the two-stage catalytic model was applied and the relation: $y = 0.885 \, (e^{-0.023t} - e^{-0.049t})$ was obtained. The frequency distribution of the microfilaria density of the population was calculated by the formula: $y = a + b \log x$, in which the values of a, b, and MfD -50 were: 3.30, 1.34, and 18.57, respectively, in 1970 before the start of the drug treatment program; 3.82, 1.39, and 7.06 in 1971 after one year; 3.83, 1.41, and 4.0 in 1972; and 3.88, 1.41, and 3.8 in 1973.

KANG et al. (1973; abstract only) conducted an epidemiological study of filariasis in Shin Shan Ri, South Cheju Goon. Of a total population of 1,678, 984 persons (58.6%) were examined at night and 86 (8.7%) were found to be positive for B. malayi microfilariae. The microfilaria rate was 9.2% (44 positives of 479 persons examined) in males and 8.3% (42 of 505) in females. The frequency distribution of the microfilaria density among the positive cases was expressed by the equation: $y = 3.45 + 1.37 \log x$, and the value of MfD-50 was 10.82 (see Section 11.B and 11.C).

KATAMINE et al. (1973) reported on the results of blood examinations and skin tests carried out in the southern part Cheju Island during 1970, 1971, and 1972. It was demonstrated that the people living in the coast regions were higher in microfilaria rates, microfilaria densities, and skin-test positive rates than those living in the inland regions. This finding is related to the local distribution of Ae. togoi, which breed mainly on the seashore. A mass treatment of microfilaria carriers was conducted in 1970, and this resulted in the reduction of the average wheal size in the skin test of the children.

A survey of mosquitoes in relation to the transmission of B. malayi on Cheju Island was conducted by WADA et al. (1973). A total of 14 mosquito species were found on this island, among which the most common species feeding on man around houses were C. p. pallens and Ae. togoi. Natural infection with mature larvae of B. malayi was demonstrated only in Ae. togoi. During 1970, 308 Ae. togoi were dissected after being fixed in alcohol on the same day they were collected; 27 (8.8%) were found to be infected (with all stages of larvae), and 5 (1.6%) contained mature larvae. In C. p. pallens, 2 of 504 had first stage larvae, but none contained mature larvae. During 1971, 292 Ae. togoi were dissected, and 12 (4.1%) were infected and 6 (2.1%) had mature larvae; only 1 out of 329 C. p. pallens was infected with first stage larvae. Anopheles sinensis was a rare mosquito on Cheju.

In experimental infections, the larvae of B. malayi ingested by Ae. togoi were estimated to reach the mature stage between six to nine days after ingestion, and this period is considered to be much shorter than that requir- ed by W. bancrofti larvae to mature. The breeding of Ae. togoi was seen mainly in rock pools on the seacoast, and only rarely in artificial water containers in the villages.

8C.4.3 Filariasis in mainland Korea

B. malayi infection has also been noted to be widely distributed in the rice-growing countries in the southeastern regions of the Korean Peninsula, especially South Ch'ungchong Do, North Cholla Do, South Cholla Do, and North Kyongsang Do. The main vector in this region is, as in the endemic areas in mainland China, *An. sinensis*. Epidemiological reports referring to malayan filariasis in the mainland of Korea have been published by Moon (1939a), Senoo & Lincicome (1951), Paik *et al.* (1957), Song *et al.* (1964), Hwang *et al.* (1965), Seo *et al.* (1965), Soh (1965), Lim Byoung-Chan (1967), Lim Han-Chong (1967), Cha (1968), Kim *et al.* (1971, 1973), Kim (1974), and Kanda *et al.* (1974).

In the mainland of Korea, Paik *et al.* (1957) conducted an epidemiological survey of filariasis in the Nonsan area.

Song & Lee (1964) reported on filariasis in Danyang District, Choongchung-Fukdo. Of 387 persons examined among 707 villagers in June 1963, 29 cases (7.7%) were positive for the microfilariae of *B. malayi*.

Hwang *et al.* (1965) found a new endemic focus of filariasis in Anchong Myon Village, Yongju-Kun, Kyongsang Pukdo. A total of 707 persons (342 males and 365 females) of all ages were examined, the microfilariae of *B. malayi* were found in 7.67% (7.97% in males and 7.37% in females). In an age distribution of the positive cases, highest rate was seen in the age-group 41 to 50 years in both sexes.

Seo *et al.* (1965) examined 3,088 soldiers who came from Kyongsang Pukdo and found 28 (0.91%) to be positive for the microfilariae of *B. malayi*.

A more detailed epidemiological survey of *B. malayi* endemic foci in the Yongju area was reported by Kim *et al.* (1971, 1973). A total of 2,178 persons were examined, and microfilaria rates of 5.0 to 18.0% were observed in villages of this area.

Soh & Kim (1974) reported on clinical findings of 72 filariasis cases detected in the above area. Five (6.9%) among them had elephantiasis but no microfilaria. Fourteen cases (19.5%) showed no clinical manifestations and only microfilaremia, but the remaining 58 cases had various clinical complaints, such as lumbago, limb pain, cold sensation, lymphoedema or elephantiasis, fever attacks, urticaria, cough, palpitation, nausea, fatigue, dizziness, and asthma, in decreasing order. Microfilarial density was not correlated with the clinical signs. Lymphoedema or elephantiasis was seen in 12 cases. No essential eosinophilia was noticed among the patients. Urine protein, sugar, and chyluria were all negative. No change was observed in body weight, blood pressure, pulse rate, or hand grips.

Kanda *et al.* (1974) conducted an epidemiological study of malayan filariasis in an inland village in Kyungpook, South Korea. Of 127 persons examined, 3 (2.4%) were found to be carrying the microfilariae of *B. malayi*. Among six species of mosquitoes dissected during September 1973, filaria larvae were found only in 6 of 98 *An. sinensis*, and out of a total of 58 filaria larvae recovered from them, 3 were identified as mature larvae of *B. malayi*. The authors conclude that *An. sinensis* is the vector of *B. malayi* in the inland endemic areas of South Korea.

8C.4.4 Control of filariasis

Trial treatments of malayan filariasis cases were conducted by KONG *et al.* (1964) and KONG (1965). A single dose of 3 mg per kg of DEC was administered to 14 elephantiasis cases without microfilaremia and to 8 cases with microfilaremia but without elephantiasis as a provocation test. This dosage was reported to be successful as provocation test in bancroftian filariasis by KATAMINE (1952), but no significant differences could be observed between the microfilarial counts before and 20 minutes after the drug administration in the malayan filariasis cases. In 13 microfilaria carriers to whom 3 mg per kg of DEC was administered, a rise in body temperature, lumbago, or headache occurred in almost everyone, but such side reactions were not encountered among the 5 control cases.

LEE *et al.* (1965) reported on the effect of various doses of DEC on microfilaria carriers on Cheju Do. Daily doses of 3 mg per kg of DEC were administered to 37 cases for periods varying from 1 to 36 days, and in general, more severe effects were observed in those treated with larger doses than in those treated with smaller doses.

SEO & LEE (1973), on Cheju Do, made a comparative study of the relative efficacy of a high dosage schedule (6 mg per kg once a day for six times, and the same schedule repeated with an interval of one or two months, totaling 72 mg per kg) and a low dosage schedule (0.5 mg per kg on the first day, 1 mg per kg on the second, 4 mg per kg on the third, 6 mg per kg on the fourth to the ninth days, totaling 37.5 mg per kg given in nine days). Of 141 *B. malayi* carriers treated with the conventional high dosage schedule, 118 (83.7%) became negative and the microfilaria reduction rate was about 99%: with the low dosage schedule, 35 (85.4%) out of 43 previously positive cases became negative, and the microfilaria reduction rate was 99.5%. The febrile reaction occurred in 80.5% of those treated with the conventional dosage schedule, while the rate was only 43.9% in those treated with the low dosage schedule. In the former group, the febrile reaction associated with headache, etc., appeared after 6 to 10 hours and lasted 48 to 72 hours, while in the latter group, the reaction appeared after 7 to 8 hours and lasted 24 to 43 hours.

8C.5 Japan

Japan consists of an island chain in the western Pacific, off the east coast of Asia. It has an area of 371,830 km², with a population of 104,665,171 (1970). The country comprises four main islands: Hokkaido, Honshu, Shikoku, Kyushu, and a number of adjacent islands. Although large parts of Japan are situated in the Temperate Zone, the island chain connecting Kyushu and Taiwan called the Amami and Ryukyu Archipelagos lie in the subtropical zone between 29°N and 24°N, and were notorious for the prevalence of filariasis until recently.

Two species and epidemiological types of human filariae were noted from Japan: the nocturnally periodic *W. bancrofti* with *Culex pipiens* s.l. as the main vector (which was once widely endemic all over Japan with the exception of the northernmost island of Hokkaido), and the nocturnally periodic *B. malayi* with *Ae. togoi* as the main vector (which was discovered rather recently from a small island south of Tokyo).

Filariasis due to *W. bancrofti* had been a serious health problem until recently, especially in southern Japan, and about one million people were estimated to be infected or suffering from the disease. However, due to the improvements of general sanitary conditions which resulted in the reduction of the vector mosquitoes, the disease has disappeared spontaneously from many of the previously known endemic areas.

A national filariasis control program was organized in Japan in 1962, covering all the prefectures concerned. As a result of extensive blood surveys followed by DEC treatment of microfilaria positive cases, remarkable reductions in filaria carriers have been achieved in all the treated areas. Assisted also by the reduction in the vector populations, filariasis is now believed to have been nearly eradicated from most of the previously known endemic areas in Japan, including the formerly notorious endemic foci in the Amami and Ryukyu Islands.

8C.5.1 Historical notes

The first record of microfilariae in the blood of a Japanese patient was made by BAELZ (1876, quoted by MIYAGAWA, 1957) who was a Visiting Professor of Medicine from Germany to the Imperial University of Tokyo. The adult worms were recovered for the first time by URAMATSU, in 1896, in Kumamoto. Later, large numbers of case reports were made from various parts of Japan, and the disease was shown to be very common in the southwestern regions, i.e., southern Shikoku, southern Kyushu, and the Amami and Ryukyu Islands. Sporadic case reports were also made from the mainland of Honshu and adjacent islands.

Meanwhile, a serious question was raised by a group of workers in Kyoto University on the filarial etiology of elephantiasis. YOSHINAGA &

CHOSA (1911) and YOSHINAGA (1912a, b) conducted epidemiological surveys on Amakusa(Kumamoto) and Hachijo-Koshima (the Izu Islands). They observed that the microfilariae were more frequently discovered from apparently healthy people than from elephantiasis cases, and they considered that the main causative agent of elephantiasis was streptococcus rather than filaria. YOSHIMURA (1912) supported the nonfilarial theory as the origin of elephantiasis on the ground that he found microfilaria carriers at a rate of 5.6% in a village in Yamanashi where clinical cases with elephantiasis and chyluria were absent. HIRATA (1939, 1940) conducted epidemiological studies on microfilaremia and elephantiasis cases and also stated that elephantiasis was not caused by filariae, but presumably by infection with streptococci in pools used for the washing by the villagers.

On the other hand, most other Japanese workers were convinced that filaria was the causative agent of elephantiasis and chyluria, mainly from epidemiological and pathologic-anatomical evidence. For example, MOCHIZUKI (1912) and MOCHIZUKI & INOUE (1912), from Kyushu University, strongly opposed the idea proposed by YOSHINAGA & CHOSA (1912a) on the etiology of elephantiasis, and claimed that the disease was primarily caused by the adult worms residing in lymph nodes.

An important contribution to the mode of distribution and prevalence of filariasis in Japan was made by the Rikugunsho Imukyoku (Bureau of the Army Surgeon: 1912), which conducted night blood examinations of the enlisted soldiers recruited from all over Japan. In this report, the numbers of persons examined and the numbers of those found to be positive for microfilariae were recorded according to the regimental districts. In this survey, 112,353 enlisted men of about age of 20 were examined, and 2,090, or 1.86%, among them were found to be carrying microfilariae in their night blood sample. The microfilaria carriers were found in 55 of 74 regimental districts. The districts showing a microfilaria rate above 3% were Okinawa (17.64%, 291 of 1,650), Omura (13.45%, 328 of 2,438), Takase (11.58%), Kagoshima (8.53%, 245 of 2,873), Yatsushiro (8.38%, 169 of 2,017), Miyakonojo (7.89%, 167 of 2,093), Nakatsu (4.50%, 103 of 1,399), Tsushima(4.00%, 2 of 50), and Kumamoto (3.55%, 72 of 2,055). Because the population surveyed may be regarded as a random sample from all the males of the age of about 20 years, this is an extremely important reference regarding the distribution and prevalence of filarial infection at that time in Japan. Based on this report, a filaria map of Japan as of 1911 was compiled by SASA (1966) (see Fig. 8-8).

Later, large numbers of papers were published by Japanese workers in reference to the clinical, epidemiological, and experimental aspects of human filariasis, but these were mostly described in Japanese and of only local interest. Reviews of the literature were made by MAEHATA (1941: bibliography), MORISHITA (1951: epidemiology), SASA & HAYASHI (1953: epidemiology), KITAMURA & KATAMINE (1953: clinical medicine), SATO (1953: clinical medicine), MIYAGAWA (1957: clinical medicine) SASA et al.

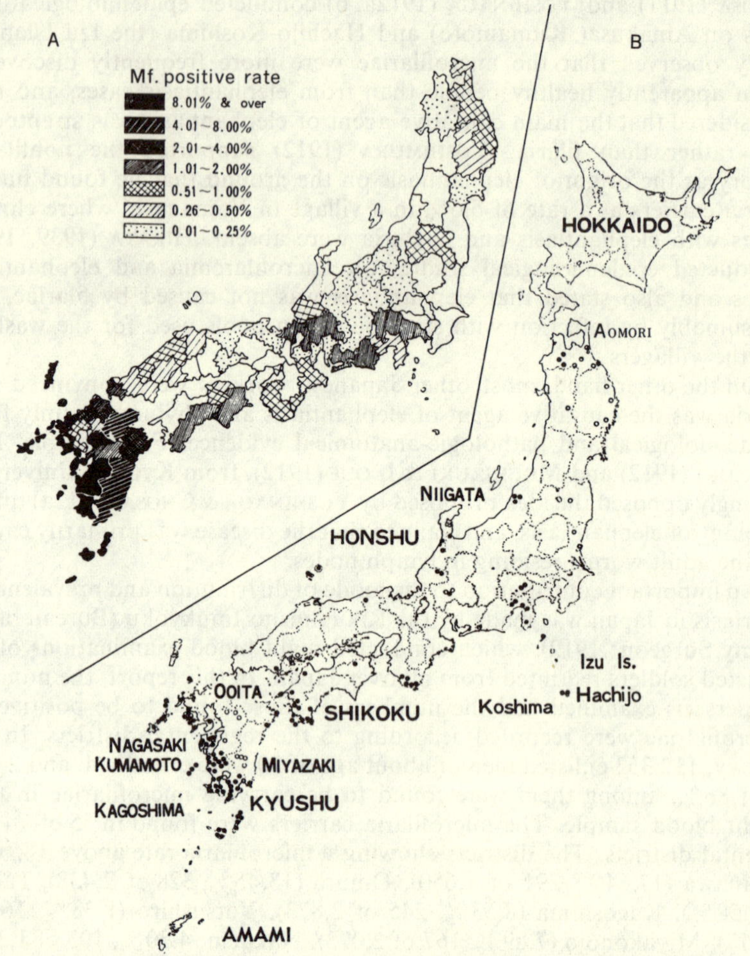

Fig. 8-8. Geographic distribution of filariasis in Japan. A. Microfilaria rate of enlisted men according to the regimental districts, 1911. B. Previous records of endemic foci; ●Area from which microfilaria cases were confirmed; ○ Area reported only by the presence of clinical cases (after Sasa, 1966).

(1959: bibliography), SASA (1962: geographic distribution), SASA (1966: epidemiology), and SASA *et al.* (1970: epidemiology and control), among which the last two reviews were published in English. SASA *et al.* (1959) listed a total of 786 papers published in Japan referring to various aspects of human filariasis.

The geographic distribution and incidence of bancroftian filariasis in Japan was illustrated by the review of previous records by MORISHITA (1951), SASA & HAYASHI (1953), and SASA (1962, 1966). Sporadic reports were made on the occurrence of large numbers of isolated endemic foci from almost all the prefectures on Honshu, Shikoku, and Kyushu Islands. The disease was shown to be prevalent in almost all villages in southern Kyushu and the adjacent islands, as well as in the Amami and Ryukyu Islands.

While it had been believed that *W. bancrofti* was the only human filaria endemic in Japan, a focus of *B. malayi* infection was discovered by HAYASHI *et al.* (1951) from a small island called Hachijo-Koshima with a total population of a little over 100. A series of studies on the epidemiology and control of this new endemic area were made by SASA *et al.* (1951, 1952, 1957) and HAYASHI (1954). The parasite was found to be a nocturnally periodic race. *Aedes togoi*, a mosquito associated with rock pools containing brackish water, was shown to be the main vector. Trial treatments with DEC were initiated in 1951.

After World War II, extensive studies on the epidemiology and control of filariasis in Japan were started by mainly three groups of workers: Kitamura, Katamine, Omori, and their associates in Nagasaki University; Sato, Fukushima, Otsuji, and their associates in Kagoshima University; and Sasa, Hayashi, Tanaka, and their associates in the Institute for Infectious Diseases (now Institute of Medical Science), University of Tokyo. Based on the results accumulated by these workers, a national filariasis control program was inaugurated in 1962, covering all the prefectures concerned. Laboratory studies using animal models, such as *Litomosoides carinii* in cotton rats in the chemotherapy and immunology of filariasis, are now in progress by Sasa, Tanaka, and their associates.

8C.5.2 Geographic distribution and prevalence

As stated previously, endemic foci of *W. bancrofti* were reported from three of the four main islands of Japan, and from a large number of adjacent islands in western and southern Japan. In general, endemic foci found from middle and northern Japan are lower in prevalence and are restricted to certain village-groups, which are isolated from each other by nonendemic zones; on the other hand, those reported from southern Kyushu and the Ryukyu Islands (including Amami and Okinawa) are higher in prevalence, and the transmission was apparently taking place in every village.

The country of Japan is administratively divided into 47 prefectures (To-

Do-Fu-Ken), and these are grouped in this text into nine districts (Chiho).
A nearly complete review of the literature referring to the distribution of
clinical filariasis and microfilaria cases was compiled by SASA (1962, in
Japanese, with 245 references), and additional information in connection
with the progress of the national filariasis control program was reviewed by
SASA (1966, 91 references) and SASA et al. (1970). The following descriptions referring to the geographic distribution of filariasis in Japan were
prepared as summaries from previous medical records.

(Note: literature published in Japanese in local medical journals are not
listed in the "List of References" attached to this book; these can be found
from the above reviews)

8C.5.2.a Hokkaido

There were no endemic foci reported from this island situated north of
Honshu, between latitudes 41°N and 46°N. In the blood surveys of military servicemen in 1911, none of 3,230 from Hokkaido were positive.

8C.5.2.b Prefectures in Tohoku (northern Honshu)

(b.1) Aomori Prefecture

Being the prefecture in the northernmost part of Honshu, at about 41°N,
the climate here is cold, and the land is covered by deep snow during the
winter season. However, at least two active endemic foci were reported from
this prefecture. In the blood surveys of military servicemen conducted in
1911, 10 of 1,216 from Aomori were found to be positive for microfilariae.
Cases with chyluria or hydrocele were reported by several workers from
1924 to 1950. SASA et al. (1953) carried out blood surveys of several villages
around Hachinohe City in the eastern part of Aomori Prefecture, and
found 3 of 89 persons from Kofunato and 13 of 117 persons from Orochi to
be positive for the microfilariae of *W. bancrofti*. The authors also reported
that at least 20 chyluria cases from several villages in this region had visited
practicing physicians.

Another group of endemic foci was discovered by KITABATAKE (1954)
from the Tsugaru region in western Aomori. Microfilariae were found in
the blood of 7 of 174 persons examined at Nozawa-Mura, and in 24 of 800
persons examined at 14 villages of this region.

(b.2) Iwate Prefecture

Sporadic case reports of chyluria were made from several villages in the
Sanriku region along the Pacific coast. Three positive cases were found
among 776 soldiers examined at Morioka in 1911.

(b.3) Akita Prefecture

A single case of chyluria was reported from this prefecture in 1930.

(b.4) Fukushima Prefecture

Three microfilaria cases were found out of 564 soldiers examined in 1911
at Wakamatsu. Four out of 53 chyluria cases examined at the University of
Tokyo Hospital before 1935 were from this prefecture. SUGAMA (1955,

quoted by SASA, 1962) stated that sporadic chyluria cases were seen in several villages around the city of Koriyama.

8C.5.2.c Prefectures in Kanto (southeastern Honshu)

(c.1) Ibaraki Prefecture

Three microfilaria cases were found among 2,979 soldiers examined in 1911 at Mito. HAYASHI (1955) conducted an epidemiological survey of several villages in Kuji-Gun, and found 4 cases with chyluria or hydrocele, but none of 187 persons examined in this region was positive for microfilaria.

(c.2) Tochigi Prefecture

One out of 2,714 soldiers examined in 1911 at Utsunomiya was positive for microfilaria. Three chyluria cases from this prefecture had been seen at the University of Tokyo Hospital as of 1935.

(c.3) Gunma Prefecture

Two microfilaria cases were found out of 2,552 soldiers examined in 1911 at Takasaki. ISHUIN (1958) examined 6,861 young men recruited from all over Japan for the National Defence Service and found 9 microfilaria cases, 1 was from Nakanojo, northern Gunma.

(c.4) The Izu Archipelago

A chain of volcanic islands in the Pacific Ocean, south of Tokyo, they lie between 32°N and 35°N, with a total population of about 42,000 as of 1965. Of ten inhabited islands, *W. bancrofti* infection has been recorded from Aogashima, Hachijoshima, Niijima, and Kozushima, while *B. malayi* infection was found in Hachijo-Koshima, Hachijoshima, and Shikinejima.

On the main island of Hachijo, MOCHIZUKI & INOUE (1912) found a total of 21 cases of elephantiasis of the legs or scrotum from four villages on the island. Since 4 cases among them were from a small settlement of 15 households, blood examinations were conducted here, and out of 33 persons examined (including 4 elephantiasis cases) microfilariae were found in 18 (including one case with elephantiasis). The authors also visited Hachijo-Koshima (the smaller island) on this occasion, and found many microfilaria and elephantiasis cases, but did not notice the difference in the filarial species between the two closely set islands.

Extensive epidemiological surveys of filariasis in the above two islands were begun by Sasa, Hayashi, and associates from 1950. While they found *B. malayi* in Hachijo-Koshima, one case of *W. bancrofti* was found among 59 high school students in Hachijo in November 1950. In the second survey carried out in September 1952, 5 of 62 high school students in Hachijo were found to harbor microfilariae of *W. bancrofti*. An island-wide blood survey was conducted in 1963 as a part of the activity of the national filariasis control program, and of 5,598 persons (about 60% of the total population) examined in Hachijo, 30 were positive for *W. bancrofti* and 2 for *B. malayi*. DEC was administered to the positive cases. In 1965, 6 out of 513 persons examined on this island were positive for *W. bancrofti* (summarized from SASA *et al.*, 1970).

On Aogashima Island, the southernmost inhabited island of the Izu Archipelago, HAYASHI *et al.* (1959) examined all the available population, and found 41 (12.9%) *W. bancrofti* microfilaria carriers out of 317 persons whose blood was examined at night. They also conducted clinical examinations on 123 adults, and found chyluria in 21, hydrocele in 23, elephantiasis of the legs in 2, recurrent fever attacks in 14, swelling of the lymph nodes in 6, lumbago in 25, and shoulder ache in 23. DEC was administered to all the microfilaria and clinical cases. In the survey conducted by members of the Tokyo Metropolitan Health Bureau in 1962, only 2 microfilaria positive cases were detected out of 269 persons examined in Aogashima island.

On Niijima Island, TANAKA *et al.* (1954) made blood and clinical surveys of the two villages. No positive case was found among 112 persons examined at Motomura, but 3 *W. bancrofti* positive cases and 10 clinical cases were discovered out of 88 persons examined at Wakago. In 1965, a team from the Tokyo Metropolitan Health Bureau visited the island and examined the blood of 211 persons, but none of them were positive for microfilaria.

On Shikine Island, 1 *B. malayi* carrier was discovered in 1964. On Kozu Island, 5 cases harboring *W. bancrofti* microfilariae were discovered among 1,400 persons examined by a team from the Tokyo Metropolitan Health Bureau.

8C.5.2.d Prefectures in Hokuriku (North-Central Honshu)

(d.1) Niigata Prefecture

Although this prefecture is situated on the north coast of Honshu and most of the land is covered by deep snow during the winter season, a fairly large endemic area of *W. bancrofti* was found from a mountainous region. SEOHARA, in 1901, presented a paper entitled "On human filariasis" and reported that he had seen several clinical filariasis cases from Higashiku-biki-Gun and the neighboring areas, and demonstrated microfilariae in a blood specimen taken from one of the cases. In the general blood surveys of soldiers conducted in 1911, microfilaria cases were found in 2 of 2,565 persons examined at Muramatsu, and 1 out of 2,400 examined at Takada. Case reports on chyluria and hydrocele patients were made later by several workers in Niigata.

KAWAMURA (1923) carried out a survey of clinical cases in Kariha-Gun and Higashikubiki-Gun, and reported that, altogether, 27 cases of chyluria and elephantiasis had been seen by practicing physicians in this region. Based on this information, TAKENOUCHI (1925) conducted a detailed epidemiological survey of this region, and found 37 cases with chyluria, 7 cases with elephantiasis of the leg, 6 cases with hydrocele, 9 cases with funiculitis, and 1 case with elephantiasis of the vulva. Microfilariae were found in 14 (14.4%) of 97 persons examined at Aizawa, 2 (9.5%) of 21 examined at Azamihira, and 3 (5.8%) of 52 examined at Onoshima of

Matsudai-Cho, Higashikubiki-Gun, 11 (12.5%) of 87 persons examined at Nakago, Takayanagi-Cho, Kariha-Gun, and 2 (8.7%) of 23 examined at Takakura, Kawanishi-Cho, Nakauonuma-Gun. These endemic areas are located at about 37° 25'N, hilly, and covered by deep snow during the winter season.

HAYASHI *et al.* (1954) carried out blood and clinical surveys of the same endemic areas in Niigata some 30 years after these were surveyed by TA- KENOUCHI (1925). Microfilariae were found in 4 (5.6%) of 72 persons examined at Azamihira, but none among 21 persons examined at Nakago, and 49 persons examined at Aizawa were positive. It was presumed that the infection had died out spontaneously from most of the previously known endemic areas due to improvements in sanitary conditions, espe- cially by the reduction in the vector populations due to the installations of pipe-water supply systems. In this survey, 15 cases of chronic filariasis (9 chyluria and 6 hydrocele) were confirmed to be still existing in this region.

During 1963, an extensive blood survey covering the whole population of these regions was conducted by health centers of Niigata Prefecture, as a project under the national filariasis control program of Japan. A total of 22,513 persons (65.2% of the registered population) were examined, in- cluding those from the previously reported endemic foci, but none of them was positive for microfilariae. Although no special treatment or control work was done in these regions, it seemed that the endemic foci had died out.

(d.2) Toyama Prefecture

In the general blood survey of soldiers in 1911, 3 microfilaria cases were found among 1,779 examined at Toyama. In a blood survey conducted by ASANO in 1913, 11 microfilaria positive cases were found out of 610 persons examined in four villages in Himi-Gun. MORISHITA (1960) and his associ- ates conducted re-examinations of the same area in 1957, and found 6 microfilaria cases in 2 of 4 villages surveyed, namely, 1 among 176 persons examined at Kumanashi and 5 among 182 persons at Kodama. Two among the microfilaria cases were under the age of 10 years. During this survey, 13 persons reported clinical symptoms presumably of filarial origin, but none of them was positive for the microfilariae.

(d.3) Ishikawa Prefecture

No microfilaria cases were discovered among 548 soldiers examined in 1911 at Kanazawa. However, FUWA, in 1913, reported that 7 cases with chyluria had been seen at Prefectural Hospital in Kanazawa during the previous three years; 1 was microfilaria positive, and it was also noted that 2 out of 173 persons examined in the suburbs of Kanazawa City were found to be harboring microfilariae.

(d.4) Fukui Prefecture

In the examination of the soldiers in 1911, 7 microfilaria cases (1.31%) were recorded out of 536 examined at Tsuruga and 17 cases (0.99%) out of 1,713 at Sabae. In 1959, TSUBOSAKA and his collaborators in 1954 conducted a survey in Katsuyama District of Ohno-Gun, and discovered 20 clinical cases in Arato-Mura, and 2 cases in Kamishihi-Mura; microfilariae were found in the blood of 10 of the above clinical cases. KASAMATSU and his associates conducted an epidemiological survey of 11 villages in this region, and detected a total of 165 microfilaria carriers among 4,116 persons examined. MORISHITA (1960) reported on the results of blood surveys conducted by his associates in 1955 in four villages in Katsuyama District, and found 50 microfilaria cases (5.4%) and 66 clinical cases (7.1%) among 932 persons examined in these villages. In another four villages of Ohno District, 12 (1.5%) of 788 persons examined were microfilaria positive, and 30 (3.8%) had some clinical symptoms suspected of having a filarial origin.

8C.5.2.e Prefectures in Chubu (Central Honshu)

(e.1) Nagano Prefecture

No endemic foci of filariasis have been reported in this prefecture.

(e.2) Yamanashi Prefecture

The central part of the Kofu Basin has been noted as the largest endemic area of *Schistosoma japonicum* in Japan. The occurrence of filariasis cases was reported from villages in valleys in the southern part of the prefecture. Microfilariae were found in 12 (1.27%) of 944 soldiers examined in 1911 at Kofu. YOSHIMURA, in 1912, reported that of 10 villages along Katsura River on the northern slope of Mount Fuji, microfilaria carriers were found in 9 villages, and 51 (5.6%) out of 969 persons examined in this area were positive. Since he did not find elephantiasis in these villages, he claimed that elephantiasis had no relation to filarial infection. However, the occurrence of chyluria and hydrocele patients was later reported from this region.

(e.3) Shizuoka Prefecture

Situated on the southern coast of central Honshu, filariasis has been reported to be endemic from a number of villages in various districts of Shizuoka. In the blood examinations of soldiers in 1911, 2 of 580 at Shizuoka and 5 of 253 at Hamamatsu were positive for microfilariae. KANEHARA, in 1917, reported that 15 (17.9%) of 84 soldiers recruited from Shizuoka Prefecture were positive for microfilariae, and that the carriers were the natives of Fuji-Gun, Sunto-Gun, Kamo-Gun, and Ehara-Gun. KAWAKAMI, in 1922, reported on the results of blood surveys carried out in five villages in Fuji-Gun on the southern slope of Mount Fuji, and in total found 39 microfilaria cases out of 503 persons.

However, in the post World War II surveys conducted in these regions, SASA & HAYASHI, in 1953, as well as ISHIZAKI *et al.*, in 1960, reported that microfilaria carriers were no longer found, although they still found some chronic clinical cases or skin-test positive cases.

(e.4) Gifu Prefecture

Although 30 microfilaria positive cases were recorded in the blood survey of 1,511 soldiers examined at Gifu, no epidemiological survey was conducted until recently. MORISHITA *et al.* (1957) reported that 31 cases with chyluria were seen at Gifu University Hospital from 1949 to 1954, and that they were from more than ten gun (counties) in the southern parts of the prefecture. These authors assumed that the disease was widely distributed in areas around the city of Gifu.

(e.5) Aichi Prefecture

Although 7 microfilaria cases were reported among 3,282 soldiers examined in 1911 at Nagoya, Kuwana, and Toyohashi, no later reports are available from this prefecture.

8C.5.2.f Prefectures in Kinki (Central West Honshu)

Previous records have shown that filariasis is probably absent from most parts of Kinki, including areas around Kyoto, Osaka, Kobe, and Nara. In Mie Prefecture, 21 of 2,351 soldiers examined in 1911 at Tsu were positive, but there have been no later report on filariasis.

In Hyogo Prefecture, endemic foci were discovered by MASUDA in 1954 from Onsen-Cho, in the north near the Japan Sea coast. They found 5 cases with chyluria, and 63 microfilaria cases out of 2,103 persons examined in seven rural communities in the hilly region.

Filariasis was also widely distributed along villages near the southern, Pacific coast of Wakayama Prefecture. Two of 236 soldiers examined in 1911 at Wakayama were positive for microfilariae. KAWAMURA, in 1914, conducted an extensive survey of villages in the southern parts of Kii Peninsula and found 329 (8.35%) microfilaria positive cases and 116 (2.97 %) clinical cases out of a total of 3,904 persons examined. MORISHITA (1960) resurveyed these previously known endemic areas, and of a total of 2,035 persons in nine villages were examined; microfilariae were found only in 5 of 219 persons examined at Wabuka Village.

8C.5.2.g Prefectures in Chugoku (West Honshu)

There have been no confirmed endemic foci reported from the mainland of Honshu, though a few microfilaria cases were found among the soldiers examined in 1911 in this region, i.e., 4 of 2,258 at Tottori, 5 of 2,019 at Matsue (including those from the Oki Islands), 10 of 1,898 at Hamada, none of 2,229 at Okayama, 9 of 1,980 at Hiroshima, none of 1,728 at Fukuyama, and 8 of 2,316 at Yamaguchi.

The Oki Islands: A group of islands in the Sea of Japan about 60 km off the north coast of Honshu, located at about 36°N. These islands belong to Shimane Prefecture, and have an area of 340 km², and a population of about 44,000. They consist of Dozen (three islands) and Dogo (one island).

The occurrence of filariasis on these islands has long been noted. WATSUJI & YAMANE, in 1894, reported that they had seen 33 clinical cases in eight villages in the Dozen Islands and 27 clinical cases in two villages on Dogo Island. These were chyluria, hydrocele, and elephantiasis, and microfilariae were found in some of these patients. They also stated that in old times about one-third of the adult population suffered from one or more of these symptoms.

NAGAHANA and his associates conducted epidemiological surveys of Oki in 1954. Microfilariae were positive in 13 of 61 persons examined at Saki (Dozen) and 17 of 83 at Tai (Dogo). Altogether, 6 cases from Dogo and 9 cases from Dozen were reported as clinical filariasis by local physicians.

8C.5.2.h Prefectures in Shikoku

Endemic areas of bancroftian filariasis were reported from 3 of 4 prefectures in Shikoku Island, with the exception of Kagawa Prefecture on the Inland Sea coast.

(h.1) Tokushima Prefecture

In the general blood survey of soldiers in 1911, 35 (1.60%) of 2,190 examined at Tokushima were positive. KOCHI & NARITA, in 1955, reported 30 chyluria cases, and ARAKAWA and his associates, in 1955, on 35 chyluria cases from Tokushima Prefecture; the patients were mostly from coastal villages or those living in the Yoshino River Basin. A total of 2,448 children in 15 schools in Tokushima were examined by DEC provocation test, and only 2 girls at Kuniyama were positive for microfilariae.

(h.2) Ehime Prefecture

In the general blood survey of soldiers in 1911, none of 2,073 examined at Matsuyama was positive. However, later studies carried out in this prefecture showed that filariasis was widely endemic, especially in villages along the western coast. Pilot experiments for the control of filariasis were initiated in 1958 in Ehime, prior to the commencement of the national program.

CHOSA, in 1913, conducted a blood survey of the western region of Ehime, and found 18 microfilaria cases among 1,090 persons examined at six localities. The highest rate was 11.8% (8 positives out of 68) at Iwanaga, Minamiuwa-Gun.

ARAKAWA, YAMAGUCHI, and their associates, in 1955, found 11 microfilaria cases among 760 persons examined at Misaki on Misaki Peninsula; 8 cases with hydrocele and 7 cases with chyluria were found among 246 adults examined in the same village. SEO, in 1958, found 4 microfilaria cases and 7 clinical filariasis cases among 369 persons examined at Matsu on Misaki Peninsula.

An extensive blood survey and control project covering all the villages on Misaki Peninsula was organized in 1958 as a joint program between the Ehime Prefecture Health Department (SHIMONO, HATANO, and associates) and the Department of Parasitology, Institute for Infectious Diseases (SASA and associates). Microfilaria cases were found in all of 12 villages surveyed in 1958 and 1959, and of a total of 9,963 persons examined, 159 (1.60%) were positive. Questionnaires were sent to all the practicing physicians and hospitals in Ehime Prefecture, and altogether, 94 chyluria cases, 4 hydrocele cases, and 7 elephantiasis cases were reported from 24 gun (counties) and shi (cities) of Ehime, which had a total population of 1,534,933 as of the 1955 census.

A filariasis control program based on the blood survey of general populations and treatment of microfilaria cases with DEC was repeated in Ehime Prefecture every year from 1958 to 1965. The population covered was expanded every year from 1958 to 1962, from 2,050 people in Misaki in 1958 to 318,898 in 1962, covering all the suspected endemic areas in the whole prefecture. Since all the positive cases were treated intensively every year, most of the microfilaria cases detected were new positives. For example, 109 of 8,507 persons examined in 1960 were positive, of whom 106 were new positive cases. The number of microfilaria cases gradually decreased after 1962, and the filariasis control program was discontinued in 1966 when the last two cases detected during 1965 became negative after treatment with DEC. Only two new positives were discovered in later surveys.

(h.3) Kochi Prefecture

Being situated on the southern coast of Shikoku and favored by warm climate and rich rainfall, filariasis has been noted to be relatively common here, especially on the offshore islands. In the survey of soldiers in 1911, 33 (1.58%) of 2,089 examined at Kochi were positive for microfilariae. MORISHITA (1951) stated that filariasis was common in the villages of the inland regions of Agawa-Gun and Takaoka-Gun, and also sporadically found in the coastal regions of Hata-Gun and Aki-Gun.

KITAMURA *et al.* (1953) reported on the results of blood and clinical surveys conducted in Hata-Gun, the western region of Kochi Prefecture. Filariasis due to *W. bancrofti* was found to be prevalent on the two offshore islands called Ukurushima and Okinoshima. In the former, 54 (23.3%) were positive for microfilariae and 25 (10.8%) had clinical filariasis signs out of 232 persons examined, with an endemicity rate (both combined) of 31.5% (73 cases had either microfilaremia or disease signs, or both); in the latter, the numbers of cases with microfilaria, disease, or either of these signs were 34 (10.1%), 47 (13.9%), and 76 (22.6%), respectively, out of a total of 337 persons examined. In seven other communities on the mainland of Shikoku surveyed at the same time, only 2 microfilaria cases and 8 clinical filariasis cases were found out of a total of 326 persons examined.

In the blood surveys conducted from 1962 to 1964 under the national filariasis control program covering all the suspected endemic areas in Kochi Prefecture, altogether, 53,653 persons were examined, and a total of 82 persons were found to harbor microfilariae during the three-year period.

8C.5.2.i Prefectures in Kyushu

(i.1) Fukuoka Prefecture

In the blood examinations of soldiers in 1911, 55 (2.32%) of 2,371 examined at Fukuoka and 10 of 2,202 examined at Kurume were positive. However, there have been no confirmed endemic foci reported from this prefecture so far.

(i.2) Saga Prefecture

Although 91 (4.88%) out of 1,904 soldiers examined in 1911 at Saga were positive for microfilariae, there have been no endemic foci reported from this prefecture, and as in Fukuoka, most of the positive cases were probably imported from other regions of Kyushu.

(i.3) Oita Prefecture

In the blood surveys of soldiers in 1911, 108 (4.50%) of 2,399 examined at Nakatsu and 68 (2.79%) of 2,439 examined at Oita were positive.

NAMIKAWA, in 1954, conducted surveys of filariasis in Minamiamabe-Gun, and found 3 microfilaria cases and 13 clinical filariasis cases among 148 persons examined in two villages of Higashinakaura; no microfilaria carriers but one chyluria case was found among 105 persons examined in Tanoura.

According to a report by SATO *et al.* in 1958, 121 clinical filariasis cases from almost all over the prefecture were seen at Kamegawa National Hospital in Oita. Microfilariae were found in 7 (1.7%) of 409 persons examined at Toyosaki, Kunisaki-Cho, but none of 187 persons examined at two other villages were positive.

Extensive blood surveys were conducted by the Oita Health Department during 1963 and 1964 under the national filariasis control program, covering all the suspected or known endemic areas within the prefecture. A total of 25,061 persons in 1963 and 22,107 persons in 1964 were examined, but no microfilaria carriers were detected among them.

(i.4) Nagasaki Prefecture

Until recently, filariasis was noted to be prevalent on both the mainland part and the adjacent islands of Nagasaki. In the general blood survey of soldiers in 1911, 328 (13.45%) out of 2,434 examined at Omura were positive for microfilaria. A large number of reports were made on the epidemiology of filariasis in Nagasaki, as reviewed by SASA (1962).

INOUE & MORI, in 1935, reported that a total of 214 chyluria patients visited Nagasaki Medical School Hospital during the previous 20 years; 199 cases were from Nagasaki Prefecture. The patients were from almost all the regions of Nagasaki, and thus the authors estimated that filariasis was widely endemic in this prefecture.

Blood and clinical surveys covering various regions of Nagasaki Prefecture were conducted by workers of Nagasaki University from 1953. In Shimabara Peninsula, the microfilaria cases were very few, but there were still many cases with chronic symptoms. In Nishisonogi Peninsula, north east of Nagasaki City, the microfilaria and disease rates were still high in some of the villages. Especially high microfilaria and disease rates were observed in the Goto Islands. Filariasis was found to be endemic also on Iki Island. On the other hand, the large islands of Tsushima in the Chosen Strait were apparently free from filariasis. The results of prefecture-wide blood surveys conducted under the National Filariasis Control Program are shown in Section 8C.5.5.3.c and Table 8-11.

(i.5) Kumamoto Prefecture

In the general blood survey of soldiers in 1911, a high microfilaria rate of 11.58% (166 positives of 1,433 examined) was reported for those examined at Takase, while among those examined at Kumamoto, there were 72 positives (3.55%) out of 2,055 persons examined.

Although a few endemic foci were reported from certain restricted areas on the mainland of Kyushu, the majority of filaria cases in Kumamoto Prefecture were people from the Amakusa Islands located south of Nagasaki. YOSHINAGA, in 1912, examined 1,353 persons in five villages in Amakusa, and obtained a high microfilaria rate of 27.6% (373 positives). The microfilaria rate of 218 elephantiasis cases was 17.9% (39 positives), while that of the apparently healthy people was 38.4% (121 positives out of 315 persons examined). For this reason, he believed that elephantiasis was not of filarial origin.

MORIGUCHI, in 1953, conducted a survey of Oe-Mura, Amakusa, and observed a microfilaria rate of 14.3%, a disease rate of 10.6%, and an endemicity rate (both combined) of 21.3% in a total of 2,272 persons examined. Of 241 cases with clinical symptoms, 186 had filarial fever, 14 had elephantiasis of the leg, 6 had chyluria, 30 had hydrocele, and 12 had swellings of the inguinal lymph nodes.

OSHIMA, in 1955, also conducted an epidemiological survey of Oe-Mura, Amakusa, and although no microfilaria or clinical cases were found among 123 persons examined at Hamazato, 68 (35.1%) microfilaria cases and 52 (26.9%) clinical filariasis cases were found among 194 persons examined at Nishi. KITAMURA & KATAMINE, in 1955, reported 18 (5.43%) of 280 persons were positive for microfilariae.

The blood survey project of Kumamoto Prefecture was begun in 1964, the third year of the national filariasis control program. The results are summarized in Section 8C.5.5.3.d.

(i.6) Miyazaki Prefecture

It is presumed that filariasis was once prevalent in large parts of this prefecture. In the general blood surveys of soldiers in 1911, 167 (7.98%) of 2,093 examined at Miyakonojo were found to be positive.

KITAHARA, in 1953, reported that he had seen a total of 24 clinical cases with chyluria or hydrocele in four municipalities (Shi-Cho-Son) in Nishi-morogata-Gun, but all of 83 persons from these areas were negative for microfilariae.

UEMURA *et al.*, in 1955, carried out a survey of Minaminaka-Gun, and among six villages where blood and clinical examinations were conducted, 1 microfilaria carrier and 21 clinical filariasis cases were found among 54 persons examined in one of the villages in Toi-Cho, near the southern extremity of the prefecture. No microfilaria carriers were found in other villages, though 3 chronic clinical cases were seen among 202 persons examined by the authors.

SATO, in 1956, reported on 4 microfilaria cases detected in examinations of 54 persons in two villages in Kitaura-Son, near the northern border of the prefecture. SATO *et al.* in 1958, reported that out of 106 practicing physicians who replied to their inquiries, 62 had seen filariasis patients and these patients were from almost all over the prefecture.

As in Oita Prefecture, filariasis, which was once distributed widely with high incidence rates in Miyazaki Prefecture, seems to have died out in recent years. In the extensive blood surveys carried out from 1963 to 1964 by the Miyazaki Health Department, covering all the suspected endemic areas, only 3 microfilaria positive cases were detected out of a total of 25,040 persons examined in 1963, and all of 3,174 persons examined in 1964 were negative.

(i.7) Kagoshima Prefecture

Being situated in the southernmost part of Kyushu, Kagoshima has the largest endemic areas of filariasis among the prefectures of Japan, and the prevalence rates in these endemic foci have been noted to be generally higher than observed in other prefectures, except those in Okinawa. For this reason, many studies were made on the epidemiology of filariasis in Kagoshima since early times. SASA (1962), in his review, listed 36 papers referring to the epidemiology of filariasis in the mainland regions of Kagoshima, 20 references on the offshore islands, and 25 references concerned with the Amami Islands. A number of additional papers referring to the epidemiology and control of filariasis in Kagoshima Prefecture were also published in later years.

Results of epidemiological surveys by previous workers indicated that filariasis was endemic nearly all over the prefecture, both on the mainland and the offshore islands at varying prevalence rates. In this sense, Kagoshima was different from all the other prefectures where the endemic foci were usually scattered and isolated from each other by filaria-free areas.

(i.7a) The mainland regions of Kagoshima Prefecture:

Since YOSHINAGA, in 1913, reported on the finding of microfilariae in 27 of 101 persons examined at Nagashima, microfilaria and/or clinical cases were reported from villages in all the counties (gun or shi) of Kagoshima, i.e., Izumi-Gun, Isa-Gun, Aira-Gun, Kagoshima-Shi, Hioki-Gun, Satsuma-Gun, Kushikino-Shi, Kawanabe-Gun, Makurazaki-Shi, Ibusuki-Gun, Soo-Gun, Kanoya-Shi, and Kimotsuki-Gun. Details of the results of microfilaria surveys conducted by previous workers were listed by SASA (1962). High microfilaria rates were reported by MATSUSHITA, in 1914, from Nagashima (28.7%, 33 of 115), by NAGAHANA *et al.*, in 1955, in Higashinagashima (26.0%, 13 of 50), by MATSUSHITA, in 1914, in Kamiideki-Mura (28.2%, 94 of 333) and Takashiro-Mura (28.2%, 68 of 241), by SATO *et al.*, in 1953, in Bonotsu-Mura (24.1%, 63 of 295), and by SAMEJIMA, in 1931, in Kiire-Mura (23.6%, 219 of 929). The overall microfilaria rate for six villages in Izumi-Gun was 26.8% (242 positives of 901) and that for four villages in Satsuma-Gun was 19.5% (108 of 554) at the time examined by MATSUSHITA in 1913.

(i.7b) Offshore islands of Kagoshima Prefecture:

All of the inhabited islands located near the mainland of Kyushu were known to be highly filarious. In Kami-Koshikijima, for example, CHOSA, in 1912, found a microfilaria rate of 26.5% (114 positives of 431 persons examined) in a survey of the general population. The rate reported by SATO *et al.* in 1953 for the people of the same island was 4.3% (27 of 630), much lower than reported previously. In three islands of Santoson (Iwojima, Takeshima, and Kuroshima), the overall microfilaria rate was reported to be 13.6% (50 of 367) by SATO *et al.* in 1950. In five village of Tanegashima, YOSHINAGA, in 1913, found 21.2% of 956 persons to be positive. In Yaku-shima, SAMEJIMA *et al.*, in 1955, reported an overall microfilaria rate of 7.9% (117 positives of 1,490). MATSUSHITA, in 1913, conducted a survey of five small islands of Juttoson, and found 115 of 655 persons to be positive (17.6%).

In the general blood surveys conducted from 1962 to 1963 by members of the Kagoshima Prefecture Health Department, the microfilaria rate was 7.19% (23 positives out of 320 persons examined) for the three islands of Santoson, 2.57% (742 of 28,883) for Tanegashima, 1.70% (214 of 12,607) for Yakushima, and 7.79% (102 of 1,310) for the Tokara Islands. All of these figures were lower than reported by previous authors (Fig. 8-9).

(i.7c) Amami Islands:

The Amami Islands are composed of five main islands: Amami-Oshima, Kikai, Tokunoshima, Okierabu, and Yoron. They are situated between latitudes 27°N and 28°30'N. All of these islands were notorious for the prevalence of filariasis, and at least 25 papers were published before 1962 in reference to filariasis surveys in this region. For example, YOSHINAGA, in 1913, conducted blood examinations in three villages on Amami-Oshima, and found 199 (27.3%) of 730 villagers to be positive for microfilariae. In a more recent sampling survey of ten municipalities of Amami-Oshima by SATO *et al.* in 1955, 298 of 1,504, or 19.8%, were positive. In four villages selected for filariasis control pilot studies, SASA *et al.*, in 1959, obtained a microfilaria rate of 11.8% (105 of 933) in Daikuma, 16.2% (32 of 198) in Nakakachi, 18.9% (36 of 192) in Ariya, and 30.2% (73 of 241) in Aminoko. In the general blood survey under the national filariasis control program in 1962, 20,054 people (41.2% of the total population) in the northern half of Amami-Oshima were examined, and 2,067 (10.3%) were positive for microfilariae. In the southern half of the island 13,797, or 51.8% of the whole population, were examined and 1,541 (11.2%) were positive.

On Tokunoshima Island, YOSHINAGA, in 1913, found 47 of 118 persons (36.8%) to be positive for microfilariae. In 1962, 10,462 persons, or 27.6% of the whole population of the island, were examined, and 1,254 persons, or 11.8%, were positive for microfilariae.

On Kikai Island, YOSHINAGA, in 1913, reported that 69 of 225, or 30.7% of the people examined, were microfilaria positive. In the general blood survey conducted from 1962 to 1963, 3,460 persons, or 33.1% of the total population, were examined, and 392, or 11.3% among them were positive for microfilariae.

On Okierabu Island, YOSHINAGA, in 1913, found 287 (30.6%) of 939 persons to be positive for microfilaria. ABE *et al.* in 1960, reported a microfilaria rate of 15.8% (112 positives out of 707) for the people in Kunigami, 16.4% (69 of 420) for Tamagusuku, and 29.4% (27 of 92) for Wadomari. In 1962 general survey, 9,598 (39.0% of the whole population) were examined, and 1,109 (11.55%) were positive for microfilariae.

On Yoron Island, ABE *et al.*, in 1960, conducted blood surveys of three villages, and found 29.6% (118 of 443) to be positive. In the general blood survey in 1962, 4,864 (61.3% of the whole population) were examined, and 749 (15.40%) were positive. This is the highest microfilaria rate observed among the Amami and the offshore islands of Kagoshima.

(i.8) Okinawa Prefecture

Okinawa is the southernmost prefecture of Japan comprising the southern part of the Ryukyu Archipelago, with a total area of 3,837 km² and a population of 945,111 (1970). There are two island groups: the Okinawa group, comprising the main island of Okinawa and a number of adjacent small islands, and the Sakishima group, comprising the Miyako Islands and the Yaeyama Islands. The former group is situated between longitudes 26°N and 27°N, and the latter group between 24°N and 25°N.

All the islands of Okinawa had been notorious for the high prevalence of filariasis until recently, and large numbers of papers were published referring to filariasis in Okinawa. KUNIYOSHI (1970a, b) compiled a comprehensive review of the studies on filariasis in Okinawa from 1949 to 1969, in which he listed 109 papers published in various medical journals.

The oldest record of filariasis in Okinawa is probably a report by Mine in 1911, on the prevalence of filaria infection among soldiers in Okinawa. In the general blood survey of soldiers in 1911, 291 of 1,650 persons examined in Okinawa were positive, and the microfilaria rate of 17.6% was the highest among all the regimental districts of Japan.

Among a number of pre-World War II studies on the epidemiology of filariasis in Okinawa, the most comprehensive one was that reported by SAIGO in 1939, who examined 7,766 persons of all ages on the mainland of Okinawa and found microfilariae in 14.24%, fever attacks in 13.99%, chyluria in 1.07%, and elephantiasis (probably including hydrocele) in 1.94%. FUJII, in 1915, reported on the prevalence of microfilaria cases among children in Okinawa, and found 14.1% of 1,001 persons under the age of 16 years positive.

(i.8a) Okinawa and adjacent islands

According to KUNIYOSHI (1970a), blood surveys were conducted by the Okinawa Prefecture Health Department from 1933 to 1937 in nine rural villages on the main island of Okinawa; of a total of 6,426 persons examined, 1,004, or 15.6%, were found to be positive for microfilaria. During the period from 1949 to 1966, extensive blood surveys of various villages were conducted by KUNIYOSHI and associates of the Ryukyu Health Laboratories, as well as by workers from the universities of Tokyo, Kagoshima, and Nagasaki. As the total figures of 46 reports made by these workers, altogether, 36,520 persons of all ages from various villages on Okinawa Island were examined, and 2,086 or 7.7% were positive for microfilaria. The microfilaria rates according to the three regions of the island were 7.0% (1,366 positives of 19,729) in southern Okinawa, 9.5% (777 of 8,158) in middle Okinawa, and 7.7% (663 of 8,633) in northern Okinawa.

In the Kumejima Islands, four surveys were conducted during the period from 1955 to 1960, and 236 (8.0%) of the total of 2,955 persons examined were positive.

On Iheya Island, two surveys were conducted in 1956 and in 1963; the middle school pupils showed a microfilaria rate of 7.9% (21 positives of 263 examined) in 1956, while the rate for the total number of people of all ages in four villages in 1963 was 15.0% (141 of 974).

On Ie Island, 1,340 persons in eight villages were examined in 1963, and 83 (6.2%) of 1,340 were positive.

Microfilaria carriers were found on all the other islands of the Okinawa group surveyed: Kouri, 9.5% (47 of 492); Kerama (total of three surveys), 6.0% (46 of 771); Henza, 11.3% (9 of 80); Miyagi, 13.0% (323 of 2,492); Ike, 16.3% (23 of 141); Tsuken, 3.8% (6 of 160); Kudaka, 1.1% (5 of 436); Kita-Daito, 2.2% (10 of 465); and Minami-Daito, 4.4% (37 of 837).

Blood examinations of pupils of 36 middle schools in the northern Okinawa region were conducted in 1969 by members of the Nago Health Center, as a preliminary survey for the planning of the filariasis control program. Altogether, 7,905 pupils (98.7% of all) were examined, and 88, or 1.2% were found to be carriers. In 12 villages where both the middle school pupils and the general population of all ages were examined, the overall microfilaria rate was 4.4% (19 positives of 435) in the pupils and 3.9 % (100 of 2,558) in the general population (excluding the pupils). The prevalence of filariasis as judged from these rates was lower than expected from the previous surveys in Okinawa.

(i.8b) Miyako Islands

The Miyako Islands include three main islands: Miyako, Irabu, and Tarama. They have a total population of 68,000 (1970). The intensity of infection of filariasis in this region was probably the highest among the island-groups of Okinawa, as indicated by the results of various surveys conducted after World War II. However, there is no prewar record on the epidemiology of filariasis in this region.

The Miyako Islands are all low and flat, being elevated coral reefs. Since there are no large rivers or streams, the people used to keep water in barrels or small tanks, which served as ideal breeding places for the vector, *C. p. fatigans*. This is probably the reason that the incidence of filariasis used to be much higher than on the neighboring Ishigaki Island, which is mountainous and has many streams.

According to the check list of literature compiled by KUNIYOSHI (1970b), a total of 14 filariasis surveys were conducted in the Miyako Islands by various workers during the period from 1958 to 1965, before the start of the drug treatment project. High microfilaria rates generally exceeding 20 % (sometimes over 30%) were reported from various villages, with the exception of a few urban areas of Hirara City. For example, TANAKA *et al.*, in 1958, examined four villages on Miyako Island and found 25.6% (169 of 661) of the people to be positive for microfilariae. Especially high microfilaria rates were reported from Hisamatsu of Miyako Island, where OMORI *et al.* (1961) found 42.4% of 290 middle school pupils, 29.8% of 650 primary school pupils, and 42.6% of 148 other villagers to be positive. In the same village, OMORI *et al.* (1962) reported 37.76% of 2,998 persons were microfilaria carriers.

On Irabu Island, KATAMINE (1962) made a survey of two villages, and found 222 positive cases (26.1%) out of 850 persons examined.

A blood survey with 30 mm^3 night samples of the whole population of the Miyako Islands was carried out in 1965, as the first-year project of the filariasis control program of the Ryukyu Islands. In this survey, 66,333 persons, or 99.0%, of the total registered population of 67,020 (excluding babies under 12 months old) of the whole area of the Miyako Islands were examined, and 12,707 persons, or 19.2%, were found to be microfilaria positive. The rates according to six municipalities were 15.9% (4,749 positives of 29,810) for Hirara-Shi, 21.0% (2,986 of 14,232) for Gusukube-Cho, 19.4% (983 of 5,074) for Shimoji-Cho, 23.9% (1,086 of 4,551) for Ueno-Son, 22.8% (2,307 of 10,104) for Irabu-Son, and 22.3% (596 of 2,560) for Tarama-Son. The distribution of microfilaria rates were all high and fairly uniform throughout the islands, with the exception of Hirara, where the urban areas showed significantly lower rates than the average.

(i.8c) Yaeyama Islands

The Yaeyama Islands comprise three large and mountainous islands, Ishigaki, Iriomote, and Yonaguni, and several other smaller, flat and low coral reef islands. Because of the prevalence of malaria until recent years (due to the breeding of many *An. minimus* in streams) both Ishigaki and Iriomote have been only sparsely populated. The prevalence of filariasis in Yaeyama was reported by YOKOGAWA & YUMOTO in 1939, OHAMA in 1939, and YOSHINO & NAKAZATO in 1940. Epidemiological surveys of various islands and villages were conducted also by a number of workers after the war, as reviewed by KUNIYOSHI (1970a). In general, *W. bancrofti* carriers and clinical filariasis cases were found all over the islands and villages of Yaeyama, but the incidence seemed to be lower than in the Miyako Islands.

A general blood survey and drug treatment program covering the whole area of Yaeyama was initiated in 1967 as the second target of the filariasis control project of the Ryukyu Islands. Of a total population of 49,432 in the Yaeyama Islands, 46,595 persons, or 94.2%, received blood examinations in 1967, and 3,400 (7.3%) among them were found to be harboring microfilariae in 30 mm^3 night blood samples. The microfilaria rate was revealed to be much lower in general than in the Miyako Islands. The rates according to the municipalities were: 7.4% (2,766 positives of 37,389 persons examined) for Ishigaki, 6.1% (200 of 3,299) for Yonaguni, and 7.3% (434 of 5,907) for Taketomi (including Taketomi, Iriomote, Hateruma, Kuroshima, Kohama, and Hatoma Islands).

Note: Prevalence of filariasis in the Ryukyu Archipelago

The Ryukyu Archipelago (in the broader sense) is a chain of islands connecting Kyushu and Taiwan, between latitudes 24°N and 32°N. The archipelago comprises the Yaeyama Islands (from Yonakuni to Ishigaki), the Miyako Islands (from Tarama to Miyako), the Okinawa Islands, the Amami Islands (from Yoron to Kikai), the Tokara Islands, the Tane-Yaku Islands (Tanegashima and Yakushima), and the Santoson Islands. The first three islands constitute Okinawa Prefecture, while the remaining northern groups of islands belong to Kagoshima Prefecture.

Blood surveys of people on these islands were conducted under the national filariasis control program of Japan (started in 1962) and the filariasis control program of the Ryukyu Islands (started in 1965). The results were compiled by SASA *et al.* (1970), as shown in Table 8-10 and Figs. 8-9, 8-10. The islands of the Yaeyama-group showed various levels of microfilaria rates, from the lowest of 3.29% in Taketomi to the highest of 20.56% in Hatoma; the big islands of Ishigaki (7.37%) and Iriomote (5.84%) had relatively lower prevalence. On the other hand, all of the three islands of the Miyako-group showed high microfilaria rates (18 to 23%). The five islands of the Amami-group showed rates of about 11%, with the exception of Yoron (15.4%). The islands situated further north and near Kyushu were much lower in general.

In general, it can be stated that the prevalence of filariasis in the Ryukyu Archipelago is highly correlated with the latitude, or with the annual average temperature, with the exception of the Yaeyama-group which comprises islands of various environmental conditions.

8C.5.3 The vectors of *W. bancrofti* in Japan

Previous studies conducted by various workers have shown that mosquitoes of the *Culex pipiens* complex (*C. pipiens pallens* in the mainland, and *C. pipiens fatigans* in the Amami and the Ryukyu Islands) are the only important vectors of *W. bancrofti* in Japan, although several other mosquito species were shown to serve as excellent intermediate hosts when infected experimentally. Reviews were made by OMORI (1962a, b) on the role of various Japanese mosquitoes in the transmission of filariasis in Japan, and by SASA (1966) on the taxonomy, biology, and insecticide resistance of filaria vectors in Japan.

8C.5.3.1 Natural and experimental infection of mosquitoes

The development of *W. bancrofti* larvae in various mosquito species in Japan was studied first by MOCHIZUKI (1911) in Fukuoka, Kyushu. Of 58

Table 8-10. Microfilarial rate observed at pretreatment blood surveys of southwestern Japanese islands, 1962–67.

Code No.	Name of island	Year of survey	Population	Number examined	Number positive	Percent positive
1	Yonakuni	1967	3,299	3,299	200	6.06
2	Hateruma	1967	1,239	1,235	109	8.83
3	Iriomote	1967	2,889	2,758	161	5.84
4	Hatoma	1967	193	180	37	20.56
5	Aragusuku	1967	91	91	11	12.09
6	Kurojima	1967	543	543	72	13.26
7	Kobama	1967	702	701	29	4.14
8	Taketomi	1967	395	395	13	3.29
9	Ishigaki	1967	40,064	37,388	2,756	7.37
10	Tarama	1966	2,579	2,560	596	23.28
11	Irabu	1966	10,201	10,104	2,307	22.83
12	Miyako	1966	52,827	52,354	9,411	17.98
13	Okinawa Isds	55–65	812,339	10,522	1,784	16.91
14	Yoron	1962	7,936	4,864	749	15.40
15	Okierabu	1962	24,591	9,598	1,109	11.55
16	Tokunoshima	1962	37,935	10,462	1,254	11.78
17	South Amami	1962	26,642	13,797	1,541	11.17
18	North Amami	1962	48,670	20,054	2,067	10.31
19	Kikai	62, 63	10,447	3,460	392	11.33
20	Tokara Isds	62, 63	1,801	1,310	102	7.79
21	Yakushima	62, 63	18,357	12,607	214	1.70
22	Tanegashima	62, 63	50,081	28,883	742	2.57
23	Santoson Isds	62, 63	515	320	23	7.19
24	Koshikijima	62, 63	19,552	8,508	569	6.69
25	Nagashima	62, 63	15,863	9,736	189	1.94

C. p. pallens which had fed on a donor carrying 3.735 microfilariae per 1 mm³ of blood and dissected 11 to 17 days after taking the blood meal, 57 (98.3%) were found to contain mature larvae. The number of mature larvae per infected mosquito was 19.14. The development to mature larvae under experimental condition was also observed in *Ae. togoi*, *C. bitaeniorhynchus*, and *C. tritaeniorhynchus*, though the rates of maturity in the last two species were very low.

YAMADA (1927) conducted comprehensive studies on the development of *W. bancrofti* larvae in 24 species of Japanese mosquitoes when experimentally fed on a microfilaria carrier. As a result, the mosquitoes were classified into various groups according to their compatibility with the parasite, as discussed in Section 2E.2. Development to the mature larvae was seen in seven species, among which the four species regarded as the most efficient vectors were *C. whitmorei*, *C. vagans*, *C. p. pallens*, and *Ae. togoi*.

KOBAYASHI (1940, 1941) conducted detailed studies on the morphology

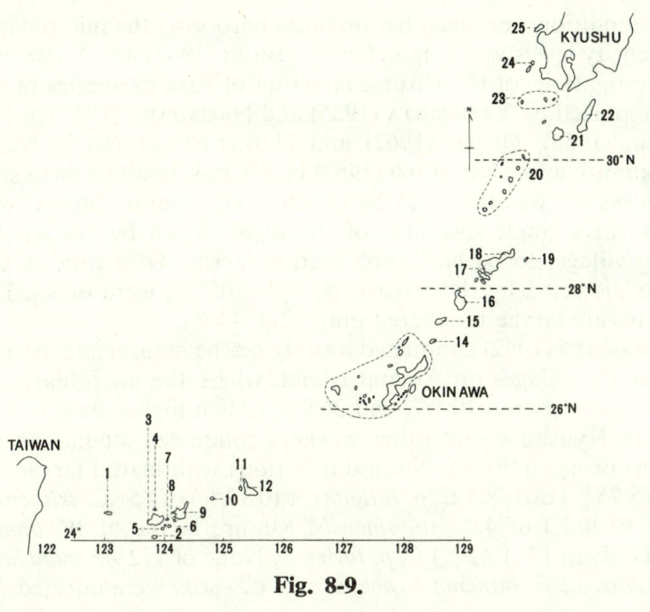

Fig. 8-9.

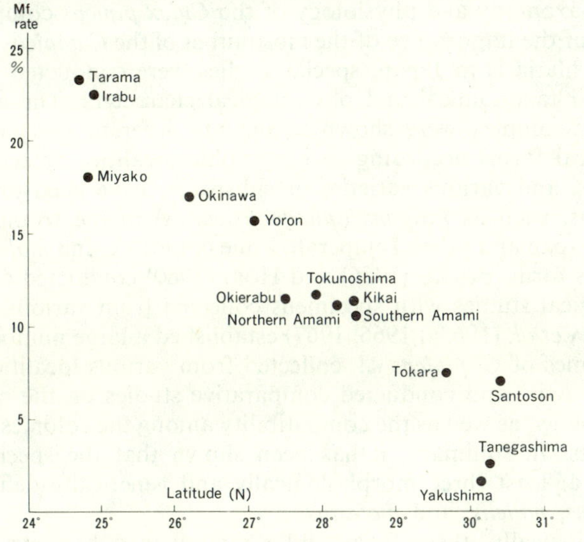

Fig. 8-10. The correlation between microfilaria rate and latitude in the islands of the Ryukyu Archipelago, southern Japan (excluding the Yaeyama Islands). Compiled from data in Table 8-10.

of *W. bancrofti* developing in *C. p. fatigans* in Taiwan.

A series of experimental studies on the development of *W. bancrofti* larvae in *C. p. pallens* and other mosquito species under different temperature conditions, or when fed on hosts harboring the microfilariae at various density levels was conducted by OMORI (1962) and YAMAMOTO (1962).

Investigations of the natural infection of various species of mosquitoes were reported by YAMASHITA (1955) and NAGAHANA (1957) in Kagoshima, OSHIMA (1956), OMORI (1962) and NAGATOMO (1960) in Nagasaki and Kumamoto, and YAMAMOTO (1962) in Amami. In all of these studies, only *C. pipiens* s.l. was found to be infected with mature larvae, with the exception of a single specimen of *Ae. togoi* shown by OMORI (1962), in a fishing village, to be harboring mature larvae. Of a total of 2,719 *C. p. pallens* dissected by these workers, 291 (10.7%) were infected, but those with mature larvae numbered only 12 (0.44%).

YAMAMOTO (1962) conducted a study on the natural infection of mosquitoes in six villages on Amami Island, where the microfilaria rate of the people was between 10.5% and 26.9% (much higher than in the endemic areas in Kyushu where other workers conducted studies on natural infections of mosquitoes). Natural infections with filarial larvae were found in 69 (5.75%) of 1,201 *C. p. fatigans*, 1 (0.12%) of 851 *C. tritaeniorhynchus*, and 2 (0.46%) of 435 *An. sinensis*. Mature larvae of *W. bancrofti* were found only in 17 (1.42%) *C. p. fatigans*. None of 172 *Ar. subalbatus*, 13 *Ae. albopictus*, 12 *C. bitaeniorhynchus*, or 1 *C. vorax* were infected.

8C.5.3.2 Taxonomy and physiology of the *Culex pipiens* complex

In view of the importance of the mosquitoes of the *C. pipiens* complex as vectors of filariasis in Japan, special studies were conducted in order to clarify their taxonomical and physiological characters. The members of this species-complex were shown to include different morphological or physiological forms according to geographic localities or ecological environments, and various varieties or subspecies have been proposed for these forms, such as *fatigans* (*quinquefasciatus*) in the tropical regions, *pallens* in Japan and other Temperate Zone countries, and *molestus* for the autogenous form. BEKKU (1956) and HORI (1960) conducted comparative morphological studies with specimens collected from various districts of Japan. SASA *et al.* (1963a, 1966, 1967) established a large number of laboratory colonies of *C. pipiens* s.l. collected from various localities in Japan and South Asia, and conducted comparative studies on the morphology and physiology, as well as the compatibility among the colonies in crossing experiments. In summary, it has been shown that the species-complex comprises at least three morphologically and genetically defined forms, i.e., *fatigans*, *pallens*, and *molestus*.

Morphologically, these forms differ mainly in a biometric character called the D/V index of the male genitalia. The form *fatigans* is distributed to the tropical and subtropical regions south of the Amami Islands. The form *pallens* includes specimens representing all the intermediate values of D/V between the typical *pallens* and *pipiens* forms. On the other hand, *molestus* in Japan is found restricted to large cities, breeding in underground sewage water from buildings and subways, and physiologically distinct from the other forms in that it is autogenous (produce eggs without taking a blood meal) and stenogamous (able to copulate in a small space). In the crossing experiments, various grades of incompatibility were shown to exist among the different colonies, and nearly complete incompatibility was shown between the *pallens* and the *molestus* colonies collected from the same localities (Sasa *et al.*, 1966, 1967). However, as reviewed by Omori (1962), all of these three forms collected and tested in Japan were shown to act as excellent intermediate hosts of *W. bancrofti* under experimental conditions.

The most important and reliable morphological character for differentiating the three forms is a biometrical index called the D/V ratio defined by Sasa *et al.* (1963a). This is the relative length (in percentage) of the distance between the tips of the dorsal arms (D) divided by the distance between the tips of the ventral arms (V) of the phallosome of male genitalia. According to Sasa *et al.* (1967), the colonies collected from Rangoon, Kuala Lumpur, and Bangkok, as well as those from the Ryukyu and the Amami Islands of Japan, had uniform values of the D/V ratio (29.1 to 35.2% in average), and are considered to represent the form *fatigans*. On the other hand, those collected from the mainland of Japan north of Kagoshima showed more or less larger values, and the ratio was found to increase as the locality of collection of the colony moved towards the north, from 49.1% in Kagoshima to 90.2% in Sapporo, Hokkaido. The form *pallens* is, therefore, regarded as a population representing all the intermediate values between the two extreme forms, i.e., *fatigans* in the tropical region and *pipiens* (*typicus*) in the arctic region. On the other hand, the colonies representing the form *molestus*, which were collected from underground waters in large cities of Japan, were differentiated from the above two forms not only by the physiological characters, such as the autogeny and stenogamy, but also by the D/V values (about 125%), which are significantly larger than even the largest form of *pallens*. (see Section 2E. 1)

Being the most common man-biting mosquito and the main vector of *W. bancrofti* in Japan, extensive studies were carried out by various authors on the behavior and bionomics of *C. pipiens* s.l. For example, Sasa *et al.* (1964, 1965) carried out observations on the biting rhythm of the females, and showed that their biting activity becomes highest at midnight, synchronizing with the peak density of the microfilariae in the circulating blood. Both males and females were found to rest in dark places in houses, and a trap for collecting the resting adult mosquitoes was devised using a cardboard box and dark cloth; this trap was useful for estimating the population density of this mosquito species. The chronological rhythm of their resting behavior and flight activity was also measured quantitatively with this type of mosquito trap. Another type of mosquito trap for collecting large numbers of the unengorged female mosquitoes was devised by Sasa *et al.* (1960), and was used for the observation of biting activities of various species of female mosquitoes in the field (see Sections 10C.1.2

and 10C.2.3). Series of investigations were conducted by HAYASHI *et al.* (1965a, b) and HAYASHI & KURIHARA (1965) on the physiological age of mosquitoes in relation to the transmission of filariasis (see Section 10C.).

8C.5.3.3 Methods for vector control

(a) Environmental methods:

Various methods have been proposed and studied in Japan for the control of vector mosquitoes, as reviewed by SASA (1966a). It has been generally accepted in Japan that the most effective and efficient method for the control of *C. pipiens* is the elimination of the breeding places by environmental sanitation measures. In fact, remarkable reductions in the transmission of *W. bancrofti* have been achieved in many endemic foci in the mainland of Japan apparently by the reduction of the breeding places after installment of pipe-water supply systems and construction of adequate sewage drains.

(b) Chemical methods:

Basic studies were made by a number of workers on the use of insecticides and other chemicals (including chemosterilants and hormones) for the control of mosquito adults or larvae. For example, IKESHOJI *et al.* (1958) tested the susceptibility of several mosquito species to chlorinated and organophosphorous insecticides; in the case of *C. pipiens* s.l., the toxicity as estimated from the value of LC-50 against the larvae was by order: parathion, dieldrin, diazinon, dichlorovos, trichlorfon, aldrin, lindane, and DDT. Developments of resistance to the chlorinated insecticides (DDT, dieldrin, lindane) were demonstrated in some colonies of *C. p. pallens* from Tokyo and *C. p. fatigans* from the endemic areas on Amami.

MIZUTANI & SUZUKI (1962), as well as SUZUKI & MIZUTANI (1962, 1963) conducted extensive surveys of insecticide resistance in the mosquitoes of Japan mainly by a topical application method in adults and by a dipping method in larvae. Remarkable differences in the susceptibility were seen especially among various colonies of the *C. pipiens* complex to chlorinated hydrocarbon insecticides. For example, the LC-50 (50% lethal concentration) of DDT against larvae of *C. p. pallens* in Kawasaki was 0.29 ppm, and was about 600 times higher than the value of 0.0005 ppm observed with the larvae of *C. tritaeniorhynchus* collected from the same locality. SUZUKI (quoted by SASA, 1963) conducted a survey of the susceptibility of *C. p. fatigans* in the endemic areas of *W. bancrofti* in the Yaeyama Islands. It was noted that the colonies collected from the formerly malarious islands where DDT residual spraying had been conducted over several years were highly resistant to DDT, while those collected from malaria-free islands were still very susceptible. The resistance of *C. pipiens* against various insecticides is a genetical character, and the mode of its inheritance and development was investigated extensively by SUZUKI *et al.* (1964a, b, 1966), UMINO & SUZUKI (1965, 1967), and UMINO (1965a, b, c; 1966). SUZUKI (1968) reported on the discovery of a colony of *C. p. pallens* in central

Honshu which had developed a multiple resistance to organophosphorous insecticides.

Because mosquitoes of the *C. pipiens* complex were shown to develop resistance to the chlorinated hydrocarbon insecticides rather easily, some organophosphorous insecticides including malathion, diazinon, fenitrothion, fenthion, and ronnel, were recommended for use in the control of filariasis vectors in Japan. Among them, fenitrothion (Sumithion) was shown to be effective as a residual indoor-spray insecticide against mosquitoes in the field studies conducted by MIZUTANI & HIRAKOSO (1962) and KURIHARA *et al.* (1965).

Studies were made by SASA *et al.* (1965b) on the comparative toxicity of various insecticides to *C. p. fatigans* larvae and to its natural enemy, *Poecilia reticulata*; most chlorinated hydrocarbons such as DDT, BHC, and dieldrin, were shown to be more toxic to the fish than to the mosquito larvae, while the relationship was reversed in most organophosphorous insecticides. For example, the LC-50 of fenitrothion to the mosquito larvae was 0.002 ppm, while the LC-50 of the mosquito-eating fish was 4.0 ppm, and thus this compound was shown to be 2,000 times more toxic to the mosquito larvae than to the fish. In this study, fenitrothion was found to loose its toxicity within a few days when mixed in polluted waters, and later laboratory studies conducted by YASUNO *et al.* (1965), HIRAKOSO & UCHIDA (1966), and HIRAKOSO (1966) have shown that this compound is a biologically degradable substance and is easily inactivated and decomposed by certain micro-organisms commonly found in polluted waters.

(c) Biological methods:

While it was believed generally that the biological control of *C. p. fatigans* by the use of fishes was impossible because the larvae breed in highly polluted waters, SASA *et al.* (1965c) discovered in Bangkok that *Poecilia reticulata*, a tropical pet fish native of South America, and commonly called the guppy, had a special ability for breeding in sewage pools and could be used as an effective, natural enemy of the filaria vector. As reviewed by SASA (1972), a series of laboratory and field studies were conducted in Japan and South Asia for the use of this and related fishes in the control of mosquito larvae. On the other hand, another viviparous freshwater fish of the same family, called the top minnow, or *Gambusia affinis*, was recently found to be breeding widely in areas in and around the city of Tokyo. This is a species introduced into Japan in 1916 from Texas for the purpose of malaria control, but it was also shown to be effective as the natural enemy of filaria vectors because it can breed in sewage waters. SATO *et al.* (1972) reported successful results in a large area control of mosquitoes breeding in ditches and swamps around the city of Tokushima on Shikoku Island by the introduction of *Gambusia affinis* from Tokyo.

KURIHARA (1973), KURIHARA & SASA (1973), and KURIHARA *et al.* (1973a, b) conducted a series of experimental and field studies on the efficiency of the guppy, *Poecilia reticulata*, in the control of *C. p. pallens* larvae. The average number of mosquito larvae eaten or killed per day by a guppy was found to differ greatly according to the age or the size of the larvae; for example, a young fish consumed about 2,000 mosquito eggs per day, 332 first instar larvae, 107 three-day-old larvae, 92 four-day-old larvae, and only 15 five-day-old larvae. Therefore, it usually requires at least a few months before the fishes released into a mosquito breeding pool reach a population density sufficient for the eradication of the larvae. On the other hand, application of insecticide such as fenitrothion at a concentration of 0.1 ppm is effective in killing all the mosquito larvae, but this must be repeated once every week in order to prevent the emergence of mosquitoes from a pool. However, the simultaneous use of the fishes and the insecticides to a pool has been shown to be effective for the permanent prevention of the mosquito breeding with a single procedure, because the insecticide at this concentration kills all the mosquito larvae but not the fishes, and the small number of the fishes can eat all the mosquito eggs subsequently deposited into the pool.

8C.5.4 *Brugia malayi* in Japan

Human filariasis in Japan had been considered to be due exclusively to *W. bancrofti* until recently. ABE (1936) conducted careful examinations of blood films collected from 915 Japanese soldiers in Taiwan recruited from various regions of southern Kyushu for the occurrence of *B. malayi* infection, but all the microfilariae found in blood specimens of 78 positive cases were those of *W. bancrofti*. On the other hand, two Japanese workers who were engaged in medical services during the war in China and Korea discovered new endemic foci of *B. malayi*, i.e., MONMA (1942, 1943, 1944) in Chekiang and Kiangsu Provinces, and SENOO (1943) in South Korea.

Incidentally, an endemic focus of *B. malayi* infection was discovered in 1950 by a team from the Institute for Infectious Diseases, University of Tokyo, on a small volcanic island called Hachijo-Koshima, and its new vector, as well as the effect of diethylcarbamazine, was reported by HAYASHI *et al.* (1951) and SASA *et al.* (1951, 1952). The island was visited frequently thereafter for studies on epidemiology and pilot control, and a series of reports were made by the same group of workers. A review was made by SASA (1966) on the progress of these studies.

8C.5.4.1 Epidemiology

Hachijo-Koshima is an island of about 3.16 km^2 in size, and is situated at 33°7′ N in latitude and 139°40′ in longitude (Fig. 8-11). It belongs to the so-called Izu-Shichito Archipelago composed of some ten islands in the Pacific south of Tokyo, and constitutes the southern group together with Hachijo and Aogashima. It is closely attached to the main island of Hachijo which has a population of about 10,000, and is separated by a channel only 4 km wide. Hachijo-Koshima is an oval-shaped volcanic island with the longer diameter of about 3 km and the shorter diameter of 1.5 km; it is steeply conical and the highest point is 616.8 m above sea level. The coast line is mostly steep rocky cliffs and there are numerous rock pools near the beach. The average monthly temperature ranges from a low of 10.0°C in February to a high of 26°C in August, and the total amount of rainfall per year reaches to over 2,400 mm on average.

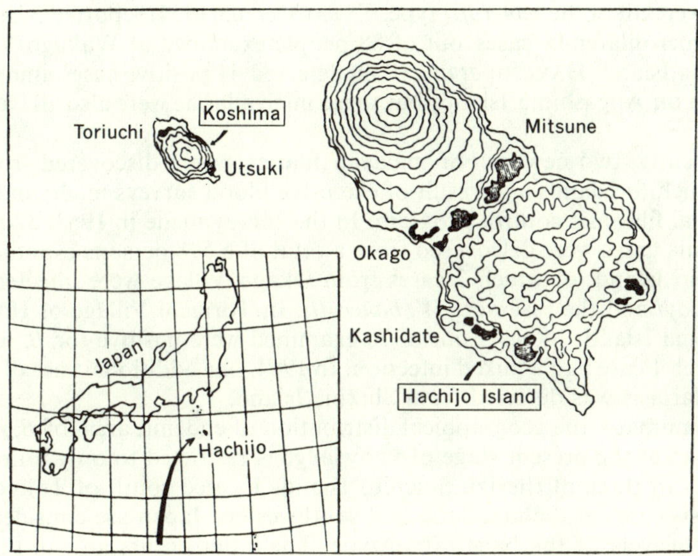

Fig. 8-11.   Map of Hachijo and Koshima

The population of the island was about 170 in 1950 when the survey was started. The people lived in two villages isolated from each other: Toriuchi on the north, with a population of about 100; and the rest in Utsuki on the southern slope. Because the island is covered by volcanic sand and rocks, there are no streams and swamps, so that each household has a large concrete tank to preserve rainwater, which also serves as a breeding place for the vector mosquitoes.

The occurrence of filariasis in the Izu-Shichito Islands has been known since old times. YOSHINAGA & CHOSA (1911) visited Hachijo and Hachijo-Koshima, and detected 76 cases of elephantiasis. MOCHIZUKI & INOUE (1912) made surveys of microfilaraemia and clinical cases in the same islands and discovered 41 microfilaria positive cases out of 88 people examined on Hachijo-Koshima. They reported that although elephantiasis cases were common among inhabitants of this island, there were no cases of hydrocele or chyluria, and that they found filarial larvae in 3 out of 15 "yabuka" mosquitoes (Japanese name for *Aedes*) collected at Toriuchi Village. This report was published 15 years before BRUG (1927) described malayian filariasis, and the authors already pointed out some unusual findings about filariasis on this island.

The investigations on the distribution of filariasis in the Izu-Shichito Islands were carried out by Sasa, Hayashi, and their associates along with the more detailed studies on malayian filariasis on Hachijo-Koshima. As was reported by Sasa & Hayashi (1953), microfilaremia positive cases detected at the surveys made in the mainland of Hachijo in 1950 and in 1952 were all of the *bancrofti* type. Tanaka *et al.* (1954) reported 3 bancroftian microfilaremia cases out of 88 people examined at Wakago Village, Niijima Island. Hayashi *et al.* (1959) detected 41 positive cases among 317 people on Aogashima Island, but these microfilariae were also all bancroftian.

Recently, two new foci of malayan filariasis were discovered from the Izu-Shichito Islands as a result of extensive blood surveys made under the national filariasis control program. In the survey made in 1963, 32 microfilaremia cases were discovered from a total of 5,598 persons examined on Hachijo Island, of which 2 cases from Okago Village were infected with *B. malayi* and the rest were *W. bancrofti*. In Toriuchi Village of Hachijo-Koshima Island, 14 cases out of 70 examined were positive for *B. malayi*, of which 1 case had a mixed infection. In 1964, one additional case of malayan filariasis was detected from Shikine Island.

In summary, the geographical distribution of endemic areas of *B. malayi* in Japan at the present stage of knowledge is restricted to only four small villages in three of the Izu-Shichito Islands located south of Tokyo, and filariasis cases in the mainland and southwestern Japan are considered to be exclusively of the bancroftian type. The latter occurs also in the Izu-Shichito Islands. All of the above endemic areas of *B. malayi* are located near the beach with large numbers of rock pools, in which *Ae. togoi* is breeding abundantly.

8C.5.4.2 Parasite carriers

The mode of distribution of microfilaria and clinical cases of malayian filariasis among inhabitants of Toriuchi Village, Koshima Island, has been repeatedly studied by the Sasa, Hayashi, and their associates since 1948. Results of the first detailed epidemiological study on this endemic focus were reported by Sasa, *et al.* (1952). Out of a total of 85 persons who were examined at this time, 29 cases (34.1%) were microfilaria positive and 44 cases (51.7%) showed some clinical signs, and the total number with either of the above filarial manifestations was 55 (64.6%). The clinical signs involved the recurrence of fever attacks associated with lymphangitis and lymphadenitis in the acute stage and elephantiasis of the legs or arms in the chronic stage, but neither chyluria nor hydrocele could be detected. The microfilaria rate was the highest in the age-group 31 to 40 years (73%, or 8 positives out of 11 examined), while the attack rate of clinical signs was 100 percent at ages above 41 years (28 cases). The experimental administration of diethylcarbamazine citrate was started in May 1950 to some of the microfilaria positive cases, and was found to be effective so long as sufficient total doses were taken, such as over 60 mg per kg of body weight. There were, however, some refusals, mainly because of the side reactions. The next survey was made four months later in September 1950, and 16.2%, or 12 cases out of 74 persons examined, were still microfilaria positive. Among 24 cases who were positive at the previous blood examination, 13 cases became negative at the second survey as a result of the drug treatment.

A total of 12 blood surveys and drug administrations were made during the 20-year period after the start of the initial trial in 1950. The drug was administered to positive cases at a rate of about 72 mg per kg of body weight (3.6 g for adults) in total. Each patient was requested to take daily doses of about 6 mg per kg. Some vector control measures were also applied occasionally, such as DDT residual spraying in houses and the application of DDT dust by helicopter in 1956, or the distribution of fishes (gold fish and medaka) in water reservoirs in 1950. Because of the lack of medical facilities on this island and the difficulties in transportation and communication, the above control measures have never been satisfactorily effective. The microfilaria rates observed in these surveys were subject to variation due to various effects, the reduction possibly owing to the drug treatments or to the vector control measures, and the increase in rates due to the occurrence of new positives and recurrent cases.

In 1962, the Izu Islands were also selected as one of the targets of the national filariasis control program, and Hachijo-Koshima was visited in 1963 by a team headed by Professor S. Hayashi. They found 14 of 85 persons still positive for the microfilariae of *B. malayi*. DEC was administered to all the people by the dosage schedule of 6 mg per kg daily for 12 days, and all the houses were sprayed with fenitrothion. When the island was again visited by the survey team in 1968, all of 68 persons examined were free from microfilaria. Because of the inconvenience of living on such a small island, in 1971, all the villagers decided to emigrate either to the mainland of Hachijo or to Tokyo and since then, Hachijo-Koshima has been an uninhabited island.

8C.5.4.3   Mosquito vectors

As was reviewed by SASA *et al.* (1952), RAGHAVAN (1961), and WHARTON (1962), there are three main groups of mosquitoes known to act as important vectors of malayan filariasis ih nature, species of *Mansonia* (*Mansonioides*), *Anopheles*, and *Aedes* (*Finlaya*). In most endemic areas in South Asia, species of the genus *Mansonia*, subgenus *Mansonioides*, are considered to be the main vectors. The malayan filariasis on Hachijo-Koshima, however, is transmitted chiefly by *Ae.* (*Finlaya*) *togoi* (THEOBALD) and thus is epidemiologically a rather unusual type, as that in southern Korea.

MOCHIZUKI & INOUE (1912), in their earliest survey of filariasis on Hachijo-Koshima, reported that among 15 'yabuka' mosquitoes collected in houses, 3 were infected with filarial larvae. These were probably *Ae.*

togoi, because this has been the only species of 'yabuka' collected from houses in Koshima at surveys made later. The first comprehensive survey of mosquito fauna of this island was made by SASA *et al.* (1952), in which six species were recorded: *C. p. pallens*, *C. vorax*, *Ae. togoi*, *Ae. albopictus*, *Ae. flavopictus*, and *Ar. subalbatus*. Among them, two species were most common, *Ae. togoi* and *C. p. pallens*. There were no swamps, streams or rice paddies on this island that allow the breeding of *Mansonia* and *Anopheles*. Larvae of *Ae. togoi* were found to be breeding abundantly in concrete water reservoirs in the village and also in rock pools near the beach. *C. p. pallens* were collected occasionally in sewage, discarded jars, and also in water reservoirs.

At the survey made in September 1950, a total of 68 mosquitoes were collected in houses, all were *Ae. togoi*, and 1 of them harbored 1 second stage and 1 third stage filarial larva; the latter was identified as an infective larva of *B. malayi*. HAYASHI (1954) further reported that 1 out of 7 *Ae. togoi* collected in houses in June 1952 harbored a second stage larva.

Results of experimental infection with local mosquitoes were also reported by HAYASHI (1954). Colonies of *C. p. pallens* and *Ae. togoi* were reared from pupae and larvae in June 1952 at Hachijo-Koshima, and were fed on a carrier of malayan filariasis whose microfilarial density was 77 per drop of blood (about 20 mm³) in average. About 40 *C. p. pallens* were successfully engorged, but unfortunately none of the *Ae. togoi* fed on the infective blood meal. The former were kept at a room temperature of 25° to 28°C, and were dissected after 13 and 18 days. Out of a total of 30 *C. p. pallens* dissected, 3 were infected; one dissected after 13 days harbored 2 third stage larvae, one dissected after 18 days harbored 1 third stage larva, and another dissected on the same day harbored 2 third stage larvae and 1 second stage larva.

8C.5.5 The national filariasis control programs in Japan

8C.5.5.1 An outline of their structures and progress

A filariasis control program for the mainland of Japan was organized in 1962, supported by budget and technical assistance from the national government. Blood surveys of suspected endemic areas and drug treatments of parasite carriers were initiated in five prefectures, i.e., Ehime, Kochi, Nagasaki, Kagoshima, and Tokyo (Izu Islands). In 1963, Miyazaki, Oita, and Niigata joined the program, and Kumamoto Prefecture participated in it in 1964. The director of health of each prefecture was responsible for the entire filariasis control activity. The blood surveys were carried out by teams dispatched from health centers to each village, while the drug administration was conducted by members of local physicians' associations. The numbers and percentages of persons examined in the target areas, and the numbers and percentages of persons found to be carrying microfilariae are as shown in Table 8-11.

Another filariasis control program for the Ryukyu Islands (Okinawa

Prefecture) was initiated in 1965 by the Government of Ryukyu, assisted by the Japanese and United States governments, with the Miyako Islands as the first target, the Yaeyema Islands as the second, and Okinawa Island as the third. The progress of this program is as shown in Table 8-13. The activity was taken over by Okinawa Prefecture when the political administration of the Ryukyus was handed over to Japan in 1971.

A critical review and comprehensive analysis of the progress of these filariasis control projects was reported by SASA *et al.* (1970). The programs in each prefecture or district proceeded roughly according to the following three phases.

(a) The preparatory phase: Collection of information on the geographic distribution of endemic foci was made in each prefectural health department by a review of published records and by the survey of clinical filariasis cases throughout the entire district. The training of health workers to engage in various activities under the filariasis control project was conducted by the Ministry of Health (for project leaders of each prefecture) and by each prefectural health department (for members of the blood survey and drug administration teams.)

(b) The attack phase: Blood survey teams were organized in each health center, and dispatched to the villages according to a schedule previously announced to the public. All the villagers above the age of one year were requested to visit a temporary filariasis clinic (usually the village hall or school) between 9 p.m. and midnight to receive a blood examination. The persons who were found to be harboring microfilariae in the blood smears (30 mm^3 in quantity) were assembled again in the village hall, and DEC was administered under the supervision of local physicians. The microfilaria carriers were examined again after completion of a course of the drug treatment, and if microfilariae were still positive in their 30 mm^3 blood samples, they were re-treated with another course of DEC administration. The entire populations of the same villages were surveyed repeatedly once a year or once in every two years until everyone became negative. Health education and vector control measures were appliedsimultaneously to the target villages.

(c) The surveillance phase: When the villages were treated repeatedly with the above control measures and judged to have become free from microfilaria carriers, they were omitted from the regular blood survey schedule, and blood examinations were conducted later with sample populations in order to check the recovery of transmission. Most of the previously known endemic foci in the mainland of Japan turned out to be practically free from microfilaria carriers after application of the control measures for a few to several years, and are now in the surveillance phase.

8C.5.5.2 Basic studies and pilot experiments

Before implementing the country-wide filariasis control project, basic studies and pilot experiments were conducted by a group of Japanese workers for a period of over ten years in order to find out the feasibility of the program and to establish a standard method by which the disease could be most effectively controlled. The successful results of this program in Japan is due largely to the introduction of effective and feasible methods established through these basic studies. The research activities during this period were directed to the following fields:

(a) Review of literature:

A bibliography referring to filariasis in Japan was compiled by SASA *et al.* (1959), in which a total of 786 papers scattered in various medical journals were collected and reviewed. A filariasis map of Japan such as shown in Fig 8-8 was prepared by SASA (1962), based on all the previous records of the occurrence of the disease. The prefectures to be involved and the areas to be covered under the national filariasis control program were selected first on the grounds of these published records.

(b) Pilot experiments for the establishment of standard methods:

Field studies were conducted from 1958 in the endemic areas of *W. bancrofti* in the Misaki district of Ehime Prefecture (Shikoku) and in the Amami district of Kagoshima Prefecture for the establishment of standard methods to be applied in epidemiological surveys and in the parasite and the vector control. The results were reported successively in separate papers, such as SASA *et al.* (1952, 1958, 1959b, 1960, 1963, 1970), SASA (1963, 1966, 1967), YAMAMOTO (1962), and KANDA & ISHII (1966). The details of methods for microfilaria survey and analysis of survey data were described by SASA (1967).

As for the methods of DEC administration, various dosage schemes were compared with respect to effectiveness, side reaction, and feasibility. The Amami Islands were especially fitted for these field studies because there were large numbers of small, isolated villages with high prevalence of microfilaria cases, and the people were very cooperative to the pilot studies. A series of comparative studies were conducted on the effectiveness of DEC administered under different dosage schemes.

At least three variables were considered to be involved in such experiments: (i) the size of the single dose; (ii) the size of the total dose, or how many times the drug should be administered; and (iii) the intervals of the drug administration, i.e., whether the drug is given three times a day, once a day, once every week, or once every month.

Since KESSEL (1957) reported that *W. bancrofti* infection in Tahiti could be effectively reduced by monthly adminstration of DEC and that the effects were less satisfactory with a daily administration scheme, it was first thought that the spaced administration, such as monthly or weekly intervals, might be the essential factor for the success of the program. However, it soon became clear through the comparative studies that the interval was not an important factor, and the effectiveness depended largely on the size of the total dose of DEC administered per person. For example, the same total dose (72 mg per kg) of DEC was administered to three groups of microfilaria carriers by 12 separate doses (all 6 mg per kg at one time) at intervals of one day, one week, and one month; the cure rates (the percentage of microfilaria carriers who became negative after the treatment) were all above 80%, and there was no significant difference in the effectiveness among the three groups. On the other hand, those who received only small total doses, such as 20 mg per kg (a standard dose in India) or 30 mg per kg, showed much lower cure rates regardless of the length of the intervals between the drug administrations (SASA, 1963; YAMAMOTO, 1965; SASA *et al.*, 1960, 1970).

Another series of comparative studies was conducted in the Amami Islands in order to understand the mode of appearance of the side effects which occur after DEC administration. By statistical analysis of the observed data, SASA *et al.* (1963, 1970) demonstrated that the so-called side effects of DEC could be classified into two syndromes with essentially different origins. A syndrome represented mainly by nausea and vomiting was caused by the toxic effect of the drug itself, dependent upon the size of the dose but with no relationship to the filaria infection; in other words this reaction occurred in almost everybody when a large single dose such as 0.6 g or more was administered. Another type of syndrome, which is called the febrile reaction, is caused mainly by the destruction of the microfilariae by the drug; it occurs about ten hours after the initial dose of DEC is swallowed, and the severity of this reaction is highly correlated with the microfilarial density in the circulating blood of carriers but rather independent of the dose of the drug. The attack rate of the febrile reaction increased as the microfilarial density became higher, and among the groups with similar levels of microfilarial density, this reaction seemed to occur more frequently among those treated with a lower dose (2 mg per kg) than those treated with a higher dose (8 mg per kg), at least in this experiment (see section 11C. 7).

From the results of these pilot experiments for effective and safe use of the drug, certain dosage schemes, such as the administration of 6 mg per kg once a day for 12 times, divided into two separate courses, were recommended for general use in Japan.

8C.5.5.3 Progress of the national filariasis control programs
(see Table 8-11)
(5.3.a) Ehime Prefecture:
Pilot experiments in the control of filariasis in this prefecture were initiated in 1958 as a joint program of the prefectural health department and the Department of Parasitology of the Institute for Infectious Diseases, University of Tokyo. Several villages in the Misaki Peninsula were selected as study areas, and comparative studies were carried out on various blood examinations and drug treatment methods for four years until 1962. The results accumulated during this period were reported by SASA *et al.* (1959c), and by SHIMONO (1961), director of the Ehime Health Department. The standard method employed by the national control program was developed during this period through experiences in this and the other pilot project in the Amami Islands.

Bancroftian filariasis was estimated to be widely distributed in this prefecture, especially in its southwestern districts, but the microfilaria rates obtained during blood surveys were lower than expected based on the number of clinical cases. Only 33 positive cases were detected in a blood survey of 2,050 persons in the pilot study area in 1958, and no districts with a positive rate exceeding 2% were found in the prefecture during later surveys. The program was expanded in 1962 to cover almost all suspected endemic areas. In connection with the start of the national project, a total of 318,898 persons were examined, and 103 positive cases (including 99 new cases) were recorded. Since all the microfilaria carriers detected at the annual blood surveys were repeatedly treated with the drug until they became negative, the reduction in the number of positive cases were remarkable, and the control project was suspended in 1966, when the last 2 positive cases became negative as a result of the drug treatment carried out during the previous year.

A follow-up blood examination was conducted in 1969 in Misaki District, where 2 cases out of 1,410 persons examined were found to be positive for microfilariae. However, in the blood survey of the same area carried out the next year, there were no positive cases detected.

(5.3.b) Kagoshima Prefecture:

The filariasis control program in Kagoshima Prefecture began in 1962 as a part of the national project. The villages designated to be covered by the control program were distributed in 64 municipalities under 15 health centers, mainly in the southern part of the prefecture and the adjacent islands. The population in the control area was 213,943 in total, or about 12% of the total population of the prefecture; 135,557 (63.4 %) received blood examinations within the fiscal year, and the overall microfilarial rate was 6.62%. The drug was distributed to all microfilaria positive cases, but its administration to individual cases was not directly supervised by health officers, except in certain model areas.

The project in the second year (1963) covered larger populations including certain new areas; a total of 167,604 persons were examined, of which 6,597, or 3.94%, were positive. The reduction in the positive rate was due mainly to the effects of the drug treatment carried out in the previous year. The control program has been applied repeatedly, either annually or once every two years, to the same villages during the period of the past seven years. Because the endemic areas in the mainland Kyushu districts of Kagoshima Prefecture became nearly free from microfilaria carriers after four years of control activity, beginning 1966, the efforts were directed to only the Amami Islands, where nearly 2,000 carriers were still detected out of a population of about 62,000 examined. The number and the rate of microfilaria cases reduced rapidly thereafter, as shown in Table 8-11.

The results of blood examinations of previously positive cases after treatment with a course of diethylcarbamazine administration are shown in Table 8-12. The so-called cure rate (percentage obtained by the number negative with the number examined after treatment of the previously

Table 8-11. Progress of the prefectural filariasis control program of Japan (compiled from reports of the prefectures).

Prefecture	Year	Population under control	Number examined	Percent examined	Number positive	Percent positive
a. Ehime	'58	2,097	2,050	97.8	33 (33)*	1.61
	'59	6,118	6,361	104.0	44 (35)	0.69
	'60	8,507	6,395	75.2	109 (106)	1.70
	'61	11,986	8,485	70.8	86 (80)	1.01
	'62	318,898	211,244	66.2	103 (99)	0.049
	'63	91,650	65,452	71.2	98 (86)	0.12
	'64	33,701	20,603	59.4	29 (24)	0.15
	'65	10,144	5,416	50.7	2 (2)	0.037
	'69	—	1,410	—	2 (2)	0.14
	'70	—	1,233	—	0	0.
b. Kagoshima	'62	213,943	135,557	63.4	8,968	6.62
	'63	295,361	167,604	56.8	6,597	3.94
	'64	186,489	99,864	53.6	4,498	4.50
	'65	161,101	81,503	50.6	2,918	3.58
	'66	138,128	61,969	44.9	1,958	3.16
	'67	154,303	68,446	44.4	1,186	1.73
	'68	—	61,116	—	755	1.24
	'69	—	66,105	—	345	0.52
	'70	—	18,118	—	134	0.74
	'71	—	11,645	—	91	0.78
c. Nagasaki	'62	340,822	202,941	59.5	2,660	1.31
	'63	258,401	165,950	64.2	1,502	0.90
	'64	230,534	138,349	60.0	887	0.64
	'65	119,623	62,789	52.5	441	0.70
	'66	83,455	42,611	51.1	255	0.60
	'67	81,067	44,814	55.3	259	0.58
	'68	52,214	27,376	52.4	151	0.55
	'69	37,718	24,531	65.0	56	0.23
	'70	12,812	9,413	73.5	30	0.32
	'71	2,855	1,449	50.8	5	0.35
d. Kumamoto	'64	456,317	41,038	9.0	111	0.27
	'65	41,707	15,486	37.1	120	0.77
	'66	16,211	5,382	33.2	43	0.80
	'67	17,097	5,414	31.7	46	0.45
e. Miyazaki	'63	48,084	25,040	52.1	3	0.012
	'64	4,730	3,174	67.1	0	0
f. Oita	'63	146,205	25,061	17.1	0	0
	'64	156,800	22,107	14.1	0	0

Table 8-11 Continued

Prefecture	Year	Population under control	Number exmined	Percent examined	Number positive	Percent positive
	'62	87,014	13,078	15.0	41	0.31
g. Kochi	'63	35,445	29,933	84.4	29	0.10
	'64	15,788	10,642	67.4	12	0.11
	'62	318	269	84.6	2	0.74
	'63	12,228	5,683	46.5	46	0.81
h. Tokyo	'64	5,187	2,592	50.0	11	0.42
(Izu Shichito	'65	4,300	2,466	57.3	11	0.45
Islands)	'66	8,680	2,399	27.6	0	0
	'67	12,100	2,250	18.6	0	0
i. Niigata	'63	34,514	22,513	65.2	0	0

*The numbers in brackets are the new positives.

Table 8-12. Results of post-treatment blood examinations as reported by prefectural health centers.

Prefecture or district	Year of survey	Number of Mf. carriers treated & examined	Number of cases became negative	So-called cure rate
	1962	6,114	4,182	68.4%
	'63	5,349	4,200	78.5
	'64	3,651	2,753	75.4
Kagoshima	'65	2,508	1,992	79.4
	'66	1,757	1,378	78.4
	'67	1,069	853	79.7
	'62	1,744	1,647	94.4
	'63	1,340	1,244	92.8
	'64	656	569	86.7
Nagasaki	'65	366	340	92.8
	'66	114	99	86.8
	'67	160	146	91.2
	'64	93	87	93.5
	'65	104	93	89.4
Kumamoto	'66	41	38	92.6
	'67	40	37	92.5
Miyako	'66	11,141	9,137	82.0
	'67	563	443	78.6

positive cases) was 68.4% in 1962, 78.5% in 1963, 75.4% in 1964, 79.4% in 1965, 78.4% in 1966, and 79.7% in 1967.

(5.3.c) Nagasaki Prefecture:

The second most important endemic region of filariasis after Kagoshima is Nagasaki Prefecture in western Kyushu; large numbers of case reports and survey records were published by various authors in the past. The prefectural-wide control program began in 1962, and areas under 15 health centers with a population of 340,822 in total were surveyed and treated during the first fiscal year. Microfilarial carriers were detected in all of the health center districts with the exception of the Tsushima Islands closest to Korea. The overall positive rate was 1.31% (2,660 of 202,941). The highest rate was observed at Oseto Health Center in Nishisonogi Peninsula, where 879 of 17,321 (5.07%) were positive. In other districts, the rates were by order: Iki Island (577 of 17,115; 2.37%), Fukue of the Goto Islands (269 of 9,392; 2.86%), and so on, to the lowest of Yoshii (5 of 17,033; 0.02%).

Blood surveys covering areas of similar size were carried out during the following two years, with observed positive rates of 0.90% (1,502 of 165,950) in 1963 and of 0.64% (887 of 138,349) in 1964. As a result, many of the villages with low infection rates became apparently parasite free, and thus the project in the following years was gradually reduced in size, as shown in Table 8-11. A total of 259 positive cases were still detected out of 44,814 persons examined in 1967, from areas under nine health centers. The cure rate reported by the prefectural health department was much higher than that reported by Kagoshima, and usually over 90% of the previously positive cases became negative within the same fiscal year (Table 8-12).

(5.3.d) Kumamoto Prefecture:

This prefecture is situated between Kagoshima and Nagasaki in western Kyushu, and has the third largest endemic areas of bancroftian filariasis in Japan, especially in the Amakusa Islands. The filariasis control project began in 1964, the third year of the national program, and a total of 41,038 persons (mainly middle and high school pupils of all suspected endemic areas) were examined, among which 111 positive cases were discovered. The control programs in the following years were directed mainly to the areas determined as active endemic foci by the presence of microfilarial carriers among the school pupils, namely, six municipalities in the Amakusa Islands and ten municipalities on the mainland of Kyushu. The numbers and percentages of microfilaria positive cases in 1965 were 95 of 9,707 (0.99%) in Amakusa, and 25 of 5,779 (0.42%) in Kyushu. The project, in 1966 and 1967, was concentrated again to more limited, active foci, and the positive cases discovered were 43 and 46, respectively. All the microfilarial carriers detected were treated with the drug within the same fiscal year so long as they were available, and the cure rates were mostly over 90%, as shown in Table 8-12.

(5.3.e) Other prefectures:

The national filariasis control program was accepted by five additional prefectures: by Kochi and Tokyo in 1962, and by Miyazaki, Oita, and Niigata in 1963. No microfilaria positive cases were detected from a survey of 34,514 persons in 1963 in Niigata. None of 25,061 examined in 1963, or 22,107 in 1964 in Oita were positive, though both prefectures were known to have had active endemic foci in the past. Rather surprising results were also obtained in Miyazaki Prefecture neighboring Kagoshima, where only 3 positive cases were discovered out of 25,040 persons in the previously known endemic areas in 1963; none of 3,174 persons examined in 1964 were positive. In all of these prefectures, it is presumed that most of the old endemic foci had become free from the infection, or had rapidly decreased in the parasite rates before the commencement of the control program.

(5.3.f) The Izu Islands (Tokyo Prefecture):

The filariasis control program in Tokyo Prefecture was directed exclusively to the Izu Islands, where both malayan and bancroftian filariasis were known to be endemic on some islands. In 1962, people were examined on the southmost island of Aogashima where HAYASHI *et al.* (1959) detected 41 microfilaria positive cases (all *W. bancrofti*) by examination of 317 persons, and treated all the parasite carries with diethylcarbamazine. The present survey showed only 2 of 269 persons who were available to be positive. In 1963, 32 positive cases (2 malayan and 30 bancroftian) were detected out of 5,598 persons on Hachijo Island with a population of 12,093, and 14 cases (13 malayan and 1 bancroftian) out of 85 persons on Hachijo-Koshima, with a registered population of 135. The numbers of positive cases detected during the survey in 1964 was 2 out of 2,069 on Niijima Island, and 9 out of 503 on Hachijo Island, all of bancroftian type; those in 1965 were 6 bancroftian positives among 513 persons on Hachijo (Okago village only), 5 bancroftian positives among 400 on Kozushima Island, none out of 211 on Niijima, and 242 in the Shikinejima Islands. The drug was administererd to all the positive cases thus detected. No positive cases were discovered on the other islands in later surveys of 1,881 persons on Miyake Island, 152 on Mikura Island, and 366 on Kozushima Island in 1966, 2,075 on Oshima Island and 175 on Toshima Island in 1967. The program was again directed to Hachijo Island in 1968, where 4 bancroftian positives were discovered out of 3,194 persons examined; none of 68 persons on Hachijo-Koshima or of 209 persons in Aogashima were positive.

(5.3.g) The Ryukyu Islands: (Table 8-12)

The filariasis control program of the Ryukyu Islands (Okinawa) was organized around the end of 1964, as a cooperative project of the governments of Ryukyu, Japan, and the United States. The Ryukyus are composed of several hundred islands with a combined population of nearly one million. High prevalence of bancroftian filariasis in all of these islands has been known for many years, and some pilot experiments in its control had been carried out previously. The present program began in January 1965 with the Miyako Islands as the initial target. A filariasis control unit composed of some 30 technicians and an administrative staff was created by the Miyako Health Center, and supervised by the United States Civil Administration of the Ryukyu Islands (USCAR). Dr. M. Sasa, and Dr. H. L. Keegan of 406 Medical Laboratory of the United States Army, acted as consultants to USCAR, and visited the Islands several times before and during the operation. A preliminary report on the initial stage of this program in Miyako was made by MARSHALL & YASUKAWA (1966), and a progress report for the years 1965 to 1970 was compiled by SASA (1970), and RYUKYUSEIFU KOSEIKYOKU (the Ryukyu Government Health Department, 1971). As stated previously, the program was extended to the Yaeyama Islands in 1967, and a program covering the northern districts of Okinawa Island was initiated in 1969. Statistical analysis of some of the microfilaria survey data was reported by SASA *et al.* (1970). The supervision of the filariasis control program was later given to the Japanese Government who then turned over the responsibility to the Okinawa Prefecture Health Department when the Ryukyu Islands were returned to the administration of Japan in 1972.

Table 8-13. Results of annual blood surveys in Miyako and Yaeyama districts, Okinawa.

District	Year	Population under control	Number examined	Percent examined	Number positive	Percent positive
	1965	67,020	66,333	99.0	12,607	19.01
	1966	63,702	63,702	100.	3,105	4.87
Miyako	1967–8	60,467	60,455	100.	1,282	2.12
	1969	12,915	12,691	98.3	177	1.40
	1970	26,605	26,238	98.6	135	0.52
	1967	49,432	46,595	94.3	3,400	7.30
	1968	50,089	41,603	83.1	1,116	2.68
Yaeyama	1969	6,635	5,855	88.2	133	2.27
	1970	16,426	12,494	76.1	160	1.28
	1971	9,223	7,811	84.7	107	1.37

(5.3.g.1) The Miyako Islands consist of eight small islands with a total population of about 73,000 divided into six municipalities and 92 villages. Previous surveys carried out in this area had shown that bancroftian filariasis was prevalent, with the microfilarial rates generally exceeding 20%. The technique of blood examination and drug administration was practically the same as that adopted on the mainland of Japan. However, much more satisfactory results were obtained here for various reasons, that is, because the program was carried out by full-time, specially trained technicians, because of the extensive health education carried out to establish better cooperation with the people, and because the budget per capita was several times higher than that allotted to most prefectures of the mainland.

In the first cycle of the blood survey in 1965, 99.0% (66,333 of 67,020) of the available population was examined, and 12,607 persons were found to be positive, with an overall microfilarial rate of 19.0%. The drug was administered only to the positive cases at daily doses of 6 mg per kg for 12 days, and the cure rate obtained by examination of 11,141 carriers was 82%. The remaining 18% of persisting positive cases received the second course of the therapy. In the second cycle of the blood survey of the whole population, carried out during the period from April to November 1966, 100% of 63,702 people were examined, of which 3,105 (4.87%) were positive. The positive cases were composed of: (A) 572 cases (18.4%) who were not examined in the previous survey; (B) 1,456 cases (46.8%) who were negative in the previous survey; (C) 778 cases (25.1%) who were positive in the previous survey, but became negative once during the posttreatment examination; and (D) 303 cases (9.8%) who continued to be positive in the three blood examinations.

The third round of blood surveys of the people in Miyako was completed during the two-year period from 1967 to 1968. Nearly 100% of the available population received the blood examination, and 2.12% (1,282 of 60,455) were still positive. The microfilaria rates observed in the fourth round survey in 1969 and 1970 were still lower, and remarkable reductions in the rates and densities of microfilaremia cases were achieved as a result of the control activity.

(5.3.g.2) The filariasis control project in the Yaeyama Islands was initiated in 1967, two years after the program was created in Miyako. In the first round of blood surveys completed during 1967, 46,595, or 94.3% of the population was examined, and 3,400, or 7.30%, were found to be carrying microfilariae. This rate was generally much lower than that observed in the Miyako Islands, and varied greatly among the individual islands, as discussed previously. The second round survey was carried out in 1968 after all the positive cases were treated with a course of DEC, and the microfilaria rate was found to have dropped to 2.68% (1,116 positives out of 41,603 persons examined). The third round blood survey was begun in 1969, and further reductions in the rates were recorded.

(5.3.g.3) The northern districts of Okinawa Island under the administration of Nago Health Center was selected as the third target of the filariasis control program of the Ryukyu Islands. In 1969, pupils of the middle school were examined as sample populations from the entire district; the total number of pupils in this district was 8,013, among whom 7,905 (98.7%) were examined, and 88 (1.11%) were found to be positive for microfilariae. Of 2,558 villagers of the same districts, 100 (3.91%) were also positive. The blood survey and drug treatment programs were in progress as of 1973.

9 | Filariasis in the Pacific region

The zoogeographic zone defined here as the Pacific region includes Australia, New Guinea and adjacent islands of Melanesia, Micronesia, and Polynesia. Human filariasis due to *Wuchereria bancrofti* is widely spread in this region, and constitutes a serious health problem in many parts of the region.

One of the characteristic features in the epidemiology of filariasis in this region is the absence of *Brugia malayi*, which is indigenous to the Asian region and is distributed eastwards up to Sulawesi (Celebes) and the Molucca Islands of Indonesia. Another interesting and important feature is the occurrence of two distinct races of *W. bancrofti* in this region which differ in microfilarial periodicity: a nocturnally periodic race common to other regions of the world, and a nonperiodic (or diurnally subperiodic) race found only in the Polynesian and the New Caledonian subregions, but not in other areas of the world.

These physiological races may be further divided into the following four ecological types according to the difference in the local mosquito vectors:

(1) The nocturnally periodic *W. bancrofti* transmitted by *Culex pipiens* s.l., and endemic in the Australian and the Micronesian subregions.

(2) The nocturnally periodic *W. bancrofti* transmitted by *Anopheles* spp., and endemic in the Papuan subregion.

(3) The diurnally subperiodic *W. bancrofti* transmitted by *Aedes (Ochlerotatus) vigilax*, and endemic in the New Caledonian subregion.

(4) The diurnally subperiodic *W. bancrofti* transmitted by mosquitoes of the *Aedes (Stegomyia) polynesiensis* group, and endemic in the Polynesian subregion.

In other words, the regions and the subregions discussed in this chapter are divided not on political or geographic grounds, but by the range of distribution of the various types of parasites and vectors. The main epidemiological features of filariasis according to the subregions are as follows:

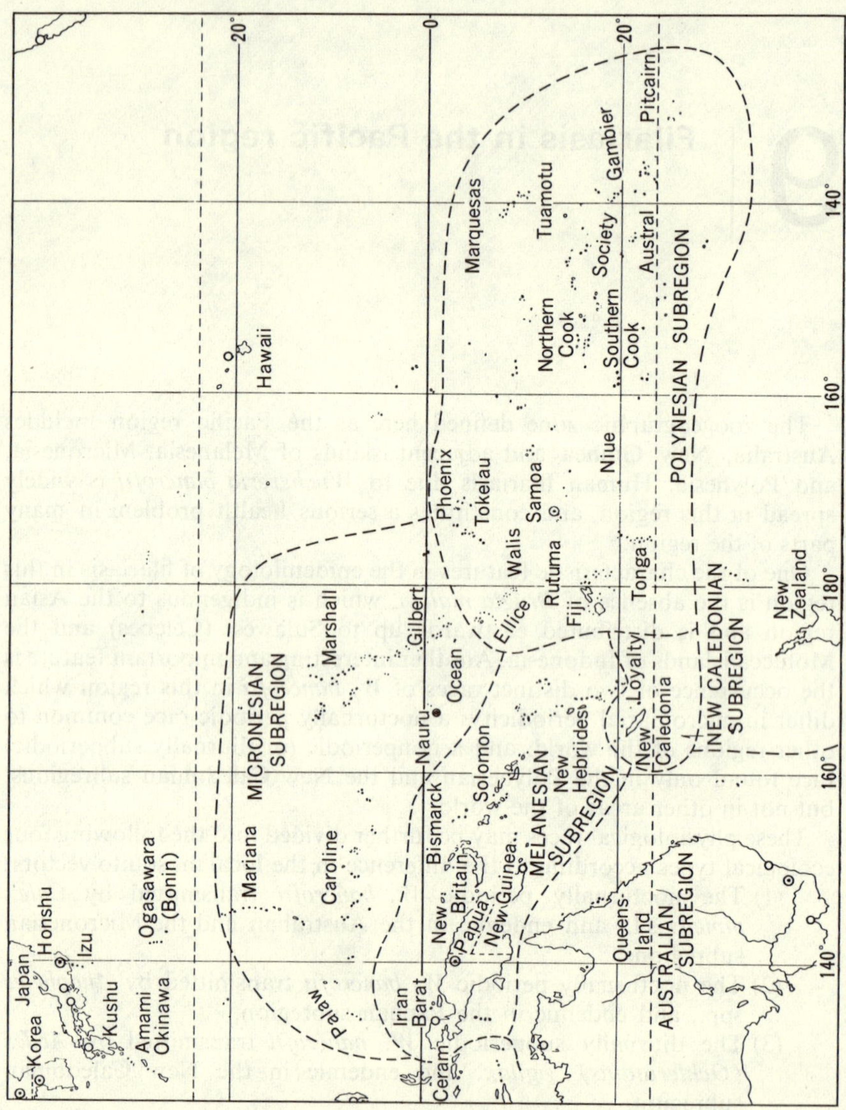

Fig. 9-1. A map of the Pacific region showing the subregions according to ecological and physiological types of filariasis.

A. The Australian subregion. The nocturnally periodic *W. bancrofti* transmitted by *C. p. fatigans* was introduced and became endemic at one time in the northeastern coastal belt of Australia, but apparently died out spontaneously before World War II.

B. The Micronesian subregion. The same type of *W. bancrofti* infection is endemic on many islands of Micronesia scattered in the northern hemisphere of the Pacific Ocean. This type of filarial infection does not extend beyond the equator except on Nauru, Ocean, and some islands of the Gilbert group.

C. The Papuan subregion. The *W. bancrofti* endemic in Papua (including Irian Barat of Indonesia), the Bismarck Archipelago, the Solomon Islands, and the New Hebrides, is nocturnally periodic, and is characterized by its principal vectors, which are members of the subgenus *Cellia* of the genus *Anopheles*. These mosquitoes also act as the main vector of malaria in this region. Some culicine mosquitoes of genera *Aedes, Culex,* and *Mansonia* have also been reported to act as vectors.

D. The New Caledonian subregion. The so-called nonperiodic race of *W. bancrofti* is endemic in New Caledonia and the Loyalty Islands. This parasite may be physiologically the same as that endemic in the Polynesian subregion, but mosquitoes of the *Ae. (Stegomyia) polynesiensis* group are absent from this zone, while a brackish water breeding mosquito, *Ae. (Ochlerotatus) vigilax,* has been incriminated as the main vector.

E. The Polynesian subregion. It has been domonstrated, since the end of last century, that the microfilariae of *W. bancrofti* found among the people on islands situated in the Pacific south of the equator, show no periodicity like that seen in people from other regions of the world. Day-biting mosquitoes of the *Ae. (Stegomyia) scutellaris* group, among which *Ae. polynesiensis* is most widely distributed, are the main vectors in this zone, but a number of other night-biting mosquitoes of the *Ae. (Finlaya) kochi* group, as well as the classical filaria vector, *C. p. fatigans,* have also been found to be acting as secondary vectors in this zone.

Historical notes

THORPE (1896) carried out an investigation of filariasis in the South Pacific Islands, and recognized, for the first time, the absence of periodicity of the microfilariae in this region. He first visited Fiji, and examined 24 slides taken at night at the hospital in Suva; he found 6 of them to be positive for microfilariae. He also obtained 100 blood smears taken at night at the same hospital, and found 24 positives. In Tonga, he examined the blood of 214 adults during the period from August to December, 1895. Thorpe stated in this article, "At first the examinations were made at night only; but in October, considering it expedient to make a few control observations in the daytime, I found to my astonishment, that the filariae exhibited no periodicity, but were swarming in the blood practically in as great numbers as at night. The parasite moreover possessed a well-marked sheath, and in general appearance resembled *F. nocturna*. 96 natives were examined both day and night, and with two exceptions, all those with filariae at night exhibited them in the daytime in equal numbers." The author obtained microfilaria rates of 34.1% (14 of 41) in males and 20.8% (5 of 24) in females of Tongatabu, 40.5% (15 of 37) in males and 18.6% (8 of 43) in females of Nomuka, 57% (18 of 31) in males and 28% (5 of 18) in females of Lifuka, and 28.6% (4 of 14) in males and 0% (0 of 6) in females of Vavau.

MANSON (1896) reported the result of blood examinations of people in Samoa. Blood films were prepared by Dr. Davis from 56 Samoans who were all suffering from some form of elephantoid disease, and micro-filariae were found in 27 slides. It became evident, therefore, that filariasis was quite as common in Samoa as it was reported so in Fiji and the Friend-ly Islands by THORPE (1896).

O'CONNOR (1923) published a comprehensive report on the results of his medical expedition to the western Pacific. During the journey of 17 months, the author visited the islands of the Ellice, Tokelau, and Samoa groups, and carried out blood and clinical surveys of filariasis prevalent in these areas. The results are summarized in Table 9-1. In Ellice Islands, eight atolls were surveyed, and a gross microfilarial rate of 40.2% (569 positives out of 1,417 persons examined) was observed, and 28.7% or 335 of 1,169 persons of age 16 years and over were found to show clinical signs of filariasis; 120 had advanced elephantiasis. The disease was found to be more prevalent in the five northerly atolls than in the three southerly atolls. In Tokelau, 330 persons on three islands were examined, and microfilariae were found in 62 (18.8%). In Samoa, the four western islands administered by New Zealand and the four eastern islands under American control were surveyed, and a high microfilarial rate of 28.7% (1,232 positives out of 4,294) was observed for the whole area. The signs of infection, either microfilaremia or clinical manifestations, were seen in 1,463 (58.3%) of 2,509 persons aged 16 years and over.

The comprehensive reports by BUXTON & HOPKINS (1927) and BUXTON (1928) entitled "Researches in Polynesia and Melanesia" consist of two volumes (seven parts), several appendices, and numerous plates; they constitute one of the most important historical contributions to the knowl-edge of filariasis and its vectors in this region. The first volume (No. 1) was published in July 1927, and contains Parts 1 to 4, which include the introduction, climate of Samoa, medical entomology, experiments per-formed on *Ae. variegatus* and *Ae. argenteus*, respectively, and four appen-dices, including "malaria and filariasis in New Hebrides." The second volume (No. 2) contains studies on filariasis (Part 5), other diseases (Part 6), "Brown man and White in Samoa" (Part 7), and seven appendices re-ferring to filariasis.

The authors left England in November 1923, and traveled through the Panama Canal and Fiji, reaching Apia in the middle of January 1924. Their headquarters was set up at Apia Hospital, and visits were made to other island-groups, such as Ellice, Tokelau, New Hebrides, and Tonga, during a two-year period. Investigations on filariasis and its vectors were conducted mainly in Western Samoa and in the New Hebrides, but some people on atolls of the Ellice and Tokelau groups were also examined.

As for the method of recording the physical signs, the author classified them into the enlargement of glands (superior or inferior inguinal and epitrochlear), epididymitis and testitis, hydrocele, and elephantiasis. In the surveys of the normal population, the author considered it best to confine his work only to males, because the filarial incidence and disease was known to be different in the two sexes, being less in females than in males. The microfilarial rates and elephantiasis rates observed in Samoa, on the atolls (Ellice and Tokelau), and the New Hebrides are shown in Table 9-1 and Table 9-2.

As for the progress of the more recent studies on epidemiology of filariasis in the Pacific region, comprehensive reviews were made by IYENGAR (1965), and HAWKING & DENHAM (1971).

Table 9-1. Showing the microfilaria rate and the mean microfilarial count per positive of male Samoans of different age-groups (after BUXTON, 1929).

Age-group (years)	Number examined	Mf. positive Number	Mf. positive %	Mean count
0–5	4	0	0.	—
6–10	65	1	1.5	23
11–15	119	22	18.5	66.2
16–20	229	72	31.4	81.1
21–25	101	42	41.6	58.9
26–35	170	88	51.8	68.2
36–45	148	70	47.3	73.2
46 & over	93	47	50.5	72.9
Total	929	342	36.8	72.9

Table 9-2. Showing percentage incidence of elephantiasis in a normal population examined in the South Pacific (after BUXTON, 1929).

Age-group (years)	Samoa No.	Samoa El.	Samoa %	Atolls No.	Atolls El.	Atolls %	New Hebrides No.	New Hebrides El.	New Hebrides %
0–20	470	0	0.	105	0	0.	100	0	0.
21–25	110	2	1.8	77	2	2.6	65	5	7.7
26–35	208	10	4.8	128	2	1.6	102	10	9.8
36–45	187	24	12.8	112	6	5.4	35	2	5.7
46 & over	128	26	20.3	106	22	20.8	16	2	12.5
Total	1,103	62	5.6	528	32	6.1	318	19	6.0

No.: Number of persons examined; El.: Number of persons with elephantiasis; %: percentage of persons with elephantiasis

9A. Australia

Australia occupies an important place in the history of filariasis studies because the adult worm (female) was first discovered by J. BANCROFT, in Brisbane (1876). Some historical contributions were made also by T. L. BANCROFT (1899), who first elucidated the mode of transmission of the filarial larvae from the mosquito to man, that is, that it was not swallowed with mosquito-contaminated water as MANSON (1877) postulated, but entered the skin from the insect's proboscis at the time of its bite on man (See Section 2B.1.). A nocturnally periodic form of bancroftian filariasis was known to be highly endemic in the eastern coastal belt of Australia, namely, in Queensland from Brisbane towards the tip of the Cape York Peninsula and the adjacent islands. However, recent investigations suggest that the disease has not been endemic in Australia since about 1940.

Filariasis due to *W. bancrofti* is known to have caused much morbidity among residents of Queensland, particularly those of Brisbane, during the last three decades of the 19th century and the early part of the 20th century. FLYNN (1903) stated that he had seen 60 cases in the previous five years. McLEAN (1910) examined unselected patients in Brisbane General Hospital during 1908 and 1909 and found 130 carriers among 1200 persons examined (that is, a 10.8% positive rate). CROLL (1919) examined 4,000 persons in Brisbane General Hospital in 1909 to 1910, and found 11.5% infected. DERRICK (1944) found 17 (6.7%) out of 252 patients at the mental Hospital in Goodna infected.

In Townsville, BREINL (1913) reported 7 (3.1%) cases of infection out of 226 patients in the General Hospital. CLIENTO & RICHARDS (1924), in the same hospital, obtained 10 (3.7%) positives in 271 persons examined. DERRICK (1940) found 3 infections in 98 patients. In a survey carried out by the staff of the Hookworn Campaign from 1922 to 1924, SWEET (1924a) reported that 373 infections were found in 14,362 persons (2.6%) in Queensland, and 199 (5.0%) in 3,962 in the Brisbane area. SWEET (1924b) also found 18 infections in 1,177 persons examined in the northwestern districts (Cloncurry, Camooweal, Normanton, and aborigines from Cape York Peninsula).

However, these endemic foci in eastern Australia seem to have died out spontaneously some years ago, presumably due to the reduction in the population of the vector mosquitoes, especially *C. p. fatigans*. DERRICK (1938) found no infections in 228 patients in Brisbane General Hospital. In the mental hospital at Goodna, where DERRICK (1944) found 17 (6.7%) positives in 252 patients, MACKERRAS & MACKERRAS (1949) saw only 2 infections in 51 patients, including the previously positive cases. ROW (1952) reported that 52 patients with chyluria had been treated between 1938 and 1950, but none had microfilaria in blood or urine. MACKERRAS (1958) also reported that there were 56 admissions for filariasis in Brisbane General Hospital in the 20 years between 1937 and 1956, but none of them showed microfilaria, and even the youngest patients gave filarial histories of 13 to 18 years. However, an acute case with high microfilaremia was reported in a Mackay resident in 1956. A survey was later carried out in the district hospitals covering the coastal region of Queensland during 1957, but it gave no positive case in 758 specimens. In the blood surveys conducted from 1949 through 1956 in various native settlements, only 2 positive cases (both aborigines) were found out of 1,094 examinees, one from Murray Island and another from Thursday Island, both islands situated in the Torres Strait between Australia and New Guinea.

There have been some questions raised as to whether endemic filariasis exists in Northern Territory of Australia. GOLDSMITH (1899) referred to 2 cases of filariasis in Darwin; one was that of an aboriginal woman with elephantiasis of the vulva, and the other that of a Japanese man with chyluria. However, according to MCMILLAN (1967), no microfilarial carriers have ever been detected despite extensive blood surveys conducted in the past under the malaria control campaign. MCMILLAN also conducted night examinations of a total of 362 aborigines and 12 Europeans over the age of 15 years in the vicinity of Darwin and in Arnhem Land, but they were all negative. Although it had been stated in some textbooks that filariasis is endemic in Northern Territory, McMillan stated that it was highly possible that Goldsmith's two cases were either of nonfilarial origin (probably *granuloma venereum* in the case of the woman), or imported (in the case of Japanese man).

As for the studies on mosquito vectors of filariasis, historical contributions to the knowledge of the mode of development of the filarial larvae and their infection to man from the mosquito were made by BANCROFT (1899–1903). It was postulated by most workers at that time that man got the infection by swallowing mosquito-contaminated water, but Bancroft showed that the larvae infected through the skin from the mosquito's proboscis. He observed the whole course of development of the larvae of *W. bancrofti* in *C. ciliaris*, the "house mosquito of Australia," which he later in 1901 recognized to be *C. pipiers fatigans* Wiedemann. He also showed that mosquitoes may live for weeks if fed and infected, and corrected the misconception of Manson that they soon die after infected by being drowned in water. In 1903, he described the precise way by which the infective larvae leave the host, breaking the labium at its tip during the time of natural biting.

WALKER (1924) observed that four species of mosquitoes were most abundant in Brisbane: *C. quinquefasciatus* (= *fatigans*), *C. annulirostris*, *Ae. vigilax*, and *Ae. aegypti*, but could not find natural infection at the dissections of "many hundreds" of naturally caught specimens. When fed on a microfilarial carrier, *C. quinquefasciatus* was demonstrated to be a very efficient host, but only partial developments were noted in *C. annulirostris*, and no development was seen in *Ae. vigilax*, and *Ae. aegypti*. HEYDON (1931) conducted further experimental infection studies with the local mosquitoes in Queensland, and concluded that: 1) *An. amictus* in North Queensland is a favorable intermediate host for *W. bancrofti*, comparable but not quite equal to *C. fatigans*; 2) *Ae. vigilax* is a rather poor host, and *C. sitiens* is a very poor host; and 3) with *Ae. argenteus*, none of 32 mosquitoes used proved to be hospitable.

9B. The Micronesian subregion

The groups of islands discussed in this text as the Micronesian subregion includes the Marianas, Carolines, Marshalls, Gilbert, Guam, Nauru and Ocean Islands. They are all small volcanic or coral reef islands situated in the tropical zone of the Pacific, either north of the equator or slightly south of it. This subregion represents area where only the nocturnally periodic *W. bancrofti* transmitted by *C. p. fatigans* is endemic. Most of the islands in this region were under the administration of Germany for about 20 years before World War I, assigned as Japanese mandates after 1919, and became trust territories of the United States in 1947. The epidemiology of filariasis in Micronesia was reviewed by PIPKIN (1953), IYENGAR (1965), and HAWKING & DENHAM (1971).

According to the *report of WHO/SPC Seminar on Filariasis* (1974), Palau and the other islands of Yap, Ponape, and Truk have a significant filariasis problem among the numerous islands of the Trust Territory of the Pacific. Palau had an microfilaria rate of 12.6% in 1967. Mass drug administration with DEC at a dosage of 5 mg per kg once every other month for two years was started in 1970. A posttreatment survey revealed a microfilaria rate of 0.3% in 1,000 persons examined. Plans are being drawn up for mass drug administration in the other three groups of islands.

9B.1 The Mariana Islands

An archipelago of the U.S. Trust Territory, the Marianas are situated between 12°N and 21°N; they comprise 15 islands. They have an area of 477 km² with a population of 12,256 (1970).

W. bancrofti infection has been noted only from the island of Saipan, where KNOTT (1944a, unpublished data cited by IYENGAR, 1965) found 13.5% of 243 natives examined by him being positive for microfilariae in blood. However, only a single case of elephantiasis was seen among the total population of about 7,000.

9B.2 Guam

Guam is a U.S. Territory island. It is the southernmost island of the Marianas, situated at about 13°N. Its area is 540 km² with a population of 86,926 (1970).

Filariasis due to *W. bancrofti* was reported to be endemic on the southeast coast of Guam by CROW (1910). Of 244 persons examined in Ynarajan Village, 13 were positive for microfilariae. KINDELBERGER (1912) stated that 11 persons in Guam were positive for microfilariae. However, KNOTT (1944b, quoted by IYENGAR, 1965) examined 517 natives of the Agana district on the west coast of Guam and failed to find positive cases. PIPKIN (1953) also reported that the Ynarajan focus had disappeared. REEVES & RUDNICK (1951) stated that filariasis did not appear to be endemic on GUAM, but the occurrence of large numbers of *C. p. fatigans* coupled with climatic factors apparently favorable for filariasis transmission would lead one to suspect that this disease could become established if human carriers were introduced.

The REPORT OF WHO/SPC SEMINAR ON FILARIASIS (1974) stated, "there are no records to indicate the occurrence of *W. bancrofti* at present."

9B.3 The Caroline Islands

An archipelago situated between 5°N and 10°N and 130°E and 166°E, the Carolines comprise about 680 islands with a total area of 1,184 km² and a total population of 66,900 (1969). They are a part of the U.S. Trust Territory. The Palau group, Yap group, Truk Islands, Ponape, and Kusaie include relatively large, high volcanic islands, while the rest are mostly coral atolls.

No record on filariasis before and during the Japanese occupation is available. PIPKIN (1953) showed that *W. bancrofti* infection was widely distributed in all of the four districts, as in Table 9-3. Natural infection was seen in 4.9% of *C. p. fatigans* examined in Palau, and 1 out of 211 *C. annulirostris* was found to be harboring a third stage larva. However, the incidence of clinical filariasis was very low.

MCNAIR *et al.* (1949) reported that filariasis was found to be endemic on four islands of the Yap District; 14 elephantiasis cases were seen in Elato, Woleai, Ulithi, and Ifalik. The microfilariae of *W. bancrofti* were seen in 4 of the 14 cases in the blood taken during daytime. *Culex p. fatigans* was found on these islands.

9B.4 The Marshall Islands

Group of 32 atolls and more than 800 reefs in the western Pacific, these islands lie between 5°30'N to 15°N and 161°E to 172°E. They have a total land area of 179 km² with a population of 20,206 (1970).

According to KNOTT (1944, quoted by IYENGAR, 1965) and PIPKIN (1953), filarial infection has been observed from only Majuro and Namorik, and microfilaria rates of 1.0% and 3.6% respectively, were recorded

Table 9-3. Microfilaria rates of the different islands of the Carolines (from PIPKIN, 1953, quoted by IYENGAR, 1965).

Island	Number examined	Microfilaria rate
Palau District:		
Tobi	81	0.0
Sonsorol	59	0.0
Angaur	102	1.0
Pelilieu	108	16.6
Keyengel	74	23.0
Babeldob	510	37.3
Koror	158	24.1
Yap District:		
Yap	205	1.0
Ulithi	203	3.4
Wolei	95	17.8
Wotegai	60	18.3
Faralep	55	18.2
Satawal	104	31.7
Ifalik	115	17.4
Lamotrek	106	17.9
Truk District:		
Moen	143	24.5
Tol	123	19.4
Fefan	71	22.5
Uman	200	24.5
Pulusuk	100	21.0
Puluwat	68	26.5
Ulul	75	20.0
Nomwin-Fenanu	67	11.9
Murillo	100	27.0
Ponape District:		
Ponape	37	8.1
Mokil	75	24.0
Nukuoro	171	0.0
Pingalap	199	0.0
Kusaie	165	0.0

by the latter author. Other islands, such as Ebon, Ailingalap, Kwajalein, Namu, Lai, and Jaluit, are apparently free from filariasis.

9B.5 The Gilbert Islands

This island-group containing 16 atolls in the western Pacific Ocean on the equator is between 4°N and 4°S, southeast of the Marshall Islands and northwest of the Ellice Islands. They have an area of 264 km², and a population of 44,206 (1968). The main islands are Tarawa (largest), Makin, Abaiang, Abemama, Tabiteuea, Nonouti, and Beru. The islands have long been densely populated.

The Gilbert Islands together with the Ellice Islands constitute a British colony, and the both island-groups are separated by an ocean gap of only about 200 miles. However, in view of the epidemiology of filariasis, this ocean gap is extremely important, because it separates the diurnally sub-periodic or South Pacific form of *W. bancrofti* in the Ellice and the southern islands from the nocturnally periodic or Micronesian form of *W. bancrofti*. Mosquitoes of the *Ae. polynesiensis* group, the main vector of the subperiodic *W. bancrofti*, are also absent from the Gilbert Islands.

The occurrence of the nocturnally periodic race of *W. bancrofti* in the Gilbert Islands was noted by LAMBERT (1928), KNOTT (1944), STEMPIEN (1944), SCHLOSSER (1944), and BYRD & ST. AMANT (1959). (as quoted by IYENGAR 1965). The nocturnal periodicity of microfilariae in carriers from Gilbert has been confirmed by SCHLOSSER (1944), BACKHOUSE & HEYDON (1950), and BYRD & ST. AMANT (1959).

According to IYENGAR (1965), filarial infection is endemic on most of the islands of the Gilbert group. In the islands of the northern group, the microfilaria rates are low; MARSHALL, in 1945, recorded 0% in Little Makin, 0.1% in Butaritari, and 0.3% in Abaiang. In the central group, microfilaria rates of 21 to 25% were recorded from Tarawa by RUDIARD in 1949, 6.5% from Maiana by MARSHALL in 1945, and 5% from Apama-ma by KNOTT (1944). In the southern Gilbert, endemic filarial infection was noted by STEMPIEN in 1944, but data on microfilaria rates are not available. Hydrocele was common among males on many of the islands of the Gilbert (BUXTON, 1928; KNOTT, 1944, unpublished data). STEMPIEN, in 1944, observed that in experimental infections with the Gilbert strain of *W. bancrofti*, complete development of the larvae to the infective stage in *C. p. fatigans* took place in 11 days.

According to MARSHALL (1956), four species of mosquitoes are found on Tarawa, namely, *Ae. aegypti, Ae. (Stegomyia) marshallensis* Stone et Bohart, 1944, *C. p. fatigans*, and *C. annulirostris. Aedes marshallensis* was very common everywhere, and its larvae were found abundantly in coconut husks. *Culex annulirostris* was very troublesome by night, and large numbers of larvae were found breeding in brackish water ponds.

Control:
The REPORT OF WHO/SPC SEMINAR ON FILARIASIS (1974) stated, "On the 17 Gilbert Islands, there does not appear to be a significant filariasis problem," and thus no control project has yet been under consideration.

9B.6 Nauru

Nauru is an island situated about 42 km south of the equator at 167° E, and west of the Gilbert Islands. Its area is 22 km² with a population of 6,603 (1970). Nauru became an independent republic in 1968. The island is famous for its rich phosphate deposits.

BRAY (1931) conducted a survey of filariasis in 1926. With the exception of infants, the entire native population numbering 1,151 Nauruans were examined, and microfilariae were found in 332 (28.8%). The microfilariae had a definite nocturnal periodicity. Elephantiasis was relatively rare; 4 males and 2 females had mild affections of legs. Six males with scrotal involvements and 2 women with breast lesions were found. Fever attack, lymphangitis, and adenitis were very common. About 10% of the male population had small hydrocele.

GRANT (1933) examined at least 20% of the population of each of the native districts in Nauru. Of 354 persons examined, 36.1% were positive for microfilariae in their night blood. Of the total population of about 1,500, there were 21 cases of elephantiasis of the legs or scrotum; hydrocele was absent. *C. p. fatigans* and *Ae. argenteus* were the common mosquitoes; natural infection with filaria larvae was seen in *C. p. fatigans*.

HEYDON & BEARUP, in 1940, (quoted by IYENGAR, 1959) also confirmed that, of three common mosquito species in Nauru, i.e., *C. p. fatigans*, *C. sitiens*, and *Ae. aegypti*, the development of filarial larvae was best in *C. p. fatigans*, less in *C. sitiens*, and not at all in *Ae. aegypti*. Natural infection was seen only in *C. p. fatigans*.

EARLE (1941) reported on 9 cases of filariasis among natives of Nauru, and the use of sulfonamides compounds in filarial complications. EARLE (1942) also conducted in Nauru a mammography study of the female breast affected by filaria.

9B.7 Ocean Island (Banaba)

Ocean is a small island about 72 km south of equator between the Gilbert Islands and Nauru, at 0°52′ S and 169°35′ E. Its area is 6.5 km² and its population is 2,192 (1968). Like Nauru, Ocean is famous for large deposits of phosphate.

No information is available on the filarial infection of people on this island. The original natives, known as the Banabans, were transferred to other islands during World War II, and those who were evacuated to Rambi Island in Fiji during 1945 were shown to be still harboring nocturnally periodic *W. bancrofti* in 1948, at a rate of 5.5% (8 positives of 146), according to MANSON-BAHR & MUGGLETON (1952).

9C. The Papuan subregion

The Papuan subregion comprises New Guinea (Papua, Irian) and adjacent islands, the Bismarck Archipelago, the Solomon Islands, and the

New Hebrides. So far as is known, the nocturnally periodic race of *W. bancrofti* is the only human filaria endemic in this subregion; the principal vectors are mosquitoes of the *An. punctulatus* group in most areas.

New Guinea (Papua, Irian) is the second largest island in the world, situated between latitudes 0° and 11°S and longitudes 131°E and 151°E, and has an area of approximately 828,000 km² (with politically attached islands, 893,360 km²) and a population of 2,968,000 (1970). The island is divided into Irian Barat (West Irian) of Indonesia, and Papua New Guinea (formerly under Australian administration, independent since 1973). From the zoogeographical point of view, Irian Barat obviously belongs to the Papuan subregion and is much different from the other regions of Indonesia.

Filariasis due to nocturnally periodic *W. bancrofti* is known to be widely endemic in Melanesia, or the Papuan subregion. The epidemiological features of filariasis in this subregion are characteristic in that filariasis is solely represented by a nocturnally periodic form of *W. bancrofti* probably adapted to a wide range of mosquito hosts, i.e., to various species of genera *Anopheles*, *Culex*, *Mansonia*, and *Aedes*. The vectors in each endemic area are thus determined by the local environments, or according to the prevalence and hospitability to the parasite of the local mosquito species. In most areas, mosquitoes of the *An. punctulatus* group have been recognized as the main vectors of both filariasis and malaria, and thus the coendemicity of the two diseases is also a characteristic feature of this subregion. No endemic area of *B. malayi* nor that of the diurnally sub-periodic form of *W. bancrofti* has ever been reported from this subregion. A review of published records of filariasis in Melanesia was made by BACKHOUSE (1950, 1953) and IYENGAY (1965).

9C.1 Irian Barat (West Irian)

West Irian is a province of Indonesia consisting of the western half of the island of New Guinea, and adjacent islands. Formerly Dutch New Guinea, West Irian has an area of 421,820 km², with a population of 957,000 (1970 estimate).

This province is discussed separately from other parts of Indonesia (Section 8B.9) because the epidemiology of filariasis in this area is basically the same as in other territories of the Papuan subregion and is better described with them. It should be noted that *B. malayi* is a parasite indigenous to the Oriental region, and does not reach beyond the Weber line which separates Irian Barat from Ceram Island. On the other hand, the anopheline mosquitos of the *An. punctulatus* group, which are the most important vectors of both malaria and *W. bancrofti* in the Papuan sub-region, have their range of distribution over the Weber line and inhabit also in the Molucca Islands.

According to COOL (1927), elephantiasis was recognized all over Dutch

New Guinea while military exploration was carried out from 1907 to 1911, and *F. bancrofti* was discovered in 10% of the healthy Papuans and 25% of the prisoners in Fak Fak. Elephantiasis was found in 21 of 453 people examined at Inawattan, and was also "many" at Manokawari in northern New Guinea.

DE ROOK (1930) made a survey of Papuans in Boven Digoel, and found microfilariae in 24 of 216 adult males, none of 22 adult females, and 6 of 145 children under the age of 17. The microfilariae were nocturnally periodic. The vector could not be determined. KARIADI (1937) carried out blood examinations and a clinical survey of the people in the Manokwari area of Vogelkop Peninsula, and obtained extremely high microfilarial rates in most villages, with an overall positive rate of nine villages (Washior, Miei, Koebiari, Wariap, Manokwari, Saosopor, Saosar, and Seged) on the main island being 41% (148 of 336) in male adults, 42% (82 of 197) in female adults, and 14% (36 of 260) in children; all of the people in five adjacent islands (Salawati, Waigeo, Gam, Noemfoor, and Amsterdam) were also highly infected. The microfilariae showed remarkable nocturnal periodocity and the overall positive rate was 33.0% (113 of 362) in adult males, 37.3% (25 of 67) in adult females and 9.2% (16 of 174) in children.

ELSBACH (1937a) carried out a survey of malaria and filariasis in the Digoel River Basin, in the southwestern plain of New Guinea. Microfilariae of *W. bancrofti* were found in 12 of 93 people (12.9%) in Koholombo, and 6 of 64 (9.3%) in Wap Village. Malaria was also endemic, with the spleen rate and parasite rate of 45% and 6.3% in 128 people in Koholombo, 31% and 8.4% in 118 people in Wap, and 57% and 10.5% in 104 people in Imahoi. ELSBACH (1937b) also made a study of the vectors of *W. bancrofti* at Tanah Merah in Boven Digoer, and obtained a natural infection rate of the filarial larvae of 10.9% (72 of 655) and an experimental infection rate of 49% (22 of 45) with *An. barbirostris bancroftii*. In Hollandia, (Djajapura) in north central New Guinea, TOFFALETI & KING (1947) observed the natural infection rates of 46.2% (6 of 13) in *An. farauti*, 8.3% (3 of 36) in *An. punctulatus*, 7.1% (11 of 154) in the intermediate form (= *An. koliensis*), and 2.2% (6 of 268) in *Ar. obturbans*.

In the more recent surveys carried out by DE ROOK (1757a) on the small island of Pam, South Waigeo District, the microfilarial rate in the 250 inhabitants was 26.8% (31.3% in males and 22.7% in females) and the filarial disease rate was 14.8%. The microfilariae were all of *W. bancrofti*, and the average number per positive case was 37 in 15 mm³ blood. Of 37 cases with clinical signs, those with hydrocele numbered 22, 14 with elephantiasis, and 6 with fibrosis of the testicles or epididymitis. At dissection of mosquitoes caught in dwellings, a natural infection rate of as high as 41.1% (192 of 476 examined) and infective rate of 6.6% (31 of 476) were obtained for *An. farauti*. Infective larvae were found also from *Ae. kochi*, *Ae. scutellaris*, and *C. annulirostris*. The importance of *An. farauti* was emphasized.

The prevalence of bancroftian filariasis as well as the importance of *An. farauti* as the vector was also demonstrated in a survey carried out by DE ROOK (1959) in the village of Inanwatan situated on the south coast of Vogelkop near the mouth of Maccluer Gulf. The whole population of 1,125 persons was examined, of which 235 (20.9%) had either microfilaria or clinical signs. Of 90 clinical cases, elephantiasis of the legs was seen in 59, and genital involvements (mainly hydrocele) were seen in 35 persons. Malaria was also prevalent, and the spleen rate as well as the parasite rate of 130 school children examined was 66% and 27%, respectively. At the examination of mosquitoes caught in dwellings, infection with the third stage filarial larvae was seen in *An. farauti, C. annulirostris* and *C. p. fatigans*. (Table 9-4).

Table 9-4. The natural infection with filarial larvae of mosquitoes in Inanwatan (adapted from DE ROOK, 1959).

Species	Number examined	Number with larvae	Number with infected larvae
An. farauti	199	55 (27.6%)	3 (1.5%)
C. annulirostris	312	77 (24.7%)	2 (0.6%)
C. p. fatigans	363	52 (14.3%)	3 (0.8%)
Ae. aegypti	45	*9 (20.0%)	0
Aedes species	72	*4 (5.6%)	0
Pardomyia aurantia	10	*1 (10.0%)	0

*Only presausage stages in the thorax.

Anopheles koliensis, another species of the *punctulatus* group and abundant in the inland parts of New Guinea, was also shown to be a suitable host of the local *W. bancrofti* in an experiment conducted by VAN DIJK (1959) in Hollandia Binnen. A donor showing 6 to 40 microfilariae in 20 mm^3 blood at the time of the mosquito bite was exposed to natural attacking of mosquitoes between 8 and 9 p.m. A total of 42 mosquitoes were caught after engorging on the infective blood meal, of which 36 were *An. koliensis*, 3 *An. farauti*, and 3 *C. annulirostirs*. Of 36 *An. koliensis*, 19 were infected; of 16 survived for 11.5 days, 9 were infected and 3 had infective larvae.

A review was made by VAN DEN ASSEM & VAN DIJK (1958) on the distribution of anopheline mosquitoes in western New Guinea. Some six Oriental species and 14 indigenous species have been recorded, of which the former group is limited in distribution to some parts of the westernmost region. Only five species are truly common and widespread. *Anopheles farauti* is the most common species and the principal vector of malaria and filariasis in many parts, and especially abundant in lowland belts and coastal zones; the larvae breed mainly in permanent water in pools and stagnant drains, and are frequently found in brackish water. *An. punctulatus* is also common and abounds in the northern and western regions, and may be the dominant species in a few inland localities; the larvae are found mostly in temporary, manmade pools without vegetation. *An. koliensis*, the third species of the *puntulatus* group, is also widespread, and recorded from lowland as well as mountain areas, even at considerable altitude; it is usually the dominant species in the Hollandia-Nimboran region, the northern plane of the Waropen area, and in other thinly populated northern interior districts. *An. longirostris* is widely distributed, and may be the most prevalent species in the south, such as in the Mimika, Asmat, and Digul areas; unlike *punctulatus*, the larvae breed in more natural waters in jungle, and its possible role as the vector of malaria or filariasis in the southern jungle areas remains to be investigated. *An. bancrofti* is also widely distributed, and is abundant and may be dominant in the southern plain; the larvae breed in rather permanent stretches of water, mostly in sheltered places.

It has thus been established, at least in several localities in western New Guinea, that bancroftian filariasis is solely or principally transmitted by mosquitoes of the *An. punctulatus* group, and occurs coendemically with malaria. IYENGAR *et al.* (1959) carried out observations on the effects of the indoor residual spraying of insecticides, originally intended for the control of malaria, on the transmission of *W. bancrofti*. Three villages near Genjem in the Nimboran district were selected for the study. They were situated about 40 miles to the southwest of Hollandia. Indoor residual spraying with dieldrin was begun in July 1955 at intervals of six months, until July 1957 then with DDT in January and July 1958. At the time this investigation started in January 1959, six months had elapsed since the last application of insecticide. At a blood survey carried out at nighttime in 1955, the microfilarial rate of a part of the population was 32.9% of 73 persons examined (41.9% of 31 adult males, 31.3% of 32 adult females, and 10% of 10 children below 15 years of age). In the blood survey conducted in January 1959, the rate was 18.6% of 285 persons examined (49.2% of 65 males 20 years and over, 28.4% of females 20 years and over, and 1.3% of 153 children of under 20 years). None of children under the age of 10 years was positive. Mosquitoes collected from the villages were examined for filarial infection. *Anopheles koliensis* was the most common species, followed by *An. punctulatus*, and other mosquitoes occurred only in very small numbers. Filarial larvae were detected in 10 of 133 *An. koliensis* and 4 of 52 *An. punctulatus*, but none in other species. All the larvae in the above infected mosquitoes were the immature stages. In another collection conducted two weeks after indoor spraying with DDT, none of 33 mosquitoes were infected except for one with sausage stage larvae. The authors concluded that evidence was furnished to show that transmission of *W. bancrofti* had been effectively interrupted by the indoor residual spraying. (The results are not persuading, and more carefully designed observations are desired to draw a conclusion.)

Bancroftian filariasis in western New Guinea has been shown, however, not solely transmitted by the anopheline mosquitoes. For instance, DE

Rook (1957b) further reported on the results of filariasis investigations in the Berau region. Of 1,179 persons examined, 20.8% were positive with microfilariae, and the density of microfilariae per 20 mm³ blood was 7.5 per total examined, or 35.5 per positive. The percentage with elephantiasis was 6.2. The investigations on the vector mosquitoes in this region have shown quite different figures. *Culex annulirostris* showed a rate of 25.5% infected and 1.6% infective at the dissection of 184 naturally caught specimens, and an 89% infection rate in 157 experimentally infected mosquitoes. In *C. bitaeniorhynchus*, 19.7% were infected and 2.1% were infective out of 142 natural samples, and the experimental infection rate was 94.2% of 97 mosquitoes.

Van Dijk (1958), working in the Bamgi-Ia area in the southwestern plain of New Guinea, presented another example of the lack of epidemiological relationship between malaria and filariasis. The region is a vast swampy area on the delta of the Digul River, and the population was estimated to be about 2,500 divided into over 13 villages. The people were practically free from malaria, and no anopheline mosquitoes were found. However, filariasis due to nocturnally periodic *W. bancrofti* was found to be hyperendemic in all of five villages surveyed, and an overall microfilarial positive rate of 25% (119 of 485 examined), and that of 55.7% (64 of 115) in those above the age of 34 years were obtained. The investigation for the determination of filariasis vectors was conducted by collecting mosquitoes that had fed on a microfilaria carrier. The total numbers thus collected during six evenings were 82 *M. uniformis*, 83 *M. papuensis*, 30 *M. longipalpis*, 7 *M. crassipes*, and 1 *C. squamosus*. They were kept in test tubes and were examined for filarial larvae when found dead, or after 15 days when they still survived. In *M. uniformis*, 51 of 56 specimens were infected, and 12 of 18 specimens that survived longer than 12 days harbored mature larvae. In *M. papuensis*, 35 of 42 specimens examined were infected, but the mortality was very high and only 1 survived 12 days; it contained 3 infective larvae. In *M. longipalpis*, 20 of 23 specimens were infected, but development of the larvae was inhibited in the presausage stage. Full development to the infective stage was seen in the single specimen of *C. squamosus*. No natural infection was seen in a small number of mosquitoes examined at that time. Although van Dijk could not obtain conclusive results in this survey, it is likely that the transmission of bancroftian filariasis in this swamp area had been maintained by mosquitoes other than anophelines, and probably by species of *Mansonia*, especially *M. uniformis*.

The above observations made by de Rook (1957) in the west part and by van Dijk (1958) in the southern part of West Irian led de Rook & van Dijk (1959) to revise the concept of *W. bancrofti* transmission in New Guinea. The authors concluded that, although there was sufficient evidence to incriminate the three major species of the *punctulatus* group, i.e., *An. farauti*, *An. punctulatus*, and *An. koliensis*, as the principal vectors in many areas, the role played by some culicine mosquitoes should also be taken into account, especially in certain nonmalarious and highly filarious areas. So far, natural infection with fully developed filarial larvae has been established in five non-anopheline mosquitoes, and experimental infection into the infective stage was observed in two other species. *Culex pipiens fatigans* was recently imported, but has established in many urban areas and was shown to be susceptible to the local filaria. Three other species of this genus, *C. bitaeniorhynchus*, *C. annulirostris*, and *C. squamosus* have also been incriminated as the vectors, together with *Ae. kochi*. At least two species of *Mansonia*, *M. uniformis* and *M. papuensis*, are now considered as the principal vectors in certain swampy areas. WILLESME (1959), in Amsterdam, carried out experimental infections of *C. p. fatigans* from western New Guinea and *Ae. polynesiensis* from Samoa with microfilariae of nocturnally periodic *W. bancrofti* in a carrier from South America, and observed the complete development only in the former, while in the latter, the mortality was high and no mosquito survived long enough to enable complete larval development.

VAN DIJK (1961) conducted a trial mass treatment of filariasis with diethylcarbamazine in the village of Inanwatan. Two surveys were made before the treatment, in June 1959 and January 1960. Of 1,206 persons examined in 1959, 128 (10.6%) had clinical manifestations, and among these, 101 (8.4%) had elephantiasis. The microfilaria rates of the population at the 1959 survey were 24% (142 of 582) in males and 20% (122 of 624) in females. The overall positive rate of the population was 21.9% (264 of 1,206) in 1959, and 21.0% (247 of 1,178) in 1960.

Diethylcarbamazine citrate (Filaricide, Nederlandsche Dieetzout Fabriek) was administered to all the persons of the village, with the exception of infants and gravely ill people, at the single daily dose of 5.5 to 6.5 mg per kg, 12 times, at intervals of four weeks. Nearly all of 1,241 eligible persons received the 12 doses, with exception of a few persons who failed to be treated for various reasons. The side effects were encountered in about 25% of the people after the first dose. At the blood examination made four weeks after the first dose, the total count of microfilariae in 225 persons decreased from 14,546 to 4,038, a reduction of 72%. At the second examination made four weeks after the second dose, the total counts of 215 originally positive cases decreased from 13,646 to 1,560, a reduction of 89%, and the microfilaria rate was reduced from 100% to 33%. At the posttreatment examination of the whole population carried out 9 to 22 days after the 12th dose, 16 of 1,280 persons were still positive, of which 4 were imported cases. Of 16 positive cases, 9 received 11 or 12 doses, and whose microfilarial count was only 1 in 7 cases, and 2 and 3, respectively, in the remaining two cases.

VAN DIJK (1964) further reported on the results of some antifilarial measures applied in New Guinea. Blood surveys were carried out in three villages in the Nimboran district, where IYENGAR *et al.* (1959) observed that the indoor spraying campaign with insecticides primarily directed towards the interruption of the transmission of malaria seemed to have interrupted the transmission of anopheline-borne filariasis. The indoor spraying operations were continued for over seven years after the first spraying cycle was completed in mid-1955. The microfilarial rates obtained in 1959, four years after the start of the operation, were 14.4% (13 of 90) in Kaitemo, 15.1% (11 of 73) in Jacotim, and 23.8% (29 of 122) in Sanggai, while the rates of the same villages in 1962, seven years after the start, were 16.1% (15 of 93), 10.1% (7 of 69), and 15.0% (15 of 100), respectively. These rates were still considerably high, though slight reductions were seen in two of the villages. In Kaitemo, new positive cases were seen in younger age-groups, while in the other two villages, gradual extinction of old infections seemed to have taken place among some adults. In conclusion, the insecticide spraying alone was considered to be not very effective in the control of filariasis even in New Guinea where the parasite is transmitted mainly by anophelines.

On the other hand, the effects of mass treatment with DEC conducted in Inawantan in 1960 were remarkable. At the presurvey made from 1959 to 60, the microfilarial rate was 21.2% (192 of 904) and the average microfilaria density was 47.7. In December 1962, only 1.9% (17 of 192) were positive, and the average count was 3.7. Of the 17 positives, all but one had already shown microfilaremia during the presurveys in 1959–60. Besides the positive cases among the villagers who had received the treatment, 12 imported microfilaria carriers were encountered at the 1962 survey. The 16 persons who were still positive at the end of the initial course of the treatment in December 1960 received another 12 doses of the drug during 1961; nine of them were re-examined in November 1961 and December 1962, and were all negative.

9C.2 Papua New Guinea

This country comprises the eastern half of New Guinea, the Bismarck Archipelago, and a number of adjacent islands. It is situated in the tropical zone between the equator and 11°S, and has an area of 473,200 km² and a population of 2,276,632 (1968). It formerly consisted of the Trust Territory of New Guinea (northern half), and the Territory of Papua (southern half) administered by Australia.

The area occupying the eastern half of New Guinea has high mountain ranges in the northwest and southeast, and large swampy areas in the south. The epidemiological characters of filariasis in this region are estimated to be essentially the same as in the western half of New Guinea, or Irian Barat.

The Bismarck Archipelago is an island-group that comprises two large islands (New Britain and New Ireland) and a number of smaller islands. The area is 49,700 km², and the population is 176,471 (1961). Most of the islands are volcanic in origin, and the native are mostly Melanesians.

Filariasis is considered to be widely endemic in Papua New Guinea, but the information is still scant. The parasite is a nocturnally periodic *W. bancrofti* and the main vectors are mosquitoes of the *An. punctulatus* group, so far as is known.

Diesing (1899) reported on a case of *Filaria sanguinis hominis* from New Guinea. The patient was a ship's engineer, who had visited the Diesing's clinic because of severe pain in the kidney area, left knee, and both hands. Embryos of *W. bancrofti* were discovered in both the urine and blood.

Breinl (1915) reported on the results of two journeys to the coastal belt of East New Guinea, which were undertaken for the purpose of mapping out the incidence and geographical distribution of tropical diseases among the natives. The first journey took place during the months of July and August 1912, and included the coastal belt of Port Moresby and north of Samarai as far as the Mambare River. During the second journey, lasting from the end of June to the beginning of October 1913, the coastal region west of Port Moresby as far as Daru was visited. During the journeys, a number of blood films were obtained in order to map out the distribution of filariasis and malaria. The blood was usuallly taken during daytime, and examined by thin smears. Out of 166 blood slides taken at random on the first journey, 24 (15%) contained microfilariae, while those taken on the second journey were positive in only 8 of 166 (5%). The microfilariae were morphologically identical with *Microfilaria nocturna*, and all of the five cases examined day and night showed the typical nocturnal periodicity. Cases of elephantiasis of the legs, arms, and scrotum were seen in varying numbers throughout the districts visited, and the patchy distribution of clinical cases and microfilaria carriers was quite marked.

An observation on filariasis and its vectors in New Guinea was conducted by Hopla (1946) while stationed in the Milne Bay area from 1944 to 1945. Nocturnally periodic *W. bancrofti* was found prevalent among the native populations, and 33 to 55% microfilarial rates was obtained. (No figures referring to the numbers examined were given.) However, 35 Europeans who had been in New Guinea from 12 to 25 years were all negative, and no clinical manifestations were evident. Mosquitoes were collected from the "boy houses" at the Sagarai Plantation. Each house contained approximately sixty natives whose microfilarial rate was 55%, with an average of 25 to 35 microfilariae per smear. (Again, the method and the number examined were not mentioned.) Of the mosquitoes dissected from these collections, 42 of 275 (15.3%) of *An. punctulatus moluccensis* were infected with various stages of filarial larvae, including the infective ones; also, 2 of 75 *C. quinquefasciatus* were infected, but none of 50 *C. annulirostris* were positive. *Culex quinquefasciatus* was more abundant at the plantation than in the surrounding villages, where *C. annulirostris* was most abundant. In night collections using human bait, the average number of bites per hour from *An. punctulatus moluccensis* was 55. Through these observations, Hopla concluded that *An. punctulatus moluccensis* was the most important and efficient vector, and *C. quinquefasciatus* was of no great importance in this area.

Bearup & Lawrence (1950) made a parasitological survey of five New Guinea villages: Busama on the Huon Gulf; Kaiapit in the valley of the Markham River; Patep, 30 miles south of Lae; Kavataria on the lagoon of Kiriwina, the largest island of the Trobriand group; and Koravagi in the Purari Delta at the junction of the Beara and Pie Rivers. Microfilariae of *W. banctofti* were found in 5 of 24 examined in the Busama area, 11 of 25 at Kaiapit, none of 15 at Patep, 11 of 65 at Kavataria, and 3 of 10 in Purari Delta. Elephantiasis was not common, but a few affected cases were seen by the authors.

A report on filariasis and its vectors at the Rabaul area (New Britain) was made by Backhouse & Heydon (1950) based on data collected between the years 1930 and 1935. At examinations of a mixed group of indentured laborers from various regions of Melanesia, 83 (19.4%) of 427 persons showed microfilaremia, 3 had elephantiasis, and 116 of 390 (29.7 %) showed enlargement of the epitrochlear glands. Among these laborers, those from northeast New Guinea (Morobe, Madang, Sepic, and Aitape) showed higher positive rates than those from New Britain; the microfilaria rate of the former group was 25.2% (44 of 174) in contrast to 7.5% (13 of 172) of the latter group. The microfilariae were nocturnally periodic; of 44 positive cases examined both night and day, 10 were positive both night and day, 34 were positive only at night, and none were positive only in the day.

Results of blood and clinical observations carried out on two small islands in New Britain were reported in the same paper. Filariasis was prevalent on both Makada and Matty Islands, and the overall positive rates of each total population were 22.7% and 25.3%, respectively, and the positive rates among the adult males were 31.1% and 40.4%, respectively. In Makada, 134 of 220 (60.9%) had enlarged epitrochlear glands. At the double blood exmination conducted day and night on the same person, all the microfilarial carriers of the two islands were either positive only at night, or had much higher counts in the night sample than in the day.

The same authors conducted investigations on the mosquito vectors in this region. Of 32 *An. farauti* collected in Makada and dissected at Rabaul, 12 were infected, and 5 of them contained mature larvae. Developments to mature larvae were also observed in experimental infections with *An. farauti* and *An. punctulatus*. In the experimental infection of *C.p. fatigans* with *W. bancrofti* in Rabaul, 5 of 67 in one experiment and 4 of 29 in another experiment contained mature larvae at dissections made 12 days after taking the infective meal (the donor showed 45 to 238 microfilariae in 20 mm³ blood in the first experiment, and 79 to 136 in the second). These results suggested that *C.p. fatigans* is less adapted for the development of *W. bancrofti* in Rabaul than that of the typical urban strains of *W. bancrofti*.

Among various culicine species tested by the same authors, full development of the Melanesian strain of *W. bancrofti* was seen in *Ae. kochi*, but *Ae. scutellaris*, *Ae. aegypti*, and *Armigeres* sp. from Madaka were all refractile.

McMillan (1960) carried out an experimental study of infection of a local strain of *C. p. fatigans* maintained at the Malaria Control Laboratory, Maprik, Sepik District, on a donor who showed a mean microfilarial count of 105 per 20 mm^3 on the first occasion and 138 on the second. A relatively low degree of infection and development was also obtained in this experiment; being kept at 64 to 76°F, 4 of 13 mosquitoes dissected on the 12.5th day contained early second stage larvae, 4 of 14 dissected on the 14.5th day had late second stage larvae only, and 4 of 20 mosquitoes dissected after 17.5 days had infective larvae.

Desowitz *et al.* (1966) carried out epidemiological surveys of filariasis of this region using blood examinations and skin tests with a purified antigen prepared from *Dirofilaria immitis* by Sawada *et al.* (1965). Three populations were surveyed; those of the Trobriand Islands and Cape Gloucester, New Britain, were exposed to endemic filariasis, while that of Gembogl in the eastern highland of New Guinea was reputedly free from filariasis. The people in the Trobriand Islands showed an overall microfilarial rate of 15.2% (47 of 310) and a skin test positive rate of 58.4% (160 of 274); these rates in Cape Gloucester were 17.2% (35 of 203) and 47.0% (94 of 200), respectively. In Gembogl, none of 62 adults and 11 children of 5 to 12 years examined had microfilaremia, and all the children, as well as 28 adult females who had never left the mountainous area, were skin test negative. However, 5 of 34 adult males gave a positive skin test reaction, and in each case the individual had been to work in a coastal endemic area for a year or longer. The results of the skin test and the blood examination were well correlated. There was a gradual increase in both rates with advancing age, but in all age-groups the percentage of skin test reactions was 3 to 4 times greater than the microfilarial rate. However, a great majority of children with demonstrable microfilaremia did not produce a positive skin reaction; some adults with microfilaremia and/or clinical signs also gave negative skin reactions.

9C.3 The Solomon Islands

The Solomons are a group of islands east of New Guinea, with an area of 39,420 km^2 and a population of 204,186 (1970). They are situated between 5°S and 12°S. The northwestern islands of Bougainville, Buka, and Green form a part of Papua New Guinea, and the remaining islands, including Guadalcanal, form the British Solomon Islands Protectorate.

According to Iyengar (1965), nocturnally periodic *W. bancrofti* infection has a wide distribution in the Solomons, but the endemic areas are restricted to lowlying coastal villages; the hilly areas in the interior are free from the disease. *Anopheles farauti, An. kolinesis*, and *An. punctulatus* are the major vectors.

A survey of filariasis in the Solomon Islands was made by Schlosser

(1945). The incidence of microfilaremia seen among the natives from various islands was 10.2% (16 of 157) in Guadalcanal, 10.2% (56 of 548) in Malaita, and 31.5% (176 of 558) in San Cristobal; the rates in immigrants from the Pacific Islands were 19.8% (29 of 146) in those from Fiji, and 16.3% (54 of 332) in those from Gilbert. The microfilariae of the Solomon Islands natives were highly nocturnally periodic, and the positive rates obtained with day and night blood were 5.4% (5 of 94) and 20.0% (180 of 880), respectively. In another observation, it was shown that of 95 Solomon natives who were positive at the blood examination made at 7:30 p.m., only 18 (19%) were positive at the examination made at 1:30 p.m. However, of 27 Gilbert natives who were positive at 7:30 p.m., 20 (74%) were also positive at 1:30 p.m.

BYRD & ST. AMANT (1959) made filariasis surveys in the central and southern Pacific islands, and recorded elephantiasis rates of 3.2% in Guadalcanal, 1.2% in San Cristobal, and 0.8% in Malaita. These authors also found that of 655 specimens of *An. farauti* collected in houses in Guadalcanal 51.9% were infected and 7.9% carried infective larvae.

A report on filariasis on two islands of the Solomon Islands was made by MATAIKA (1965). In Guadalcanal, a total of 245 persons in five coastal villages were examined, and 28.5% of them were found to be positive for microfilariae and 0.8% with elephantiasis. In three bush villages, 25% of 88 persons examined had microfilariae but none had elephantiasis. In immigrant villagers from Gilbert and Ellice, 1.5% of 64 persons were microfilaria positive. In Rennel and Bellona Tenaru, 1.3% of 77 persons examined were microfilaria positive, but none had elephantiasis. On Florida Island, 40.2% of 266 persons examined had microfilariae and 3% had elephantiasis.

9C.4 New Hebrides

A group of islands northeast of New Caledonia and west of Fiji, situated between 12°S–21°S and 165°E–170°E. Area, 14,760 km²; population, 86,000 (1971). A British and French condominium.

BUXTON (1927) reported on the results of malaria and filariasis surveys in the New Hebrides. Of 209 children from various islands examined, 17 (8%) were positive for *Plasmodium falciparum* and 23 (11%) for *Pl. vivax*, with a total number of positives of 38 (18%). Blood examinations for filarial infection were made on 318 male natives over 12 years of age from 16 islands of the New Hebrides, and 100 (31.4%) were found microfilaria positive in 20 mm³ night blood samples. At clinical examinations of the same population, 19 had elephantiasis, 23 had hydrocele, and 53 had palpable epitrochlear glands. The microfilariae were nocturnally periodic. *Anopheles punctulatus*, which breed in swamps and stagnant surface water, was the only species of the genus known to occur in the New Hebrides.

Although he could not confirm the mosquito vectors, Buxton concluded that "possibly the carrier of filariasis in the New Hebrides is *Anopheles punctulatus*, and cannot be *Culex fatigans*, which is a recent importation only known from Vila."

The Buxton's idea was later confirmed by an experimental study of BACKHAUS (1934) in Rabaul, New Britain. By feeding on a microfilarial carrier, *Anopheles punctulatus* var. *mollucensis* (now referred to as *An. farauti*) showed full development of the filarial larvae in 14 of 20 mosquitoes that survived 14 days and longer. In *An. punctulatus punctulatus*, the laboratory rearing was more difficult, the induced feeding was poor, and the mortality was higher than the former, but 3 of 4 mosquitoes that survived 14 days after the feeding contained mature larvae.

PERRY (1949) carried out studies on *M. xanthogaster* in the New Hebrides, in view of the fact that other species of this group are known to be the vector of *B. malayi*. Although microfilarial carriers of *B. malayi* existed among the Tonkinese immigrants in the South Pacific Islands, no evidence of transmission by this mosquito was obtained. The author gave accounts on its biology and description of the larvae and pupae. The host plant for the larvae was determined to be a soft-rooted dwarf water plant, which was found abundantly in freshwater swamps.

9D. The New Caledonian subregion

Filariasis endemic in the geographic subregion consisting of New Caledonia and the Loyalty Islands is different from that in the nearby islands of the New Hebrides, in that the parasite is a diurnally subperiodic race of *W. bancrofti*, the same as that found in the Polynesian subregion. The main vector in this subregion is *Ae. (Ochlerotatus) vigilax* (Skuse, 1889), which is a day-biting mosquito that breeds in brackish waters. Mosquitoes of the *Ae. (Stegomyia) polynesiensis* group, the main vectors in the Polynesian subregion, as well as *An. farauti* and allied species acting as the main vectors in the Papuan subregion, are absent from the New Caledonian subregion.

The islands in this subregion are situated between latitudes 20°S and 23°S, and longitudes 164°E and 169°E. Although most of the islands lie south and east of the New Hebrides and the distance between Aneityum of New Hebrides and Mare of the Loyalty Islands is only about 200 km, the parasite and the vectors have been shown to be completely different.

New Caledonia is a French overseas territory in the southwest Pacific, east of Queensland, Australia. It includes the main island of New Caledonia, the Loyalty Islands, Ile des Pins, and several other island-groups. The total area is 19,080 km², with a total population of 113,680 (1971). The islands are situated in the subtropical zone between 20°S and 23°S.

The main island of New Caledonia is situated between 20°S and 23°S, and has an area of 16,900 km² and a population of 84,000 (1963). It is a mountainous island about 400 km long and 50 km wide. The higher peaks reach over 1,600 meters above sea level. Rich in precipitation, there are many small rivers and streams here. The natives are Melanesians of the Papuan type.

The Loyalty Islands (Îles Loyauté) are an island-group located 100 km east of New Caledonia and about 260 km southwest of the southern end of the New Hebrides group. Their area is 1,955 km² with a population of 11,409 (1956 census). Chief islands are Lifou, Maré, and Uvea; the islands are mostly low coral upheavals.

Historical notes:

The occurrence of elephantiasis in this region has been noted since early days.

BOYER (1878), in his general account on the diseases in the South Pacific, stated that hydrocele of the scrotum was very common in Noumea of Tahiti and also in Liou of the Loyalty Islands; elephantiasis was common all over Oceania, and numerous victims were seen in New Caledonia. LANG & NOC (1903) reported on human and animal filariasis in New Caledonia. They stated that manifestations of filariasis among people in New Caledonia had long been noted, and the occurrence of cases with elephantiasis was recorded by VINSON in 1892. The authors examined the blood of 117 (including natives and Europeans) over the age of 20, and discovered the microfilariae of *Filaria sanguinis hominis* in 4, and observed 3 cases of elephantiasis without microfilaremia among them. The authors found *Dirofilaria immitis* in dogs and *Filaria mansoni* in chickens. PERRY (1950) gave an historic account on mosquitoes and mosquito-borne diseases in New Caledonia, and reported on his own observations of filariasis. Microfilariae of *W. bancrofti* were found in 3 (5.7%) of 52 natives of New Caledonia and 16 (11.9%) of 135 natives of the Loyalty Islands, but none of 6 French, 25 Javanese, or 9 people from Indochina. The author emphasized the importance of *C. quinquefasciatus* (= *fatigans*) as the probable vector of *W. bancrofti* in this region.

The more recent information on filariasis in New Caledonia has been published or recorded mainly in local periodicals or government records which are difficult to obtain outside of the region, but IYENGAR (1965) gives an excellent review of the available records.

Microfilarial periodicity:

IYENGAR (1954a) made microfilaria counts in his study on the microfilarial periodicity of *W. bancrofti* in New Caledonia (Table 9-5), and concluded that it showed the lack of periodicity. However, SASA & TANAKA (1972) made statistical analysis of his data, and demonstrated that the New Caledonian *W. bancrofti* is a typical example of the diurnally subperiodic, Polynesian form of *W. bancrofti*, with a periodicity index of 22.8 and the peak hour at 3 p.m. (see Section 11F.5).

Table 9-5. Average microfilaria counts in 20 mm³ of peripheral blood in carriers from Mou Village, New Caledonia (average of six cases, after IYENGAR, 1965).

Hour	900	1100	1300	1500	1700	1900	2100	2300	100	300	500	700	900
Count	37.3	41.3	58.2	58.7	52.2	53.5	42.7	39.0	31.8	27.7	39.3	37.0	48.7

Geographic distribution:

According to IYENGAR (1965), the main foci of filarial infection in New Caledonia are: (1) Balade, Pouebe, Touho, Mou, and Ouasse on the east coast; and (2) Koumac, Gomen, Voh, and Nepou on the west coast. In the Loyalty Islands, cases of filarial infection have been recorded from Lifou and Ouvea. The recorded microfilaria rates for these foci are shown in Table 9-6. It should be noted that unusually high microfilaria rates were observed in these areas.

Endemic filarial infection in New Caledonia has been observed to be restricted in its distribution to only some foci along the coast, i.e., to certain areas close to mangrove swamps where *Ae. vigilax* breeds abundantly. MERLET (1950) observed that in communities living even a few miles into the interior from a coastal focus, the infection was practically absent. IYENGAR (1954b) stated that in Nassirah Village, situated four miles into the interior from the coastal marshes of Bouloupari, none of the local inhabitants showed filarial infection, though *Ae. vigilax* occurred in fair numbers at certain periods of the year. Also, coastal villages not situated close to mangrove swamps had little or no filarial infection.

Clinical filariasis cases:

According to IYENGAR (1965), cases of elephantiasis and other filarial diseases were very common in New Caledonia judging by early medical records during the 18th and 19th centuries. The islands were annexed by the French in 1853, and a shift of the coastal native populations to the interior took place during the period from 1880 to 1918, as a measure for the prevention of various communicable diseases. In recent surveys conducted by MERLET (1950) and IYENGAR (1954a, 1965), only very small numbers of elephantiasis cases were observed in the coastal villages in New Caledonia and the Loyalty Islands, though high microfilaria rates were recorded from the same areas.

Mosquito vector:

Aedes (Ochlerotatus) vigilax (SKUSE, 1889) has been shown to be the vector of the diurnally subperiodic *W. bancrofti* of the New Caledonian subregion by IYENGAR (1954a). A natural infection rate of 5% was recorded by IYENGAR (1954a) in Mou Village, and 2.2% for the areas investigated by LACOUR & RAGEAU (1957). Complete development to the infective stage larvae were observed in experimental infections by IYENGAR (1954a), IYENGAR & MENON (1956), and BACKHOUSE & WOODHILL (1956). Under experi-

Table 9-6. Microfilaria rates of the main endemic foci of filarial infection in New Caledonia and Loyalty Islands (after IYENGAR, 1965).

Area	Number of persons examined		Micro-filaria rate	Observer
New Caledonia				
(a) East Coast				
Ponerihouen				
Mou village	57	adults	49.1	Merlet (1950)
Mou village	86	all ages	37.2	Iyengar (1954a)
Mou village	—	—	42.0	Lacour & Rageau (1957)
Touho	—	—	25.0	Lacour & Rageau (1957)
Pouebo	81	adults	59.3	Kerrest (1951)
Pouebo	—	adult males	56.0	Merlet (1950)
Pouebo	—	adult females	41.0	Merlet (1950)
Pouebo	—	—	28.3	Lacour & Rageau (1957)
Balade	—	—	13.0	Lacour & Rageau (1957)
Ouasse	—	—	25.0	Lacour & Rageau (1957)
(b) West Coast				
Koumac	24	adults	16.6	Kerrest (1951)
Koumac	—	—	4.0	Lacour & Rageau (1957)
Gomen	13 adults		7.7	Kerrest (1951)
Gomen	—	—	1.4	Lacour & Rageau (1957)
Voh: Gatope	45	all ages	22.2	Merlet (1950)
Voh: Gatope	—	—	16.3	Lacour & Rageau (1957)
Voh: Oundjo	129	all ages	24.8	Merlet (1950)
Voh: Oundjo	—	—	9.3	Lacour & Rageau (1957)
Loyalty Islands				
Lifou	—	adults	3.0	Perry (1950)
Ouvea	—	adults	11.0	Perry (1950)
Ouvea: Fayaoue	—	—	9.0	Lacour & Rageau (1957)
Ouvea: St. Joseph	—	—	21.0	Lacour & Rageau (1957)

mental conditions, *C. p. fatigans* and *Ae.* (*Finlaya*) *notoscriptus* were also shown to be hospitable to the New Caledonian race of *W. bancrofti* by the above authors.

Detailed accounts were made by IYENGAR (1965) on the bionomics of *Ae. vigilax* in New Caledonia. It is prolific in stagnant, shallow, brakish water pools along the coast line, well exposed to direct sunshine. Clearance of mangrove vegetation and interference with tidal flow of salt marshes are important factors which favor intensive breeding of *Ae. vigilax*. Adult females of this mosquito species are vicious human biters, active only during daytime, exophilous (rarely come inside houses), and rest in low vegetation near damp soil.

9E. The Polynesian subregion

A zoogeographic subregion where the diurnally subperiodic race of *W. bacnrofti* is endemic, with mosquitoes of the *Ae.* (*Stegomyia*) *polynesiensis* group as the main vectors. The subregion includes large numbers of small islands in the tropics and subtropics of the southern hemisphere in the Pacific Ocean.

9E.1 Fiji

An island-group in the southwestern Pacific Ocean, Fiji is east of New Hebrides between 16°S to 19°20′S in latitude and 178°W to 177°E in longitude. It has a total area of 17,970 km² and a population of 524,457 (1970). Fiji includes some 100 inhabited islands, of which Viti Levu and Vanua Levu are the largest. Most of the islands are high and of volcanic origin, and consist of mountainous area and fertile valleys either well cultivated or densely covered with tropical forests.

9E.1.1 Epidemiology

Filariasis has long been noted to be prevalent in Fiji.

MESSER (1876), who was the medical officer of the British frigate "Pearl," gave general accounts on health condition and disease in Fiji, and described that "elephantiasis is very common among indigenous people in certain localities, especially in low and marshy parts. The lower limb is more often affected than the scrotum. So long as we know, only two Europeans cases have been observed. One was resident for 5 years and another for 15 years. In both cases, the legs were affected."

SAFFRE (1884) also gave general accounts on the health conditions of the islands of Tonga, Samoa, Wallis, Futuma and Fiji, and mentioned that "féfé" or elephantiasis was very prevalent here as in all Oceania, and that the residence on low land, poor illumination, humid soil on which the natives sleep, and the diet of essentially vegetable origin would probably be the cause of development of such a disease.

BOISSIERE (1904), a medical officer in Bua, Fiji, reported briefly on filariasis and yaws in Fiji. He stated, "Filariasis is extremely prevalent in Fiji, and in my own province, Bua, it is especially so. The individual adult who has not been attacked in some way or other by this disease is the exception. The most common manifestation of the disease is the condition of variose groin glands, with occasional attacks of fever. Owing to the very severe rigor which commonly accompanies the early stages of filarial fever, this has frequently been mistaken for malaria by the laity."

LYNCH (1905), the resident medical superintendent of Colonial Hospital, Fiji, reported on his experiences with filariasis of the islands. During a period extending over 13 months, the blood of 608 Fijian natives who visited the hospital for various reasons were examined both day and night at the Colonial Hospital; embryos were present in 156, or 25.7%. They were present in 125 day specimens and 136 night specimens, and 105 showed them in both day and night specimens. The 608 cases had come from 15 different provinces of Fiji, and the positive rate according to the provinces varied from the lowest of 8.3% in Naitasiri to the highest of 35.5% in Kadavu.

BRUNWIN (1909), the government medical officer in Fiji, also gave general accounts on the condition of filariasis in Fiji, which he recognized as one of the most common pathological conditions from which the natives were suffering.

BAHR (1912), who stayed in Fiji during a period from January 12, 1910 to February 21, 1911, compiled a comprehensive report on filariasis and elephantiasis of this area. The report includes various important and interesting observations on filariasis in Fiji. In a summary, the following observations were made by the author:

(1) A large proportion of Fijians harbor microfilariae in their blood. Of 1,320 people (804 males and 516 females) examined, 358 persons (27.1%) were found positive, of whom 245 (30.4%) were males and 113 (23.8%) were females. The rate was lower in males than in females in the age-groups younger than 20 years, but the relation was reversed in the older age-groups.

(2a) Adult filariae were found in the lymphatics without the presence of microfilariae in the blood. The author found numerous adult filariae by surgical biopsy of the lymph glands, even in those whose blood did not show microfilaremia, and pointed out that the absence of microfilariae in circulating blood did not mean the freedom from the filarial infection.

(2b) A large proportion of Fijians were found affected with the filarial disease. Clinical signs were found in 446 (55.5%) of 804 males and 128 (24.8%) of 516 females examined. However, 287 males and 95 females among those with clinical signs had no demonstrable microfilaremia, while

77 males and 81 females had demonstrable microfilaremia without clinical signs. In total, 523 (65.0%) out of 804 males and 209 (40.5%) out of 516 females examined had some signs of filarial affections.

Elephantiasis was seen in 47 (3.56%) of 1,320 people examined. Of these 47 with elephantiasis, 18 (38.2%) had microfilariae. The elephantiasis rate was 4.8% in males and 1.5% in females. The author also stated that the number of microfilariae in the blood had no relation to the severity of the lesions present.

(2c) All Fijians, as well as foreigners resident in Fiji for some time, exhibited a well-marked eosinophilia, even in the absence of infection with other parasites. Fecal examinations were made on 156 persons, of whom 77 (37.2%) harbored *Ancylostoma* or *Necator* eggs, 21 (27.2%) had *Trichocephalus* eggs, but *Ascaris* eggs were encountered only in 3 cases.

(2d) Patients with microfilariae in the blood had lost their microfilariae while under observation. The author observed the loss of microfilaremia in 7 cases while he stayed in the Islands.

(3a) No periodicity was seen in microfilaria of Fiji, as was observed by some previous workers in some South Pacific Islands. Measured quantities of blood were taken from 372 Fijians, Samoans, and Tongans, of whom microfilariae were found in 114; 91 had microfilariae in both day and night samples, 48 had more at nighttime, 43 had more in daytime; 17 had microfilariae at night only, and 6 had microfilariae by day only, usually very scant in both cases. On the other hand, immigrants from India and the Solomon Islands had microfilariae of nocturnal periodicity, except for some who were old residents. Of 35 Europeans examined, 6 (17.1%) had microfilariae without periodicity, and 5 suffered from filarial disease.

(3b) The development in *C. fatigans* was not so efficient as in *Stegomyia pseudoscutellaris* (now *Ae. polynesiensis*), the common mosquito in Fiji. Seven species of mosquitoes were collected in the neighborhood of the author's laboratory in Suva; they were, in the order of prevalence, as follows: *Stegomyia pseudoscutellaris, C. fatigans, C. jepsoni, Finlaya poecilia, Stegomyia fasciata, C. nocturnus,* and *Phoniomyia* sp. The results of experimental infection in the first two species were described in detail.

(3c) Leiper examined adult worms obtained by Bahr, and confirmed that they were identical with those of *F. bancrofti*.

(4) Surveys were made on filariasis in different islands of Fiji. The microfilarial rate and the elephantiasis rate were 12.5% and 0% in Bau, 32.8% and 1.8% in Loma-Loma, 22.5% and 1.5% in Oneata, and 36.5% and 8.7% in Lakemba.

KNOTT (1944, unpublished report, quoted by IYENGAR, 1959) stated that filariasis was very common in small coconut-growing islands but rare on large sugar cane-growing islands; the disease was also rare at Nandi located on the dry side of the island of Viti Levu, but 5 of 25 in one village and 24 of 50 in another village on Suva Peninsula showed microfilariae. According to NELSON & CRUIKSHANK (1956, unpublished report, quoted by

IYENGAR, 1959, 1965), 14.2% of 57,888 persons of all ages examined in Fiji by Knott's concentration method were positive for microfilariae, with the rate of 17.5% in males and 11.2% in females; elephantiasis was seen in 511 (0.9%) of the people examined. The microfilaria rates varied from zero to 44% in areas on Viti Levu Island, and from 20% to 30% on Tavenui Island. On Vanua Levu Island, much higher microfilaria rates with an average of 24.7% were seen on the windward wet side than on the leeward dry side, where the average rate was 7.5%.

9E.1.2 Vectors

The first comprehensive study on the transmission of filariasis in Fiji was conducted by BAHR (1912), who incriminated *Ae. (Stegomyia) pseudoscutellaris* (Theobald, 1910) as the main vector of the nonperiodic *W. bancrofti*, and found *C. p. fatigans* to be less efficient for its transmission. However, MARKS (1951) demonstrated that two species had been confused as *Ae. pseudoscutellaris* in all previous filariasis studies in Fiji and other South Pacific Islands, and indicated that the proven vector in most areas in this region was a new species, which she named *Ae. polynesiensis*.

In Fiji, SYMES (1955, 1960a, 1960b), as well as BURNETT (1960), showed that both *Ae. polynesiensis* and *Ae. pseudoscutellaris* were efficient vectors of *W. bancrofti*, and that a third species, the night-biting *Ae. (Finlaya) fijiensis* Marks, 1947, a member of the *kochi* group, was the main vector in certain *Pandanus*-growing villages. SYMES (1955) demonstrated that besides *Ae. polynesiensis* and *Ae. pseudoscutellaris*, three other mosquito species, i.e., *C. p. fatigans*, *C. annulirostris*, and *Ae. (Aedimorphus) vexans*, were also naturally infected with mature larvae of presumably *W. bancrofti*.

According to IYENGAR (1965), two species of the *Ae. (Stagomyia) scutellaris* group, i.e., *Ae. polynesiensis* Marks, 1951 and *Ae. pseudoscutellaris* (Theobald, 1910), are the most important vectors of *W. bancrofti* in Fiji. The former is common to many other Polynesian islands, while the latter is a vector only in Fiji. The two species are morphologically closely related, and early records of dissection for *Ae. pseudoscutellaris* were not separated from those of *Ae. polynesiensis*. MATAIKA *et al.* (1970, mimeographed report) stated that the former species is common in coastal areas, while the latter replaces the former in inland areas.

9E.1.3 Control

BURNETT & MATAIKA (1961) conducted a pilot experiment of DEC mass administration to the people in the Rewa area of Fiji for prevention of transmission of filariasis. The total population of the area at the 1956 census was 1,180, but more people were found to have homes there. Two courses of drug administration were given to everyone, approximately 6 mg per kg per dose, six doses at weekly intervals as a course; 1,226 persons completed the first course, and 911 the second. The microfilaria rate was reduced from 12.1 % to 2.7 % five months after end of the second course, and the mean microfilarial density from 4.084 to 0.360. There was a considerable movement of the people in and out of the area, which reduced the apparent effect of the drug. Before the treatment, 4.6 % were found infected and 0.66 % had mature larvae among 1,208 bush vectors (*Ae. pseudoscutellaris* and *Ae. polynesiensis*) collected and dissected in this area. After the first course, 8 (0.95 %) were infected and 1 (0.12 %) had mature larvae among 841 bush vectors. After the second course, only 1 out of 832 bush vectors were found infected with immature larvae.

The REPORT OF WHO/SPC SEMINAR (1974) stated, "Due to the geography of the islands and the population distribution, simultaneous mass drug administration for the entire country (Fiji) has not been feasible. Thus, the following five stage mass treatment programme with DEC was begun in 1969: Stage I. 1969–71: Southern part of Northern Island and Rotuma Islands. II. 1970–72: Northern part of Northern Island and Lau group. III. 1971–73: Eastern Division and Yasawa group. IV. 1972–74: Central Division. V. 1973–75: Western Division.

The programme continued for two years in each of these five areas. The DEC dosage was 5 mg/kg body weight weekly for 6 weeks and then monthly for 22 months, with a total dosage of 140 mg/kg body weight. Post-treatment surveys of the 16–60-year age group only will be carried out, as this group showed the highest microfilaria rate before treatment. Since the inception of mass drug administration, there has been a dramatic reduction in the hospital admissions due to filariasis. Post-treatment surveys show a decrease in microfilaria rate to 1 % or less."

9E.2 Tonga

Known also as the Friendly Islands, Tonga is a kingdom in the southwest Pacific Ocean, with an area of 700 km² and a population of 87,406 (1970). It comprises an archipelago of about 150 islands, divided into three groups: Tongatabu, Vavau, and Haapai, together with Niuafoo and Niuatobutabu further to the north. The Vavau group and Tofua of the Haapai group are high and mountainous and of volcanic origin. The other islands are lowland and of coral formation. Tonga became British protectorate in 1900, and achieved independence in 1970. The Tonga Islands are scattered over a vast area in the tropical zone, between latitudes 15°S and 23°S, and longitudes 173°W and 177°W.

9E.2.1 Epidemiology

Filariasis has long been noted to be prevalent in Tonga. According to IYENGAR (1965), Captain Cook, in his note in 1785 on his voyage in the South Pacific, already mentioned the common occurrence of enormous swelling of the leg, arm, and scrotum among the natives of Tonga. Elephantiasis was also reported to be common in Tonga by SAFFRE (1884), MANSON (1896), THORPE (1896), and LEBER & PROWAZEK (1914).

As stated before, the absence of nocturnal periodicity of the microfilariae of the South Pacific race of *W. bancrofti* was discovered first in Tonga by THORPE (1896). Based on examination of adults, he observed a microfilaria rate of 28.8% in Nomuka, 46.9% in Lifuka (Haapai group), 20% in Vavau, and 29.2% in Tongatapu. HOPKINS (1925, quoted by BUXTON, 1927) examined boys and young men residing in a college in Tongatapu, and found microfilaria rates of 13.5% among those from Tongatapu, 14.3% among those from Haapai, and 46.2% among those from Vavau. TAPA (1957, quoted by IYENGAR, 1965) examined hospital patients, and found microfilaria rates varying from 28.2% to 48.5% among those in Vaiola Hospital in Tongatapu and 49.6% in those in Ngu Hospital in Vavau.

9E.2.2 Mosquito vectors

Two species of the *Ae.* (*Stegomyia*) *scutellaris* group have been reported from Tonga: *Ae. tongae* EDWARDS, 1926 and *Ae. tabu* RAMALINGAM & BELKIN, 1965. The former is known only from the Haapai and Vavau groups, while the latter occurs in the Tongatapu group and also in the Haapai group. Both species had been confused in the past and reported as *Ae. tongae* until RAMALINGAM & BELKIN (1965) established the presence of the two distinct species in the Tonga Islands. To date, the two species have not been recorded outside the Tonga islands. BUXTON (1927) assumed on epidemiological grounds that "*Ae. tongae*" was the vector of filariasis in Tonga. RAMALINGAM & BELKIN (1964, 1965) and RAMALINGAM (1968), working in Tongatapu, observed that 16 (5.8%) of 274 *Ae. tabu* collected on human bait were positive for all stages of larvae, and 1 (0.4%) among them had infective larvae, but that none of 19 *Ae.* (*Stegomyia*) *aegypti*, 13 *Ae.* (*Finlaya*) *oceanus*, 3 *Ae.* (*Aedimorphus*) *nocturnus*, 76 *C. p. fatigans*, or 1 *C. annulirostris* was infected; in experimental infections with reared adults, 8 (66.7%) were found infected, and 6 (50%) had mature larvae out of 12 *Ae. tabu* dissected 14 to 16 days after taking the blood of microfilaria carriers.

9E.2.3 Control

The REPORT OF WHO/SPC SEMINAR (1974) stated: "It is planned to start an anti-filariasis programme in 1975 or 1976. Blood and clinical surveys were started in 1968."

9E.3 Rotuma

A small isolated group of islands of volcanic origin, Rotuma is situated

390 km north of Fiji, at 12°30'S and 177°E. The main island is about 13 km long and 36 km² in area. The original Rotumans are the Polynesians. Rotuma has been administratively part of Fiji since 1881.

Filariasis is known to be prevalent among the inhabitants of Rotuma. THORPE (1896) stated, "Rotuma is a hotbed of elephantiasis." BRUNWIN (1909) reported, "In Rotuma, nearly all the inhabitants seem to be affected, white as well as native." LAMBERT (1929) examined 2,020 persons on Rotuma and found 185 of them with clinical signs of filariasis, including 29 cases of elephantiasis (leg, 20; arm, 7; mamma, 2) and the rest mostly with genital lesions. Microfilariae were found in 28.7% of 171 persons examined, and they were the nonperiodic race of *W. bancrofti*. AMOS (1946, quoted by IYENGAR, 1959, 1965) examined 1,938 persons of all ages in Rotuma, and found elephantiasis in 2.1%, and microfilariae in 28.7%. Microfilaria rate among young age-group of 5 to 20 years was 5.7% in males and 7.9% in females.

Aedes (*Stegomyia*) *rotumae* BELKIN 1962, a member of the *Ae. scutellaris* group and the only species of this group occuring on this island, is suspected as the vector (IYENGAR, 1965).

9E.4 The Ellice Islands

The Ellice Islands consist of nine coral atolls situated between 6°S and 11°S, and 176°E and 180°E. All of the nine islands are inhabited, but are all small and low, not higher than 20 feet above sea level. The total area is only 23 km², and the population is 5,782 (1968). The islands have been administered under the British Colony of the Gilbert and Ellice since 1915.

From the epidemiological point of view, the Gilbert Islands belong to the Micronesian Subregion where the nocturnally periodic race of *W. bancrofti* is endemic, while the so-called nonperiodic race of *W. bancrofti* occurs in the Ellice group of the islands.

9E.4.1 Epidemiology

According to IYENGAR (1965), the Ellice Islands are composed of two groups with different topographical characters. The five islands of the northerly group, namely, Nanumea, Niutao, Nanumanga, Niu, and Vaitutu, are broad reef islands and are densely forested, while the three islands of Nukufetau, Funafuti, and Nukulailai, are narrow atolls encircling deep lagoons. The density of vector mosquitoes, as well as the incidence of filariasis, have been shown to be higher in the former group of islands than in the latter.

The so-called nonperiodic race of *W. bancrofti* infection has been noted to be highly endemic in all of the inhabited islands of the Ellice group. MCNAUGHTON (1919) made a census of elephantiasis cases in the Ellice

Islands, and recorded 90 cases (2.6%) out of 3,434 persons examined. O'CONNOR (1923) conducted a very detailed survey in the entire group of the Ellice Islands, and obtained an overall microfilaria rate of 46.0% and an elephantiasis rate of 10.3% among 1,169 persons of 16 years of age and over. In the different islands, the microfilaria rates varied from 28.6% to 53.9%, and the elephantiasis rate was lowest in Nukufetau (1.1%) and was between 5% and 30% in other islands. BUXTON (1928) examined 333 males over the age of 20 years, and found 38.1% to be positive for microfilariae, 8.1% with elephantiasis, and 23.0% with hydrocele. VENNER (1944) examined 65 persons from Nanumea and recorded a microfilaria rate of 50.8 %. LEWIS (1945) examined 173 persons of all ages from Nukufetau and observed a microfilaria rate of 34.1%. On Nukulailai, 19.0% of 258 persons examined were microfilaria positive (*Annual Report of Medical Department*, quoted by IYENGAR, 1965).

9E.4.2 Vector

Aedes (*Stegomyia*) *polynesiensis* has been considered as the sole vector of *W. bancrofti* in the Ellice Islands. O'CONNOR (1923) observed that the larvae developed to the mature stage 14 days after ingested by this mosquito. The vector density was found to vary considerably according to the islands, namely, extremely high in the northern Ellice group where the islands are broad coral reefs and the villages are surrounded by dense bush and plantations, and usually much lower in the southern Ellice group of atolls, devoid of dense vegetation. In the atoll island of Funafuti, the main breeding places of *Ae. polynesiensis* are the containers for storing water, coconut shells, and tin cans around houses. Detailed studies on the bionomics of mosquitoes were carried out by BYRD & ST. AMANT (1959) and by IYENGAR (1965).

LAIRD (1956) carried out a survey of mosquitoes of Funafuti, Ellice Islands, and recorded the occurrence of four species, namely, *Ae.* (*Stegomyia*) *aegypti*, *Ae.* (*Stegomyia*) *polynesiensis*, *Ae.* (*Aedimorphus*) *vexans*, and *C. annulirostris*. Both *Ae. marshallensis* and *C. p. fatigans*, which he found in the Gilbert Islands, were absent from Funafuti.

9E.4.3 Control

The REPORT OF WHO/SPC SEMINAR ON FILARIASIS (1974) stated, "Filariasis is a major public health problem on the eight Ellice Islands. Mass drug administration was started in 1972 with the assistance of the WHO intercountry filariasis advisory team. Pre-treatment surveys in Funafuti indicated an microfilaria rate of 14.7% and an average microfilaria count per carrier of 85.5 per 20 mm^3 blood. A preliminary post-treatment survey shows reduction of the microfilaria rate to 0.96%."

Annex: Fanning Island

Fanning is an atoll of the Line Islands in the central Pacific Ocean, south of Hawaii, situated at latitude 3°52′N and longitude 159°W. It has an area of 39 km², and has been administered under the British Colony of Gilbert and Ellice since 1916. Ross (1947) gave accounts on the health status of Fanning Island. There are no anophelines, but *Ae. scutellaris* is present. There are apparently no infectious diseases, except for sporadic cases of dengue fever. The inhabitants are mostly laborers, about 200 in number, who come to Fanning for a two-year term.

9E.5 The Tokelau Islands

Formerly called the Union Islands, these islands are situated north of American Samoa, between 8°S and 10°S, and 171°W and 173°W. They include Atafu, Fakaofo, and Nukunonu Islands. They have an area of 10 km², with a population of 1,687 (1970). They have been administered as part of New Zealand since 1948.

9E.5.1 Epidemiology

Nonperiodic *W. bancrofti* infection is endemic on all of the inhabited islands, but clinical manifestations have been observed to be rare. O'Connor (1923) examined 320 persons of all ages, about one-third of the population, and found 18.8% to be positive for microfilariae, but failed to find even a single case of elephantiasis. The rate among 245 persons aged 16 years and over was 22.4% (18.5% to 23.3% for the three atolls). Buxton (1928) examined 17 males under 20 years of age and 90 males over 20, and obtained microfilaria rates of 5.9% and 22.2%, respectively. Laird (1955) found none of 31 persons under 20, and 25.8% of 66 persons above the age of 20 years to be positive for microfilariae. Laird & Colles (1959, quoted by Iyengar, 1965) obtained microfilaria rates of 0% among 31 persons aged 1 to 9 years, 4.5% for 67 persons aged 10 to 19 years, and 25.2% for 226 persons aged 20 years and over. The rates of persons aged 20 years and over were higher in males than in females, i.e., 28.1% of 32 males and 12.5% of 40 females in Nukunonu, 46.9% of 32 males and 14.3% of 42 females in Fakaofo, and 38.9% of 36 males and 18.2% of 44 females in Atafu.

9E.5.2 Vector

Only two species of mosquitoes have been recorded from Tokelau: *Ae. polynesiensis* and *Ae. vexans nocturnus*. The former was recorded by Laird (1956) as the only mosquito he found in Tokelau at that time. Later, Laird

& COLLES (1959, quoted by IYENGAR, 1965) found a small focus of the latter species on Fanuafala islet of Fakaofo Atoll. According to IYENGAR (1965), *Ae. polynesiensis* was breeding abundantly all over the islands, and there was no doubt that it was the vector of filariasis. The people in Tokelau reside on "village islets" where the environment is kept relatively clean and open, and the density of mosquitoes is comparatively low. The other islets, used for coconuts plantations are more favorable for the breeding of *Ae. polynesiensis* and large numbers of larvae are found in coconut shells damaged by rats.

9E.6 The Wallis and Futuna Islands

These are a French overseas territory in the southwest Pacific Ocean, with a total area of 166 km² and a population of 8,546 (1969). They are situated west of western Samoa, between latitudes 14°S and 16°S and longitudes 176°W and 178°W. The main islands are high and of volcanic origin.

9E.6.1 Epidemiology

Filariasis has long been known to be prevalent on Wallis Island. REYNAUD (1876), CLAVEL (1884), and SAFFRE (1884) reported that elephantiasis was very common among the islanders, even among the white people. VIALA (1909) stated that nearly half of the adult population of Wallis suffered from elephantiasis of the legs or scrotum. BRONCHARD (1910a,b) found nonperiodic *W. bancrofti* to be the causative agent, and observed 20% of the population to be suffering from elephantiasis. High incidence of elephantiasis was reported also by DAVID in 1939 and ESTIENNE in 1959 (quoted by IYENGAR, 1965).

High microfilaria rates were recorded also from Wallis. TOUZE, in 1954, found 40% of the natives of Wallis to be positive, and RAGEAU & ESTIENNE, in 1959, observed 20.4% of 1,029 persons of all ages to be harboring microfilariae. The periodicity of microfilariae were examined by collecting blood samples at two-hour intervals by BYRD & ST. AMANT in 1945 and by RAGEAU & ESTIENNE in 1959; and the peak microfilarial density was observed at about 4 p.m. in both cases (quoted by IYENGAR, 1965).

Elephantiasis was reported to be very common on Futuna Island of the Hoorn group islands by VIALA (1909) and by DAVID (1939, quoted by IYENGAR, 1959, 1965).

9E.6.2 Vector

On Wallis Island, *Ae. polynesiensis* was shown to be the sole vector. BYRD & ST. AMANT examined 770 mosquitoes collected from different villages and found 6 to 38% of them to be infected, with an overall infection rate of 12.2%; those collected outside of the native habitations were rarely infected. RAGEAU & ESTIENNE recorded a natural infection rate of 3.7% among 1,435 mosquitoes collected from different villages (quoted by IYNEGAR, 1965).

In the Futuna Islands (Hoorn Islands), two species of the *Ae.* (*Stegomyia*) *scutellaris* group are known to be present, *Ae. polynesiensis* Marks, 1951, and *Ae. futunae* Belkin 1962. BELKIN (1962) considered the latter species to be the main vector in the Futuna group because it was more abundant than *Ae. polynesiensis*.

9E.7 Western Samoa

An independent state in the southwest Pacific situated at about 14°S and 172°W, Western Samoa is composed of the two main islands (Upolu and Savaii) and several small islands. It has an area of 2,935 km² and a population of 148,565 (1971). Administered by Germany before World War I, and then by New Zealand from 1914, it became independent in 1962.

9E.7.1 Epidemiology

A high incidence of filariasis has been noted since early times. The frequent occurrence of patients with elephantiasis of the legs or scrotum, often of enormous sizes, was described by KÖNIGER (1878), HIRSCH (1886, in "Handbook of Geographical and Historical Pathology"), WISE (1893), MANSON (1894, 1896), KRAEMER (1903, in "Die Samoan Insel"), and LEBER (1914).

O'CONNOR (1923) examined 4,294 persons of all ages from Eastern (American) and Western Samoa, and recorded 115 cases (2.7%) of elephantiasis; the microfilaria rate was 28.7% for Eastern and Western Samoa combined. BUXTON (1928) examined 1,103 males of all ages in Western Samoa, and recorded an elephantiasis rate of 5.6% (9.8% for males 20 years and over, nil for under 21 years, 1.8% for 21 to 35 years, 4.8% for 26 to 35 years, 12.8% for 36 to 45 years, and 20.3% for over 45 years). The hydrocele rate was 16% for all ages (nil for ages under 16, 4.7% for 16 to 20 years, 14.5% for 21 to 25 years, 23.6% for 26 to 35 years, and 31.7% for over 35 years). The microfilaria rate was 23.7% for the island of Upolu and 41.0% for Savaii, and the overall hydrocele rate was 13.5% for Upolu and 17.1% for Savaii.

In another survey conducted by IYENGAR (1954c), the overall elephantiasis rate was 3.6%, and from 15% to 20% of the people in Western Samoa were subject to periodical attacks of lymphadenitis; the microfilaria rate was 19.2% for Upolu and 24.1% for Savaii. McCARTHY & FITZGERALD (1955, 1956) recorded an elephantiasis rate of 2% and a microfilaria rate of 17.1% in Laulii Village of Upolu, and a microfilaria rate of 33% in Tuasivi Village of Savaii. LOPDELL (1953) recorded a microfilaria rate of 14.8% in school children aged 11 to 20 years.

9E.7.2 Vector

Aedes polynesiensis has been incriminated as the main vector of *W. bancrofti* in Western Samoa. O'CONNOR (1923) examined 100 specimens caught in a bungalow, and found 7 to be infected with *W. bancrofti* larvae. Under experimental conditions, the larvae completed their development in the mosquitoes in 13 days. PHILIPPS (1954, quoted by IYENGAR, 1965) observed an infection rate of 7.4%, and IYENGAR (1954) found an infection rate of 11.1% in *Ae. polynesiensis* caught in villages. Both LOPDELL (1953) and IYENGAR (1954) considered that transmission occurred primarily in villages, since infected mosquitoes were found mostly in or around residential areas and only rarely in areas away from habitations, while MCCARTHY & FITZGERALD (1956) stated infection of the human host occurs mainly in the plantation and along bush paths.

More detailed studies on the mosquito fauna and the transmission of filariasis in the Samoan region were reported by BELKIN (1962), RAMALINGAM & BELKIN (1964), and RAMALINGAM (1968). Besides *Ae. polynesiensis*, another species of the *Ae. scutellaris* group indigenous to this region, *Ae. upolensis* Marks, 1957, as well as two species of the *Ae. (Finlaya) kochi* group, i.e., *Ae. samoanus* (GRÜNBERG, 1913) and *Ae. tutuilae* Ramalingam et Belkin, 1965, were shown to be naturally infected. According to RAMALINGAM (1968), the positive rates for all stages of larvae and that for mature larvae of naturally caught mosquitoes were respectively, 8.4% and 2.4% of 407 *Ae. polynesiensis*, 11.9% and 1.1% of 59 *Ae. upolensis*, 4.5% and 0.3% of 380 *Ae. samoanus*, and none of 60 *Ae. (Finlaya) oceanicus,* 2 *Ae. (Aedimorphus) vexans nocturnus,* 51 *C. p. fatigans,* and 8 *C. annulirostris* was found to be naturally infected.

SUZUKI & SONE (1974) carried out observations by the human-bait collection method on the biting activity and seasonal prevalence of the two main filariasis vectors in Western Samoa, *Ae. polynesiensis* and *Ae. samoanus.* The former was shown to be a day-biting mosquito with two peaks in its biting density on man, one in the morning and another in the afternoon, of which the afternoon peak was usually higher. This mosquito species was, however, found to be biting on man also at night under bright moonlight. Of the three biting collection stations selected for this study, the highest catches were obtained in the bush outside of houses rather than indoors, while the mosquito was more abundant in a Samoan house than in an European house. *Ae. samoanus* was shown to be a night-biting mosquito with a peak usually during the third quarter of the night; there were no differences between the biting densities of indoor and outdoor stations. The two species were found to bite man throughout the year, and seasonal changes in their biting density were correlated with the amount of precipitation among various climatic factors tested.

9E.7.3 Control

As reported briefly by WHO (1974, *Report on the Fourth Joint WHO/ SPC Seminar on Filariasis and Vector Control*, Apia, W. Samoa), the WHO/UNICEF assisted pilot filariasis control project was established in 1965, and the first round of mass drug administration with DEC at 5 mg per kg once a week followed by a monthly dose for 12 months was completed in 1967. The average 18-dose covering was 21%. Volunteers of the Women's Health Committee assisted in the distribution of the drug. The microfilaria rate was reduced from 19.06% to 1.63% and the average count from 58 per 20 mm³ blood of positive carriers to 9. The second round with DEC at 6 mg per kg body weight, monthly for 12 months, was undertaken from January to December 1971 and it reduced the microfilaria rate from 2.26% in 1969 to 0.14% in 1973 and 0.11% in April 1974. A detailed report of the microfilaria survey data and statistical analysis for evaluation of the control work was submitted to WHO by SASA (1972, assignment report) but unfortunately still remains unpublished.

9E.8 American Samoa (Eastern Samoa)

American Samoa is a group of islands situated east of Western Samoa, at about 14°S and 171°W. It includes the islands of Tutuila, Manua Islands, Aunuu, Rose, and Swains. The total area is 197 km², with a population of 27,769 (1970). It has been administered by the United States since 1899.

9E.8.1 Epidemiology

Filariasis has been noted to be prevalent. O'CONNOR (1923) found 47.3% of 422 persons above the age of 15 years had either microfilaremia or some clinical signs. PHELPS *et al.* (1930) obtained microfilaria rates of 44 to 64% in adult populations of American Samoa. DICKSON (1943, quoted by BYRD & ST. AMANT, 1969) examined 2,171 persons above the age of four years from 31 villages on Tutuila, and found microfilaria rates ranging from 12.5% to 38.7%, with an overall positive rate of 19.1%. JACHOWSKI & OTTO (1955) examined 2,421 persons of all ages from ten villages, and obtained an overall microfilaria rate of 20.3%. KENNEDY (1959, quoted by IYENGAR, 1965) found 15.9% of 5,398 persons of all ages to be microfilaria positive.

As for the incidence of clinical filariasis, PHELPS *et al.* (1930) reported that at least 669 cases out of the total population of about 10,000 at that time had elephantiasis; of these, 394 were from the main island of Tutuila and 273 were from the islands of Manua group. Dickson in 1943, recorded elephantiasis in 5.8% among 978 adults, or 2.6% among 2,171 persons of all ages examined, and hydrocele in 6.3% of males of all ages.

MURRAY (1948) conducted epidemiological surveys of filariasis in American Samoa. Blood smears (volume unmeasured) were taken from 5,144 Samoans five years of age and older, of whom 982 (19.1%) showed microfilariae, and the average number of microfilariae per positive slide was 41.3. There was an increase in the amount of microfilariae in the population from the age-groups 5 to 9 up to 50 to 54, after which there was a steady drop to the upper age limit. There was little difference in incidence of microfilaremia until the age of puberty between males and females, but from that period on the rate in the two sexes diverged, males being far higher than females (Table 9-7). The incidence of elephantiasis increased steadily as the age increased, and males had a much higher rate of elephantiasis than females even when the scrotum was not considered. Samoans with elephantiasis had a considerably higher rate of microfilaremia and average microfilaria count than did Samoans without elephantiasis, when comparable age and sex-groups were considered.

Table 9-7. Sex and age incidence of microfilaremia of Samoans (after MURRAY, 1948).

Age-group (years)	Males				Females			
	No. exam.	No. pos.	% pos.	Average Mf. per pos.	No. exam.	No. pos.	% pos.	Average Mf. per pos.
5–9	336	16	4.4	16.8	351	21	6.1	21.5
10–14	534	27	5.1	24.5	434	34	7.8	19.0
15–19	441	39	8.8	43.1	410	54	13.2	20.4
20–24	309	70	22.7	34.1	243	44	18.1	24.0
25–29	241	71	29.5	24.5	243	24	11.1	27.8
30–34	232	96	41.4	44.5	186	39	21.0	23.2
35–39	185	88	47.6	52.0	143	32	22.4	49.2
40–44	122	52	42.6	68.0	84	21	25.0	55.5
45–49	121	60	49.6	63.5	100	31	31.0	41.4
50–54	72	39	54.2	90.1	70	22	31.4	38.3
55–59	47	21	46.8	57.5	38	9	23.7	55.4
60–64	48	18	37.5	67.2	41	11	26.8	18.5
65–69	28	15	53.6	44.8	15	4	26.7	12.8
70–74	10	5	50.0	29.6	9	2	22.2	8.0
75	13	9	69.2	24.0	11	3	27.2	16.6

Abbreviations: *No.*: number; *pos.*: positive; *exam.*: examined *Mf.*: microfilaria

9E.8.2 Vector

Aedes polynesiensis was shown to act as the vector of *W. bancrofti* in American Samoa by a number of workers. On Tutuila Island. JACHOWSKI

& OTTO (1952, 1953) found 3.6 to 4.6% of the naturally caught female mosquitoes to be infected, BYRD & ST. AMANT (1959) reported 13.2% to be infected and 2.6% to be carrying mature larvae out of 3,468 specimens examined, and IYENGAR (1959, quoted by IYENGAR, 1965) found 9.6% to be infected. On Swain's Island, JACHOWSKI (1955) recorded an infection rate of 2.9% in this species of mosquito. The bionomics of *Ae. polynesiensis* in American Samoa was studied in detail by JACHOWSKI (1954).

The mosquito fauna and the mode of transmission of filariasis in American Samoa are considered to be essentially the same as in the neighboring islands of Western Samoa. RAMALINGAM (1968) reported that the rates of naturally caught mosquitoes with all stages of larvae and with mature larvae were 5.2% and 1.3%, respectively, of 1,274 *Ae. polynesiensis*, 6.3% and 2.1% of 48 *Ae. upolensis*, 5.4% and 1.9% of 371 *Ae. samoanus*; however, none of 76 *Ae. oceanicus*, 18 *C. p. fatigans* or 3 *C. annulirostirs* were found infected, and also, 1 of 2 naturally caught *Ae. tutuilae*, all of 10 *Ae. samoanus*, and 1 *Ae. tutuilae* experimentally fed on a microfilaria carrier were found to be harboring mature larvae.

As for the site of transmission of filariasis, BYRD *et al.* (1945) and BYRD & ST. AMANT (1959) considered that the infection to man occurred mainly in the villages, because the natural infection rates of *Ae. polynesiensis* were much higher in those caught in the residential areas than in those collected outside of the villages. However, JACHOWSKI & OTTO (1952, 1953, 1955) considered, based on their calculated "index of transmission" (a combination of the vector density and the vector infection rate), that transmission of filarial infection occurred primarily outside of the villages, for example, in the bush, along the trails, and on the plantations. IYENGAR (1965) presented a critical review on the problem of relative importance of the environments in relation to the transmission of the nonperiodic *W. bancrofti* in the Pacific islands.

9E.8.3 Control

As in Western Samoa, it was noted before the start of a systematic filariasis control program in American Samoa that the incidence of clinical filariasis was gradually receding probably due to the improvements of sanitation, leading to the reduction of breeding places of *Ae. polynesiesnsis*. The incidence of elephantiasis was reported to be about 6.7% of the total population in 1930, 2.4% in 1942, and 1.0% in 1959 (IYENGAR, 1965).

The results of filariasis control projects in American Samoa were reviewed by CIFERRI *et al.* (1969) and KESSEL *et al.* (1970). As mentioned previously, surveys made in American Samoa soon after the war indicated that about 20% of the villagers in Tutuila above the age of five years showed microfilariae, and some 2.6% among them had elephantiasis. A filariasis pilot control program was initiated in 1962 by the Medical Services of American Samoa and the University of California School of Medicine, Los Angeles. During the first three years, four villages were surveyed by MURRAY in 1945, another village was surveyed by JACHOWSKI in 1948, and five new villages were surveyed under this program. In the first five villages, previous surveys showed that the overall microfilaria rate in examination of two thick blood films of 20 mm³ each was 20% (129 positives of 653 persons examined) and the median microfilaria density was 22; in the survey in 1963, the rate was 26% (247 of 966) and the density was 29. Preliminary treatment with a single total regimen of 72 mg per kg given in 12 doses of 6 mg per kg each was administered in several villages over a period of six months. At the end of three years, the microfilaria rate was 7.3% and the median density was 2. Since these results appeared to be inadequate for a successful control program, a periodic mass treatment project of two or more regimens of 72 mg per kg to be administered every two years was instituted on the island of Tutulia.

Surveys made two years after the second mass treatment in seven villages, in which 1,407 persons were examined, showed that three villages were totally negative for microfilariae, and the average microfilaria rate in all the villages was 0.4%. These villages were also negative in intensive mosquito surveys for infective stage larvae of *W. bancrofti*.

According to the REPORT OF WHO/SPC SEMINAR (1974), mass blood and clinical surveys were conducted from 1970 to 1972, involving 79.7% of the total population of American Samoa. An overall microfilaria rate of 0.9%, a mean microfilaria density in positive films of 10.7 per 20 mm³ of blood, an elephantiasis rate of 0.9%, a recurrent lymphangitis rate of 1.1%, and a hydrocele rate of 2.1% were obtained. All persons found to be positive were treated.

9E.9 Niue

Niue (also called Savage Island) is an island situated east of Tonga and about 560 km southeast of Samoa, at 19°S and 170°W. Its area is 260 km² and its population is 5,128 (1971). Niue is a New Zealand dependency. It is an upheaved coral island forming two limestone terraces about 30 m and 70 m above sea level, respectively. The soil is porous and there are no streams or marshes; the people collect rainwater from the roofs and store it in barrels and cisterns.

9E.9.1 Epidemiology

SIMPSON (1957) examined 748 adults during 1954 on Niue, and found 22.1% of them to be harboring microfilariae in their blood. Mass administration of DEC to the entire population at monthly doses was begun in January 1956. A second blood survey was conducted during November-December 1956, and 2.9% of 2,791 persons of ages six years and over were still positive. IYENGAR (1958, quoted by IYENGAR, 1959, 1964) examined

586 persons of all ages on Niue, and found that 2.6% had elephantiasis, 1.9% of males of all ages and 3.4% among adult males had hydrocele, and 7% of the population was subject to periodical attacks of filarial lymphangitis. He concluded that in comparison with the majority of the Polynesian islands, the general incidence of filariasis in Niue was low. Microfilaria counts made at two-hour intervals from a microfilaria carrier showed that the filaria was a nonperiodic *W. bancrofti*. According to the official report for the year 1957, 36 cases of elephantiasis of the legs were found among the total population of 4,600. McCarthy (1959b) stated, "In Niue, some 20% of the adult population of the village of Mutalau demonstrated microfilariae, but indigenous clinical filariasis was extremely uncommon."

9E.9.2 Vector

According to Iyengar (1965), *Ae. cooki* Belkin, 1962, is the only mosquito of the *Ae. scutellaris* group in Niue, and is probably the vector of nonperiodic filariasis on Niue. He examined 87 naturally caught specimens, but the results were all negative. *Aedes cooki*, like its allies, breeds in cisterns and barrels for storing rainwater, coconut shells, and tin cans. The breeding of this species is subject to great variation on Niue; high during the summer months when the temperature is high and rainfall is more frequent, but low during the cool and dry winter season.

9E.9.3 Control

According to the Report of WHO/SPC Seminar on Filariasis (1974), a mass drug administration program was launched in mid-1972 on Niue with the assistance of WHO Inter-Country Filariasis Advisory Team. DEC was given at a dosage of 6 mg per kg, once a week for 12 weeks, followed by once a month for 12 months. Pretreatment surveys revealed microfilaria rate of 16.3% and an average microfilaria count per carrier of 30.6 per 20 mm³ blood. Posttreatment surveys have just begun.

9E.10 The Cook Islands

The Cook Islands are a group of 15 islands in the South Pacific Ocean, west of French Polynesia, situated between 8°S and 23°S, and 156°W and 167°W. The total area is 238 km², with a population of 22,000 (1970). They have been under self-government in free association with New Zealand since 1965. The islands falls under two topographically distinct groups. The northern group comprises seven small, low islands of coral origin: Penrhyn, Rakahanga, Manihiki, Palmerston, Pukapuka, Nassau, and Suwarrow, of which first five are inhabited. The southern group consists of eight large, high islands of volcanic origin, six of which are inhabited, namely, Aitutaki, Atiu, Mangaia, Mauke, Mitiaro, and Rarotonga. Rarotonga, the largest islands, has an area of 67 km² and a population of 10,853 (1968).

9E.10.1 Epidemiology

A. The Southern Cook Islands

Filariasis has been noted to be prevalent in this region. McKenzie (1925), for example, reported an elephantiasis rate and an microfilaria rate of 2.0% and 40.1%, respectively, for 197 persons examined in Rarotonga, and 5.6% and 50.7%, respectively, for 71 persons examined in Aitutaki; the microfilariae showed no periodicity.

Lambert (1926, quoted by Iyengar, 1959) recorded 22 cases (2.4%) of elephantiasis out of a population of 900 on Atiu Island, 23 cases (4.1%) out of 560 on Mauke Island, and no case in 180 persons on Mitiaro Island. Blood examinations were conducted on five islands, and the microfilaria rates observed were 35.5% on Rarotonga, 26% in Mangaia, 46.2% on Mauke, 54.8% Mitiaro, and 49.1% on Aitutaki. In 218 persons examined both during daytime and at night, 98 (45%) were positive for microfilariae by day and 90 (41.2%) by night, indicating that the microfilariae did not exhibit nocturnal periodicity. He concluded that filariasis could not be treated with present knowledge, and that prophylaxis, or the suppression of the mosquito vectors (*Stegomyia pseudoscutellaris* = *Ae. polynesiensis*), probably out of the range of the Cook Islands Treasury.

Davis (1949) conducted epidemiological and entomological surveys in the southern Cook Islands. In Aitutaki, 102 (42.5%) of 240 persons (over nine years of age) examined were positive for microfilariae. In Rarotonga, 12% of hospital admissions were due to filariasis. The elephantiasis rate, as well as the microfilaria rate, recorded by Iyengar (1957) were 4.3% and 23.3%, respectively, of 554 persons of all ages examined on Rarotonga, and 3.7% and 20.9%, respectively, of 1,297 persons examined on Aitutaki. McCarthy (1959a) reported an elephantiasis rate of 2.9% in 358 persons and a microfilaria rate of 22.3% in 1,890 persons (all ages) examined on Rarotonga, and an elephantiasis rate of 4.2% in 528 persons and microfilaria rate of 29.2% in 609 persons (all ages) examined on Aitutaki.

B. The Northern Cook Islands

According to Iyengar (1965), the low coral islands comprising the northern Cook group can be further classified into two distinct types: the broad reef islands of Pukapuka where the incidence of filariasis is very high, and narrow ring-form atolls where the incidence is relatively low. In Pukapuka, McCarthy (1959a) found 29.4% of 218 persons to be carrying microfilariae, and the New Zealand Medical Research Report (quoted by Iyengar, 1965) recorded a microfilaria rate of 28.4% and elephantiasis rate of 3.8% among 498 persons examined. On the atoll islands, McCarthy (1959a) observed microfilaria carriers in 5.8% of 274 persons on Penroman, 8.4% of 226 persons on Rakahanga, 8.7% of 69 persons on Palmerston, and 19.7% of 371 on Manihiki, but he did not find any elephantiasis case on these islands.

9E.10.2 Vector

The sole vector of *W. bancrofti* in the entire Cook Islands has been reported to be *Ae. polynesiensis* (*Ae. cooki* occurs only on Niue and not on the Cook Islands). High infection rates have been recorded from Aitutaki and Rarotonga, 6.0% by McKenzie (1925), 9.1% by Satchel (1950), 13.4% by Iyengar (1957); McCarthy (1959a) observed an infection rate of 11.3% in Aitutaki and 2.8% in Rarotonga. According to Amos (1946), Davis (1949), and Iyengar (1957), the main breeding sites of *Ae. polynesiensis* are discarded tin cans, bottles, coconut shells in the bush adjoining habitations, and rat-damaged coconuts on plantations. On Rarotonga, the vector density is low during the dry and cool season from April to November, and higher during the hot and rainy season from December to March. Satchell (1950, quoted by Iyengar, 1959), on Rarotonga, recorded infection rate of 9.1% (115 of 1,258) in *Ae. polynesiensis* collected in houses, 6.9% (35 of 503) in those caught outside houses, and 1.6% (8 of 495) in those caught on plantations. The infection rate of mosquitoes in a village was 13.0% and the density was 16.6 per catch during December following a period of dry weather, but about ten days after heavy rainfall, the average number of mosquitoes per catch rose to 38.7, but the infection rate dropped to 1.6%.

Iyengar (1957), from studies in Rarotonga and Aitutaki, also found that the transmission of filariasis occurred primarily in and around houses, and mosquitoes caught only 100 yards from habitations were rarely infected. McCarthy (1959) obtained in Aitutaki an infection rate of 25.9% in *Ae. polynesiensis* collected in the vicinity of houses, but none of those caught 200 yards from houses were infected.

According to Iyengar (1965), the vector density is quite different between the reef islands of Pukapuka and the atoll islands, and this accounts for the remarkable difference in the incidence of filariasis between the two groups. In Pukapuka, the villages, as well as the plantations, are heavily infested with *Ae. polynesiensis*. The main breeding sites of its larvae are coconut shells opened for copra, coconuts opened for coconut water, and rat-damaged coconuts. The heavy rainfall (120 inches annually) keeps these breeding sites constantly filled with water. In the atoll islands, on the other hand, communal cisterns are installed and the people do not have to store rainwater in domestic receptacles. The village areas are clean and free from litter such as coconut shells.

According to Laird (1955), three mosquito species are found in Aitutaki, Southern Cook, namely, *Ae. polynesiensis*, *C. p. fatjgans*, and *C. annulirostris*. A mosquito-eating fish, *Gambusia*, was introduced into Rarotonga in 1935; it soon increased by millions, and greatly reduced the mosquito pest.

9E.10.3 Control

The REPORT OF WHO/SPC SEMINAR (1974) stated, "Mass drug administration started on the island of Aitutaki in 1968 reduced the microfilaria
rate from more than 30% to 0.8% in 1969 and 0.2% in 1971.

9E.11 The Society Islands

An island-group in the western part of French Polynesia, these islands
have a total area of 1,608 km² and a population of 81,424 (1967). They
comprise two groups: the Windward Islands (Tahiti, Moorea, and several
islets) and the Leeward Islands. Mostly volcanic in origin and mountainous, eight islands among them are inhabited. The Society Islands lie
between latitudes 16°S and 18°S and between longitudes. 148°W and
150°W. Because the climate is tropical-oceanic and rich in rainfall which
favors the breeding of the vector mosquitoes, filariasis has been noted to
be prevalent among the inhabitants. The parasite is the diurnally subperiodic race of *W. bancrofti*, and the main vector is *Ae. polynesiensis*. Basic
studies on the control of filariasis have been conducted here as pilot experiments by Prof. Kessel and his coworkers, and have contributed a great
deal to the establishment of the present knowledge about the use of DEC in
mass treatments.

9E.11.1 Epidemiology

High incidences of filariasis have been noted in the Society Islands since
early times, as reviewed by IYENGAR (1965); the prevalence of elephantiasis
was reported by LESSON in 1839, BENNETT in 1840, HERCOUET in 1880,
CLAVEL in 1884, GROS in 1892, and TRIBONDEAU in 1900. The last author,
for example, mentioned that in the districts of Afareaitu and Haapiti on
Moorea, about half of the population was affected with the disease.

DUBRUEL (1909 a,b) reported on his observations on elephantiasis and its
treatment while staying at the hospital of Papeete from 1906 to 1909. The
author recognized that elephantiasis was not uniformly distributed among
the people of the area but the islands of Sous-le-Vent (the Leeward Islands)
were more affected than the Society Islands; also, the island of Huahine
was very high in incidence, and 1 out of 8 inhabitants were affected, and
the situation was almost the same in Tahaa; Moorea had the incidence of
1 per 12, and was more contaminated than Tahiti. However, since he could
not find microfilaria in the blood of most elephantiasis cases, and found it
more frequently in healthy people, he concluded that filaria was probably
not the cause of elephantiasis as Manson attributed, but that elephantiasis
was due to the repeated attack of erysipelas caused by microbes.

GALLIAD *et al.* (1949), in Tahiti, reported on the results of a survey carried out from 1947 to 1948 in the district of Paea. The whole population,

except those of ages under five years were examined; of 916 persons, 280 (30.3%) showed microfilaremia, of whom 211 had no clinical signs; elephantiasis was seen in 83 (9%), of whom 25 were microfilaria positive and 58 were negative; lymphangitis was seen in 173 (18.8%), of whom 69 were microfilaria positive and 105 were negative; the total of cases with clinical manifestations was 182, of whom 72 had microfilariae in peripheral blood and 110 were negative. The authors incriminated *Ae. pseudoscutellaris* (now *Ae. polynesiensis*) as the principal vector, and found the natural infection in about 50% of the mosquitoes of this species dissected.

GALLIARD & MILLE (1949) made a trial treatment of microfilaria carriers in Tahiti with DEC (Hetrazan). The drug was given at the single dose of 2 mg per kg of body weight, three times a day, for seven consecutive days, to 96 microfilarial carriers. Clearance of microfilariae were seen in all cases after 2 to 7 days. Of 65 cases who were examined four months after the treatment, 14% showed a relapse but the microfilariae were never resistant, and of 12 cases treated with the second course of the drug administration, 3 were negative after two months and the remaining 9 showed only 1 to 5 microfilariae per 20 mm³ blood.

Extensive blood surveys have been conducted in the Society Islands in connection with the filariasis control program. BEYE *et al.* (1953) carried out blood examination in 15 rural villages in Tahiti from 1949 to 1950, and obtained an overall microfilaria rate of 32.3% for the total of 8,537 persons examined; the rates by the villages varied from 25.2% (119 positives of 472 persons examined in Afaahiti) to 43.6% (101 positives of 231 persons examined in Hitiaa). According to MARCH *et al.* (1960), the microfilaria rate observed in 1949 in examination of 3,390 persons in 15 rural districts in Tahiti was 37.9%. LAIGRET (1959, quoted by IYENGAR, 1965) reported microfilaria rates of 11.8% in examination of 13,608 persons in 1955 in Papeete (urban area) of Tahiti, 26.8% of 2,133 persons examined in Moorea in 1955, 24.7% of 230 persons in Bora Bora in 1954, 27.7% of 166 persons in Maiao in 1949, 20.5% of 657 persons in Raiatea in 1956, 25.0% of 304 persons in Huahie in 1956, 27.5% of 342 persons in Tahaa in 1956, and 26.6% of 514 persons in Maupiti in 1956.

In general, the microfilaria rate was found to be higher in rural areas than in the urban area of Papeete. As will be discussed separately, the rates have dropped considerably as the result of mass drug administration programs in the villages concerned.

LAGRAULET *et al.* (1974) reported on the prevalence of filariasis on Tahaa Island (Leeward Islands, French Polynesia). Microfilariae were found in the blood of 16.6% of the population, and elephantiasis in 1.3% of the total population or 11.1% of those aged above 50 years. Elephantiasis was very rarely associated with positive microfilaremia and most often localized to the inferior limb.

9E.11.2 Vector

Various authors have confirmed that *Ae. polynesiensis* is the main vector of *W. bancrofti* in the Society Islands. GALLIARD *et al.* (1949) reported that 50% of this species (identified as *Ae. pseudoscutellaris*) which they examined in Tahiti were infected. BEYE *et al.* (1952) found 6.7% of 445 specimens collected from Tahiti and 3.4% of 88 specimens from Maiao carried full-grown larvae of *W. bancrofti*. ROSEN (1955) found 233 (9.7%) of 2,390 specimens of this species caught in Tahiti and Maktea were infected, and 43 (1.80%) among them were carrying third stage larvae. The infection rates in other mosquito species were 11.9% (126 out of 1,061) in *C. quinquefasciatus*, 1.2% (1 of 81) in *C. atripes*, 0% (none of 446) of *C. annulipes*, 1.7% (1 of 58) in *C.* sp., 20.0% (16 of 80) in *Ae. aegypti*, and 0% (0 of 47) in *Ae. edgari*. However, none of these species had live mature larvae. In a more recent study conducted by LAIGRET (1959, quoted by IYENGAR, 1965), *Ae. polynesiensis* was found to be infected at a rate of 5.8% of 2,290 from Moorea, 11.2% of 732 from Raiatea, 12.7% of 150 from Tahaa, 16.5% of 103 from Bora Bora, 6.0% of 284 from Huahine, and 21.3% of 155 from Maupiti.

ROSEN (1955) conducted comprehensive studies on the transmission of *W. bancrofti* in the Society Islands. In experimental infections of *Ae. polynesiensis* fed on a carrier of nocturnally periodic *W. bancrofti* who acquired the infection in the West Indies, it was found that the development of this form was clearly different from that of the Tahitian, nonperiodic strain; the maturation of larvae required 16 days as compared with 13 days for the Tahitian strain under the same conditions, and about 80% of the third stage larvae of the periodic strain found in this mosquito were abnormal, i.e., only half the length of the third stage larvae of the Tahitian strain. On the other hand, *C. quinquefasciatus* in Tahiti was shown to be a poor vector of the nonperiodic *W. bancrofti*, and the percentages and the numbers of mature larvae found to have developed in this mosquito were much lower than those found in *Ae. polynesiensis* experimentally infected under similar laboratory conditions. A detailed study was conducted to see the survival rate, the percentages of infection, and the numbers of larvae found in *Ae. polynesiensis* fed on 23 microfilaria carriers showing various levels of microfilarial density from 0.4 to 555.1 per 20 mm^3 (see Section 10A). The prevalence of microfilaria positive cases by age and sex groups was determined, and higher microfilarial rates were found among male adults than among female adults. The variation over a 48-hour period in the density of microfilariae in the peripheral blood of ten individuals were observed (the results of statistical analysis of the microfilarial periodicity are as discussed in Section 11F). The density of microfilariae in the peripheral blood of 261 cases before and after a three-year interval was recorded.

9E.11.3 Control

The control of the vector mosquitoes by removal of their breeding sites, and the control of parasite by mass administration of DEC have been carried out in the Society Islands.

ACCORDING to IYENGAR (1965), the main breeding sites of *Ae. polynes-*

iensis are rainwater barrels, coconut shells, rat-damaged coconuts, tin cans, tree holes, and crab holes. During the past 50 years, nearly all of the inhabited areas on Tahiti and Moorea, and the majority of the villages on the Leeward Islands have been provided with a pipe-water supply system, and domestic containers for storing rainwater have been almost completely eliminated from these areas. However, as pointed out by ROSEN (1955) and IYENGAR (1965), rat-damaged coconuts are another important breeding site of the vector, and thus, extensive banding of coconut trees against rats has been carried out. In Tahiti, significant reductions in the elephantiasis rates were noticed before commencement of the drug administration programs as compared with that reported in early days.

Trial treatments of microfilaria carriers or clinical filariasis cases with DEC were conducted by BEYE *et al.* (1952), GALLIARD & MILLE (1953), and KESSEL *et al.* (1953). THOORIS *et al.* (1956) and KESSEL (1957) reported on successful results in the control of filariasis in certain villages in Tahiti by mass administration of the drug. The dosage schedule tested were: A–1: 2 mg per kg of body weight, three times a day for one week (42 mg per kg in total); A–2: same as above, plus a second similar dose at the beginning of the second year (84 mg per kg in total); and B: 6 mg per kg of body weight, once a month for 24 months (144 mg per kg in total). The most satisfactory result was obtained by the monthly administration method (B), and only 2 out of 94 previously positive cases were still positive for microfilariae at the end of 24 months, and their microfilaria counts were only 1 or 2. The infection of the vector mosquitoes also reduced remarkably.

The filariasis control program in Tahiti, from November 1967 to January 1968, was reviewed by KESSEL (1971). Three districts were selected for the review: Vairao, with a population of 825, where DEC treatment was withheld as the control area; and Mataiea and Tautira, with a combined population of 1,200 and among the 15 rural districts included in the mass treatment program that began in 1953. In the control area, 255 out of 825 persons examined in 1950 were positive for microfilariae with a rate of 30.9%, and the MfD–50 of the positive cases was about 30 per 60 mm³ blood samples. The rate and the density remained practically unchanged when examined again in 1953 and from 1954 to 1956. In Mataiea, where the mass drug administration with monthly doses was given, the microfilaria rate of 39% and the median density of 23 observed in 1949 before the treatment dropped to 4.9% and 4.5, respectively, at the survey conducted in 1958, or four years after mass treatment; and the rate and the density was 5.2% and 3.5, respectively, in 1966, or 11 years after the treatment. In Tautira, where the people received the similar 24-month treatment beginning in 1953, the microfilaria rate and the median density, respectively, were 27% and 18 in 1950 (before the treatment), 3.3% and 4.0 in 1958, and 4.0% and 3.5 in 1966. In other words, the single-course mass drug administration program was effective in reducing the rates of microfilaria carriers in the population, as well as the density of microfilariae in the positive cases, for periods of over ten years, but could not achieve the complete eradication of the parasite from the communities.

A recent report from the WORLD HEALTH ORGANIZATION (1974) stated, "In French Polynesia, mass drug administration with DEC commenced between 1950 and 1960 and has reduced the mf rate from 34% to 4% and the mf density from 78 to 11 per 20 mm³ blood in positive films. In 1963, only mf carriers were treated, resulting in an increase in prevalence to 7% and in density to 80 mf/20 mm³ of blood. Between 1966 and 1968, mass drug administration was carried out only in certain areas. From 1968 to 1972, quarterly mass drug administration and monthly distribution of the drug in schools was tried out but the incidence remained static. From 1973 up to present, quarterly mass drug administration has been undertaken. The mf rate is now 4.5% and the density is 20 per 20 mm³."

9E.12 The Tubuai Islands (Austral Islands)

The Tubuai are a group of small volcanic islands in southern French Polynesia, south of the Society Islands, forming a chain of islands about 1,400 km long, between latitudes 21°50′ and 27°41′S and longitudes 144° 22′ and 155°W. They have an area of 140 km² and a population of 5,053 (1967). The climate is a temperate-oceanic type, and the seasons are well marked, namely cool weather from May to September and warm weather from November to March.

9E.12.1 Epidemiology

According to IYENGAR (1965), nonperiodic *W. bancrofti* infection is known to be endemic in 4 of the 5 inhabited islands, namely, Rimatara, Rurutu, Tubuai, and Raivavea, while no information is available from Rapa, the southernmost island. However, elephantiasis has been reported to be very rare (GROS, 1892; VILLARET, 1938; KERREST, 1954; INSTITUT DE RECHERCHES MÉDICALES DE LA POLYNÉSIE FRANÇAISE, 1961, 1962; all quoted by IYENGAR).

BEYE *et al.* (1953) recorded a microfilaria rate of 19.1% in 235 persons examined in Tubuai. KERREST (1954) obtained microfilaria rates of 25.8% in 62 persons examined in Tubuai, 33.3% in 45 persons in Rurutu, and 30.1% in 289 persons in Raivavae.

An extensive survey of filariasis was conducted by Institut de Recherche Médicales de la Polynésie Française from 1961 to 1962. Microfilariae were found in 11.1% of 607 persons examined in Rimatara, 15.5% of 1,281 persons in Rurutu, 8.8% of 927 persons in Tubuai, and 22.8% of 901 persons in Raivavae (IYENGAR, 1965). In 1969, after control measures, the microfilaria rate was only 1.5% (HAWKING & DENHAM, 1971).

9E.12.2 Vector

According to IYENGAR (1965), *Ae. polynesiensis* is prevalent and is probably the vector of filariasis in the Austral Islands.

9E.13 The Tuamotu Archipelago

These are a group of about 80 small islands of French Polynesia, situated east of the Society Islands and south of Marquesas, between 14°S–23°S, and 134°W and 149°W. Their area is 857 km², and the population is 6,148 (1967). The island of Makatea has a large phosphate deposit, and its population is made up of imported laborers from the Society, Cook, and other Tuamotu Islands.

BEYE *et al.* (1953) examined 276 persons in Makatea and found 41.6% of them to be positive for microfilariae. ROSEN (1955) recorded a natural infection rate of 9.7% among 2,390 *Ae. polynesiensis* collected from Tahiti and Makatea taken together.

As for the other islands of Tuamotu, Dr. E. MASSAL and his associates of Institut de Recherches Médicales de la Polynésie Française conducted blood surveys of some 90% of the total population of 30 islands, and found microfilariae in 260 (5.8%) of 4,489 persons examined (quoted by IYENGAR, 1965). *Aedes polynesiensis* is the only mosquito of the *Ae. scutellaris* group in the Tuamotu Archipelago, and there is little doubt that this is the local vector (IYENGAR, 1965).

Elephantiasis and other filarial diseases have been reported to be very rare in the Tuamotu Archipelago, including Makatea and the Gambier Islands.

9E.14 The Marquesas Islands

A group of ten islands in French Polynesia, the Marquesas are situated north of the Tuamotu Archipelago between 8°S and 11°S and at about 140°W. They have an area of 1,240 km² and a population of 5,174 (1967). They are rocky and mountainous islands of volcanic origin.

9E.14.1 Epidemiology

The Marquesas have a tropical-oceanic climate with little seasonal variation and heavy rainfall, and thus filariasis has been noted to be prevalent. BUXTON (1928) noted that members of the St. George Expedition found elephantiasis cases on each of the three islands they visited, i.e., Hiva-oa,

Nukuhiva, and Fatuhiva. ROLLIN (1929, quoted by IYENGAR, 1965) stated that elephantiasis was seen in every valley, especially at Hapatoni on Tahuata Island. BENOIT (1932, 1937, quoted by VILLARET, 1938) reported that 50 to 60% of the populations of Hapatoni (Tahuata), Nahae (Hiva-oa) and Hakaui (Nukuhiva) suffered from elephantiasis, and 50 to 90% of the people from different areas were carrying microfilariae. VILLARET (1938) stated that elephantiasis was rife on all the islands of the Marquesas, especially in the islands of the southern group.

ROSEN (1954) reported that at least 5% of the total populations on each of the six inhabited islands had gross manifestations of elephantiasis, and several Europeans had also acquired elephantiasis; microfilariae were found in 33.7% of 59 persons examined on Fatuhiva Island. BAMBRIDGE (1956, quoted by KESSEL, 1957) recorded an elephantiasis rate of 3% and a microfilaria rate of 33.7% in the Marquesas.

According to LAGRAULET et al. (1972a), clinical filariasis of the advanced stages are very common in the Marquesas Islands. Elephantiasis was found in 1.5% of the population and in 8.2% of those aged between 40 and 69 years. The lower limbs were most commonly affected (89%), and inguinal adenopathy was found in 30%. Of the cases of elephantiasis, recurrent lymphangitis occurred in 80% and 16.6% showed microfilaremia.

LAGRAULET et al. (1972b) conducted epidemiological survey of filariasis in the Marquesas Islands; of 2,706 inhabitants examined, microfilariae were found in 18.4%, elephantiasis in 2.8%, and lymphangitis attacks in 3.6%.

A more detailed report on the epidemiology of filariasis in the Marquesas was published by LAUGRET et al. (1972c). The islands have a population of 5,600, and the microfilarial rates were from 6 to 34% according to the villages. In addition many people without microfilariae showed clinical signs; elephantiasis occurred in 5% of persons aged more than 20 years, adenolymphoceles in 3% and hydrocele in 9% of adult men. One man had 1,203 microfilariae in 20 mm^3 blood. Comparison was made with the numbers of microfilariae in 20mm^3 blood samples taken from five body sites of 22 carriers (ear, deltoid region, index finger, iliac crest and calf); the largest numbers were found in blood from the finger and the average figures from the other sites were 64 to 81% of those from the finger.

LAGRAULET et al. (1973) further discussed on the epidemiology of filariasis in the Marquesas. In certain of these islands no control work had ever been done and thus provided a useful area for the study of natural conditions. Studies on filariasis had been carried out on a modest scale from 1960, since travel facilities became improved by introduction of light aircraft. In 1962, 17% of 4,227 inhabitants were found to be infected. Treatment with DEC was carried out in 1966 and 1969, and 97% of those involved became negative for microfilariae. The percentage of mosquitoes infected varied greatly from one area to another, and there was good correlation between the mosquito infection rates and the human microfilarial rates.

9E.14.2 Vector

Aedes polynesiensis is reported to be abundant in the Marquesas (MUMFORD & ADAMSON, 1933; STONE & ROSEN, 1953; ROSEN, 1954).

9E.14.3 Control

According to IYENGAR (1965), there were appreciable improvements in recent years in the condition of inhabited areas in the Marquesas. The population is largely concentrated in two main settlements, Taiohae on Nukuhiva and Atuona on Hiva-oa, which are provided with a pipe-water supply system, schools, and hospitals. Reductions in the local vector density and a regression of filarial disease has been noted.

9E.15 Pitcairn

A volcanic island situated at 25°04′S and 130°05′W, Pitcairn is about 4 km long and 3 km wide, with a population of 91 (1971). It is a British colony.

Neither clinical filariasis nor microfilaria cases have been noted from Pitcairn. BEYE *et al.* (1953) examined 54 persons, but found no microfilaria carriers. *Aedes polynesiensis* was present, but the density was low.

Part **3** | **Methodology in Filariasis Study**

10

Methods for survey and control of filariasis

10A. The dynamics of transmission of filariasis

10A.1 The transmission cycle

The life cycle of parasites causing human filariasis consists of two parts: the reproductive stage in the definitive host, and the growth stage in the intermediate host. One of the most important aspects of the epidemiology of filariasis is to study the dynamics of transmission of the parasites through the above two stages under particular environmental conditions. However, this is not an easy task, because a great number of factors which influence the transmission of the parasite are involved. It should be noted further that filariasis in an endemic area can be controlled, or the transmission of the parasite can be interrupted, if certain sanitary measures are applied effectively at one or more points in the life cycle of the parasites or their carriers.

The various factors involved in the force of transmission of filariasis have been studied by a number of researchers in the past. Table 10-1 shows some of the important parameters involved in the dynamics of transmission of filariasis, which should be investigated through field and laboratory observations for evaluating the intensity of infection in various phases of the life cycle. As shown in this table, the dynamics of transmission of filariasis may be evaluated by parameters related to at least five phases of the transmission cycle, i.e., parameters relating to (1) the human population as the source of infection of the vector population, (2) the infection of the vectors, (3) the development of filarial larvae in the vectors, (4) the efficiency of vectors in infecting human populations, and (5) the efficiency of development and reproduction of the parasite after being transferred from the vector to the human population. Since many of these parameters can be measured or estimated by epidemiological, parasitological, and entomological surveys discussed in the

565

previous sections, mathematical models can be constructed for at least certain phases of the transmission.

Table 10-1. Parameters for analysis of the dynamics of transmission of filariasis (revised from Paragraph 3.3, the Third Report, WHO Expert Committee on Filariasis, 1974).

(1) Parameters relating to the status of infection of human populations
    (1–a) the clinical manifestation rate (see Section 10B.1)
    (1–b) the microfilarial rate (see Section 10B.2.2 and 11B)
    (1–c) the microfilarial density (see Section 11C)
    (1–d) the skin test positive rate, etc. (see Section 10B.3)
(2) Parameters relating to the infection of the vector population
    (2–a) the infectivity potential of the human population (see Section 11E)
    (2–b) the rate of ingestion of microfilariae by the vector (whether microfilariae are ingested randomly by the vector at a rate corresponding to the density in the blood, or whether they are concentrated or diluted while feeding; see Section 10C.2)
    (2–c) the circadian rhythm of the microfilariae and the vector (see Section 10C.3 and 11F)
    (2–d) the biting density of the vector per man per year (see Section 10C)
    (2–e) the proportion of human blood among the blood meals taken by the vector (human blood index; see Section 10A.2.2.5)
(3) Parameters relating to the development of filarial larvae in the vector
    (3–a) the rate of development of ingested filaria larvae to maturity in the vector (see Section 10C.1)
    (3–b) the time required for completion of larval development under the local condition (see Section 10A.3, and 10C.1.4)
    (3–c) the gonotrophic cycle of the vector under local condition (see Section 10A.2.3C)
    (3–d) the survival rate of vector (per day, per gonotrophic cycle, or per maturation time; see Section 10C.2.4)
    (3–e) the proportion of vector with all stage larvae (the infection rate) and with mature larvae (the infective rate) (see Section 10C.2.1 and 10C.2.2)
    (3–f) the frequency distribution of the number of mature larvae found in the infective vectors (see Section 10C.2.1)
(4) Parameters relating to infection of man
    (4–a) the number of infective bites per man per year (see Section)
    (4–b) the rate of transfer of infective larvae to man while the vector is taking a blood meal (see Section 10A.3, DE MEILLON *et al.*, 1967e)
(5) Parameters relating to the development and reproduction of filaria in human host
    (5–a) the proportion of filaria larvae to reach adults of the reproductive stage (see Section 10A.2.5)
    (5–b) the efficiency of adult filariae in producing microfilaremia in man (see Section 10A.2.5)

10A.2 Parameters in the dynamics of transmission

10A.2.1 Parameters relating to the status of infection in human populations

The status of filarial infection in human populations may be evaluated by various measures, such as the proportion of persons showing various clinical manifestations, the proportion and density of microfilaremia cases, and the proportion and titer of certain immunological reactions. These signs of filarial infection are usually correlated with each other, i.e., when the microfilarial rate of a population is high, the clinical manifestation rate or skin test positive rate of the same population is also high, as a rule. However, these signs are reflections of different aspects or phases of filarial infections, and therefore the distribution of each of these signs among human populations is usually quite independent, so that there exist many people who show only one or two of these signs, but are negative for other evidence of infection.

The clinical manifestation rate of a population is measured by methods discussed in Section 10B.1. Each filarial species causes certain specific or nonspecific clinical signs in persons infected with the parasite. Because the ultimate purpose of a filariasis control program is the reduction and extermination of suffering from clinical affections by the prevention of new infection and by the treatment of already established infection, the survey of clinical filariasis cases is an important task. However, since most filariasis signs are difficult to be strictly differentiated from those of nonfilarial origins except for those in the advanced stages, the results of clinical surveys are subject to great variation according to the methods and criteria employed by individual surveyors. It should also be pointed out that the persons who show clinical manifestations are not always the source of infection to other persons, nor are they always susceptible to the drug treatment.

In the practical aspects of a filariasis control program, a more important and effective target is the number of people showing microfilariae in the blood or in the skin. They are not only the main source of infection of the vectors, but also represent the population susceptible to treatment with DEC. Two parameters are involved in the force of transmission: the proportion of persons showing microfilariae in a survey, and the density of the number of microfilariae per unit volume or weight of blood or skin. The details of quantitative aspects of these parameters are discussed in Sections 11B and 11C.

Unfortunately, most immunological diagnostic methods for filariasis are still of little practical usefulness because of the ambiguity in specificity and/or sensitivity (see Section 12C.2).

The occurrence of various filarial signs in the human population can be evaluated from two aspects, the prevalence rate and the incidence rate. If

100 persons in a village are surveyed, and 45 persons are found to be positive for a filarial sign (such as microfilaremia or skin test reaction), the prevalence rate is 45%. On the other hand, if 15 among the positive cases were negative at the examination made one year ago, the incidence rate per year is regarded roughly to be 15%. The analysis of human populations both by the prevalence and by the incidence provides much more valuable information in the epidemiology than the simple observation of the prevalence rates.

10A.2.2 Parameters relating to the infection of the vector population

10A.2.2.1   The proportions, as well as the intensities of infection of filaria vectors are determined by various factors, as shown in Table 10-2. The infectivity potential of a human population is determined mainly by the microfilarial rate and the microfilarial density, and a method has been developed for estimating the theoretical infection rate of the vector population when the average amount of blood ingested at one meal is known (see Section 11-E). In this case, it is postulated that microfilariae are contained in the blood meal of a vector in the same density as found in the circulating blood of a host. A correction factor is necessary if the vector concentrates or dilutes the microfilariae while taking the blood meal. In the case of mosquitoes, it is known that the contents of blood in the midgut of a vector is concentrated because they discharge fluid (serum) while taking a blood meal, and thus, the observed number of microfilariae in the midgut is usually larger than expected from the amount of blood, as estimated by the difference in body weight before and after the engorgement.

10A.2.2.2   Various authors have reported on the results of infection of mosquito or other filaria vectors when taking blood (or skin fluid) containing various density levels of the microfilariae (see Section 10A.3).

10A.2.2.3   The relationship between the circadian rhythm, called the microfilarial periodicity (the daily change in the density of microfilariae in the blood or body fluid of host), and that of the biting activity of the vectors is another important factor determining the possibility of infection of vector populations. In general, both are more or less synchronized. The nocturnally periodic races of *Wuchereria bancrofti* and *Brugia malayi* are usually transmitted by nocturnally biting mosquitoes, such as *Culex pipiens fatigans, Anoheles* spp., and *Mansonia uniformis*. The diurnally subperiodic race of *W. bancrofti* in the South Pacific islands is transmitted by the day-biting mosquito of the *Aedes polynesiensis* group, and also by the night-biting species of the *Aedes kochi* group. Such a coincidence is probably not accidental, but is a result of the evolution and adaptation of the filarial races for better survival and reproduction. However, there also exist examples of inefficient relationships, such as the occurrence of the nocturnally periodic race of *B. malayi* transmitted by *Ae. togoi*, which is primarily a day-biting mosquito (see Sections 10C.3.1; 11F).

The relationship between the biting rhythm of *C. p. fatigans* and the microfilarial periodicity (the circadian rhythm of the microfilaria density in the circulating blood) of nocturnally periodic *W. bancrofti* was discussed by SASA *et al.* (1964, 1965a) in southern Japan and Bangkok, and by DE MEILLON & SEBASTIAN (1967b) in Rangoon (see Section 10A.3).

10A.2.2.4   The biting density of a bloodsucking insect species in an area per man per year is an important parameter determining its vectorial capacity. A rare species cannot be an important vector even when it is physiologically highly adapted for the transmission, as *Ae. togoi* is in most endemic areas of *W. bancrofti* in Japan. A number of observations have been made on the biting density per year or during a season of various vector species in endemic filariasis areas (see Section 10C.2.3).

10A.2.2.5   The man-biting habit is another important factor for determining the vectorial capacity of an insect vector. As discussed by MACDONALD (1957), this habit has been extensively studied for various anopheline mosquitoes in relation to the transmission of malaria. Because most human filariae are also transmitted exclusively from man to man by a bloodsucking insect, its efficiency as the vector is highly dependent upon its man-biting index. If a species will feed on man at a rate of 90%, the probability of taking human blood twice (at the time of ingesting microfilariae and at the time of inoculating mature larvae) becomes 81%, while in another species which only 5% takes human blood, the efficiency as a filaria vector in this relation is found to be 0.25%. In other words, the former species is 320 times more efficient as a human filaria vector than the latter, even when the physiological capacity as the intermediate host is the same. In other words, at least a 320-times greater population density is necessary for the latter species in order to maintain the same level of transmission as the former species.

10A.2.3 Parameters relating to the development of filarial larvae in the vector

10A.2.3.1 The rate of development of filaria larvae in the vector

There are, again, a number of factors involved in this phase of the transmission. First of all, there exist various grades of compatibility between the parasite and the intermediate host, as discussed in detail by YAMADA (1927, see Section 2E.2). The microfilariae ingested by a bloodsucking insect may develop to mature and infective larvae at high rates, or the development may be delayed or hampered at certain stages, or the insect host may be completely refractory for the development of the filarial larvae.

The rate and the speed of development to the mature stage may also be affected by the density of infection per insect host; the rate of maturity is usually high when the number of larvae per intermediate host is small, while the rate of maturity gradually drops, and also the survival rate of the host at the time when the larvae reach mature stage becomes lower as the density of filarial larvae per insect increases. Such relationships have been investigated extensively for various filarial and vector species (see Section 10A.3).

10A.2.3.2 The time required for the larval development in vector

The time required for the development of filaria larvae to reach the mature stage differs greatly according to the environmental conditions (especially by the atmospheric temperature), by the species of filaria, and by the intermediate host.

In general, the speed of development of the larvae in an intermediate host is retarded as the temperature drops, and becomes faster as the temperature rises. However, such a relationship is effective only for a certain temperature range, such as between 15°C and 30°C. A comprehensive study on the effects of temperature on the development of *W. bancrofti* larvae in *C. p. pallens* was made by OMORI (1958c; see Section 2E.3).

The climatic factors other than the temperature, such as humidity, precipitation, wind, illumination, and day length, are also important since they affect the activity and the survival rate of the vectors. The intensity of transmission of filariasis is thus subject to great seasonal variations in most endemic areas. In the Temperate Zones, the temperature is usually the main limiting factor of transmission, while in the tropical zones, the transmission is greatly hampered during the dry season by reduction in the vector populations and also by the increase in the mortality rate of the vectors.

10A.2.3.3 The gonotrophic cycle

A gonotrophic cycle of a blood-sucking insect consists usually of the three phases: (1) the search for a host and taking of a blood meal; (2) the blood digestion and development of the ovaries; and (3) a search for a suitable oviposition site, the oviposition, and the search for another host. As reviewed by DETINOVA (1962), the duration of the gonotrophic cycle of anopheline mosquitoes in the tropics may be as short as 48 hours, but the time may differ among different vector species, or may be delayed according to the climatic and other environmental conditions, especially when the temperature is low. A filaria vector passes usually two or more gonotrophic cycles during the time required for the full development of the filaria larvae. The daily survival rate of a vector population can be estimated by the gonotrophic cycle and the physiological age composition, as discussed in the next section.

10A.2.3.4. The survival rate of vector

The survival rate of vectors in relation to the days required for completion of development of filarial larvae to the infective stage is a crucial factor for determining the efficiency of transmission. If the period required for a filarial larva to complete development is n days and the daily survival rate of the vector is p, the probability of an infected vector surviving through n days is p^n, the expectation of life is $1/(-\log e^p)$, and the expectation of life after survival through n days is $p^n/(-\log e^p)$, as discussed in detail by MACDONALD (1957) in connection with the epidemiology of malaria. When the daily survival rate of a vector species in an endemic area is 0.95, and the minimum period of the filaria larvae for the full development in the vector is 12 days, the probability of a vector that had fed on a carrier surviving through 12 days is $(0.95)^{12} = 0.54$. If another vector species had a daily survival rate of 0.8, the probability is $(0.8)^{12} = 0.069$. This means that the former species is about eight times more efficient as a vector of filariasis than the latter, provided that the compatibility with the filarial parasite is the same. In other words, the latter species requires an eight-times higher population density than the former in order to maintain the same level of transmission.

Various methods have been proposed for estimating the life span of arthropod vectors of human diseases. In mosquitoes and other blood-sucking insects of the order Diptera, methods were developed mainly by Russian workers for determination of the physiological age (either nulliparous or parous, and if parous the number of times of oviposition), as described by DETINOVA (1962) and in Section 10C.2.4 of this book. In general, a mosquito population with a higher parous rate is considered to be longer in average life span than one with a lower parous rate if the environmental condition is the same. These techniques may also be applied in evaluating the effects of vector control measures, since the parous rate of the vector population must drop if the mortality of adult females increases by some imagocidal measures, such as the use of residual insecticide sprays, while the rate increases when some larval control measures are effectively practiced and the supply of new adult population is decreased.

If the average period in days (d) required for a gonotrophic cycle (the number of days from the time of taking a blood meal to oviposition and the next blood meal) is known, the daily survival rate (p) of a mosquito population can be roughly estimated from the parous rate (q) by the equation: $p = {}^d\sqrt{q}$. For example, if the parous rate of a mosquito species in an area is 33% and the gonotrophic cycle is 5 days, the daily survival rate is estimated as 0.8, because $(0.8)^5 = 0.33$.

10A.2.3.5 & 6 The proportion and density of infection in vectors

The proportions of vectors with all stages of larvae (the so-called infection rate of vector) and those with mature larvae (the so-called infective rate of vector) are two important indices reflecting the intensity of transmission of filariasis in an endemic area. The methods for determination of these indices are shown in Section 10C.2. The indices often vary greatly by the season of year according to the changes in the survival rate. As is the observation of filarial infections in human populations, the density of infection of filarial larvae in the vector populations is another important factor. The frequency distribution of the numbers of infective larvae found in infected mosquitoes has also been shown to be roughly logarithmically normal, as shown in Section 10C.2.1.

10A.2.4 Parameters relating to infection of man

The quantity of filarial infection in man is dependent on various factors, including the proportion and density of vectors with infective filarial larvae, the number of infective bites per man per year, and the rate of transfer of infective larvae to man while the vector is taking a blood meal.

The proportion and density (by frequency distribution of the number of infective larvae per vector) can be estimated for each endemic area by the methods described in Sections 10C.1 and 10C.2. It should be noted that both the infection and the population density of vectors may differ greatly in the Temperate Zones by climate, or in tropical areas where the dry and rainy seasons are well defined.

When the average number of vectors biting per man per year is (a), the average proportion of infective individuals among the vector population per year is ($b\%$), the average number of infective larvae per infective vector is (c), and the average proportion of infective larvae inoculated into man at one bite is ($d\%$), then the average number of infective larvae transferred from the vector population to the human population is expressed by a simple formula: $a \times b \times c \times d \times e$, where e is the human blood index (the proportion of the vector taking a human blood meal when biting a host, see Section 10A.2.2.5).

10A.2.5 Parameters relating to the development and reproduction of filarial parasites in human hosts

The main factors involved in this phase of the transmission cycle are the percentages of filaria larvae which become mature and reproductive adult worms, the longevity of the reproductive life of the adult worms, the efficiency of production of microfilariae by the adult worms under various host and parasite conditions, and the proportion and longevity of microfilariae in the circulating blood (or in the skin) of the host. Most of these factors are difficult to estimate in human filarial infections, and thus various indirect approaches to the problem have been made by previous workers.

In human infection with *W. bancrofti*, or other filariae, it is difficult to estimate the proportion of infective larvae which develop to mature adults after inoculation by mosquito bites. However, these proportions can be estimated in animal experiments, when known numbers of infective larvae are inoculated and the adult worms are recovered by autopsy of the hosts after certain periods; such studies were reported by EDESON & WHARTON

(1957) and LAING *et al.* (1961) with *B. malayi* infection in cats, by ASH &
RILEY (1970a, b) with *B. malayi* and *B. pahangi* infection in jirds, and by
DUKE (1960a, b) in experimental *Loa loa* infection in drills.

The efficiency of adult filariae in producing microfilaremia in man is
another factor difficult to estimate directly, because there are no means of
estimating the number of adult worms present in human hosts. However,
such an estimate can be made directly in animal experiments, such as with
B. malayi infection in cats or *L. loa* infection in monkeys. The course of
microfilaremia after infection with known numbers of infective larvae
have been observed in a number of cases in these animal experiments, and
it has generally been accepted that the level of the peak density of microfilaremia is correlated with the number of parasites inoculated, or the
number of adult females present in the hosts. However, because such a
relation is highly variable, we have no means of estimating the number of
adult worms in a host from the level of microfilaremia (HAYASHI & TANAKA,
1965; WILSON & RAMACHANDRAN, 1971). It has also been observed in
human and animal infections with various filariae that the microfilarial
density changes according to the time course of infection, even within the
same hosts; the microfilariae become detectable after a certain incubation
period, then increase gradually until the density reaches a peak after several months to several years, and then decreases in density rather rapidly,
probably due to the development of immunity in the host. Therefore, it
has frequently been observed in patients in the chronic stage of filarial
infection that conspicuous filarial disease signs are present, or adult worms
are recovered, in hosts whose blood is negative for the microfilariae.

10A.3 Some theoretical and field studies relevant to the dynamics of transmission

A comprehensive discussion and review referring to the various factors
involved in the dynamics of transmission of *W. bancrofti* and *B. malayi*
was made by BEYE & GURIAN (1960). As crucial factors in the life cycle,
the following problems were discussed:

"HAWKING (1954) estimated that an adult *Litomosoides carinii* produces
12,000 to 22,000 (average 15,000) microfilariae per 24 hours. RAGHAVAN
et al. (1956) indicated that an adult *Conispiculum guindiensis* gives birth to
some 19,517 (range 1,350 to 87,660) microfilariae per 48 hours. RAO (1933)
concluded the life span of microfilariae of *W. bancrofti* to be as long as 70
days, and KNOTT (1935), in transfusion experiments, observed their persistence no longer than 14 days. BEYE *et al.* (1952) and KESSEL (1953) reported that carriers in Tahiti had microfilarial densities of 79 to 128 per 20
mm^3 blood, or some 2×10^7 in whole blood. Using Knott's microfilaria
survival time, such a carrier would harbor 150 adult female worms; if

Rao's time were used, such a carrier would harbor 30 female worms.

The probability of a carrier host being bitten by a suitable vector, and the rate of ingestion of microfilariae are other crucial factors. WHARTON (1957), for example, reports that 2.5 mm³ blood is ingested by a biting *M. longipalpis*. The infection rate of mosquitoes when fed on carriers harboring a low microfilaria density of 0.4 to 0.5 per 20 mm³ blood was 5.3% in *Ae. polynesiensis* according to ROSEN (1955), 11.6% in *M. longipalpis* according to WHARTON (1957), and 2.6% in *C. p. fatigans* according to JORDAN (1959). Increased vector mortality after feeding on human carriers with heavy microfilaria densities was recognized by BAHR (1912), BRUYNING (1953), and BYRD & ST. AMANT (1959)."

Various results have been reported on the relationship between the number of microfilariae ingested by insect vectors and the microfilarial density in the blood of donors. KERSHAW *et al.* (1953) reviewed the literature and stated that, "though previous reports in the literature on filariasis have stressed the wide variation in intake by individual mosquitoes, most prominence has been given to the fact that occasional mosquitoes take in surprisingly large numbers of microfilariae." In their own observation on *Dirofilaria immitis* in *Ae. aegypti*, however, they found that most *Ae. aegypti* ingested fewer microfilariae than might have been expected, and that the ingestion of large numbers of microfilariae was exceptional.

WHARTON (1957) studied the intake of microfilariae of *B. malayi* by *M. longipalpis* (now *M. bonneae/dives*), and found that the mosquito ingested an average of 3.1 mg (2.4, 2.9, and 3.4 mg in three series of experiments) of blood, but the average numbers of microfilariae actually ingested by the mosquito were about 1.5 times greater than the numbers expected from the volume of the blood meal. The author assumed that this might be due to the effect of concentration of the blood meal after ingestion by the mosquito through the discharge of fluid from the midgut. Similar observations on *Ae. aegypti* and *Ae. albopictus* showed that both species usually ingested about the same number of microfilariae as would be expected.

GUBLER *et al.* (1973) compared the microfilarial density of periodic *W. bancrofti* in venous blood, finger prick blood and blood ingested by *C. p. fatigans*. Blood samples were taken by venipuncture and finger prick over a 24-hour period, and fully engorged female mosquitoes were collected from each of two carriers for 15 minutes before and after each blood sample was taken during the night. There was no difference between the microfilarial density in venous and finger prick blood during the study period, suggesting that there was no obstruction nor blockage of the microfilariae by the capillary bed. Mosquitoes feeding on the carrier with a high microfilaremia ingested, on the average, fewer microfilariae than expected, whereas those feeding on the carrier with a lower density ingested, on the average, about the expected numbers of the microfilariae.

The relationship between the microfilarial density of human donors' blood and the number and percentage of mature larvae found in the mosquito vector was investigated in detail by ROSEN (1955), in the Society Islands, with the nonperiodic *W. bancrofti* and its vector, *Ae. polynesiensis*. The mosquitoes were fed on 23 donors harboring the microfilariae at varying densities from 0.4 per 20 mm³ blood to 555.1 per 20 mm³ blood, and were dissected after the larvae had developed to the third stage. At the lower densities of microfilariae, the ratio between the mean number of microfilariae in the 20 mm³ blood and the mean number of third stage larvae per mosquito was approximately 5 to 1, i.e., the mosquito took microfilariae found in about 4 mm³ of the donor's blood. As the microfilarial density of the blood increased, this ratio also increased, so that in the experiment with the highest blood densities of over 500 per 20 mm³, the ratio was more than 25 to 1, probably due to the crowding effect. The relationship between the microfilarial density of the donor's blood and the average number of filaria larvae found per mosquito is shown in Fig. 10-1. Also, the survival rate of *Ae. polynesiensis* after taking the infective meal was not affected by the infection with the worm for at least 7 days, but after 9.5 days, high mortality of the mosquitoes was observed in the groups which had ingested large numbers of microfilariae.

The efficiency of *M. longipalpis* (=*bonneae/dives*) as an experimental vector of *B. malayi* was investigated in detail by WHARTON (1957, 1962) in East Pahang, Malaya. The relation between the microfilarial density in man and the percentages and numbers of filarial larvae found in the mosquito were studied in 22 cases with the density ranging from 0.025 per mm³ to 25.0 per mm³. The number of larvae in *M. longipalpis* dissected 10.5 to 11.0 days after feeding on a *B. malayi* carrier was directly proportional to the number of microfilariae in the peripheral blood at the time of feeding, and the mean number of larvae per mosquito was approximately five times the number of microfilariae per mm³ in the carrier's blood (Fig. 10-1). The percentage of mosquitoes which became infected was also found to be related to the microfilarial density; whereas 12% became infected after feeding on a carrier with only 0.025 microfilariae per mm³, 100% became infected after feeding on carriers with 2.0 or more microfilariae per mm³. It follows that there can be a noninfective microfilarial level in the blood (other than zero), but that when microfilariae are few, then few mosquitoes will become infected. When the mosquitoes were fed on two carriers with very high densities, the larval development was retarded, and only 12 or 10% of the larvae had reached maturity. As for the survival rate of the infected mosquitoes, there was no difference between those fed on carriers with 2.3 microfilariae per mm³ or less and those fed on uninfected persons; the mosquitoes fed on carriers with 10.7 microfilariae per mm³ or more survived normally during the first week, but died rapidly from the eighth day onwards when the filarial larvae were reaching maturity. An index of experimental infection was defined, representing an estimate of the number of mature larvae produced in each mosquito which had fed on a carrier 11 days previously. The index rose as the density of microfilariae in the donor increased, reached a peak in the 3 to 11 micro-

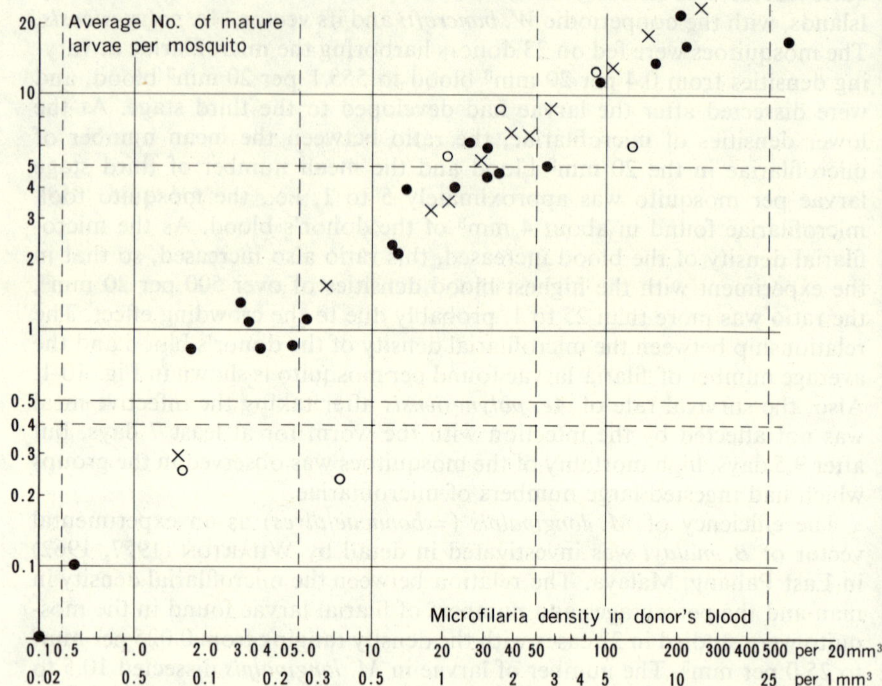

Fig. 10-1. The relationship between the density of microfilariae in the donors' blood and the average number of mature filarial larvae found in mosquito vectors.

● *W. bancrofti* (the Pacific race) in *Ae. polynesiensis* (after ROSEN, 1955).

○ *W. bancrofti* (nocturnally periodic race) in *C. p. pallens* (after OMORI, 1962).

× *B. malayi* (subperiodic race) in *M. annulata* (after WHARTON, (1962).

filariae per mm³ range, and fell away when the density was higher because of the crowding and lethal effects of very large numbers of larvae.

A comprehensive study was conducted by Omori and his associates on the relationship between the infection and the infective rates of mosquitoes and the rates of maturity and the indices of infective larvae per mosquito under experimental conditions by feeding *C. p. pallens* on human carriers harboring *W. bancrofti* microfilariae at densities ranging from 0.092 per mm³ to 6.125 per mm³. These and other results of experimental infection studies conducted in Japan were reviewed by OMORI (1962). The results obtained in experiments conducted from 1953 to 1955 were as follows (Table 10-2).

The development of filaria larvae in mosquito intermediate hosts is

Table 10-2. The relationship between the microfilarial density of the donors' blood and the status of infection of *Culex pipiens pallens* dissected 12 or more days after the experimental infection (after OMORI, 1962).

Mf. density per mm³	No. of mosquitoes dissected	Infection rate of mosquito	Mature rate of filaria larvae	No. of mature larvae per mosquito
0.092	118	19.5%	93.3%	0.24
0.375	33	15.2	100.0	0.21
1.090	99	91.9	94.4	5.28
1.165	104	96.2	90.1	8.74
4.600	49	89.2	64.3	11.41
6.125	24	87.5	70.9	5.58

greatly affected by various environmental factors, especially by temperature and humidity. The speed of development of filaria larvae after ingestion by mosquitoes is highly dependent upon the temperature of the environment. Humidity, on the other hand, probably has little effect on the speed of development, but is an important environmental factor determining the longevity of the mosquito hosts.

OMORI (1957, 1958a, b, c, d) carried out a series of experimental studies on the role of *C. p. pallens* as the intermediate host of *W. bancrofti*. In experiments in which the mosquitoes were kept at constant temperatures after ingesting the microfilariae, it was shown: (a) that almost no development beyond the first stage occurred at 16°C or lower; (b) that the period required for the *W. bancrofti* larvae to reach the mature stage became shorter as the temperature was set higher, such as 48 days at 18°C, 26 days at 20°C, 21 days at 22°C, 16 days at 24°C, 14 days at 25°C, 11 days at 27°C, and 10 days at 30°C; and (c) that a rise in temperature above 30°C was harmful to the development of filaria larvae as it caused both degeneration of the developing parasites and high mortality of the host mosquitoes. The results are summarized in Table 10-3.

OMORI (1958b) conducted a series of studies on the effects of temperature on the longevity of filaria larvae and of host mosquitoes. Batches of some 40 to 80 *C. p. pallens* were reared at 25°C or 27°C until the ingested *W. bancrofti* larvae reached maturity, and were then exposed to various degrees of constant temperatures. The mosquitoes were dissected as soon as they were found dead in each cage. Under the low temperatures (at 10°C and blow, including the mosquitoes kept in room temperature of the winter in Nagasaki), the mosquitoes generally survived five months or longer, but the filaria larvae in the mosquitoes died between 30 to 60 days after being exposed to the cold temperature. The results suggested, therefore, that although the host mosquitoes may survive through the winter, they are unable to carry over the filaria larvae until next summer. At higher temperatures, such as 16°C and above, the filaria larvae were shown to

Table 10-3. The periods (in days) required for the development of *W. bancrofti* larvae after ingestion by *C. p. pallens* under constant temperatures (after OMORI, 1958c).

Temperature (°C)	Developmental period (days)		
	First stage	Second stage	Total
16	40	x	x
18	28	20	48
19	17	10	27
20	16	10	26
22	15	6	21
24	12	4	16
25	9	5	14
27	6	5	11
30	6	4	10
33	7	3	10

survive so long as the host mosquitoes remained alive. However, the longevity of mosquitoes became shorter as the temperature was set to higher levels. A comprehensive review was made by OMORI (1966) referring to the results of experimental studies on the effects of temperature on the development and survival of *W. bancrofti* larvae in mosquito hosts.

The relationship between the biting rhythm of vector insects and the microfilarial periodicity (the circadian rhythm of microfilarial density in the peripheral blood of the host) is a crucial factor for determining the efficiency of microfilariae being ingested by the intermediate hosts. Although the microfilarial periodicity has been studied in a number of endemic areas of various races and species of human filariae by many workers (see Section 11F), its relation to the biting rhythm of the local vector insects has been investigated quantitatively in only a few instances. For example, SASA *et al.* (1964, 1965a) observed that the biting density of *C. p. pallens* and *C. p. fatigans* was a nocturnally periodic form with a peak at about midnight, and was quite similar to the periodicity of the density of *W. bancrofti* microfilariae in the circulating blood of man, as shown, in Fig. 10-2. Similar results were obtained by De MEILLON & SEBASTIAN (1967b) in their observations of *C. p. fatigans* and *W. bancrofti* microfilariae in Rangoon. Likewise, DUKE (1958, 1964) have shown that the microfilariae of *L. loa* in man are diurnally periodic and are transmitted by the day-biting *Chrysops* species, while those in monkeys are nocturnally periodic and their vectors are crepuscular-biting *Chrysops* species.

ZIELKE (1973) conducted experimental studies on the quantitative aspects of transmission of *Dirofilaria immitis* by mosquitoes. The intake of microfilariae by mosquitoes was directly proportional to the number of microfilariae in the blood of host and the amount of blood taken by the insect. However, this infectious potential was considerably reduced by the

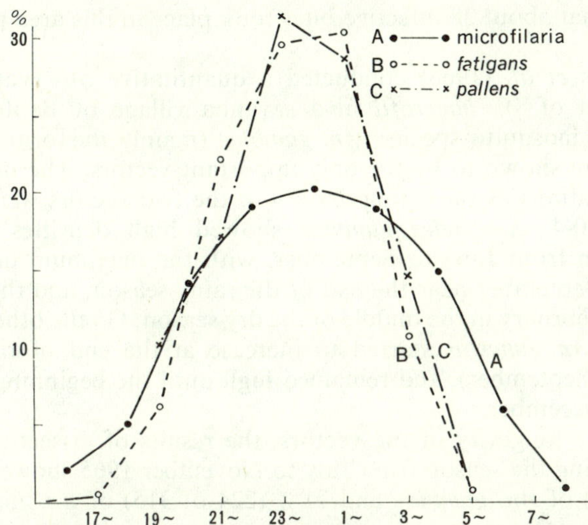

Fig. 10-2. Showing nocturnal periodicities of A: microfilarial densities in the blood of human carriers, B: biting rhythm of *Culex pipiens fatigans* in Koniya,C: biting rhythm of *Culex pipiens pallens* in Omiya, in percentage distributions (SASA *et al.*, 1964).

increased mortality rates of the infected mosquitoes; 80% of *Anopheles atroparvus* and 20% of *Aedes togoi* females being infected with three filarial larvae each, on an average, died before the filariae reached the infective stage. With only 20 to 30% of the infective larvae leaving the mosquito during the blood meal, and only 10% of them being capable of penetrating the skin, not more than 3% of all infective larvae eventually reached the final host. Infective larvae were not found to escape when the mosquitoes were feeding on sugar or 0.9% sodium chloride solutions.

There have been several studies conducted for estimating the intensity of transmission of filariasis in particular endemic areas. WHARTON (1962), for example, conducted a year-round observation on the intensity of *B. malayi* transmission by *Mansonioides* species in a village in Malaya. Regular trapping of mosquitoes were made in stable traps baited with goats. The goat was chosen as bait because comparative trapping experiments had indicated that goat and man were about equal in attraction to *M. dives/ bonneae* mosquitoes. The number of infective bites per month (or per year) was calculated from the number of mosquitoes caught per night and the mature larva rate. In this endemic area, the transmission was shown to take place throughout the year, with apparently two peaks, one in December and another in May. The average number of mosquito bites per day per host was 20.7, and with an average mature larva rate of 0.80, it was estimated that about 38 infective bites took place in this area per year per person.

BRENGUES *et al.* (1968) conducted a quantitative observation on the transmission of *W. bancrofti* in a savanna village of Banfora, Upper Volta. Two mosquito species, *An. gambiae* (mainly the form A) and *An. funestus* were shown to be the only important vectors. The monthly and annual variations of the biting density of the two vectors were as shown in Table 10-4. *Anopheles gambiae* showed high densities during the rainy season from June to September, with the maximum density from August to September near the end of the rainy season, and the minimum density in February in the middle of the dry season. On the other hand, the density of *An. funestus* started to increase at the end of rainy season (August to September), and remained high until the beginning of the dry season in December.

As for the longevity of the vectors, the results of dissections of mosquitoes during the season from July to November 1965 showed that 82% (290 of 354) of *An. gambiae* and 71% (224 of 315) of *An. funestus* were

Table 10-4. The biting density and the filaria infective rate of *An. gambiae* and *An. funestus* according to months; at Tingrela, Upper Volta (after BRENGUES *et al.* 1968).

(A): mean number of biting mosquitoes per man per night;

(B) percentage of mosquitoes containing infective larvae calculated from dissections of all mosquitoes collected directly on human bait, those of daytime collections in houses, and those collected from outdoor shelters; (C): Number of infective bites per man per month, calculated from the human bait collections only.

Year & month	No. of night catches	*An. gambiae*			*An. funestus*		
		(A)	(B)	(C)	(A)	(B)	(C)
1964 8	2	40.5	0.3	0	5.5	0.3	0
9	16	57.1	0.6	14	12.2	1.0	6.6
10	4	8.9	0.9	0	6.5	0.3	0
11	3	3.0	0.5	5	36.5	0.2	0
12	6	2.1	0	0	22.6	0	0
1965 1	1	4.5	0	0	18.5	0	0
2	4	1.3	0	0	12.9	0	0
3	11	3.7	0	0	4.2	0	0
4	8	1.4	0	0	0.6	0	0
5	9	3.2	0	0	0.7	0	0
6	2	18.5	0	0	0.7	0	0
7	9	14.3	0.3	1.7	6.6	0.2	1.7
8	8	31.2	0.6	5.6	8.5	0.3	1.9
9	9	15.3	0.8	5.0	8.5	0.4	3.3
10	8	4.2	0.4	3.8	10.8	0.3	3.8
11	4	2.9	0	0	13.4	0.2	3.8

parous. From the gonotrophic cycle of two days generally observed for these species, the daily survival rate was estimated to be 0.95 for *An. gambiae* and 0.92 for *An. funestus*.

The biting rhythm was observed with two collecters, one indoors and another outdoors. In *An. gambiae*, the peak was between 2 a.m. and 4 a.m, and 80% of the biting mosquitoes were collected after midnight. The biting rhythms observed indoors and outdoors were not significantly different. In *An. funestus*, more than 80% of the biting also occurred after midnight. The biting rhythm, however, showed a significant difference, being highest near the end of the night between 3 a.m. and 5 a.m. inside of houses, but showing two peaks outside of houses, one near the end of the night and another at about midnight.

In comparison of the indoor and outdoor collections on human bait, 57.3% (1970 of 3474) of *An. gambiae* and 66.6% (1266 of 1901) of *An funestus* were from inside of houses. It was also shown in examination of blood contained in the midgut of engorged mosquitoes by precipitin test conducted at Lister Institute, London, that 93% (125 of 135) of *An. gambiae* and 100% (36 of 36) of *An funestus* captured indoors, as well as 82% (79 of 96) of *An. gambiae* and 80% (80 of 100) of *An. funestus* captured outdoors had ingested human blood.

The mosquitoes collected on human bait, as well as those captured from other sources, were dissected for examination of infection with filaria larvae. The percentages of infective mosquitoes from all sources were as shown on column B of Table 10-4, and the numbers of infective bites per man per month were as in column C. It was estimated from these results that an average of 20.7 infective bites by *An. gambiae* and 8.3 infective bites by *An. funestus* took place in this village during the one year period from August 1964 to July 1965.

HAIRSTON & JACHOWSKI (1968) made analytical studies on the *W. bancrofti* population in the people of American Samoa. Based on the records of microfilarial counts repeated on many people over four and half years, these authors set up certain hypotheses and calculated the duration of patency for single infections (two and half years), the maximum density of microfilariae achieved by one female (70 per 60 mm³ of peripheral blood), the average output of larvae by a female during her lifetime (1.32×10^7), the death rate of mated females (0.02 to 0.05 per month), the average load of reproducing female worms per blood positive person (6.91 for men, 6.07 for women, 2.93 for children), and the average total load of worms in infected people (11.18 for men, 7.70 for women, 4.02 for children).

These figures were mainly derived from analysis of long-term fluctuations in microfilarial counts in persons re-examined at intervals over a period of four and half years. The counts tended to increase over a period of about 24 months to their peak and then to decrease more rapidly, the whole pattern requiring two to four years. When the peak counts of individual cases were adjusted to the values corresponding to the blood volume of adult males, these were found to fall mostly into multiples of 70 (this conclusion was supported by Chi-square test). For this reason, these authors assumed that a female worm produced microfilariae to a maximum level corresponding to 70 per 60 mm³ of peripheral blood of adult males, and estimated the worm load of reproducing female worms per positive person. They also considered that overlapping infections were relatively rare and that there must be long intervals between the few infective bites.

HAIRSTON & DE MEILLON (1968) discussed the inefficiency of transmission of *W. bancrofti* from *C. p. fatigans* to the human host based on observations in Rangoon. They considered that the efficiency of transmission was best regarded as the fraction: number of people becoming positive per year ÷ total number of bites by infective mosquito per year. It was observed by DE MEILLON, GRAB & SEBASTIAN (1967) in Rangoon that an average of 18 bites per man per hour was taking place for the first half of the night, and that this accounted for approximately 47% of the whole night; by applying this to the whole year, a person was estimated to receive 82,873 bites by *C. p. fatigans* per year. The overall proportion of *C. p. fatigans* carrying the third stage larvae of *W. bancrofti* was 0.0036, thus a person in Rangoon (Kemmendine experimental area) was estimated to receive 298 infective bites per year. (In a poor sanitation area in Calcutta, ROZEBOOM *et al.*, 1968, estimated with the same method that there were, on average, 50 bites by infective *C. p. fatigans* per year). On the other hand, the annual rate of the people in this area becoming microfilaria positive was calculated as 0.0094 using the reversible catalytic model, or 0.012 using the two-stage catalytic model (from data of the age distribution of microfilaria rate, by the method shown in Section 11B). It was further observed by DE MEILLON, HAYASHI & SEBASTIAN (1967) that *C. p. fatigans* containing infective larvae would lose 41.4% of them at one feeding. It was finally estimated from these figures that the efficiency of the parasite from third stage larvae in the mosquito to the production of microfilariae was as low as 6.04 to 6.71 × 10⁻⁵, indicating that an average of around 15,500 bites by infective mosquitoes was necessary to produce one case of microfilaremia.

WILSON & RAMACHANDRAN (1971), in East Malaysia, also conducted long-term observations on microfilaremia and made estimates of the efficiency of transmission from mosquito vector to definitive host in *Brugia* infections in man and animals. Annual blood surveys were conducted on the people in Kampong Ubai, Pahang, from 1953 to 1960. The rise to a peak count often took three to four years, while the subsequent decline to a low level or to zero might take five to six years. On the basis of infective bites per person per year related to microfilaria rates in the local population, subperiodic *B. malayi* in East Pahang was at least 200 times more efficient in producing microfilaremia in man than was periodic *W. bancrofti* in Rangoon, reported by HAIRSTON & DE MEILLON (1968).

The results of mosquito catches and dissections in the same area by WHARTON (1962) indicated that the infective bites per person per year were

57.9 in 1954, 28.3 in 1955, 16.6 in 1956, and 21.8 in 1957, with an average for the four-year period of 31.2 (dieldrin house spraying was begun in 1954 twice every year). Two-thirds of these infective bites were from *M. dives/bonneae* and one-third from *M. annulata*. The average number of mature larvae per infective mosquito was about 5.0 in Pahang and 4.5 in Rangoon; the estimated number of infective bites of 298 in Rangoon was nearly ten times higher than in Pahang, but the microfilarial rates in Pahang (*B. malayi*) and in Rangoon (*W. bancrofti*) were, respectively, 31% and 0.3% for the age group of 0–4 years, and 54% and 2.2% for the age group of years 5–9. WILSON & RAMACHNANDRAN (1971) also pointed out from results of experimental infections of large numbers of cats with *Brugia* spp., that there was no consistent relationship between the worm load and the peak microfilaria count, and thus suggested that the method of estimating the adult worm loads from the peak counts reported by HAIRSTON & JACHOWSKI (1968) could not be relied upon.

As for the parameters relating to the transmission of onchocerciasis, a series of laboratory and field studies were carried out by Duke and associates (1962–73: Studies on factors influencing the transmission of onchocerciasis, Parts 1–8). For example, DUKE (1962d, Part 1) compared the survival rates of the four groups of *S. damnosum* fed on four groups of volunteers harboring the microfilariae of *O. volvulus* at densities of nil, three, nine and 20 per fly, and observed that there was no significant difference except for those taking 20 microfilariae per fly showed a slightly lower survival rate. DUKE (1962e, Part 2) compared the intake of *O. volvulus* microfilariae by *S. damnosum* and the survival rate of the larvae when the flies were fed on volunteers harboring the microfilariae at various densities. DUKE & LEWIS (1964, Part 3) observed the effect of the peritrophic membrane on limiting the development of *O. volvulus* microfilariae in *S. damnosum*. DUKE (1968f) studies the biting cycle, infective biting density and transmission potential of 'forest' *S. damnosum* at the Cameroon forest village of Bolo. The daily biting cycle of the fly was one-peaked, with the peak in the afternoon at about 4 p.m. in the nulliparous flies and that in the morning at about 10 a.m. in the parous flies. On the other hand, the annual biting densities showed two-peaked curves, one in about June and another in October. The biting density of infective flies also showed similar seasonal changes.

MILLS (1969) conducted a study for quantitative approach to the epidemiology of onchocerciasis. The variables relating to the transmission of onchocerciasis were gathered from the literature, and were arranged into the three parameters, i.e. those relating to man as the source of infection, those relating to the *Simulium* vector, and those relating to the parasite. By using these parameters, it was estimated that the number of infective larvae received per man per day in West Africa was 0.72 in the forest zone, 20.2 in the guinea savanna zone, and 58 in the sudan savanna zone. Thus the time taken for an individual to acquire 400 infective larvae, giving a probability of infection of 0.96, was estimated to be 1 year three months in the forest zone, 20 days in the guinea savanna zone, and 7 days in the sudan savanna zone. Similar statistical treatments were made on the force of transmission of onchocerciasis in Guatemala by using data reported by DALMAT (1955) and DE LEON & DUKE (1966).

GARMS (1973) carried out a quantitative study on the intensity of transmission of *O. volvulus* by *S. damnosum* in the Bong Range, Liberia. The biting densities of *S. damnosum* throughout the year were observed regularly at seven catching stations, and the flies caught on the human baits were dissected to determine the parous rate and the infections of *O. volvulus* larvae and other parasites. In all the stations, there were distinct seasonal patterns, and the biting densities were highest in the rainy season and lowest in the dry season of February and Mrach, and were closely related with the water levels of the river. The flies were found biting from dawn to dusk, ar.d the daily feeding cycle showed two peaks, one in the morning and another in the afternoon, the latter being the more pronounced. From a total of 67,758 flies dissected, 7,077 were parous, with an average parous rate of 10.9%. Of the parous flies examined for the filarial infections, 1,215 (17.2%) were carrying filaria larvae, and 186 (2.6%) had infective larvae of *O. volvulus*, while 211 (3.0%) had infective larvae of other filariae. The arithmetic mean of *O. volvulus* infective larvae per infective flies was 5.8. There were two seasonal peaks of the intensity of transmission, one between May and July at the beginning of the rains and the other between November and January at the end of the rainy season. Although the biting density was highest at the peak of the rains in August and September, the transmission was almost absent in this season because parous flies were almost absent. The number of *S. damnosum* bites per man per year, the number of infective *O. volvulus* larvae per man per year were estimated to be 150,000, 550 and 3,500 at station B, 54,000, 120 and 640 at station A, and 12,000, 20 and 50 at station F. These figures corresponded to a microfilaria rate of 63% in the human population of this area.

10B. Epidemiological survey methods of human populations

The diagnosis of filariasis is made by various methods, such as clinical, parasitological, and immunological measures. In general, each method has both advantages and disadvantages with regard to sensitivity and specificity. For example, the parasitological method for the demonstration of microfilariae is highly specific, but is usually poor in sensitivity (i.e., there are many people among the infected populations who are negative for microfilariae in a test). Some immunological tests may be more sensitive, but there usually exist a number of people who are infected yet turn out to be immunologically negative, or the test may show positive reactions in uninfected persons. Each of the clinical, immunological, and parasitological tests have merits and demerits according to the purposes, and the selection of diagnostic methods in a filariasis survey program is an important decision for the efficiency of the project.

10B.1 Clinical survey methods

As stated previously, different filarial species cause various clinical signs specific to each type of filariasis (Section 1.3.1). For example, the adult worms of *W. bancrofti* and *B. malayi* are parasites of the lymphatic systems and cause fever attacks and lymphangitis in the acute stage, and elephantiasis of the legs or hands in the chronic stage. However, the involvement of the genital or urinary systems is a sign peculiar to *W. bancrofti*, and if hydrocele, funiculitis, or chyluria is found it can be almost surely stated that it is not malayan filariasis (Section 2B.5.1. and 2C.5.1). *Onchocerca volvulus* causes peculiar changes or swellings of the skin, and also certain eye lesions, by which experienced physicians can easily make diagnosis (Section 5.4.1). *Loa loa* infection may be diagnosed by the appearance of the adult worm in the eye, or by the inflammation of the skin called "fugitive swelling" or "Calabar swelling" (Section 3.4.1). *Mansonia ozzardi*, *D. perstans*, and *D. streptocerca* are considered to be usually nonpathogenic, or may cause some nonspecific allergic symptoms, and are difficult to diagnose by clinical signs.

The clinical symptoms of filariasis stated above may be characteristic to each type of filariasis, but it should always be taken into consideration that similar or the same signs can be caused by other diseases. For example, hydrocele of chronic, traumatic origin is commonly encountered among "samrau" (tricycle) drivers in the tropical countries. Swellings of inguinal lymph nodes are common symptoms accompanied by *W. bancrofti* and *B. malayi* infections, but these alone cannot be utilized as criteria for diagnosis of filariasis. In some areas in Africa, especially in Ethiopia and Sudan, the common occurrence of nonfilarial elephantiasis has been reported by a number of workers.

In organizing a filariasis control program, the search for the presence of clinical filariasis cases is the most important task for locating and delimiting the endemic areas. This initial survey can be made by visiting individual villages and questioning village chiefs or local health workers, or by distributing questionnaires to all practicing physicians, asking whether they have seen patients suspected of filariasis. The systematic collection of information by the latter method was adopted in all the prefectures concerned before initiating the filariasis control program in Japan, as stated previously (Section 8C.5).

The survey of clinical filariasis cases among the people in an endemic area is a useful measure in the practice of filariasis control project, especially in evaluating the importance of the program. However, it is always difficult to set up criteria for clinical diagnosis of filariasis, because there exist a number of people showing more or less ambiguous signs. The results may differ greatly according to the personal experiences of the physicians, and by the methods employed for the diagnosis. Since the standard of diagnosis is difficult to determine, the results of clinical surveys are usually only an auxiliary measure for comparison of the intensity of infection among different endemic areas, or for evaluation of filariasis control activities.

10B.2 Parasitological survey methods

The diagnosis of a filarial infection can be made definitely by demonstration of adult worms or microfilariae in a host. Because the adult worms can be recovered only on special occasions, the search for microfilariae is the only practical measure in the diagnoses of individual patients or in epidemiological surveys. As previously stated, it should be noted that the detection of microfilariae is highly specific, but rather poor in view of the sensitivity as a diagnostic measure of infection (especially in *W. bancrofti*), so far as the routine thick smear method is concern. Various devices have been proposed for increasing the rate of detection by concentration or purification of microfilariae from larger volumes of blood samples.

Because microfilariae of different species of filaria show various physiological behaviors with respect to the site of appearance and the circadian rhythm of the biting activity, different diagnostic methods fitted to each parasite species must be applied. As shown in Table 1-4, the microfilariae of *W. bancrofti*, *B. malayi*, *L. loa*, *M. ozzardi*, and *D. perstans* appear in the circulating blood, while those of *D. streptocerca* and *O. volvulus* reside in the skin. In the nocturnally periodic or the nocturnally subperiodic forms of *W. bancrofti* and *B. malayi*, the blood examination should be conducted at night, preferably around midnight when the microfilarial density is highest, while in the human strain of *L. loa*, the examination should be made at around noon because its microfilariae are diurnally periodic. In the Pacific race of *W. bancrofti*, and in *M. ozzardi* and *D. perstans*, blood examination may be made at any time of day, because their microfilariae are nearly nonperiodic.

The skin-dwelling microfilariae of *O. volvulus* and *D. streptocerca* are known to be nearly nonperiodic and thus can be examined at any time of day. However, it has been shown in Africa that the microfilariae of *O. volvulus* are found more frequently or at higher densities in the skin of legs below the knee than on the trunk, while in those of *D. streptocerca* this relationship is reversed (KERSHAW *et al.*, 1954 a; DUKE, 1954,1956,1962; see Section 5.4.3).

10B.2.1 Survey of skin microfilariae

The microfilariae of *O. volvulus* and *D. streptocerca* are recovered by skin scarification or from skin snips. The details of the methods and discussions are presented in Section 5.4.3 (Onchocerciasis). Various scarification procedures have been used both for laboratory diagnoses and epidemiological surveys (WANSON, 1950; HUGHES & DALY, 1951; NELSON, 1955; ONORI, 1963; BASSET & LACAN, 1967). After the skin surface is scarified with a razor blade, impression smears are made on slide glass and examined directly or after being stained with Giemsa or hematoxylin.

Most workers prefer the skin snip method to the scarification. A needle or mounted entomological pin is used to raise a small cone of skin, which is then cut off with a sharp razor blade to a diameter of about 3 mm. A corneo-scleral punch was introduced recently for taking skin snips for diagnosis of onchocerciasis, and is now widely used, as reviewed by Buck (1974, WHO Publication). The skin snip is placed in a drop of physiological saline or water. In the standard method recommended by the WHO EXPERT COMMITTEE (1966), the skin snips are allowed to stand 10 to 15 minutes before being examined under low-power magnification of a microscope. Some workers recommend teasing the skin snips in saline in order to facilitate the release of microfilariae. TADA *et al.* (1973), in a quantitative study of the microfilariae of *O. volvulus* recovered by various methods, stated that skin snips should not be teased into small pieces because such procedures often kill the microfilariae and reduce the number to be recovered, and that intact skin snips should be incubated for longer periods, such as four to six hours, in order to recover maximum numbers of microfilariae.

10B.2.2 Survey of blood microfilariae

Various methods have been proposed for the demonstration of microfilariae from the blood. These may be classified into the three categories: (a) direct examination of fresh blood, (b) examination of blood smears after staining, and (c) microfilariae concentration methods.

10B.2.2.1 Examination of fresh specimens

The microfilariae in blood can be detected directly, by taking a drop of blood (diluted with a few drops of water) on a slide and examining under low-power magnification of a microscope. The microfilariae in fresh specimens are easily recognized as they move actively in the blood. However, because such specimens are not preservable, and because it is difficult to identify species with the fresh, unstained blood, this method is used only for special purposes, such as the rapid diagnosis of outpatients.

Counting chamber method:

DENHAM *et al.* (1971) constructed a simple glass chamber for counting microfilariae in fresh specimens, and compared the results with the thick smear method. The chamber consists of a well, approximately 1 mm deep, 25 mm in length, and 15 mm wide (for a 20 mm³ blood sample), constructed by fixing cut strips of slide glass on another slide glass with a mounting medium. To facilitate counting, the base of the chamber contains parallel lines (etched or diamond cut) spaced at 3 mm intervals. Approximately 100 mm³ of water is placed in the well, and the fresh blood collected with a 20 mm³ pipette is discharged into the water. Microfilariae are counted under a dissecting microscope (about 35 x magnification) without using a cover glass. The authors found that in the case of the microfilariae of *B. pahangi* in cats' blood, the mean microfilaria count obtained by the chamber count method always exceeded that obtained by thick smear methods, and that between 30 and 40% of the microfilariae were lost in the latter method during the processes of dehemoglobinization and staining.

CRANS (1972) described a counting chamber method for epidemiological surveys of filariasis. He used a disposable blood diluting pipette, Unipipette, and a Sedgewick-Rafter counting cell. In surveys carried out in Africa, he found that the Unipipette technique revealed a microfilaria rate of 31.9% with 50 mm³ blood samples and 32.7% with 100 mm³ blood samples, while examination of 25 mm³ stained blood films gave a 26.2% microfilaria rate. SOUTHGATE (1973), in Fiji, found that 29.5% more persons were positive by the counting chamber method than by the stained blood film method.

10B.2.2.2 Examination of blood smears

The examination of blood smeared on microscopic slides is the most basic and common procedure for detection of microfilariae in diagnosis or survey of filariasis due to *W. bancrofti, B. malayi, L. loa, M. ozzardi,* and *D. perstans*. The microfilariae can be detected in unstained blood smears under low-power magnification of a compound microscope, and such a method may be useful in the quantitative study of the microfilarial density, or in diagnosis in countries where staining reagents are difficult to obtain. However, the blood smears are examined usually after hemolysis in water (or other media) and stained with dyes, because the microfilariae are more easily detected and identified when properly stained.

In many countries, the conventional methods, such as taking a drop of blood from a finger prick on a slide, are still practiced in filaria surveys. However, it is recommended to collect measured blood samples for the routine microfilaria survey, such as one 20 mm³, three 10 mm³, or three 20 mm³ samples from each person. For trained technicians, the collection of measured blood samples with a pipette is a simple and easy task, and the results obtained with the measured blood sample surveys are much more valuable than those collected with the conventional unmeasured methods.

Various types of micropipettes have been used for collecting measured blood samples. The most commonly available type is the 20 mm³ Melangeur micropipette for hematological examination. In Japan, a type called "Filaria Pipette", which is calibrated in three 10 mm³ levels, (Ikemoto

Rikakikai Co., Bunkyoku, Tokyo) has been used. The same pipette can be used repeatedly for taking blood from a number of persons, if the pipette is washed every time with 0.1 % benzalconium chloride solution in water, which acts as both detergent and disinfectant (SASA, 1963, 1967). There are also various types of disposable capillary micropipettes used in hematological examinations.

In making a blood smear on a slide, it is recommended to collect at least three samples of 10 mm³ or 20 mm³ each from the same individual rather than taking only one sample per person. When multiple samples are collected, the efficiency of the detection of microfilariae can be estimated by statistical analysis of the microfilaria positive grades (SASA, 1967; Section 11D.4). The blood films are sometimes lost or damaged while rinsing or staining in water and making more than one smear is a safeguard against such problems.

Various methods have been used by different workers for preparing blood smears on a slide. The blood may be smeared on a round area to the size of a coin on a slide, as in making a thick blood smear for the examination of malaria parasites, but this method is not recommended for filariasis study because it is difficult to examine the whole field without duplication. The blood smears may be spread into a square shape. A method of making linear smears of 10 mm³ or 20 mm³ each on a slide to strips of about 3 mm in width and 70 mm in length, such as described by SASA (1963, 1967), is most convenient because the entire field of the blood smears can be more efficiently and easily examined under low-power magnifications of a microscope.

The examination of thick blood smears after hemolysis and staining is the usual method in the blood survey of most filariasis control program because of its simplicity and reliability. However, as pointed out by DENHAM et al. (1971) in their study in animal filariae, it is suspected that considerable numbers of microfilariae may be lost from the thick smears while rinsing in water or staining when the technique is inadequate. DESOWITZ (1974) obtained higher microfilaria rates with his membrane filter concentration method in surveys of filariasis in the South Pacific than expected from the results of examination of thick blood smears. Since the examination of microfilariae in thick blood smears has been the routine method in most filariasis surveys, it is necessary to re-evaluate its efficiency and to develop reliable techniques with which the loss of microfilariae from the smears can be minimized.

Blood smears on microscopic slides may be stained individually, by placing them on a pair of metal or glass bars fixed on a staining dish. However, in the staining of large numbers of slides with the same dye, it is more convenient and timesaving to use a slide box deviced for the mass staining of slides. These boxes are provided with grooves to fix individual slides by distances of a few millimeters from each other, and the dye, such as diluted Giemsa's solution, is filled in the box while staining.

A more convenient and timesaving method for carrying and staining large numbers of slides was described by SASA (1963, 1970). In this method, microscopic slides (76 mm long and 26 mm wide) are placed on a desk, and after all the blood samples smeared on them have dried in the air, a pair of cut rubber rings (about 20 mm long and 1 mm in thickness) are placed near both ends of every other slide. After the rubber pieces are placed on half of all the slides, the remaining half of the slides are placed on them with the smeared surface downwards, so that the blood smears of each pair face each other at a distance of about 1 mm separated by the rubber pieces. Usually 15 pairs of such slides are collected and fixed with plastic tape, into a bundle of 30 slides. These slide bundles are immersed in tap water for a few minutes for hemolysis, and then transferred into a staining box containing diluted Giemsa or Azeo-stain. A commercially available plastic butter case, 17 cm long, 10.7 cm wide, and 4 cm deep takes 4 of such slide bundles. After staining for about one hour, the slide bundles are dipped in water in order to remove the dyes, and are then dried in the air. This method does not require any special slide boxes for transportation, and saves a lot of labor in hemolysis, staining, and washing as compared with the conventional method of handling individual slides.

10B.2.2.3 Microfilaria concentration methods

There have been various devices made for the detection of microfilariae from larger blood samples (1 ml or more) than to be examined directly with the thick smears (maximum of about 60 mm³ per slide). In these methods erythrocytes are hemolysed first by chemical or physical means, and then the microfilariae are concentrated either by sedimentation or filtration. A number of studies were conducted by previous workers on the efficiency of the detection of microfilariae in comparison to that by the thick blood smears. A review was made by Ho THI SANG & PETITHORY (1963) on the techniques for concentration of microfilariae in blood.

(a) The sedimentation methods

In the early days, SMITH & RIVAS (1914) and SUGANUMA (1921) used 2% acetic acid solution as the hemolytic agent, and collected microfilariae after centrifugation. KNOTT (1939) used 2% formalin for the destruction of erythrocytes, and because of its simplicity and practical usefulness, this method was followed by a number of later workers in epidemiological surveys. HARRIS & SUMMERS (1945) and FRANKS & STOLL (1945) used a saponin solution for the hemolysis. WAKASUGI (1957) compared various hemolytic agents for their efficiency and the effects on microfilariae, and concluded that the freezing and thawing method or the 20% ethanol method gave the best results in the concentration of microfilariae.

Knott's technique: The original description of the microfilaria concentration technique by KNOTT (1939) is as follows:

> One c.c. of blood is drawn from the cubital vein with a 2 c.c. all-glass
> syringe fitted with a 1 inch 22 gauge needle. The blood is immediately

discharged into 10 c.c. of 2% formalin solution in a 15 c.c. conical-tip centrifuge tube. The blood and solution are thoroughly mixed by inverting the tube and shaking it. The solution lakes the blood and kills the microfilariae, which die in a stretched out attitude. The tube is set aside for 12 to 24 hours. A small compact sediment collects at its tip, consisting of luecocytes and microfilariae, the formalin solution preventing any clotting or clumping of the constituents of the sediment.

The supernatant fluid is carefully decanted by a quick tipping of the tube so that any bubbles floating on the top of the fluid will be poured away. The tube is held inclined, and after all the fluid has drained away from the sediment a long capillary pipette, fitted with a rubber tube and mouthpiece and having a small quantity of clean water in it, is passed to the tip of the tube and the sediment carefully taken up. Its contents are then discharged on to a glass slide, stirred into a smooth mixture, and spread with the tip of the pipette over an area of 2 × 3 cm. The slide is placed on a level surface until dry. If one wants an immediate diagnosis on a single patient, the blood can be laked and centrifuges and the sediment examined in the wet unstained state.

The dry spread is stained for 2 or more minutes with Loeffler's methylene blue, and then counterstained for 1 or 2 minutes with 0.5% aqueous solution of eosin.

Working on nocturnally periodic *W. bancrofti* carriers in St. Crois, KNOTT (1939, see Section 6Bc. 1) found that the number of microfilariae in the sediment from 1 ml of day blood taken between 9 and 10 a.m. and the number in a standard 20 mm³ drop of night blood taken between 9 and 10 p.m. were so close and comparable that this method could replace the night blood examination when necessary.

WAKASUGI (1957) and SASA (1963) conducted comparative studies on the efficiency of various measures for hemolysis in microfilaria sedimentation methods. In this method, 1 ml or more of blood is taken from the cubital vein into a syringe containing anticoagulant (10% potassium succinate or 3.8% sodium citrate), transferred to a centrifuge tube, and after centrifugation and removal of the supernatant, the sediment containing red blood cells, white blood cells, and microfilariae are hemolysed by either of the following measures. Thereafter, the hemolysed fluid is again centrifuged (1,500 rpm for ten minutes), and the sediment is collected on a slide with a micropipette. The sediment may be examined directly under low-power magnification of a microscope, but it is usually dried, fixed in methanol, and stained with Giemsa or other dyes for examination of the detailed structure.

Freezing and thawing method: This method was reported by SASA (1944) for purification of fresh malaria parasites. The sediment in the centrifuge tube is placed in a mixture of ice and sodium chloride (3:1) or dry ice in acetone for more than ten minutes, or stored overnight in a freezer. Complete hemolysis is achieved when the frozen sediment is thawed at room temperature or in a water bath at about 37°C. About 5 ml of physiological saline is added and then this mixture is centrifuged for ten minutes at 1,500 rpm. (The washing with saline is repeated for the collection of hemoglobin-free microfilariae to be used in chemical or immunological studies.) The microfilariae collected from the sediment are generally actively moving, and their morphological structure remains intact.

Hemolysis with saponin: Excellent hemolysis is achieved by adding 5 volumes of 1% saponin solution in water to the sediment. The microfilariae are usually active.

Hemolysis with alcohol: Pure ethanol or methanol is a good fixative of erythrocytes when applied directly on the blood smears, but both act as powerful hemolysers at concentrations of about 20% in water. Complete hemolysis is obtained within a few minutes by adding 5 volumes of 20% methanol (or ethanol) to the sediment, while the same amount of distilled water does not provide such complete hemolysis. Although the microfilariae are generally dead, they retain perfect morphological characters when fixed on a slide with pure methanol and stained with Giemsa or other dyes.

Hemolysis with formalin: As originally reported by KNOTT (1939), formalin in concentrations between 2 and 10% in water destroys erythrocytes, and the microfilariae can be concentrated in the sediment. However, formalin produces a considerable amount of coagulants, and thus the sediment becomes very dirty. The microfilariae are only pooly stained after exposure to formalin. However, because the sediment is easily formed without centrifugation, this method may be useful in field laboratories where electricity is not available.

Other hemolysing agents: Many other chemicals, including acetic acid, benzalconium chloride (invert soap), and various detergents, are known to act as hemolysers, and although some of them may be useful in special studies ,they were found to yield less satisfactory results in the staining of microfilariae than the freezing and thawing or the 20% methanol methods described above.

The Hematocrit centrifuge methods

A method for laboratory diagnosis of hematozoa with the hematocrit centrifuge was described by BENNETT (1962). A standard heparinized hematocrit capillary tube (outside diameter 1.3 to 1.5 mm; length 75 mm) is filled with 40 to 50 mm³ of blood. One end of the tube is sealed with a plug of plasticine. The hematocrit tube is now centrifuged for eight minutes at 11,500 rpm. in an microcapillary centrifuge. Following centrifugation, the capillary tube is examined, under low-power magnification of a compound microscope, for motile parasites. Then the tube is cut 2 to 3 mm above the buffy layer. By pushing on the plasticine plug with a thin wire, the buffy layer and top 2 to 3 mm of the red cell layer are forced out of the tube. A thin blood film made from this material is fixed, stained, and examined under a compound microscope for blood protozoa and microfilaria. This method was originally described for the examination of blood parasites of birds. COWER (1967) used a similar method for the routine examination of human microfilariae. GOLDSMID *et al.* (1972) also reported on a technique for processing finger prick samples with a microhematocrit.

(b) The filtration methods

Methods for collecting microfilariae in blood on a filter were also reported by various workers.

GORDON & WEBBER (1955) constructed an apparatus for collecting microfilariae from a large amount of blood on a conical filter made of a wire fabric with a mesh size of 23 μ. The sample of blood is taken from a cubital vein and squirted into a test tube containing a few drops of diluted heparin. The blood is hemolysed by adding nine parts of distilled water to one part of whole blood, and the microfilariae are fixed by adding an equal part of 5% formalin to the hemolysed blood. This solution is further diluted by addition of nine parts of distilled water, thereby giving a final dilution of one part whole blood to 200 parts dilute formalin. This fluid is filtered on a conical wire fabric, and about 10 ml of the sediment and the washings are centrifuged, and the sediment is transferred on a slide after washing with human serum. The smear is fixed with alcohol and stained with hot hematoxylin for 50 seconds.

BELL (1967) devised a method for the concentration of microfilariae with a membrane filter "Millipore" (Millipore Filter Cooperation, Bedford, Mass., U.S.A.). The procedure is as follows: One ml of blood, 9 ml of physiological saline, and 1 ml of Teepol (Shell Chemicals Ltd) are added, in turn, to a 15-ml graduated centrifuge tube, and thoroughly mixed. The tube is emptied onto the filter and filtration is done by vacuum. The membrane filter is washed with saline, and then by boiling in distilled water to fix the microfilariae. The membrane is then removed from the metal holder and stained in hot Ehrlich's hematoxylin for 2 to 5 minutes or in 1:25 dilution of Giemsa's stain for 30 to 60 minutes. The membrane is washed and dried, and then mounted on a slide in a few drops of microscope immersion oil for examination under a microscope.

CHULARERK & DESOWITZ (1970) further simplified the membrane filtration technique. Their method requires no electiricity and needs only a syringe and a syringe-filter holder. The procedure is:

> One ml of venous blood is drawn into a heparinized syringe. Nine ml of a 10% solution of Teepol (Shell Chemicals) in physiological saline is then taken into the syringe, and mixed with the blood by gentle rotation for 1 to 1.5 minutes until the blood is completely hemolyzed. The needle is removed and replaced by a 25-mm circular holder containing a 25-mm membrane filter (Millipore Corperation) of 5μ in porosity placed over a circular piece of filter paper (Whatman No. 1) of the same size. The latter acts as a supporting pad for the membrane filter. Gentle

steady pressure is exerted on the syringe piston until all the hemolyzed blood is forced through the filter. The membrane is washed by passing 5 ml of physiological saline through it. Ten ml of formol-saline is then passed through the filter to fix any microfilariae present. Following fixation, the filter is washed twice with 10 ml of distilled water. It is then removed from the folder and placed in 1:25 Giemsa stain for 1 hour, washed rapidly in distilled water, and allowed to dry thoroughly. The membrane is placed on a glass microscope slide and a few drops of immersion oil applied to clear it. Alternatively a clearing-mounting medium such as Permount (Fisher Scientific Company) may be used to make permanent preparations. The cleared stained membrane can be scanned with the 10 × objective for the presence of microfilariae.

This membrane filtration technique was further improved and modified by DESOWITZ (1971) for the use in field studies (an apparatus for easier pressing of the syringe; staining for five minutes with hot hematoxylin of Harris, in which mercury oxide and acetic acid act as the fixatives and the use of formalin can be omitted). DESOWITZ & SOUTHGATE (1973) and DESOWITZ (1973,1974) conducted extensive surveys of various populations in the endemic areas of *W. bancrofti* in the South Pacific, and obtained much higher microfilaria rates with the membrane filter concentration method than with 60 mm³ thick smear method.

10B.2.2.4 Microfilaria provocation methods

Most microfilariae of the nocturnally periodic race of *W. bancrofti* and *B. malayi* are absent from the peripheral blood and are not detectable in daytime blood surveys. However, KATAMINE *et al.* (1952) reported that an oral administration of a small dose of DEC (such as 2 mg per kg) during the daytime mobilized the nocturnally periodic microfilariae into the circulating blood, and this method might be utilized for daytime diagnosis of *W. bancrofti* infection. This phenonenom was further studied by TAMURA (1954) and was adapted for daytime blood surveys by SASA *et al.* (1963). Such provocative effects of DEC on microfilariae were also confirmed by SULLIVAN & HEMBREE (1970), MANSON-BAHR & WIJERS (1972), and PARTONO *et al.* (1972).

The time course of the appearance of microfilariae after administration of DEC was observed by KATAMINE *et al.* (1952). In all of the four cases with *W. bancrofti* infection, the microfilariae were not detectable by day before the drug administration, but large numbers of them began to appear in the circulating blood five minutes after the drug was swallowed, reached the peak density after some 15 to 30 minutes, and remained detectable even after five hours. However, the peak counts observed in daytime after the DEC administration are usually about one-third to one-half of the counts observed in blood examinations conducted in the previous night.

The efficiency of the DEC provocative test conducted by day as compared to the standard midnight blood examinations was studied by SASA *et al.* (1963). The results are summarized in Table 10-5. In Ashiken Village, 48 persons were found to be carrying microfilariae in the first night-blood survey. In the second night-blood survey conducted on the same persons some two months later, 42 of 48 (87.5%) were again positive, but 6 of them were negative even though no control measures were applied during this period. In a daytime blood examination conducted at 2 p.m. on the next day, only 8 of 48 (16.7%) were positive. Then, DEC was administered to these persons at a rate of about 2 mg per kg (100 mg to adults), and the blood samples were collected about 30 minutes after the drug was swallowed; in this test, 34 of 48 persons examined were positive (70.8%), and the average microfilaria count per 30 mm³ blood sample was 29.2% of that of the previous night-blood survey. Similar results were obtained in the other two villages. It should be noted that the efficiency of detection of microfilariae became much less in the following nights when the DEC provocative test was once applied; the microfilariae apparently lost the character of periodicity and appreciable numbers remained in the peripheral blood even during the daytime.

When DEC was administered to the microfilaria carriers at about midnight (when the microfilarial density in the circulating blood was at

Table 10-5. Observations on the provocative effects of diethylcarbamazine on the microfilariae of *Wuchereria bancrofti* in the Amami Islands (after SASA *et al.*, 1963).

VILLAGE Experiment number	Date of examination	Time examined	No. of cases examined	No. of cases positive	Percent positive	Average Mf. count (30 mm³)	Ratio of Mf. count (%)
ASHIKEN							
1. Night I	2 Aug.	21 p. m.–	48	48	100.0	29.9	67.3
2. Night II	13 Oct.	21 p. m.–	48	42	87.5	44.4	100.0
3. Day	14 Oct.	14 p. m.–	48	8	16.7	0.3	0.7
4. Day-Prov.	14 Oct.	15 p. m.–	48	34	70.8	13.0	29.2
YUWAN							
1. Night I	2–3 Aug.	21 p. m.–	49	49	100.0	29.3	88.0
2. Night II	13 Oct.	21 p. m.–	49	44	89.8	33.3	100.0
3. Day	14 Oct.	6 a. m.–	49	22	44.9	2.9	8.8
4. Day-Prov.	14 Oct.	7 a. m.–	49	41	83.7	17.1	51.5
5. Night III	14 Oct.	21 p. m.–	49	35	71.4	4.7	14.0
SUKO							
1. Night I	3 Aug.	21 p. m.	34	34	100.0	25.1	100.0
2. Night II	15 Oct.	21 p. m.	34	26	76.5	25.1	100.0
3. Night-Prov.	15 Oct.	22 p. m.	33	25	75.8	22.3	88.6
4. Day	16 Oct.	18 p. m.	30	24	80.0	3.6	14.2
5. Day-Prov.	16 Oct.	19 p. m.	28	17	60.7	6.3	25.0

its highest level), the drug caused an immediate reduction of the micro-filariae in the circulating blood in place of the immediate increase seen in the daytime. Therefore, it is useless or rather harmful to make the DEC provocative test as an aid to diagnosis in the regular night-blood surveys.

As discussed previously, the numbers of microfilariae found in blood samples collected after the daytime administration of DEC are usually much smaller than those obtained in regular night-blood surveys, and therefore the efficiency of detection of microfilaria carriers is more or less lower in the former than in the latter. Hence, the use of the daytime provocation method should be restricted to areas where the regular night-blood survey is impracticable for some reason. It should also be noted that the administration of some 2 mg per kg of DEC is sufficient to provoke severe fever reactions in persons containing microfilariae at high densities, especially in *B. malayi* cases. This test should be performed with extreme care in areas where *L. loa* or *O. volvulus* is endemic, because the drug may cause serious side effects in some cases.

10B.2.3 Methods of staining microfilariae

Although the microfilariae may be detected and differentiated in fresh specimens, the staining with adequate dyes and appropriate procedures is necessary in order to examine the structure for identification of the species. Various dyes and staining methods have been proposed according to the purposes and requirements. The use of Giemsa or allied stains is the most common practice in clinical diagnoses and epidemiological surveys of filariasis, but some other methods have been recommended in special studies.

10B.2.3.1 Giemsa and allied stains

The dyes used in Giemsa and related stains consist of a mixture of methylene blue and its derivatives, and eosin. The former stains better in alkaline media, while the latter stains well in acid media. When the two groups of dyes are dissolved in water and mixed, they form precipitates within a few hours to a few days, and thus loose the staining effect. Various devices have been made by previous workers in order to produce stable, well-staining, more standardized, and less expensive dyes and methods.

The first report on the use of these sorts of dyes was made by ROMANOW-SKY, in 1891, who used a mixture of eosin and methylene blue for staining malaria parasites in blood films. It was later found that compounds of dyes produced by oxidizing methylene blue in an alkaline solution, such as with potassium dichromate, stain nuclei better than methylene blue, and various improved methods were reported by later workers, such as NOCHT in 1898, LEISHMAN in 1901, and WRIGHT in 1902. A stable and standardized dye which is now called Giemsa's solution was invented in 1904 by GIEMSA; it is an alcohol-glycerine solution of the mixture of the alkaline oxidation product of methylene blue, eosin, and methylene blue itself.

Later workers, who were not satisfied with the use of Giemsa's stain in their work for some reason, invented a variety of modifications more fitted to their purposes, such as saving time in the staining process, economy, or for better differentiation of the morphological structures. The following are the representative methods recommended for the staining of microfilariae by previous workers.

(a) *Giemsa's stain*

This stain is available from various companies as a solution of the dyes in alcohol-glycerine. The staining quality sometimes differs greatly according to the company and the product lots, and care must be taken to select good samples. Powdered stain (mixture of dye crystals) is also available, from which the stock solution is made by dissolving 1 g of the crystals in 60 ml of glycerine and 66 ml of methanol.

Procedure: 1. Thin blood smears or tissue smears are fixed in methanol; thick blood smears are dried overnight, dehemoglobinized by soaking in water (or better, in 20% methanol in water) for a few minutes, and fixed in methanol if necessary (this fixing can usually be omitted). 2. The stock solution is diluted with 20 to 25 times the volume of distilled water, which is adjusted to a proper pH by adding a phosphate buffer (see Table 10-6). The slides are soaked in the diluted Giemsa's solution for 20 to 60 minutes. For individual staining of the slides, about 3 ml of the diluted solution is placed on the slide surface with a pipette. 3. After the staining, the slides are rinsed gently in water, and dried in the air.

Remarks: Microfilariae are differentiated better when stained at a slightly acid condition, such as pH 6.7; however, this author prefers to stain the smears with an alkaline medium, from pH 7.4 to 7.8 for about one hour, then to remove the excess of blue dyes by rinsing the overstained slides for a few seconds in 1:1,000 dilution of acetic acid in water, and to wash them finally in water. The nuclei of microfilariae are stained blue or purple and give good contrast to the pink background. The smears take more eosin in the acid media and more azur in alkaline media. Azur dyes stained in the smears are dissolved in water and removed by rinsing with a slightly acid medium.

The pH values of water used for diluting Giemsa's stain can be adjusted to the desired level by adding a small amount of phosphate buffer solution prepared according to the ratios given in Table 10-6.

Table 10-6. The pH values of phosphate buffer solutions at various mixing ratios of 1/15 mol sodium phosphate bibasic, and potassium phosphate monobasic.

	Ratio of solutions A and B.										
A. Na_2HPO_4	0	1	2	3	4	5	6	7	8	9	10
B. KH_2PO_4	10	9	8	7	6	5	4	3	2	1	0
pH	4.53	5.91	6.24	6.47	6.64	6.81	6.98	7.17	7.38	7.73	8.30

A. 11.876 g of $Na_2HPO_4 \cdot 2H_2O$ dissolved in 1 liter of distilled water;
B. 9.078 g of KH_4PO_2 dissolved in 1 liter of distilled water.

(b) *The Azeo-stain*

It has been well known among specialists in hematology and protozoology that the combined use of azur II (purple, basophilic dye) and eosin (red, acidophilic) is useful for differentiation of leucocytes and blood protozoans. The Azeo-stain reported by SASA & HAYASHI in 1943 as a standard method for mass staining of malaria parasites, and later recommended by SASA (1963) for the mass staining of microfilariae is a modification of these techniques. Azur II is a dye with a special affinity to the nuclei, and stains better in an alkaline medium, but dissolves more from tissue into water in an acid medium, while eosin has the reverse staining characteristic. Therefore, excellent staining of the microfilariae for differentiation of the structures is made by excessive staining in an alkaline medium and differentiation with a slightly acid medium. The two dyes should be preserved separately in stock solutions because they form precipitates when mixed together in water.

Procedures: The stock solutions are prepared by the following prescriptions. Stock solution A: take 2 g of azur II (crystal) and dissolve in 500 ml of ethanol or methanol (0.4% solution). Stock solution B: take 1 g of eosin Y (crystal) and dissolve in 500 ml of ethanol or methanol (0.2 % solution). The stock solutions can be preserved semipermanently at room temperature. When staining the thick blood smears, take 9 volumes of deionized water adjusted to pH 7.4, and add 0.5 volumes of solution A and 0.5 volumes of solution B, to make 10 volumes. The blood films are stained with this diluted Azeo-solution (0.02 % azur II and 0.01 % eosin solution) for one hour. The slides are then washed in water, rinsed half a minute in weak acid water (1:1,000 dilution of acetic acid) for differentiation, again washed in water and air dried.

Remarks: The microfilariae properly stained with this method are easily differentiated under low-power magnifications as purple wormlike bodies in pink fields, showing an excellent contrast. The fine structures of the fixed points and nuclear arrangements can be demonstrated under high-power magnification, since azur II selectively stains the nuclei, while eosin stains the contents of the anal and excretory pores. According to a commercial catalogue of chemicals in Japan, 50 g of azur II costs 2,400 yen (about U.S.$ 8) and 25 g of eosin is available for 460 yen (U.S.$ 1.50). This amount is enough to prepare 250,000 ml of diluted Azeo-solution, with which about 100,000 slides can be stained. In the case of Giemsa's stain, 12,500 ml of the concentrated solution is required for preparing the same amount of staining media; according to the same catalogue, 100 ml of Giemsa's solution costs 520 yen (U.S.$ 1.70) or 65,000 yen for 12.5 liters. Hence, Giemsa's stain is 22.7 times more expensive than the Azeo-stain. If necessary, more concentrated stock solutions can be prepared in order to save alcohol. The shipment of dyes to the field laboratories is much easier when the Azeo-staining method is employed, because 50 g of azur II and 25 g of eosin is comparable to more than 10 l of Giemsa's solution.

(c) *J.S.B. stain*

A stain introduced by SINGH & BHATTACHARJI (1944), and slightly modified later by SINGH *et al.* (1953) and SINGH & MISRA (1956). The stain consists of solution I, which is prepared in each laboratory from methylene blue, and solution II, which is a 0.2% solution of water-soluble yellow eosin in water. According to SINGH & MISRA (1956), Solution I is prepared as follows.

"Methylene blue, medicinal (0.5 g) is dissolved in water (500 ml), and 1% sulphuric acid (3 ml) is added gradually with stirring to ensure thorough mixing. Potassium dichromate (0.5 g) is then added which forms a purple precipitate. Disodium hydrogen phosphate dihydrate (3.5 g) is added next, and after stirring the solution for some time, the precipitate appears to get dissolved. This solution is boiled in a flask with a reflux condenser for one hour when the blue color of the solution deepens. This solution is ready for immediate use as J.S.B. solution I.

A review was made by SINGH (1956) on various modified methods for the preparation of the stain, including a method for preparing solution I in powder form, their chemical properties, and merits and demerits of the use of this stain.

Procedure: In the staining of thick smears: 1. immerse the slide in solution I for 10 seconds; 2. wash in a jar containing acidulated water (pH 6.2 to 6.6) for 2 seconds; 3. stain in solution II for one second; 4. wash in the same jar for 5 seconds; 5. immerse in solution I again for 10 seconds; 6. wash as above for 2 seconds or till the smear gives pink background; 7. dry and examine (according to the original description by SINGH & BHATTACHARJI, 1944).

A modified and more simplified technique proposed by SINGH *et al.* (1953) for thick blood smears is as follows: 1. immerse the slides in a jar containing solution II for 1 to 2 seconds; 2. excess of eosin stain is removed by dipping the slides in a jar containing buffered wash water; 3. transfer to solution I and keep 10 to 15 seconds; wash again in the same buffered water for 3 to 4 seconds; dry and examine.

Remarks: J.S.B. stain was introduced mainly to save cost and time in the examination of malaria parasites, and has been used widely in India and Ceylon. The stain has been used also in microfilaria surveys in India and Ceylon since it was recommended by RAGHAVAN & KRISHNAN (1949). According to SINGH *et al.* (1953), J.S.B. stain is about 50 times cheaper than Giemsa. However, difficulties have been experienced in standardizing the dye samples to be prepared in each laboratory. The microfilariae are only poorly stained with this method, and thus it is not fitted for the study of detailed structure for identification of species.

10B.2.3.2 Hematoxylin stains

Hematoxylin (haematoxylin) is an almost colorless crystal extracted from a Central American plant, *Haematoxylon campechianum* Linnaeus.

This substance becomes hematein when oxidized, and exhibits a strong and specific staining character on the nuclei.

Various hematoxylin preparations and staining methods have been employed for the staining of microfilariae. Some workers prefer hematoxylin to Giemsa's stain even in routine examinations. Since hematoxylin stains the nuclei selectively, the microfilariae show their structural details very clearly, and this is especially valuable for demonstrating the caudal nuclei of *B. malayi*. Hematoxylin is also useful in demonstrating the sheath of *W. bancrofti* and the Timor microfilaria, which is hardly visible when stained with Giemsa.

A method recommended by FENG (1933) is as follows: The dried blood smears are dehemoglobinized in normal saline for about ten minutes. The smears are then fixed in 70 % alcohol heated to 50 to 60° C. The slides are transferred into hemalum solution and stained from five hours to overnight, and then destained in 70 % alcohol containing 1 % hydrochloric acid until the desired degree of differentiation is obtained. The slides are then passed through various grades of alcohol and finally to xylol and mounted in balsam.

The following preparations are commonly used in the staining of parasites and histological specimens.

Mayer's acid hemalum: The solution is composed of the mixture of 1 g of hematoxylin, 1,000 ml of distilled water, 0.2 g of sodium iodate $NaIO_3 \cdot 5H_2O$, and 50 g of potassium alum $KAl(SO_4)_2 \cdot 12H_2O$; after these are thoroughly mixed and dissolved, 50 g of chloralhydrate $CCl_3CH(OH)_2$ and 1 g of citric acid crystal $C_3H_4(OH)(COOH)_3 + H_2O$ are added.

Ehrlich's acid hematoxylin: Dissolve 2 g of hematoxylin in 100 ml of ethyl alcohol; add 100 ml of distilled water, 100 ml of glycerin, 3 g of potassium alum and 10 ml of glacial acetic acid.

In staining thick blood smears with Mayer's hemalum, DAVID & EDESON (1965) employed the following method: the slides are dehemoglobinized in tap water, fixed with methyl alcohol, stained for ten minutes in hot hemalum, washed, and dried. (With this method, the authors clearly demonstrated the sheath of Timor microfilaria, which was hardly stained with Giemsa's solution.)

Faust's iron-hematoxylin stain: The method described by FAUST (1937, quoted by FAUST *et al.* 1970) is as follows: 1. Fix smears in Schaudinn's solution to which glacial acetic acid has been added, and heat to a temperature of 60°C, for two minutes; 2. Immerse smears in 70% alcohol, then in 70% alcohol to which enough iodine has been added to give a port wine color, then in 70% and 50% alcohol, leaving in each two minutes; 3. Wash in running water for two minutes; 4. Immerse smears in 2% aqueous iron-alum solution at 40°C for two minutes; 5. Wash in running water for three minutes; 6. Stain in 0.5% aqueous hematoxylin for 10 to 15 minutes; 7. Wash in running water two minutes; 8. Differentiate in a saturated solution of picric acid for five minutes; 9. Wash in running water 10 to 15 minutes.

Bullard's hematoxylin: According to FAUST *et al.* (1970), the procedure is as follows: 1. Mix 144 ml 50% alcohol, 16 ml glacial acetic acid, and 8 g hematoxylin crystal; 2. Heat the above, and add 250 ml distilled water and 20 g ammonium alum; 3. Heat to boiling and slowly add 8 g of mercuric oxide; 4. Cool quickly, filter and add: 275 ml 95% alcohol, 330 ml glycerol, 18 ml glacial acetic acid, 40 g ammonium alum; 5. Keep in bright light for about one week for ripening, and filter again before using; 6. In the staining, immerse the smear in the full-strength staining solution for 12 to 15 minutes, wash in tap water or 1% lithium carbonate solution until the film is distinctly blue, then dry.

10B.2.3.3 Other stains
Methylgreen-pyronin stain:

This method was specially recommended by FENG (1933) and HAYASHI (1954) for examination of the fixed points of microfilariae. The procedures are relatively simple, and permanent preparations can be obtained. The ordinary nuclei are stained green, the excretory and anal pores, as well as the G-cells, are stained red, and the cuticle and the sheath are stained grey.

Procedures: After the thick blood smears are dehemoglobinized in water (or preferably in 20% methanol in water), the blood films are fixed in ethanol for a few minutes, and are stained in the methylgreen-pyronin solution for 12 to 24 hours. The slides are passed quickly through the following grades of ethanol: 70%, 5 seconds; 85%, 10 seconds; 95%, 15 seconds; 100% I, 20 seconds; 100% II, 1 to 3 minutes. The smears are then cleared in xylol, and mounted in balsam.

The methylgreen-pyronin solution is prepared by dissolving 0.2 g of methylgreen and 0.3 g of pyronin in 100 ml of normal saline. It is usually necessary to purify methylgreen with chloroform.

Vital staining methods:

Vital staining has been recommended, especially by classical workers, for demonstration and study of certain specified structures in the microfilariae. For example, the staining of microfilariae by adding a few drops of blood into 0.04% solution of azur II in water has been recommended by RODENWALD (1908), FÜLLEBORN (1913), and FENG (1933) for the study of detailed structure of G-cells, excretory, and anal pores. Counterstaining with eosin gives better contrast to other structures. Vital staining with neutral red was also used by FÜLLEBORN (1913) for the demonstration of the external apparatus of microfilariae.

10B.3 Immunological survey methods

In the diagnosis of infections with certain tissue-dwelling parasites, such as schistosomiasis and paragonimiasis, it has been well recognized that immunological methods offer very useful and valuable information.

However, in the case of human filariasis, most workers consider that immunological means of diagnosis are still of little practical usefulness, although a large number of reports and devices were made for this purpose. For example, WILSON (1961), in his review stated, "most published accounts of other aids to diagnosis, such as skin reactions and complement fixation tests indicate that they are not sufficiently specific and that false-negatives are common."

All diagnostic tests must be evaluated from at least two different aspects, i.e., specificity and sensitivity. It is obvious that the diagnosis of filarial infections by clinical signs is poor both in specificity and sensitivity, although the results may be practically very important. Most of the clinical symptoms which appear as the result of filarial infections may also be caused by other agents or diseases. There are also many persons who are actually infected, but do not exhibit any clinical symptoms. The demonstration of microfilariae is a specific sign of infection, but it is also very poor in sensitivity, because, as is well known, there are many persons who are really infected, but fail to show microfilariae.

Likewise, most immunological tests so far reported are considered to be unsatisfactory in sensitivity and/or specificity. The results of epidemiological surveys conducted with various immunological tests have usually yielded higher positive rates than those obtained by examination of microfilariae in thick blood smears, and thus, they may be more sensitive than the parasitological test; however, there were also considerable numbers of persons who were parasitologically or clinically positive but immunologically negative.

Because of difficulties in collecting homologous antigens in sufficient amounts, the immunological diagnosis of human filariasis has been usually done with heterologous antigens derived from animal filariae, such as *Dirofilaria immitis* in dogs, and it has always been suspected that the reaction might be a nonspecific one.

Practically important is the significance of a positive reaction in various immunological tests. From the mode of infection of filariasis, it can be assumed that large proportions of the people living in endemic areas of filariasis are infected with varying numbers of the parasite, although most of them may be parasitologically or clinically negative. In areas of high endemicities, nearly all of the inhabitants are considered to be infected. Since the strength of most immunological reactions is usually not correlated with the parasite load, a positive result in man in an immunological test may not be as valuable as his personal history, such as the length of years he had lived in the endemic area.

Although most immunological methods proposed by previous workers are considered to be still of little practical usefulness in the treatment and control of filariasis, this does not mean that immunology is useless in filariasis studies. The involvement of immunological reactions is considered to be an important factor for the development of various clinical signs of filariasis. Analytical studies of the mode of effects of DEC have shown that development of immunity in the hosts is an essential factor in the release of its filaricidal effects (Section 12B). It has also been shown in recent studies with animals that so long as immunological tests are adequately made with the homologous adult antigens, the development of antibodies can be detected at high specificities and sensitivities (Section 12C.2).

Examples of the use of the skin test for the assessment of filariasis control programs as reported by HAYASHI *et al.* (1967) and YAMAMOTO *et al.* (1968) are discussed in Section 11G.1.3.

An excellent review was made by KAGAN (1963) on the immunological methods for the diagnosis of filariasis. He quoted a total of 148 papers published during the period from 1916 to 1962 referring to the skin test, complement fixation reaction, precipitin test, hemagglutination, and bentonite flocculation, and to the Prausnitz-Kuestner test in the diagnosis of various filarial infections in man and animals. He was of the optimistic opinion that "with standardization of techniques, immunological methods can be made to furnish a reliable means of diagnosis, notwithstanding the past unreliability of such methods."

10C. Entomological survey methods of vector populations

10C.1 Methods for determination of filariasis vectors

10C.1.1 Criteria for a natural vector of human filariasis

The known vectors of human filariae are bloodsucking insects of the Order Diptera, i.e., mosquitoes (for *W. bancrofti* and *B. malayi*), black flies (for *O. volvulus* and ?*M. ozzardi*), biting midges (for *D. perstans*, *D. streptocerca*, and *M. ozzardi*) and horse flies (for *L. loa*). In most endemic areas of filariasis, more than one species of insects are responsible for the transmission, although one of them usually acts as the main vector. It should also be noted that the role played by various insect species as the vectors of filariasis may differ according to geographic sites or local environmental conditions of endemic areas, and thus determination of the vectors must be made for each area by the standard entomological survey methods described below.

When incriminating an insect species as a vector of filariasis in an area, it is necessary to confirm at least the following three facts:

(1) that the species is a bloodsucking arthropod commonly found attacking man in the endemic area concerned,

(2) that natural infection with mature stage larvae of the particular human filarial species are found in specimens caught in the endemic area, and

(3) that mature stage larvae of morphologically identical structure have developed in the specimens (preferably those of clean, laboratory-reared colonies) experimentally fed on a human microfilaria carrier.

In studies for determination of vectors of a filarial species whose mature stage larvae are morphologically well known and can be differentiated from those of other human or animal filarial species, such as in the case of *W. bancrofti* in mosquitoes, or *O. volvulus* in black flies, the experimental infection study can be omitted and the vector may be determined simply by demonstration of the mature larvae in naturally caught specimens. In areas where natural infections of filariae are occurring among animals, careful examination of morphological structures of filaria larvae must be made in order to differentiate the vectors of animal filariae from those of the human filaria species being studied. In the case of *B. malayi* in mosquitoes or *L. loa* in *Chrysops* flies, mature larvae of certain animal filariae may be identical with those of the human race or species, and thus an experimental infection study with human donors is indispensable for determination of the real vectors of human filariasis.

On the other hand, successful results in experimental infection with human donors alone do not necessarily mean that the insect species tested is a natural vector. The species may be too short-lived under natural conditions, or may be too scarce to maintain the transmission. The demonstration of immature stage larvae in naturally caught specimens does not necessarily imply that it is a natural vector. In any event, differentiation of the filarial species by morphological examination of the structure of the mature stage larvae by the methods such as shown in Sections 2A.2.4 and 5.3.3 is a crucial technique for vector identification.

In an endemic area of filariasis where the vector is yet unknown, a method of experimental infection under seminatural conditions such as employed by BRUG & DE ROOK (1930) is often very useful for rapid determination of the vectors. In an endemic area of *B. malayi* in Sumatra, these authors exposed human microfilaria carriers to the bites of mosquitoes and other bloodsucking insects, and collected the individual specimens into test tubes when they fully engorged on the blood containing microfilariae. These bloodsucking insect specimens were dissected as soon as they died, or after 14 days if they were still alive. With this method, these authors found that mosquito species of the subgenus *Mansonia*, which had never been incriminated as vectors of human filariasis before, were the most abundant human biters in this region and also that excellent development of the filarial larvae to the mature stage was seen in them. The same method was used by JURGENS (1932) for determination of *An. barbirostris* as the main vector and *M. annulipes* as the secondary vector of *B. malayi* in Mamoedjoe, Sulawesi. This simple and efficient method was employed by a number of other Dutch workers in Indonesia for determination of local filarial vector species, as described in Section 8B.9.

Successful results were obtained with similar seminatural experimental infection studies by SHARP (1928) for the determination of *Culicoides austeni* as the vector of *D. perstans* in Cameroon, Africa, and by BUCKLEY (1934) for the determination of *Culicoides furens* as the vector of *M. ozzardi* in St. Vincent, West Indies.

10C.1.2 Collection of bloodsucking insects for vector indentification

Various methods have been used for the collection of bloodsucking insects occurring in filariasis endemic areas. In areas where *C.p. fatigans* and some anopheline species act as the main vectors, the specimens may be efficiently collected from the wall of human dwellings by sucking tubes. In the case of an exophilic species, such as most *Aedes* and *Mansonia* mosquitoes or simuliid and tabanid flies, the collection must be made outdoors at the right time of day by human or animal baits, or with certain insect traps.

The collection of bloodsucking insects on human baits with test tubes or sucking tubes provides especially important information on the dynamics of transmission of filariasis. The number of specimens caught per day (or per year) per person with these methods is an important index of the prevalence of the species as a bloodsucker of man. If the collection is made every hour for 24 hours, the biting rhythm can also be obtained for each bloodsucking insect species. If microfilaria carriers are used as the baits, the engorged specimens can be used for an experimental infection study.

Collection of bloodsucking insects with animal baits or in animal sheds may be more efficient for collecting large numbers of specimens, but it should be noted that the species attracted to animals are not necessarily the human biters. By comparison of insect species attracted to man, domestic animals, and birds, we can estimate the host preference of various species of mosquitoes and other bloodsucking flies occurring in the same areas (see Section 10C.2.5).

Various traps have been developed for the collection of bloodsucking arthropods. The following are the main types of devices commonly used by entomologists.

Mosquito light traps:

Light traps are composed of an electric bulb or fluorescent lamp (especially black light), a sucking fan, and a collecting cage. The efficiency of attraction of various species of insects differs greatly according to the light source. Both males and females of certain mosquito and biting midge species are collected with these types of traps together with various nonbloodsucking insects. The light traps must have a screen of about 5 mm mesh size in order to separate small insects from large insects which would otherwise destroy the small specimens. Several types of light traps are commercially available e.g., CDC light trap, New Jersey type mosquito trap, etc. As reported by SASA *et al.* (1965a), NEWHOUSE *et al.* (1966), CARESTIA & SAVAGE (1967), MILLER *et al.* (1969), and HERBERT *et al.* (1972), the use of carbon dioxide remarkably increases the number of female mosquitoes attracted to the light traps. Portable light traps operated by automobile batteries are also available for field use.

It should, however, be noted that the species and sex composition of mosquitoes and other bloodsucking insects attracted by a light trap may be quite different from that actually attacking man in the same areas. Most day-biting insects (including *Aedes*-mosquitoes and horse flies) are not collectable with light traps. The ratio of female *C. tritaeniorhynchus* to female *C.p. fatigans* collected by light traps is much larger than that collected on human bait in the same areas. On the other hand, more males of *C. p. fatigans* are collected than those of *C. tritaeniorhynchus* in the light traps (SASA *et al.*, 1965a).

Dry ice traps:

The dry ice traps are a very useful and powerful means of collecting some species of bloodsucking insects. A simple method using dry ice and mosquito net was reported by TAKEDA *et al.* (1962) and has been used widely in Japan for the collection of mosquitoes in the field. A single-bed mosquito net is put up outdoors, and a small opening of about 30 cm high and 50 cm wide is made on one side of the net for the entrance of attracted mosquitoes. About 1 kg of dry ice is placed on the floor near the center of the mosquito net. With this simple method, large numbers of unengorged female mosquitoes (often several thousands or more) are attracted and trapped into the mosquito net, especially within a few hours after sunset. The mosquitoes may be collected with sucking tubes, or more efficiently with a small vacuum sweeper operated by battery or portable electric generator.

Horse flies, including *Chrysops* species, were also found to be collected efficiently with a Malaise trap baited with CO_2, as reported by TOWNES (1962). Detailed studies were conducted on the relationship between the amount of CO_2 to be released and the efficiency of collection of horse flies by ROBERTS (1970, 1975).

Animal bait traps:

Certain species of bloodsucking insects can be collected efficiently by traps baited with various animal species, including man, and such methods can be used also for estimating the zoophilism of various bloodsucking insects occurring in certain areas. The traps can be constructed simply by putting up single-bed mosquito nets with a small opening on one side (about 30 cm high and 50 cm wide) over an animal cage, same as those used for the dry ice traps. The construction of window-trap huts to take animal or human baits has been preferred by other workers.

10C.1.3 Dissection of insect specimens

Dissection of insect specimens for demonstration of infection with filaria larvae is usually made under a binocular dissecting microscope. The individual specimens are placed on a slide in a drop of physiological saline (0.6% for insect tissue) and first separated into head, thorax, and abdomen with a pair of fine needles mounted on metal holders. Each body part is then teased into small pieces. Filaria larvae of various stages may be found in tissues of particular insect organs, i.e., the microfilariae and first stage larvae in the midgut contents, the developing stage larvae in the thoracic muscle (*Wuchereria* and *Brugia*) or in the Malpighian tubules (*Dirofilaria immitis*), and the third stage larvae in the proboscis, head, or any part of the body cavity, sometimes even in the legs.

The filaria larvae isolated from fresh insect tissues are usually actively moving in the saline. The third stage larvae are easily differentiated from other immature larvae by the body being long and slender, and by the motion being more active. The species can be identified by the body length and by the morphological structure, especially by the shape of the tail. (See Section 2A.2.4 for structures in mosquitoes, and Section 5.3.3 for those in black flies.)

The insect specimens collected in the field are usually kept alive in paper cups or small cages until they are dissected in the laboratory. In case these cannot be examined immediately, the specimens may be preserved in an icebox (for several days), in a deep freezer (several months), or in 70% ethyl alcohol (indefinitely). It should be noted that identification of insect hosts sometimes becomes difficult when they are preserved in alcohol. The filaria larvae in fresh specimens are more easily differentiated than those in preserved specimens since they move actively, though the differentiation of filaria larvae and host tissues is not difficult even after fixing in alcohol. The filaria larvae in insect tissue can be beautifully stained while preserved in alcohol by adding a small amount of Giemsa's stain or 1% azur II solution in alcohol a few hours before being dissected.

NELSON (1958) recommends the following method for the preservation and staining of mosquitoes when examining for filaria larvae.

(1) Mosquitoes collected alive are transferred to 80% pure ethyl alcohol where they may remain indefinitely.

(2) Alcohol is removed by taking the mosquito specimens through descending dilutions to water; they are then stained for three days in Mayer's acid hemalum, differentiated for three days in distilled water, and transferred to glycerol to await dissection. (Fresh acid hemalum should be prepared every 2 to 3 months because the stain gradually deteriorates.)

(3) Stained mosquitoes are dissected in glycerol. All larval stages in the thorax are readily seen, and mature larvae can be picked up and transferred to a fresh slide under a coverslip for examination under high magnification.

10C.2 Methods for estimating the vectorial capacity

10C.2.1 The natural infection rate

The natural infection rate of a vector species with a particular filarial larvae is obviously the most important measure of the vectorial capacity, and large numbers of reports have been made from various regions of the world referring to the infection rate of various naturally caught insect specimens, as stated in the previous chapters.

In these studies, some classical workers referred only to the infection rate with all stages of filaria larvae. However, most important is the rate of an insect species with mature stage larvae. The infection with only the immature stage larvae does not necessarily indicate that the species is a real vector, because the larvae may die out before reaching mature stage, or the insect host may be too short-lived to allow full development of the larvae.

In studying the natural infection of bloodsucking flies with filaria larvae, it is essentially important to identify the filarial species at least by their mature stages by morphological examination of the body structure, especially by the shape of tail part. It has almost always been observed that more than one species of animal filariae are endemic in the same areas (those in dogs, cattle, horses, birds, reptiles, and amphibians) and their larvae appear in the same or different insect vectors collected in the same areas.

The status of infection of bloodsucking insects in a filariasis endemic area is usually surveyed by examination of large numbers of naturally caught specimens. The percentage of specimens containing all stages of filaria larvae is usually called "the infection rate," while that with mature (third stage) larvae is referred to as "the infective rate."

The intensity of transmission of filariasis in an endemic area is evaluated by examinations of the vector population at least by two parameters: the percentage of the infective (or infected) specimens, and the numbers of mature (or of all stages) larvae found in the individual specimens. The worm burden among the vector populations is best expressed by showing the frequency distribution of specimens according to the number of filaria larvae found in individual specimens, such as shown in Table 10-7.

From this table, one finds out that the patterns of distribution of filarial larvae among vector populations are extremely skewed, especially when the noninfected specimens are taken into consideration. However, the distribution among the infected population is nearly a logarithmic normal type, as that seen with the microfilarial density among the infected human populations (see Section 11C.). The intensity of infection of mature larvae among the vector population can also be expressed by a simple equation: $y = a + b \log x$, where y is the probit of the cumulative percentage of specimens containing x or more filaria larvae among the

Table 10-7. Frequency distribution and cumulative percentages of naturally caught infective mosquitoes according to the number per mosquito of the mature filaria larvae.

No. of mature larvae per mosquito	(1) *W. bancrofti* in *C. fatigans* Rangoon			(2) *W. bancrofti* in *C. fatigans* Sri Lanka			(3) *B. malayi* in *Mansonia* spp. Pahang		
	Obs. No.	Cumulative No.	%	Obs. No.	Cumulative No.	%	Obs. No.	Cumulative No.	%
1	32	32	32.0	54	54	19.5	26	26	20.0
2	23	55	55.0	69	123	44.4	27	53	40.8
3	10	65	65.0	61	184	66.4	14	67	51.5
4	6	71	71.0	35	219	79.1	12	79	60.8
5	3	74	74.0	12	231	83.4			
6	3	77	77.0	8	239	86.3			
7	4	81	81.0	12	251	90.6	32	111	85.4
8	5	86	86.0	6	257	92.8			
9	2	88	88.0	7	264	95.3			
10–14	6	94	94.0	9	273	98.6	11	122	93.8
15–19	3	97	97.0	1	274	98.92	3	125	96.2
20–29	2	99	99.0	2	276	99.64	5	130	100
30+	1	100	100.	1	277	100.	0	130	100
Total larvae	454			1,020			(not recorded)		
Mean per mosquito	4.54			3.68			about 5		

(1) after HAIRSTON & DE MEILLON (1968); (2) after ABDULCADER & SASA (1966); (3) after WHARTON (1962)

infected population. Comparison of the arithmetic mean of the filaria larvae among the infected or the total vector population is also meaningless in this case, while the median density can be regarded as a more significant measure of the intensity of infection. The median density of mature larvae as estimated from the regression line turned out to be about 1.8 in Rangoon (*W. bancrofti* in *C. p. fatigans*), 2.2 in Sri Lanka (*W. bancrofti* in *C. p. fatigans*), and 2.8 in Pahang (*B. malayi* in *Mansonia* spp.).

10C.2.2 The experimental infection rate

The vectorial capacity of an insect vector is also dependent upon the efficiency of transmission of a filarial species when infected under various host and environmental conditions. Various parameters are involved in this phase of the transmission cycle, such as the efficiency of intake of microfilariae when fed on donors with various levels of microfilarial density, the efficiency in supporting their development to the infective stage under the various environmental conditions, and the efficiency of discharging the infective larvae at the time of feeding on a new host.

When conducting an experimental infection study, it is necessary to measure the density of microfilariae in the blood (or in the skin) of donors at the time of the experimental feeding. It is recommended to collect multiple samples of measured specimens, such as six specimens of 10 mm³ (or 20 mm³), so that the average and the variance of the microfilarial counts can be estimated. The average amount of blood taken by the insects can be measured by weighing their bodies on a microbalance either individually, or as a mass. Mosquitoes usually discharge serum from the anus while taking blood into the midgut, and therefore ingest more blood than obtained as the difference between the body weights before and after the blood meal.

Mosquitoes, black flies, and other bloodsucking flies must be preserved alive for about ten days in order to see whether the experimentally ingested microfilariae will develop to the infective stage (third stage) larvae, or whether the insect host is not fitted as the vector and the larvae cease the development at certain immature stages. For this purpose, the insect specimens engorged with the donor's blood are either kept individually in test tubes together with moist filter paper, or they can be kept in mass in paper cups covered with gauze or in mosquito cages. As a rule, the temperature should be kept constant, between 25°C and 30°C, otherwise development of the filaria larvae is retarded (at lower temperature), or mortality of the host increases (at higher temperature). Most insects require high humidity for survival, such as between 75 to 90%. However, the mortality increases when the humidity is too high as they may be drowned in the dew or killed by the growth of fungi. In the case of mosquitoes, better results are usually obtained by keeping them at a relatively low humidity such as 75%, and by providing syrup (5% sugar solution in water) soaked in cotton pads. For a detailed study of the development of filaria larvae, it is recommended to keep the insects individually in test tubes covered with gauze, so that the specimens can be dissected at varying intervals.

10C.2.3 The population density of the vectors

The population density of the vectors constitutes a parameter directly proportional to the force of transmission of filariasis. As stated previously, various methods have been used by different workers for collecting vector insects in various endemic areas, and the numbers collected by a standard method can be regarded as indices for comparison of the population densities. For example, the seasonal prevalence of certain anopheline and culicine mosquitoes, as well as biting midges, can be estimated by operating mosquito light traps once every week throughout a year. The average numbers of mosquitoes caught at fixed stations (usually human or animal dwellings) per day per working hour (such as ten minutes of collection in each house) have been recorded as indices of the effects of larval control measures against *C. p. fatigans* in the filariasis control programs in Sri Lanka (ABDULCADER & SASA, 1966) and in Brazil (RACHOU, 1960). The numbers of mosquitoes biting per man per hour have been used as measures for determining the vector density in the filariasis control program in India (INDIAN COUNCIL OF MEDICAL RESEARCH REPORT, 1971).

A mosquito trap useful for estimating the population density of *C. p. fatigans* was described by SASA *et al.* (1965a). It is constructed from a cardboard box, commercially available anywhere for the shipment of canned food, and is set inside houses with the top covers left partly open, as shown in Fig. 10-3. Both males and females of *C. p. fatigans* enter into the trap using it as a daytime resting shelter; they can be collected by injecting chloroform or ether into the box after closing the top covers. Several hundred mosquitoes are usually collected every morning in areas where the mosquito density is high, such as in Bangkok. The trap was used in estimating the effects of mosquito control measures (indoor spraying of fenitrothion, or larval control with insecticides), or for comparison of the population density of *C. p. fatigans* among different areas or at different heights above ground level (SASA *et al.*, 1965a; KURIHARA *et al.*, 1965). Table 10-8 shows a result of observations on the effects of an adult control operation by the indoor spraying of Sumithion (fenitrothion), by that of larval control by extensive spraying of the same insecticide into

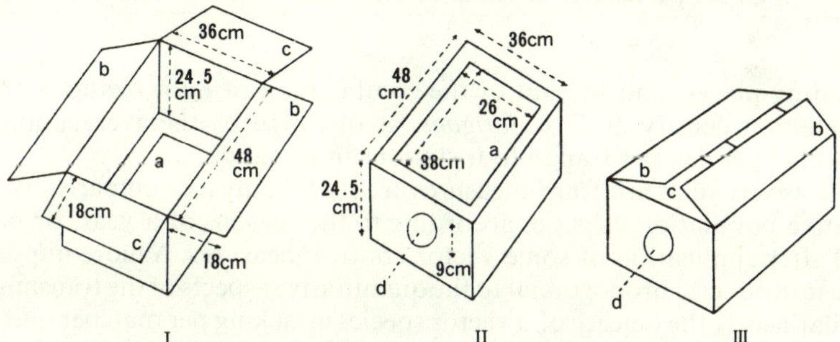

Fig. 10-3. Cardboard box trap for the indoor collection of *Culex pipiens fatigans* (SASA *et al.*, 1965a).

I. Box trap with the top covers *b* & *c* open. II. Box trap in upside-down position, with X-ray film window (*a*) above, and showing the hole *d* for introducing chloroform. III. Box trap set for the collection of mosquitoes. The covers *c* are closed leaving an entrance of 12 cm width between them, and the covers *b* are partly opened with a bamboo stick supporter to make the entrance for the mosquitoes. A sheet of black cotton cloth 40 cm long and 52 cm wide is distended in the box.

Table 10-8. Observations on the effects of mosquito control operations on the density of adult *fatigans* as estimated by the average numbers collected per day per trap by the cardboard box traps set in four wards in Bangkok, 1964 (after KURIHARA *et al.*, 1965).

Ward	Method of treatment		Weeks after start of the treatment						
			0	1	2	3	4	5	6
T	Adult	No.	39.8	5.0	8.1	19.1	20.2	8.3	3.0
	control	%	100	13	20	47	50	21	8
	only	Ratio	197	100	58	76	158	127	125
W	Larval	No.	56.0	61.1	14.1	6.1	8.8	7.0	3.6
	control	%	100	109	25	11	16	13	6
	only	Ratio	139	153	123	117	103	40	83
R	Larval &	No.	31.3	14.4	11.4	9.2	15.8	3.0	5.0
	adult	%	100	45	37	29	50	10	16
	control	Ratio	154	97	128	146	131	350	200
C	None	No.	155.8	143.8	159.6	107.7	116.1	181.5	137.5
		%	100	91	102	69	75	116	88
		Ratio	195	230	276	247	218	292	307

Note: No.: Average number of mosquitoes (both males and females combined) collected per day per trap. %: Percentage of the average number by taking the precontrol density as 100. Ratio: Sex ratio of the mosquitoes trapped, percentage of males by taking the number of females as 100.

breeding places, and by that of the combination of both methods on the population density of *C. p. fatigans*, as observed by the average number collected per day per trap in four stations in Bangkok.

However, such arbitrary measures are useful only for comparison of the relative population densities according to the seasons of a year, or before and after application of some vector control measures. A more important measure directly proportional to the quantitative aspects of the transmission of filariasis is the density of a vector species attacking per man per unit time (such as ten minutes, or one hour) at a certain hour of the day. By repeating these observations with human bait exposed to the bite of vectors over 24-hour periods, one can obtain the pattern of the biting rhythm of each vector species, and also the average numbers of vectors attacking per day, per month, and per year. From these figures, together with the seasonal changes in the rates and densities of infective stage larvae found in the vector species, one can estimate the force of transmission of filaria from the vector population to the human population, for example, "a person in Rangoon receives an average of 298 infective bites of *C. p. fatigans* per year" (DE MEILLON *et al.*, 1967), or "a person in a village in Pahang,

Malaya, had received 57.9 infective bites of *Mansonia* species in 1954, 28.3 in 1955, and 16.6 in 1956" (WHARTON, 1962).

10C.2.4 The longevity

The age-grouping methods for estimating the physiological age of mosquitoes and other bloodsucking flies (including Simuliidae and Tabanidae) of the order Diptera have been developed by Russian workers (GILLES, 1958; POLOVODOVA, 1959) and described in detail by DETINOVA (1962). The techniques are based on the fact that a small thickening called a follicular relic is formed on the pedicles of ovarioles after each oviposition, and that the number of times of oviposition can be determined for each female fly by dissecting her ovaries. The females which have never deposited eggs, i.e., the nulliparous group, have no relic, while those with a maximum of 1, 2, 3, and n relics on one pedicle indicate that they have already deposited eggs at least 1, 2, 3, and n times, respectively. Under tropical climate, a blood meal is taken a few days after the emergence, and the first batch of eggs are deposited at least three days thereafter. The second blood meal may be taken on the same day soon after the oviposition, or one to several days thereafter. Therefore, the age composition of a mosquito population can be determined by dissecting a large number of specimens collected in an area, and their average life span can be estimated by their physiological age composition. Because it requires at least ten days for filaria larvae to complete development in the mosquito body, the mosquitoes which harbor the infective stage larvae are nearly always parous and contain at least one, usually two or more, relics.

The age-grouping method based on the number of relics on the ovariole tubules was developed first by Russian workers, mainly with *An. maculipennis* in relation to the transmission of malaria. The same technique has been applied successfully for the age-grouping of vectors of filariasis by various workers, such as by BERTRAM & SAMARAWICKREMA (1958) with *Mansonioides*, by LIE *et al.* (1960), SAMARAWICKREMA (1963), HAYASHI & KURIHARA (1965), HAYASHI *et al.* (1965 a,b), and KURIHARA & HAYASHI (1965) with *C. pipiens* complex, and by HAYASHI *et al.* (1965a) with *Ae. togoi.*

The age grouping by examination of follicular relics is, however, a very time-consuming job and requires skill and patience. Some workers prefer a simpler method also described by DETINOVA (1962) for differentiation of the nulliparous and the parous groups by examination of the structure of tracheoles on the ovaries or on the midgut. In nulliparous females, the end of the fine tracheoles is closely wound up into coils or bundles, while in the parous females, the end of fine tracheoles is extended, because both the ovaries and midgut have once been expanded by the eggs or by the blood meal.

HAYASHI *et al.* (1965a) conducted a comparative study on the relationship between the results obtained with the ovariole-relic examination and the tracheole examination methods in *C. p. pallens* and *Ae togoi*. DE MEILLON *et al.* (1967f) used the simple age-grading method for the assessment of the effects of larval control measures on the age composition of *C. p. fatigans* in Rangoon.

YAMAMOTO *et al.* (1966) conducted observations on the effects of indoor residual spraying of fenthion in one village and fenitrothion in another two villages on the population density and the age composition of various mosquito species in endemic areas of *W. bancrofti* filariasis on Amami Island, southern Japan. The collection of mosquitoes was conducted with a sucking tube in several designated houses for 30 minutes (between 8 to 10 p.m.) The insecticides were diluted in water to a concentration of 0.5%, and were sprayed on the walls of all houses in the villages at a rate of 50 ml per m². Altogether, 17 species of mosquitoes were collected in the villages before the insecticides were sprayed. *C. p. fatigans*, the major vector of *W. bancrofti* transmission in this region, was shown to have disappeared completely for three weeks after the spraying in all of the three villages, and remained extremely rare for a period of two months, after which the observation was suspended. The age composition of this mosquito species before the insecticide spray, as obtained by dissection of 279 females, was 54.1% nulliparous, 42.3% uniparous, and 3.58% biparous, while the ratio observed by dissection of 21 females after the spraying was 57.1% nulliparous and 42.9% uniparous. Therefore, it was estimated that the insecticide spraying remarkably reduced the population densities of *C. p. fatigans*, but caused no significant change in their age composition. On the other hand, no appreciable changes in age composition or reductions in the population densities were seen in other common mosquitoes, such as *C. tritaeniorhynchus*, *C. pseudovishnui*, or *An. sinensis*.

10C.2.5 The anthropophilism

The insect vectors of human or animal diseases always select host species when taking a blood meal, and such a behavior is expressed by the term 'anthropophilism' contrary to the term 'zoophilism.' There are various grades of anthropophilism or zoophilism according to the blood-sucking arthropod species. As already discussed in Section 10A.2.2.5, the grade of anthropophilism as expressed by the human blood index (the percentage of human blood among the blood meals taken by an insect population in nature) is an important figure in estimating the vectorial capacity.

The anthropophilism or zoophilism of various mosquito species in an area can be estimated by the simultaneous use of mosquito-net traps baited with various animals (such as man, goat, chicken, etc.), by the method such as reported by SASA & SABIN (1950). It can also be determined by precipitin test of large numbers of blood samples collected from midgut of freshly engorged insect populations.

10C.3 Entomological surveys relevant to the vector control

10C.3.1 The behavior of vectors

Effective control of a vector species can be achieved, in general, only after its behavior in nature is fully understood through basic studies. These include: The behavior of larvae, such as the type of breeding places, habitats, and food; the behavior of pupae, their habitats, and emergence to the adults; the behavior of adults, especially the place and time of copulation of adults; the gonotrophic cycle, biting rhythm, host preference, time and place of oviposition, the daytime resting place, the flight range, etc.

> For mosquitoes: see Section 2E
> For biting midges: see Section 4D
> For horse flies: see Section 3.5
> For black flies: see Section 5.5

10C.3.2 The insecticide susceptibility

The tests for insecticide susceptibility of larvae, pupae, and adults of the vector population are necessary for the selection of insecticides to be used in the vector control program, and large numbers of studies were conducted by various workers with respect to the effects of insecticides against different stages of vector species. Certain standard methods have been proposed by the WHO EXPERT COMMITTEE ON INSECTICIDE (1963, 1970) for the assessment of the susceptibility level of larvae and adults of vector insects (including mosquitoes, biting midges, black flies, and horse flies) to organochlorine, organophosphorous, and carbamate insecticides.

10C.3.2.1 Laboratory test methods

When selecting insecticides to be used in vector control, and in determining the dose of insecticide in practical applications, it is necessary to standardize methods for laboratory tests of the toxicity of chemical compounds against various stages of vectors. Various methods have been used by previous workers, among which the following are outlines proposed as standards by the WHO EXPERT COMMITTEE ON INSECTICIDES (1963, 13th Report; 1970, 17th Report).

(a) Mosquito larvae

For a test with one insecticide, about 300 third or early fourth stage larvae of the same species are collected from a breeding place. Lots of 20 to 25 larvae are distributed with a pipette in each of 12 small beakers, each beaker containing 25 ml of water. Into each of 12 glass vessels, approximately 7.5 to 10 cm in diameter (jars, bottles, or 500 ml beakers), 225 ml of water (free from chlorine and organic contaminants) is placed. The test should be made at about 25°C. Test insecticides dissolved in ethanol at given serial concentrations are prepared, and 1 ml each of insecticide solution is added to each vessel, and mixed well by stirring vigorously with a pipette. Then mosquito larvae in 24 ml of water are added to each vessel, giving a final volume of 250 ml.

Mortality counts are made after 24 hours of exposure to the given concentrations of insecticides. The larvae that have pupated during the test are discarded. Moribund larvae showing various signs of intoxication are counted as dead.

A series of two-fold dilution is used usually for each insecticide, and there should be two replicates for each concentration. When the titer of LC-50 is roughly known, additional intermediate concentrations may be prepared in order to obtain more precise values of LC-50. In general, it is important to obtain not less than three mortality counts between 10% and 90% in a final test. The standard solutions of insecticides for these tests are available in test kits from WHO. The results are recorded on the forms provided by WHO, and also on a logarithmic probability paper to draw regression lines for obtaining the LC-50 or LC-90 from the graph.

(b) Adult mosquitoes

A test kit for determining the susceptibility of adult mosquitoes to certain insecticides has been designed by WHO. It is composed of: (1) 20 plastic tubes (125 mm long by 44 mm in diameter, each fitted at one end with a 16 mesh screen; half of these tubes are used for pre-test sorting and post-exposure observation, and another half for exposing mosquitoes to insecticides, including the control exposure without insecticide; (2) ten slide units, each with a screw-cap on either side and provided with a 20 mm filling hole; (3) five packages of papers impregnated with DDT in mineral oil (Risella 17, Shell) at concentrations of 0.25%, 0.5%, 1.0%, 2.0%, and 4.0%, respectively, one package treated with oil only, seven packages of papers impregnated with dieldrin in mineral oil at two-fold series of concentrations from 0.05% to 3.2%; similar series of papers impregnated with malathion, fenthion, and fenitrothion are also available; (4) sheets of clean paper for lining the holding tubes; (5) clips to hold the papers in position; (6) glass aspirator tubes, 12 mm in internal diameter, connected with 60 cm rubber tube.

Procedure: Approximately 200 female mosquitoes are collected with the aspirator, and are transferred to the holding tubes, 15 to 25 mosquitoes per tube. The holding tubes are set upright, screen end up, for one hour, and at the end of this time the damaged insects are removed. A sheet of impregnated paper is introduced into each tube, rolled into a cylinder to line the wall, and is fastened with a clip. The mosquitoes are introduced into the exposure tube from the holding tube by the aid of the slide. The mosquitoes are exposed to the impregnated paper for one hour under diffuse illumination, and are again transferred to the holding tube or other suitable containers, such as a paper cup. A pad of wet cotton wool is placed on the top screen of the container. Mortality counts are made after 24 hours. Such a test is usually repeated four times with the same population of mosquitoes, and the results are listed in a table and also plotted on a logarithmic probability graph paper to obtain the LC-50 and LC-90. In cases where the control mortality is between 5% and 20%, the percentage mortality should be corrected by Abbott's formula

$$\frac{(\% \text{ test mortality} - \% \text{ control mortality})}{(100 - \% \text{ control mortality})} \times 100.$$

(c) Black fly larvae

Tentative instructions for determining the susceptibility or resistance of black fly larvae to insecticides were given by the WHO EXPERT COMMITTEE ON INSECTICIDES (1963). Larvae are taken from natural breeding places by collecting the submerged and trailing grasses to which they are attached. For transport to the laboratory, the vegatation with attached larvae is kept wet in a bucket or plastic bag, but must not be immersed in water. In this way the larvae will stay in good condition for two or three hours.

Twelve glass cylindrical jars of about five liters capacity are used, six for separating larvae and six others for exposure of larvae to insecticides. For the extraction of larvae from the field material, six jars are filled with clean stream water, and a vertical glass plate (approximately 10 cm × 30 cm) is inserted on one side of each jar. By means of an electric pump, a steady stream of compressed air is directed against the foot of the glass plate through a glass tube drawn out into a fine point, thus producing a stream of air bubbles rinsing vertically to the top of the glass plate. When grass with attached larvae is immersed in these jars, larvae are induced to leave the vegetation and congregate on the glass plate along the stream of bubbles in the course of a few hours.

While this extraction of larvae is proceeding, the second set of six containers is filled to the five-liter mark and the required amount of insecticide solution is added to five of them to produce a series of concentrations from 0.01 to 0.25 ppm. In the sixth jar, used as a control, an equal amount of solvent only is placed.

Each of the glass plates in the first series of jars containing a standard number of attached larvae (only fourth stage; early stages and excess larvae are removed by forceps) is quickly transferred to the corresponding position in one of the insecticide testing jars, and a continuous stream of air bubbles is immediately directed onto it.

After 30 minutes of exposure, the plates with attached larvae are quickly removed from the testing jar and placed back in their original positions in the first series of jars. The mortality counts are usually made after 24 hours.

In an alternative method, twelve enamel or glass trays are used in place of the glass jars, stream water is introduced to a depth of 1.0 to 1.5 cm, and compressed air is injected into the water with a drawn-out pipette along one side of the tray; 25 to 50 first instar larvae collected from vegetation by gentle handling with forceps are introduced onto each tray. When the larvae have attached themselves to the trays, the water is removed gently and is replaced by an equal amount of diluted insecticide solution. Two replicates should be done at each concentration, and two control replicates. After 30 minutes of exposure, the insecticide solution is removed gently, and the trays are rinsed gently with river water, and refilled with the same amount of river water as before. The water in each tray is changed every 4 to 6 hours, and the mortality counts are made after 24 hours.

(d) Adult black flies

Tentative instructions for determining the susceptibility or resistance of adult black flies to insecticides was also presented by the WHO EXPERT COMMITTEE ON INSECTICIDES (1963). The test kit used in this test and the procedures are almost the same as that in the test of adult mosquitoes. The same or similar kits and procedures may be applied in the tests for determining the susceptibility of adult *Culicoides* and *Chrysops*.

10C.3.2.2 Field test methods

The laboratory tests for determining the susceptibility of various stages of filaria vectors to insecticides are useful in collecting baseline data for standardizing the methods to be applied in the fields, but the effectiveness of various insecticides in the field must be evaluated by field studies. For example, the toxicity level of various insecticides obtained in laboratory tests against mosquito larvae are based on exposure in clean, stagnant water for certain time periods, but in the field, the insecticides may be applied on the mosquito larvae in highly polluted waters, or in running waters. Likewise, the toxicity level obtained with the filter paper surface of WHO test kits of various insecticides to adult mosquitoes may not be applicable to the walls of houses.

Large numbers of reports have been made on the results of field tests with various methods with respect to the effectiveness of insecticides against disease vectors, including those transmitting filariasis.

As reviewed by WRIGHT (1971), the World Health Organization established in 1960 a program for evaluating and testing new insecticides with the special objective of finding new compounds that would overcome the problem of insecticide resistance and not lead to further contamination of the environment. The procedure for the screening of insecticides is composed of the following seven stages.

Stage I: screening of compounds by the insecticidal activity; criteria for acceptance are either a 24-hour mortality of 50% at 16 μg per cm^2 after exposure of adult mosquitoes for one hour as residue, or 50% kill at 0.1 ppm in 24-hour exposure of mosquito larvae, or 24-hour mortality of 50% at 1 μg per fly in topical application.

Stage II: further laboratory tests of toxicity to laboratory animals and various other insects of medical importance.

Stage III: simulated field trials of insecticides against adult mosquitoes, larval mosquitoes, lice, and fleas.

Stage IV: tests of compounds on naturally occurring insect populations at various field laboratories.

Stage V: includes village-scale testing of compounds against anophelines by the *Anopheles* Control Unit in Nigeria, and also against various other mosquito vector species, including *C.p. fatigans* and *Ae. aegypti*; toxicological observations on operators.

Stage VI: trials involving human populations up to 25,000 living in several thousand houses; four rounds of spraying are carried out, and the effectiveness and toxicity are evaluated.

Stage VII: compounds passing Stage VI may then move to a full epidemiological evaluation involving populations of up to 100,000 persons; so far, only malathion, propoxur, and fenitrothion have passed these seven stages of evaluation.

By the end of 1970, almost 1,400 compounds of all types had passed through Stage I; of this total, 1,265 were insecticides, the remainder were rodenticides, chemosterilants, synergists, and growth-inhibiting compounds. In tests against adult anophelines, 41 compounds were evaluated in huts; 19 failed to meet the criteria for effectiveness and 2 were considered unsuitable because of lachrymatory effects. Twenty were assessed in villages at Stage V; of these, 3 compounds were considered to be unsafe, 6 compounds were proposed for large-scale field trials, of which trials of malathion, propoxur, and fenitrothion have been completed. In tests against mosquito larvae, 18 compounds were evaluated at Stage IV for the control of *C.p. fatigans* in polluted water; carbamates were generally ineffective as mosquito larvicides, and most of organophosphorous compounds were rapidly decomposed; only diazinon, fenthion, and Dursban were found to withstand such decomposition. In the tests with *Ae. aegypti* larvae, Abate was shown to be by far the best in effectiveness and safety.

10C.3.2.3 Some observations on the toxicity of insecticides

One of the prerequisites of insecticides to be used in vector control is the high toxicity to the vectors in contrast to the relative safety to other living organisms, including their natural enemies. In selecting insecticides in the control of mosquito larvae in certain environments, such as most of the sewage pools containing stagnant waters, it is desired to use an insecticide which is safe to the mosquito-eating fishes. SASA *et al.* (1965b), for example, tested the toxicity of 12 kinds of chlorinated hydrocarbon and organophosphorous insecticides to the larvae of *C. p. fatigans* and *Ae. aegypti*, as well as to the guppy, *Lebistes*, and obtained the results summarized in Table 10-9. These authors calculated the safety index for each insecticide, which is the ratio between LC-95 (the concentration at which 95% of test animals are killed) for mosquito larvae and LC-05 (the concentration at which 5% of test animals are killed) for the fish. In this case, the concentration of fenitrothion required for killing 95% of *C. p. fatigans*

Table 10-9. Relative toxicity of insecticides to larvae of *Culex pipiens fatigans*, *Aedes aegypti* and to a mosquito-eating fish guppy, *Lebistes reticulatus* (Provisional estimates of lethal concentrations in ppm with the respective percent mortality, based on laboratory experiments at 28 to 30°C in 24-hours exposure, for wild colonies collected at Din Dang, southeast Bangkok, after SASA *et al.*, 1965b).

Insecticides	*fatigans*		*aegypti*		*Lebistes*	Safety
	LC-95	LC-50	LC-95	LC-50	LC-05	index
1. *p, p′*-DDT	1.5	0.3	0.2	0.05	0.01	0.007
2. tech. DDT	1.0	0.2	0.2	0.06	0.01	0.01
3. Lindane	0.6	0.1	0.05	0.5	0.3	0.5
4. Chlordane	1.6	0.3	0.2	0.3	0.1	0.06
5. Dieldrin	0.16	0.04	0.03	0.02	0.005	0.03
6. Diazinon	0.05	0.03	0.07	0.3	0.2	4.0
7. Malathion	0.08	0.03	0.05	1.0	0.3	4.0
8. Sumithion	0.006	0.003	0.004	5.5	4.5	750.
9. Fenthion	0.006	0.003	0.004	5.0	4.0	670.
10. Ronnel	0.008	0.005	0.04	2.5	1.5	200.
11. Dichlorvos	0.05	0.025	0.03	7.0	3.0	60.
12. Trichlorfon	0.06	0.03	0.07	10.0	4.0	67.

Safety index: LC-05 (or maximum safety concentration) against *Lebistes* divided by LC-95 (or minimum effective concentration) against *fatigans*.

larvae was about 750 times lower than the concentration slightly toxic to the fish, while the relation was reversed for DDT and other chlorinated hydrocarbon insecticides. In the field tests, it was also shown that application of fenitrothion in sewage pools at a concentration between 0.1 and 1.0 ppm kills all mosquito larvae, but none of the fishes were killed at this concentration.

The acute toxicity of various compounds to man is usually estimated from the results of tests with laboratory mice or rats. Table 10-10 shows LD-50 values of various insecticides in oral and cutaneous administration to mice and rats.

10C.3.3 Survey of natural enemies and pathogens

Field studies of natural enemies, parasites, and pathogens of disease vectors comprise an important but so far rather neglected aspect of information to be collected as baseline data for orientation of the control activities. As reviewed by JENKINS (1964), large numbers of species of microorganisms, protozoans, plants, and invertebrate, as well as vertebrate animals are known to act as natural enemies (pathogens, parasites, or predators) of various disease vectors. However, most of the previous reports contain only sporadic records, and the role of natural enemies in

Table 10-10.   LC-50 values (mg per kg of body weight) of various insecticides (after UEDA & NISHIMURA, quoted by SUZUKI & OGATA, 1968).

Insecticides	In mice		In rats	
	oral	cutaneous	oral	cutaneous
Chlorinated hydrocarbons:				
DDT	258	2,050	390	—
lindane	96	140	204	—
chlordane	290	480	534	—
dieldrin	45	76	140	370
Organophosphorus:				
parathion	6	22	10	—
diazinon	53	115	132	—
malathion	570	2,300	910	—
dichlorvos	70	200	110	—
trichlorfon	600	1,900	890	3,600
Dibrom (naled)	180	600	360	—
ronnel	875	—	—	—
fenitrothion	780	2,730	340	—
fenthion	74	170	—	—
Pyrethroids:				
allethrin	445	1,200	—	—

population control of the vectors or their possibility for use as a biocontrol measure have generally remained unclarified.

As reported by SASA *et al.* (1965c) and SASA (1972), some poeciliid fishes introduced from the New World have established in breeding places of *C. p. fatigans* or other filariasis vectors in South Asia rather naturally or after being artificially released, and careless use of some insecticides which are toxic to fishes was found to increase the breeding of mosquitoes while reducing the larvae for only a short period.

While engaged in field studies on the bionomics of mosquito vectors of Japanese encephalitis in Okayama, this author was deeply impressed by the presence of large numbers of their natural enemies, both in adult and larval stages (SASA *et al.*, 1968). It was suggested that destruction of the naturally balanced fauna in waters of rice paddies and swamps by application of broad-spectrum insecticides such as BHC, which kills almost all animals in rice paddies, would result in the increase of insect pests of both rice and man. The high mortality of mosquito and black fly larvae in nature is mainly due to the occurrence of predators, parasites, and pathogens.

In collecting baseline data referring to the bionomics of the vectors, it is recommended to study the natural enemies and their significance in the population control of the vectors, and to explore possible measures of vector control without causing destruction of these biocontrol agents. It should also be noted that some of them might be used as biocontrol agents when methods are established for the mass breeding, as discussed in Section 10D.3.2.3.

10D. The control of filariasis

10D.1 Present status of filariasis control programs

As stated in the previous chapters, regional or national programs for the control of filariasis are in progress or now being organized in a number of endemic areas. The present status of these programs may be classified roughly into the following three categories.

(1) Where a country-wide filariasis control program has been organized:

    Pacific Islands: The Society Islands, American Samoa, Western Samoa, Fiji, etc.

    Asia: India, Sri Lanka, Thailand, West Malaysia, China, Japan

    Central and South Americas: Brazil

(2) Where pilot control programs in restricted areas are in progress:

    Pacific Islands: Tonga

    Asia: Burma, Philippines, Indonesia, Korea

    Central and South Americas: Guyana, Surinam, French Guiana

    Africa: Egypt

(3) Where control programs may be in preparation, but are not yet organized:

    The endemic areas not included in the above categories: include most parts of Africa; Nepal, Bangladesh, Laos, Khmer, Vietnam; Papua New Guinea, Micronesian islands.

10D.2 Planning and organization of filariasis control programs

In planning a malaria eradication/control program on a national scale, the WHO EXPERT COMMITTEE ON MALARIA (1957, Sixth Report) defined four consecutive phases: the preparatory phase, the attack phase, the consolidation phase, and the maintenance phase. The same or similar processes are required for planning and pursuing a filariasis control program, though the extent of area to be covered and the length of years necessary for each phase, and the techniques to be employed may differ greatly between the two diseases.

The need for establishment of a filariasis control program is decided by the administrative authorities based on information accumulated during the precontrol survey period. The surveys during this period are usually arbitrary and do not cover the whole areas to be investigated. A systematic survey of the extent of distribution and the prevalence of the disease is undertaken as an activity of the preparatory phase. Both antiparasite measures and antivector measures are practiced, so far as feasible, in the attack phase. When the microfilaria rate and density of the human population are reduced below a certain level as the result of control activities, and the control measures which have been directed to the whole population and the whole area are judged to be no longer necessary, the program may go into the surveillance phase. However, the blood surveys, case detection, and entomological surveys are still necessary, at least on sample populations in order to detect the recovery of transmission.

The procedures to be followed in each of the phases were defined in detail for the malaria control/eradication program by E. PAMPANA (1963, *A Textbook of Malaria Eradication, Oxford Univ. Press, 508 pp.*). The following is an outline of the plans and procedures to be followed in a filariasis control program as modified and adapted from the malaria programs.

10D.2.1 Preparatory phase

(a) Geographic reconnaissance of the country's filarious area.
(b) Completion of an epidemiological and entomological study of the same.
(c) Organization of a national filariasis control service (NFCS): recruitment, procurement of equipment and supplies; establishment of offices, stores, workshop, laboratories in the headquarters and the peripheral centers; organization of logistic and reporting systems.
(d) Training of personnel.
(e) Organization of health education of the public in filariasis control.
(f) Carrying out of pilot studies for the control program.

10D.2.2 Attack phase

The attack phase consists of two main parts: the attack operations, and the evaluation operations.
(a) The attack operations: In filariasis control programs, the operations have been directed to various aspects, such as
(a–1) The parasite control: chemotherapy of human parasite carriers by administration of DEC (or other drugs), either nonselectively to the whole population of the target areas, or selectively to only the microfilaria positive cases detected in mass blood surveys.
(a–2) The vector control:
The control of larval breeding places by physical methods (clearing or

management of water), chemical methods (mainly the use of insecticides), and biological methods (mainly the use of natural enemies).

The control of adults by Residual insecticide spray and/or other measures

In contrast to malaria control programs in which the main operation consists of spraying with residual insecticides (such as DDT) to all houses in the target areas, the efforts in most of the successful control programs against *Wuchereria* and *Brugia* infections have been directed mainly to the chemotherapy of human parasite carriers with DEC. The control of adult stage vectors with chlorinated insecticides such as DDT has proved to be ineffective in most filariasis control programs.

In the control of onchocerciasis, the experiences of most previous workers have shown that DEC and other drugs are either too toxic or ineffective for the use in mass administration, while the treatment of rivers and streams with insecticides for the control of black fly larvae has turned out to be successful in some endemic areas (see Section 5.5.3). In other types of filariasis, including the mosquito-borne *Wuchereria* and *Brugia* infections, no satisfactory results have ever been obtained by larval control operation alone, although it was the main part of programs in some countries, such as India (see Section 8A.2).

(b) The evaluation operations:

This is the responsibility of the epidemiological section of the filariasis control program. The operations consist of:

The survey of human populations (examination of incidence and prevalence of microfilaria carriers, clinical cases, skin test positives, etc.; see Section 10B and Chapter 11).

The survey of vector populations (the density of adults and larvae, the infection and infective rates of the adults, the survival rates of adults and larvae, the insecticide susceptibility of adults and larvae, etc.; see Section 10C).

10D.2.3 Surveillance phase

This phase begins when the parasite rate or the vector density has been reduced to a negligible level, and it is judged that the infection will probably die out spontaneously even after all or a majority of the attack operations are stopped. Because filariasis is an extremely slow-developing disease, it is difficult to determine whether the transmission has already ceased or is still in progress from the results of parasitological or entomological survey data accumulated at one time. Therefore, it is desirable, for the sake of safety, to continue the attack operations as long as possible until the parasite or the vector is completely eradicated. However, in filariasis control programs in which the control activities are effective, the time comes, sooner or later, when the project leader must decide that all or a part of the attack operations should be suspended, at least for some period. In the surveillance phase, examinations of sampled human populations for the detection of new microfilaria carriers, as well as the entomological assessments of the density and infection rate of the vector population, are the main operations. It should be noted that the attack operations may have to be resumed, at least in areas where significant numbers of new or recurrent cases have appeared.

10D.3 Methods in control operations

The filariasis control operations are directed, as a principle, both to the reduction of human parasite carriers by chemotherapy, and to the reduction of infected vector populations by physical (or environmental), chemical (mainly insecticidal), biological, or genetic measures.

10D.3.1 Methods in parasite control

(a) The drugs to be used in chemotherapy
As discussed in Section 10E.1, several groups of compounds have proved to be effective as chemotherapeutics against various species of human or animal filariae. At the present stage, however, the only drug which can be commonly used in the mass treatment of infected human populations is DEC; all the others were shown to be either too toxic for general use, or unsatisfactory in efficacy. In *Wuchereria* and *Brugia* infections in man, DEC has been shown to be effective and safely administered so long as the drug administration program is adequately organized. However, special care should be taken for administration of DEC in areas where *L. loa* or *O. volvulus* is endemic, because the drug may cause severe side reactions in those who harbor the microfilariae of *L. loa* or *O. volvulus* at high densities. Other drugs, including arsenical or antimonial compounds and suramine, should be administered in hospital under careful observation for side effects.

(b) The populations to be treated (mass treatment or selective treatment?)
There have been two different methods employed in the control of parasite carriers, namely, the mass treatment of entire populations of the endemic areas, and the selective treatment of microfilaria positive cases detected in blood surveys of the whole population. Both methods have merits and demerits. In areas where the prevalence of filariasis is high, it is generally recommended to treat the whole population with DEC, regardless of the presence or absence of microfilariae in the examinations of blood samples, because there usually exist many people among the microfilaria negative group who are actually infected and need to be treated with the drug.

Mass treatment of the whole population is usually practicable and effective in areas where the human populations to be treated are clearly differentiated from those of nonendemic areas, such as the islands in the South Pacific. In countries like India, mass drug administration was once tried but soon abandoned for various reasons. In Japan, Sri Lanka, and Brazil, effective filariasis control programs are in progress, not by the mass treatment method, but by the selective treatment of the microfilaria positive cases, mainly because the endemic areas are so widespread and have varying prevalence rates.

(c) Dosage regimens of the treatment

Various dosage regimens were employed in the mass or selective treatments with DEC. In the treatment of *Wuchereria* and *Brugia* infections, it has been shown that daily doses of 6 mg per kg of DEC citrate at daily, weekly, or monthly intervals for 12 doses (72 mg per kg in total) is an effective and practicable schedule. About 80 to 90% of microfilaria positive cases turn out to be negative after completion of this treatment. With lower dosages, such as a five-day treatment of 4 mg per kg per day employed in India, the cure rates are lower, though the attack rate of the febrile reactions may be the same as with the above larger dosages. The administration of DEC at monthly intervals for 12 or more months has been employed in the mass treatment of whole populations in the South Pacific islands (see Section 9E). The weekly administration method has been recommended by workers in Malaya in the treatment of *Brugia* infection. The daily administration method has been practiced widely in the treatment of *Wuchereria* cases in Japan, Sri Lanka, Brazil, China, etc.

(d) Distribution of the drug

In endemic areas of *Wuchereria* or *Brugia* only, DEC can usually be administered safely to the public even by nonmedical workers, such as has been practiced in many countries in Asia and the Pacific. However, the attendance and supervision of a physician or a medical officer is desirable at least on the occasion of administration of the first dose, because it is expected that the persons showing microfilaremia at high densities may have fever reactions which could be dangerous when combined with other, already existing diseases. The attack rate and the grade of fever reaction due to DEC is highly correlated with the microfilarial level of individual cases, and is a sign of cure from the infection, as stated previously (Section 2B. 5. 3). Therefore, health education of the public on the mode of effects and side reactions of the drug must be practiced before the drug is administered in order to have the full cooperation of the people.

In some countries, the drug is distributed by house-to-house visit of health workers, and the amount necessary for the full course of the treatment is handed over to the households at one time. In such a system, it is difficult to supervise the treatment. So far as possible, the tablets should be delivered by the hand of health workers into the mouth of individual cases and it should be confirmed that they are really swallowed. This was the practice in Okinawa (Section 8C.5).

(e) Administration of DEC by medicated salt, food, or drink

Since DEC citrate is a compound soluble in water, colorless, almost tasteless (only slightly sour and bitter in high concentration), and stable at high temperatures, it can be administered mixed in cooking salt, food, or drink. The procedure for controlling malaria by incorporating antimalarial compounds in cooking salt was introduced by PINOTTI, in Brazil, in 1952, and was reported to be successful at least in some regions under certain conditions, such as reported by GIGLIOLI *et al.* (1967) in Guyana.

One of the earliest trials of this sort in the treatment of filariasis was the administration of the drug mixed in orangeade in the treatment of infant carriers in Amami beginning August 1958. Samples of the drug were prepared by mixing diethylcarbamazine citrate into commercial orangeade powder at the ratios of 5%, 10%, and 15%. Two grams of the powder are dissolved in a cup to make a medicated drink, containing 0.1 g, 0.2 g, and 0.3 g of DEC, respectively. These samples were especially useful in the treatment of infants under school age, or primary school pupils. In a blood survey of primary school pupils in Koniya Town, 67 were positive for microfilariae of *W. bancrofti* out of 655 persons examined. The positive pupils were assembled in a classroom every day for 14 days at lunch time to take a cup of medicated orangeade, which contained DEC at a rate of 2 mg per kg for the first three days and 6 mg per kg for the remaining 11 days, with a total dose of 72 mg per kg. At a posttreatment blood examination conducted five months thereafter, all of the previously positive cases became negative for the microfilariae except for a boy who had only one microfilaria in a 30 mm^3 blood sample. No unpleasant side effects occurred in the children thus treated, except that four among them had fever on the second day only. Because infants of primary school age or younger generally refuse or are unable to take drug tablets, this method was also useful in the treatment of children in the villages.

KANDA *et al.* (1967) conducted trial treatments of microfilaria carriers in a dormitory by providing DEC medicated "miso soup" every morning at a rate of about 2 mg per kg for 32 successive days. Of 14 cases with microfilariae, four were still positive in a blood examination conducted four weeks after the start of the treatment, but all of them were found to be negative one year later. The same medicated "miso" containing 50 g of DEC per 1 kg was distributed to all households in three villages of Amami Island, and the housewives were instructed to add one spoonful (about 2 g) of the medicated miso per person to their miso soup every morning for 32 days. In a blood survey carried out six months after the treatment, the microfilariae disappeared from all of 31 previously positive cases with the exception of one person who had only one microfilaria in his 30 mm^3 blood sample. Because miso (fermented soy bean) is taken as soup every morning by almost everybody in the endemic areas of filariasis in Japan, this method also proved useful in the mass treatment.

HAWKING & MARQUES (1967) carried out a pilot trial at Recife, Brazil, of the use of DEC-medicated salt for the mass treatment of *W. bancrofti* filariasis. Laboratory trials showed that cooking DEC in food did not make it toxic for rats or diminish its antifilarial activity. Cooking salt containing 0.4% DEC (corresponding to a daily intake of 100 mg per day) was given to 1,000 adults for 40 days, and then, salt containing 0.1% of the compound for a year. This medication was simple to administer; it was quite acceptable to the subjects; it caused no untoward effects; and it removed almost all the microfilariae from the blood. Administration of medicated salt (0.3%) for 18 days to another group of 1,300 adults was well tolerated and produced a considerable reduction of the microfilarial load, but this short period was insufficient to remove all the microfilariae.

DAVID & BAILEY (1969) reported on results of a trial conducted in Tanzania on the effect on *W. bancrofti* microfilariae of DEC-medicated salt (0.1%) given to a closed population (prisoners) of 600 to 700 with a known salt intake. In a pretreatment survey of 672 persons, 148 or 22.0% were positive; in the second pretreatment survey, 71 (35.0%) of 203 new admissions were positive. Blood examinations of the previously positive cases were repeated once every month for six months after the start of medication. The mean microfilarial densities fell steadily, being reduced by 73% at three months and 90% after six months. The intake of DEC in a ration of 14 g of salt per person per day is estimated to be 14 mg, or about 2.52 g (42 mg per kg) as a total of six months. The authors suggested that a trial with salt containing 0.2% DEC may achieve optimum results.

According to a report of the INDIAN COUNCIL OF MEDICAL RESEARCH (ICMR) (1971) on assessment of the National Filaria Control Program, pilot studies were conducted in two villages in India for the control of *W. bancrofti* filariasis by instituting regimes of common salt medicated with 0.1% DEC. In the field study undertaken in Parbatpur Village, Uttar Pradesh, it was shown that (a) the regime covering eight weeks was found acceptable to the population, (b) 94% reduction in a number of circulating microfilariae was achieved in the index population and considerable reduction was also seen in the vector infection rate, and (c) the reactions noted were mild, and from the third week onward there were no complaints of reactions.

In another study at Nelaturu Village, Andhra Pradesh, the medicated salt regime was started so as to cover 1,227 persons of all age-groups in 350 human dwellings. The medicated salt was distributed to each family on a regular weekly visit basis for 12 weeks (January to April 1969). The regime was interrupted for a period of nine weeks, and resumed by distribution of the medicated salt from grocers in the villages, which continued for another period of 33 weeks. In the precontrol survey, 26.32% of 1,227 persons of all ages were positive for microfilariae, and the average microfilarial den-

sity per 20 mm³ of blood was 47.48. In a postcontrol survey, only 3.7%
of 913 persons examined were positive, and the average microfilarial density was 2.5. The results indicated about an 86% reduction in the number
of microfilaria carriers and about a 95% reduction in the average microfilarial density. Marked decline was also noted in the vector infection.

10D.3.2 Methods in vector control

In the control of filariasis vectors, there is no general method which
can be applied effectively to all the species or to all types of endemic areas.
Sometimes, entirely different methods are recommended in the control of
even the same species of vectors according to the environment.

In contrast to malaria control programs in which control of adult mosquitoes by residual house spraying of insecticides is usually the operation
of primary importance, the main operation in filariasis control has been the
drug-treatment of human parasite carriers, and the vector control operations were usually of only secondary importance. The house spraying with
residual insecticides has been shown to be almost ineffective in the control
of *C. p. fatigans*, the main vector of *W. bancrofti* in large parts of the world.
Except for certain Temperate Zone countries where general improvements
of sanitary conditions have resulted in the reduction of vector mosquitoes
and further, to spontaneous reduction or disappearance of filariasis cases,
no successful results have been obtained in the tropical countries by vector
control alone.

Methods in filariasis vector control may be classified into three categories, namely, (a) the physical measures (mainly, clearing of breeding
places by environmental sanitation methods), (b) the chemical measures
(mainly, the use of insecticides against adults or immature stages), and (c)
the biological measures (mainly, the use of natural enemies or pathogens,
or by genetic manipulations).

10D.3.2.1 Physical measures in vector control

There have been ample examples of trials in vector control by physical
measures, especially by the clearing of breeding places by various environmental sanitation methods

In mosquitoes of the *C. pipiens* complex, the immature stages develop in
sewage water pools and artificial containers, and thus, construction of adequate sewage systems obviously reduces the population density. However,
as frequently seen in the semiurban areas in Japan, inadequate construction of open sewage ditches has increased the breeding of mosquito larvae.
The installation of a pipe-water supply system also reduces the breeding of
the mosquitoes, because the main breeding places such as wells (in Egypt,
see Section 7A.1) or various rainwater containers (in Japan, see Section
8C.5) become unnecessary for the people.

In areas where swamp-breeding mosquitoes act as filariasis vectors, construction of adequate drainage systems for drying up the swamps and converting the land for agricultural use is also effective for the purpose of filariasis (or malaria) control. In endemic areas of *B. malayi* where *Mansonioides* mosquitoes serve as the main vectors, removal by hand of their host plants, such as *Pistia*, has been recommended as a measure of filariasis control (Sectons 8A.2; 8A.4).

The so-called nonperiodic race of *W. bancrofti* in the Polynesian islands is transmitted mainly by day-biting mosquitoes of the subgenus *Stegomyia*, genus *Aedes*. Their larvae breed mainly in small rainwater containers, and thus the removal of empty cans, discarded bottles, used tires, coconut shells, and various other breeding places around houses is effective in reducing the vector population. However, complete eradication of the mosquitoes by manpower only is usually difficult, because the larvae also use other natural water containers for the breeding, such as tree holes in the jungle, the leaf axils of various wild plants, and crab holes in sandy beaches (see Section 2E.3).

10D.3.2.2 Chemical measures in vector control

The use of insecticides in vector control has been extensively investigated, especially in connection with malaria eradication programs, such as reviewed by MACDONALD (1957) and PAMPANA (1963). Although promising results have been reported on the use of chemosterilants and insect hormones in vector control, there still exist a number of problems to be solved before these can be approved for general use in the control of filariasis vectors.

The insecticides which have been commonly used in vector control fall into four groups: (1) the naturally occurring substances or their allies synthesized artificially (especially the pyrethroids); (2) the chlorinated hydrocarbon insecticides including DDT, BHC, chlordane dieldrin, etc.; and (3) the organophosphorous insecticides or phosphoric acid esters of various organic compounds, including the "notorious" parathion, but also safer compounds such as malathion, diazinon, dichlorvos, trichlorfon, fenthion, fenitrothion, and Abate; and (4) other miscellaneous compounds, including some carbamates. Because of the usefulness of insecticides in the control of insects pests of agricultural and medical importances, tremendous numbers of studies have been conducted in this field of the sciences.

Methods for testing the effects of various insecticides on filariasis vectors are discussed in Section 10C.3.2 of this book. The problems of insecticide resistance were reviewed in detail by BROWN (1958) and the WHO EXPERT COMMITTEE ON INSECTICIDES (13th Report, 1963; 17th Report, 1970, etc.). In general, chlorinated hydrocarbon insecticides (including DDT) have been shown to have little effect and their use contraindicated in the control of the mosquito vectors of filariasis, mainly because of the development of resistance. DDT was once used in the control of black fly larvae in onchocerciasis endemic areas, but is now not recommended for this purpose because of its destructive and cumulative effects on the environment. As alternative insecticides, a number of organophosphorous compounds or pyrethroids have been tested and some of them have proved to be useful. An extensive review on the alternative insecticides for vector control was published by various authors in *Bul. Wld Hlth Org.* Vol. 44, Nos. 1, 2, 3, pp. 1–470. A detailed description of the modern equipment to be used in vector control was also published by the WORLD HEALTH ORGANIZATION (1974).

(a) Control of adult vectors by indoor spraying of residual insecticides:
This is a method widely used and highly effective in most malaria control programs. The treatment of walls with 5 % DDT suspension in water, sprayed at a rate of 40 ml per m^2 (2g of DDT per m^2) has been a routine procedure in malaria vector control operations. There has been some evidence of the reduction or disappearance of filariasis in connection with the progress of DDT house-spraying programs for the control of malaria, such as observed with *B. malayi* infection in Sri Lanka (see Section 8A.4). Several workers have attempted the control of filariasis vectors by indoor spraying of residual insecticides (KOHLER, 1949, and BROWN & WILLIAMS, 1949, in St. Croix; WHARTON & SANTA MARIA, 1958, in Malaya; IKESHOJI *et al.*, 1959 and SASA *et al.*, 1959, 1960, in Japan; IYENGAR *et al.*, 1959, in New Guinea), but the results were mostly unsatisfactory and the spraying operations have been abandoned in most endemic areas. The reason for failure was either the development of resistance to the insecticides or the absence in the vectors of the behavior of coming in contact with the walls of houses.
The insecticide most commonly used for the indoor spraying has been DDT, because of its long-lasting effects when deposited on the wall surface. However, most insects, including *C. p. fatigans*, house flies, bedbugs, and fleas, easily develop resistance to DDT, and thus the operations become ineffective against these pests. Dieldrin was used by SASA *et al.* (1959, 1960) in the endemic areas of *W. bancrofti* in southern Japan but it was shown to become ineffective after several weeks. The development of resistance to DDT and to dieldrin in *pipiens* complex was demonstrated in analytical studies by SUZUKI *et al.* (1964) and UMINO & SUZUKI (1964) in Japan. On the other hand, promising results in the use of fenitrothion for indoor spraying against *C. p. fatigans* were reported by KURIHARA *et al.* (1965) in Bangkok. Malathion (3 % solution in kerosene) was used in the initial stage of the filariasis control program in Okinawa, as reported by MARSHALL & YASUKAWA (1966), but the effects of this operation on the control of *C. p. fatigans* and on the transmission of filariasis were not adequately evaluated.
In general, the method of indoor spraying of residual insecticides is effective against disease vectors which are endophilic (coming to bite man inside houses, and staying on walls before and after taking a blood meal), and those which do not develop insecticide resistance at least for periods of greater than several years. Most malaria vectors, including *An. minimus*

in Southeast Asia, are examples of this type of bloodsucking insect. Mosquitoes of the *An. gambiae* complex, the main vectors of malaria and *W. bancrofti* in Africa, are known to develop resistance to DDT rather easily. As demonstrated in a series of studies conducted by SUZUKI and associates (1962–1967) in the author's laboratory, mosquitoes of the *C. pipiens* complex are also examples of vectors which easily develop insecticide resistance and thus their control by indoor spraying is difficult. It has also been experienced in many areas where DDT spraying is repeated that the people complain about the increase of other insect pests by this operation, especially of bedbugs, fleas, house flies, cockroaches, which apparently have developed resistance.

It has also been demonstrated by various workers that insects develop resistance more easily to chlorinated hydrocarbon insecticides (including DDT, BHC, dieldrin and chlordane) than to most organophosphorous insecticides (including parathion, malathion, diazinon, fenthion, ronnel, fenitrothion, dichlorvos, and trichlorfon).

Most *Simulium* vectors of human onchocerciasis and the *Chrysops* vectors of human loiasis are exophilic biters, and thus the indoor spraying operations will probably have no effect. However, some of the *Culicoides* flies that transmit *Dipetalonema* and *Mansonella* infections in man are known to be endophilic and therefore, effective control may be achieved if an insecticide, such as fenitrothion, is extensively used in residual spraying of the whole area.

(b) Control of immature stage vectors with insecticides:
Various insecticides have been used in the control of larval stage vectors of human filariasis. In some countries, including India, the use of mosquito larvicides still constitutes the main operation of the antifilariasis campaign. In Sri Lanka, a very systematic treatment of the larval breeding places of *C. p. fatigans* has been conducted, together with the treatment of human microfilaria carriers with DEC (ABDULCADER & SASA, 1966). In some endemic areas of onchocerciasis in East Africa, the control of black fly larvae by application of DDT into rivers resulted in successful control of the disease (see Section 5.5.3).

Crude petroleum is used as a cheap mosquito larvicide in many tropical countries even now. However, petroleum is not recommendable as a mosquito larvicide because its effect is not satisfactory even when large doses are sprayed, it causes environmental pollution, and costs much more than other adequately used insecticides.

Some chlorinated hydrocarbon insecticides, including DDT, BHC, and dieldrin, have been used extensively as mosquito larvicides in many countries. However, as demonstrated by SASA *et al.* (1965b), in Bangkok, most chlorinated hydrocarbon insecticides are less toxic to mosquito larvae than to the mosquito-eating fishes. At the present stage, the use of this group of insecticides as larvicides is not generally recommendable, because they are not only the sources of environmental pollution as cumulative toxicants, but they also destroy the natural balance by killing more of the natural enemies of insect pests than the pest insects themselves.

Most of the so-called low-toxicity organophosphorous insecticides, such as malathion, diazinon, ronnel, fenthion, fenifrothion, and Abate, were shown also by Sasa *et al.* (1956b) to be much more toxic to the mosquito larvae than to the mosquito-eating fishes and, therefore, can be used safely as larvicides without killing their natural enemies when applied under adequate dosages (Section 10C.3.2.3). Fenitrothion, for example, kills mosquito larvae at a concentration of 0.01 ppm, but is harmless to the fishes at concentrations of 1 ppm or less (both in 24-hour exposure tests). Further studies conducted in the author's laboratory by Yasuno *et al.* (1965) and Hirakoso (1966a, b, 1968) have shown that this and related organophosphorous insecticides are decomposed and inactivated by microorganisms in water, and thus do not accumulate in the environment as do most chlorinated compounds.

10D.3.2.3 Biological means of vector control

Large numbers of pathogens, parasites, and predators have been recorded as natural enemies of insect pests, and some of them have been utilized successfully or are being studied as promising biological agents in the control of insect pests and disease vectors. A comprehensive catalogue of pathogens, parasites, and predators of medically important authropods was published by Jenkins (1964). The microorganisms, animals, and plants recorded as parasites or predators of mosquitoes, horse flies, biting midges, and black flies include viruses, rickettsiae, bacteria, spriochetes, fungi, protozoa, rotatoria, nematodes, trematodes, molluscas, crustaceans, insects, mites, spiders, fishes, amphibians, reptiles, birds, and mammals. However, most of these records which appeared in previous literature refer to sporadic reports of the occurrence of the parasites or predators, and our present knowledge on the significance of these biological agents in the population control of insect vectors, as well as the methods of their applications in the control of diseases, is still meager. The following are some of the promising or already established methods in the biological control of mosquitoes and black flies.

(a) The use of fishes in the control of mosquito larvae:

It has been known since old times that certain fishes act as excellent natural enemies of mosquito larvae when released into their breeding sites, and as reviewed by Gerbrich & Laird (1966, 1968), large numbers of reports were made on the use of fishes in mosquito control. Most small fishes breeding in swamps, pools, and lakes are predators of mosquito larvae when both are coexistent. Burton (1960), for example, conducted a comprehensive study on the relative efficiency in larvivorous activity of various fish species in India.

Besides fish species indigenous to swamps and lakes in filariasis endemic areas in Asia and Africa, certain imported fish species have been bred and artificially introduced into ponds, swamps, and rice paddies for the purpose of the control of mosquito larvae. These include the gold fish (*Carassius auratus*), "medaka" (*Oryzias latipes*), and several species of minnows. Among them, the most popular fish used in this purpose since old times is *Gambusia affinis* (Baird et Girard, 1853), which is commonly called "top minnow" or "mosquito fish." This is a species of the ovoviviparous fish family Poeciliidae, and is a native of the southern United States. It was introduced into Europe, Africa, and Asia as early as in the beginning of this century, mainly for the purpose of malaria control, and has established itself in many areas. According to NAKAGAWA & IKEDA (1969), *G. affinis* was introduced from Texas to Hawaii in 1905 and has established wild colonies in all of the Hawaiian Islands. According to OKADA (1957), *G. affinis* was shipped from Hawaii to Taiwan in 1911, and then to Japan in 1916.

The guppy, or *Poecilia* (*Lebistes*) *reticulata* (Peters, 1859), is another member of the family Poeciliidae, and was discovered by SASA *et al*. (1965c) to be breeding massively in sewage pools around houses in Bangkok. Effective control of the larvae of *C. p. fatigans* could be achieved by releasing the fishes into ground pools containing sewage water. The guppies were also reported to be breeding as wild colonies in Malaya by JOHNSON & SOONG (1963), and in Nagpur, India, by KALRA *et al*. (1967). As reviewed more recently by SASA (1972), this fish species is especially adapted for breeding in polluted waters and is an excellent predator of mosquito larvae; it can be used in the control of mosquito larvae in wells, coconut husk pits, and various types of sewage pools. However, in contrast to *G. affinis* which can survive through winter in the Temperate Zone, such as in the Tokyo area, the lowest temperature which *Poecilia reticulata* can tolerate is about 13°C, and therefore, it is difficult to use in the Temperate Zone. In Japan, *P. reticulata* has been found to be breeding in sewage ditches in a number of hot spring towns. The northern most region where *P. reticulata* is breeding in natural environment in Asia is the city of Naha on Okinawa Island, southern Japan.

BAY & SELF (1972) carried out observations on the guppy in *C. p. fatigans* breeding sites in Bangkok, Rangoon, and Taipei. In Bangkok, they also observed that the guppy controls mosquito larvae effectively in many accumulations of domestic wastewater where conditions are favorable. However, it was also recognized that there were many pools where the guppies did not breed well and their effects as natural enemies were unsatisfactory. The fish was released in Rangoon to see the effects in the control of *C. p. fatigans*. In this city, however, many of the breeding sites of *C. p. fatigans* larvae were unstable and too temporary for the survival of the fish colony. The guppies were also found in the city of Taipei, and were shown to be effective in the control of mosquito larvae when introduced into garbage-contaminated drainage ditches throughout the city. In Rangoon, spraying of a pyrethroid insecticide (tetramethrin) at a concentration of 1.0 ppm was shown to kill the guppies along a ditch, but the fish population recovered to the original level about one month later. In Taipei, the guppies once introduced into a sewage ditch had reached a heavy population and were harvested by the people to feed domestic ducks.

The use of fish in the control of mosquito larvae has both advantages and disadvantages as an alternative measure to other methods, such as the environmental or insecticidal control. It usually takes at least several weeks for the released fish colony to reach a population density sufficient for appreciable reduction or complete eradication of mosquito larvae from the pools. Under certain environmental conditions, especially where water plants are abundant or where the water is not suited for breeding of the fish species, the effect of the released fishes often remains insufficient and either the fishes die out or they coexist with mosquito larvae. However, when fish species especially fitted for breeding in the target areas are used, such as the guppy (*Poecilia reticulata*) in polluted sewage pools or *G. affinis* in swamps around residential areas, permanent eradication of mosquito larvae can often be achieved by the single procedure of their release, such as reported by SASA (1972). KURIHARA *et al.* (1973, a) further demonstrated that the simultaneous application of a low-toxicity insecticide (fenitrothion) and the fish to mosquito-breeding sites is more effective than the single application of either of the control measure, because the insecticide at a concentration of about 0.1 ppm kills all mosquito larvae within a few hours, and the small number of fishes released into the water feed on all mosquito eggs subsequently deposited (a young guppy can consume only about twenty 4th stage mosquito larvae per day, but eats as many as 2,000 mosquito eggs per day; see Section 8C.5; Japan; Part 3.3.c).

The efficiency of fish as mosquito eaters differs greatly by the species. SATO *et al.* (1972) observed in Tokushima, southern Japan, that *G. affinis* introduced from Tokyo had been established in many swamps, ditches, and ponds in and around the city, and achieved practically complete eradication of mosquito larvae which had been breeding in enormous numbers in coexistence with the native fish species, "medaka" or *Oryzias latipes*.

One of the merits of the fish (especially those of the family Poeciliidae) in the control of mosquito larvae is the fact that they can breed and maintain high population density even after the mosquito larvae are all killed. This is a character essentially different from other predators or parasites which are solely dependent on mosquitoes and must die out when the hosts are completely eradicated.

The use of fish in the control of mosquito larvae, so far as it is feasible and effective, is a very economical, labor-saving, and nonpolluting measure. In Sri Lanka, for example, this author estimated that at least two-thirds among several thousand potential mosquito breeding places sprayed so far at weekly intervals with malathion in diesel oil could have been made free from mosquito larvae by the release of the guppy. These potential breeding sites were numerous abandoned wells (after installation of a pipe-water supply system), coconut husk pits, certain sewage pools, and ditches.

(b) The use of parasites in vector control

The occurrence of nematode parasites in various groups of insects has been noted since old times, and promising results have been reported recently on their uses in the control of insect pests, including mosquitoes and black flies. A review of entomophilic nematodes was compiled by WELCH (1965), NICKLE (1973) and STOFFOLANO (1973).

According to NICKLE (1973), the nematodes parasitic in insects fall into three groups: the sphaerulariids (Sphaerulariidae and Entaphelenchidae), the mermithids (Mermithoides: Tetradonematidae and Mermithidae), and the neoaplectanids (the genus *Neoplectana*). The species known to be parasitic in mosquitoes and black flies belong to the family Mermithidae. Over 50 genera are already described in this family, though many of these are poorly or inadequately known. Mermithids are known to parasitize at least 15 orders of insects.

PETERSEN (1973b) reviewed the role of mermithid nematodes in the biological control of mosquitoes. They have been reported to be parasitic in at least 63 species of mosquitoes from North America, Mexico, Europe, India, Sumatra, and Australia. The species of mermithids parasitic in mosquitoes were known mostly by immature stages in the mosquito larvae and thus it was difficult to identify the nematode species until recently; however the taxonomic studies conducted recently based on the morphology of laboratory-reared adult nematodes have indicated that at least 20 species of mermithids are parasitic in mosquitoes.

The life cycle of mermithid parasites of mosquitoes and other aquatic insects is generally as follows. The eggs deposited by free-living adults in water begin to develop soon after they are laid. Then, after hatching, the free-swimming nematode larvae gain entry to the insect larvae by penetration of the cuticle. Some species of mermithids develop little until the host reaches the adult stage; thereafter, the nemas migrate to the abdomen of the hosts, mature rapidly, and generally kill the hosts on emergence. Other species develop rapidly in the larval hosts, prevent pupation, and kill the hosts as they emerge. After emergence, the postparasitic nemas burrow into the soil where they mature to adults, mate, and lay eggs. The life cycle of some species can be completed in 4 to 6 weeks, but may take a year in species parasitic on univoltine mosquitoes.

As for the host specificity, it has generally been observed that mermithids that develop only in adult mosquitoes are usually specific for a single species, and that most species that develop in larval hosts are parasitic on several to many insect species. For example, *Reesemermis nielseni* was found to be parasitic in 16 mosquito species in nature, and 57 of 61 mosquito species experimentally exposed to the infection, with the exception of 4 mosquito species resistant to the infection. On the other hand, *Diximermis peterseni* was shown to develop only in anopheline mosquitoes both in nature and in laboratory experiments.

PETERSEN (1973b) further stated that several factors make mermithids prime candidates as biocontrol agents: they have adapted to the life cycle of the hosts, they are host specific for one or several mosquito species, they kill their hosts, they produce high levels of parasitism, they do not feed after emerging from the host which makes for ease of handling, they have a high reproductive potential, they are free swimming and can be dis-seminated easily in the preparasitic stage, and they can be used against mosquitoes in an inandative manner (dissemination of the nemas to give immediate control) or in an inoculative manner (establishment of the pra-site to give continuous partial control).

A method for mass production of *R. nielseni* was established by PETERSEN & WILLIS (1970, 1972a), and PETERSEN (1973a) and field applications were conducted by PETERSEN & WILLIS (1972b) in Louisiana and elsewhere in the United States, where at least partial parasitism of mosquito larvae has been observed. Since *C. p. fatigans* and most anopheline species were shown to be suitable hosts for *R. nielseni*, both in laboratory and field ex-periments, the use of this parasite in the control of filariasis vectors is con-sidered promising and worthy of being explored in future studies.

PETERSEN (1973a) studied various factors affecting mass production of *R. nielseni* in the laboratory by using *C. p. fatigans* as the host. The parasite was shown to be reared most rapidly and economically in 51 × 137 × 5 cm trays containing 20,000 mosquito larvae per tray. When hosts were exposed to the preparasitic nematode larvae at a ratio of 12:1 parasites to hosts, the hosts fed on 0.30, 0.45, 0.60 g of food (finely ground and sieved rabbit chow) per host on the first, second, and third days, respectively, and 0.90 g each day thereafter. About 80% of the hosts were parasitized under this condition. Higher parasitism reduced the ultimate production of preparasitic nemas because multiple parasitism favored the production of male nematodes.

Mermithid nematodes have also been recorded from black flies, or bloodsucking flies of the family Simuliidae, and a review was prepared by WELCH (1964) and GORDON *et al.* (1973) on their potential for the biocon-trol of onchocerciasis vectors. Reports on accidental findings of larval mer-mithid nematodes in black fly larvae have been made beginning 1911 by STRICKLAND and a number of later workers, but the taxonomic assignment of these mermithids in black flies have mostly remained uncertain until recently. Taxonomically valid descriptions of mermithids in black flies were made by WELCH (1962), who recorded new species of *Gastromermis*, *Isomermis*, and *Mesomermis* from black flies from North America. Addi-tional and more comprehensive studies on the distribution and taxonomy of mermithids in black flies were conducted in the USSR and Europe by RUBTSOV and associates from 1963 to 1970, and no less than 12 additional species of *Gastromermis*, 6 of *Mesomermis*, and 1 of *Isomermis* have been recorded; several of these species were subdivided into subspecies and even morphologically distinct varieties.

Mermithids are also known to be widely distributed in tropical regions of the world, as reviewed by WELCH (1964), but little is known about the prevalence of these parasites in black flies of the onchocerciasis endemic regions. The possibility of the use of this and related parasites in the control of onchocerciasis vectors still awaits studies in order to draw a conclusion.

Black flies of all three common genera (*Simulium, Prosimulium,* and *Cnephia*) are known to be the victims of mermithids. The life cycle of mermithid parasites of simuliids is known only partially for *Gastromermis viridis* and *Isomermis wisconsinensis* taken from *Simulium vittatum* in Wisconsin, U.S.A. (PHELPS & DEFOLIART, 1964, *Univ. Wisconsin Research Bull.* No. 245, 78 pp.). The infective stage larvae that have hatched from eggs develop in the hemocoel of the black fly larvae after infection, and molt at least once before completion of parasitic development and eventual emergence from the host. Within the stream bed, free-living, postparasitic mermithid larvae molt to adults, copulate, and lay eggs, which embryonate, and hatch to release the preparasitic larvae.

Mermithid nematodes have undoubted potential as biological control agents of black flies, because they are relatively host-specific and kill or sterilize the host. These nematodes are known to exert a natural control over black fly populations as evidenced by the numerous field reports of the percentages of parasitism. However, our present knowledge is not sufficient to allow the experimental redistribution of these parasites from infested to uninfested streams. Field experiments of this nature have been greatly hampered by the difficulty in the mass production of the host black flies in the laboratory. Trials to produce large numbers of the infective, juvenile nematodes by *in vivo* techniques are yet unsuccessful. The development of an axenic *in vitro* culture method of mermithids is considered as another possibility for their use in the biocontrol of black flies (abstracted from a review by GORDON *et al.*, 1973).

(c) The use of pathogens in vector control

Coelomomyces is a group of fungi (Blastocladiales; Phycomycetes) which are often found to be parasitic in mosquito larvae. A review of previously recorded species and hosts was compiled by JENKINS (1964). They have oval sporangia 18 to 127 μ long and 10 to 65 μ in diameter, surrounded by a thick, yellowish wall. The mycelium apparently lacks a true cell wall, the nonseptate hyphae being easily overlooked in early infections prior to sporangium formation. Infection may become evident in the first instar larvae, and sporangia attain full development in the third and fourth instars. Infected larvae rarely develop into adult mosquitoes and nearly always die before pupation. Egg development is inhibited in parasitized females. Some 30 species of *Coelomomyces* had been recorded from various species of mosquitoes prior to 1964. MUSPRATT (1946), for example, found in Rhodesia that as high as 95% of *An. gambiae* larvae had the fatal infection with *Coelomomyces*. LAIRD (1959a, b, 1760, 1971) gave accounts on the taxonomic status of the genus *Coelomomyces* and the possibility of this and other microorganisms being used in the biological control of mosquitoes.

Some Microsporidia are also known to cause fatal infection in mosquito larvae, and their potentials in mosquito control were discussed by KELLEN (1960, 1962). Microsporidia are single-celled Protozoa of the Class Sporozoa and thus closely related to the malaria parasites. However, Microsporidia require only one host to complete their life cycle; about 90% of the known species of Microsporidia parasitize invertebrates, while the remainder have been reported from cold-blooded vertebrates, but none from warm-blooded vertebrates. The typical life cycle of a microsporidian, as exemplified by members of the genus *Thelohania*, consists of the resting stage spent as a resistant spore which is deposited by the host in the soil or water; members of this genus form eight spores, which are dissociated as the host succumbs to the disease and decomposes. The infection of new hosts takes place by ingesting the resting spores. Field and laboratory studies by KELLEN (1962) in California have shown that various sporidian species of the genus *Thelohania* and *Rosema* are found in mosquito larvae, and probably all species of mosquitoes are hosts to one or more species of Microsporidia.

10D.3.2.4 Genetic means of vector control

Genetics comprise an important part in the taxonomy, biology, and control of disease vectors, and a comprehensive review was published by WRIGHT & PAL (editors, 1967). Genetic measures in vector control are discussed separately here because these are based on entirely different ideas from those presented in the previous sections. From the standpoint of methodology, the genetic control measures involve physical means (such as by gamma radiation), chemical means (such as the use of chemosterilants), or biological means (such as cytoplasmic incompatibility and hybrid sterility). Genetic control has been defined as "the use of any condition or treatment that can reduce the reproductive potential of noxious forms by altering or replacing the hereditary material" (WLD. HLTH. ORG. TECH. REP. Ser. No. 268, 1968).

In the control of filariasis vectors, most genetic methods are still in the experimental stage or only of theoretic or academic interest, though at least some of them may be promising as future control measures.

As reviewed by a WHO Scientific Group on "Cytogenesis of Vectors of Disease of Man" (WHO TECH. REP. Ser. No. 398, 1968), insect sterility can be produced by various genetic methods. These may be classified into the two categories: (1) the induced sterility, and (2) the genetic sterility.

(1) Sterility of various insects may be induced by exposure during the late pupal or adult stages to either ionizing radiation or chemosterilants at adequate dosages. Such treatment induced dominant lethal mutations in all the mature sperm contained in the insect, as the result of chromosomal changes. Successful results have been obtained at least in certain cases in reducing or eradictating insect pests by releasing large numbers of sterile males.

(2) On the other hand, there also exist many cytogenetic mechanisms that result in varying degrees of sterility in vector insects. Such genetic

sterility involves the following types, and some of them have also proved to be effective in reducing vector populations when applied with adequate methods under certain environmental conditions:
Reciprocal translocations, Inversions, Deletions (deficiencies), Aneuploidy, Polyploidy, Hybrid sterility, Cytoplasmic incompatibility.

(a) The sterile-male technique

This technique consists of inducing dominant lethal mutations in male gametes by radiation or chemosterilants, and reducing the production of viable offsprings by overwhelming the natural populations with such sterilized males. The most successful example of this sort of trial is the eradication of the screwworm fly from the island of Curacao and the southern United States through the release of males sterilized by gamma radiation, as reported by KNIPLING (1959). This or a similar technique has been applied with success to several other insects in various countries. The status of the use of sterile-male technique for mosquito control was reviewed by RAI (1969).

In the case of mosquitoes, the sterile-male technique has been tried, for example, with *An. quadrimaculatus* by WEIDHAAS *et al.* (1962), with *Ae. aegypti* by MORLAN *et al.* (1962), and with *C. p. fatigans* by RAMAKRISHNAN *et al.* (1962) and KRISHNAMURTHY *et al.* (1962). However, none of these trials were successful in terms of reductions in natural populations. In the case of *An. quadrimaculatus*, the failure of the field experiment using this technique was due probably to behavior differences between the native females and the sterilized males which were obtained from stocks having a long history of laboratory colonization. In the case of the *Ae. aegypti* field trial, males sterilized by irradiation of the pupae with doses ranging from 11,000 to 18,000 rad were shown to have reduced vigor and mating competitiveness. In the case of the *C. p. fatigans* trial in India, 24,000 sterile males were released over a period of 35 days, and a reduction of 6% in the ability of egg rafts to hatch was observed. However, the experiment was discontinued because of objections from the villagers at the site of release.

A feasibility study was conducted by RAI (1966), in Ceylon, on the application of the sterile-male technique for the control of filariasis vector, *C. p. fatigans*. The World Health Organization has established a field research unit on the genetic control of mosquitoes in New Delhi, India, in order to investigate the feasibility of various genetic methods in the control of *C. p. fatigans* and *Ae. aegypti*. Reviews on the activities and achievements made by WHO/ICMR Research Unit were published by SHARMA *et al.* (1973), RAJAGOPALAN *et al.* (1973), RAO (1974), GROVE & SHARMA (1974) SHARMA (1974) and REUBEN (1974).

(b)   The use of chemosterilants

As shown separately in Section 10E.2.4, it has recently been found that certain groups of chemicals have the ability of sterilizing insects and other animals when absorbed by contact or by ingestion; furthermore, some of them were shown to be effective, at least under experimental conditions, in reducing the insect pest populations. A review was made by LABREQUE & SMITH (1968) on the compounds to be used as insect chemosterilants, and the methods of their applications.

The insect chemosterilants may be used in two ways, one for the mass production of sterile males in the laboratory to be released in the field, and another for the direct applications in the field to produce sterility in natural populations. These compounds are effective as chemosterilants at certain dosage; they usually act as insecticides in higher doses or concentrations, while the sterilizing effect become lost in lower doses or concentrations. Therefore, it is difficult to expose all the target insect populations to adequate doses of chemosterilants in the field, and this is a reason that the field use of chemosterilants still remains unpopular.

MULLA (1964) conducted laboratory studies on the toxicity and sterilizing effectiveness of three ethylenamine derivatives (apholate, tepa, and metepa) against larvae and adults of the mosquito, *C.p. quinquefasciatus*. Apholate, at the concentration of 0.01 %, as well as tepa and metepa at the concentration of 0.05%, killed the larvae. The adults emerged at high percentages from larvae exposed to apholate at the concentration of 0.0001 %, those exposed to tepa at 0.005%, and those exposed to metepa at 0.01 %; the eggs produced by these adults were very low in the ability to hatch, being 4%, 54%, and 5%, respectively. It was assumed that the effective concentration of apholate and metepa for inducing sterility through larval exposure would be in the range of 0.001 to 0.003%. It was also observed that the adults fed for 24 hours with sugar solution containing 0.01 % apholate, 0.1 % tepa, or 0.1 % metepa produced eggs with very low hatching rates.

BROWN (1967, quoted by RAI, 1969) reported the development of traps into which male mosquitoes could be attracted either through light or other specific attractions. This provides a means for autochemosterilization and represents an important advance. Using a battery-operated CDC trap fitted with ultraviolet light, *C. p. fatigans* adults were drawn into a chamber treated with tepa. The escaping adults showed about 87 to 93% sterility. WHITE (1966) has reported chemosterilization by thiotepa of *Ae. aegypti* through pupal treatment.

SAITO & HAYASHI (1967) conducted observations on the sterilizing effects of metepa and hempa on *C. p. molestus*. When the larvae were exposed to the chemosterilants at various concentrations, the inhibition of egg production or that of hatchability was observed at the concentration of 0.01 % in metepa and 0.1 % in hempa, but the effects became lost at lower concentrations, while these chemicals exhibited larvicidal effects at higher concentrations. When these compounds were fed to the adults by mixing in a sugar solution, a high sterilizing effect was seen with metepa at the concentrations of 0.1 % and 0.01 %, as well as with hempa at the concentration of 0.1 %.

SAITO & HAYASHI (1968) further conducted laboratory studies on the effects of hempa and metepa on the adults of *C. p. molestus* when they were exposed in contact with the chemicals impregnated on filter paper. The chemicals were dissolved in acetone to a given concentration, and were spread evenly with a pipette at a rate of 50 ml per m². Both hempa and metepa caused nearly 100% sterility when applied at a concentration of 1.0% (0.5 g per m²), but lost the activity at 0.1% or lower concentrations. The effective exposure time was shorter with hempa than with metepa. The filter paper treated with 1.0% hempa solution gave 95% sterility even after 11 weeks.

It has been shown from these and other studies that at least some compounds are effective in producing sterile insect vectors under certain conditions, and provide promising tools in the control of vector-borne diseases. For example, chemosterilants were shown to be useful in producing sterile males in the laboratories. However, much more study is needed before these methods can be used effectively in the field as a means of chemosterilization of natural vector populations. Their potential hazards as mutagens or carcinogens should also be considered in their field application.

(c)   The use of genetic sterility

Some of the cytogenetic mechanisms causing sterility were shown to be promising or actually effective in the control of vector insects. Basic and field studies along this line have been conducted most extensively with three groups of mosquitoes; *Ae. aegypti* and related *Stegomyia* species, the *An. gambiae* complex, and the *C. pipiens* complex.

LAVEN (1967), for example, reported on "Eradication of *C. p. fatigans* through cytoplasmic incompatibility" from Village Okpo in Burma. This was a pilot experiment sponsored by WHO at the Filariasis Research Unit in Rangoon. A strain of *C. p. fatigans* with the cytoplasm from a strain from Paris and the genome from a strain of Fresno, California, was used. Cage experiments showed that males of this strain was incompatible with the females of Rangoon *fatigans*; of 1,472 egg rafts with a total of 130,445 eggs produced by these couples, only 180 (0.14%) larvae hatched. The incompatible males were released between February and May 1967. From March 16 until May 6, 5,000 incompatible males were released. Soon after the release of the optimum number of 5,000 incompatible males per day, the percentage of inviable rafts started to increase, reached 39.0% from April 11 to 17 (week 8), 70.4% during April 25 to May 1 (week 10), and on May 9 and 10, 100% sterile rafts were obtained. However, the monsoons started on May 11 and the experiment had to stop.

10E. Properties of main chemicals to be used for the control of filariasis

As stated in previous sections, certain chemicals have been shown to be effective in the control of filariasis, either for the cure of human parasite carriers as chemotherapeutics, or for the control of filaria vectors as insecticides, chemosterilants, etc. In view of the importance of these chemicals in the control of filariasis, a special review is made in this section on the chemical and biological properties of the main compounds to be used for these purposes.

10E.1 Chemicals for parasite control

There have been several groups of compounds which have proved to be effective as filaricides or chemotherapeutics in the treatment of filariasis. These include diethylcarbamazine (DEC), antimonial compounds, arsenical compounds, cyanine compounds, and suramine. Their efficacies as well as side effects may differ considerably according to the filarial species or host animals. Methods in chemotherapy of various species of human filariasis were described separately in each chapter of this book. Review on the chemotherapy of filariasis were published by SEWELL & HAWKING (1950), HAWKING (1955), SINGH & RAGHAVAN (1957), and HAWKING (1962, 1963, 1966a, b, 1973).

10E.1.1 Diethylcarbamazine (DEC)

This is the most important compound for the treatment of human filariasis and it has widely been used in the control of *Wuchereria* and *Brugia* infections.

Chemical structure: 1-diethylcarbamyl-4-methylpiperazine

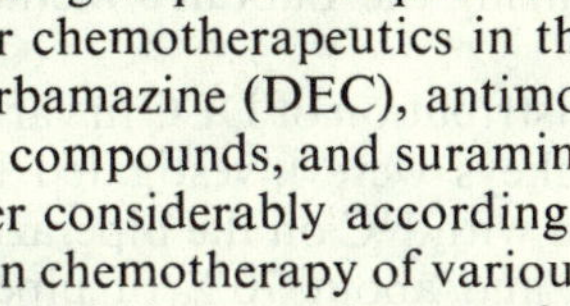

$$H_3C-N\begin{array}{c} H_2\ H_2 \\ C-C \\ \\ C-C \\ H_2\ H_2 \end{array}N-\overset{\overset{\displaystyle O}{\|}}{C}-N\begin{array}{c} C_2H_5 \\ \\ C_2H_5 \end{array}$$

Trade names: Hetrazan, Banocide, Notezine, Supatonin, Caricide, Carbilazine

Chemical and physical properties:
Colorless, oderless powder, and issued usually as the dihydrogen citrate which contains about half in weight as base. Therefore, it should be indicated in giving reports whether the dose refers to the base or the citrate salt; it is usually expressed by the dose of the citrate. The citrate of DEC is freely soluble in water, and tastes only slightly bitter, and therefore can be accepted willingly by infants when mixed with orangeade powder (KANDA et al., 1967). It is usually sold as tablets, each containing 50 mg of citrate, and thus one tablet corresponds roughly to 1 mg per kg of body weight in adults. The compound is stable under usual conditions. HAWKING & MARQUES (1967) showed that it is stable to autoclaving even if mixed with diet, and can be used by incorporation into cooking salt.

Absorption and excretion:

It has been demonstrated that DEC is a compound rapidly absorbed through the alimentary canal into the blood, and is again rapidly excreted from the body. LUBRAN (1950) developed a method for colorimetric determination of DEC in the biological fluid, and observed that when DEC is administered to man at an oral dose of 10 mg per kg (as base) of body weight, a peak blood level of 4 to 5 μg per ml is produced in three hours, and this falls to zero within 48 hours. A detailed study on the relationship between the dose of DEC and the time course of the blood level, as well as the effect of the drug on the microfilariae in the blood, was conducted by HUJIMAKI (1956), by utilizing the Lubran's method for the determination of DEC.

The metabolism and distribution of DEC in various organs when administered to rats and monkeys were investigated by BANGHAM (1955a, b) with a compound labeled with ^{14}C on the piperazine ring. This was shown to be rapidly absorbed, and about 70% of piperazine metabolites were excreted in the urine in the first 24 hours. About 10 to 20% of the dose appeared as unchanged compound, and the rest appeared as four different metabolites, in which the piperazine ring remained intact but the side chain underwent various degradations. The compound was distributed almost equally throughout all the organs of the body. There was no significant concentration of the drug in microfiariae or in adult worms. Excretion took place almost entirely by the urine. There was little tendency to accumulate when repeated doses were given (also quoted by HAWKING, 1963).

The chronological changes in the distribution of DEC in various organs were observed directly by an autoradiography method by SAKUMA *et al.* (1967). A tritium-labeled DEC was produced by exposing a commercially available sample (Supatonin, Tanabe Co.) to tritium gas under high voltage electric discharge in a chamber, and was purified by repeated crystallization. The compound was injected into the peritoneal cavity of mice; and whole body sections of 30 μ in thickness were preparared by a freezing microtome after 10, 20, 40, 60 minutes, 3 hours, 6 hours, and 24 hours. The chronological distribution and density of DEC in various organs of mice was illustrated clearly in this experiment. The tritium-labeled compound was shown to be absorbed rapidly from the peritoneal cavity and distributed to various organs, especially to the liver after ten minutes, but dropped rapidly thereafter. The compound was shown to accumulate, especially in the brain, body muscles, and various glands, for a few hours after the injection. The excretion of the compound was noted through the stomach wall into the alimentary canal, and also with the bile into the gall bladder. The radioactivity associated with DEC disappeared almost completely from the whole body after 24 hours. The unusual affinity of the compound to the stomach wall cells was clearly demonstrated, which probably accounted for its side effect of gastric irritation.

The fact that DEC is rapidly absorbed when administered orally is also clear from the evidence that the microfilarial density in the daytime blood samples increases conspicuously within a few minutes after the tablet is swallowed by human microfilaria carriers. (see Section 10B.2.2.4). The compound is rapidly excreted, and there seems to be, at least pharmacologically speaking, no cumulative effects on the mammalian hosts of filariasis. However, the compound is very unusual in that it exhibits cumulative chemotherapeutic effects on the filarial parasites, as is well known to workers in this field.

Toxicity:

The toxicity of DEC itself to man and mammals is very low. According to HARNED *et al.* (1948, quoted by HAWKING, 1973), the acute LD-50 in mice is 240 mg per kg by intraperitoneal injection, and 560 mg per kg by oral administration. In rats, the oral LD-50 is 395 mg per kg and there is little accumulation and no signs of chronic toxicity even when high doses such as 170 mg per kg are repeatedly given (all doses refer to the base).

DEC is remarkably safe when given to man. HAWKING (1973) stated, "Although hundreds of thousands of people have been treated, no case of death proved to be due to diethylcarbamazine has been reported. The untoward reactions in man (when they occur) may be annoying but they are never dangerous."

As stated in detail in Section 2B.5.3.2 (a), the adverse effects of DEC which may occur when administered to *W. bancrofti* carriers take two essentially different forms each with different origins; the symptoms caused by the toxic effect of the drug itself, i.e., nausea and vomiting; and the others caused as a result of the death of microfilariae or adult worms, i.e., fever, lymphangitis, and lymphadenitis. The degree of the former type of reaction is mainly dependent upon the amount of the drug administered at one time, while the occurrence of the latter type of reaction is highly correlated with the microfilarial density in the blood of patients before the drug administration (SASA *et al.*, 1963b; see Table 2*B*-4 and Fig 2*B*-1).

The occurrence of the first type of the reaction, that is, nausea and vomiting, is independent of whether the persons are infected with filaria or not. The attack rate was 9.3% of 118 persons who received 2 mg per kg, 15.6% of those who received 8 mg per kg, and 75.9% of those who received 16 mg per kg of DEC at one time (SASA *et al.*, 1963b). In connection with the treatment of filariasis with large single doses of 1.0 to 1.5 g per person (roughly 20 to 30 mg per kg) which was conducted in China, CH'EN (1964) stated that the dose was best administered in the evening, otherwise vomiting occured in many persons.

The second type of reaction occurs only in filaria carriers as a result of the death of microfilariae or adult worms. It should be noted that the symptoms and the severity of these reactions differ greatly according to the filarial species. In *W. bancrofti* and *B. malavi* infections, these are represented mainly by an acute rise of body temperature which starts several hours after the first dose of DEC is swallowed. In general, the reactions are more severe in *B. malayi* carriers than in *W. bancrofti* carriers. In both cases, typical swelling of the lymph nodes occurs after a few days, which is apparently connected with the death of adult worms (CH'EN TSU-TA *et al.*, 1959b). In any case, these reactions are usually transient, subside within a few days even when additional doses of DEC are continuously administered, and never turn into a dangerous form such as collapse or shock (see Sections 2B.5.3.2 and 2C.5.3).

In patients with *O. volvulus*, there is usually a violent reaction which begins a few hours after administration of the first dose of DEC and becomes well marked in about 16 hours. It includes swelling and edema of the skin, intense itching, enlargement and tenderness of lymph nodes, papular rash, and rise of body temperature. These symptoms persist for a few days to a week, and then subside, after which the patients can tolerate quite high doses. The severity of the reaction is proportional to the density of microfilariae in the skin, but not to the size of the initial dose of the drug, as in *W. bancrofti* infection. In severe cases, the patients collapse and lapse into coma, which may be irreversible and death ensues several days after the first dose. Of 327 onchocerciasis patients treated with DEC by OOMEN (1969d) in Ethiopia, for example, seven died in circumstances suggestive of a fatal effect of the drug (see Section 5.4.4.2).

According to SALAZAR-MALLÉN *et al.* (1962, quoted by HAWKING, 1973), this "therapeutic shock" differs from anaphylactic shock in various ways, since true urticaria or angioneurotic edema are not seen, blood pressure remains normal, there is no respiratory obstruction, and pyrexia and prostration are marked. Blood histamine and complement are not changed during the reaction, but serotonin increases significantly and a "reactive-protein C" also appears in the blood. This reaction was diminished by the previous administration of cortisone, etc., or, to a lesser extent, by antihistamines. HAWKING (1973) stated also that the reaction was prevented more effectively by antagonists of serotonin, such as cryptoheptazine, or by combinations such as Tacryl plus metisergide dimaleate, or triamcinalone plus methdilazine.

In patients infected with *L. loa*, the occurrence of a syndrome of meningoencephalitis has also been noted after administration of DEC, especially among those who harbor large numbers of microfilariae in the circulating blood (see Sections 3.4.1 and 3.4.3).

DEC frequently causes an acute shocklike symptom when administered to dogs infected with *Dirofilaria immitis* which may sometimes be fatal to the host. This is a type of reaction which has never been encountered in man in the treatment of filariasis.

Antifilarial effect:

As stated previously, this compound was first demonstrated to be effective in clearing or remarkably reducing microfilariae of *Litomosoides carinii* in cotton rats by HEWITT *et al.* (1947). Later studies on its effect and the mode of action in experimental filariasis are reviewed in Section 12B. In general, DEC is effective against the microfilariae of *L. carinii* in cotton rats, but hardly effective against its adult worms; the drug is nearly non-effective against microfilariae and adults of *Dipetalonema witei* in jirds, only slightly effective against the microfilariae but not effective against the adult worms of *Dirofilaria immitis* in dogs.

In *W. bancrofti* and *B. malayi* infections in man, DEC is effective against both microfilariae and adult worms when sufficient doses such as over 72 mg per kg in total are successfully administered. The reaction of patients due to destruction of the parasite may be severe, especially in *B. malayi* cases, but is transient and never dangerous (see Sections 2B.5.3 and 2C.5.3).

Loa loa in man is apparently very susceptible to treatment with DEC, and results of previous studies conducted in Africa suggest that both the microfilariae and the adult worms can be cleared when sufficient doses are administered (LAGRANGE, 1949; WANSON, 1949; WOODRUFF, 1951; DUKE & MOORE, 1961; also see Section 3.4.3). However, sporadic reports were made from its superendemic areas that a serious syndrome of a type of meningoencephalitis was occasionally observed after administration of DEC to persons with the microfilariae of *L. loa* at high densities (see Section 3.4.1). Therefore, special care should be taken in the treatment of *L. loa* patients for the possible occurrence of such a dangerous reaction. It was further demonstrated by DUKE (1961, 1963) that prophylaxis against infection with *L. loa* can be achieved by DEC when the drug is administered continuously at daily doses of 5 mg per kg (see Section 3.4.4).

According to HAWKING (1963), DEC has little action against adults of *D. perstans*. On the other hand, DUKE (1973) has shown that both microfilariae and adult worms of *D. streptocerca* are susceptible to DEC, and the drug can produce a radical cure (see Section 4B.4).

The chemotherapy of human onchocerciasis with DEC should be conducted under special care and supervision, since the drug provokes violent reactions, as stated in the previous section. After the initial side reactions have subsided, subsequent doses of the drug can be administered safely, without causing additional reactions. In such cases, DEC is effective in clearing the microfilariae from the skin and usually from the eyes, causing remarkable improvements in the skin and eye complications of onchocerciasis. However, DEC is usually not effective against adult worms of *O. volvulus*, and thus the microfilariae become re-established in the skin or eyes after DEC administration is suspended. Therefore, combined use of drugs effective against the adult worms, such as suramine, is necessary if radical cure is desired (see Section 5.4.4.2).

10E.1.2 Suramin

Physical and chemical characters:
Suramin is a complex derivative of urea with the above chemical structure. It is a white, finely crystalline powder, slowly but freely soluble in water. It is a cumulative drug, excreted via the kidney. The compound is administered usually by intravenous injection as a 10% solution in distilled water, and at a dose of 0.5g to 1.0g at one time for an average adult.

Trade names: Bayer 205, Germanin, Antrypol, Moranyl, Naganol, Belganin

Antifilarial activity: (also see Section 5.4.4.2b).

Suramin was introduced first in 1921 as an effective remedy for human trypanosomiasis and has been used extensively in Africa for its treatment. Its effect on onchocerciasis was discovered by VAN HOOF *et al.* (1945) while conducting treatments for trypanosomiasis in patients infected simultaneously with *O. volvulus*. Later, a number of workers confirmed that suramin is an effective chemotherapeutic for radical cure of onchocerciasis when adequate doses are administered. The drug is given intravenously, usually at weekly intervals, starting from 0.5 g as the initial dose for an average adult, followed by an injection of 1.0 g at one time for a total of five times as a course (4.5 g in total).

So far as our present knowledge is concerned, *O. volvulus* is the only human filaria species against which suramin is effective. As reviewed by HAWKING (1973), it has little effect on *W. bancrofti*, *L. loa*, *D. perstans*, or *D. streptocerca* in man, *D. immitis* in dog, or *L. carinii* in cotton rats. Its action on *O. volvulus* is exerted mainly upon the adult female worms, which die or degenerate after four or five weekly doses. The male adults are more resistant. The microfilariae are cleared some weeks after the death of adult females. The dead worms excite inflammatory reactions round them and then they are gradually absorbed.

Reports on the use of suramin in the treatment of human onchocerciasis were made by VAN HOOF *et al.* (1947), WANSON (1950), BURCH & ASHBURN (1951), MASSEQUIN *et al.* (1954), NELSON (1955), DUKE (1962, quoted by DUKE, 1968c), WHO EXPERT COMMITTEE ON ONCHOCERCIASIS (1966), DUKE (1968c, 1974), and HAWKING (1963, 1966, 1973).

DUKE (1968c) conducted quantitative observations on the effects of suramin on the microfilariae and adults of *O. volvulus* when administered under various dosage regimens. A group of patients was treated with weekly 1.0 g doses to totals varying from 9.5 g to 2.2 g, and skin snips (usually 11 samples from each person) were examined two weeks, eight months and 25 months after treatment. In general, the microfilarial density dropped gradually by the lapse of time until it became almost zero after 25 months in most cases who received a total dose of 7.5 g or more, but the rate of reduction of the microfilarial density became less marked as the total doses became smaller. The average microfilarial concentration at the examination made 2 to 3 weeks after taking total dosages of 9.5 g, 8.5 g, 7.5 g, 4.5 g, and 2.2 g to 3.2 g were reduced to 8%, 19%, 32%, 46% and 71% respectively, of their pretreatment levels. However, none of the suramine dosage schedules that were subsequently shown to be lethal to the adult worms resulted in all the microfilariae being killed. Other patients were treated with varying dosage regimens, such as (1) courses of 0.1 g doses weekly to totals of from 2.2 g to 9.5 g, (2) courses of 0.5 g doses weekly to totals of 3.5 g to 4.0 g, (3) a course of daily injections of 0.2 g, 0.5 g, 1.0 g, 0.5 g, and 0.5 g, making a total of 2.7 g in five days, or the same dosage at weekly intervals, and (4) a course of 0.25 g weekly to a total of 2.0 g. In general, the effect of the drug in view of the reduction of microfilarial density in skin snips was higher as the total dose was increased. The treatments at weekly intervals were better tolerated by the patients than at daily courses.

Toxicity and side effects:

According to a report by the WHO EXPERT COMMITTEE ON ONCHOCERCIASIS (1966), the side reactions encountered during treatment of onchocerciasis patients with suramin are classified into the following types:

(1) Toxic reactions attributable to the action of the drug:

(1-a) Immediate reaction of collapse. This occurs very rarely and may be avoided by giving a very small initial test dose.

(1-b) Irritation of the kidney. This is revealed by albumin and granular casts in the urine, and is the drug's most common toxic manifestation. A slight temporary albuminuria is often encountered during treatment, which clears in a few weeks as the drug is excreted. However, the occurrence of much albuminuria and granular casts should be taken as an indication to suspend the injection of further doses.

(1-c) Tenderness of the soles of the feet and palms of the hands.

(1-d) Degeneration of the adrenal cortex. Fatalities from this reaction have been reported when very large doses were administered in animal experiments, or in humans for the treatment of penphigus.

(2) Reactions attributable to the death of the parasite:

(2-a) Reactions to the death of microfilariae. These comprise fever, itching, swelling, and heat affecting the skin, fine or coarse papular eruptions, and ensuing desquamation. When microfilariae in the eye are involved, conjunctivitis and blepharitis may result. These signs however, are milder as a rule than those encountered after treatment with DEC.

(2-b) Reactions due to the death of adult worms: Pain and tenderness in nodules are common during treatment when the adult worms are killed by the drug. Occasionally, tender spots develop in the tissues around the joints and over bony prominences, or deep intramuscular abscesses are formed, which may be attributable to dead adult worms.

(2-c) Reactions of obscure pathogenesis. A feeling of general weakness continuing for eight to ten weeks after treatment is common. Reactions, sometimes fatal, have also been recorded in patients who developed prolonged high fever, prostration, arthritis, true exfoliative dermatitis, and ulceration of the buccal mucosa extending down the bronchial tract. The pathogenesis of these reactions is by no means clear, and together with severe diarrhea, they are all danger signals that indicate the need for immediate cessation of treatment.

10E.1.3 Antimony compounds

Various organic compounds containing antimony have been used in the treatment of trypanosomiasis and schistosomiasis since about 1920, and some of them were also shown to be effective against *D. immitis* in dogs or *W. bancrofti* in man. Comprehensive reviews were made by HAWKING (1963, 1973) on the effects of various antimony compounds on filariasis reported by previous workers. For example, ROGERS (1920) showed that tartar emetic had some effect on *W. bancrofti* in man. BROWN & AUSTEN (1939) showed that a compound called Stibsol acted on *D. immitis* in dogs. CULBERTSON & ROSE (1744) and CULBERTSON (1947, 1948) conducted systematic studies on the effects of various antimony compounds on *L. carinii* in cotton rats, and also on *W. bancrofti* in man. Neostibosan, a compound containing quinquevalent antimony, was the best of those studied in man, sterilized *W. bancrofti* in 25 of 35 patients treated. Neostibosan was effective also against *Loa*, but not against *Onchocerca*. Another compound, anthiomalin, was used against *W. bancrofti* in man by BROWN (1948). However, all of these compounds used by early workers were too toxic for general use in the treatment of human filariasis.

FRIEDHEIM (1962c, d) showed that an antimony compound, MSbB, was effective against *W. bancrofti* in man, though it had some side effects. CH'EN TZU-TA (1964) reported that urea stibamine, one of the compounds introduced by CULBERTSON *et al.* (1945) in treatment of filariasis, was used in China in the treatment of *W. bancrofti* and *B. malayi* cases and was shown to be effective in killing adult filaria worms, but it produced various side effects.

DUKE (1968b) reviewed the trial experiments on the use of various antimony compounds in the treatment of *O. volvulus* in man reported by

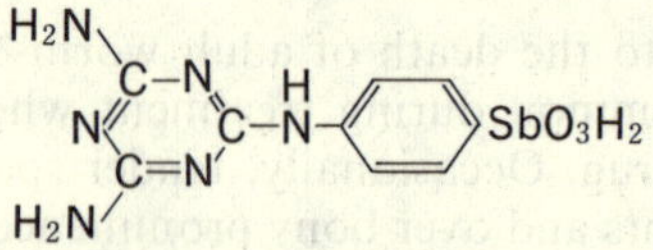

$$\begin{array}{c} H_2N \\ \end{array} \quad C-N \quad \begin{array}{c} H \\ \end{array} \quad C-N-\!\!\!\bigcirc\!\!\!-SbO_3H_2$$

(MSbB, FRIEDHEIN & BERMAN, 1946)

various workers, and also tested the effects of TWSb and MSbE on patients in West Africa. Both compounds, which were presumed to be most promising in view of effectiveness and safety, were shown to be still too toxic to be used generally in the treatment of human onchocerciasis.

10E.1.4 Arsenic compounds

The organic compounds of arsenic provided the first effective chemotherapeutics in the treatment of syphilis and trypanosomiasis introduced by Ehrlich and Hata. The first systematic study on the effects of various arsenicals on experimental filariasis was conducted by OTTO & MAREN (1947, 1949), who showed that phenylarsenoxide derivatives such as Arsenamide were very effective filaricides. This compound was suitable for the treatment of *D. immitis* in dogs, especially in that it kills adult worms; however, it was found to be too toxic for the treatment of human filariasis.

$$(HOOC \cdot CH_2S)_2 = As - \langle \rangle - CO - NH_2$$

(Arsenamide)

Melarsen derivatives, another series of arsenical compounds, were once considered to be hopeful for the treatment of human filariasis. A compound called Mel W was introduced by FRIEDHEIM (1962a,b) as a drug effective against *W. bancrofti* and *O. volvulus* in man. The compound was shown to be remarkably effective against adult worms of these filarial species, and radical cure of filariasis by killing apparently all adult worms was achieved in a number of cases who received intramuscular injections of the drug in one to five doses of 10 mg per kg. The drug had no direct effect on microfilariae, and it took about nine months before the blood or skin became free from the microfilariae.

(Mel W)

The effectiveness of Mel W against *W. bancrofti* filariasis was confirmed also by McCARTHY *et al.* (1962) in the Pacific and VAN DIJK (1963) in New Guinea. However, reports were subsequently made by various authors from a number of areas that the compound occasionally caused serious, sometimes irreversible or fatal, encephalopathy among those who were treated with the drug (JONES & EDWARD, 1967; HAWKING, 1973). The rare occurrence of such fatal cases may be admissible in the treatment of highly fatal diseases such as African trypanosomiasis, but most physicians responsible for the treatment or control of human filariasis consider, at present, that any arsenical compound, including Mel W, should not be used for the treatment or control of apparently nonfatal diseases such as filariasis.

10E.1.5 Other compound

Trichlorfon (trichlorophone, dipterex, Metrifonate, Bilancil)
This is an organophosphorous compound effective as an insecticide (see Section 10E.2.3), and also as a chemotherapeutic against certain helminthic parasites in man and animals. Its effect in the treatment of onchocerciasis in man was demonstrated in Mexico by Salazar Mallén *et al.* (1970), Salazar Mallén & Gonzalez Barranco (1971) and Salazar Mallén (1974). The compound was administered at first by the doses of 10 to 15 mg per kg of body weight at intervals of two weeks for a total of 5 to 16 doses, and later by doses of 10 mg per kg daily for six days. The treatment was well tolerated, remarkably reduced the microfilariae in the skin, and cured the clinical symptoms in at least in some cases. Duke (1972) tested the compound on human onchocerciasis in West Africa, and Duke (1974) further conducted experimental treatment of *O. volvulus* infection in chimpanzees, and demonstrated that the drug was a microfilaricide, but that even at doses as high as 22 mg per kg daily for six days, no action could be detected on the adult worms (see Section 5.4.4.2: b4).

10E.2 Chemicals for the vector control

10E.2.1 General remarks

Chemicals being used or studied for the control of filariasis vectors are classified into various groups according to the mode of action, for example, insecticides, chemosterilants, insect hormones, insect attractants, etc. In the practical aspects of filariasis control programs, only some of the chlorinated hydrocarbon and the organophosphorous insecticides have been integrated into control operations with more or less successful results. The other groups of chemicals are mostly still in the stage of academic interest as potential tools in the vector control operations.

The insecticides are used under various formulations and for different purposes. The active ingredients are rarely used as pure chemicals, but are issued usually mixed with solvents, detergents, or inactive carriers in forms such as wettable powder (to be suspended in water), emulsifiable concentrate (to be diluted with water to make an emulsion), solution in petroleum (for direct spraying), or soaked in powder (to be applied as dust). In special purposes, such as ultralow volume application (ULV) with airplanes, some insecticides are used as pure chemicals.

Insecticides are used for various purposes, such as larvicides (to be applied into breeding places of larvae), and imagocides or adulticides (to be applied for the purpose of killing adult forms). The most common method of the use of insecticides for the control of adult stage vectors is the indoor residual spraying. In this case, insecticides are suspended or emulsified in water (such as suspension of DDT wettable powder at a concentration of 5% of the active ingredient), and are sprayed on the wall of houses at a rate of 50 ml per m². The indoor residual spraying of DDT has constituted the main operation in most malaria control programs and has contributed to the complete eradication of the disease from such areas as Taiwan and Yaeyama. However, this method has been only poorly effective for the control of filariasis in most areas tested, mainly because of the differences in the mode of development of the disease (much more chronic and persistent in filariasis), by the difference in the behavior of mosquito vectors (such as the absence of the habit of resting on the walls of houses), or by the rapid development of insecticide resistance.

Each insecticide has both merits and demerits when used for certain purposes under certain environmental conditions. The following are the main factors to be taken into consideration in the selection of insecticides to be used in filariasis control operations.

10E.2.1.1 Toxicity to the target insects

The toxicity of a compound is expressed usually as LD-50 (50% lethal dose), or LC-50 (50% lethal concentration) as calculated from the tests of exposure of the target insects to insecticides under various conditions. It should be noted that the toxicity of most modern insecticides to insects is extremely high, and mosquito larvae are killed by exposure to concentrations of the order of ppb (parts per billion) in the case of most organophosphorous compounds. In most larviciding operations, excessive amounts of insecticides, such as several hundred or thousand times more of the active ingredients than necessary, are estimated to be used by the operators. Methods for biological assay of the effectiveness of insecticides are given in Section 10C.3.2.

10E.2.1.2 Toxicity to man and other nontarget animals

The insecticides to be used in vector control operations must be, first of all, safe to man (both operators and people in the controlled areas). The compound such as parathion cannot be used in this purpose because of its high mammalian toxicity, even though it is highly effective as an insecticide. Most chlorinated hydrocarbon insecticides, including DDT, lindane, and dieldrin, were shown to be more toxic to fishes, amphibians, and reptiles than to the target insects when applied in the field, and thus frequently caused unusual increases in the vector populations as a result of high toxicity to their natural enemies. Some insecticides exhibit special toxicity to certain groups of animals, such as the death of large numbers of birds as a result of field applications of fenthion as a mosquito larvicide.

The relative toxicity of insecticides to fishes is an important factor to be considered in the selection of mosquito or black fly larvicides. In a study on the comparative toxicity of various insecticides against larvae of *C. p. fatigans* and a mosquito-eating fish *Poecilia reticulata* (the guppy) conducted by SASA *et al.* (1965b) in Bangkok, it was shown that all the hydrocarbon insecticides tested were more toxic to the fish than to the mosquito larvae, while some organophosphorous insecticides, including fenitrothion, were several hundred times more toxic to the mosquito larvae than to the fishes. It has therefore been demonstrated by KURIHARA *et al.* (1973a) that the integrated use of the release of mosquito-eating fish and applications of an adequate amount of such insecticides is a more effective method of the control of mosquito larvae than individual uses of either the fish or the insecticides (see Section 10C.3.2.1; Tables 10C-3, 10C-4; Section 10D.3.2.3).

10E.2.1.3 Residual effects versus degradability

When insecticides are used in residual house spraying for the control of adult mosquito vectors, it is hoped that the effectiveness lasts as long as possible in order to save the labor and cost of reapplication. DDT and dieldrin were shown to be effective for at least several months when applied to wall surfaces. Fenitrothion was shown to be useful and sometimes more effective than the chlorinated hydrocarbon insecticides as a residual spray insecticide. The compounds used for residual spraying must be stable to exposure to the air (resistant to oxidation), and low in vapor tension.

On the other hand, most chlorinated hydrocarbon insecticides are highly stable in nature, and are accumulated easily in fat bodies of plants and animals in connection with the succession of food chains. Although most of them are low in the acute toxicity, their extensive use in the field is now considered to be undesirable. Most organophosphorous insecticides are biologically degradable, and thus never accumulate as toxicants in nature. Compounds like parathion and fenitrothion were shown to be rapidly deteriorated when mixed in sewage waters by the activity of some microorganisms, as discussed in the following sections.

10E.2.1.4 Development of insecticide resistance

The development of insecticide resistance in vector insects is sometimes a serious problem which nullifies a vector control program with that insecticide. The speed of development of resistance differs greatly by the insect species; the house fly, *Musca domestica*, and the house mosquito, *C. pipiens* s.l., are the two representatives which readily develop resistance to insecticides. Mosquitoes of the *An. gambiae* complex, which are the main vectors of malaria and *W. bancrofti* filariasis in tropical Africa, are also known to develop resistance to insecticides rather easily. The problems re-

ferring to the insecticide resistance in disease vectors were reviewed by
BROWN (1958).

It has also been demonstrated by a number of workers that insects develop resistance to chlorinated hydrocarbon insecticides more easily than to organophosphorous insecticides, and the grade of resistance is usually much higher in the former than in the latter group of insecticides.

10E.2.2 Chlorinated hydrocarbon insecticides

DDT (dichlorodiphenyltrichloroethane)

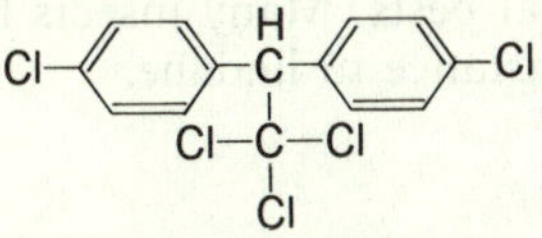

2,2-Bis-(p-chlorophenyl)-1, 1, 1-trichloroethane(p,p'-DDT)

p,p'-DDT is a white crystal with a melting point of 108°C, a specific gravity of 1.3, and a vapor tension of as low as 1.5×10^{-7} mm at 20°C and 3×10^{-7} mm at 25°C. It is almost insoluble in water, and issued usually as 75% wettable powder, 5% solution in diesel oil, 30% emulsifiable concentrate, or 10% dust. DDT is relatively low in the mammalian toxicity, but is highly toxic to reptiles and fishes. It is therefore not recommendable for the control of mosquito or black fly larvae in water, because it is more toxic to the fishes than to the insects, and also acts as an environmental pollutant which gradually accumulates in the fat bodies of man and animals. On the other hand, DDT sprayed on the walls of houses is chemically stable and has a long residual effect, and thus has been used extensively for the control of malaria vectors.

One of the serious problems encountered almost always in the use of DDT for vector control is the development of insecticide resistance in various insect species, such as in house flies, some mosquitoes (especially *C. pipiens* s.l.), bedbugs, and fleas. This is a reason that DDT house spraying has been shown to be ineffective in the control of filariasis in a number of trials.

Lindane

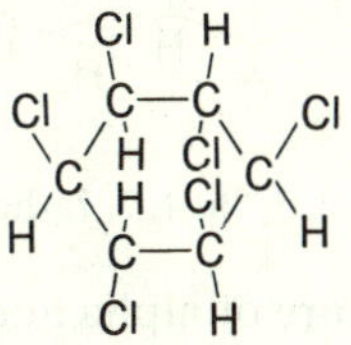

(1, 2, 3, 4, 5, 6-hexachlorocyclohexane)

Lindane is a product containing not less than 99% of gamma-BHC. BHC (benzene hexachloride) or HCH (hexachloro-cyclohexane) has seven isomers, among which gamma isomer is the active ingredient as the insecticide. It is a white crystal with a melting point of 112.9°C and a vapor tension of 3.17×10^{-2} mm at 20°C and 0.116 mm at 30°C. It has a strong effect as a contact insecticide and as a vapor insecticide. Its residual effect is, however, less than that of DDT because it is gradually lost from the wall surface as vapor. Lindane is also highly effective as a larvicide against mosquitoes and black flies. However, it is highly toxic to fishes, and its mammalian toxicity is higher than DDT. Benzene-hexachloride is a serious environmental pollutant after it was extensively used in some countries in the control of agricultural pests. Many insects have been shown to have developed insecticide resistance to lindane.

Dieldrin

1, 2, 3, 4, 10, 10-Hexachloro-6, 7-epoxy-1, 4, 4a, 5, 6, 7,
8, 8a-octahydro-1, 4-endo, exo-5, 8-dimethanonaphthalene

Dieldrin is a yellowish crystal with a melting point of 176°C and a vapor tension of 1.8×10^{-7} mm at 25°C. Because of its extremely low vapor tension and chemically stable nature, dieldrin has been used as a residual insecticide for house spraying as a substitute of DDT, especially after insect pests had developed DDT resistance. However, dieldrin is higher in mammalian toxicity than DDT, and is also highly toxic to fishes. It has been experienced in many areas where dieldrin was extensively used that house flies and some other insect pests easily develop resistance to this insecticide, too.

Chlordane

2, 3, 4, 5, 6, 7, 8, 8-Octachloro-2, 3, 3a, 4, 7, 7a-hexahydro-9, 7-methanoindene

Chlordane is usually a mixture of alpha and beta isomers. It differs from the previous three chlorinated hydrocarbon insecticides in that it is a sticky liquid and can be easily emulsified in water. Its vapor tension is relatively low (about 10^{-5} mm at 25°C). Chlordane has been used also as a residual insecticide for indoor spraying, or as a mosquito larvicide. Its mammalian toxicity is the lowest among the four chlorinated hydrocarbon insecticides (LD-50 of 290 mg per kg in oral administration to mice). In various insects cross resistance develops to the three compounds, lindane, dieldrin, and chlordane.

10E.2.3 Organophosphorous insecticides

Certain phosphoric acid esters have been shown, since 1938, to be toxic to mammals or insects as cholineesterase inhibitors, and some of them were introduced as insecticides for agriculture or public health uses. The compounds used in the early stages, such as parathion and TEPP, were highly toxic to man and caused a number of casualities, but those introduced recently for vector control are usually low in toxicity to mammals and fishes and have largely replaced chlorinated hydrocarbon insecticides in view of effectiveness and safety. Most organophosphorous insecticides are more or less unstable in nature and biologically degradable, but are effective as insecticides at extremely low dosages. The development of insecticide resistance to the organophosphorous compounds is much less frequent and the degree of resistance is usually less conspicuous than in the chlorinated hydrocarbon insecticides.

In connection with the extensive use of organophosphorous insecticides in the control of various agricultural pests and disease vectors, large numbers of reports were made, especially during the past ten years, on the chemistry, toxicity, and pharmacology of this group of compounds. O'BRIEN (1960) compiled a monograph on "toxic phosphorous esters." Methods for analysis and chemical characters were described by GUNTHER & BLINN (1955). An extensive review of studies on this group of compounds were made in by the sponsorship of WHO (1971) under the common title of "Alternative Insecticides for Vector Control" (BULL. WLD HLTH ORG. Vol. 44, pp. 1–470).

Parathion

$$\begin{array}{c} C_2H_5O \\ \\ C_2H_5O \end{array}\!\!\!>\!\!\overset{\overset{\textstyle S}{\|}}{P}\!\!-\!\!O\!\!-\!\!\bigcirc\!\!-\!\!NO_2$$

(O,O-diethyl-O-p-nitrophenyl thiophosphate)

Parathion is a compound with a melting point of 6.0°C and a vapor tension of 3.78×10^{-5} mm at 20°C. Parathion, or its allied compound methylparathion, was once used extensively as an insecticide for the control of agricultural pests but its use has now been almost entirely abolished because of high toxicity to man. The LD-50 value of parathion is about 7 mg per kg in oral administration to mice. Under field conditions, parathion is readily decomposed to nontoxic compounds, especially by the activity of microorganisms in water (YASUNO *et al.*, 1965; HIRAKOSO, 1966; HIRAKOSO & UCHIDA; 1966, MIYAMOTO *et al.*, 1966).

Malathion

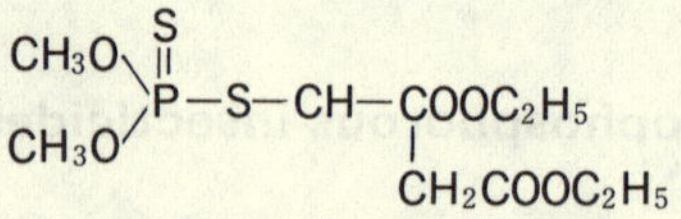

$$CH_3O\diagdown \underset{\displaystyle P}{\overset{\displaystyle S}{\|}}-S-CH-COOC_2H_5$$

$$CH_3O\diagup \qquad\qquad CH_2COOC_2H_5$$

O, O-Dimethyl-*S*-(1, 2-dicarboethoxyethyl) dithiophosphate

Malathion is a yellowish brown liquid with a melting point of 3°C, a boiling point of 156°C at 0.7 mm, and a vapor tension of about 10^{-5} mm at 30°C. Its toxicity to mammals and birds is very low (570 mg per kg in oral administration to mice) and this is the earliest compound introduced into disease vector control operations as a low-toxicity organophosphorous insecticide. It can safely be sprayed on the walls of houses or directly on the body of animals, but its residual effect is inferior to DDT and fenitrothion. Malathion was used as a mosquito larvicide in filariasis control programs in Sri Lanka (ABDULCADER & SASA 1965) and Okinawa, and also as a residual house spray insecticide in Okinawa from 1965 (MARSHALL & YASUKAWA, 1966).

Diazinon

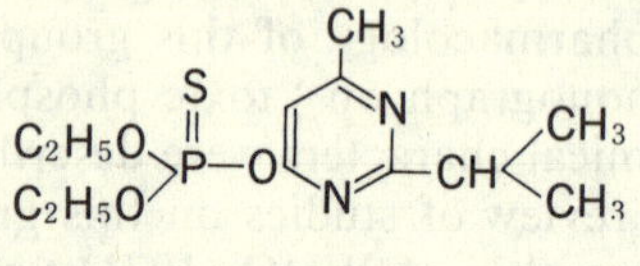

O, O-Diethyl *O*-2-isopropyl-4-methyl-6-pyrimidyl thiophosphate

Diazinon is an organophosphorous insecticide with a wide range of effectiveness to various insect pests, especially to adults of house flies and mosquitoes, and to mosquito larvae. The compound is a liquid with a boiling point of 83°C at 0.002 mm, and a vapor tension of 1.4×10^{-4} mm at 20°C and 1.1×10^{-3} mm at 40°C. It has a medium grade mammalian toxicity with an LD-50 value of about 50 mg per kg in oral administration to mice.

Dichlorvos (DDVP)

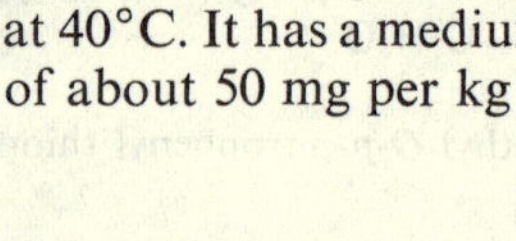

$$CH_3O\diagdown \underset{\displaystyle P}{\overset{\displaystyle O}{\|}}-O-CH=CCl_2$$

$$CH_3O\diagup$$

O, O-Dimethyl *O*-2, 2-dichlorovinyl phosphate

This is a liquid and volatile compound with a medium mammalian toxicity. It is highly effective as a space insecticide when applied as a mist, fog, or aerosol. A type of plastic plate containing dichlorvos at high concentrations is also sold commercially, and is effective against mosquitoes and other insects when placed in air-conditioned rooms, closed toilets, cisterns, and manholes because of the spontaneous evaporation of the insecticide.

Trichlorfon

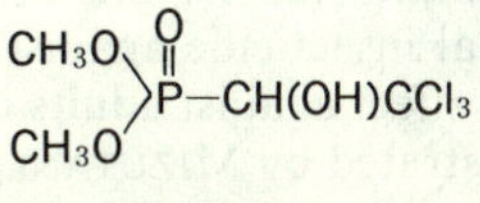

$$CH_3O \\ CH_3O {\Large>} \overset{\overset{O}{\|}}{P}-CH(OH)CCl_3$$

O, O-Dimethyl-1-hydroxy-2-trichloromethyl-phosphonate

A white crystal with a melting point of 78 to 80°C, soluble in water and most other solvents. The mammalian toxicity is relatively low and the LD-50 in oral administration to mice is about 600 mg per kg. Under natural environments, trichlorfon gradually changes to dichlorvos and effects the insecticidal activity. Therefore, it is effective as a residual insecticide when sprayed on walls. The compound also decomposes to dichlorvos when ingested by insects, and thus can be used as an insecticidal bait.

This compound is also effective as a chemotherapeutic against *O. volvulus* and some other helminthic parasites of man and animals (see Section 10E.1.5).

Fenthion (Trade name: Baytex)

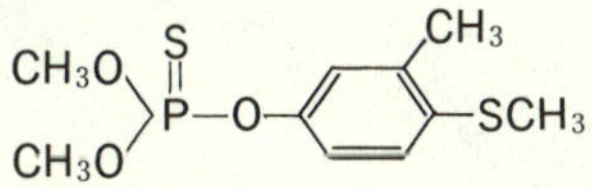

$$CH_3O \\ CH_3O {\Large>} \overset{\overset{S}{\|}}{P}-O-\text{(ring)}-SCH_3 \;\; CH_3$$

O, O-Dimethyl-*O*-4(methyl mercapto)-3-methyl phenyl thionophosphate

This is a brown-colored liquid, hardly soluble in water. It is highly effective as an insecticide against both adult and larval stage vectors. Because the compound is stable even when mixed in highly polluted waters, it has been used as larvicide for the control of *C. p. fatigans* larvae in sewage waters in the *W. bancrofti* endemic areas of southern Asia. However, because

Fenitrothion (Trade name: Sumithion)

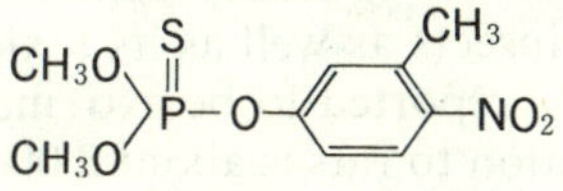

$$CH_3O \\ CH_3O {\Large>} \overset{\overset{S}{\|}}{P}-O-\text{(ring)}-NO_2 \;\; CH_3$$

O, O-Dimethyl *O*-(3-methyl-4-nitrophenyl) phosphorothioate

of its relatively high toxicity to man, mammals, and especially to birds, special care should be taken for in any wide application as a mosquito or black fly larvicide, or as an indoor spray.

The chemical structure of fenitrothion differs from parathion only by the presence of a methyl radical on the benzene ring. However, its mammalian toxicity is surprisingly low (about 800 mg per kg for LD-50 in oral administration to mice), while the insecticidal activity is nearly the same or higher than parathion. Fenitrothion is stable and hardly volatile when sprayed on walls in houses and stables. The compound was shown to be highly effective as a residual insecticide against cockroaches by pest control operators in Japan. Its effect against adults of *C. p. fatigans* in residual house spraying was demonstrated by MIZUTANI & HIRAKOSO (1962), KURIHARA *et al.* (1965), and YAMAMOTO *et al.* (1966). Operational evaluation of fenitrothion for the control of adult anophelines in Kenya, East Africa, was issued in a WHO report (WHO/VBC/72.391).

On the other hand, this compound was shown to be easily decomposed when mixed in sewage water, mainly by the activity of microorganisms, such as *Bacillus subtilis* (YASUNO *et al.*, 1965; MIYAMOTO *et al.*, 1966; HIRAKOSO, 1966; HIRAKOSO & UCHIDA, 1966). Such a characteristic may be a disadvantage in view of the residual effects when used as a mosquito larvicide, but is obviously a safeguard against environmental pollution with artificially synthesized chemicals. Since the toxicity of fenitrothion to mosquito-eating fishes is several hundred times lower than that to mosquito larvae, the combined use of the natural enemy (*Lebistes* or *Gambusia*) and the insecticide (fenitrothion) at the same time to mosquito breeding places was demonstrated to be more efficient and effective than the use of either of the two methods alone (KURIHARA *et al.*, 1973a).

Abate

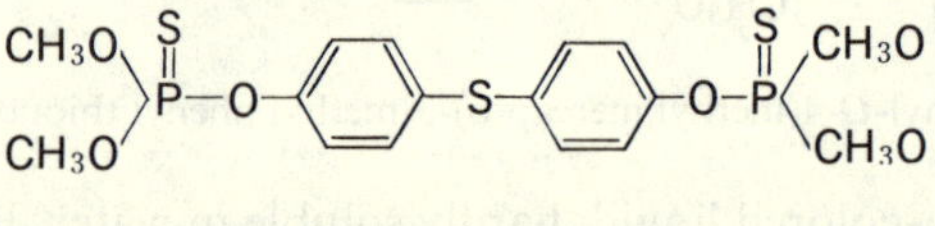

$$CH_3O\diagdown \overset{\overset{S}{\|}}{P}-O-\langle C_6H_4 \rangle -S-\langle C_6H_4 \rangle -O-\overset{\overset{S}{\|}}{P}\diagup CH_3O$$

O, O, O′, O′-Tetramethyl *O, O′*-thiodi-*p*-phenylene phosphorothioate

This is an organophosphorous insecticide introduced recently for the control of mosquito and black fly larvae. It is white crystal when purified, but technical samples are yellowish, sticky liquids. The compound is highly effective as a mosquito larvicide, and the LC-50 against larvae of *C. p. fatigans* was reported to be as low as 0.0005 to 0.0007 ppm. Its insecticidal effect on mosquito adults and other insects as well as its toxicity to man, other mammals, birds, and fishes was reported to be extremely low. The acute toxicity dose in oral administration to rats is about 2,000 mg per kg.

Because of its low toxicity to man, and its fairly stable character when added to water, Abate has been recommended as the choice mosquito larvicide for the treatment of drinking water. According to LAWS *et al.* (1968), the compound did not cause any ill effects nor detectable change in blood choline-esterase levels when given under controlled conditions to volunteers at a dosage of 64 mg per man per day for 30 days. It has also been demonstrated by BROOKS *et al.* (1965, 1967) and LAWS *et al.* (1968) that treatment of water containers (drums, barrels, cisterns, etc.) with Abate sand granules at a nominal rate of 1 ppm was highly effective in the control of mosquito larvae, and no toxic effects were observed among the people who used the Abate-treated waters for drinking.

10E.2.4 Other insecticides

Pyrethroid insecticides.
A group of compounds including the pyrethrins (the active ingredients of *Chrysanthemum cinerariaefolium*) and allied synthesized insecticides, such as allethrin and phthalthrin, have strong insecticidal characters when used as space sprays. Their mammalian toxicity is usually very low. Pyrethroids have been used commonly for personal protection from mosquito bites in the forms of mosquito coils or aerosols. It has also been used in *Ae. aegypti* control programs in urban areas, such as in the city of Singapore.

Compounds effective as insecticides have been screened out among a number of other groups of chemicals, and some carbamates (such as dimetilan and sevin) are considered to be promising in the control of insect vectors, at least under certain conditions. A comprehensive review was made by various authors in a symposium on "Alternative Insecticides for Vector Control" (BULL. WLD HLTH ORG. 1971, Vol. 44, pp. 1–470).

10E.2.5 Insect chemosterilants

Insect chemosterilants are chemicals which make insects reproductively sterile. As stated in Section 10D.3.2.4, these may possibly be used as a means of genetic control of insect vectors, either for the production of sterile males to be released in the field, or for applications in the field for sterilizing natural vector populations. A comprehensive review was made in a book compiled by LABREQUE & SMITH (1968, *Principles of Insect Chemosterilization*, 345 pp.).

The insect chemosterilants may be classified by their mode of action into the following groups:

Alkylating agents: These include tepa, tretamine, apholate, metepa (mapo), and aphamide. Most of these compounds are water soluble, and easily decomposed in nature.

Antimetabolites: A large number of compounds have been shown to act as antimetabolites in microbial and mammalian systems, and some of them were also proved to have antifertility effects. These include aminopterin (apga), 5-fluorouracil, and 5-fluoro-orotic acid.

Organotin compounds: Some organic compounds containing tin (Sn) were shown to have strong antifertility activity. These include triphenyl tin chloride, and triphenyl tin acetate.

Phosphoric triamide derivatives: Among these, hempa (hexamethyl-phosphoric triamide) is best known because of its high sterilizing activity. This compound is fairly stable in nature, easily absorbed by insects, and is considered to be one of the most promising chemosterilants.

Table 10-11.   Chemical structure of three chemosterilants.

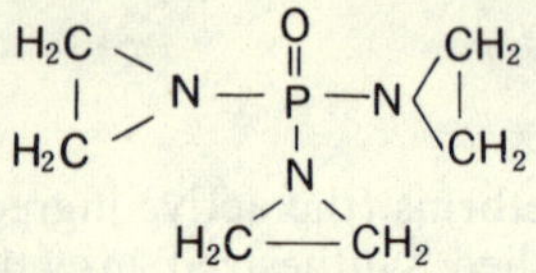

Tepa:
   tris (1-aziridinyl)-phosphine oxide

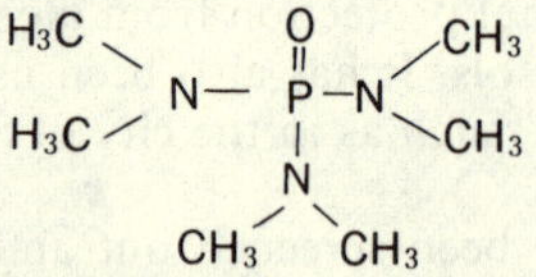

Hempa:
   hexamethyl-phosphoric triamide

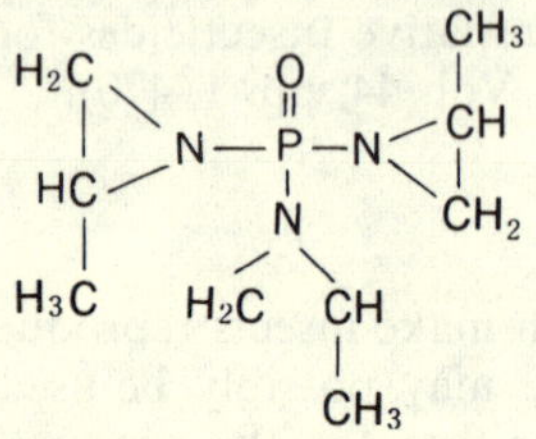

Metepa:
   tris (2-methyl-1-azidinyl)-phosphine oxide;

<table><tr><td style="font-size:3em">11</td><td><h1>Analysis and evaluation
of filariasis survey data</h1></td></tr></table>

11A. Statistical methods in the epidemiology of filariasis

11A.1 The use and misuse of statistics

Statistics is useful and valuable in many ways in the epidemiology of filariasis. Although most workers in filariasis are not mathematicians, they must make decisions or evaluations based on results of some statistical treatment of the observed data; either the procedures could involve simple arithmetic computations, or could be very sophisticated mathematics. On the other hand, most mathematicians or statisticians are not filariologists, and cannot assist in the epidemiology of filariasis unless the data are collected using appropriate form and technique.

Statistics is useful, first of all, in that it provides quantitative information in place of qualitative information drawn by simple impressions from the observed data. For example, instead of saying, "filariasis is wide spread in this village," after very simple mathematical treatment of the survey data, it can be stated that "the persons examined in this village showed a microfilaria rate of 35% and a clinical filariasis rate of 24%."

As discussed in detail in Section 11F, the microfilariae found in the circulating blood of human hosts have been shown to exhibit various types of periodicity, and by this character were classified into several forms, such as the nocturnally periodic form, the nocturnally subperiodic form, the diurnally subperiodic form, etc. A method was proposed by SASA & TANAKA (1972, 1974) with which the patterns of the periodicity can be expressed by two parameters: the periodicity index, and the best estimate of peak hour. The so-called nocturnally periodic form of *B. malayi* shows a periodicity index of about 70 and a best estimate of the peak hour of about

24 (midnight), while the so-called nocturnally subperiodic form of *B. malayi* has an index of about 30 and a peak hour of about 23 (11 p.m.). Both forms are thus clearly differentiated by the value of the periodicity index, and no intermediate forms have ever been discovered. A new form of *W. bancrofti* was recorded from Thailand by HARINASUTA *et al.* (1970) and was described as a nocturnally subperiodic form. Results of the statistical analysis of data reported by the original authors have shown that it differs clearly from the classical nocturnally periodic form of *W. bancrofti* by having a periodicity index of about 50 in contrast to that of about 100 in the classical form. Furthermore, it was pointed out that the periodicity index of Harinasuta's subperiodic form is larger than that of the subperiodic *B. malayi*, though both were called by the same name.

By convention, the periodicity of microfilariae of *Loa loa* is called "diurnally periodic," and that of the South Pacific race of *W. bancrofti* is "diurnally subperiodic." The periodicity index of the two forms are quite different, the former being about 90 and the latter only about 22. As for the peak hour, both are called "diurnal," but they are quantitatively quite different, and the best estimate of the peak hour is about 12 (noon) in the former, but about 16 (4 p.m.) in the latter. From this evidence, it is clear that statistics provides a new language by which results of scientific studies can be expressed quantitatively, in place of the conventional qualitative descriptions.

The second merit of the use of statistics is the introduction of the idea of reliability or significance of a conclusion, in place of "yes-or-no", or "all-or-none" expressions. For example, if a drug is given to 15 microfilaria positive cases and 16 microfilaria negative cases and a reaction was observed in 12 persons (80%) of the former and 5 persons (32.3%) of the latter group, can it be stated that the reaction rate is higher in the microfilaria positive cases? Some workers may say by impression that this is true, because the difference in the percentages is fairly big. Others may say that such a test is unreliable because the numbers tested were too small to draw a conclusion. However, the result of a statistical treatment called the "Chi-square test" suggests that the difference is statistically significant even with such a small numbers of samples, and the risk of making a mistake by drawing the conclusion is only about 2%. By simple statistical treatment of the observed data, the reliability or significance level of both the arithmetic means and the proportions can be obtained.

The adequate use of statistics can very often save time, labor, and money in conducting experiments or surveys for certain purposes. In general, it can estimate how many samples are necessary in order to draw a conclusion at the reliability level of 95% or 99%, if the differences in the means or proportions among the groups are roughly anticipated. The minimum number of samples necessary to draw a conclusion differs according to the reliability level and by the size of differences between the means or proportions.

The test of significance of the difference between the two averages can be made, as a rule, only when the frequency distribution of the numbers of both groups are nearly normal. If the frequency distribution is skewed, such as the distribution of microfilarial counts among the infected human populations, it is necessary to convert the distribution to near normal by some statistical treatment. It this case, the frequency distribution of the microfilarial density was found to be roughly logarithmically normal, and therefore the median density (which is the logarithmic mean) can be used for comparison of populations in place of the arithmetic mean (discussed in Section 11C).

Statistics sometimes provide a conclusion which is apparently different from that being drawn by impression or intuition. For example, as discussed in Section 11D-2, the microfilarial counts observed in the same volume of blood samples collected every day at the same time from the same persons were shown to be quite variable and apparently irregular. In one of the series, the counts fluctuated from 0 to 9 in the same person. It was therefore considered that such a variable and irregular measure could not be used for the statistical studies. However, in a test of goodness of fit to the Poisson distribution, the same data were shown to be regarded as not irregular, but a random distribution with a probability of higher than 30%.

In one of the South Pacific islands where filariasis due to the non-periodic race of *W. bancrofti* was prevalent, an extensive control program by mass administration of DEC to the whole population was carried out, and the microfilarial rate of the sampled population dropped from over 20% of the pretreatment level to 1.74%. On the other hand, the microfilarial rate of emigrants from the same islands turned out to be 3.49% and was apparently twice as high as that of the sampled villages. It was therefore suspected by the administrators that the difference in the rate might have been due to poor coverage of the drug treatment program in some villages, where many microfilaria carriers were still present but had remained unexamined. However, a study of the age and sex composition of the two populations demonstrated that the difference in the microfilarial rate was simply caused by the much higher proportion of the adult males among the emigrants than among the people of the sampled villages, and not by the difference in the endemicity of the disease. In other words, the results of statistical analysis indicated that the coverage of the drug treatment operation in unsurveyed villages was probably as good as that in the villages selected for the sample surveys (see Section 11B.3).

Statistics often provides valuable advice to decision makers. For example, in one of the South Pacific islands, a filariasis control program was in progress, and as a result of a mass drug administration program, the microfilarial rate obtained in 1967 by examination of 20 mm^3 blood samples dropped to 1.63% after completion of a course of treatment. From the next year, the method of blood survey was modified in order to increase the efficiency of detection of microfilariae, and three 20 mm^3 smears (60 mm^3 in total) were examined. The microfilarial rate obtained with this new method was 1.74%. If this rise in the microfilarial rate implied that the transmission of filariasis was still taking place, it would have been considered necessary to resume the drug administration program. However, the results of statistical analysis of the blood survey records indicated that the correction factor for converting the rate obtained with 60 mm³ to that with 20 mm³ was 0.834 in this case, and thus the rate observed in the second survey was actually about 1.46% if 20 mm³ films were examined. This means that the rate was lower than that of the previous year. (see Section 11D.5).

Most health workers (including this author) engaged in the epidemiology and control of filariasis do not like to introduce statistics into the field because some of the mathematics used is difficult to understand. In the experience of this author, statistics is misused by many filariologists in two ways: first, by making statistical judgements without understanding statistics, and second, by expecting too much from statistics and wanting to collect rather useless data. In both of these cases, the introduction of statistics into the filariasis epidemiology/control programs might be more harmful than useful.

For example, when this author visited a South Asian country in 1965 as a consultant to the antifilariasis campaign, he found out that the methods for blood surveys needed to be improved, if possible, in several aspects. However, it took a few weeks to a few months before these recommendations were understood by the project leader. There was too much parasitological and entomological work imposed on technicians and laborers in order to obtain meaningless statistics. On the other hand, collecting measured blood samples in place of the conventional method of taking one drop of blood was not accepted, because the project leader said that he was interested only in whether a person had microfilaria or not, but not in the amount of microfilariae harbored by individual cases. He probably was not aware that positive or negative depended upon the size of blood samples examined.

When visiting a South Pacific country as a consultant to the filariasis control program in 1971, this author was again impressed by the fact that an international medical officer who was in charge of this project was very poor in mathematics and too statistically minded; he had been requesting the national staff to collect too much complicated and meaningless data. The national health workers were apparently too busy working on jobs requested by the medical officer for meaningless statistics, and had no time to conduct more important health activities.

There are a number of other examples in which statistics is misused and as a result lead to erroneous or misleading decisions. There have also been a number of cases where the administrators were too interested in the statistics without having appropriate understanding of their real meaning, and imposed too much work on assistant health workers in collecting meaningless data.

Excellent examples of the use of statistics in the epidemiology of parasitic diseases were presented by UEMURA (1973; in "Epidemiology and Control of Schistosomiasis," ed. by ANSARI, WHO, pp. 704–739). A review was made by SASA (1967) on the methods for the statistical analysis of microfilaria survey data. There are a number of textbooks on statistics for medical and biological workers, among which the following are especially useful:

> G. W. SNEDECOR & W. G. COCHRAN (1967: sixth edition): *Statistical Methods*, 593 pp., Iowa State University Press.
>
> F. E. CROXTON (1953): *Elementary Statistics, with application in Medicine and the Biological Sciences*: 376 pp. Dover Publications, Inc., New York.

11A.2 The sampling methods for examination of blood microfilariae

For practical purposes, the method of examination for microfilariae must be as simple and easy as possible, but at the same time it should be standardized so that the results can be used for statistical analysis. Therefore, the following method has been recommended as a routine procedure of blood examination for microfilaria survey of human populations (SASA, 1967):

(a) Collect measured blood samples (either 10 mm^3 or 20 mm^3) in place of the conventional unmeasured blood samples,

(b) take three (or more) samples from everybody in place of taking only one sample at one time, and

(c) make linear smears such as described in Section 10B.2.3, in place of making circular smears, for the purpose of counting the number of microfilariae exactly.

The blood smears are examined under low-power magnification of a compound microscope after being dehemoglobinized and stained with Giemsa or Azeo-dyes. The number of microfilariae in each of the three smears should be recorded separately for each person, such as (8, 6, 9/23), (0, 1, 0/1), or (0, 0, 0/0).

Notes:

(1) Some field workers believe that the collection of measured blood samples with micropipettes is much more time-consuming and troublesome than the collection of unmeasured blood samples, such as a drop of blood on a slide. However, it is true that after a few days' training, a technician can collect the measured blood samples almost as easily and fast as collecting the unmeasured ones. In Japan and Okinawa, the method of making three 10 mm^3 blood smears has been practiced by more than 100 technicians on over one million people.

(2) The thick blood smears for examination of blood parasites were usually prepared on a slide in the shape of a coin. However, this shape is not adequate for counting microfilariae in the total field of thick blood smears.

The method of making three linear (or bandlike) smears of about 3 mm wide has been a standard in the filariasis control program in Japan.

(3) To make three blood smears on a slide has various advantages. The efficiency of detection of microfilariae by examination of thick smears of a given volume of blood can be estimated from the positive grade (see Section 11D.4). With this method, the risk of losing all the blood films while rinsing in water or staining is avoided, which may be a problem when only one smear is collected from a person.

11A.3 Criteria for evaluation of the microfilaria survey data

The results of examination for microfilariae can be statistically analyzed and evaluated from various standpoints. There are at least the following three measures as indices of the intensity of infection of human populations.

(a) The microfilarial rate (Mf-rate): This is expressed simply by the percentage obtained by dividing the number of microfilaria positive persons with the total number of persons examined. In this case, only the presence or absence of microfilariae in the specimens examined is of interest, not the number of microfilariae found in each sample. It can be roughly stated that a human population which shows a higher Mf-rate is more intensely infected with the filaria than one showing lower rate. However, there always exist considerable numbers of persons in all filariasis endemic areas who are infected but whose blood sample is negative for microfilaria. It should also be pointed out that the Mf-rate is subject to variation according to various conditions, such as the time of day at which the examination is undertaken (especially in the periodic races of *W. bancrofti*, *B. malayi* and *L. loa*), the standard amount of blood or skin being examined at the survey (the rate is higher in larger samples), and the age and sex composition of the samples of persons examined (Section 11B).

(b) The microfilaria positive grade (Mf-grade): When two or more samples are examined for each individual, the results may be classified into groups according to the number of positive samples. In the scheme of collecting three 10 mm³ blood samples from individual cases, such as practiced in the filariasis control program in Japan, the results of blood examination can be classified into the following four groups: the persons with all the three smears positive (group 3:3), those with two smears positive and one negative (group 2:3), those with only one smear positive (group 1:3), and those with all the three smears negative (group 0:3). The numbers and the ratios of these groups are also dependent upon the intensity of infection of a human population, and statistical methods were developed for estimating the efficiency of detection of microfilariae from the study of the microfilaria positive grade (Section 11D.4).

(c) The microfilarial density (Mf-density): The microfilarial density in a blood or skin sample is usually expressed by the number of microfilariae found per unit weight (or volume) of the sample. This is, therefore, an index of the parasite load of the host and a quantitative measure of the intensity of infection. It has been observed by a number of workers that the microfilarial count is highly variable even when almost the same amount of samples are collected at the same time from the same host, and, therefore, some authors stated that it is not a statistically useful measure (Section 11D.2). Some workers calculated the mean microfilarial counts of various human populations for the purpose of comparing the intensity of infection, but other workers claimed that such a measure is meaningless because the distribution of the density in a population is highly skewed. However, it has recently been demonstrated that the studies of microfilarial density provide various useful information both in theory and in practice on the epidemiology and control of filariasis (Section 11C).

11B. Comparison and evaluation of the rates

11B. 1 Introduction

As stated previously, various rates are obtained as results of epidemiological surveys of human populations, such as the microfilarial rates, clinical manifestation rates (this may be subclassified into the ratios of persons with fever attacks, filarial lymphangitis, elephantiasis, hydrocele, chyluria, etc.), and the skin-test positive rates. When these rates are compared with the intensity of infection with filariae among different human populations, the interest is simply in whether a person is positive or negative in a test, but not in the quantitative aspects of the test results.

Among various criteria for evaluation of the intensity of infection, the problems referring to the statistical treatment of the microfilarial rates (Mf-rates) are discussed mainly in this section. As stated in the previous section (11A.3), the Mf-rate is a simple but very important index for comparison of the status of filarial infection. However, it is subject to variation, even within the same human populations, by the sampling methods, such as by the hour of day at which the blood sample was collected, by the volume of blood collected from individual persons, and by the age and sex distribution of the sampled populations. The problems referring to the microfilarial periodicity are discussed in Section 11F, and those relating to the efficiency of detection of microfilariae by the blood sample sizes are presented in Section 11D. In this section, the problems in variation in the rates by the age and sex compositions are discussed.

11B. 2 The difference in Mf-rate by age and sex-groups

It has generally been observed since the early times of filariasis research that the microfilarial rates differ greatly by the age-group, even within people in the same endemic areas, the rate being very low in ages under five years, gradually increasing by age until about 30 to 40 years, and remaining at nearly the same high level thereafter. Furthermore, there exist differences between the males and females, as pointed out by BAHR (1912) in Fiji, JACHOWSKI & OTTO (1952) in American Samoa, SINGH *et al.* (1956) in India, BEYE & GURIAN (1960; a review), and SASA *et al.* (1970) in Japan.

As shown in examples in Table 11-1 and Fig 11-1, it has been noted in almost all previous surveys of *W. bancrofti* endemic areas that there exists a remarkable difference in the age distribution patterns of the Mf-rate between the two sexes. With regard to the pre-adult age-groups (under 20 years), there is usually not much difference in rates between the sexes, or more frequently, the females show slightly higher rates than the males. On the other hand, there usually exists a remarkable difference in the rates between the two sexes after the age of 20 years, and the rates in adult males turn out to be sometimes more than 50% higher than those in the adult females. It is further interesting that the difference in Mf-rates between the two sexes usually become inconspicuous in the older age-groups, such as over 60 years.

The difference in the age and sex distribution patterns of Mf-rates has been reported also in *B. malayi* endemic areas in East Malaysia by WILSON (1961). In the endemic area of the nocturnally periodic form in Kedah/Penang, where the prevalence is of a medium grade, the Mf-rate in the males reaches the highest level of nearly 50% in the age-group of 25 to 29 years, and the rate stays at almost the same level thereafter. There was a well-marked tendency to lower rates in females of the reproductive age-groups. In the endemic area of the nocturnally subperiodic race of *B. malayi* in Pahang, where the disease is hyperendemic, the Mf-rate reaches the highest level of about 60% in the age-group of 5 to 9 years in the females and 10 to 14 years in the males, and the speed of reduction in Mf-rates in the older age-groups was higher in the females than in the males, thus causing considerable differences between the rates of the two sexes in the adult age-groups.

In many endemic areas of onchocerciasis in Africa, extremely high microfilarial rates have also been recorded by skin snip examination of the people. The age and sex distribution of the Mf-rates of *Onchocerca volvulus* has been shown to be similar to that of *W. bancrofti* and *B. malayi* infections in that it increases almost linearly from near zero in the youngest age-group of 0 to 4 years to the young adult ages of 20 to 24 years, but after this, the rate stays on almost the same level, and also in that female adults show lower rates than male adults through all age-groups, as shown

Table 11-1. Age and sex distribution of the microfilaria rate in three endemic areas of *W. bancrofti* in Japan (after SASA *et al.*, 1970).

Age-group	A. Amami, 1962				B. Kagoshima, 1962				C. Nagasaki, 1962			
	Male		Female		Male		Female		Male		Female	
	No. exam.	% pos.	No. exam.	% pos.	No. exam.	% pos.	No. exam.	% pos.	No. exam.	% pos.	No. exam.	% pos.
0–4	2061	1.94	1868	2.41	3364	0.54	3362	0.42	7377	0.52	7177	0.65
5–9	3146	6.61	3293	8.17	6424	0.93	6094	0.74	13579	0.66	13518	0.80
10–14	4470	10.02	5073	11.41	7847	2.01	7625	2.79	21846	0.82	22078	0.90
15–19	1359	12.36	1521	14.86	1449	2.14	1325	2.19	6839	0.72	7207	1.11
20–24	490	17.35	784	13.01	1003	4.49	1555	2.12	3263	1.65	5246	0.97
25–29	877	18.47	1209	11.50	1652	5.81	2353	1.40	4344	2.05	6754	0.98
30–34	1036	19.11	1474	11.13	1850	5.14	2791	2.58	5265	2.07	7810	1.32
35–39	1079	19.46	1601	14.93	1855	5.82	3147	3.28	5299	2.42	8042	1.38
40–44	915	17.05	1382	11.72	1572	5.66	2742	2.92	3960	2.30	6758	1.39
45–49	901	19.20	1334	12.82	1535	6.71	2546	3.14	3782	2.51	5829	1.24
50–54	822	17.27	1194	13.57	1590	5.91	2295	3.09	3701	2.76	5540	1.68
55–59	675	16.44	937	16.22	1350	5.56	1838	3.48	3169	2.71	4435	2.21
60–64	606	17.16	926	16.41	1114	5.21	1427	3.78	3020	2.85	3810	2.28
65–69	490	20.41	621	14.98	805	5.84	1057	3.50	2286	2.76	2852	1.26
70+	676	14.20	906	12.31	812	3.94	1155	3.12	2125	3.25	2992	1.94
Total	19605	12.45	24213	11.51	34222	3.24	41312	2.29	89855	1.50	110048	1.18

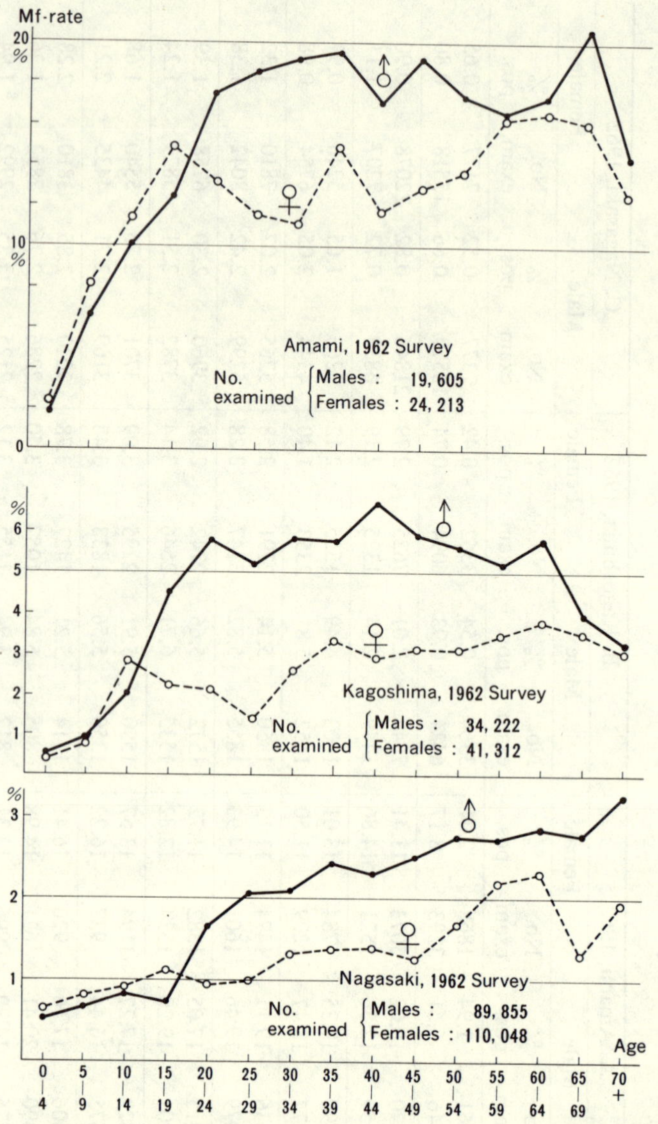

Fig. 11-1. Age and sex distribution of microfilarial rate in three endemic areas of *W. bancrofti* in southern Japan (data from SASA *et al.*, 1970).

Amami, 1962 Survey	No. examined	Males: 19,605
		Females: 24,213
Kagoshima, 1962 Survey	No. examined	Males: 34,222
		Females: 41,312
Nagasaki, 1962 Survey	No. examined	Males: 89,855
		Females: 110,048

in Table 11-2. Table 11-3 is an example showing the age or sex distribution of *Dipetalonema perstans* microfilariae in the blood of an African population.

Table 11-2. Age and sex distribution of *O. volvulus* microfilaria rate in Ethiopia (combined results of 31 places where transmission was found to occur; after OOMEN, 1969).

Age group (years)	Total	Males pos.	% pos.	Total	Females pos.	% pos.
1–4	67	0	0	64	0	0
5–9	203	19	9.4	166	7	4.2
10–14	338	76	22.5	142	18	12.7
15–19	311	81	26.1	92	16	17.4
20–24	209	96	46.0	103	20	19.4
25–29	268	115	43.0	130	34	26.2
30–34	258	91	35.2	125	21	16.8
35–39	202	87	43.1	71	16	22.7
40–44	144	71	49.4	76	14	18.4
45–49	68	30	44.2	32	3	9.7
over 50	278	97	35.0	83	22	26.7
Total	2346	763	32.6	1084	171	15.7

Table 11-3. Age and sex distribution of microfilaremia cases (*Dipetalonema perstans*) in a blood survey of people in the Lunda district, Angola (summarized from MOURA PIRES *et al.* 1959).

Age group (years)	Males			Females		
	No. exam.	No. pos.	% pos.	No. exam.	No. pos.	% pos.
1	197	3	1.5	235	1	0.4
1–4	467	60	12.8	533	48	9.0
5–14	954	242	25.4	1,010	254	25.1
15–24	390	231	59.2	939	516	54.9
25–44	1,154	863	74.8	3,316	2,330	70.3
45–64	466	394	84.5	848	666	78.5
65	28	23	82.1	35	28	80.0
Total	3,656	1,816	49.7	6,916	3,843	55.6

11B.3 Interpretation with catalytic models

The peculiar pattern of the age distribution of the Mf-rate can be simulated with a catalytic model, which was introduced first by MÜNCH (1959)

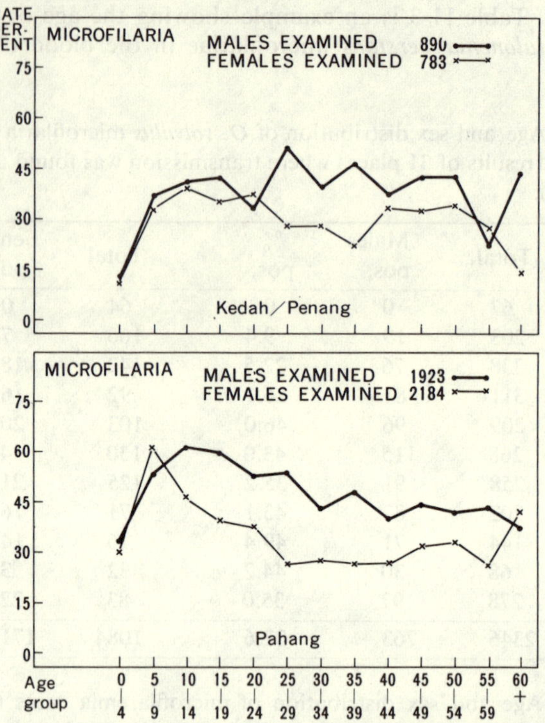

Fig. 11-2.   Age and sex distribution of the microfilarial rate of the people in the endemic areas of *B. malayi* in Kedah/Penang (the periodic form) and in Pahang (the subperiodic form) (redrawn from data by Wilson, 1961).

for interpretation of the age distribution of various signs of infection in the epidemiology of communicable diseases. Three basic models were proposed: (a) the simple catalytic curve (b) the reversible catalytic curve (two-way reactions), and (c) the two-stage catalytic curve (successive reactions).

(a) In the simple catalytic model, the proportion of persons showing the sign of infection can be expressed by the equation:

$$y = 1 - e^{-rt}$$

where y is the percentage of persons showing the sign of infection at the age of t years in an area where the rate of infection per person per year is r. In this case, it is assumed that the people in the endemic area are exposed to the risk of infection by the same rate, and that all those who have been infected are diagnosed as positive by the given test method.

(b) In the reversible catalytic model, it is assumed that the persons in an endemic area are exposed to a constant risk of infection and those who are negative for a sign of infection turn out to be positive at a rate of $a\%$ per year, while those who are positive for the sign of infection turn out to be negative at a rate of $b\%$ per year. In this case, the proportion y of persons at the age of t years showing the sign of infection is expressed by the equation:

$$y = \frac{a}{a+b}(1 - e^{-(a+b)t})$$

(c) In the two-stage catalytic model, it is assumed that persons living in an endemic area of an infectious disease are exposed to a constant risk of infection and those who are negative for a sign of infection turn out to be positive at a rate of $a\%$ per year, while those who once were positive lose the sign of infection at a rate of $b\%$ per year and never become positive again. In this case, the percentage y of the persons aged t showing the positive sign of the infection is expressed by the equation:

$$y = \frac{a}{a-b}(e^{-bt} - e^{-at})$$

It is obvious that all of these mathematical models are constructed on simple hypotheses neglecting the effects of various minor and complicated biological factors. In the cases of interpretation of the age distribution of microfilarial rates, it is obvious that the simple catalytic model (1) is not applicable because the rate does not reach to near 100% even in hyperendemic areas. HAYASHI (1962) analyzed survey data based on relatively small samples collected in Japan using the two-stage catalytic model, but HAIRSTON & JACHOWSKI (1968) adopted the reversible catalytic model for interpretation of data collected by them in American Samoa. In this report, HAIRSTON & JACKOWSKI (1968) stated, "The two-stage catalytic model of Münch assumes that an indivudual who has lost his infection never becomes positive again. Ample evidence shows that this model is not appropriate to the Samoan data, as there are 14 cases went from positive to negative and back to positive. More appropriate is the reversible catalytic model which assumes a constant rate of infection and a constant rate of loss of infection." (BULL. WLD. HLTH. ORG. 1968, Vol. 33, p. 50)

The problem of which of the two catalytic models is better for the theoretical interpretation of the age distribution of the microfilarial rate of people in filariasis endemic areas seems to be not so simple as could be solved by such simple mathematical formulae. As pointed out by these authors, the microfilarial density in the circulating blood fluctuates for various reasons even within the same carriers, and thus it is not surprising that the same individuals sometimes become positive and sometimes negative. However, this does not mean that the same persons once infected become free from the parasite, and then become reinfected, such as postulated in applying the reversible catalytic model. In the cases of *W. bancrofti* and

B. malayi infections, it has been commonly accepted by medical workers that patients in the chronic stage become permanently negative for the microfilariae. In this context, it is unconceivable that those who once lost the sign of infection become positive again as easily as the uninfected persons, and thus the application of the two-stage catalytic model sounds more logical.

As stated previously, there have been a number of studies conducted in various endemic areas on the pattern of the age distribution of microfilarial rates. In general, it seems that the curve keeps on increasing towards the oldest age-group in areas where the force of infection is low (such as Kumamoto and Nagasaki of Japan), the curve reaches an equilibrium level in areas where the intensity of infection is medium (such as Amami and Kagoshima of Japan or Kedah/Penang of Malaya), and the curve shows a peak at young adult age-groups and declines thereafter in older age-groups in hyperendemic areas (such as Pahang of Malaya or Western Samoa before the commencement of the control program). The appearance of a peak and the reduction in the rate in older age-groups can be interpreted only by the two-stage catalytic model.

There has been no adequate explanation given to the question of why the microfilarial rates in adult females are conspicuously lower than those in adult males. JACHOWSKI & OTTO (1955) conducted microfilaria surveys of people in American Samoa, found remarkable differences in the prevalence of microfilaremia between male adults and female adults, and attributed this to the more frequent exposure to infection in males in bushes outside villages. However, the same relationship has been observed in all forms of *Wuchereria* and *Brugia* infections in man regardless of the biting habits of the main vectors, whether indoor or outdoor biters, or whether day-biting or night-biting species. The microfilarial rates in adult females are not only lower than those of the males but also lower than that of the prepuberty age-group of 15 to 19 years. It is therefore possible that some physiological factors appear in females when they reach puberty or reproductive age, which inhibit the appearance of microfilariae in the circulating blood, or increase the value of b (the rate per annum of the loss of the sign of infection) in the two-stage catalytic model. In other words, the value of b is considered to be a variable (not constant) parameter at least in the case of females.

11B.4 Comparison of Mf-rates between populations with different age or sex compositions

As previously stated, the incidence of microfilaria carriers differs greatly by the age and sex-groups, even within the same populations, and therefore results of blood surveys which are presented without reference to the age and sex composition of the samples of persons examined, or those calculated by combining both sexes, are considered rather meaningless. The overall Mf-rate (all ages and both sexes combined) can be utilized as a measure for comparison of the intensity of infection among different populations only when the age and sex composition is nearly the same.

However, it often becomes necessary to compare the intensity of infection among populations with different age and sex compositions. For example, in one of the South Pacific islands where the overall Mf-rate before application of a mass drug administration program was about 20%, the rate observed in blood surveys of people in sampled villages after completion of the treatment was found to have dropped to 1.74% (129 positives out of 7,393 persons examined); on the other hand, results of blood examinations of emigrants who came from all over the island for passport applications showed that 3.49% (107 of 3,064 examined) were positive during the same period. Since the Mf-rate of the latter population was about twice as high as that of the people in selected villages, statistical analysis was made in order to clarify what was the cause of such a difference.

The results of blood examinations of the villagers and the emigrants were classified into age and sex-groups, as shown in Table 11-4. It is clear from this table that the two populations differ greatly in age and sex composition. The villagers are much higher in the ratio of younger age-groups than the emigrants, and are composed of more females than males, while the sex ratio is reversed in the emigrants. By comparing the incidence of microfilaria cases according to the age and sex-groups, it is further found that the two populations are nearly the same in the intensity of infection, and that the big difference in the observed Mf-rates is mainly due to the difference in the age and sex structure of the two populations.

Comparison of the overall Mf-rates of the two populations can be made more reasonably by converting the age and sex composition of the emigrants to that of the standard population (villager), and by obtaining the theoretical number of the sum of microfilaria cases in the emigrants as expected from the standard population. For this purpose, the theoretical number of positive cases is calculated for each age and sex-group (column L) by multiplying the observed number (column J) with the index I (obtained by dividing the ratio D with the ratio H). The sum of the theoretical numbers of all age and sex-groups, 66.48 in this case, is then divided with the total number of persons examined (3,064), and a theoretical Mf-rate of 2.17% based on the standard population is obtained for emigrants. This value is much lower than the crude Mf-rate of the emigrants, and is closer to the observed Mf-rate of the villagers.

There is, however, a simpler method for comparison of the two populations, which this author believes to be more practical and sufficiently reliable. Each population is classified into three groups: males over 20 years of age, females over 20 years, and children of both sexes under 20 years. The adult males, as well as the adult females, are considered to be roughly homogenous in view of Mf-rates, and thus comparison can be made by the rates calculated for both groups. In this case, the rate of adult males is

Table 11-4.   An example of analysis of age and sex distribution of Mf-rate; comparison of blood survey data of different samples.

| A & B | VILLAGERS | | | | EMIGRANTS | | | | | L. |
Sex & Age group	C. No. exam.	D. Ratio (%)	E. No. posit.	F. % posit.	G. No. exam.	H. Ratio (%)	I. Index (D/H)	J. No. posit.	K. % posit.	(J×I) Relative No. posit.
Male 0–4	675	9.13	2	0.30	26	0.85	10.74	0	0.00	0.00
5–9	891	12.05	0	0.00	45	1.47	8.20	0	0.00	0.00
10–14	685	9.27	5	0.73	70	2.28	4.07	0	0.00	0.00
15–19	269	3.64	6	2.23	270	8.81	0.41	10	3.70	4.10
20–29	383	5.18	33	8.62	560	18.28	0.28	31	5.54	10.64
30–39	223	3.02	12	5.38	213	6.95	0.43	16	7.51	6.88
40–49	187	2.53	17	9.09	207	6.76	0.37	11	5.31	4.07
50 +	238	3.22	15	6.30	200	6.53	0.49	14	7.00	6.86
Total	3,551	48.03	90	2.53	1,591	51.93	0.92	82	5.15	32.55
Fem. 0–4	645	8.72	3	0.47	25	0.82	10.63	0	0.00	0.00
5–9	936	12.66	4	0.43	41	1.34	9.45	2	4.88	18.96
10–14	650	8.79	2	0.31	67	2.19	4.01	1	1.49	4.01
15–19	311	4.21	5	1.61	372	12.41	0.35	5	1.34	1.75
20–29	485	6.56	17	3.51	400	13.05	0.50	8	2.00	4.00
30–39	366	4.95	5	1.37	194	6.33	0.78	3	1.55	2.34
40–49	225	3.04	3	1.33	197	6.43	0.47	5	2.54	2.35
50 +	224	3.03	0	0.00	177	5.78	0.52	1	0.56	0.52
Total	3,842	51.97	39	1.02	1,473	48.07	1.08	25	1.70	33.93
TOTAL	7,393	100.	129	1.74	3,064	100.	1.00	107	3.49	66.48
M+F0–19	5,062	68.47	27	0.53	916	29.90	2.29	18	1.97	41.22
M 20+	1,031	13.95	77	7.47	1,180	38.51	0.36	72	6.10	25.92
F 20 +	1,300	17.58	25	1.92	968	31.5w	0.56	17	1.76	9.52

(Data compiled from laboratory records of the Filariasis Control Pilot Project, Western Samoa, 1969; Sasa, M., WHO Assignment Report, 1972).

7.47 % in the villagers and 6.10 % in the emigrants, and that of adult females is 1.92 % in the villagers and 1.76 % in the emigrants. It is again clear that the two populations are nearly the same in the prevalance of filariasis, though the observed overall Mf-rates were much different.

As for standardizing the age and sex composition of the population to be surveyed, McCarthy (1959) used a "standard population group" and compared the prevalence of filariasis in various Pacific islands. His standard group consisted 100 males and 100 females divided into age-groups according to the latest local census returns. On the other hand, Wilson (1962) proposed a standard population to be applicable commonly to the tropical countries by combining the census figures of Ceylon (for 1953) and the Federation of Malaya (for 1957). The age and sex distribution of this standard population distributed to equal 10,000 persons, as well as the method for calculating a standardized elephantiasis rate from an observed data, was described in this report.

11C. Analysis of the microfilarial density

11C.1 Introduction

The microfilarial density is generally expressed by the number of micro-filariae found per unit volume of blood samples examined. This is an important measure in the treatment, control, and epidemilogy of filariasis. In individual cases, persons harboring high densities of microfilariae are considered to be higher in the risk of developing clinical symptoms, and to developing more severe fever reactions when treated with diethylcar-bamazine. They are more dangerous as the source of infection to the vectors than those with lower densities. However, it should be noted that the dentity of microfilariae in the circulating blood is not always correlated with the worm burden (number of adult worms per person) or with the severity of clinical affections. The density of microfilariae usually becomes extremely low or they disappear from the circulating blood when a patient develops chronic symptoms, such as elephantiasis or chyluria, even though they may still harbor large numbers of adult worms. The high densities are seen more frequently in persons still in the subclinical or acute stage of filarial infection.

In studying the microfilarial density of a human population, it is recommended to compile the data of a blood survey according to a form such as shown in Table 11-5 which is a classification of persons according to the observed microfilarial counts. From this table, one can easily calculate the microfilaremia rate, the mean microfilarial count per positive case, as well as that per total cases examined.

11C.2 The mean microfilarial density

The mean microfilarial density is obtained by dividing the sum of all microfilarial counts with the number of positive cases, or with the total number of cases examined, and has been used by some workers as a measure for the comparison of densities among different populations or that before and after application of a control measure. It is true that the mean density decreases remarkably when an effective control measure is applied to an infected population. However, as shown in Table 11-6, the frequency distribution of the microfilarial counts is always extremely skewed, or far

Table 11-5. An example of the method for recording the microfilaria count (after SASA, 1966a).

RECORD OF MICROFILARIAL COUNT   No. *Su-3*

Area surveyed: *Setouchi & Ukon District*   Date: *Sept. 1964*
Population: *22,698*   Blood sample: *30* mm³

FREQUENCY DISTRIBUTION ACCORDING TO Mf-COUNT

Mf No.	1	2	3	4	5	6	7	8	9	10	Total	Cum.
0	57	48	30	25	16	14	11	13	11	11	236	236
10	9	9	9	4	1	2	6	1	3	2	46	282
20	2	3	2	5	2	3				1	18	300
30	1	1		1	1	1	1	1	1	1	9	309
40			1				1			2	4	313
50		1							1		2	315
60		1					1			1	3	318
70							1				1	319
80		1	1								2	321
90	1						2			1	4	325
101–200	104, 105, 105, 117, 117, 126, 123											
	151, 154, 181, 195										11	336
201–300	258											
											1	337
301–400											1	338
401–500												
501–600												
601–700												
701–800												
801–900												
901–1,000												
1,001– over												

Number negative: _9,644_   No. positive & Mf count unknown: _____
Number examined: _9,990_   Total Mf count: _5,216_
Percent examined: _44.0_   Percent positive: _3.46_
Average Mf count: per positive _15.43_   per total _0.522_
Remarks: *Result two years after start of drug treatment programme*

from the normal distribution pattern. In such a case, the simple "arithmetic mean" is subject to great variation by chance, especially by the counts obtained from small numbers of cases with extremely high densities. It is therefore necessary to apply some statistical treatment with which the frequency distribution be converted to near a normal pattern.

Table 11-6. Frequency distribution of microfilaria positive cases classified by density per 30 mm³ blood sample, South Amami District (Setouchi & Uken) 1964 (Sasa, 1967).

Mf. count (A)	Frequency (B)	Cumul. freq. (C)	Cumul. percent (D)	Probit (E)
1	57	57	16.9	4.14
2	48	105	31.1	4.51
3	30	135	39.9	4.74
4	25	160	47.3	4.93
5	16	176	52.1	5.05
6	14	190	56.2	5.16
7	11	201	59.5	5.24
8	13	214	63.3	5.34
9	11	225	66.6	5.43
10	11	236	69.8	5.52
11–20	46	282	83.4	5.97
21–30	18	300	88.8	6.22
31–40	9	309	91.4	6.37
41–50	4	313	92.6	6.45
51–60	2	315	93.2	6.49
61–70	3	318	94.1	6.56
71–80	1	319	94.4	6.59
81–90	2	321	95.0	6.65
91–100	4	325	96.2	6.77
101–200	11	336	99.4	7.14
201–300	1	337	99.7	7.32
301–400	1	338	100.	—
401+	0	338	100.	—

11C.3 The logarithmic normal distribution of micro-filarial density

After testing with various mathematical formulae, it was eventually demonstrated that the frequency distribution of positive cases by the microfilarial density is generally a logarithmically normal type (Sasa, 1967). In order to confirm this, it is convenient to prepare a table such as shown in Table 11-6, which can be easily prepared from data compiled in Table 11-5. When a frequency distribution is logarithmically normal, the cumulative percentages plotted on a graph paper with a logarithmic scale on the X-axis and a probit scale on the Y-axis fits on a linear regression line generally expressed by a simple formula:

$$y = a + b \log x$$

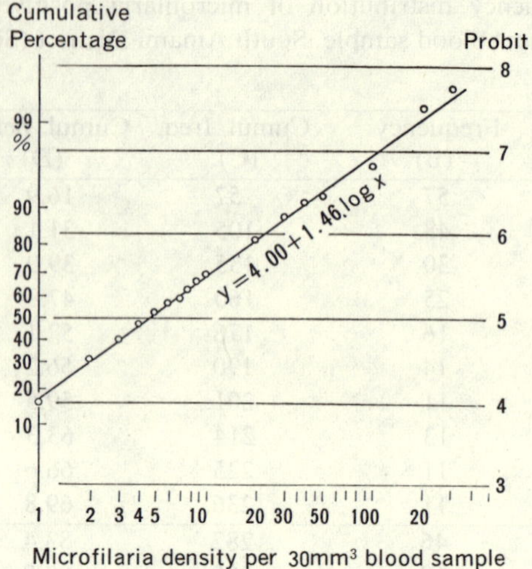

Fig. 11-3. Showing regression line of cumulative frequency distribution of microfilaria positive cases, southern Amami district, 1964 survey (after SASA, 1966).

An example of the regression line obtained from data in Table 11-6 is shown in Fig. 11-3. The two parameters, *a* and *b*, are obtained from this figure. The value of *a* corresponds to the percentage of persons harboring 1 microfilaria per unit of blood sample (since log 1 is 0), and *b* is the slope of the regression line. The same statistical treatment has been widely used in obtaining the dose-response relationship, such as in the test of toxicity of insecticides or drugs. When log-probability graph paper is not available, the conversion of percentages to the probits can be made from a mathematical table. (In the case of a simple normal distribution, the same linear relation can be obtained on a section paper with an arithmetic scale on x-axis and a probit scale on Y-axis.)

It should be pointed out here that the number of negative cases (with no microfilaria) is entirely omitted from the group, and only the positive cases are taken into the account. If we include the negatives, the regression line takes a form of Polya-Eggenberger distribution, and does not fit the logarithmic normal type. Also, the regression lines drawn from data collected from populations with high intensities of infection tends to be curved upwards in the zone of high microfilarial densities. This may be interpreted as due to the crowding effect on the microfilariae in the circulating blood.

Note: SOUTHGATE (1974) applied the above method for obtaining the regreesion lines from his blood survey data collected in Fiji by using four different techniques (20 mm³ smear, 60 mm³ smear, counting chamber, and membrance filtration), and concluded also that the data presentation deviced by SASA (1967) was extremely valuable for comparing the intensity of transmission between different human populations with the same survey method, or for comparing the efficiency of detection of microfilariae from the same human populations with different survey methods. SOUTHGATE (1974) further proposed to calculate three additional parame ters in order to validate the use of this formula; namely, r, which is the correlation coefficient of the regression line of the cumulative percentage of microfilaria positive cases against microfilaria density on a log-probit scale; SE(r), which is the standard error of r; and the ratio r: SE(r). When this ratio exceeds 3 in value, such as in all of the four techniques used by this author, we can be confident in handling log-probit regression lines as close approximations to straight lines, and in attaching significance to the values of a, b and MfD-50.

11C.4 Method of comparison of microfilarial density

Since it has become clear that the density in a population is distributed on a log-normal type, comparison of densities among different populations can be made with the "median," or the "geometric mean," which are the measures corresponding to the arithmetic mean of a normal distribution. If a distribution is precisely log-normal, these two measures take the same value. For practical purposes, it is much simpler to obtain the median (the density corresponding to 50% level) than to calculate the geometric mean. Because of the involvement of a crowding effect in the high density zone, it is also more logical to use the median than the geometric mean. The median microfilarial density of a population is called MfD-50, which is a value comparable to LD-50 or TLM in toxicity tests.

In obtaining the MfD-50 from blood survey data, it is convenient to draw a regression line by the visual fitting of the observed values, and to find the density on x-axis corresponding to the level at which the regression line crosses the 50% (probit 5) horizon. However, more valuable information on the density of a population can be presented by giving the values of a and b obtained from the chart, rather than with the single value of MfD-50.

11C.5 Comparison of the microfilarial density among various endemic areas

Examples of comparison of microfilarial density among different endemic areas are shown in Figs. 11-4 and 11-5. It should be noted that where the intensity of infection was high, such as Tahiti (before treatment), the microfilaria rates as well as Mf-rate. showed larger values, and both a and b showed smaller values than in areas with lower intensity of infection. These indices (MfD-rate, a, b) are usually highly correlated, but are basically independent from each other. In other words, it can be said that the

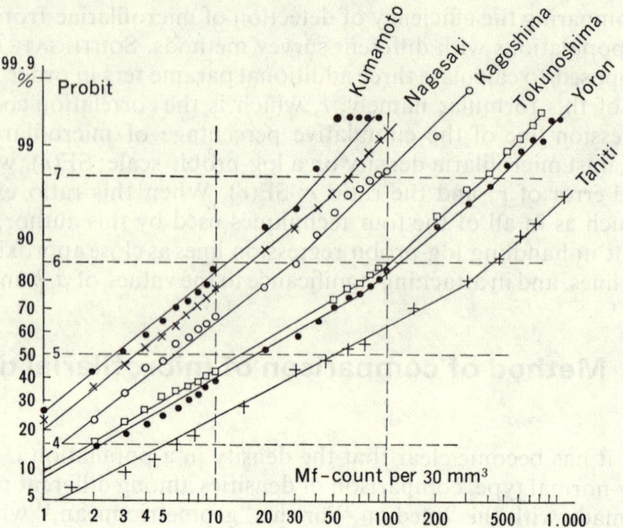

Fig. 11-4. Cumulative percentage distribution of microfilaria positive cases by microfilaria density in various endemic areas (SASA, 1967).

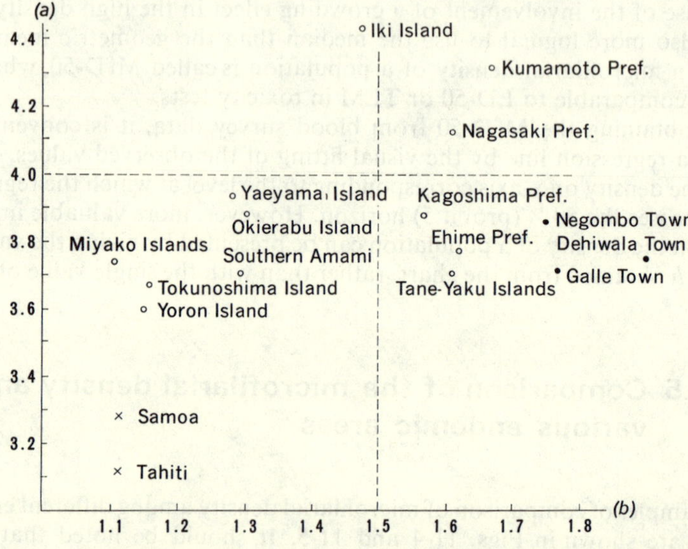

Fig. 11-5. Values of *a* and *b* of the regression lines: y = a + b log x; according to the endemic areas (before control).
× : South Pacific Islands (KESSEL, 1957).
● : Ceylon (ABDULCADER & SASA, 1965).
○ : Japan, (SASA, 1967).

intensity of infection may not be the same even when the microfilaremia rate or the value of MfD-50 is the same. Therefore, it is necessary to present at least the three indices (Mf-rate, a, and b) for all blood survey data.

It has been noted that in endemic areas where filariasis is more evenly distributed at low densities, the values of MfD-50 are lower than in areas where the disease is endemic in certain restricted foci at high intensities, even when the Mf-rate is the same or higher. Such evidence was shown,

Table 11-7. Comparison of frequency distribution of microfilarial density before and after DEC administrations (after SASA, 1967).

| Mf. density | Tahiti[a] | | | | North Amami[b] | | | |
| | Before treatment | | After treatment | | Before treatment | | After treatment | |
	Freq.	Cum.%	Freq.	Cum.%	Freq.	Cum.%	Freq.	Cum.%
1	14	5.5	11	14.7	10	4.5	47	21.4
2	10	9.4	6	22.6	4	6.4	32	35.5
3	8	12.5	6	30.6	5	8.6	26	47.7
4	8	15.7	4	36.0	11	13.6	3	49.1
5	7	18.4	2	38.6	6	16.4	15	55.9
6	4	20.0	5	45.2	7	19.1	10	60.4
7	15	25.9	1	46.6	2	20.4	5	62.7
8	3	27.1	3	50.6	2	20.9	9	66.7
9	3	28.3	1	52.0	4	22.8	4	68.5
10	4	29.8	1	53.3	2	23.6	5	70.8
11–20	36	44.0	10	66.6	35	39.6	31	85.0
21–30	10	47.8	7	76.0	15	46.4	12	90.5
31–40	12	52.5	3	80.0	20	55.5	4	92.3
41–50	6	54.9	5	86.6	13	61.3	3	93.6
51–60	12	59.5	5	93.3	11	66.3	1	94.1
61–70	6	61.9	1	94.7	11	71.2	3	95.5
71–80	10	65.8	1	96.0	7	74.5	2	96.8
81–90	6	68.1	9	96.0	8	78.0	1	96.8
91–100	6	70.6	0	96.0	5	80.4	0	96.8
101–200	23	79.6	3	100	26	92.3	3	98.2
201–300	20	87.5			8	95.9	3	99.6
301–400	9	91.0			6	98.6	0	99.6
401–500	7	93.7			0	98.6	1	100
501–600	6	96.1			3	100		
601–900	7	98.8						
901–	3	100						
Total	255		75		220		220	

[a]After KESSEL (1957), density per 20 mm^3.
[b]From records of Naze Health Center, Amami, 1963, density per 30 mm^3.

for example, from a comparison of data collected from the whole Nagasaki Prefecture (with restricted foci) and from Iki Island (even distribution).

11C.6 Comparison of the microfilarial density for evaluation of filariasis control measures

The same method can be applied for the assessment of effects of control measures applied to a human population. As shown in Table 11-7 and Fig. 11-6, both the Mf-rate and Mf-density drop when effective control measures (such as mass administration of diethylcarbamazine) are applied to a population in an endemic area, and the degree of reduction of these indices is regarded as an indication of the effectiveness of the work. Again, the results may be evaluated from various aspects by utilizing the statistical methods discussed before.

In areas where mass administration is made to the whole population, it is expected that the work not only reduces the Mf-rate, but also reduces the value of MfD-50, because those who are still positive harbor only small amounts of microfilariae. On the other hand, if a considerable number of microfilaria carriers are left untreated and the rest of the population is extensively treated, the MfD-50 may be still high, even though the Mf-rate drops significantly. Thus, the analysis of the distribution of the Mf-density is very useful in the assessment of the effects of mass drug administration programs.

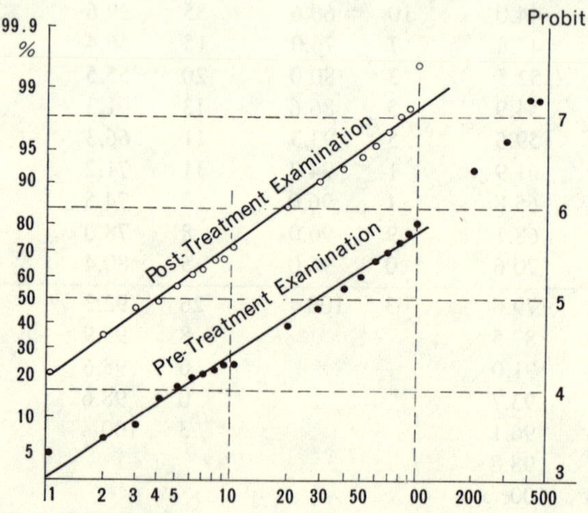

Fig. 11-6. Frequency distribution of microfilarial density among cases positive at both pretreatment and posttreatment blood surveys (northern Amami district, 1963).

11C.7 Correlation between the microfilarial density and the attack rate of fever reaction after DEC administration

Observations on the microfilarial density of individual cases are not only of academic interest in the epidemiology of filariasis, but are also of practical importance in conducting the mass treatment of parasite carriers with DEC. For example Sasa *et al.* (1963c) treated 105 cases of microfilaria carriers with daily doses of 2 mg per kg of DEC, and 187 cases of carriers with daily doses of 8 mg per kg, given once a day, in endemic areas of *W. bancrofti* in the Amami Islands. Body temperatures of all of these cases were taken three times a day for three days after the initial dose, and those who showed a fever reaction of over 37.3°C or over 38.1°C were classified according to the microfilarial density observed at a blood examination conducted just before the treatment. The results were as shown in Table 2-6 and Fig. 2-2 on page 67. It is clear that the attack rate and the severity of the fever reaction caused by administration of DEC is highly correlated with the level of the microfilarial density. It was rather surprising that those treated with a lower dosage of 2 mg per kg per day showed higher attack rates of fever than those treated with the higher dose of 8 mg per kg per day. This relationship is important, since the attack rate and severity of fever reactions can be predicted to individual cases before the drug administration according to the microfilarial level observed at the pretreatment blood survey.

11D. The efficiency of detection of microfilariae

11D.1 Introduction

As stated previously, the detection of microfilariae is the most important and the only specific means of diagnosis of a filarial infection at the present time, but at the same time, it is a poor diagnostic method in the sense that there always exists a number of persons among the microfilaria negative group who are actually infected but whose microfilariae do not show up in the blood or skin samples examined at one time. If we repeat blood or skin surveys on the same population with the same method at nearly the same time, we almost always find new positive cases in the second examination among those who were negative in the first examination, while nearly the same number among the previously positive groups turn out to be negative in the second examination. The microfilarial rate (Mf-rate) of an infected population is dependent upon the volume (or weight) of the standard samples collected from each person, and becomes higher as the standard volume is increased. It is therefore necessary to know the efficiency of detection of microfilariae when a certain volume of blood or skin sample is examined, or to develop a method for estimating a correction factor for the comparison of results obtained by the examination of different amounts of blood or skin samples.

In the past, some workers tried to develop a common mathematical solution for the correction factors applicable to certain positive rates and to certain volumes. For example, if a microfilarial rate of 10% is obtained by examination of 20 mm³ blood samples, what would be the rate if 60 mm³ samples were examined? The answer is, as discussed by SASA (1967, 1974), that there is no common correction factor applicable to a certain microfilarial rate because the efficiency of detection of microfilariae is not dependent upon the microfilarial rate of the population but upon the pattern of distribution of the microfilarial density in the population concerned. In other words, since the microfilarial density may differ greatly among the populations showing the same microfilarial rates, the answer may be 12% in one population but could be 15% in another population. The following are summaries of the results of studies reported by SASA (1967, 1974).

11D.2 The variation of microfilarial counts in blood samples

The numbers of microfilariae found in apparently the same volume of blood is highly variable. For example, EDESON (1959) examined microfilariae in 60 mm³ blood samples collected every day at about 9 p.m. for about 30 days from 13 cases of *B. malayi* carriers, and stated that "there was a considerable and apparently irregular variation in numbers." Many other workers have experienced similar trouble in blood examinations, and considered such a test to be an unreliable diagnostic measure.

It should, however, be noted that the numbers of microfilariae found in small samples are always subject to variation even when they are randomly distributed in the circulating blood. In such a case, there is a mathematical method of testing whether the variation in the counts can be expected simply as error by chance, or whether the microfilariae are not randomly distributed in the circulating blood.

In one of the cases (No. 9) examined by EDESON (1959), for example, the microfilarial counts in 29 examinations varied from 0 to 9; or more precisely, his data shows that the frequency of samples showing 0, 1, 2, 3, 4, 5, 6, 7, 8, and 9 microfilariae were 2, 4, 4, 6, 6, 2, 1, 3, 0, and 1, respectively. The mean microfilarial count in this case is:

$$m = [(0 \times 2) + (1 \times 4) + (2 \times 4) + (3 \times 6) + (4 \times 6) + (5 \times 2)$$
$$+ (6 \times 1) + (7 \times 3) + (8 \times 0) + (9 \times 1)] \div 29 = 100 \div 29$$
$$= 3.448$$

As a general rule, it can be stated that if the microfilariae are randomly distributed in the circulating blood at an average density of m per unit volume of the blood (60 mm³ in this case), the probability of obtaining n microfilariae in a blood sample is expressed by the following equation of the Poisson distribution:

$$P_{(n)} = e^{-m}m^n/n!$$

where e is the base of natural logarithms ($e = 2.7182$).

In this case, the probability of the occurrence of 4 microfilariae in a blood sample is:

$$P_{(4)} = (2.7182)^{-3.448} \times (3.448)^4/(4 \times 3 \times 2 \times 1) = 0.1874$$

Likewise, the probabilities of the occurrence of all the numbers from 0 to 7 can be calculated, as shown in Table 11-8. The theoretical frequencies (X') of samples containing n microfilariae are calculated by multiplying these probabilities $P_{(n)}$ by 29. The value of Chi-square turns out to be 7.06. With the degree of freedom of $8 - 2 = 6$, this value lies between 25% (Chi-square $= 7.84$) and 50% (Chi-square $= 5.35$). This means that such a variation in the microfilarial counts could occur by chance at a probability of higher than 25%.

Table 11-8. Test of fitness of microfilaria counts to the Poisson distribution. Data compiled from reports by EDESON, 1959, case No. 9, microfilaria counts in 60 mm³ blood samples collected every day at 9 p.m. for 29 consecutive days. The probabilities are calculated from the formula:
$$P(n) = e^{-m}m^n/n!,\ e = 2.781,\ m = 3.448 = (100/29),\ e^{-m} = 0.03181$$

Mf-count (n)	Observed frequency (X)	m^n	$m^n/n!$	Probability P(n)	Theoretical frequency (X)	$\dfrac{(X-X')^2}{X'}$
0	2	1	1	0.0318	0.92	1.27
1	4	3.448	3.448	0.1097	3.18	0.21
2	4	11.890	5.945	0.1891	5.48	0.40
3	6	41.002	6.834	0.2174	6.30	0.01
4	6	141.386	5.891	0.1874	5.43	0.06
5	2	487.54	4.062	1.1292	3.75	0.82
6	1	1681.17	2.335	0.0743	2.15	0.62
7	3	5797.14	1.150	0.0366	1.06	3.55
8	1	—	—	0.0246	0.71	0.12
Total	29	—	—	1.0000	29.00	7.06

Chi-square test: 50% > P > 30% (Degree of freedom $= 6$).

11D.3 The probability for positive or negative

In the examination of microfilariae in thick blood smears, our primary interest is whether a person is positive or negative, and the percentage of positive cases among the populations surveyed. In the diagnosis of filariasis, using the result of a blood examination to determine whether a person is positive or negative is sometimes considered to be as contradictory as the decision of a judge as to whether the person is guilty or innocent. In the filariasis control programs so far implemented in Japan, Sri Lanka, Brazil, etc., only the persons who were found to be positive were treated with the drug, and those who were negative in a blood examination were left untreated.

However, it should be noted that the difference between positive or negative can not be categorized as clearly as black or white. Even with the same method of blood examination, the same person can be positive at one time and negative at another, as shown in the previous section. The probability of obtaining a positive result becomes higher as the microfilarial density is larger, or the amount of blood collected for the examination is increased. From equations it can be stated that the probability of obtaining a negative (n = 0) result at the examination of a person harboring an average of m microfilariae per unit volume of blood sample is e^{-m}, and that for a positive result is $1 - e^{-m}$, because both m^0 and O! are equal to 1.

Table 11-9 shows the values of e^{-m} for various values of m. Because $e^{-(a+b+c+d)} = e^{-a} \times e^{-b} \times e^{-c} \times e^{-d}$, the value of such as $e^{-1.347}$ can be calculated by the equation:

$$e^{-1.347} = e^{-1} \times e^{-0.3} \times e^{-0.04} \times e^{-0.007} = 0.367879 \times 0.740818$$

$$\times 0.960789 \times 0.993024 = 0.2600.$$

Table 11-9. Values of negative exponentials, e^{-m}.

m	e^{-m}	$e^{-0.1n}$	$e^{-0.01m}$	$e^{-0.001m}$
0	1.000 000	1.000 000	1.000 000	1.000 000
1	0.367 879	0.904 837	0.990 050	0.999 000
2	0.135 335	0.818 731	0.980 199	0.998 002
3	0.049 787	0.740 818	0.970 446	0.997 004
4	0.018 316	0.670 320	0.960 789	0.996 008
5	0.006 738	0.606 531	0.951 123	0.995 012
6	0.002 479	0.548 812	0.941 765	0.994 018
7	0.000 912	0.496 585	0.932 116	0.993 024
8	0.000 335	0.449 329	0.923 116	0.992 032
9	0.000 123	0.406 570	0.913 931	0.991 040
10	0.000 045	0.367 879	0.904 837	0.990 050

Some workers in filariasis control may consider that a person harboring an average of 1 microfilaria per 20 mm³ should show 1 microfilaria in all 20 mm³ blood samples collected from him. However, this is not the case in theory and also in practical experience. As seen in Table 11-10, some 36.8% of those who have the average density of $m = 1$ are expected to be negative, and only 63.2% among them can be diagnosed as positive at one examination. Among the positive cases, those showing 1 microfilaria ($n = 1$) in this case is also 36.8%, and the other 26.4% are expected to show 2 or more microfilariae in the blood sample. Even in those who harbor the microfilariae at an average density of 2 per unit, as many as 13.5% of them are expected to be "misdiagnosed" as negative, by a single examination of the unit volume of blood. From this table, we can also estimate the grade of increase or decrease of the efficiency of detection of microfilariae in relation to the increase or decrease of the size of blood samples. In persons harboring an average of 1.0 microfilaria per 20 mm³, the efficiency of detection of microfilariae in examination of 20 mm³ blood is $(1 - 0.367879) = 0.632121$, but the rate increases to $(1 - 0.049787) = 0.950213$ if 60 mm³ of the blood is examined, because the average count per unit increases three times ($m = 3$).

11D.4 A direct method for estimating the correction factor from Mf-grade

When microfilaria surveys are conducted by examination of multiple blood samples and the numbers or ratios of cases with various positive grades are recorded, the correction factors to be applied among Mf-rates obtained with examination of different units can be easily estimated. For example, the national filariasis control program of Japan accepted this author's idea and carried out microfilaria surveys by collecting three blood samples of 10 mm³ from each person. The numbers of persons showing microfilariae in all of the three samples (N_3), those with two samples positive and one negative (N_2), those with only one sample positive and two samples negative (N_1), and those with all of the three samples negative (N_0) were recorded separately. In these cases, the numbers of cases to be diagnosed as positive by examinations of 30 mm³, 20 mm³ or 10 mm³ can be estimated by the following simple formula:

For 30 mm³: $N_1 + N_2 + N_3$
For 20 mm³: $\frac{2}{3}N_1 + N_2 + N_3$
For 10 mm³: $\frac{1}{3}N_1 + \frac{2}{3}N_2 + N_3$

The correction factors for the conversion of Mf-rates observed with 30 mm³ to those with 20 mm³ or 10 mm³ can be calculated for each endemic area by utilizing the above direct conversion method, as shown in Table 11-10.

Table 11-10. Some results of blood surveys under the national filariasis control program of Japan: (A) survey before start of control, (B) posttreatment blood surveys, N_3: number of persons with all three films positive, N_2: those with two films positive, N_1 those with only one film positive, N: total number examined (from SASA *et al.*, 1970).

Area	Year	Number with positive grades				Percent positive	Correction factor for		MfD-$_{50}$	a	b
		N_3	N_2	N_1	N		20 mm$_3$	10 mm$_3$			
(A) Miyako	1965	8,144	1,827	1,992	47,342	20.17	0.945	0.838	18.8	3.73	1.10
Yoron	1962	564	91	88	4,825	15.40	0.961	0.864	16.6	3.60	1.15
Tokunoshima	1962	840	191	189	10,357	11.78	0.949	0.845	14.1	3.67	1.16
Tanegashima	1962	185	59	45	6,848	4.22	0.948	0.858	7.1	3.71	1.61
Kagoshima	1962	205	85	67	15,432	2.43	0.937	0.800	5.2	3.88	1.56
Nagasaki	1962	540	462	484	113,435	1.31	0.894	0.678	3.4	4.12	1.62
Iki	1962	124	184	201	42,066	1.21	0.864	0.616	2.3	4.47	1.48
Kumamoto	1964	111	102	127	82,927	0.41	0.876	0.651	2.5	4.43	1.67
(B) Miyako	1965	557	502	1,000	12,352	20.31	0.840	0.599	1.3	4.57	1.12
Amami	1963	140	81	105	695	46.91	0.893	0.723	7.2	4.07	1.11
Tokunoshima	1963	68	59	103	1,988	11.57	0.851	0.616	3.3	4.13	1.29
	1964	111	89	58	1.538	16.78	0.925	0.745	4.3	3.77	1.67

It has been demonstrated that the correction factors are highly correlated with the median density of microfilariae (Mf-50) in the population, and become smaller as the density decreases. The efficiency of detection of microfilariae by examination of a unit volume of blood sample is dependent also on the density of microfilariae among the infected populations, and becomes much less after the people are treated with diethylcarbamazine. In Miyako, for example, Mf-rate of the population in the pretreatment blood survey was 20.17% in examinations of three units (30 mm^3) of smears, and as high as 83.8% of the positive cases are estimated to be diagnosed also to be positive in examination of only 1 unit (10 mm^3). However, in the posttreatment blood surveys of the previously positive cases, the Mf-rate was about the same level (20.31%), but the conversion factor of the rate from three units to one unit became as low as 59.9% because the density among the population became much lower.

11D.5 Comparison of microfilarial rates obtained by examinations of different amount of blood samples

In Western Samoa, where *W. bancrofti* was highly prevalent and more than 20% of the population were microfilaria positive in the pretreatment blood examination, a mass administration program of DEC to the whole population was effected in 1964 by the dosage regimen of 5 mg per kg given 18 times at weekly and monthly intervals; in a posttreatment blood survey carried out in 1967 by taking 20 mm^3 blood samples, 42,697 persons were examined and 696 or 1.63% were positive for the microfilariae. Because the efficiency of detection of microfilariae with 20 mm^3 samples was considered to be unsatisfactory, the project leader decided to increase the amount of blood samples to 60 mm^3 (three smears of 20 mm^3) beginning August 1968; in the blood examinations carried out with this method, 129 out of 7,393 persons were positive, with the microfilarial rate of 1.74%. A question was raised by the project leader at this point whether this increase from 1.63% to 1.73% meant that filariasis was increasing again after the mass drug administration was suspended and thus another course of drug administration was necessary, or whether the difference was merely a result of an increase in the efficiency of detection of microfilariae.

A statistical analysis was conducted by this author in 1972 from original records; of the total of 129 cases found to be carrying microfilariae in 60 mm^3 blood samples, 87 had microfilariae in all of the three 20 mm^3 films, 20 had them in two of the three films, and 22 had them in only one film. Therefore, the number of microfilaria cases expected to be detected when only 20 mm^3 blood samples are examined would be:

$$87 + 20 \times (2/3) + 22 \times (1/3) = 107.6$$

This led to an adjusted microfilarial rate of 1.46% (107.6/7,393), which was smaller than the 1.63% in 1967. This meant that the increase in the microfilarial rate from 1.63 in 1967 to 1.74% in 1968–9 was presumably due to the change of the blood survey method, and not to the recovery of transmission as was feared by the administrators.

11D.6 A method for estimating the efficiency of detection of microfilariae from the frequency distribution of microfilaria counts

In the pretreatment blood survey conducted in the Miyako District of Okinawa in 1965, a total of 59,212 persons were examined with the three 10 mm³ blood smear method, and 11,889 persons among them were found to be positive, with a microfilaria rate of 20.08%. The frequency distribution of Mf-counts in 30 mm³ among the positive cases was as shown in Table 11-11.

In such a case, if another survey is conducted with the same method at the same time on exactly the same population, it can be expected that the rate would be almost the same. However, some of the cases who were positive in the first blood survey would not show microfilaria in the second survey, and about the same number of new positive cases would be expected to be detected in the second survey from the group of persons who were negative in the first survey.

By adopting the idea presented in Section 11D.3, the number of persons who would be diagnosed as negative if a second blood examination be performed can be calculated for each class of microfilaria density. For example, 1,236 cases among the total of 11,889 positives were showing only one microfilaria ($m = 1$), and thus 36.79% (e^{-1}) among them or 465.82 are estimated to be negative if a second survey were conducted. Likewise, 13.53% (e^{-2}) among 864 cases showing 2 microfilariae, or 116.93 persons of this class, are considered to fall into the negative group in the second survey. The numbers of these "new negatives" rapidly decrease as the Mf-count (m) becomes higher, because both the observed number of cases (N) and the probability (e^{-m}) reduce rapidly. The theoretical numbers of new negatives become small and negligible over a certain Mf-level, such as above 10 per 30 mm³ in this case. The sum of N e^{-m} calculated for every class of Mf-counts is 627.45 in this case. This means that if another blood examination were performed on the same population with the same method, 627.45 persons are estimated to be detected as "new positives" from the group diagnosed as negative at the blood survey conducted in Miyako in 1965. It can be further stated that, if 60 mm³ (2 units) are examined on this population, the total number of positive cases will increase to 11,889 + 627.45 = 12,516.45, and the Mf-rate will change from 20.08% to 21.14%, with a correction factor of 1.0527.

Table 11-11. The frequency distribution and cumulative percentages of persons by the microfilaria count in 30 mm³ blood samples, and the numbers of new positives to be detected if the same blood examination is repeated. Data from records of Miyako Health Center (after SASA, 1974).

Pretreatment survey: Number examined-59.212, number &% postive-11889(20.08%)

Postreatment survey: Number examined-12,352, number &% positive-2,052(16.61)

m	A. Pretreatment survey							B. Posttreatment survey						
	N	Cum.%	Ne^{-m}	Ne^{-2m}	Ne^{-3m}	Ne^{-4m}	Ne^{-5m}	N	Cum.%	Ne^{-m}	Ne^{-2m}	Ne^{-3m}	Ne^{-4m}	Ne^{-5m}
1	1236	10.4	465.82	167.27	61.54	22.64	8.33	807	39.3	296.88	109.22	40.18	14.18	5.44
2	864	17.7	116.93	15.83	2.14	0.29	0.04	371	57.4	50.21	6.80	0.92	0.12	0.02
3	627	22.9	31.22	1.15	0.08	0.00	0.00	174	65.9	8.66	0.43	0.02	0.00	0.00
4	500	27.1	9.16	0.17	0.00	—	—	112	71.3	2.05	0.04	0.00	—	—
5	426	30.7	2.87	0.02	—	—	—	73	74.9	0.49	0.00	—	—	—
6	389	34.0	0.96	0.00	—	—	—	37	76.7	0.09	—	—	—	—
7	381	37.2	0.35	—	—	—	—	43	78.8	0.04	—	—	—	—
8	297	39.7	0.10	—	—	—	—	64	81.9	0.02	—	—	—	—
9	273	42.0	0.03	—	—	—	—	63	85.0	0.01	—	—	—	—
10	249	44.1	0.01	—	—	—	—	17	85.8	0.00	—	—	—	—
11+	6647	100.	—	—	—	—	—	291	100.	—	—	—	—	—
Total	11889	—	627.45	184.84	63.76	22.93	8.37	2052	—	358.42	116.49	41.12	14.90	5.46
Mf-rate	20.08	—	21.14	21.45	21.56	21.60	21.61	16.61	—	19.51	20.46	20.79	20.91	20.96
Ratio	1.00	—	1.053	1.068	1.074	1.076	1.076	1.00	—	1.175	1.249	1.252	1.259	1.261

Table 11-12. Conversion of Mf-rates observed by examination of 30 mm³ blood samples to that expected when 10 mm³ samples are examined; Data from microfilaria surveys in Miyako District, 1965 (after SASA, 1974).

	$m=$			A: $y = 3.74 + 1.10 \log x$ Pretreatment survey*					B: $y = 4.77 + 1.29 \log x$ Posttreatment survey**				
x	$(1/3)\,x$	e^{-m}	$\log x$	y	Cu-R (%)	R (%)	n (N×R)	$n \times e^{-m}$	y	Cu-R (%)	R (%)	n (N×R)	$n \times e^{-m}$
1	0.333	0.7168	0.0000	3.74	10.4	10.4	1236	886.0	4.77	40.9	839.3	40.9	601.6
2	0.667	0.5138	0.3010	4.07	17.6	7.2	856	439.8	5.16	56.4	15.5	318.1	163.4
3	1.000	0.3679	0.4771	4.27	23.3	5.7	678	249.4	5.39	65.2	8.8	180.6	66.4
4	1.333	0.2637	0.6021	4.40	27.4	4.1	487	128.4	5.55	709.	5.7	117.0	30.9
5	1.667	0.4890	0.6990	4.51	31.2	3.8	451	85.2	5.67	74.9	4.0	82.1	15.5
6	2.000	0.1353	0.7782	4.60	34.5	3.3	392	53.0	5.77	77.9	3.0	61.6	8.3
7	2.333	0.0970	0.8451	4.67	37.1	2.6	309	30.0	5.86	80.5	26	53.3	5.2
8	2.667	0.0695	0.9031	4.73	39.4	2.3	273	19.0	5.93	82.4	1.9	39.0	2.7
9	3.000	0.0498	0.9542	4.79	41.6	2.2	262	13.0	6.00	84.1	1.7	34.9	1.7
10	3.333	0.0357	1.0000	4.84	43.7	2.1	250	8.9	6.06	85.5	1.4	28.7	1.0
11	3.667	0.0256	1.0414	4.89	45.6	1.9	226	5.8	6.11	87.6	1.2	24.6	0.6
12	4.000	0.0183	1.0792	4.93	47.3	1.7	202	3.7	6.16	87.7	1.0	20.5	0.4
13	4.333	0.0131	1.1139	4.97	48.8	1.5	178	2.3	6.21	88.7	1.0	20.5	0.3
14	4.667	0.0094	1.1461	5.00	50.0	1.2	143	1.3	6.25	89.4	0.7	14.4	0.1
15	5.000	0.0067	1.1761	5.03	51.2	1.2	143	1.0	6.29	90.1	0.7	14.4	0.1
16–20	6.000	0.0025	1.2553	5.12	54.8	3.6	428	1.1	6.39	91.8	1.7	34.9	0.1

| 21–30 | 8.000 | 0.0003 | 1.3974 | 5.27 | 60.7 | 5.9 | 701 | 0.2 | 6.57 | 94.2 | 2.4 | 49.2 | 0.0 |
| 31+ | — | — | — | — | 100. | 39.3 | 4674 | — | — | 100. | 5.8 | 119.0 | — |

Total of negatives:	$\sum (n \times e^{-m}) = 1928.1$	$\sum (n \times e^{-3}) = 898.3$
Total of positives:	$11889 - 1928.1 = 9960.9$	$2052 - 898.3 = 1153.7$
Correction factor	$9960.9/11889 = 0.8378$	$1153.7/2052 = 0.5622$

*Survey of the people before the drug administration; number of persons examined: 59212; number of persons positive: 11889; Mf-rate: 20.08 %.

**Survey of previously positive cases after the drug administration; persons examined: 12352; persons positive: 2052; Mf-rate: 16.61 %.

x:Mf-count in 30 mm³ sample; m: Mf-density in 10 mm³, or (1/3) x; y: Probit of cumulative percentage obtained from the regression line $y = a + b \log x$; Cu-R: cumulative percentage for corresponding value of y, obtained from the conversion table of percentages-probits in FISHER & YATES. 1954; R: theoretical percentage for each class of x: n: theoretical frequency of each class of x (total number positive × R); $n \times e^{-m}$; theoretical number of negative cases in each class in examination of 10 mm³.

This idea can be further extended to the results expected to be obtained if a third, or subsequent blood surveys were conducted. The probability of detecting new positive cases in the third blood examination is obtained for each class of Mf-counts by calculating the values of e^{-2m}. In this case, another 184.84 positive cases are estimated to be detected if a third blood survey is conducted, or 90 mm³ of blood smears were examined at that time. The numbers of new positives to be detected by repeating r times of blood surveys with the same procedure can be estimated by multiplying the probability $e^{-(r-1)m}$ by the observed numbers of cases in each class of m. In this case, no new positive cases are expected to be detected after 10 samples (300 mm³) are examined.

The same statistical treatment was applied to the results of the posttreatment blood surveys conducted in the same year in Miyako. Because the density of microfilariae among the positive cases were much lower than in the pretreatment phase, the rates of increase in Mf-rates to be obtained by repeating the blood examinations turned out to be much higher, as shown in Table 11-11B. In such a case, the efficiency of detection of microfilariae by examination of a single unit of blood sample is much lower than in the pretreatment blood examinations, and thus it is recommended to examine as large blood volumes as possible.

11D.7 Correction factors for smaller volume blood samples

The method described in the previous section refers to the conversion of Mf-rates obtained by examination of a single sample to that expected when multiple samples are examined. A similar idea can be applied for estimating Mf-rates to be observed if smaller blood samples are examined, by using the Poisson distribution formula for obtaining the efficiency of detection of microfilariae at various density levels.

For example, 11,889 cases among 59,212 persons examined with the 30 mm³ thick smear method in Miyako District were found to be positive in the pretreatment survey. What would be the rate if 10 mm³ samples were examined? In this case, the persons showing x microfilariae per 30 mm³ are regarded as a group harboring $\frac{1}{3}x$ micofilariae per 10 mm³. Therefore, the numbers of persons expected to be diagnosed as negative can be obtained by multiplying $e^{-(\frac{1}{3})x}$ by the observed numbers of each class of x. Of 1,236 cases who had 1 microfilaria in 30 mm³, $e^{-0.33} = 71.68\%$ (886 cases) are estimated to be deleted from the positives if only 10 mm³ samples were examined. Likewise, these numbers for all the classes of Mf-count can be calculated, and the sum of these numbers are used for calculating a new Mf-rate.

The frequency distribution of microfilaria cases according to Mf-counts in 30 mm³ samples is given in Table 11-12. By drawing a regression line from the observed data, an equation: $y = 3.74 + 1.10 \log x$ is obtained for the probit of the cumulative percentage of cases with x microfilariae per 30 mm³. The theoretical numbers (n) of cases with x microfilariae per 30 mm³ are calculated from the equation. A mathematical table for conversion of the probits to percentages is used for obtaining the cumulative percentage (Cu-R) of each class of Mf-count. As a result, a sum of 1,928.1 cases are estimated to be diagnosed as negative among 11,889 microfilaria cases, if 10 mm³ samples are examined. The correction factor in this case is therefore $(11,889 - 1,928.1) \div 11,889 = 0.8378$. The correction factor obtained with the same method for the posttreatment examination shown in Table 11-12B is 0.5622, which is much lower than in the pre-treatment survey because the Mf-density is remarkably reduced.

11D.8 Comparison of the efficiency of detection of microfilariae between different diagnostic techniques

SOUTHGATE (1974) compared the efficiency of detection of the microfilariae of *W. bancrofti* in Fiji among four different blood survey methods. (1) the traditional 20 mm³ blood samples collected from finger tip and smeared in a circle of 2 cm in diameter, dried overnight, dehemoglobinized for 10 minutes in distilled water, fixed in methanol, and stained for 30 minutes in a 10% solution of Giemsa. (2) Sixty mm³ blood samples collected with a pipette reported by HITCHCOCK & LEWIS (1970), smeared on a slide making three circular films each 20 mm³, stained by the same method as in (1). (3) Counting-chamber examinations of 60 mm finger-prick blood by the method described by SOUTHGATE (1973). (4) Membrane-filtration examinations carried out by the method described by DESOWITZ & SOUTHGATE (1973). A total of 366 persons of all ages and both sexes in two villages on the south coast of Viti Levu were examined by all four techniques. The number and percentage of microfilaria positive cases, and the values of a, b, MfD-50, r, SE(r) and the ratio r: SE(r) obtained from the same population by each of the four blood survey methods were as in Table 11-13 (also see Sections 10B.2.2 and 11C.5).

It is a rather surprising fact that the microfilarial rates obtained from survey of the same population at the same time by different techniques showed such remarkable differences. By applying the correction factors calculated with the mathematical method described in Section 11D.7 to the original data reported by SOUTHGATE (1974), the difference in rates observed with the two blood smear methods (20 mm³ and 60 mm³) was found to be exactly the same as that expected from the difference in size of the blood samples. However, the differences between the rates observed by the blood smear methods and those obtained by the counting chamber or membrane filtration methods were much larger than that expected from the volume of blood samples. The results suggest that considerable proportions of microfilariae would have been lost in this case during the staining process of the blood smears, as was previously pointed out also by DENHAM (1971).

Table 11-13. The descriptive epidemetrons of microfilaremia in a community of 366 persons in Fiji produced by four different survey techniques (after SOUTHGATE, 1974).

Technique	No. posit.	% posit.	MfD-50	a	b	r	SE(r)	r: SE(r)
20 mm³ smear	81	22.1	3.2	4.353	1.182	0.983	0.224	4.398
60 mm³ smear	109	29.8	3.9	4.321	1.172	0.984	0.209	4.719
Counting chamber	142	38.8	19.0	3.370	1.260	0.993	0.196	5.061
Membrane filtration	248	68.8	34.0	3.423	1.045	0.993	0.183	5.438

11E. The infectivity potential of human populations

The potential force of infection of a human population to the vector population can be estimated from the blood or skin survey data, if the average amount of blood (or skin fluid) ingested by the vector and the rate of ingestion of microfilariae by the vector are known. The method for calculating "the infectivity index" from blood survey data is shown in Table 11–14. This index is the theoretical rate of infection of a vector population that have once ingested the blood of a human population, on the presumption that people are evenly exposed to the bite of the vector, and that the density of microfilariae in the blood ingested by the vector is the same as that in the circulating blood. The method for calculating this index is based on the same idea as that for estimating the microfilarial rate when smaller blood samples are examined (see Section 11D.7). In Western Samoa, for example, a total of 10,129 persons were examined in the pretreatment survey in 1965 by the 20 mm³ blood smear method, and the numbers (r) of persons showing the respective microfilarial counts were recorded as in Table 11-14. Since it is known that *Ae. polynesiensis*, the local vector, ingests an average of about 2 mg of blood, the probabilities of occurrence of one or more microfilariae in this volume of blood sample are estimated as in column (3) by the formula: $P_{(+)} = 1 - e^{-m}$. In this case, for example, 141 persons had one microfilaria in 20 mm³ blood sample. This density corresponds to 0.1 microfilaria per 2 mm³. The probability of occurrence of one or more microfilariae when the mosquito has ingested 2 mm³ blood from one such person is: $1 - e^{-0.1} = 0.0952$. Therefore, it is estimated that if 141 persons with this density are attacked by one vector each, a total of $13.42 = (141 \times 0.952)$ infected mosquitoes are produced from this population. Likewise, the theoretical numbers and percentages of vector mosquitoes being infected from this human population can be calculated. In this case, the infectivity index of microfilaria positive cases (IIP) is obtained by dividing the sum of column 5 (1,401.82) with the total number of positive cases (1,932), which comes out to be 72.6%. The infectivity index of the total population (IIT) is obtained by dividing the sum of column 5 with the total number of persons examined (including negative cases), which is 13.8% in the pretreatment population of Western Samoa.

Comparison of the infectivity potential by means of the rate of reduction in the infectivity indices is especially useful as a measure of evaluating the effects of filariasis control programs. In Western Samoa, for example, 42,697 persons were examined by the same method after completion of a course of mass administration of DEC to the whole population, and 691 persons (1.63%) were still positive for microfilariae. The frequency distribution of positive cases according to the microfilarial counts in 20 mm³ blood samples was as shown in column (6) of Table 11-14. The values of the infectivity index of microfilaria positive cases was 38.2% and that of the total population was 0.62%. It is shown from this statistical analysis of the two surveys' data that the mass drug administration not only reduced the microfilarial rate of the human population from 19.1% to 1.63% (reduction to 8.53% of the original level), but also the infectivity potential of the whole human population from 13.8% to 0.62% (reduction to 4.49% of the original level).

The method for calculating the infectivity index shown in Table 11-13 is based on the observed frequency distribution of the microfilarial counts. Since the frequency distribution of the microfilarial density in a population is essentially a logarithmically normal type, especially in the range of relatively low microfilarial density, it is more logical to use the theoretical frequency distribution for the respective densities from the equation: $y = a + b \log x$ (see Section 11C. 3). Table 11-15 shows an example of the results obtained with this "indirect method." The values of IIP and IIT obtained with this method are 70.60% and 13.5% for the pretreatment survey of Western Samoa and are very close to 72.6% and 13.8% obtained by the former "direct method." The IIP and IIT values for the posttreatment survey of Western Samoa are 1.63% and 0.60%, respectively, and are also nearly identical with that obtained by the direct method. The results of the pretreatment survey reported from Tahiti by KESSEL (1971) indicate that people here had a higher infectivity potential to the vector mosquitoes than the people in Western Samoa, since the IIP and IIT were 73.32% and 22.7%, respectively.

11F. Analysis of the microfilarial periodicity

11F.1 Introduction

Since MANSON (1879) observed that the microfilariae of *W. bancrofti* in Amoy (South China) were found numerously in the blood of infected patients at night but became rare or absent from the blood during the

Table 11-14. A direct method of calculating the infectivity index of a human population*

Microfilaria density per 2 mm³ blood meal	Probability infective	Pretreatment		Posttreatment	
		No. of cases[b]	No. infective	No. of cases[b]	No. infective
(1)	(2)	(3)	(2) × (3)	(5)	(2) × (3)
0.1	0.0952	141	13.42	173	16.47
0.2	0.1813	90	16.32	117	21.21
0.3	0.2952	79	23.32	77	22.73
0.4	0.3297	66	21.76	42	13.85
0.5	0.3935	79	31.09	36	14.17
0.6	0.4512	54	24.36	34	15.34
0.7	0.5034	44	22.15	22	11.07
0.8	0.5507	45	24.78	20	11.01
0.9	0.5934	39	23.14	12	7.12
1.0	0.6321	30	18.96	11	6.95
1.1	0.6671	34	22.68	13	8.67
1.2	0.6988	33	23.06	9	6.29
1.3	0.7275	24	17.46	12	8.73
1.4	0.7534	31	23.36	6	4.52
1.5	0.7769	30	23.31	3	2.33
1.6	0.7981	29	23.14	2	1.60
1.7	0.8173	22	17.98	3	2.45
1.8	0.8347	28	23.37	6	5.01
1.9	0.8504	23	19.56	5	4.25
2.0	0.8647	21	18.16	4	3.46
2.2	0.8892	31	27.57	3	2.67
2.4	0.9093	38	34.55	5	4.55
2.6	0.9257	39	36.10	6	5.55
2.8	0.9398	37	34.77	3	2.82
3.0	0.9502	26	24.71	0	0
3.2	0.9592	31	29.74	3	2.88
3.4	0.9666	31	29.96	3	2.90
3.6	0.9727	25	24.32	2	1.95
3.8	0.9776	30	29.38	5	4.89
4.0	0.9817	21	20.62	1	0.98
4.2	0.9850	21	20.69	6	5.91
4.4	0.9877	22	21.73	1	0.99
4.6	0.9900	20	19.80	1	0.99
4.8	0.9918	19	18.84	1	0.99
5.0	0.9933	20	19.87	1	0.99
>5.0	0.998+	579	577.84	1	42.91
Total		1932	1401.82	691	269.20

No. of people examined	10129	42697
Microfilaria rate (%)	19.1	1.63
Infectivity index (%) of microfilaria-positive persons (IIP)	72.6	38.2
Infectivity index (%) of total population (IIT)	13.8	0.62

*This index is an expression of the infectivity potential of a human population for the vector population, or, in other words, the theoretical infection rate of mosquitoes that have ingested microfilariae once from man, on the presumption that people were evenly exposed to the mosquito bites, and that all filarial larvae and mosquitoes survived until the time of capture and dissection. The calculation is based on blood survey data from the Filariais Control Programme in Western Samoa; the pretreatment survey was made in 1965, the posttreatment survey in 1967.

[a]It is postulated that the vector ingests 2 mm³ of blood during a blood meal. In the particular surveys referred to here this unit blood meal corresponds to one-tenth of the 20 mm³ blood sample taken from the people examined.

[b]Peope found positive for microfilariae.

*This table was compiled by SASA & SUZUKI for the Third WHO Expert Committee on Filariasis, from blood survey data collected by the Health Department, Western Samoa; modified from Table 2, *WHO Tech. Rep. Ser. No.* 542, 1974)

daytime, a large number of articles dealing with this very interesting biological phenomenon have appeared in reference to various species or forms of human or animal filariae. As reviewed by HAWKING (1960), it is admitted by most workers that the periodicity occurs as the result of retention of larger numbers of microfilariae in the lung capillaries during certain hours of the day and their release into the circulating blood during other hours. Various hypotheses or theories have been proposed as to the host or environmental factors responsible for such a circadian rhythm. In most instances, the periodicity of a form of microfilaria is closely correlated with the biting activity of the insect species which act as the intermediate host.

Previous studies by a number of workers in various regions of the world have revealed that there exist different forms even within the same species which differ in the pattern of the microfilarial periodicity. According to the nomenclature recommended by a WHO EXPERT COMMITTEE ON FILARIASIS (1962), there exist at least two species and five forms of human filariae in the Asiatic-Pacific region: (1) the nocturnally periodic *W. bancrofti* (NPWb) which is a cosmopolitan form, (2) the nonperiodic (or more precisely, the diurnally subperiodic) *W. bancrofti* (DSWb) endemic in certain South Pacific islands, (3) the nocturnally subperiodic *W. bancrofti* (NSWb) discovered recently from West Thailand, (4) the nocturnally periodic *B. malayi* (NPBm) widely distributed in South and East Asia, and (5) the nocturnally subperiodic *B. malayi* (NSBm) found from swampy areas in Malaysia, Indonesia, and the Philippines. In Africa, the microfilariae of *L.*

loa in man are known to be diurnally periodic and develop in certain day-biting *Chrysops* fly species, while those parasitic in monkeys are nocturnally periodic and are transmitted by another night-biting *Chrysops* species. Both *D. perstans* in Africa and *M. ozzardi* in the Americas have been referred to as nonperiodic forms.

Table 11-15 An indirect method for calculating the infectivity index of a human population from the distribution of microfilaria density among carriers (SASA & SUZUKI, 1973)

Microfilaria density per 2mm³ unit blood meal	Probability of unit volume of blood meal being infective (p)	Western Samoa pretreatment (1965)			Western Samoa posttreatment (1967)			Tahiti pretreatment (1954)		
		$c(\%)$	$d(\%)$	$p\times d$	$c(\%)$	$d(\%)$	$p\times d$	$c(\%)$	$d(\%)$	$p\times d$
0.1	0.0952	6	6	0.57	32	32	3.05	6	6	0.57
0.2	0.1813	11	5	0.91	49	17	3.08	12	6	1.09
0.3	0.2952	16	5	1.48	58	9	2.66	16	4	1.18
0.4	0.3297	20	4	1.32	64	6	1.98	20	4	1.32
0.5	0.3935	24	4	1.57	69	5	1.97	23	3	1.18
0.6	0.4521	27	3	1.36	73	4	1.81	26	3	1.36
0.7	0.5034	30	3	1.51	76	3	1.51	28	2	1.01
0.8	0.5507	33	3	1.65	79	3	1.65	30	2	1.10
0.9	0.5934	35	2	1.19	81	2	1.19	32	2	1.19
1.0	0.6321	37	2	1.26	83	2	1.26	33	1	0.63
1.1–2.0	0.7484	52	16	11.97	90	7	5.24	46	13	9.73
2.1–3.0	0.9057	62	9	8.15	93	3	2.72	53	7	6.34
3.1–4.0	0.9660	68	6	5.80	94	1	0.97	59	6	5.80
4.1–5.0	0.9875	72	4	3.95	95	1	0.99	63	4	3.95
$\geqslant$	0.9967	100	28	27.91	100	5	4.98	100	37	36.88
IIP(%)				70.60			35.05			73.32
Mf-rate (%)				19.1			1.63			30.9
ITT (%)				13.5			0.60			22.7
Natural (observed) vector infection rate (%)				8.35			0.61			13.2

*Calculated using the regression line of the cumulative percentage of microfilaria positive cases against the microfilaria density in the log probit scale, $y = a + b \log x$ (see Section 11C. 3).

c = Cumulative percentage of microfilaria positive cases; d = difference between the cumulative percentages, or percentage of each class.

IIP: Infectivity index of microfilaria positive persons

IIT: Infectivity index of total population

A mathematical method for quantitative analysis of the circadian rhythm such as the microfilarial periodicity was developed recently by SASA & TANAKA (1972, 1974). These authors interpreted what has been called the periodicity of microfilariae as a wave of the density of microfilariae in the circulating blood in relation to the hour of day. In this case, the conventional terms "periodic," "subperiodoc" and "nonperiodic" can be replaced by the size of the relative amplitude of the wave, and the terms "nocturnal" and "diurnal" is expressed by the position of the peak hour of the wave. Further postulating that the wave profile is basically a harmonic type (sine or cosine curve), the microfilarial periodicity can be expressed by the following mathematical formula:

$$Y = 100 + 1.347\ D \cos 15\ (h - K)°$$

where Y is the relative microfilarial density (the percentage by taking the average density of 24 hours to be 100%) at the hour h, K is the peak hour, and D is the coefficient of variation (in percentage) of 24 hours' microfilarial counts.

11F.2 A critical review of the previously reported methods

11F.2.1 Methods for observation of the microfilarial periodicity

A large number of papers have been published by various workers referring to the periodicity of microfilariae of different filarial species and forms with a variety of methods. Most classical workers recognized the presence or absence of the periodicity by comparison of the results of blood examinations carried out both by day and by night. For example, the discovery of the "nonperiodic" form of *W. bancrofti* in the South Pacific islands was made by THORPE (1896), who examined blood of 96 natives in Tonga both day and night and found that, with two exceptions, all of those with microfilariae at night exhibited them in the daytime in almost equal numbers. BUXTON (1927), on the other hand, reported that filariasis in New Hebrides was a nocturnally periodic form because out of 32 cases who were positive at night, only 11 were positive in daytime examination, and the microfilarial counts in the latter was much lower than at night even when they were present.

However, such simple and nonquantitative methods obviously harbor the risk of causing various misunderstandings of the real nature of the periodicity. For example, ASHBURN & CRAIG (1908) examined the blood of three microfilarial carriers in the Philippines both day and night with unmeasured thick smears, and considered that the filaria was a new nonperiodic form because the microfilariae were present in both day and night samples. This idea was probably a mistake, because all the later reports from the Philippines, including detailed studies by AFRICA *et al.* (1935) and by CABRERA & ROZEBOOM (1965), as well as those from the surrounding regions, have indicated that the so-called non-periodic *W. bancrofti* in the South Pacific does not extend to areas north of the equator, and the type found in the Asian region all belong to the nocturnally periodic type.

More valuable information can be obtained with a two-point observation by taking larger blood samples during the day when the density is low, such as reported by ERBER (1927) and VAN SLEE (1930). These authors examined 20 mm³ night blood samples and 1 ml day blood samples taken from microfilarial carriers of *B. malayi* in Sulawesi, and found that the average counts were about three times larger in the former than in the latter. As will be discussed later, the ratio between the daytime and the nighttime densities can be estimated with more reliable statistical background with such a method than with the conventional methods of taking the same amount of small blood samples both day and night.

On the other hand, most modern workers, adopted more comprehensive and quantitative methods for the study of periodicity, with which the chronological trend of the change of microfilarial density during a 24-hour period can be expressed on a curve. There are ample records of the results of such studies conducted by various workers with different species and forms of human filariae. For example, MANSON (1881, 1882) in his historical study of the discovery of the nocturnal periodicity of the microfilariae of *W. bancrofti*, recorded microfilaria counts in the blood continuously at three-hour intervals for a period of 23 days in one case, 16 days in another, 27 days in the third case, and 20 days in the fourth case. Since it has become clear from these studies that the periodicity of the microfilariae is repeated every day in a similar pattern, observations for a period of 24 hours at certain time intervals (such as every hour, two hours, three hours, four hours, etc.) are considered to be sufficient for determination of the estimating characters. In general, the reliability of the observed data as a representative of the natural trend of the periodicity of a filaria in an endemic area depends upon various factors, such as the accuracy of the technique, the amount of blood samples examined at one time, the interval of the blood examination, and the number of cases examined at one time in the same endemic areas.

11F.2.2 Methods for analysis of the observed data

As stated previously, most workers in the early stages judged whether a filarial form was periodic or nonperiodic by comparison of the microfilarial positive rates observed by day and at night in examination of the same individuals, or by comparison of the counts between the two examinations. A more quantitative idea was introduced by BRUG (1931) who compared the microfilarial periodicity of *W. bancrofti* and *B. malayi* in a case of mixed infections by recording the counts in one ml of blood samples collected at four hour intervals. In both species, the peak counts were at 24 hour (midnight). He took the peak count of each species as 100%, and calculated the percentages of the other counts to the peak. The lowest counts were at 12 hour (noon) in both species, and was 1.7% of the peak in *B. malayi* and 0.5% in *W. bancrofti*. It is however difficult to judge whether such a difference is significant, because the individual counts are subject to great variations, as will be discussed later. In this case, the periodicity index calculated by the present author's method of utilizing all the observed counts came out to be 112% for *W. bancrofti* and 69% for *B. malayi*, and thus it can be stated, with higher reliability, that the grade of periodicity is higher in the former that in the latter species.

Most later workers who studied the periodicity of microfilariae in certain endemic areas judged whether the form was a periodic or a subperiodic form by simple impressions from crude data or from the periodicity curves, because there was no adequate method for further statistical analysis. A method for obtaining "relative periodicity curves" from data collected from a number of cases infected with the same form of filaria was proposed by TURNER & EDESON (1957), who demonstrated the difference in the periodicity characters of *B. malayi* in Penang and that in Pahang, the former being nocturnally periodic, and the latter being nocturnally subperiodic. These authors recorded the microfilarial counts in measured blood samples collected at two-hour intervals from a number of cases in the same endemic areas, computed the percentages of all the counts by taking the peak count of individual cases as 100%, and obtained the averages of these percentages for each hour. This method was adopted by CABRERA & ROZEBOOM (1965) for comparison of the periodicity of *W. bancrofti* and *B. malayi* in Palawan, and by HARINASUTA *et al.* (1970) in concluding that a form of *W. bancrofti* discovered from Sankla-buri, West Thailand, was a nocturnally subperiodic form.

Another approach for obtaining a common periodicity curve from data collected from multiple samples was reported by DUKE & WIJERS (1958) and DUKE (1964). These authors studied the periodicity of microfilariae of *L. loa* in man and monkeys, and when multiple samples were available for the same populations, calculated the geometric mean (average of log [x + 1]) for counts of each hour, and obtained its percentage to the sum of all the means for drawing each plot of the periodicity curves. From various reasons, this method is considered to provide more reliable periodicity curves than with the method utilized by TURNER & EDESON (1957).

In general, it is considered that although these methods may be useful for drawing relative periodicity curves based on multiple samples, there is no means of obtaining quantitative measures for comparison of different populations from these curves. Because the individual microfilarial counts are subject to great variations, especially when the values are small, the use of single counts such as those of the peak hour is not recommendable from a statistical standpoint, so far as other more reliable measures such as the mean and the standard deviation are available for this purpose.

11F.3 Mathematical approaches to the microfilarial periodicity

11F.3.1 The nature of microfilarial periodicity

As stated previously, the circadian rhythm commonly called the microfilarial periodicity can be interpreted as a wave of the density of microfilariae in the circulating blood of vertebrate hosts in relation to the hour of day.

In general, a wave formula is determined by various factors, such as the amplitude, the wave length, the period, the phase, and the wave profile, and various wave formulae have been developed for simulating the naturally occurring wave processes. General mathematical accounts are given in textbooks on waves, such as those complied by COULSON (1955; *Waves*, University Mathematical Text, Oliver & Boyd, Ltd, Edinburgh, pp. 159). In the case of microfilarial periodicity, the factors involved are much simplified because its wave length and speed are fixed to 24-hour rhythms. Therefore, the only three factors necessary to determine the characters of such a wave, are: the relative amplitude (the grade of difference between the maximum and minimum densities), the phase (the hour of day at which the density becomes maximum and minimum), and the wave profile.

11F.3.2 Mathematical formulae to be applied to the microfilarial periodicity

In general, a wave process such as the microfilarial periodicity can be expressed by the following simple formula:

$$y = m + a\,\mathrm{f}(x) \tag{1}$$

where y is the height (microfilarial density) of the wave at phase x (hour), m is the average height through one period of the wave, a is a constant related to the amplitude, and $\mathrm{f}(x)$ is the factor that determines the wave profile. The simplest example of such a wave is the harmonic form (sine or cosine curve), and if it is assumed that the microfilarial periodicity occurs according to this form, the following formula can be applied to this circadian rhythm.

$$y = m + a \cos x; \qquad x = 15(h - k)^\circ = 0.2618(h - k)\,\theta \tag{2}$$

In the above formula, k is the peak hour, and y is the microfilarial density at the angle x or at the hour h. In this case, the hour can be converted to the degree (°) by multiplying with 15, because 24 hours correspond to 360°, or to the radian (θ), because $1° = 0.0174533\ \theta$. This relation is illustrated in Fig. 11-7.

When it is further postulated that the chronological pattern of the percentages of the microfilariae that appear in the circulating blood is a character common to each filarial race and is independent of the microfilarial load of individual hosts, a race-specific periodicity curve can be developed by dividing both sides of the formula (2) with the mean count (m). In this case, the ratio Y (in percentage) of the microfilarial density to the mean can be expressed by the formula (3).

$$Y = 100\ y/m = 100 + 100\ (a/m) \cos 15\ (h - k)° \tag{3}$$

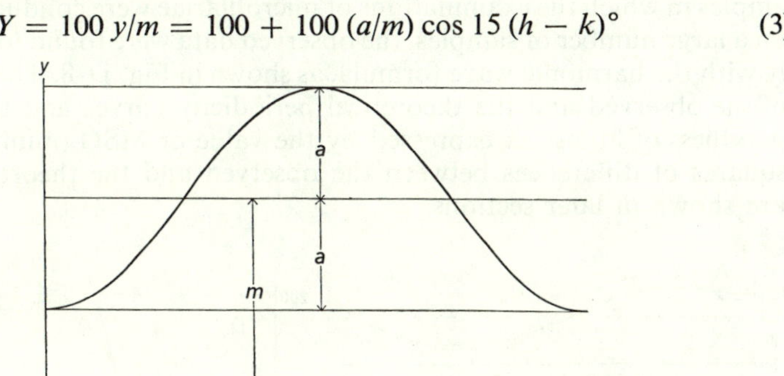

Fig. 11-7.   A graph of the harmonic wave: $y = m + a \cos [(h - k) \times 15]$.

The value a/m is called the relative amplitude, and in the case of a harmonic wave the size of a (half amplitude) can be estimated from the standard deviation of microfilarial counts observed during a 24-hour period. When 12 blood examinations are made at two hour-intervals, the size of a is 1.347 times larger than the standard deviation s, or "$a = 1.347\ s$." Therefore, if a constant $D = 100\ s/m$ is introduced, the formula (3) can be converted to formula (4), which is called "the relative periodicity formula." The constant D is the value obtained by dividing the standard deviation with the mean, or is the coefficient of variation (in percentage), and was named "the periodicity index," by SASA & TANAKA (1972), because it represents a quantitative measure for the conventional concept such as "periodic" or "subperiodic."

$$Y = 100 + 1.347D \cos 15(h - k)° \tag{4}$$

11 F.3.3 Is the microfilarial periodicity harmonic?

Formula (4) is a mathematical model which can be generally applied to circadian rhythms of a harmonic wave type. It has only two parameters, D and k, which can be estimated from the observed data by the method described in the next section. One of the basic problems in application of this formula to the microfilarial periodicity is whether this circadian rhythm is a harmonic form or it follows other more complicated wave formulae. At present, there is no theoretical background for estimating the real nature of the wave profile from the physiology of microfilariae. Actually, the results of observations on the periodicity of various forms of filariae reported by previous workers have shown a variety of deformities from the harmonic wave form, but it can be stated that, in general, they are closer to the harmonic form than to any other more complicated wave forms. In some examples in which the examinations of microfilariae were conducted carefully on a large number of samples, the observed data were found to fit excellently with the harmonic wave formula, as shown in Fig. 11-8. The comparison of the observed and the theoretical periodicity curves and the results of goodness of fit test as expressed by the value of MSQ (minimum sum of squares of differences between the observed and the theoretical values) are shown in later sections.

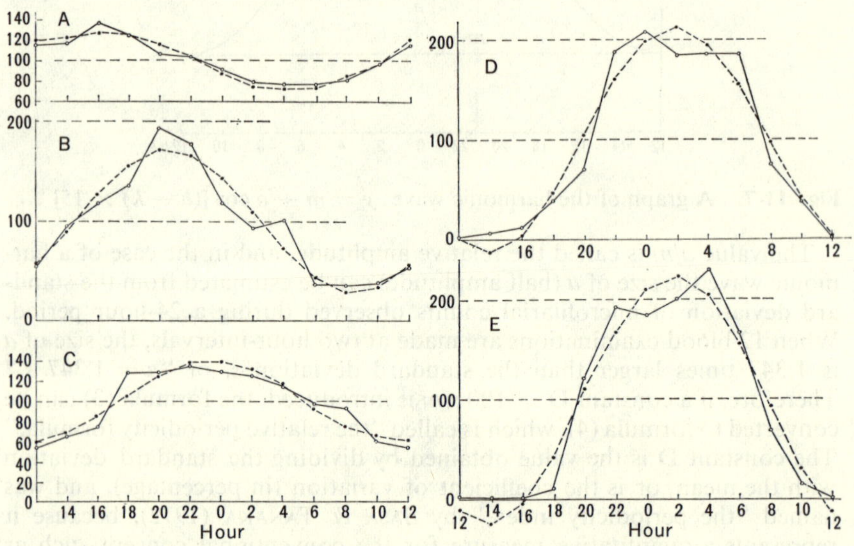

A. Diurnally subperiodic *W. bancrofti*, Rosen, 1955 South Pacific

B. Nocturnally subperiodic *W. bancrofti*, Harinasuta *et al.*, 1970 West Thailand

C. Nocturnally subperiodic *B. malayi*, Cabrera & Rozeboom, 1965 Ralawan, Philippines

D. Nocturnally periodic *B. malayi*, Turner & Edeson, 1957 Penang, Malaya

E. Nocturnally periodic *W. bancrofti*, Ramachandran *et al.*, 1964 Bukit Lanjan, Malaya

Fig. 11-8.   Comparison of the observed and the theoretical periodicity curves
of various filarial forms.

11F.3.4 Some basic characters of the harmonic wave formula

If the microfilarial periodicity is basically a rhythm of the harmonic wave, the relative periodicity formula (4) can be applied in order to make quantitative evaluation of the observed data, and the parameters D and K are considered to represent the type specific characters of a filarial race.

In this formula, the value of D (the periodicity index) is a measure of the relative amplitude, and is a quantitative expression for the conventional concept such as periodic, subperiodic, or nonperiodic. Because it is the value obtained by dividing the standard deviation with the mean, it is more reliable than other measures of the amplitude, such as obtained from the difference between the minimum and the maximum counts. The value of D is independent of the wave profile, and can be used as a measure of the relative amplitude in any form of the wave phenomenon.

The theoretical peak count of the microfilariae occurs at the hour when $h = k$, and the minimum count occurs at the hour when $h = k \pm 12$. The theoretical maximum count during a 24-hour period is "$m \times (1 + 1.347\ D/100)$" and the minimum count is "$m \times (1 - 1.347\ D/100)$." In the cases of the periodic forms, the values of the theoretical minimum counts often come out to be below zero, but this is probably due to errors in the observed counts.

The slope of the periodicity curve (dy/dh) is smallest at the hours of the peak and the minimum counts, and is largest at the hours $h = k \pm 6$. This means that the peak hour is the most variable (or unreliable) point for estimating the phase of the wave from observed data. It has also been demonstrated that the observed peak hours are highly variable even among the cases examined at the same time in the same endemic areas. Therefore, a method for obtaining the best estimate of the peak hour by the minimum sum of squares has been developed by SASA & TANAKA (1972), in which all the data collected during a 24-hour period are utilized for estimating the peak hour.

11F.3.5 The relationship between the variability and the mean count

The variability in ratios of the observed counts is dependent upon the microfilarial density of the blood of a host at the time of the examination, and decreases as the density becomes larger. From the table of Poisson distribution, one can easily calculate, for example, the probability of picking up two times or more microfilariae than the mean count for various density levels. In a person carrying an average of 1 microfilaria per unit volume, the probability of picking up two or more microfilariae in a unit volume of blood sample is 0.26434 (26.434%), and that of picking up no microfilaria is 0.36788. When the average density is 2, the probability for 4 or more is 0.14287, and that for 0 (negative result) is 0.13534. Both probabilities become smaller as the average density increases, and at the density of 15, the probability of picking up 30 or more microfilariae in a blood sample becomes to 0.00041, and that for negative specimens is practically 0.

In the statistical analysis of the microfilarial periodicity survey data, our concern is with the chronological change of the ratio of the individual counts to a standard value (the mean count in 24 hours in the present section, or the peak count in the method of TURNER & EDESON, 1957). Therefore, it can be stated that the periodicity curves (in ratios) drawn from data obtained from carriers with higher microfilarial densities are more reliable than those with lower densities.

11F.4 Methods for statistical analysis of survey data

11F.4.1 The periodicity curves

The first step for analysis of the periodicity survey data is the conversion of observed microfilarial counts to ratios in order to obtain a periodicity curve representing a type-specific character of a filarial form. BRUG (1931) and TURNER & EDESON (1957) used the observed peak count of individual cases as the common denominator, but by various reasons, the mean of 24-hour counts is recommended for this purpose. When multiple cases infected with the same form of filaria are examined by the same method, the hourly counts of individual cases may be added for obtaining group data. DUKE & WIJERS (1958) calculated the geometric mean of individual counts of each hour by the "log $(x + 1)$" method.

An example of statistical analysis of periodicity survey data is shown in TABLE 11-16. The material was cited from a report by ROSEN (1955), who conducted examination of microfilariae in 60 mm³ blood samples collected at two-hour intervals over a period of 48 hours from 10 cases of *W. bancrofti* carriers in the Society Islands, South Pacific. The sum of microfilarial counts in 20 samples is obtained for each hour of the blood examination (column: Total count, n). The mean count $m = 1426.2$ is obtained by dividing 17114 (total of all counts) with 12, and the ratio Y is calculated for each hour as the percentage of n divided by m. The relative periodicity curve is drawn by plotting these ratios on a section paper.

The curves showing the relative density of microfilariae at different hours of day obtained by this method are considered to represent the type-specific characters of various filarial forms, and are useful for differentiating filarial species or forms by simple comparison of their shape, as shown in Fig. 11-8. With such a statistical treatment as the first step, theoretical periodicity curves and various numerical indices useful for comparison of microfilarial periodicity survey data can be obtained, as will be discussed later.

Table 11-16. Statistical analysis of the microfilarial periodicity survey data; Goodness of fit test of the formula: $Y' = 100 + 1.347D \cos 15(h - k)°$, with $D = 20.62$, $k = 16.4$ (Data from ROSEN, 1955; total counts of 10 cases of *W. bancrofti*, the Society Islands).

Hour (h)	Total count (n)	Ratio (%) $Y = n/m$	$(Y - 100)$	$(Y - 100)^2$	Theoretical ratio (Y')	$(Y - Y')$	$(Y - Y')^2$	$(Y - Y')^2/Y'$
8	1158	81.2	−18.8	353.44	83.7	−2.5	6.25	0.075
10	1398	98.0	−2.0	4.00	97.1	0.9	0.81	0.001
12	1531	107.3	7.3	52.29	113.1	−4.0	16.00	0.141
14	1691	118.6	18.6	354.96	122.5	−3.9	15.21	0.124
16	1980	138.8	38.8	1505.44	127.6	11.2	125.44	0.983
18	1787	125.3	25.3	640.09	125.4	−0.1	0.01	0.000
20	1520	106.6	6.6	43.56	116.3	−9.7	94.09	0.809
22	1473	103.3	3.3	10.89	102.9	0.4	0.16	0.002
24	1290	90.5	−9.5	90.25	88.7	1.8	3.24	0.037
2	1120	78.5	−21.5	462.25	77.5	1.0	1.00	0.013
4	1091	76.5	−23.5	552.25	72.4	4.1	16.31	0.232
6	1075	75.4	−24.6	605.16	74.6	0.8	0.64	0.009
Total	17114	1200.	0	4675.58	1200.	0.	279.66	2.426

Mean count: $m = 1426.2$; Periodicity index: $D = \sqrt{4675.58/(12 - 1)} - 20.62$.

11F.4.2 The periodicity index

One of the differentiating characters in the microfilarial periodicity whether a filarial form is periodic, subperiodic, or nonperiodic is a matter which refers to the relative amplitude, and can be expressed quantitatively by the size of the periodicity index defined by SASA & TANAKA (1972). This index is the coefficient of variation of microfilarial counts observed at certain time intervals during a period of 24 hours, or the standard deviation of their ratios to the mean of 24-hour counts. In order to obtain the periodicity index from observed data, it is convenient to calculate the ratios by dividing the hourly counts with the mean count, and then obtain the sum of squares of the balance $(Y - 100)$; the periodicity index is the square root of "the sum of squares divided with 11." In the example shown in TABLE 11-16, the sum of squares came out to 4675.58, and therefore the periodicity index (D) is 20.62. This means that in this observation with the subperiodic *W. bancrofti*, the standard deviation of the hourly counts was about 20% of the mean count.

The periodicity indices obtained with various cases of filariae have been shown to differ greatly among the forms, from some 20% in subperiodic forms to over 100% in most periodic forms, but were found to be fairly uniform within the same forms, irrespective to the microfilarial load of individual cases, the geographic location of the endemic areas, or the methods of blood examinations adopted by individual workers. In other words, the periodicity index is a type-specific character of a filarial form, and its value is expected to be the same whether the blood examinations are conducted at two-hour or four-hour intervals, or whether the volume of blood samples examined is 20, 30, or 60 mm^3. It should also be pointed out that in contrast to the value of K (best estimate of the peak hour) which is determined by the assumption that the periodicity is a harmonic wave, the periodicity index is a value independent of the wave profile whether it is harmonic or not. From statistical point of view it is better index of the relative amplitude than that estimated from any other method (such as taking the difference between the maximum and the minimum ratios), because the factors involved are only the mean and the standard deviation of the observed data.

11F.4.3 Goodness of fit to the harmonic wave formula

If we postulate that the microfilarial periodicity is a circadian rhythm of a harmonic wave type, one can calculate the theoretical density of microfilariae of a given hour of day by providing adequate values of D and k to formula (4). In the example shown in TABLE 11-16, the theoretical ratios Y' are calculated with the equation: $Y' = 100 + 1.347 \, D \cos 15(h - k)°$, by giving the values $D = 20.62$ and $k = 16.4$. The value of k was tentatively set by visual fitting of the observed and the theoretical curves on section paper.

Since there are 12 pairs of observed and theoretical ratios, a test of fitness with the Chi-square method can be made. In this case, the sum of the squares of the difference between the observed and theoretical ratios is 279.66, and the value of Ch-square is 2.426. The degree of freedom is 9 in this case. From the table of Chi-squares this value is smaller than 2.532 of 98% confidence level. Therefore, the periodicity curve obtained from data presented by ROSEN (1955) fits nearly completely a harmonic wave.

The goodness of fit test has been conducted on data accumulated by other workers with various filarial forms. In general, the periodicity curves referring to subperiodic forms were found to fit well to the harmonic types, though the values of Chi-square were usually more or less larger than observed with the Rosen's example. However, in the case of the periodic forms, the sum of squares came out to much larger values and the Chi-square test was generally impracticable, because the values of the theoretical ratios at low density hours showed extremely small or even minus values so far as the present method of taking some 20 to 60 mm³ blood samples is concerned. Therefore, the grade of fitness to the theoretical curves is estimated simply by comparison of the values of the sum of squares $\Sigma(Y - Y')^2$.

11F.4.4 Methods for estimating the peak hour

The term "nocturnal" or "diurnal" has been used commonly by previous workers in order to express a character of the microfilarial periodicity, whether their density increases at night or during the daytime. However, it has also been recognized that the hour at which the density reaches the peak differs even among the nocturnal or diurnal forms. In *L. loa* infection in man, in which the microfilarial periodicity is called diurnally periodic, the highest counts are observed at about noon, while the peaks in the cases of the so-called diurnally subperiodic *W. bancrofti* in the South Pacific islands are usually seen in the afternoon at about 4 p.m. In the nocturnally periodic form of *W. bancrofti*, the peak hour is usually at about midnight, while that of the nocturnally subperiodic *B. malayi* has been observed at earlier time, such as at about 10 p.m.

One of the methods for estimating the peak hour of a form of filaria is to obtain the average of the observed peak hours. However, the peak hours are highly variable according to the individual cases, especially in the subperiodic forms, and thus their standard deviations are usually very high. In the observations of 26 cases of the nocturnally periodic *B. malayi* in Penang by TURNER & EDESON (1957), the peak hour was at 0.96 hour (about 1 a.m.) in average with the standard deviation of 3.06 hours, while that of 20 cases of the subperiodic *B. malayi* in Pahang examined by the same authors was 21.46 hours (about 9:28 p.m.) in average with the standard deviation of 4.59 hours.

A mathematical method for estimating the peak hour was proposed by SASA & TANAKA (1972, 1974), with which, by the aid of a computer, it can be determined even with a single case observation. The hypothetical periodicity curve is obtained from the formula: $Y' = 100 + 1.347\ D \cos 15(h - k)°$, and the values of Y' are calculated for various values of k tentatively provided to the formula. The term "best estimate of the peak hour" is the value of k with which the sum of squares of the difference between the observed and the calculated densities (Y and Y') becomes minimum. In the example given in TABLE 11-16, the sum of squares of 279.66 with the tentative peak hour of 16.4 was obtained. Further, repeat the same procedures for the values of $k = 16.5$ and larger, and also that of 16.3 or less, and finally find out which of these values provides the minimum sum of the squares. In this case, it was fortunate that the tentative peak hour of 16.4 simply estimated from the observed periodicity curve was the correct answer, but in general it probably requires hours or days of time before one can obtain the solution, if a computer is not available. However, make rough estimate of the peak hour can be made usually by the visual fitting of the theoretical curve to the observed data.

11F.4.5. A computer program for the statistical analysis of the observed data

A computer program was developed by Tanaka, for obtaining the periodicity index (D), the best estimate of the peak hour (K), and the minimum sum of squares (MSQ) from the observed data. A 4 kiloword minicomputer programmed with BASIC-3000 level was used for this purpose. The program is as shown in TABLE 11-17, and an example of its operation is shown in TABLE 11-18.

11F.5 Comparison of the periodicity index and the peak hour of various filarial species and races

Literature referring to the field observations on the microfilarial periodicity of various species or forms of human filariae were surveyed, and statistical treatment with the above described methods were conducted with the materials reported by the original authors. Only the data collected at two-hour (or every hour) intervals over a period of 24 hours were used for the study. The materials were available for all of the six species of human filariae whose microfilariae appear in the circulating blood. The results are summarized in TABLE 11-19 and Fig. 11-9.

11F.5.1 *Wuchereria bancrofti*

Three distinct forms are differentiated by the values of the periodicity index and the best estimate of peak hour, i.e., the nocturnally periodic (NPWb), the nocturnally subperiodic (NSWb), and the diurnally subperi-

Table 11-17.   A computer program for calculating the periodicity index and the best estimate of the peak hour with a 4-kiloword minicomputer of Basic-3000 level.

```
C-AICAL, 1971
01.10 T "ESTIMATE OF MF PERIODICITY STP 4-10"!!
01.20 S A = O;S B = O;S C = O;S D = O;S E = O;S G = O;S MI = 999999
01.30 A "MF 'RATIO' OR 'COUNT' ? "CO
01.40 IF (CO-OCOUNT)2.1,1.5,2.1
01.50 T !! "O'CLOCK MF COUNT"
01.60 F H = O,11;T !%2,H*2; A" "X(H);S A = A + X(H)
01.70 S M = A/12;T !!%5.02,"MEAN "M
01.80 F H = O,11;S X(H) = (X(H)*100)/M
01.90 GOTO 2.31
02.10 T !!"O'CLOCK MF RATIO"
02.20 F H = O,11;T !%2.,H*2;A" "X(H)
02.30 T !
02.31 F H = O,11;S B = B + X(H);S C = C + X(H)*X(H)
02.40 S SD = FSQT (C-B*B/12)/11)
02.41 T !"SD (MF RATIO) "%5.02,SD,!!
02.50 A "TENTATIVE PEAK HOUR "K
02.60 T !!"HOUR EXM. SUM SQUARE"
03.10 F I = 10*(K-1),10*(K + 1);F H = O,11; DO 5.0
03.20 T !!"PEAK HOUR"%3.01,J/10,
03.21 T "MINIMUM SUM SQR "%6.02, MI,!!
03.30 A "ANOTHER TENTATIVE PEAK HOUR "K
03.50 IF (K-ONO)3.6,3.7,3.6
03.60 S MI = 999999; GOTO 2.6
03.70 T !!"O'CLOCK MF RATIO OBS. MF RATIO CALC."
03.80 S I = J
03.90 = F H = O,11; DO 6.0
04.10 T !"TOTAL "%5.01,E," "%6.02,G
04.20 T !!!!; QUIT
05.10 MH = 100 + SD*1.347*FCOS( (H*2-I/10)*0.2618)
05.20 S D = D + (X(H) − MH)'2
05.30 IF (H-11)5.9,5.4,5.9
05.40 T !%3.01,I/10," "%6.02,D,
05.50 IF (D-MI)5.6,5.6,5.7
05.60 MI = D;S J = I
05.70 S D = O
05.90 RETURN
06.10 DO 5.1
06.40 T !%2.,H*2," "%5.01,X(H)," "%6.02,MH,
06.50 S E = E + X(H);S G = G + MH
06.60 RETURN
```

Table 11-18.   An example of "the estimate of microfilarial periodicity" by the computer program (data from Turner & Edeson, 1957, subperiodic *B. malayi* cases).

```
*GO
ESTIMATE OF MF PERIODICITY STP 4–10
1. MF 'RATIO' OR 'COUNT' ? :COUNT
```

2. O'CLOCK	MF COUNT
0	:3108
2	:3196
4	:3470
6	:2902
8	:3157
10	:2251
12	:2119
14	:2000
16	:2587
18	:3212
20	:4277
22	:4426

```
MEAN    3058.8
SD (MF RATIO)    25.10
3. TENTATIVE PEAK HOUR    :23
```

HOUR EXM.	SUM SQUARE
22.0	3274.04
22.1	3185.95
22.2	3105.13
22.3	3031.62
22.4	2965.48
22.5	2906.75
22.5	2855.47
22.7	2811.69
22.8	2775.43
22.9	2746.70
23.0	2725.54
23.1	2711.96
23.2	2705.97
23.3	2707.56
23.4	2716.75
23.5	2733.52
23.6	2757.86
23.7	2789.75
23.8	2829.18
23.9	2876.12
24.0	2930.54

PEAK HOUR 23.2   MINIMUM SUM SQR 2705.97
4. ANOTHER TENTATIVE PEAK HOUR? :NO

O'CLOCK	MF RATIO OBS.	MF RATIO CALC.
0	101.6	133.06
2	104.5	125.12
4	113.5	110.45
6	94.9	92.97
8	103.2	77.38
10	73.6	67.85
12	69.3	66.94
14	65.4	74.88
16	84.6	89.56
18	105.0	107.03
20	139.8	122.62
22	144.7	132.15
TOTAL	1200.0	1200.00

odic form (DSWb). As shown in TABLE 11-19, records of occurrence of NPWb are available from Asia (Japan, China, Malaya, the Philippines), some Pacific islands (Solomon), Africa (Liberia), and South America (Brazil). In all of these examples, the periodicity index calculated from the original data was over 90%, and the peak hour was around midnight (from 10 p.m. to 2 a.m.). This almost cosmopolitan form of human filaria is considered to be composed of a fairly uniform population in view of the periodicity pattern.

A form of *W. bancrofti* reported by HARINASUTA *et al.* (1970) from West Thailand as to be "nocturnally subperiodic" is really distinct from other groups in that the periodicity index is only a little over 50%. However, it should be pointed out that this value is about two times larger than those of the previously known "subperiodic" forms of *W. bancrofti* and *B. malayi*, which are usually between 20% and 30%.

The Pacific form of *W. bancrofti* so far commonly called the nonperiodic or diurnally subperiodic type is peculiar in that the periodicity index is only about one-fifth of the periodic form, and that the peak hour is situated in the afternoon at about 4 p.m. The values of MSQ are all small, especially in the examples reported by ROSEN (1955) from the Society Islands and by EYLES *et al.* (1947) for the American soldiers infected in the South Pacific fields, indicating that the periodicity curves are close to the harmonic wave form.

11F.5.2 *Brugia malayi*

Two forms are clearly differentiated, both nocturnal in the peak hour but differ greatly in the size of the periodicity index, around 30% in the sub-

Table 11-19. Comparison of the periodicity index (D), the peak hour (K) and the minimum value of the sum of squares of the differences between the observed and the theoretical ratios (MSQ) of various species and forms of human filaria (after SASA & TANAKA, 1974).

Sp. No.	Filarial group	Locality of observation	D (%)	K (hour)	MSQ (%)	Author (senior only) and year
1)	NPWb	Amami, Japan	102.53	2.4	17689	Ibusuki, 1957
		Kagoshima, Japan (A)	100.08	22.8	14847	Otsuji, 1958
		Kagoshima, Japan (B)	111.17	0.8	11723	Otsuji, 1958
		Kagoshima, Japan (C)	106.59	1.1	10511	Otsuji, 1958
		Kagoshima, Japan (D)	110.61	0.7	12772	Otsuji, 1958
		Nagasaki, Japan	103.01	2.1	6997	Fukamachi, 1960
		Taiwan	138.48	0.1	75121	Tanaka, 1934
		Tioman, Malaya	115.92	22.3	24319	Balasingam, 1967
		Bukit Lanjan, Malaya	92.10	1.8	5614	Ramachandran, 1964
		Ulu Trengganu, Malaya	97.16	1.8	8857	Ramachandran, 1970
		Selangor, Malaya	106.65	1.7	11858	Wharton, 1960
		Palawan, Philippines (A)	112.36	22.9	16777	Cabrera, 1965
		Palawan, Philippines (B)	104.96	23.7	9789	Cabrera, 1965
		Solomon Islands	95.23	0.6	10212	Schlosser, 1945
		Liberia, Africa	96.89	0.8	8904	Poindexter, 1950
		Liberia, Africa (A)	92.61	2.0	5193	Burch, 1950
		Liberia, Africa (B)	95.65	1.6	8707	Burch, 1950
		Florianapolis, Brazil	107.30	1.9	24098	Rachou, 1954
		Belem, Brazil	101.25	1.0	6209	Rachou, 1954
	NSWb	Sangkla-buri, Thailand	59.24	20.5	2899	Harinasuta, 1970
	DSWb	South Pacific	22.00	13.3	375	Eyles, 1947
		New Caledonia	22.78	15.0	1003	Iyengar, 1954
		Society Islands	20.62	16.4	280	Rosen, 1955
		Wallis Islands	27.24	17.0	4495	Rageau, 1959

		Selangor, Malaya	95.01	2.1	5572	Wharton, 1960
		Bukit Lanjan, Malaya	103.76	3.0	8730	Ramachandran, 1964
		Ulu Trengganu, Malaya	97.26	2.9	4913	Ramachandran, 1970
		South Thailand	103.27	22.9	15194	Nair, 1961
		Kerala (hill), India	86.08	1.0	6404	Raghavan, 1963
		Kerala (plane), India	92.77	23.4	5230	Raghavan, 1963
		Sulawesi, Indonesia	86.87	23.5	7317	Oemijati (pers. comm.)
		Huchow, China	110.16	0.2	16551	Feng, 1935
	NSBm	Pahang, Malaya	22.79	23.3	1625	Turner, 1957
		Malaya (in cat)	29.21	21.9	1067	Edeson, 1959
		Palawan, Philippines (A)	34.36	22.8	2003	Cabrera, 1965
		Palawan, Philippines (B)	29.36	23.5	993	Cabrera, 1965
3)	Timor-Fil.	Portuguese Timor	102.82	23.7	10571	David, 1965
4)	Mans. ozz.	Amazonas, Brazil	14.85	11.6	1857	Rachou, 1954
5)	D. perst.	Cameroon, Africa	22.69	9.6	2391	Kershaw, 1950
6)	DPLl	Cameroon (in man)	92.53	11.6	6470	Kershaw, 1950
		Cameroon (in man)	93.65	11.6	6527	Duke, 1958
		Human race in drill (A)	108.80	13.6	15586	Duke, 1958
		Human race in drill (B)	101.60	13.5	9038	Duke, 1958
	NPLl	Monkey, Cameroon (A)	105.34	23.1	17255	Duke, 1958
		Monkey, Cameroon (B)	91.06	0.8	6660	Duke, 1958
		Monkey, Cameroon (C)	131.16	22.4	69141	Duke, 1958
	Hybrid-Ll	ND-F-1	92.22	15.3	10116	Duke, 1964
		DN-F-1	89.77	15.5	16242	Duke, 1964
		ND-F-2	84.93	16.7	10834	Duke, 1964
		Optional hybrid F-2	67.16	16.6	10121	Duke, 1964
		Back cross DN/DD	88.86	13.5	15003	Duke, 1964
		Back cross DN/NN	105.39	19.2	18867	Duke, 1964

NPWb: nocturnally periodic *Wuchereria bancrofti*; NSWb: nocturnally subperiodic *Wuchereria bancrofti*; DSWb: diurnally subperiodic *Wuchereria bancrofti*; NPBm: nocturnally periodic *Brugia malayi*; NSBm: nocturnally subperiodic *Brugia malayi*; Mans. ozz.: *Mansonella ozzardi*; D. perst.: *Dipetalonema perstans*; DPLl: diurnally periodic *Loa loa*; NPLl: nocturnally periodic *Loa loa*.

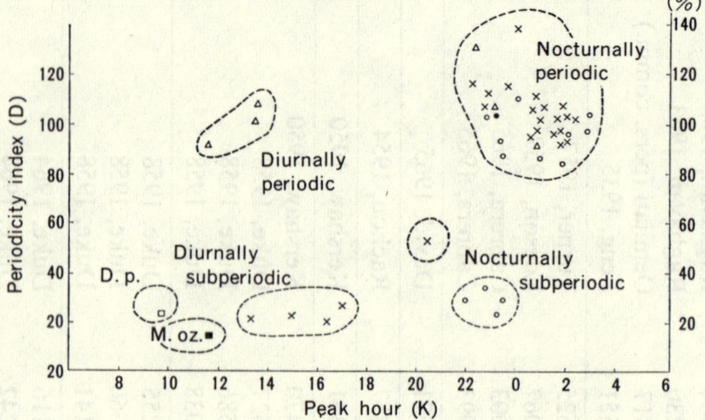

Fig 11-9.   Scatter diagrams of various filarial forms according to the periodicity index (D) and the best estimate of peak hour (K); (from SASA & TANAKA, 1974)

periodic form but are above 80 % in the periodic form. There have been no intermediate types observed in any locality in South and East Asia. The periodic form has been recorded from Malaysia, Indonesia, Thailand, India, and China (also from Japan and Korea), while the subperiodic form is known from Malaysia, Indonesia (Kalimantan), and the Philippines. The subperiodic form of *B. malayi* reported from South Thailand by GUPTA-VENIJ *et al.* (1971) is unusual in that the counts observed with three cases showed a periodicity index of 40.71 and the peak hour of 13.0 1 p.m.; additional observations based on larger samples are required in order to confirm whether this example represents a new subperiodic form of *B. malayi*, or such an unusual result was caused by errors of chance.

11F.5.3 The Timor filaria

The study of periodicity reported by DAVID & EDESON (1965) indicates that the Timor filaria is a typical "nocturnally periodic" form, with the periodicity index of 103 % and the peak hour of 23.7 (18 minutes before midnight).

11F.5.4. *Mansonella ozzardi*

This filarial species is known to be endemic among the natives of South and Central Americas as well as in certain islands of the West Indies, as reviewed by SASA (1974), and has been considered to be a "nonperiodic" form. However, statistical analysis of data reported by RACHOU & LACERDE (1954) has shown that it is probably a diurnally subperiodic form, with the periodicity index of as small as about 15 %, and with the peak hour at around noon (11.6 hour in this case).

11F.5.5 *Dipetalonema perstans*

This species is widely distributed among the people in the tropical region of Africa, and also in the Guianas of South America, and has also been called a nonperiodic type. However, statistical analysis of the data recorded by KERSHAW (1950) from nine cases of carriers (including five cases of mixed infections with *L. loa*) shows that it is probably a diurnally subperiodic type, with the periodicity index of 23.7 % and the peak hour of about 10 a.m. in this case.

11F.5.6 *Loa loa*

Loa loa is a filarial parasite indigenous to the rain forest zone of tropical Africa, and its microfilariae in the peripheral blood of human hosts are known to be diurnally periodic. KERSHAW (1950) recorded microfilarial counts in 50 mm³ blood samples collected over 24-hour period from nine prisoners in Kumba, British Cameroons; the microfilariae of *L. loa* were found from five cases, and those of *D. perstans* from all of the nine cases. By statistical analysis of the data according to the previously described method, the sums of counts of the microfilariae of *L. loa* in these five cases were found to show a periodicity index of 92.53 and the peak hour of 11.6 (24 minutes before noon). Similar results were obtained by analysis of data cited by DUKE & WIJERS (1958).

11G.   Methods for evaluation of filariasis control programs

The efficacy of a filariasis control program can be evaluated by various scales related to the intensity of infection of the human or vector populations being covered by the control operations. When certain effective control measures are applied, various changes occur in these scales, and the overall efficacy can be assessed from the degrees of changes in these scales. The methods available for this purpose may be classified into the following categories.

1. Survey of human populations:
    1.1 Clinical survey methods: Reduction in the morbidity rate
    1.2 Parasitological survey methods
        1.2.1 Comparison of the microfilarial rates
        1.2.2 Comparison of the microfilarial densities
    1.3 Immunological survey methods
2. Survey of vector populations:
    2.1 Reduction in the vector density and the longevity
    2.2 Reduction in the infection rate of vector populations

2.3 Reduction in the infectivity potential of vector populations

11G.1 Evaluation from survey of human populations

11G.1.1 Evaluation from clinical survey data

Because the ultimate purpose of a filariasis control project is the reduction or eradication of any illness due to filarial infections from a human community, the survey of prevalence and incidence of various clinical affections comprises an important part of epidemiological survey programs, as discussed in Section 10B.1. However, most of the chronic signs of filarial infections, such as elephantiasis, hydrocele, and chyluria, are not directly influenced by drug treatment or vector control operations, and thus cannot be utilized as criteria for evaluation of efficacy unless the changes in the prevalence or incidence are compared on a long-range scale, such as an interval of ten years. It should also be pointed out that most acute clinical signs caused as a result of filarial infections such as fever, lymphangitis, and lymphadenitis may also be caused by other pathogenic agents and thus cannot be used as specific signs for comparison of the efficacy of control operations.

BEYE *et al.* (1952), for example, conducted clinical and microfilarial surveys of people in Tahiti and Maiao, the Society Islands, southern Pacific, before and one year after a filariasis control operation. The control program constituted mainly of mass administration of DEC to the whole population at a dosage of 2 mg per kg, three times a day for seven days, and the control of mosquitoes with DDT and sanitary measures. In comparison of the survey data collected before application of the control measures and at six and 12 months after the start of the operations, the microfilarial rate of the treatment areas dropped from 34.4% to 21.5% and 19.6%, and the average number of microfilariae per 20 mm³ blood was also reduced from 103.3 to 6.8 and 7.1, respectively. However, there were no significant differences in the prevalence of clinical filariasis rates, such as in those of lymphangitis and elephantiasis.

However, the results of clinical and blood surveys reported by MARCH *et al.* (1960) for the same area revealed conspicuous differences even in the clinical filariasis rates. A systematic, islandwide filariasis control program was implemented in 1954 in Tahiti, as described by KESSEL (1957). The whole population was covered by a mass drug administration program of monthly doses of DEC at 6 mg per kg for 12 months. In comparison of the surveys of all male populations conducted in 1949 and in 1959, the microfilaremia rate was reduced from 37.9% to 6.5% and the elephantiasis rate from 6.9% to 2.2%. The elephantiasis rate of males of the laboring age-group of 20 to 40 years fell from 5% to 0.6%. The total hydrocele rate was reduced from 9.8% to 3.2%, and the acute lymphangitis rate of males above the age of 20 years fell from 36.0% to 4.0%. Most remarkable was the fact that no new cases of hydrocele and elephantiasis developed following application of the control measures (also see Section 9E.11).

CIFERRI *et al.* (1969), in American Samoa, also compared the distribution of clinical filariasis before and after two years of treatment with DEC in 160 male microfilaria carriers, and observed that acute lymphagitis fell from 10% to 0%, and adenopathy from 31.3% to 15.6%. However, the rate of elephantiasis was 5.0% and 5.6%, and that of hydrocele was 6.2% and 5.0%, and there were practically no reductions in the attack rate of both signs during this period.

11G.1.2 Evaluation from microfilaria survey data

As stated previously, the detection of microfilariae in blood or skin of man is the only specific means of diagnosis of filarial infection, and thus it constitutes the most important aspect of the evaluation program. The methods for microfilaria survey should be standardized such as discussed in Section 10B.2. When the examination of microfilariae is made with a standardized method on measured samples, the results can be assessed from at least two different aspects, i.e., the proportion of positive cases (the microfilarial rate), and the density per unit weight or volume of samples (the microfilarial density). The efficiency of detection of microfilariae becomes higher as the size of samples examined is increased, as discussed in Section 11D.

11G.1.2.1 Comparison of the microfilarial rates

The microfilarial rate is usually expressed by the percentage obtained by dividing the number of persons who are positive for microfilariae with the total number of persons examined in a survey. This is a simplest index of the prevalence of filariasis in a human population, and an important scale for comparison of the efficacy of filariasis control programs. Remarkable reductions in the microfilarial rates have been observed after application of effective filariasis control measures, such as reported by KESSEL (1957, 1971) and MARCH *et al.* (1960) from Tahiti, CIFERRI *et al.* (1966, 1967) from American Samoa, ABDULCADER & SASA (1966) from Sri Lanka, and SASA *et al.* (1970) from Japan.

Although the microfilarial rate is a very simple statistical measure, it involves a number of complicated problems to be considered in its use for evaluation of epidemiological survey data, as discussed in Sections 11B and 11D. Various criteria are also available in the use of microfilarial rates for the assessment of filariasis control operations.

(a) Comparison of the gross microfilarial rate
In most instances where large numbers of people in the same endemic

areas are repeatedly surveyed by the same method, the efficacy of a filariasis control program may be evaluated by comparison of the microfilarial rates obtained before start of the program with those observed during the operation period or at various intervals after its cessation.

The relative efficacy of filariasis control programs implemented in different administrative regions may roughly be compared by the speed of reductions in the microfilarial rates observed in annual blood surveys, such as shown in Fig. 11-10. In this figure, the microfilarial rates reported annually from four districts in Japan are plotted on a semi logarithmic paper, for a five-year period for districts in Okinawa (Miyako and Yaeyama, where the control programs began in 1966 and 1967) and for a ten-year period for two prefectures in Kyushu (Kagoshima and Nagasaki, where the control programs began in 1962). The percentages are quoted from Tables 8-11 and 8-13 in Section 8C.4.

In these four districts in Japan, filariasis control programs had been in progress under the same principles, that is, they were aimed at examining all the people above the age of one year living in the target areas, and to treat only the microfilaria positive cases with DEC by the dosage schedule

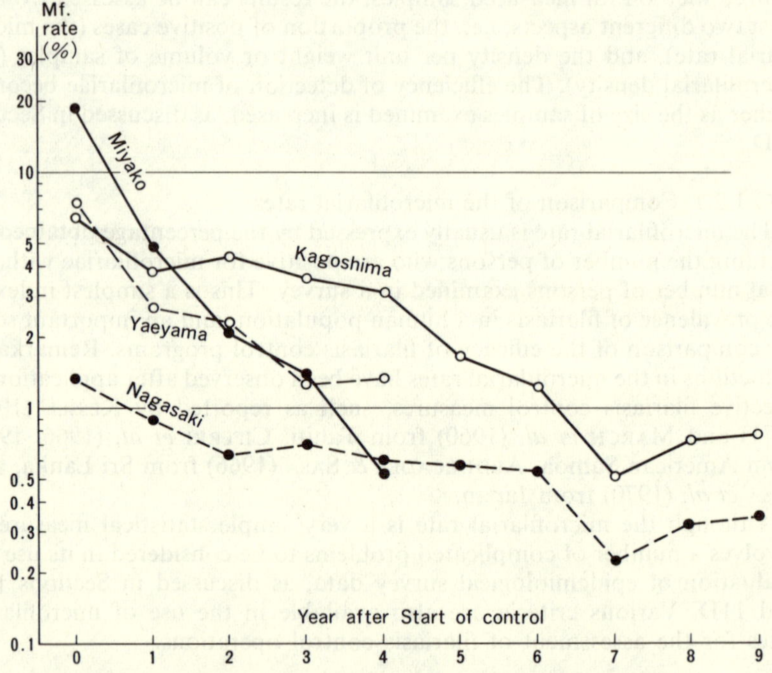

Fig 11-10.   Microfilarial rates observed in annual blood surveys conducted in four districts in Japan before and after start of filariasis control programs.

of 6 mg per kg once a day for at least 12 doses. However, the efficiency of the blood survey, as well as the drug treatment operations, differed greatly among the districts for various reasons. As a result, the relative efficacy of the control operations as shown in this figure was quite different, and was largest in Miyako and smallest in Nagasaki.

There is another interesting example of the efficacy of a vector control operation on the prevalence of filariasis as assessed from a comparison of the gross microfilarial rates. SASA (1963) showed microfilarial rates observed in four villages on Ishigaki Island in 1955 and from 1960 to 1961. This island is located in the southernmost part of Japan with a total population of about 50,000, and was notorious for the prevalence of both malaria and *W. bancrofti* filariasis. It was noted that at least several hundred, and often nearly two thousand people died of malaria on this small island every year. A malaria control program was organized on this island in 1955, and a DDT house spraying operation was repeated twice a year; this resulted in a complete eradication of malaria by about 1961. However, the repeated application of DDT house spraying which was so effective in the control of malaria on this island was shown to have no effect on the reduction of microfilarial rate, as shown in Table 11-20.

Table 11-20. Comparison of the microfilarial rates in four villages on Ishigaki Island, Yaeyema, as observed before and after the DDT residual house spraying operation for malaria control was practiced (SASA, 1963).

Village	Before spraying (1955)			After spraying (1960, 1961)		
	No. examined	No. positive	Percentage positive	No. examined	No. positive	Percentage positive
Heishin	497	94	18.9	294	57	19.4
Ohama	161	40	24.8	255	51	20.0
Miyara	201	25	12.4	164	41	25.0
Shiraho	255	41	16.1	315	67	21.3

(b) Evaluation from paired blood examination data

Evaluation of the efficiency of a blood survey method, as well as that of the effectiveness of a filariasis control operation, can be made more precisely by comparison of the paired blood examination data collected subsequently from the same human populations in an endemic area. For example, SASA *et al.* (1963) compared the results of two blood surveys made over an interval of two months on the residents of two villages in Amami, an endemic area of bancroftian filariasis in southern Japan (Table 11-21). The registered population of these villages at that time was 659. In August 1962, 533 persons (80.9% of the registered population) were examined, and 101 cases were microfilaria positive, with the gross positive rate of 18.9%. At the second blood survey carried out two months later, 496 persons (75.3% of the registered population) were examined, and 112 cases were positive, with the gross positive rate of 22.6%. No control measures were practiced during this period.

Further analysis of the results were made by grouping the persons according to the paired data. As shown in Table 11-21, they were classified into nine groups by the combination of three categories: positive, negative, and absent. Of 659 registered population of these villages, 428 persons (64.9%) received the two consecutive blood examinations, and 111 among them were found positive in either or both of the examinations, with a positive rate of 25.9%. The efficiency of detection of microfilariae was 76.6% (85 of 111) at the first and 90.1% (100 of 111) at the second examination. It should be noted here that a significant number of new positive cases were discovered at the second examination from the previously negative persons

Table 11-21. Classification of the people in an endemic area of *W. bancrofti* filariasis in Amami, southern Japan, according to the coupled results of two consecutive blood surveys conducted over an interval of two months (after SASA *et al.*, 1963). (+: microfilaria positive; —: microfilaria negative; o: not examined)

1st survey	+	+	+	—	—	—	o	o	o	Total
2nd survey	+	—	o	+	—	o	+	—	o	
No. observed	74	11	16	26	317	89	12	56	58	659
Percent	11.2	1.7	2.4	3.9	48.1	13.5	1.8	8.5	8.8	100.

Table 11-22. Classification of microfilaria cases detected during the course of the filariasis control program in Miyako District, Okinawa (from data compiled by Miyako Health Center, quoted by SASA, 1970). A: Microfilaria cases who did not receive blood examination in the previous year. B: Microfilaria cases who were negative in the previous year blood survey. C: Microfilaria cases who were positive in the previous year blood survey and became negative after treated with a course of DEC (12 doses of 6 mg per kg each), but were found positive again at the mass blood survey of this year. D: Microfilaria cases who were positive in the previous year blood survey, and always remained positive despite treatment with two courses of DEC administration (altogether, 12 doses of 6 mg per kg each).

Year after start of control	Period		Total number percent Mf. cases	Classification of Mf. cases			
				A	B	C	D
2nd year	April	1966–	3,105	572	1,452	778	303
	Nov.	1966	100%	18.4%	46.8%	25.1%	9.1%
3rd year	Jan.	1967–	1,282	168	678	351	85
	Oct.	1968	100%	13.1	52.9	27.4	6.6
4th year	Mar.	1969–	174	25	71	64	14
	Dec.	1969	100%	14.4	40.8	36.8	8.0

(26 of 343, 7.6%), and also that a considerable number of previously positive cases were negative at the second examination (11 of 85, 12.7%), while no drug treatment was conducted during this period.

Analysis was also made with the paired blood survey data collected by Miyako Health Center during the course of the control program. As shown in Table 11-22, microfilaria positive cases detected at the second and subsequent blood surveys were classified into four categories: A, persons absent at the previous survey; B, persons who were negative at the previous survey, and therefore received no drug treatment between the present and the previous surveys; C, persons who were positive at the previous survey, and therefore treated with a course of DEC administration with a total dose of about 72 mg per kg, then became negative at the posttreatment blood examination, but were positive again at the present mass blood survey; and D, persons who were positive at the previous survey, then treated with the same dosage scheme as in C, but remained to be positive at both the posttreatment and present mass blood survey.

The persons under category A should be excluded from evaluation of the effect of the control measure because they are imported cases. Among those who received the previous blood examination, those who were under the category B were highest in the ratio in all these three surveys, indicating that the method of selective treatment of only the microfilaria positive cases such as applied in Miyako and elsewhere in Japan is less efficient than that of the mass treatment of the whole population. The numbers and ratios of persons under the categories C and D reflect the efficiency of the present drug treatment method. It should be noted that some 80% to 90% of the microfilaria positive cases become negative after administration of 72 mg per kg of DEC in 12 divided doses, and also that apparently recurrent cases (category C) are not uncommon among the treated carriers.

(c) Comparison of microfilarial rates among populations with different age or sex compositions.
See examples shown in Section 11B.4

(d) Comparison of microfilarial rates observed by examination of different size of samples.
See examples shown in Section 11D.5.

11G.1.2.2 Comparison of the microfilarial densities (also see Section 11C)
The microfilarial density and the microfilarial rate of human populations in filariasis endemic areas are highly correlated, that is, where the rate is high, the density is usually also high. However, the two indices are independent factors, and the effects of filariasis control programs should be assessed from both aspects.

When a filariasis control program, such as with mass administration of DEC, is initiated in an endemic area, it causes not only the reduction of microfilarial rate of the population, but also changes the pattern of distribution of microfilarial density of the infected people, causing a reduction in the value of MfD-50 and the increase in the values of a and/or b of the regression line. The grade of reduction in MfD-50 or that of increase in a

Table 11-23. Microfilaria positive rate, positive grade, and density obtained at blood surveys of people in Miyako, compiled from records of Miyako Health Center. (SASA *et al.*, 1970).

Type of blood survey	A. All people, before control 1965		C. All people, second year 1966		B. Previously positives, post-treatment, 1965	
I. Mf-positive rate	No.	%	No.	%	No.	%
No. & % examined	59212	99.1	60411		12352	98.3
No. & % positive	11963	20.20	2956	4.89	2079	16.83
II. Mf-positive grade	No.	%	No.	%	No.	%
No. & % $\lbrace$ N₃	8144	68.1	1083	36.6	577	27.8
N₂	1827	15.3	673	22.8	502	24.1
N₁	1992	16.7	1200	40.6	1000	48.1
Index	0.838		0.743		0.599	
Detection rate p	0.774				0.449	
III. Mf-density	No.	Cu.%	No.	Cu.%	No.	Cu.%
No. of persons 1	1236	10.4	1029	33.4	807	39.3
and cumulative 2	864	17.7	409	47.2	371	57.4
percentage 3	627	22.9	263	55.8	174	65.9
4	500	27.1	163	61.2	112	71.3
5	426	30.7	122	65.2	73	74.9
6–10	1589	44.1	387	77.8	219	85.6
11–20	1855	59.7	244	85.9	139	92.3
21–30	1030	68.4	112	89.5	59	95.2
31–40	735	74.5	61	91.5	30	96.7
41–50	567	79.3	52	93.2	19	97.6
51–100	1257	89.9	126	97.4	35	99.3
101–200	860	97.1	60	99.3	11	99.85
201–300	209	98.9	9	99.6	2	99.95
301–400	68	99.4	8	99.90	0	99.95
401–500	37	99.8	2	99.97	0	99.95
501+	29	100	1	100	1	100.0
Total No.	11889		3048		2052	
MfD-50	13.8		2.3		2.5	
a & b	3.74 & 1.10		4.57 & 1.12		4.77 & 1.29	
Mf-count, total	459193		29012		15036	
Average, per positive	38.62		9.52		7.33	
Average, all person	7.76		0.48		1.22	

or *b* value is another measure of the effectiveness of a control program than the simple comparison of the microfilarial rates. For example, it was observed in a filariasis control program in Miyako district that as a result of one year's course of selective treatment of microfilaria cases detected at the initial pretreatment survey of the whole population (Survey A), the microfilarial rate dropped at the posttreatment general survey (Survey C) from 19.16% to 4.87% as shown in Table 11-23; at the same time, analysis of microfilarial density by the method shown in Table 11-6 and Fig. 11-3 indicates that MfD-50 decreased from 13.8 per 30 mm³ to 2.3 per 30 mm³, and also that the values of *a* and *b* of the regression line changed from 3.74 and 1.10 to 4.57 and 1.12, respectively. There occurred a remarkable reduction in both rates and densities of microfilariae by this control measure. A posttreatment blood survey of only the previously positive cases (Survey B) was conducted also between these two general surveys, and a microfilarial rate of 18.0% (2,004 positives out of 11,141 previously positive cases examined) was observed. The so-called cure rate of this course of DEC treatment (12 daily doses of 6 mg per kg each) was 92.0%.

The patterns of distribution of microfilarial density observed at the above three surveys were quite different. From data shown in Table 11-22, regression lines were drawn as in Fig. 11-11, and the values of MfD-50, *a*, and *b* were obtained by simple visual fitting of the lines on the log probit section paper. As stated above, the microfilarial rate was by the order of A, B, and C (19.16%, 18.0%, and 4.87% respectively). However, the MfD-50 was by order of A, C, and B (13.8, 2.3, and 1.5). The values of *a* and *b* were 3.74 and 1.10 in the Survey A, 4.77 and 1.29 in B, and 4.57 and 1.12 in C. It should be noted here that the lines of A and C differ greatly in the values of *a* but are similar in the values of *b*, and thus make almost parallel

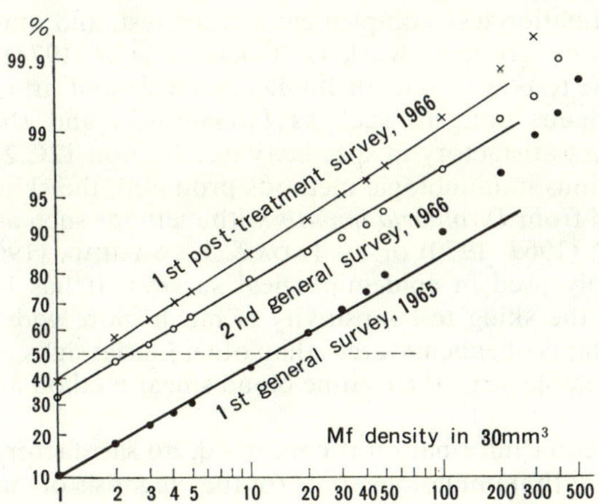

Fig. 11-11. Curmulative percentage distribution of Mf-positive cases (Miyako Island) (from Sasa, 1967)

lines distant from each other, while the line B is close in the value of a to the line C, but differ greatly from the other two lines in the angle against X-axis due to the larger value of b.

Such differences in the pattern of distribution of microfilarial density can be explained by the composition of the positive cases detected at the respective blood surveys. Because the microfilaria carriers in the Survey B were represented by only the treated cases, their densities were naturally low even when still positive. On the other hand, the positive cases found at the general Survey C included a considerable number of untreated cases (imported, or previously negative), as shown in Table 11-22 and therefore many of them were still harbouring microfilariae at relatively high densities. Comparison of data collected from different filariasis control programs with such a statistical analysis is considered to provide more valuable information for the assessment than with simple methods, such as comparison of the speed of reduction of microfilarial rates.

11G.1.3 Evaluation from immunologic survey data

As reviewed in Section 10B.3, many studies have been reported on immunologic methods for the diagnosis of human filariasis, but their practical usefulness is still disreputed by most workers. As stated previously, WILSON (1961) concluded that such tests were not satisfactory because "most published accounts of other aids to diagnosis, such as skin reactions and complement fixation tests indicate that they are not sufficiently specific and that false negatives are common." On the other hand, TANAKA *et al.* (1970) demonstrated in *L. carinii* infection in cotton rats that infected and noninfected hosts can be clearly differentiated by the development of antibodies in the latter against the homologous adult worm antigens in the hemagglutination test, complement fixation test, and immunodiffusion test, but the same group or workers (TAKAOKA *et al.*, 1974) observed that results of these tests with sera of human filariasis and antigens prepared from heterologous antigens such as *Litomosoides* and *Dirofilaria* were more or less unsatisfactory in specificity (see Section 12C.2).

Among various immunologic methods proposed, the skin test with antigen prepared from *Dirofilaria immitis* with methods such as described by SAWADA *et al.* (1967, 1970) or by TADA & KAWASHIMA (1964) have been most commonly used in epidemiological surveys. It has been generally accepted that the sking test sensitivity is much more widely distributed among inhabitants of endemic areas than other filarial signs, such as microfilaremia detectable with the routine blood smear method and the clinical manifestations.

So far as present information is concerned, no satisfactory results have been reported with immunologic tests for the diagnosis of cure from filariasis. The skin reaction, for example, is known to persist long periods after the patients are practically cured by drug administration. However, the skin test may be a useful tool in long-term observations on the status of filarial transmission, because the positive rate has been found to be very high in active foci, lower in areas where the disease had once existed but already disappeared, (especially in young age-groups), and extremely low in filariasis-free areas (DESOWITZ *et al.*, 1966; ISHIZAKI *et al.*, 1960, 1963, 1964; KATAMINE *et al.*, 1970; SATO *et al.*, 1970).

In view of the fact that the skin test reaction is more sensitive as a sign of filarial infection than other methods, such as detection of microfilariae, HAYASHI *et al.* (1967) proposed a method for comparing the force of transmission of filariasis among different endemic areas or before and after the application of control measures. They selected certain age-groups (usually 10 to 15 years) in an area, conducted skin tests with Sawada's FST antigen on the same persons at an interval of about three months, and regarded the difference of a wheal size of over 4 mm as significant. One of the results of surveys conducted with this method was reported by YAMAMOTO *et al.* (1968) in Amami. A filariasis control program was in progress in this district, and the microfilaria rates at the pretreatment survey in 1961 and the posttreatment survey in 1966 were 10.4% and 0.85%, respectively, in urban areas, and 18.2% and 1.2%, respectively, in rural areas. The mosquito infection rate before control was seven times higher in the rural area than in the town. At the skin tests carried out in 1966 and 1967, the percentages of persons who showed a significant increase in the reaction were 18.3% in the urban area and 17.6% in the rural areas. It was concluded from these results that although filariasis was more prevalent in the rural area than in the urban area before the treatment, the force of transmission in the two areas dropped to almost to the same level in 1967, after application of the control measures.

11G.2 Evaluation from survey of vector populations

11G.2.1 Comparison of the vector density and the longevity

The efficacy of various vector control operations is usually evaluated by comparison of the density and longevity of the vector populations before and after start of the program. Various methods used for this purpose were described in Section 10C. There have been various measures utilized as indices of the vector density, such as the average number per man per day (or hour) of biting females collected on man or animal, the average number of resting females per house (in case of an endophilic vector species), the average number of females collected per day with a trap, and the average number of larvae per unit surface of breeding places. Among these, the most important index as that directly related to the intensity of transmission of filariasis is the biting density per man per day or per year. In the filariasis control programs in India, for example, tremendous effort and manpower are apparently devoted to collect the density per man per hour from all the control units in operation.

As discussed in Section 10C.2, the changes in the average longevity (or daily survival rate) of the vector population after taking an infective blood meal cause significant effects on the efficiency of transmission of the parasites. Therefore, observations on the vector longevity by methods such as described by DETINOVA (1962) constitute an important aspect of the assessment of vector control operations.

11G.2.2 Comparison of the vector infection rate

The effects of parasite control measures such as by mass or selective administration of DEC to human populations obviously appear as changes in the infection rates of vector populations with the filarial parasite. As discussed in Section 11E, the infection rate of the vector population is directly dependent upon the infectivity index of the human population, which is determined by the mode of distribution of microfilariae among the infected people. Therefore, the efficacy of drug treatment operations can also be assessed indirectly from the changes in the rate of filarial infection of the vectors, and such a method often constitutes an important operation in the evaluation program especially when the blood or skin survey of human populations is impracticable for various reasons. In Western Samoa, for example, the infectivity index of the human population, as well as the infection rate of vector population, were 13.5%, and 8.35%, respectively, in the pretreatment survey, while they fell to 0.60% and 0.61%, respectively, in a survey conducted after completion of a mass drug administration program, as shown in Table 11-14 and 11-15.

11G.2.3 Comparison of the infectivity potential of the vector population

As already discussed in Section 10A, various parameters are involved as factors in the dynamics of transmission of filariasis in each endemic area. The infectivity potential of human populations to vector populations is determined mainly by the rate and density of the distribution of microfilariae among people in endemic areas, such as shown in Section 11E. Likewise, the infectivity potential of vector populations to human populations is also determined mainly by the rate and density of the infection of vectors with mature filaria larvae, and the biting density of the vectors on man. In this case, not the mere infection with all stages of larvae but the infection with only the mature stage larvae is of interest. The force of infectivity of the vector population in an area may be expressed by an index such as obtained by multiplying the percentage of vector insects harboring mature filaria larave, the average number of mature larvae per infective vector, and the density of biting vector per man per year, as shown in Section 10A.3. WHARTON (1962), for example, showed in an endemic area of *B. malayi* in Malaya that the infective bites per man per year was 57.9 in 1954, but fell to 28.3 in 1955, and 16.6 in 1956 after the houses in the village were treated with dieldrin residual spraying.

12 | Experimental methods in filariasis studies

Most filarial species parasitic in man are not transmissible to laboratory animals, and therefore experimental studies in filariasis have usually been made with certain nonhuman filariae easily maintained in laboratory animals, such as *Dirofilaria immitis* in dog, *Litomosoides carinii* in cotton rat, and *Dipetalonema witei* in jird. So far as our present information is concerned, the only filarial parasite naturally occurring in man and easily transmissible to animals is the subperiodic form of *B. malayi* endemic in certain rural areas in Southeast Asia. Another species closely related to it, *B. phangi*, has also been shown to be maintained in some laboratory animals. It has also been reported that *Loa loa* in man can be transmitted to some African monkeys, and certain strains of *Onchocerca volvulus* to chimpanzees, as discussed in the previous sections.

A considerable amount of information has been accumulated on the chemotherapy and immunology of filariasis with laboratory animal experiments. However, a number of problems are involved when implicating these results as models of human filariasis. For example, some drugs showing remarkable effects in certain animal filariasis were shown to have no action on human filariasis, while a drug such as diethylcarbamazine (DEC) has been shown to be effective in the treatment of human filariasis but is only slightly effective or completely ineffective in some laboratory animal filariae. Similar or more difficult problems are involved in immunological studies. In some animal models, such as *L. carinii* infection in cotton rats, it has been demonstrated that specific antibodies against the homologous adult antigens develop after certain periods of infection, and thus diagnosis of the disease can be made with immunologic methods, such as indirect hemagglutination test, complement fixation test, fluorescent antibody tests, and immunodiffusion test. However, more or less ambiguous results were obtained with heterologous filarial antigens. Dogs infected with *Dirofilaria immitis* failed to show positive reactions in complement fixation test even with the homologous antigens. In human filariasis, homologous antigens are difficult to prepare and most serological or skin sensitivity tests so far proposed were unsatisfactory in specificity and/or sensitivity.

Each filarial species as well as its host exhibits species-specific characters in susceptibility to drugs as well as in immunologic reactions. However, it should be emphasized also that filariae have general characters common to this group of parasites, and there has been much to learn from animal filariasis experiments for the treatment and diagnosis of human filariasis. In this connection, a review is made on the species of filariae maintained in laboratory animals, and their uses in chemotherapeutic and immunologic studies.

12A. Experimental filariasis in laboratory animals

12A.1 Species of laboratory animal filariae

Among over 500 species of filariae recorded from various animals, only several species have been introduced into laboratories and successfully maintained. The filarial species which are commonly used for experimental studies are listed in Table 12-1, together with their final and intermediate hosts.

12A.2 Maintenance of laboratory animal filariae

12A.2.1 *Litomosoides carinii* (Travassos, 1919)

High rates of natural infection of the parasite have been observed in the cotton rat, *Sigmodon hispidus*, a rodent native to the southern United States. This was used by CULBERTSON & ROSE (1944) for chemotherapeutic tests. HEWITT *et al.* (1947a, b, c) also utilized naturally infected cotton rats and discovered the effects of diethylcarbamazine (DEC) on the parasite. Experimental transmission in the laboratory using the tropical rat mite, *Ornithonyssus bacoti*, was achieved by SCOTT *et al.* (1947), BERTRAM (1947), and WILLIAMS (1948). Later, a large number of studies were carried out on the host-parasite relationships, as reviewed by BERTRAN (1966). It was utilized also for chemotherapeutic studies by HAWKING & SEWELL (1948), SEWELL & HAWKING (1950), WAGNER (1956), SATO (1959), RHODE (1960), TANAKA (1965), TASAKA (1965), and KOBAYASHI *et al.* (1969). Extensive studies on the development of antibodies after infection of *L. carinii* in cotton rats have been made by TANAKA *et al.* (1968, 1969, 1970), ISHII *et al.* (1968, 1969, 1970), and FUJITA *et al.* (1969a, b).

The cotton rat filariasis has various advantages over filariasis in other

Table 12-1. Species of filariae and their hosts commonly used in experimental studies.

Species of filaria	Final hosts	Intermediate hosts
Litomosoides carinii	cotton rat (*Sigmodon*) jird (*Meriones*), *Mastomys*	tropical rat mite (*Ornithonyssus bacoti*)
Dipetalonema witei	jird (*Meriones*)	tick (*Ornithodoros tartakovskyi* & *O. moubata*)
Dirofilaria immitis	dog	mosquito (*Aedes togoi, Armigeres subalbatus, Culex pipiens*, etc.)
Dirofilaria repens	dog	mosquito
Dipetalonema reconditum	dog	dog flea (*Ctenocephalides canis*)
Brugia malayi	cats, dogs, monkeys, jird (*Meriones*)	mosquito (*Aedes togoi, Aedes aegypti, Mansonia* spp., *Anopheles* spp. etc.)
Brugia pahangi	dog, cat, monkey, jird (*Meriones*)	mosquito (*Armigeres subalbatus, Aedes togoi, Mansonia* spp., etc.)

laboratory animals and has been used most extensively as an experimental model of human filariasis. A large number of animals can be maintained in a small laboratory space as compared with the use of dogs and monkeys, the adults are easily recovered from the pleural and peritoneal cavities, the microfilariae reach high densities and are easily examined by bleeding from the tail, and the parasite is susceptible to drugs such as DEC, arsenicals, and antimonials, which were also shown to be effective in human filariasis. However, cotton rats are very nervous and aggressive animals and they are more difficult to handle and breed in the laboratory than mice, rats, jirds, and hamsters. This is the principal reason that their use as a laboratory animal has been nearly abolished in the U.S.A., their native country. However, laboratory colonies are still maintained in Europe and Japan. A strain of cotton rat was imported into Japan and has been bred in this author's laboratory since 1954 and is now quite domesticated as a laboratory animal; it has become almost as easy to handle and breed as albino rats. Its susceptibility to *L. carinii* infection is excellent, and seems to be higher than the wild colonies.

12A.2.1.1 Method of laboratory infection of *Litomosoides carinii*

Methods for laboratory infection of the cotton rat filaria using the tropical rat mite as the intermediate host, and the course of infection in cotton rats and other laboratory animals have been reported by various workers, as reviewed by HAWKING & SEWELL (1942), HAWKING (1963), and BERTRAM (1966). With the Japanese strain of the cotton rat and *L. carinii*, detailed studies were made by WAKASUGI (1955, 1958), TANAKA (1964, 1965), TANAKA *et al.* (1963), KANDA & TASAKA (1966), and KOBAYASHI *et al.* (1967).

In this author's laboratory, stock colonies of the tropical rat mite are maintained on thick layers of cotton placed in desiccator jars (30 cm in diameter), kept in a room regulated at 25°C. The desiccators contain a saturated solution of KCl in order to keep the humidity at about 85%, and are each placed on a pan containing 0.1 solution of detergent in water in order to prevent the escape of the tropical mite and invasion of predacious mites. A mouse is fixed between two sheets of wire screen and is placed into each jar twice a week for the feeding and breeding of the stock colony mites. Care should be taken to prevent the tropical rat mite colonies from being invaded by cheyletid mites, since the latter are predacious on other mites and often cause destruction of the stock colonies, especially in the summer season.

For infection of the mites, about 1,000 unengorged females are collected with a sucking tube and are released on an infected cotton rat kept in a small cage with about 50 g of cotton mat. The rat cage is placed on a vessel containing water, and the mites are allowed to feed for a week. The engorged mites are then isolated again with a sucking tube, and are transferred to a plastic tube containing small amount of cotton. The mouth of the tube is stopped with 200 mesh wire screen in order to allow the mite larvae to escape through it. The tubes containing infected mites are kept for two weeks at 28°C in a jar regulated at 85% relative humidity, until most of the filarial larvae develop to the infective stage. The numbers of microfilariae ingested by the mites are only about 4.7% to 13.8% of those expected from the amount of blood ingested and the density of microfilariae in the host's blood, and their frequency distribution among mites is a negative binominal type (TANAKA *et al.*, 1963). The numbers of infective larvae found among mites of the infective colonies are also very variable, and roughly follow a logarithmically normal distribution.

The tropical rat mite passes five stages in its life history: egg, larva, protonymph, deutonymph, and adult. The mite takes blood meals only in the protonymph and adult stages, and passes the other stages without taking food. According to KANDA & TASAKA (1966), the average amount of blood ingested was 0.015 mg in protonymphs, 0.05 mg in males and 0.12 mg in females; efficient development of the filarial larvae was seen only when the microfilariae were ingested by the adult mites.

Infection of cotton rats with *L. carinii* can be made either by inoculating known numbers of infective larvae dissected from mites into subcutaneous tissue, or by allowing certain numbers of infective mites to feed on clean cotton rats. For producing large numbers of infected animals, the latter method is easier and less time-consuming. In most experiments it is necessary to standardize the number of larvae to be inoculated into each animal. For this purpose, about 30 mites are taken as samples from the infective colony, the number of infective larvae found in each mite is recorded, and its frequency distribution is obtained. Since the arithmetic mean is subject to great variation, the geometric mean is used to determine the number of mites to be fed on one animal. A constant and reasonable infection of cotton rats could be achieved by releasing a colony of mites on each rat containing 60 infective larvae as its geometric mean. With this method, fairly constant infections in all of 84 cotton rats tested have been obtained. Before adopting this method, the number of mites to be used for infection of cotton rats was determined by the arithmetic mean of 60 infective larvae per rat, but since the actual numbers of infective larvae contained per lot estimated with this method were so variable, failure of infection occurred 40 (15.6%) out of 257 rats exposed to the infection.

The mites on cotton rats after the infection are then removed by spraying a 0.1% emulsion of malathion or fenitrothion on the rat body, since contamination of the animal house with the tropical rat mite may cause spontaneous transmission of the parasite. Among various insecticides tested against tropical rat mites, the above two compounds were found to be most effective and practically nontoxic to the rats (KOBAYASHI *et al.* 1967).

The incubation period from infection to the appearance of microfilariae at detectable levels in the circulating blood of infected rats was shown to vary from five weeks to over ten weeks, and the microfilarial density in the blood also varied a great deal according to the number of worms inoculated. In observations with quantitative inoculation made by KANDA & TASAKA (1966), 2 of 5 rats inoculated with 5 infective larvae remained microfilaria negative, and the remaining 3 showed microfilariae 8, 9, and 10 weeks after the inoculation; of 7 rats inoculated with 10 infective larvae,

1 remained negative, and the rest became positive after 8 to 25 weeks; all animals inoculated with 20 or more infective larvae became positive after an incubation period from about 8 weeks. Therefore, it was recommended to inoculate roughly 30 to 60 infective larvae per rat, as a rule, in order to obtain a stable infection and also to avoid the death of the rats due to a heavier worm load.

The time course of the microfilaremia level in the infected cotton rats was observed with the Japanese strain by WAKASUGI (1958) and TANAKA (1964), and more quantitatively by HAYASHI & TANAKA (1965) and by KANDA & TASAKA (1966). The microfilariae once appearing in the circulating blood after a certain incubation period, increase in density on a logistic curve: $Y = K/(1 + me^{-at})$, and reach a maximum level after several weeks. In the chronic stage of infection after several months from the appearance of microfilariae, the density gradually becomes lower and finally drops to one-tenth or less of the peak density, but complete disappearance of microfilariae from the circulating blood such as seen in the chronic stage of human filariasis has been rare. When 30 or more females are parasitizing in a host, the microfilarial density of the peak reaches as high as 1,000 to several thousand per 2.5 mm^3. When the worm burden is 30 females or less per rat, there is a positive correlation between the microfilarial density and the number of parasitizing worms, but infections of larger numbers of worms apparently cause crowding effects on the growth of adults and the production of microfilariae. The adult worms in the pleural cavity cause pleuritis and pericarditis of a peculiar nature, and frequently kill the host, especially when the infection is heavy.

12A.2.1.2   Experimental infection of *L. carinii* to other laboratory
             animals

Successful results of the maintenance of *L. carinii* in albino rats were reported by ROHDE (1959, 1960) RAMAKRISHNAN *et al.* (1961), DALIP SINGH & RAGHAVAN (1962), and BAGAI & SUBRAHMANYAM (1968). However, as pointed out by HAWKING (1963), white rats are usually unsuitable animals for maintaining *L. carinii* and the above results were probably favored by particularities in their strains of rat or parasite. The rates of successful infection, as well as the levels and durations of microfilaremia, observed by these authors in white rats were generally lower than in cotton rats. KOBAYASHI *et al.* (1967) conducted experimental infections of *L. carinii* in several species of rodents, and obtained no development in a squirrel (*Tamias sibiricus*), only poor development of adults and microfilariae in white rats and mice, fair development in hamsters, in a field mouse (*Apodemus speciousus*), in field voles (*Microtus montebelli* and *Clethrionomys gapperi*), and excellent development in both cotton rats and Mongolian jirds (*Meriones unguiculatus*). Because of these results, this author has been using jirds for maintenance and experimental studies of *L. carinii* together with the cotton rats. SCHNEIDER *et al.* (1968) also compared early infections of *L. carinii* in cotton rats and Mongolian jirds, and observed remarkable similarity in the susceptibility of the two species of rodents.

The use of a multimammate rat *Praomys* (*Mastomys*) *natalensis* as experimental host of *L. carinii* was commenced by LÄMMLER *et al.* (1968) and PRINGLE & KING (1968), and the development of the parasite in this new host was reported to be as efficient as in the cotton rats. KING (1968) described a quantitative method for routine transmission of *L. carinii* to *Praomys* with the tropical rat mite. This system was utilized for experimental chemotherapeutic studies by FOSTER *et al.* (1969) and LÄMMLER *et al.* (1971).

12A.2.2 *Dipetalonema witei* (Krepkogorskaya, 1933)

A laboratory infection of *D. witei* was established by BALTAZARD *et al.* (1953) using the Libyan jird (*Meriones libycus*) as the final host and the argasid tick (*Ornithodoros tartakovski*) as the intermediate host. The life history and method for laboratory infection were described in detail by WORMS *et al.* (1961), who also reported that *Ornithodoros moubata* served as excellent intermediate host. A strain of *D. witei* was received in 1967 from Dr. P. Weinstein, National Institute of Health, U.S.A., and has been maintained in this author's laboratory with the Mongolian jird *Meriones unguiculatus* as the final host and *Ornithodoros moubata* (a strain received from Dr. Weyer, Tropeninstitut, Hamburg) or *O. tartakovski* (received from Dr. Weinstein, NIH) as the intermediate host. A quantitative study on the infection of *O. tartakovskyi* upon feeding on the blood of jirds containing various levels of microfilaremia was reported by PACHECO *et al.* (1972).

12A.2.2.1   Method of laboratory infection of *D. witei*

The breeding and maintenance of ticks *O. moubata* and *O. tartakovskyi* is fairly easy as compared with other arthropod vectors. Stock colonies are kept at 29°C in small plastic cylinders with a piece of tissue paper and plugged with cotton, placed in desiccators with the humidity adjusted to about 75% with saturated sodium chloride for the former, or to 85% with saturated potassium chloride for the latter. The ticks are fed once a week on shaved rats or mice (hairless mice are most convenient) fastened between metal wire screens or under anesthesia with Nembutal. The females deposit large numbers of eggs, and the life cycle of the ticks is completed in three to four months.

Infected jirds showing about 10 microfilariae per 2.5 mm^3 of blood are used for the source of infection of the ticks. The jirds are also fixed between wire screens or anesthetized, and deutonymphs or young adults of the ticks are allowed to feed until fully engorged. Feeding of too many ticks kills the jirds, and also, the ingestion of blood containing too many microfilariae causes high mortality of the ticks. Larvae of *D. witei* develop to the infective stage in about three weeks at 29°C. The infective larvae remain alive in the ticks for several months.

When infecting clean jirds with *D. witei*, the ticks harboring infective larvae are dissected in normal saline, and 30 larvae per jird are injected, as a rule, subcutaneously into the inguinal region. The number of infective larvae recovered from a tick is roughly from 50 to 100. Microfilariae appear in the peripheral blood of jirds after prepatent periods from 7 to 11 weeks, and the density of microfilariae in the jirds have varied from 6 to 190 per 2.5 mm³. The adult worms can be recovered from the subcutaneous tissue at a ratio of 10 to 50 % to the number of infective larvae inoculated.

Laboratory maintenance of *D. witei* is generally easier and less time-consuming than that of *L. carinii* in cotton rats. Jirds are easier to handle and breed than cotton rats. However, recovery of adult worms are more difficult and less accurate than those residing in the body cavity or in the heart as in *L. carinii*. The use of *D. witei* for immunologic or chemotherapeutic studies is also handicapped, since either the parasite or the host is often refractile to drugs (such as DEC) and/or development of antibodies, as discussed later.

12A.2.3 *Brugia malayi* (Brug, 1927) and *Brugia pahangi* (Buckley & Edeson, 1956)

The use of *Brugia* species in experimental studies is of special significance since they are the same as or closely related to those found naturally infecting in man. EDESON *et al*. (1955) observed that two filarial species apparently indistinguishable from human *B. malayi* in the morphology of the microfilariae were commonly found in some wild and domestic animals in Malaya. Later, BUCKLEY & EDESON (1956) report that one of them was identical to human *B. malayi* and the other to be a new species, *B. pahangi*. EDESON & WHARTON (1957) successfully transmitted a subperiodic form of *B. malayi* in man to domestic cat by direct inoculation of infective larvae after feeding laboratory-reared *Mansonia uniformis* on a human carrier. EDESON *et al*. (1960) succeeded in transmitting *B. pahangi* from cats to cats and other animals with *M. annulata*, *An. barbirostris*, and *Ar. obturbans*.

Both *B. pahangi* and subperiodic *B. malayi* are highly adapted for developing in a wide range of hosts, and LAING *et al*. (1960) in East Pahang, Malaya, found *B. malayi* in man, dusky leaf monkey, domestic and wild cats, civet, long-tailed macaque, and pangolin, and *B. pahangi* in domestic and wild cats, dog, slow loris, palm civet, tiger, pangol, moon rat, and giant squirrel. LAING *et al*. (1961) carried out experimental infections of *B. malayi* and *W. bancrofti* (a periodic form) to various animals, and successful transmission as judged from the appearance of microfilariae and recovery of adult worms was obtained with subperiodic *B. malayi* in 2 of 6 hamsters, none of 6 rats, none of 6 mice, one of 2 dogs, and in one leaf monkey; with periodic *B. malayi*, slight infection was found in cats, rhesus monkeys, and leaf monkeys, but not in any other animal tested (golden hamster, rat, mouse, long-tailed macaque, or slow loris); and with *W. bancrofti*, no worms were found in cats or rhesus monkeys.

With these findings as a base, *B. malayi* (subperiodic form) and *B. pahangi* have been brought into a number of laboratories as useful tools in experimental filariasis studies. RAMACHANDRAN *et al*. (1960) demonstrated that *B. malayi* could be transmitted by *Ae. aegypti*, a mosquito easily maintained in the laboratory, and MACDONALD (1961, 1962) succeeded in selecting a strain of *Ae. aegypti* susceptible to infection of *B. malayi*. RAMACHANDRAN *et al.* (1963) further found that *Ae. togoi*, another mosquito easily maintained in the laboratory and larger in size than *Ae. aegypti*, was a very efficient vector of various filarial species including *B. malayi* and *B. pahangi*.

Trails were made by several workers to transmit *B. malayi* or *B. pahangi* to animals smaller than cats, dogs, and monkeys. Recently, ASH & RILEY (1970a,b) succeeded in transmitting both *B. pahangi* and *B. malayi* in the Mongolian jird (*Meriones unguiculatus*) from cats or dogs with *Ar. subalbatus* as the vector for the former and with *Ae. aegypti* or *Ae. togoi* for the latter. Microfilaremia developed in 25 of 33 jirds in *B. pahangi*, and 13 or 19 jirds in *B. malayi*. Adult worms of both species were found in the heart and lung, and more numerously in the testes. Transmission and maintenance of the two parasites could be achieved from jirds to jirds. Preferential susceptibility of male jirds to infection with *B. pahangi* was studied in more detail by ASH (1971). The mode of distribution of developing and mature *B. malayi* was investigated in cats, rhesus monkeys, and jirds by EWERT (1971) and ELBIHARI & EWART (1971).

12A.2.4 *Dirofilaria immitis* (Leidy, 1856)

This is a filarial parasite of dogs, cats, and other carnivores, and is commonly called canine heartworm. The adult worms usually reside in the pulmonary artery and left ventricle of the heart, and often causes serious or fatal heart disorders on the hosts. Microfilariae are found in the circulating blood of the infected hosts, and are nocturnally subperiodic in the circadian rhythm of activity. Various species of mosquitoes belonging to genera *Anopheles*, *Culex*, *Aedes*, and *Armigeres* have been shown to serve as natural or experimental vectors.

Natural infection of dogs with *Dirofilaria immitis* is found commonly in the tropical and Temperate Zones of the world, and most experimental studies on dog filariasis have been conducted with these naturally infected animals. Experimental infections of clean dogs by inoculating infective larvae collected from laboratory-reared mosquitoes have also been practiced in certain laboratories where the facilities are available for keeping dogs in mosquito-free environments. It should be noted that dogs are also often infected with *Dirofilaria reconditum* (Grassi, 1890), whose microfilariae also appear in the circulating blood. In the United States, for example, NEWTON & WRIGHT (1956) reported for the first time the occurrence of *Dirofilaria reconditum* which had been confused with *D. immitis* by previous workers. As reviewed by OTTO (1972), both *D. immitis* and *D. reconditum* have been noted to be coendemic in most states in the United States.

Dirofilaria immitis in dogs is a useful animal model in filariasis studies for various purposes. In many countries, the naturally infected animals are easily available in large numbers, and can be used in chemotherapeutic and immunological tests. The adult worms can be recovered from the heart at necropsy of stray dogs, and have been used by many workers as material for preparing filarial antigens.

Experimental infection of *D. immitis* to clean dogs can be made rather easily by using certain mosquito species as the intermediate hosts. In Japan, *Ae. togoi* and *Ar. subalbatus* have been used by most workers as laboratory vectors, because both are easily bred and efficient intermediate hosts. In the United States, most workers use *An. quadrimaculatus*, which is also an efficient vector. Infective larvae develop in the mosquito intermediate hosts within two weeks when kept at a temperature above 25°C. The larval development takes place in the Malpighian tubules of mosquitoes. The infective larvae can be isolated from the mosquitoes by dissection or by crushing with pressure of the side wall of test tube, and are injected subcutaneously. It usually takes about 25 weeks (six months) for the appearance of microfilariae in the circulating blood.

Dirofilaria immitis has been used extensively in experimental filariasis studies in many laboratories, and was practically the only filarial parasite being maintained in laboratory animals until recently. *D. immitis* in dogs has both merits and demerits as a laboratory animal filaria. In many countries it is easily available from stray dogs, but at the same time it is rather difficult and expensive to secure large numbers of filaria-free dogs in the naturally endemic areas, and to produce infected animals under strict experimental conditions. The susceptibility to some chemotherapeutic drugs of either the parasite or the host may be essentially different from that in human filariasis; the adult worms in dogs are refractory to DEC, while the microfilariae of *D. immitis* are killed by some compounds (such as dithiazanine) which are entirely inactive against the microfilariae or adult filarial worms in man. There seem to exist some essential differences in the immune response systems in man and dog, as discussed in Section 12.C.2.

Dirofilaria immitis infection is a serious, often fatal disease in dogs. The prevention and treatment of dirofilariasis is therefore an important problem in itself in veterinary medicine. *Dirofilaria immitis* also causes disease in man by accidental infection in various organs, especially granulomas in the lung. In this connection, large numbers of studies have been published referring to the epidemiology, pathology, treatment, prevention, and experimental infection of this parasite. A symposium on the current knowledge of the canine heartworm disease was published recently by BRADLEY (editor, 1972), in which the following papers are included:

Epidemiology:

OTTO, G. F.: "Epizootiology of canine heartworm disease"

Pathology and immunology:

CASEY, H. W. *et al.*: "Immunopathology studies on canine heartworm disease"

PIERSON, K. K.: "Gumma like pulmonary granulomas due to *Dirofilaria* sp. in man"

SIMPSON, C. F *et al.*: "Alterations of glomerular capillaries in canine heartworm disease

AH, H. S. *et al.*: "Studies on *Dirofilaria immitis* infections in dogs relative immunizations and antigen antibody interactions"

ALLAIN, D. S. *et al.*: "Serologic studies on dogs experimentally infected with *Dirofilaria immitis*"

WEINER, D. J. & BRADLEY, R. E.: "Serologic changes in primary and secondary infections of beagle dogs with *Dirofilaria immitis*"

Chemotherapy:

BURKHART, R. L. & ALFORD, B. T.: "Pharmacology and mode of action of diethylcarbamazine"

WALLACE, C. R. & SCREWS, R.: "Preliminary study of microfilarial embolization after filaricidal therapy"

CASEY, H. W. *et al.*: "Results of a two-year field evaluation of diethylcarbamazine as a heartworm chemoprophylactic"

TULLOCH, G. S. & ANDERSON, R. A.: "Tetramisole and canine dirofilariasis"

GERBERG, E. J. *et al.* "Preliminary evaluation of *l*-tetramisole as an antifilarial in a mosquito test system"

TULLOCH, G. S. *et al.*: "Diethylcarbamazine chemoprophylaxis for canine dirofilariasis experimentally induced by multiple infections"

JACKSON, R. F.: "Some new chemotherapeutic agents for dirofilariasis—A preliminary report"

PACHECO, G.: "Synopsis for Dr. Seiji Kume's reports at the first international symposium on canine heartworm disease"

Miscellaneous:

ALTMAN, N. H.: "Laboratory diagnosis of *Dirofilaria immitis*: Evaluation of current tests"

TULLOCH, G. S. *et al.*: "Scanning electron microscopy of adult male *Dirofilaria immitis*"

BISGARD, G. E. & LEWIS, R. E.: "*In vivo* arteriography in canine heartworm disease"

12B. Experimental chemotherapy

Methods and results of experimental chemotherapeutic studies with laboratory animal filariasis were described by SEWELL & HAWKING (1950) and HAWKING (1955, 1963). Several groups of compounds have been demonstrated to be effective either or both *in vivo* and *in vitro* against various stages of the filarial parasites. However, some of them, such as most compounds containing arsenic or antimony, were found to be too toxic for general use in the treatment of human filariasis. Differences in susceptibility of various filarial species to some compounds have been also pointed out; for example, certain cyanine compounds were shown to be effective on *Litomosoides* infection in cotton rats, but had no effect on *Wuchereria* infection in man, and dithiazanine was shown to be effective against microfilariae of *Dirofilaria immitis* in dogs, but was ineffective against its adult worms, as well as on microfilariae and adults of other filarial species tested.

It is admitted by most workers that DEC is the only compound now available for mass treatment of human filariasis, both in effectiveness and safety. However, the use of this drug has met with difficulties in many countries, as it causes various types of side effects, and requires ten or more doses for the effective treatment. Therefore, development of new antifilarial drugs with higher efficacy and fewer side effects are necessary before filariasis as a world health problem can be solved.

12B.1 *In vitro* tests

Adults and microfilariae of most filarial species so far tested are known to be maintained alive *in vitro* in certain culture media for at least several days, and prolonged production of microfilariae by female worms can be obtained, as reported by HAWKING (1954), TAYLOR (1960), and MATSUDA *et al.* (1968). The action of various drugs against adult worms and/or microfilariae *in vitro* was studied by HAWKING (1940) for arsenicals and other compounds, CULBERTSON & ROSE (1944) for antimonials, ROSE *et al.* (1944) and OTTO & MAREN (1949) for arsenicals, etc., PETERS *et al.* (1949) for cyanine dyes, HAWKING *et al.* (1950) for DEC, KULANGARA & SUBRAMANIAM (1960) for fluorides, etc., AHLUWALIA & DALIP SINGH (1961) for potassium permanganate, and MATSUDA *et al.* (1968) for DEC, arsenicals and suramine.

The filaricidal tests *in vitro* provide valuable information on the mode of effects of drugs on various stages of the parasites, such as whether a drug has direct action on certain organs, or is ineffective when tested *in vitro*. It could probably be a useful technique for the screening of certain groups of compounds. However, since drugs such as DEC were found to be completely inactive on adults and microfilariae at *in vitro* tests, simultaneous tests *in vivo* are essentially required for general screening of antifilarial drugs.

12B.2 *In vivo* screening test

To date, systematic screening tests have been done almost exclusively on *L. carinii* infection in cotton rats or *Mastomys* rats. There are several reasons for this; the animals can be kept in a small space, the mite vector is easily bred in large numbers, both are not expensive to maintain, the infection can be fairly well standardized and can be carried out in mass, both microfilariae and adult worms are easily recovered quantitatively, and the susceptibility of the parasite and/or host can be interpreted in most cases to be closer to human filariasis than most other animal filariae. However, since it has been known that every parasite or host species exhibits its own susceptibility to drugs, such as experienced with some cyanine compounds (effective on *Litomosoides* but ineffective on human *Wuchereria* infection) or suramine (effective on human *Onchocerca* infection but not on *Litomosoides*), care should be taken on interpretation of the results of such screening tests.

The technique for screening test with *Litomosoides* was described by HAWKING & SEWELL (1948) and SEWELL & HAWKING (1950). In this author's laboratory, the following are routine procedures with the Japanese strain of *Litomosoides* and cotton rats.

Young cotton rats of about one to two months in age are exposed individually to infection for one week with a mite colony harboring about 60 infective larvae. The rats are examined after 12 weeks to confirm that the infection has been successful and sufficient numbers of microfilariae are present in the circulating blood. The numbers of microfilariae found in 2.5 mm³ blood taken from a tail vein are recorded for two consecutive days, and the drug to be tested is injected intraperitoneally once a day for five consecutive days, two to five animals for each lot. The daily dose is usually fixed to 100 mg per kg of body weight, because compounds showing toxic or lethal effect on rats at this dose are likely to be dangerous for use on human filariasis. In certain instances when the toxicity is known or more detailed study is desired, various doses of the drugs are administered with the maximum of one-fifth LD-50 as the single dose. The rats' blood is examined one or two weeks after injection of the initial dose, and rats are sacrificed two weeks after the initial dose to examine whether the adult worms in the pleural cavity are intact or affected by the drug treatment. Drugs like diethylcarbamazine cause remarkable reductions in the microfilarial density at this test, but the adult worms usually remain intact, while some arsenicals kill most of the adult worms without causing appreciable reductions in the microfilarial density.

12.B.3 The mode of action of DEC

The drug DEC (diethylcarbamazine, or 1-diethylcarbamyl-4-methylpiperazine) is the principal weapon in the campaign against human filariasis, and effective control of the disease has been achieved in a number of areas where the drug treatments were conducted with good population coverages and under adequate dosage regimens. However, as stated before, there still exist a number of difficulties for its extensive use in developing areas, and also, little is known about why the drug is effective against the filarial parasites.

The compound DEC was demonstrated to be effective in reducing microfilariae of *L. carinii* in naturally infected cotton rats by HEWITT *et al.* (1947), and also in the treatment of human bancroftian filariasis cases by SANTIEGO-STEVENSON *et al.* (1947). HAWKING *et al.* (1950) demonstrated that the drug had no direct action *in vitro* on either microfilariae or adult worms of *L. carinii*, but when administered to cotton rats infected with the parasite, the microfilariae rapidly decreased from the circulating blood and were mostly trapped in the sinusoids of the liver, where they were destroyed by phagocytosis; such a peculiar action of DEC was interpreted as "opsoninlike."

The trapping of microfilariae in the living liver of cotton rats was observed directly under an ultrapak microscope by TAYLOR (1960). It has also been confirmed by MITSUI *et al.* (1966) that the density of microfilariae in the liver of cotton rats is only about one-tenth of that in the circulating blood, while the relation becomes reversed after administration of large doses of DEC; and upon autopsies after 30 minutes, the density in the liver and the lung becomes several times higher than that in the blood. The histopathological changes of microfilariae in the liver were studied in detail chronologically at various time intervals after DEC administration by TASAKA (1965) and KOBAYASHI *et al.* (1969). SCHARDEIN *et al.* (1968) studied ultrastructural changes in *L. carinii* microfilariae in the liver of jirds sacrificed 20 minutes and four hours after DEC administration, and observed the loss of the sheath, and subsequent lysis by phagocytes. DEC is rapidly absorbed from the gut when administered by mouth, and the blood level reaches a peak within a few hours. It is discharged rapidly into the urine generally within 24 hours, as demonstrated by LUBRAN (1950). A more detailed study on the fate of DEC in animals was reported by BANGHAM (1955a, b) with a C^{14}-labelled compound. The distribution of DEC in the animal body after intraperitoneal infection of tritium-labelled DEC was shown by SAKUMA *et al.* (1967), with the whole body-section autoradiography method, and its rapid discharge, as well as temporary accumulation in the gut wall has been noted. The mode of occurrence of side effects in man was analytically studied by SASA *et al.* (1963). They administered various doses of DEC to people in endemic areas of bancroftian filariasis in Amami, southern Japan, and demonstrated that there occurred side effects of the drug of two essentially different origins: one caused by the toxic effect of the drug itself, i.e., nausea and vomiting appearing soon after the drug is taken, which is dependent on the dose and independent from the filarial infection; and another caused presumably by the destruction of microfilariae, appearing several hours after the drug administration only in those who had high microfilaria density, and rather independent from the dose administered. Both of these side effects were shown to be only transient and had never been dangerous.

The absence of filaricidal effect in DEC *in vitro* was also confirmed by MATSUDA *et al.* (1968), who exposed female worms of *L. carinii* to various concentrations of DEC dissolved in culture media, and found that production of microfilariae, as well as the viability of adults and microfilariae, were not affected even at the highest concentration of 1,500 μg per ml, whereas an arsenical compound, Mapharsol, killed adults at concentrations 0.2 μg per ml and above.

The mode of action of DEC *in vivo* on various filariae in experimental animals has been investigated also by a number of workers, but the results are rather puzzling. The drug was shown to be effective in clearing, or at least reducing, microfilariae for certain periods in most filarial species, including those parasitic in man, but the effects were variable according to the species of filariae and hosts, and was almost inactive against microfilariae of *D. perstans* in man (HAWKING, 1950) and those of *D. witei* in jirds (WORMS *er al.* 1961). Past experiences in filariasis control programs carried out in many areas have shown that when sufficiently high doses are administered, human carriers of both *W. bancrofti* and *B. malayi* can be permanently cured by DEC at least by rates of 80% or higher. In *L. carinii*, clearance of microfilariae was reported to be achieved by DEC in naturally infected cotton rats (HEWITT *et al.* 1947) or in albino rats (RAMAKRISHNAN *et al.* 1963), but these probably refer to infections with low microfilarial density; moreover, as observed by SATO (1959) and TANAKA (1965), the drug cannot achieve complete clearance of microfilariae from experimentally infected cotton rats showing high levels of microfilaremia, even when nearly lethal doses (200 mg to 500 mg per kg at one dose) are repeatedly administered for long periods.

The problem of whether DEC kills adult filarial worms or not is still much debated. In *Wuchereria* and *Brugia* infections in man, it is presumed, mainly from epidemiological evidence, that the drug kills or sterilizes the adults when sufficient doses are administered, and this was confirmed in cats infected with *B. malayi* by EDESON & LAING (1959), and in man infected with *W. bancrofti* and *B. malayi* by CH'EN (1964) in China (see Section 8C.1). In *Dirofilaria immitis* in dogs, the drug is considered to be ineffective against adult worms in the heart. RAMAKRISHNAN *et al.* (1963) observed in *L. carinii* infection in albino rats that all adult worms collected after treatment with DEC were alive, and produced microfilariae after being transplanted into the peritoneal cavity of normal rats. HAWKING *et al.* (1950) found some dead adult worms of *L. carinii* in cotton rats after DEC treatments, but doubted its adulticidal effect because dead worms were also found in untreated animals. According to SATO (1960), the drug does not kill adults at relatively small doses, such as below 180 mg per kg in total, or in treatments for short periods even with large doses, but certain numbers of dead worms at proportions significantly higher than in the untreated animals were always found in animals treated with DEC at 10 or more doses during one to several-month periods, with the total doses from 280 mg to 6,000 mg per kg. The dead worms in DEC-treated animals were almost always found adherent to the wall of the pleural cavity and isolated from each other, while those killed by treatment with Mapharsol were free in the pleural cavity, often forming conglomerates of worms together with fibrinous substance. Certain histological changes were observed in female reproductive organs in worms exposed to DEC, which were also different from those found in worms treated with Mapharsol.

Because of its peculiar mode of action of DEC against microfilariae *in vivo*, it has been suspected that some immune response might be involved in activating the microfilaricidal activity. Actually, microfilariae which have been exposed to DEC *in vivo* but are still circulating in the blood of hosts are shown to be viable when cultured *in vitro*, or can develop to infective stage larvae when ingested by invertebrate hosts, as demonstrated by HAWKING *et al.* (1950), KUME *et al.* (1954), and DALIP SINGH (1962) for *Dirofilaria* in dogs, or by KANDA *et al.* (1967) for *L. carinii* in cotton rats and *W. bancrofti* in man. Therefore, neither DEC alone nor in combination with the circulating antibodies has direct microfilaricidal activity.

In this connection, KOBAYASHI *et al.* (1967) carried out a series of experiments with *L. carinii* in cotton rats. In summary:

(1) Microfilariae produced *in vitro* by female worms, as well as infective larvae collected by dissection of tropical rat mites, and cultured *in vitro* in media containing one of the four kinds of cotton rat sera, i.e., those collected from normal rats, those from infected rats, those from normal rats 30 minutes after injection of 200 mg per kg of DEC, those from infected rats also 30 minutes after injection of the same dose of DEC, showed no significant differences in the survival rates in 1 to 24-hour periods of exposure.

(2) Microfilariae collected *in vitro* from female worms and kept for 24 hours in culture medium (Simms' solution containing 30% horse serum) containing 1,500 μg per ml of DEC were injected intraperitoneally into a clean cotton rat, but the level and duration of microfilaremia were nearly the same as in another animal injected with untreated microfilariae.

(3) Microfilariae produced *in vitro* by female worms or those collected from the pleural cavity of infected animals were injected intraperitoneally into 11 clean cotton rats, at rates of 350,000 to 930,000 per animal, and the microfilariae appeared in the circulating blood within 24 hours and microfilaremia lasted for at least several months; DEC was injected at a single dose of 200 mg per kg to the animals 3 days, 5 days, and 40 to 48 days after inoculation of microfilariae, but neither appreciable reduction nor clearance of microfilariae were seen in any of the animals.

(4) Serum was collected from a cotton rat which had passed 32 weeks after infection and harbored microfilariae at a count of 487 in 2.5 mm³ blood sample, and was injected into three of the above rats already inoculated with microfilariae, 1.5 ml of the immune serum per animal; after one hour from this "passive immunization," DEC was injected into the animals at a dose of 200 mg per kg; in this case, an apparently significant but transient reduction of microfilaremia was observed in all the animals, but the microfilaremia level recovered to the original levels after two to three days.

(5) Adult worms collected from the pleural cavity of infected cotton rats were transplanted into the peritoneal cavity of 5 clean cotton rats, 20 to 40 worms per animal; microfilariae became detectable from about the second day and all reached to appreciable levels on the fifth day. DEC injected at a dose of 200 mg per kg did not cause significant reductions of microfilariae in any of the animals, and even increased later in one of the animals; however, the same dose of DEC injected to the same animals 15 days after the transplantation caused rapid and remarkable reductions, which lasted for periods of over 30 days thereafter and complete clearance of microfilariae was seen in two animals after 20 and 30 days, respectively. New microfilariae collected *in vitro* were injected into one of the above treated animals, and another dose of 200 mg per kg of DEC was again effective in clearing the microfilariae from the circulating blood.

The above series of experiments suggest that the presence of some kind of immunity is required for the release of the microfilaricidal activity of DEC, since microfilariae passively introduced into clean animals were not affected by the drug, and those circulating in the blood of rats soon after transplanted with adult worms were also not susceptible to the drug. The remarkable effects of clearance of microfilariae such as seen in normally infected animals were seen only after 15 days from transplantation of adult worms. These results apparently coincide with the observations made by FUJITA & KOBAYASHI (1969), who used the same lot of animals and found that hemagglutination (HA) antibodies became detectable in sera of cotton rats from ten days after transplantation of adult worms, but not in animals transfused only with microfilariae. However, as stated previously, circulating antibodies are probably not the principal factor which activates the microfilaricidal action of DEC, since it has only a slight and transient effect in the passive immunization test.

Further analytical studies are in progress by TANAKA *et al.* (*loc. cit.*) in this author's laboratory in order to clarify the relationship between the activity of DEC and immunity. As a principle, reduction of microfilarial density for periods of over two or more days, such as seen after injection of a standard dose of 200 mg per kg is considered to be significant, because its temporary reduction together with rapid and transient drop of body temperature is often encountered in cotton rats at an intraperitoneal injection of even normal saline. The sera collected from infected cotton rats soon after injection of DEC were found to be inactive when injected into another infected animal either intraperitoneally or intravenously. Likewise, spleen cells collected from the infected and DEC-treated rats were also inactive when transfused into another infected animal. However, when spleen cells collected from normally infected animals were transfused intravenously into cotton rats to which microfilariae had been inoculated artifically by the previously stated method, a slow but steady reduction of microfilaremia level was observed and the hosts became free from microfilariae after four weeks. DEC injected at the standard dose into the same lot of animals exhibited significant levels of activity only two days and three weeks after inoculation of the spleen cells, but not on animals tested in a similar way after one and two weeks from the inoculation. HA antibody titer does not rise in animals simply transfused with microfilariae, as stated previously, but it rapidly rises when spleen cells from infected animals are inoculated into clean animals, and stays at high levels for periods of over four weeks. Therefore, this is interpreted as another piece of evidence that the presence of circulating antibodies is not the essential factor for the release of action of DEC. Also, injections of 0.5 ml of immune sera collected from infected animals twice a day for five days into animals thus passively inoculated with microfilariae were not effective in reducing the microfilaremia levels, such as seen in groups injected with the spleen cells from the infected animals. This and previously stated evidence suggest that release of the activity is not primarily dependent on the circulating antibodies, but could be a cell mediated response, if immunity is ever involved.

Treatments with some immunosuppressive measures were found to be effective in inhibiting the action of DEC at least in certain cases. For example, the effect of DEC given at a dose of 100 mg per kg was apparently inactivated in infected cotton rats after treated with prednisolone at daily doses of 120 mg per kg for 4 days, but administration of 200 mg per kg of DEC to the same lot of animals caused a significant reduction of microfilaremia. Previous treatments with 6-mercaptopurine and cyclophosphamide at similar doses were apparently ineffective in view of the inactivation of DEC. However, the inhibitory effects of antilymphocyte serum (ALS), and antithymus serum (ATS) on the release of the microfilaricidal action of DEC in infected animals are apparently conspicuous. ALS was prepared by injecting 10^7 to 10^8 lymphocytes isolated from lymph nodes of cotton rats into two rabbits, once a week for three weeks. The titers of ALS measured by the cytotoxicity test were 1:60 and 1:120. Ten clean cotton rats were treated continuously with injections of 0.5 ml of ALS three times a week, and *L. carinii* was infected to the animals by the standard method of the mite bite one week after commencement of ALS treatments. Only two cotton rats survived through these intensive ALS treatments, and microfilariae became detectable from seven weeks after the infection. No antibody as measured with the HA test was detected and DEC was also ineffective in reducing microfilariae during the period of continous treatments with ALS. However, production of antibody began soon after the ALS treatment was suspended, and in another test of administration of DEC one month after the ALS treatments had been suspended, the drug was shown to be still ineffective, while the HA titer of the serum rose to 1:4000. This again suggests that the mere presence of humoral antibody is not sufficient for disclosure of the action of DEC.

Another interesting aspect of the mode of action of DEC was disclosed through experimental filariasis in jirds. As stated previously, microfilariae of *D. witei* in Libyan jirds were shown to be refractory to DEC (WORMS *et al.* 1961). Since the Mongolian jird is susceptible to both *D. witei* and

L. carinii, they were infected with either or both of the filarial parasites. In mixed infections, microfilariae of the two species appear in the same blood samples, but can be easily differentiated by a remarkable difference in morphology. So far as observations to date are concerned, DEC is apparently ineffective against microfilariae of both *D. witei* and *L. carinii* in the jirds. Since the latter is known to be susceptible to DEC when infecting in cotton rats, it is probable that this particular host rather than the parasite is refractory to the action of DEC.

12C. Experimental immunology

12C.1 Natural and acquired resistance

It is a well-known fact that certain filariae can develop to adults or to infective larvae only in certain vertebrates or arthropod vectors, and the host-parasite relationships are rather strict in the filarial infections. In this sense, natural resistance to infection is considered to exist in all animals in reference to certain groups of filariae. Partial resistance is also common, especially when a filarial species have infected an animal which is closely related to its natural host, such as in the case of infection of cotton rat filaria, *L. carinii*, to rat, mouse, or hamster. When a host is partially resistant, the growth of infective larvae to adults are mostly unsuccessful or retarded, and production of microfilariae is poor or lasts for only a short period.

However, development of acquired resistance is usually poor when the host is susceptible to infection of a filarial species, and repeated infections of large numbers of filariae during long periods of exposure are common events in both human and animal filariasis. Nevertheless, development of acquired resistance at repeated infections has been confirmed from various aspects, such as the retardation of growth, reduction of rates of successful development to adults, reduction or clearance of microfilariae in circulating blood, and finally the death of adult worms. Extensive studies were conducted by several groups of workers on the mode of development of acquired immunity with cotton rat filariasis and other animal models, as reviewed by SCOTT *et al.* (1958) and BERTRAM (1966).

12C.2 Immunodiagnosis of filariasis

Immunologic studies in human and animal filariasis are faced with a number of difficult problems, and although quite a few papers have been reported in this field, the reliability of immunologic methods for the diagnosis of filariasis has been much debated, in view of both specificity and sensitivity. KAGAN (1963) presented an excellent review on the immunologic studies in the diagnosis of filariasis reported up to 1962. Altogether, 148 papers were available for the skin test, complement fixation test, precipitin test, hemagglutination test, bentonite flocculation test, or Prausnitz-Küstner test of filarial infection. The reviewer suggested, "with standardization of techniques, immunologic methods can in future be made to furnish a reliable means of diagnosis, notwithstanding the past unreliability of such methods."

The essential weak point of the immunodiagnosis of human filariasis is the difficulty in obtaining the homologous antigen, especially in wuchereriasis, and the antigens were prepared mostly from animal filariae, such as *Dirofilaria immitis* in dogs. However, it is questionable how far filariae possess group-specific antigens independent from other commonly occurring parasites. In this connection, the common occurrence of other nematode parasites causes another difficult problem in the diagnosis of filariasis.

12C.2.1 Antibody response in experimental and human filariasis

Litomosoides carinii infection in cotton rats is considered to be an ideal model for the immunologic studies is filariasis, since large numbers of infected animals with different history are available, the infection can be easily controlled, the hosts are free from other nematode infections, the homologous antigen can be amply supplied, and the reaction of the hosts are immunologically not unusual. Recent improvements in immunological techniques, especially the introduction of microtiter method, had made repeated examinations from such small hosts feasible. A series of experimental studies were carried out in this author's laboratory in order to clarify the mode of development of antibodies in the cotton rat filariasis. The principal methods used were hemagglutination (HA), complement fixation (CF), immunodiffusion (ID), and fluorescent antibody test (FA). A portion of the results were reviewed by TANAKA *et al.* (1970b).

12C.2.1.1   Hemagglutination test

The method applied for the indirect hemagglutination test of cotton rat sera was described by TANAKA *et al.* (1968a). A buffered saline extract of adult worms was used as the antigen. Rabbit sera, collected after immunizing with adult *Litomosoides* extracts, were used as the standard for determining the optimum condition of the HA test. Formalinized and tanned sheep red blood cells were used as the indicator, and the test was made usually in microtiter wells. Sera which showed 3-plus agglutination at 1:32 dilution were regarded as positive. In a series of preliminary tests conducted with stock sera collected from cotton rats with a known history of infection, 85 (92.4%) of 92 samples from infected rats were positive with the highest titers over 1:16384 in 8 animals, while all of 68 clean rats were negative. The test was shown to be excellent in specificity, and good in sensitivity. There was no significant correlation between the numbers of adult worms found in the hosts and HA titers, but the difference between the logarithms of microfilarial densities and HA titers was statistically significant. In the similar tests with an antigen prepared from *Dirofilaria immitis*, only 20% of 75 infected cotton rat sera showed positive results.

A study for purification and recovery of antigen from adult *Litomosoides* extracts was reported by TANAKA *et al.* (1968b). The worms were homogenized, lyophilized, delipided, extracted with buffered saline at pH 7.4, and centrifuged. The supernant was fractionated on DEAE cellulose, or filtered on Cephadex G-200. The quantities of antigen in all the fractions were measured by the HA test, and the rates of purification were estimated by the ratios of antigen unit to protein concentration. As a result, it was demonstrated that the antigen was not distributed evenly with the protein concentrations, but was limited to certain fractions of relatively high molecular weights. The most purified fraction showed 42.9-fold concentration and 12.5% recovery with Cephadex G-200, 6.0-fold and 3.1% at a gradient ellution with NaCl on DEAE, 14.7-fold and 9.4% at stepwise ellution with NaCl on DEAE. Little loss of antigen was observed at delipidation and centrifugation, but about half of the antigen was lost by lyophilization.

12C.2.1.2 Complement fixation test

A method of the complement fixation test (CF) on cotton rat filariasis with adult *Litomosoides* antigens was described by TANAKA *et al.* (1969, 1970a). The extract with Coca's solution was found to be more active than that with buffered saline or the alcohol extract. The CF test was made on microtiter plates following modified Kolmer's technique. The sera showing titers 1:16 or higher with the described technique were regarded positive. Of 116 cotton rat sera collected 11 weeks after exposure to the infection, 112 (96.6%) were positive, while only 1 (2.1%) of 48 sera of clean cotton rats were positive. There was a significant correlation between CF and HA titers of the same sera, with a correlation coefficient of 0.842, but only slight or no correlation was seen between the CF titer and the number of parasitizing adults, the number of females, or the density of microfilariae. So far as the *Litomosoides* infection in cotton rats is concerned, serodiagnosis with the CF test was also shown to be satisfactory both in sensitivity and specificity.

12C.2.1.3 Fluorescent antibody test

Methods for application of the indirect fluorescent antibody test (FA) for diagnosis of *L. carinii* infection in cotton rats were presented by ISHII & TANAKA (1968) and ISHII *et al.* (1969). Frozen sections of adults, microfilariae, and infective larvae of *L. carinii*, prepared by cold microtome, were used as the antigens. Since tremendous numbers of antigens can be prepared with this method, the FA test was considered to have advantages over other immunologic tests if it turned out to be satisfactory both in specificity and sensitivity, especially if it could be used for diagnosis of human filariasis. The antibody against cotton rat globulin was produced by immunizing rabbits with the antigen purified from 37 cotton rat sera and the adjuvant. The globulin fraction of the immunized rabbit serum was labelled with fluorescein isothiocyanate, and purified on cephadex G-25 and on DEAE cellulose following Kawamura's method. The FA test was conducted first by exposing the test sera at various dulutions on the frozen section antigen, and after washing, by demonstrating the conjugated antibody with the fluorescent antibody.

When the infected cotton rat sera were applied on the sections of adult worms, specific fluorescence was most conspicuously seen on subcuticular muscle layers, and also on lateral glands, and on the contents of digestive canal. Of 7 cotton rat sera collected 11 weeks after exposure to infection, all showed positive reactions at titers 1:125 to 1:3125, while the titers were up to 1:25 in clean cotton rat sera, with an exception of a sample which was positive to 1:125. On the other hand, the antigenicity of the microfilariae and infective larvae was much weaker than the adults, especially in the latter, and the highest titer seen with the microfilariae was 1:64.

The results of the FA test reported in these papers have provided important information on the distribution of antigens in tissues of various stages of the parasite, but its use in diagnosis of filariasis still awaits further improvements in the technique, because with the present technique, certain grades of false positive reactions were seen even with sera from clean animals, probably due to the presence of cotton rat antigen in the section of the worms.

More recently, BARBOSA *et al.* (1972) carried out indirect immunofluorescent tests using fragments of adult *O. volvulus* from a nodule as antigen. Tests were made on seven sera from loiasis cases, seven from onchocerciasis cases, five from bancroftian filariasis cases, and one from tropical eosinophilia case. When reactions at 1:40 or higher dilutions were taken as positive, the test was positive in 19 of 20 sera. In sera from 50 ancylostomiasis or stronglyloidiasis and those from 50 healthy control subjects were all negative.

ROMBERT *et al.* (1972) also conducted similar indirect fluorescent antibody tests with eggs of *D. immitis* and *L. loa* as the antigens. The results with *D. immitis* eggs were rather doubtful in diagnosis of human filariasis, but with the eggs of *Loa* all of nine loiasis cases were positive at 1:160 dilution, and ten normal sera and four from ancylostomiasis were negative.

AMBROISE-THOMAS & TRUONG (1974) reviewed recent advances in the immunodiagnosis of human filariasis with various techniques, and also reported on results of a indirect fluorescent antibody test carried out on a frozen section of *Dipetalonema witei* adults.

12C.2.1.4   Immunodiffusion test

Among various methods of precipitin tests so far proposed, the double diffusion test by Ouchterlony's method is considered to be simplest and specific. In the gel-diffusion test on agar plate conducted by TAKAOKA *et al.* (1973) in this author's laboratory using antigen extracted from adult *Litomosoides*, all of 88 cotton rat sera collected 11 weeks after exposure to infection showed one to four bands, with the exception of 2 samples which were negative. None of 82 serum samples collected from clean cotton rats showed precipitation bands. When an extract from adult *Dirofilaria immitis* was used as the antigen, only 8 of 88 infected sera samples showed 1 or 2 bands. However, 15 serum samples from filariasis cases in Okinawa and 38 samples from filariasis cases in Tahiti were all negative in the test with the *Dirofilaria* antigen, and only 2 were positive with the *Litomosoides* antigen. The precipitin test with the double diffusion method is considered to be excellent in specificity and sensitivity in the homologous antigen-antibody system of the cotton rat filariasis, but was poor in sensitivity for the diagnosis of heterologous or human filariasis.

Further analysis of the species-specific and group-common antigens with immunoelectrophoresis with the technique such as reported for filarial infections by CAPRON *et al.* (1968) is being reported by the same group of workers.

12C.2.2 The time course of production of antibodies

Since it has been established from previous studies that specific antibodies can be detected with various immunologic methods in the case of cotton rat filariasis, studies were made by ISHII *et al.* (1968) on the time course of the production of antibodies by the infected animals. Ten cotton rats of four weeks in age were used, and 7 of them were exposed to infection by the mite bite with estimated average of 75 infective larvae per rat, and the remaining 3 were kept uninfected. Examinations of microfilariae and tests of sera with the HA and CF techniques were made from all the rats every two weeks. All the infected cotton rats died during the period from 8 to 32 weeks after exposure to the infection, while all the uninfected rats survived through 32 weeks. In all the infected rats, microfilariae became detectable from 8 weeks after the infection, and remained positive until they died. In the CF test, all of the three uninfected rats remained negative (below 1:16), but an increase in the titers above 1:32 was seen in the infected rats, one from six weeks, and the others from eight weeks or 10 weeks after the exposure. The highest CF titer observed was 1:128. There was apparently no correlation between microfilarial density and CF titer, and the latter often dropped when microfilarial density increased. In most animals, CF titers dropped in the period just before they died of the infection. The results of the HA test were more sensitive, and increase in titers began from four to six weeks, and the maximum titer reached 1:32800. In one rat which survived through 30 weeks after exposure to the infection, a peak titer of 1:1078 was observed after ten weeks, such as reported by PACHECO (1966) in an HA test on dogs infected with *Dirofilaria immitis*, but the titers remained on high levels throughout the life span in most other infected rats.

The sequential appearance of 19S and 7S antibodies in cotton rats after exposure to *L. carinii* infection was confirmed by FUJITA & KOBAYASHI (1969a). Altogether, 49 four-week-old cotton rats were exposed to infection of about 80 infective larvae by the mite bites, and were sacrified at intervals of three or four days during the period from 2.5 to 51 weeks from the infection. The serum samples were fractionated by gel-filtration on Cephadex G-200, and the HA titer of each fraction was examined for all the sera. Identification of 19S and 7S globulins was made with ultracentrifugation, and also by simultaneous gel-filtration with ^{131}I-labelled 7S immunoglobulin. The HA activity of the infected cotton rat sera appeared first in the 19S fractions from six to seven weeks after exposure to infection, lasted until about the 12th week, and then disappeared in most cases, while the activity in the 7S fractions became detectable later from about the tenth week, and persisted for long periods thereafter. This was also confirmed by treatment of the sera with 2-mercaptoethanol.

The development of antibodies in cotton rats after transplantation of adult *L. carinii* into the peritoneal cavity was also observed by FUJITA & KOBAYASHI (1969b). In this case, production of antibodies began much earlier than the exposure to infection with the infective larvae, and HA activity appeared first in the 19S fractions in the sera collected ten days after transplantation, while the 7S antibody became detectable somewhat later, gradually increased, persisted thereafter, and became dominant over 19S from about 18th day. As stated previously, the effect of DEC on microfilariae in the transplanted animals also became active from about two weeks after the adults were inoculated, roughly coincident with the appearance of antibodies.

12C.2.3 Immunodiagnosis of filariasis with heterologous antigens

The above series of studies with the homologus antigen-antibody system have shown that so far as *L. carinii* infection in cotton rats is concerned, the infected animals can be clearly differentiated from uninfected animals by various immunological methods. It should also be mentioned that the animals tested were free from other parasites. However, similar tests with heterologous filarial antigens were more or less unsatisfactory either in specificity or sensitivty, or in both. As stated previously, immunodiffusion test was poor in sensitivity, and usually failed to show positive reactions with *L. carinii* or *Dirofilaria immitis* antigen when tested on sera from cases infected with other filarial species, at least using the present method. On the other hand, the HA test is too sensitive in general, and false positives have been obtained with nonfilarial sera. As reported by TANAKA *et al.* (1970a), more promising results were obtained with the CF test. Among various methods of preparation of antigens from adult worms compared, Chaffee's antigen was shown to be most satisfactory in the pattern of the block titration and in sensitivity. Antigens extracted with this method from *L. carinii*, *D. immitis*, and *Setaria cervi* were tested with the CF technique against sera from cotton rats infected with *L. carinii*, those from dogs with *Dirofilaria immitis*, cattle with *S. cervi*, men with *W. bancrofti*, cats with *B. malayi*, jirds and *Apodemus speciosus* with *D. witei*, and rabbit sera immunized with *L. carinii* and *Dirofilaria immitis* extracts. Sera from uninfected hosts were also tested. All dog sera were refractory to the CF test. In all other cases, various grades of cross-reactions were observed between the antigens and the sera from hosts infected with other filarial species. For example, sensitivity and specificity of *L. carinii* antigen was excellent for diagnosis of *L. carinii* infection, good for *Dirofilaria immitis* and *W. bancrofti* infections, fair for *D. witei*, and poor for *S. cervi* infection. *Dirofilaria immitis* antigen was excellent for *S. cervi*, good for *W. bancrofti*, fair for *L. carinii* and *D. witei* infection. *S. cervi* antigen was good for *S. cervi* and *D. witei*, fair for *L. carinii*, and poor for *W. bancrofti* infection. Sawada's FPSD$_4$ antigen fractionated from *Dirofilaria immitis* extract was fair for *D. witei* and poor for *W. bancrofti*, *L. carinii*, and *S. cervi* infections.

REFERENCES

Abdalla, R. E. (1974): *Trans. Roy. Soc. Trop. Med. Hyg.* **68**:53.
Abdulcader, M. H. M. (1961): *J. Ceylon Publ. Health Assoc.* **2**:101.
   (1962): *J. Trop. Med. Hyg.* (London) **65**:298.
   (1965): *Bull. Indian Soc. Malaria Comm. Dis.* **2**:201.
   (1967a): *Bull. Wld Hlth Org.* **37**:245.
   (1967b): *J. Trop. Med. Hyg.* **70**:199.
   (1971): *WHO Chronicle,* **25**:61.
Abdulcader, M. H. M. & Padley, R. (1960): *Indian J. Malariol.* **14**:521.
Abdulcader, M. H. M. & Sasa M. (1966): *Jap. J. Exp. Med.* **36**:609.
Abdulcader, M. H. M., Rajakone, P., Fernando, W. B. & Siriwardene, S. (1965):
 Ceylon. J. Med. Sci. **14**:49.
Abdulcader, M. H. M., Antonipulle, P., Jeyaratinam, P. G. & Rajendran, K. (1966b):
 Bull. Indian Soc. Malaria Com. Dis. **3**:345.
Abdulcader, M. H. M., Rajakone, P., Pajendran, K. & Aponso, L. (1966): *Amer. J.*
 Trop. Med. Hyg. **15**:519.
Abe, S. (1935): *Taiwan Igakkai Zasshi.* **35**:2833. (in Japanese)
  (1937): *Taiwan Igakkai Zasshi* (*J. Taiwan Med. Assoc.*) **36**:483.
Acton, H. W. & Rao, S. S. (1930): *Indian Med. Gaz.* **65**:620.
   (1933): *Indian Med. Gas.* **68**:305.
Adams & Maegraith (1964): "Clinical Tropical Diseases." pp 555. Blackwell Scientific
 Publications Oxford, London.
Adolph, P. E., Kagan, I. G., & McQuay, R. M. (1962): *Amer. J. Trop. Med. & Hyg.* **11**:
 76.
Africa, C. M., Garcia, E. Y. & Layco, J. (1935): *J. Philipp. Med. Assoc.,* **15**:407.
Aguirre, G. H., Serafim, E. M., Barbosa, J. A. & Rachou, R. C. (1956): *Rev. Brasil.*
 Malariol. D. Trop. **8**:433.
Ah, H. S. & Thompson, P. E. (1973): *Expl. Parasit.* **34**:393.
Ah, H. S., Peckham, J. C., Mitchell, F. E. & Thompson, P. E. (1972): Studies on *Diro-*
 filaria immitis infections in dogs relative to immunizations and antigen-antibody
 interactions. In Bradley's "Canine Heartworm Disease," Bradley, R. E. (ed.) 55–
 67 pp.
Ahluwalia, G. S. & Dalip Singh. (1961): *Indian J. Malariol.* **15**:301.
Ahmed, S. S. (1966): *J. Trop. Hyg.* **69**:291.
Aikat, T. K., Sen, T. & Singh, N. N. (1974): *J. Com. Dis.* **6**:284.
Allain, D. S., Kagan, I. G. & Schlotthauer, J. C. (1972): "Canine Heartworm Disease,"
 Bradley, R. E. (ed.) 69–76 pp.

[A more comprehensive list of references, including the title of each paper, is being
published separately from "Nihon Nettaiigaku Kyokai (Japan Association for Tropical
Medicine), Togin Building, 1-4-2, Marunouchi, Chiyodaku, Tokyo."]

Almeida, C. L. de (1952): Filariase e elefantiase na Guiné Portuguesa, Bissau (Memorias do Centro de Estudos da Guine Portuguesa, No. 17); quoted by Hawking, 1957

Alves, R. D. & Van WYK. A. (1960): *Cent. Afr. J. Med.* **6**:431.

Amaral, A. (1919): Filariose de Bancroft. *Memorias Inst. Butantan* 1918–19, 89.

Ambroise-Thomas, P. (1974): *Acta Trop.* **31**:108.

Ambroise-Thomas, P. & Kien Truong, T. (1974): *Ann. Trop. Med. Parasit.* **68**:435.

Anderson, J. (1924): *London School Hyg. Trop. Med. Res. Memoir Series.* **5**:20.

Anderson, J. & Fuglsang, H. (1973a): *Trans. Roy. Soc. Trop. Med. Hyg.* **67**:544.

Anderson, J. & Fuglsang, H. (1973b): *Trans. Roy. Soc. Trop. Med. Hyg.* **67**:710.

Anderson, J., Fuglsang, H., Hamilton, P. J. S. & Marshall, T. F. C. (1974): *Trans. Roy. Soc. Trop. Med. Hyg.* **68**:190; 209.

Anderson, R. C. (1956): *Canad. J. Zool.* **34**:485.

Anjaria, P. D., Basantani, G. K. & Mehta, J. K. (1972): *J. Ass. Phys. India.* **20**:55.

Annett, H. E., Dutton, J. E. & Elliot, J. H. (1901): *Liverpool Sch. Trop. Med. Mem.* **4**:67.

Antani, J. A., Srinivas, H. V., Krishnamurthy, K. R. & Borgaonkar, A. N. (1972): *Amer. J. Trop. Med. Hyg.* **21**:178.

Antonipulle, P., David, H. V. & Karunaratne, M. D. R. (1958): *Bull. Wld Hlth Org.* **19**:285.

Aoki, Y. (1971a): *Trop. Med.* **13**:7.
       (1971b): *Trop. Med.* **13**:170.

Arends, T. (1966): *Trans. Roy. Soc. Trop. Med. Hyg.* **60**, Correspondence, 418.

Ariaratnam, V. & Brown, A. W. A. (1969): *Bull. Wld Hlth Org.* **40**:561.

Armstrong, J. A. & Hawking, F. (1964): *Trans. Roy. Soc. Trop. Med. Hyg.* **58**:9 (Abstr.)

Ash, L. R. (1971): *J. Parasit.* **57**:777.

Ash, L. R. & Little, M. D. (1964): *J. Parasit.* **50**:119.

Ash, L. R. & Riley, J. M. (1970a): *J. Parasit.* **56**:962.

Ash, L. R. & Riley, J. M. (1970b): *J. Parasit.* **56**:969.

Ash, L. R. & Schacher, J. F. (1971): *J. Parasit.* **57**:1043.

Ashburn, L. L., Burch, T. A. & Brady, F. J. (1949): *Bol. ofic. sanit. panam.* **28**:1107.

Ashburn, P. M. & Craig, C. F. (1906): *J. Med. Sci.* **132**:435.

Ashburn, P. M. & Craig, C. F. (1907): *Philipp. J. Sci.* B **2**:1.

Ashcroft, M. T. (1965): *Ann. Trop. Med. Parasit.* **59**:478.

Ashford, B. K. (1903): *Medical Record,* Nov. **7**:1903.

Ashford, B. K. & Snyder, H. Mc C. (1933): *Puerto Rico J. Pub. Hlth Trop. Med.* **8**:375.

Aslamkhan, M. & Salman, C. (1969): *Pakist. J. Zool.* **1**:183.

Aslamkhan, M. & Wolfe, M. S. (1972): *Amer. J. Trop. Med. Hyg.* **21**:30.

Assem, J. van den & Dijk, W. J. O. M., van (1958): *Trop. Geogr. Med.* **10**:249.

Assem, J. van den & Metselaar, D. (1958): *Trop. Geogr. Med.* **10**:51.

Assis-Masri, G. & Little, M. D. (1965): *Trans. Roy. Soc. Trop. Med. Hyg.* **59**, Correspondence, 717.

Ata, A. A. (1967): *J. Trop. Med. Hyg.* (London) **70**:113.

Ata, A. E. H. A., Raziky, E. S. H., El-Abdin, A. Z., Kaliouby, A. H. El. & Meshriky, S. (1967): *J. Trop. Med. Hyg.* **70**:113.

Athias, S. P. & Gueiros, Z. M. (1963): *Rev. Brasil. Malariol.* **15**:593.

Augustine, D. L. (1951): Filariasis. In "Gradwohl, et al. Clinical Tropical Medicine," *Mosby Ch., St. Luis.* 781.

Austin, W. C., Lunts, L. H. G., Potter, M. D. & Taylor, E. P. (1959): *J. Pharm. & Pharmacol.* **11**:80.

Avery, J. L. (1946): *J. Parasit.* **32**:497.

Azarova, N. S., Miretsky, O. Y., & Sonin, M. D. (1965): *Med. Parasitol. & Parasit. Dis.* (Moscow), **34**:156. (Russian, English summary.)

Azevédo, R. J. S. de (1955): Contribuicao ao estudo da bancroftose. 525 pp., Recife, Brasil.

Backhouse, T. C. (1934): *Trans. Roy. Soc. Trop. Med. Hyg.* **27**:365.

Backhouse, T. C. (1953a): *Proc. 7th Pac. Sci. Congr.*, New Zealand (1949): **7**:239.
 (1953b): *Wuchereria bancrofti* in Melanesia and Polynesia, in "Filariasis in the Pacific" 1–7 pp. *South Pacific Commission, Noumea*
 (1954): *Trans. Roy. Soc. Trop. Med. Hyg.* **27**:365.

Backhouse, T. C. & Heydon, G. A. M. (1950): *Trans. Roy. Soc. Trop. Med. Hyg.* **44**:291.

Backhouse, T. C. & Woodhill, A. R. (1956): *South Pacif. Comm. Tech. Inf. Circ.* No. 17.

Bagai, R. C. & Subrahmanyam, D. (1968): *Amer. J. Trop. Med. Hyg.* **17**:833.

Bagai, R. C. & Subrahmanyam, D. (1970): (Correspondence). *Nature*. London, Nov. 14, 228:682.

Bagai, R. C., Subrahmanyam, D. & Singh, V. B. (1968): *Indian J. Med. Res.* **56**:1064.

Bahr, P. H. (1912): *London Sch. Trop. Med. Res. Mem.* Ser. **1**:1.
 (1914): *Parasitology.* **7**:128.

Bain, O. (1968): WHO mimeograph. WHO/Oncho/68.70 pp.
 (1971): *Ann. Parasit. Hum. Comp.* **46**:613.

Bain, O. & Brengues, J. (1972): *Ann. Parasit. Hum. Comp.* **47**:399.

Bain, O., Durette-Desset, M. C. & De Léon, R. (1974): *Ann. Parasit. Hum. Comp.* **49**:467.

Baisas, F. E. (1958): *Philipp. J. Sci.* **86**:71.

Baker, N. M., Baldachin, D. J., Rachman, I. & Thomas, J. E. P. (1967): *Cent. Afr. J. Med.* **13**:23 (Hawking 73).

Balasingam, E., Ramachandran, C. P., Heyneman, D. & Wong, M. M. (1967): *Med. J. Malaya.* **21**:261.

Baltazard, M., Chabaud, A. G., Mofidi, C. & Minou, A. (1953): *Ann. Parasit.* **28**:388.

Bancroft, T. L. (1877): *Lancet,* London **2**:70.
 (1898): *Austr. Med. Gaz.* 20(6).
 (1899): *J. Proc. Roy. Soc. N. S. Wales* **33**:48.
 (1901): *J. Proc. Roy. Soc. N. S. Wales* **35**:41.
 (1903): *J. Proc. Roy. Soc. N. S. Wales* **37**:254.

Bangham, D. R. (1955a): *Brit. J. Pharm. Chemoth.* **10**:397.
 (1955b): *Brit. J. Pharm. Chemoth.* **10**:406.

Barber, M. A., Rice, J. B. & Brown, J. Y. (1932): *Amer. J. Hyg.* **15**:601.

Barbosa, W., Rombert, P. C. & Rocha, R. P. M. (1972): *Revta Patol. Trop.* **1**:93.

Barclay, R. (1965): *Ann. Trop. Med. Parasit.* **59**:340.
 (1969): *Ann. Trop. Med. Parasit.* **63**:473.
 (1971): *Med. J. Zambia,* **5**:201.

Barnes, J. M., Hayes, W. J. & Kay, K. (1957): *Bull. Wld Hlth Org.* **16**:41.

Barnley, G. R. (1949): *East African. Med. J.* **26**:308.
 (1953): WHO/Onchocerciasis/18. Geneva. Report to the first Expert Committee on onchocerciasis.
 (1958): Control of *Simulium* vectors of onchocerciasis in Uganda. *In Proceedings of the 10th International Congress of Entomology, Montreal,* 1956. Ottawa, **3**:535.

Barnley, G. R. & Prentice, M. A. (1958): *E. Afr. med. J.* **35**:475.

Barreto, P., Trapido, H. & Lee, V. H. (1970): *Amer. J. Trop. Med. Hyg.* **19**:837.

Barry, C., Ahmed, A. & Abdul Quadir Khan (1971): *Amer. J. Trop. Med. & Hyg.* **20**:592.

Basave Gowda, N. & Jeevandhara Kumar, S. A. (1961): *Nat. Soc. India for Malaria and other Mosquito-borne Dis. Bul.* **9**:171.

Basset, A. & Lacan, A. (1967): *Méd. Afr. Noire,* **10**:497.

Basu, P. C. (1957): *Indian J. Malariol.* **11**:293.
 (1958): *Bull. Nat. Soc. India Malaria Mosquito Diseases.* **6**:193.

Basu, P. C. & Rao, S. S. (1939): *Indian J. Med. Res.* **27**:233.

Basu, P. C., Ras, V. N. & Pattanayak, S. (1967a): *Bull. Indian Soc. Malaria Com. Dis.* **4**:296.

Basu, P. C., Raghavan, N. G. S., Sundaresuwaran, T. V., Singh, B., & Bedi, K. M. S. (1967b): *Bull. Indian Soc. Malaria. Com. Dis.* **4**:375.

764   REFERENCES

Basu, P. C., Singh, B., Raghaven, N. G. S. & Gaur, M. P. (1968): *Bull. Indian Soc. Malaria. Com. Dis.* **5**:105.
Basu, P. C., Raghaven, N. G. S. & Gaur, M. P. (1971): *J. Comm. Dis.* **3**:113.
Bauche, J. & Bernard, N. (1912): *Bull. Soc. Pathol. Exot.,* **5**:622.
Baumgartner, J. (1953): *Bol. Indigenista Venez.* **1**:379 (quoted by Restrepo *et al.* 1962).
Bay, E. C. & Self, L. S. (1972): *Bull. Wld Hlth Org.* **46**:407.
Baylis, H. A. (1942): (Correspondence). *Trans. Roy. Soc. Trop. Med. Hyg.* **35**:333.
Baz, I. I. (1946): *J. Roy. Egypt. Med. Assoc.* **29**:280.
Bearup. A. J. & Lawrence, J. J. (1950): *Med. J. Aust.,* **1**:**22**:724.
Beaver, P. C. (1970): *Am. J. Trop. Med. Hyg.,* **19**:181.
Beaver, P. C., Fallon, M. & Smith, G. H. (1971): *Am. J. Trop. Med. Hyg.* **20**:661.
Beckett, E. B. (1965): *Trans. Roy. Soc. Trop. Med. Hyg.* **59**:461.
          (1971a): *Parasitology* **63**:119.
          (1971b): *Parasitology* **63**:365.
          (1973): *Ann. Trop. Med. Parasit.* **67**:455.
Beckett, E. B. & Macdonald, W. W. (1970): *Parasitology.* **61**:211.
                    (1971a): *Ann. Trop. Med. Parasit.* **65**:271.
                    (1971b): *Trans. Roy. Soc. Trop. Med. Hyg.* **65**:339.
                    (1972): *Ann. Trop. Med. Parasit.* **66**:135.
Becquet, R., Gasteau-Strobel, T. & Happi, C. (1961): *J. Sci. Med. de Lille.* **79**:196.
Bedier (1925): *Bull. Med. Chir. Indochine,* **12**:626.
Bekku, H. (1956): *Nagasaki Igakkai Zasshi.* **31**:956. (in Japanese)
Belkin, J. N. (1962): "The Mosquitoes of the South Pacific." Vol. 1: 608 pp. Vol. 2; 411 Pl. Univ. California Press, Berkeley & Los Angeles.
Belkin, J. N., Knight, K. L., & Rozeboom, L. E. (1945): *J. Parasitol.* **31**:241.
Bell, D. (1967): *Ann. Trop. Med. Parasit.* **61**:220.
Bellefontaine, L. (1949): *Ann. Soc. Belge de Med. Trop.* **29**:251.
Ben-Sira, I., Ticho, U. & Yassur, Y. (1972): *Trans. Roy. Soc. Trop. Med. Hyg.* **66**:296.
Bennett, G. (1831): London Med. Gaz. 9:434, 628.
Bennet, G. F. (1962): *Canad. J. Zool.* **40**:124.
Bequaert, J. (1928): *Proc. 4th Int'l Congr. Entomol.* **2**:605.
Bequaert, J. C. (1938): *Amer. J. Trop. Med.* **18**:Suppl, 116.
Bercovitz, Z. T. & Shwachman, H. (1946): *Puerto Rico J. Pub. Hlth & Trop. Med.* **22**:66.
Berghe, L., van den (1941): *Ann. Soc. Belge Med. Trop.* **21**:63–82; 167–87; 261.
Berghe, L., van den & Chardome. M. (1951): *Amer. J. Trop. Med.* **31**:411.
                    (1952): *Trans. Roy. Soc. Trop. Med. Hyg.* **46**:99.
Berghout, E. (1973): *Trop. Geogr. Med.* **25**:233.
Bern, H. A. & Hansen, M. F. (1950): *J. Parasit.* **36**:103.
Berre, R., le (1966): "Contribution à l'étude écologique de *Simulium damnosum* Theobald, 1903 (Diptera, Simuliidae)." 204 pp. Bondy (Seine): Office de la Recherche Scientifique et Technique Outre-Mer, Route d'Aulnay, France.
Berre, R. le, Balay, G., Brengues, J. & Coz. J. (1964): *Bull. Wld Hlth Org.* **31**:843.
Bertram (1947): *Ann. Trop. Med. Parasit.* **41**:253.
Bertram, D. S. (1959): *Internatl. Cong. Zool. Proc.* **15**:686.
              (1966): *Advances in Parasitology* **4**:255.
Bertram, D. S. & Samarawickrema, W. A. (1958): *Nature.* **182**:444.
Bertram, D. S., Unworth, K. & Gordon, R. M. (1946): *Ann. Trop. Med. Parasit.* **40**:228.
Bertram, D. S., McGregor, I. A. & McFadzean, J. A. (1958): *Trans. Roy. Soc. Trop. Med. Hyg.* **52**:135.
Beye, H. K. (1959): Report on review of problems in filariasis control programme in British Guiana. *Pan American Health Organization* No. ZI-5198-59.
          (1960): *Indian J. Malariol.* **14**:503.
Beye, H. K. & Gurian, J. (1960): *Indian J. Malariol.* **14**:415.
Beye, H. K., Edgar, S. A., Mille, R., Kessel, J. F. & Bamridge, B. (1952): *Amer. J. Trop. Med. Hyg.* **1**:637.

Beye, H. K., kessel, J. F., Heuls, J., Thooris, G. C. & Bambridge, B. (1953): *Bull. Soc. Path. Exot.* **46**:144.

Beye, H. K., Milles, R., Thooris, G. & Tapu, J. (1956): *Amer. J. Hyg.* **64**:23.

Beye, H., Brooks, C. & Guinn, E. (1961): *Amer. J. Pub. Health.* **51**(12):1862.

Beytout, M. (1952): *Bull. Soc. Path. Exot.* **45**:704.

Bhattacharya, N. C. & Gubler, D. J. (1973): *Indian J. Med. Res.* **61**:8.

Bhattacharya, N. C., Rozeboom, L. E. & Chowdhury, A. B. (1966): *Bull. Calcutta Sch. Trop. Med.* **14**:78.

Biagi, F. (1956a): *Medicina* (Mexico) **36**:521.

      (1956b): *Medicina* (Mexico) **36**:545.

      (1957): *Medicina* (Mexico) **37**:145.

Biagi, F. & Castrejou. O. (1957): *Medicina* (Mexico) **37**:125.

Biglieri, R. (1923): *Com. Ren. Soc. Biol.* **88**:362.

Biguet, J., D' Haussy, R., Aubry, M. & Rosé, F. (1964): *Bull. Soc. Path. Exot.* **57**:1098.

Biswas, S. K., Saha, S. C. & Choudhury, M. (1975): Lancet Feb. 1, 285.

Blackburn, C. R. B. & Ma, M. H. (1971): *Trop. Geogr. Med.,* **23**:272.

Blacklock, D. B. (1922): *Ann. Trop. Med. Parasit.* **16**:107.

      (1926a): *Ann. Trop. Med. Parasit.* **20**:1.

      (1926b): *Ann. Trop. Med. Parasit.* **20**:203.

      (1930): Abstracted in *Trop. Dis. Bull.* **28**:756.

Blatin, M. & Joyeux, C. (1908): *Arch. Parasit.* **12**:28.

Bloss, J. F. E. (1949): *Trans. Roy. Soc. Trop. Med. Hyg.* **43**:236.

Blumberg, B., McGiff, J. & Guicherit, I. (1951): *Doc. Med. Geogr. Trop.* **3**:368.

Boase, A. J. (1935): *East African Med. J.* **11**:326.

Boissière, R. de (1904): *J. Trop. Med.* **7**:179.

Bonne. C., Lie Kian Joe., *et al.* (1941): *Geneesk. Tijdschr. Nederl.-Indie.,* **81**:1487.

Bonnet, D. D. & Chapman, H. (1956): *Mosq. News.* **16**:301.

              (1958): *Amer. J. Trop. Med. Hyg.* **7**:512.

Bonne-Wepster, J. (1937): "*Geneesk. Tijdschr. Nederl.-Indie.* **77**:1055.

      (1938): *Meded. Dienst Volks. Nederld-Indie.* **27**:206.

Bonne-Wepster, J. & Brug, S. L. (1937): *Geneesk. Tijdschr. Nederl.-Indie.* **77**:515.

Bose, A. K. & Singh, V. P. (1965): *Patna J. Med.* **39**:555..

Bouillez, M. (1916): *Bull. Soc. Path. Exot.* **9**:143.

Bourguignon, G. C. (1937): *Ann. Soc. Belge Med. Trop.* **17**:1.

Boyer (1878a): *Arch. Med. Nav.* **29**:61.

      (1878b): *Arch. Med. Nav.* **30**:224.

Bradley, R. E. & Pacheco, G. (1972): *The current knowledge.* 148 pp. (Dpt. Veterinary Science, Univ. Florida, Gainesville).

Bray, G. W. (1931): *Proc. Roy. Soc. Med.* **24**:673.

Breinle, A. (1913): *Rep. Austr. Inst. Trop. Med.* 1911–18.

      (1915): *Ann. Trop. Med. Parasitol.* **9**:285.

Bremont, E. & Léger, M. (1917): *Bull. Soc. Path. Exot.* **10**:896.

Brengues, J. (1973): La filariose de Bancroft en Afrique de l'Ouest. Thèse présentée à l'Université de Paris-Sud, 463 pp.

Brengues, J. & Coz, J. (1972): *Cah. ORSTOM Entom. Méd. Parasit.* **10**:207.

Brengues *et al* (1965):

Brengues, J., Subra, R., Mouche, J. & Nelson, G. S. (1968): *Bull. Wld Hlth Org.* **38**(4):595.

Brengues, J., Subra, R. & Bouchite, B. (1969): *Cah. ORSTOM Entom. Méd. Parasit.* **7**:279.

Briceno Rosi, A. L. & Mayer, M. (1949): *Arch. Venez. Pat. Trop. Maras. Med.* **1**:92.

Brinkmann, U. K. (1972): *Ztschr. Tropenmed. Parasit.* **23**:369.

Brinkmann, U. K. (1973): *Ztschr. Tropenmed. Parasit.* **24**:397.

      (1974): *Ztschr. Tropenmed. Parasit.* **25**:160.

Brochards, V. (1910a): *Bull. Soc. Path. Exot.* **3**:138.

Brochards, V (1910b): *Bull. Soc. Path. Exot.* **3**:401.
Brooks, G. D., Schoof, H. F. & Smith, E. A. (1965): *Mosquito News.* **25**:423.
Brooks, G. D., Smith, E. A. & Miles, J. W. (1967): *Mosquito News.* **27**:164.
Broquet, Ch. et Montel, R. (1909): *Bull. Soc. Pathol. Exot.* **2**:4.
Brown, A. W. A. (1958): *W. H. O. Monograph Ser.* **38**:240.
    (1960):
    (1962a): *Bull. Wld Hlth Org.* **27**:511.
    (1962b): *Bull. Wld Hlth Org.* **27**:632.
    (1967): *Bull. Wld. Hlth. Org.* **37**:297.
Brown, H. P. & Austin, J. A. (1939): *J. Amer. Bet. Med. Assoc.* **95**:566.
Brown, H. W. (1948): *Ann. N. Y. Acad. Sci.* **50**:51.
Brouwn, H. W. & Williams, R. W. (1949): *Public Health Rep.* **64**:863.
Browne, S. G. (1954): *J. Trop. Med. Hyg.* **57**:229 (loiasis).
    (1959a): *Ann. trop. Med. Parasit.* **53**:421.
    (1959b): *Trans. Roy. Soc. Trop. Med. Hyg.* **53**:506.
    (1960a): *Bull. Entomol. Res.* **51**:9.
    (1960b): *Cent. Afr. Med.,* 513.
Brug, S. L. (1920): *Geneesk. Tijdschr. Nederl.-Indie.,* **60**:612.
    (1927): *Geneesk. Tijdschr. Nederl.-Indie.* **67**:750.
    (1928): *Geneesk. Tijdschr. Nederl.-Indie.* **68**:681.
    (1931a): *Geneesk. Tijdschr, Nederl.-Indie.* **71**:210.
    (1931b): *Proc. Roy, Soc. Med.* **24**:663.
    (1937): *Geneesk. Tijdschr. Nederl.-Indie.* **77**:1462.
    (1938): *Mededeel. Dienst Volksgezondheid Nederl.-Indie.* **27**:88.
Brug, S. L. & de Rook, H. (1930): *Geneesk, Tijdschr. Nederl.-Indie.* **70**:451.
Brumpt, E. (1904): *Comp. Rend. Seance Mem. Soc. Biol.* **56**:758.
    (1919): *Bull. Soc. Path. Exot.* **12**:442, 446.
Brumpt, L. C. & Tirouvenziam, J. M. (1973): *Bull. Soc. Path. Exot.,* **66**:307.
Brunhes, J. (1969a): *Bull. Wld Hlth Org.* **40**:763.
    (1969b): *Cahiers O. R. S. T. O. M. sér. Ent. Mét. et Parasitol.* **7**:155.
    (1973): Thèse présentée a l'Université de Paris-Sud, 274 pp.
Brunhes, J. & Brengues, J. (1973): *WHO/FIL/WP*/73.10, 7 pp. (unpublished document).
Brunhes, J., Rabenirainy, L. & Ravaonjanahary, C. (1969): *C. R. Seanc. Soc. Biol.* **163**: 1009.
Brunhes, J., Rajaonarivelo, E. & Nelson, G. S. (1972): *Cah. ORSTOM Sér. Ent. Méd. Parasitol.* **10**:193.
Brunwin, A. D. (1909): *J. Trop. Med. Hyg.* **12**:365.
Bruyning C. F. A. (1953): *Doc. Med. Geogr. Trop.* **5**:333.
Bruyning, C. F. A. (1961): *Ann. Soc. Belge Med. Trop.* **41**:255.
Bryant, J. (1935): *Trans. Roy. Soc. Trop. Med. Hyg.* **28**:523.
Brygoo, E. R. (1951): Notes sur la Conference Internationale de la Filariose et de l'Elephantiasis, tenue a Tahiti en 1951. *Inst. Pasteur de Saigon,* 41 pp.
    (1953): Epidemiology of filariasis in the South Pacific. In "Filariasis in the South Paciffic" South Pacific Commission, Nouea, 17–52 pp.
    (1958): *Arch. Inst. Past. Madagascar.* **26**:34.
Brygoo, E. R. & Brunhes, J. (1971): *Arch, Institut Pasteur Madagascar.* **40**:47.
Brygoo, E. R. & Escolivet, J. (1955): *Bull. Soc. Path. Exot.* **48**:833.
Brygoo, E. R. & Grejebine, A. (1957): *Mém. Inst. Scient. Madagascar,* **9**:252.
    (1958): *Mém. Inst Tech. Scient. Madagascar,* série E. **9**:307.
Buck, A. A. (1973): *Ztschr. Tropenmed. Parasit.* **24**:336.
    (1974a): In 'Research and Control of Onchocerciasis in the Western Hemisphere, Pan Amer. Hlth. Assoc., 3–9 pp.
    (1974b): Epidemiologic features of Onchocerciasis. *ibid.* 35–45 pp.
    (editor: 1974): Onchocerciasis: Symptomatology, pathology, diagnosis. 80 pp. World Health Org., Geneva.

Buck, A. A., Anderson, R. I., Kawata, K. & Hitchcock, I. C. Jr. (1969): *Amer. J. Trop. Med. Hyg.* **18**:217.
Buck, A. A., Anderson, R. I., Sasaki, T. T. & Kawata, K. (1970): Health and disease in Chad. Epidemiology, culture and environment in five villages. The Johns Hopkins Press, Baltimore (quoted by Hawking, 1973).
Buck, A. A., Anderson, R. I. & Macrae, A. A. (1973): *Ztschr. Tropenmed. Parasit.* **24**:21.
Buckley, J. J. C. (1933): *J. Helminth.* **11**:257.
     (1934): *J. Helminth.* **12**:99.
     (1938): *J. Helminth.* **16**:121.
     (1946): *J. Helminth.* **21**:111.
     (1949): *J. Helminth.* **23**:1.
     (1951): *J. Helminth.* **25**:213.
     (1952): *Trans. Roy. Soc. trop. Med. Hyg.* **46**(3): 321.
     (1958a): *Trans. Roy. Soc. Trop. Med. Hyg.* **52**:39.
     (1958b): *Trans. Roy. Soc. Trop. Med. Hyg.* **52**:335.
     (1960): *Ann. Trop. Med. Parasitol.* **54**:75.
Buckley, J. J. C. & Edeson, J. F. B. (1956): *J. Helminth.* **30**:1.
Buckley, J. J. C. & Singh, S. N. (1965): *J. Helminth.* **39**:127.
Buckley, J. J. C. & Wharton, R. H. (1961): *J. Helminthology,* Suppl. 1961:17.
Buckley, J. J. C., Nelson, G. S. & Heisch, R. B. (1958): *J. Helminth.* **32**:73.
Budden, F. H. (1956): *Trans. Roy. Soc. Trop. Med. Hyg.* **50**:366.
     (1957): *Br. J. Ophthal.* **41**:214.
     (1958): *Trans. Roy. Soc. Trop. Med. Hyg.* **52**:500.
     (1962): *Brit. J. Ophthalmol.* **46**:1.
     (1963a): *Trans. Roy. Soc. Trop. Med. Hyg.* **57**:64.
     (1963b): *Trans. Roy. Soc. Trop. Med. Hyg.* **57**:71.
Bull, C. & Cockett, S. A. (1972): *Trans. Roy, Soc. Trop. Med. Hyg.* **66**:916.
Bun, J. C. (1939): *J. Chosen Med. Assoc.* **20**:1426.
Burch, T. A., & Ashburn, L. L. (1951): *Am. J. Trop. Med.* **31**:617.
Burch, T. A. & Greeenville, H. J. (1955): *Amer. J. Trop. Med. Hyg.* **4**:47.
Burch, T. A., Qualls, D. M. & Greenville, H. J. (1955): *Amer. J. Trop. Med. Hyg.* **4**:923.
Burke, A. (1928): *Puerto Rico J. Public Health & Trop. Med.* **4**:169.
Burkgart, R. L. & Alford, B. T. (1972): Pharmacology and mode of action of diethyl-carbamazine in Bradley, R. E. "Canine Heartworm Disease," 17–26 pp.
Burkitt, D. P. (1951): *Lancet* **1**:1341.
Burnett, G. F. (1960): *J. Trop. Med. Hyg.* **63**:153–62; 208.
Burnett, G. F. & Mataika, J. U. (1961): *Trans. Roy. Soc. Trop. Med. Hyg.* **55**:178.
Burnett, G. F. & Mataika, J. U. (1964): *Trans. Roy. Soc. Trop. Med. IIyg.* **58**:545.
Burton, G. J. (1959): *Indian J. Malariol.* **13**:75.
     (1960 a, b, c): *Indian J. Malariol.* **14**:81; **14**:107; **14**:131.
     (1960d): *Indian J. Malariol.* **14**:593.
     (1964a): *Ann. Trop. Med. Parasitol.* **58**:333.
     (1964b): *U.S. Pub. Health Rpts.* **79**:137.
     (1967): *Bull. Wld Hlth Org.* **37**:317.
Burton, G. J. & McRae, T. M. (1965): *Ann. Trop. Med. Parasit.* **59**:405.
Butts, D. C. A. (1947): *Amer. J. Trop. Med.* **27**:607.
Buxton (1927): Malaria and filariasis in the New Hebrides. in "Researches in Polynesia and Melanesia" Appendix II, pp. 225–37
Buxton, P. A. (1927, '28): Researches in Polynesia and Melanesia. Mem. London Sch. Hyg. Trop. Med. 1927, Parts 1–4 (Relating principally to Medical Entomology) 260 pp. 1928, Parts 5–7 (Relating to human disease) 139 pp.
Byrd, E. E. (1945): *J. Parasitol. 31* Supp.:13.
Byrd, E. E. & St. Amant, L. S. (1950): Studies on the epidemiology of filariasis on Central and South Pacific islands. Department of Navy, Wash., 220 pp. Mimeographed.

768   REFERENCES

Byrd, E. E. & St. Amant, L. S. (1959): Studies on the epidemiology of filariasis on
    Central and South Pacific Islands. *South Pacific. Comm. Tech. Pep.* 125, 90 pp.
Byrd, E. E. & St. Amant, L. S. (1950):
Byrd, E. E., St. Amant, L. S. & Promberg, L. (1945): *U. S. Naval Med. Bull* 44:1.
Cabrera, B. D. (1966a): *Acta Med. Philipp.* 3:77.
                    (1966b): *Acta Med. Philipp.* 3:107.
                    (1968): *J. Philipp. Med. Ass.* 44:117.
                    (1970): *Southeast Asian J. Trop. Med. Pub. Hlth.* 1:496.
                    (1971): *Acta Med. Philipp.* 7:95.
Cabrera, B. D. & Arambulo, P. V. III. (1973): *Acta Med. Philipp.* 9:160.
Cabrera, B. D. & Cruz, I. (1968): *Acta Med. Philipp.* 5:1.
Cabrera, B. D. & Rozeboom, L. E. (1964): *Nature* 202(4933):725.
                                  (1965): *Amer. J. Epidemiol.* 81:192.
Cabrera, B. D. & Tamondong, C. T. (1966a): *Acta Med. Philipp.* 3:Ser. 2, 20.
                                  (1966b): *Acta Med. Philipp.* 3:Ser. 2, 86.
                                  (1970a): *J. Philipp. Med. Ass.* 46:74.
                                  (1970b): *Acta Med. Philipp.* 6:102.
Cabrera, B. D. & Tubangui, M. (1951): *Acta Med. Philipp.* 7:221.
Cabrera, B. D. ; Valeza, F. (1972): *Acta Med. Philipp.* 8:145.
Callot, J., Ratignier, A. & Kremer, M. (1967): *Bul. Soc. Path. Exot.* 60:184.
Calvalho, G. de (1955): *Rev. Brasil. Med.* 12:209.
Calvert, W. J. (1902): *Bull. Johns Hopkins Hospital,* 13:23.
Canet, J. (1950): *Bull. Soc. Path. Exot.* 43:216; 332.
          (1952): *Ann. Parasit. Hum. Comp.* 27:286.
Canet, J. & Jahan, P. (1949): *Bull. Soc. Pathol. Exot.* 42:408.
Capponi, M. (1949): *Med. Trop.* (Marseille) 9:442.
Capron, A., Gentilini, M. & Vernes, A. (1968): *Pathologie-Biologie.* 6:1039.
Carayon, A. & Datchary, A. (1962): *Med. Trop.* (Marseille) 22:215.
Carayon, A., Courbil, L. J. & Colomar, R. (1968): *Med. D'Afr. Noire.* 15:21.
Carestia, R. R. & Savage, L. B. (1967): *Mosquito News* 27:90.
Carter, .F. (1948): *Ann. Trop. Med. Parasit.* 42:312.
         (1950): *Ceylon J. Sci.* B. 24:1
Carter, J. F., Ingram, A. & Macfie, J. W. S. (1920): *Ann. Trop. Med. Parasit.* 14:
    187.
Carvalho, C. de (1955): *Rev. Brasil. Med.* 12:209.
Casaca, V. M. R. (1966a): *An. Inst. Med. Trop.* (Lisbon) 23:127.
                 (1966b): *An. Inst. Med. Trop.* (Lisbon) 23:133.
                 (1967a): *Rev. Brasil. Malariol. D. Trop.* 19:5.
                 (1967b): *Rev. Brasil. Malariol. D. Trop.* 19:33.
Casey, J. W., Fineg, J., Tulloch, G. S. & Davis, H. C. (1972): year field evaluation of
    diethylcarbamazine as a heartworm chemoprophelactic. *In* 95–9 pp. Bradley, R. E.
    (ed.) "Canine Heartworm Disease," (Univ. Florida).
Castellani, A. (1908): *Lancet* 4, July, p. 15
               (1917): *J. Trop. Med.* 20:209.
Causey, O. R., Deane, M. P., Costa, O. R. & Deane, L. M. (1945): *Amer. J. Hyg.* 41:
    143.
Cavier, R., Leger, N., Harichaux, J. M. & Lonne, M. C. (1971): *Ann. Parasit. Hum.
    Comp.* 46:497.
Cerqueirq, N. L. (1959): *J. Brasil. Med.* (Rio). 1:885.
Cha, C. W. Seo, B. S. & Song, M. Z. (1968): *Korean J. Parasit.* 6:53.
Chabaud, A. G. (1952): *Ann. Parasit.* 27:250.
Chakravartty, T. N. (1927): *Indian Med. Gaz,* 62:295.
Chandra, S., Chandra, R., Katiyar, J. C., Govil, P., George, P. A. & Sen, A. B. (1973):
    Indian J. Med. Res. 61:1127.
Chandra, R., Govila, P., Chandra, S., Katiyar, J. C. & Sen, A. B. (1974): *Indian J. Med.
    Res.* 62:1017.

Chardome, M. & Peel, E. (1949): *Ann. Soc. Belge Med. Trop.* **29**:99
               (1951a): *Ann. Soc. Belge Med. Trop.* **31**:571.
               (1951b): *Inst. Roy. Col. Belge, Sect. Sci, Nat. Med. Mém. Coll.* **19**:1.
Chari, M. V. & Hiremath, R. S. (1967): *J. Indian Med. Assoc.* **48**:543.
Charles, L. J. (1953): *Ann. Trop. Med. Parasit.* **47**:113.
Charoenlarp, P., Sucharit, S. & Harinasuta, C. (1964): *Trans. Roy. Soc. Trop. Med. Hyg.* **58**:580.
Chassaniol, A. & Guyot, F. (1878): *Arch. Méd. Nav.* **29**:61.
Chatterjee, K. C. (1954): *Indian J. Med. Ass.* **24**:146.
Chatterjee, A. & Chowdhury, A. B. (1964): *Bull. Calcutta School Trop. Med.* **12**:3.
Cháves Nuñez, M. (1963): *Boln Epidem. Méx.* **27**:17.
Chen, K. C. (1948): *J. Lingnan Sci.* **22**:85.
Chen, Tsu-Ta (1964): *Chin. Med. J.* (Peking) **83**:624.
Ch'en Tsu-Ta, Ch'en Ching-Ts'ai, *et al.* (1959a): *Chin Med. J.* **68**:173.
               (1959b): *Chin. Med. J.* **68**:174.
Cheong, W. H. & Abu Hassan bin Omar (1965): *Med. J. Malaya* **20**:74.
Cheong, W. H., Omar, H. A. & Sivanadam, S. (1965): *Singapore Med. J.* **6**:43.
Chin, Ta-Hsiung, Ho, Kuo-Ping & Li, Ming-Kao (1959): *Chin. Med. J.* **78**:176.
Chinese Medical Journal (1959): *Chin. Med. J.* **78**:226.
Choisser, R. M. (1923): *U.S. Naval Med. Bull.* **18**:56.
Choyce, D. P. (1958): *Trans. Roy. Soc. Trop. Med. Hyg.* **52**:112.
               (1966): *Trans. Roy. Soc. Trop. Med. Hyg.* **60**:720.
Chow, C. Y. (1973): *Zeitschr. Tropenmed. Parasit.* **24**:404.
Chow, C. Y. & Thevasagayam, E. S. (1957): *Bull. Wld Hlth Org.* **16**:609.
Chow, C. Y. Lie, K. J., Winoto, R. M. P., Rusad, M. & Soegiarto (1959): *Bull. Wld Hlth Org.* **20**:667.
Chowdhury, A. B. & Schiller, E. L. (1968): *Amer. J. Epidemiol.* **87**:299.
Chu Feng-I (1958): *Indian J. Malariol.* **12**:109.
Chu, I. H. (1963): *Korean J. Parasit.* **1**:7.
Chu Shin-Huei, Shen Chen-huang, *et al.* (1959a): *Chin. Med. J.* **78**:177.
Chu Shin-huei, Shen Chen-huang & Ch'en Shao-hsiun (1959b): *Acta Microbiologica Sinica* **7**:25 (Abstract in *Chinese Med. J.* **80**:191, 1960).
Chuiton, le (1923): *Arch. Méd. Pharmac. Navales* (1923): 294 pp.
               (1924): *Bull. Soc. Path. Exot.* **17**:405.
Chularerk, P. & Desowitz, R. S. (1970): *J. Parasitol.* **56**:623.
Chzuvet, G., Davidson, G. & Coz, J. (1969): *Entom. Med. et Parasit.* **7**:9.
Ciferri, F. E. & Kessel, J. F. (1967): *Amer. J. Trop. Med. Hyg.* **16**:321.
Ciferri, F. E., Kessel, J. F., Lewis, W. P. & Rieber, S. (1965): *Am. J. Trop. Med. Hyg.* **14**:263.
Ciferri, F. E., Siliga, N., Long, G. & Kessel, J. F. (1969): *Amer. J. Trop. Med. Hyg.,* **18**:369.
Cilento, R. W. (1924): *Dept. Health Serv. Publ.* (Trop. Dic.) **4**:1.
Cilento, R. W. & Richards, R. E. (1923): *Austr. Med. Congr. Trans.* **1**:325.
Clarke, V. de V., Harwin, R. M., Macdonald, D. F., Green, C. A. & Rittey, D. A. W. (1971): *Central African J. Med.* **17**:1.
Clavel (1884): *Arch. Méd. Nav.* **42**:194.
Cloitre, J. (1928): *Bull. Soc. Path. Exot.* **21**:722.
Cobban, K. McC. (1954): *J. Trop. Med. Hyg.* **62**:129.
Cobbold, T. S. (1864): An Introduction to the study of Helminthology with Reference more particularly to the Internal Parasites of Man. London, 480 pp.
               (1877a): *Lancet,* July 14, 1877:70.
               (1877b): *Lancet,* Oct. 6, 1877: 495.
Cohen, L. B. (1960): *East African Med. J.* **37**:53.
Colbourne, M. J. & Ng, W. K. (1972): *Southeast Asian J. Trop. Med. Pub. Hlth* **3**:40.

Colbourne, M. J., Edington, G. M., Hughes, M. H. & Ward-Brew, A. (1950): *Trans. Roy. Soc. Trop. Med. Hyg.* **44**:271.

Colles, D. H. (1957): *Ann. Trop. Med. Parasit.* **51**:87.

(1959): *Ann. Trop. Med. Parasit.* **53**:166.

(1971): *Ann. Trop. Med. Parasit.* **65**:245.

Collomb, J., Camerlynck, P., Dumas, M., Tap, D. & Vieillard, J. J. (1969): *Bull. Soc. Path. Exot.* **62**:907.

Coluzzi, M. (1968): *Parasitologia,* **10**:179.

Coluzzi, M. & Sabatini, A. (1967): *Parasitologia.* **9**:73.

Colwell, E. J., Armstrong, D. R., Brown, J. D., Duxbury, R. E., Sadun, E. H. & Legters, L. J. (1970): *Amer. J. Trop. Med. Hyg.* **19**:227.

Condy, J. B. & Hill, R. R. (1970): *Cent. Afr. J. Med.* **16**:249.

Coni, A. C. (1967): Rev. Brasil Malariol. D. Trop. **19**:91.

Connal, A. & Connal, S. L. M. (1922): *Trans. Roy. Soc. Trop. Med. Hyg.* **16**:64.

Connor, D. H. (1974): *Pan Amer. Hlth Org.* 11 pp.

Conor, A. (1911): *Bull. Soc. Path. Exot.* **4**:47.

Conran, O. F. & Conran, A. (1956): *J. Trop. Med. Hyg.* **59**:285.

Convit, J. (1974): in "Research and Control of Onchocerciasis in Western Hemisphere," *Pan Amer. Hlth Org.* 105

Convit, J., Quintero, C. S. & Ibáñez de Aldecoa, R. (1961): *Revta Venez. Sanid. Asist. Soc.* **26**: Suppl. 1, 260.

Cool, P. (1927): *Gen. Tijdschr. Ned. Indie.* **67**:314.

Cornet, M. (1969): *Cahiers O. R. S. T. O. M. Ser. Entom. Med. Parasit.* **7**:341.

Corredor, A. A. (1974): in "Research and Control of Onchocerciasis in Western Hemisphere," *Pan Amer. Hlth Org.* 116.

Corson, J. F. (1925): *Ann. Trop. Med. Parasit.* **19**:381.

Coudert, J., Ambroise-Thomas, P., Kien Troung, T. S. (1968): *Bull. Soc. Path. Exot.* **61**: 435.

Coulson, C. A. (1955): "Waves" (University Mathematical Text) 159 pp. Oliver & Boyd, Ltd. Edinburgh.

Courmes, E., Fauran, P. & Lespinasse, J. J. (1968): Bull. Soc. Path. Exot. **61**:234.

Courtney, B. J. (1923): *J. Trop. Med. Hyg.* **26**:87.

Couzineau, P., Bouree, P. & Molimard, R. (1973): *Bull. Soc., Path. Exot.* **66**:553.

Cowper, S. G. (1967): *West Afr. Med. J.* (N. S.) **16**:3.

Cowper, S. G. & Jackson, H. (1964): *J. Trop. Med. Hyg.* **67**:69.

Cowper, S. G. & Woodward, S. F. (1960): *West African Med. J.* **9**:123.

(1961): *West African Med. J.* **10**:366.

Coz, J. (1973a): *Cah. O. R. S. T. O. M. Ent. Med. Parasit.* **11**:3.

(1973b): *Cah. O. R. S. T. O. M. Ent. Med. Parasit.* **11**:33.

(1973c): *Cah. O. R. S. T. O. M. Ent. Med. Parasit.* **11**:41.

Coz, J. & Brengues, J. (1967): *Med. D'Afr. Noire* **14**:301.

Coz, J. & Hamon, J. (1964): *Riv. Malariol.* **43**:233.

Crans, W. J. (1969) Mosquito News 29:563.

(1972): A rapid technique for the determination of microfilaremia in filariasis carriers. (Unpublished document WHO/FIL/92.98).

(1973): *J. Med. Entomol.* **10**:189.

Crewe, W. (1954): *Ann. Trop. Med. Parasit.* **48**:216.

(1955): *Trans. Roy. Soc. Trop. Med. Hyg.* **49**:106.

(1961a): *Ann. Trop. Med. Parasit.* **55**:211.

(1961b): *Ann. Trop. Med. Parasit.* **55**:357.

Crewe, W. & Williams, P. (1961): *Ann. Trop. Med. Parasit.* **55**:363.

Crisp, G. (1956a): *Ann. Trop. Med. Parasit.* **50**:260.

(1956b): *Ann. Trop. Med. Parasit.* **50**:444.

(1956c): Simulium and onchocerciasis in the Northern Territories of the Gold Coast. British Society for the Blind. H. K. Lewis, London. 171 pp.

Croll, D. G. (1919): *Brit. Med. J.* **1**:28.

Crosskey, R. W. (1954): *Ann. Trop. Med. Parasit.* **48**:152.
     (1955): *Ann. Trop. Med. Parasit.* **49**:142.
     (1956): *Trans. Roy. Soc. Trop. Med. Hyg.* **50**:379.
     (1957a): *Ann. Trop. Med. Parasit.* **51**:80.
     (1957b): *Trans. Roy. Soc. Trop. Med. Hyg.* **51**:541.
     (1958): *Bull. Entomol. Res.* **49**:715.
     (1959): *Bull. Wld Hlth Org.* **21**:727.
     (1962): *Bull. Wld Hlth Org.* **27**:483.
     (1962): *Ann. Trop. Med. Parasit.* **56**:141.
     (1968): *Trans. Roy. Soc. Trop. Med. Hyg.* 62, Discussion, 44.
     (1973): Simuliidae (Black-flies), in Insects and other Arthropods of
Medical Importance, (K. G. V. Smith, ed.), pp. 109–154, British Museum, London.
Crosskey, R. W. & Crosskey, M. E. (1958): *Nature* **181**:713.
Crosskey, R. W. & Crosskey, M. E. (1959): *Ann. Trop. Med. Parasit.* **53**:10.
Crow, G. B. (1910): *J. Amer. Med. Assoc.* **55**:595.
Cruickshank, A. (1936): *East African Med. J.* **13**:172.
Cruickshank, J. A. & Wright, R. E. (1914): *Indian J. Med. Res.* **1**:741.
Cruickshank, J. A., Cunningham J. & Iyer, T. S. (1923): *Indian J. Med. Res.* **11**:79.
Culbertson, J. T. (1947): *Trans. Roy. Soc. Trop. Med. Hyg.* **41**:18.
     (1948): *Ann. N.Y. Acad. Sci.* **50**:73.
Culbertson, J. T. & Rose, H. M. (1944): *J. Pharm. Exptl. Therap.* **81**:189.
Culbertson, J. T., Rose, H. M. & Demarest, G. R. (1943): *Amer. J. Hyg.* **39**:156.
Dalip Singh & Raghaven, N. G. S. (1962): *Indian J. Malariol.* **16**:193.
Dalmat, H. T. (1955): The black flies (Diptera, Simuliidae) of Guatemala and their role
 as vectors of onchocerciasis. Smithsonian Misc. Pub. vol. 125, No. 1, 425 pp.
Danaraj, T. J., Schacher, J. F. & Colless, D. H. (1958): *Med. J. Malaya.* **12**:605.
Danaraj, T. J., Da Silva, L. S. & Schacher, J. F. (1959): *Amer. J. Trop. Med. Hyg.* **8**:151.
Daniels, C. W. (1896): *British Guiana Medical Annual.* **8**:62.
     (1897): *British Guiana Medical Annual* **9**:28.
     (1898): *Brit. Med. J.* April 16, 1898:1011.
     (1899): *Brit. Med. J.* June 17; 1899:1459.
     (1901): *J. Trop. Med.* **4**:193.
     (1908): "Animal parasites in man and some of the lower animals in
Malaya.," *Stud. Inst. Med. Res. F.M.S.* **3**(Pt. 1):1–18
Daniels, C. W. & Conyers, J. H. (1896): *British Guiana Medical Annual,* **8**:42–61.
Dassanayake, W. L. P. (1938): *J. Trop. Med. Hyg.* **41**:141.
     (1939): *J. Trop. Med. Hyg.* **42**:145.
     (1950): J. Ceylon Br. Brit. Mcd. Assoc. **45**:27.
     (1954a): *Ann. Trop. Med. Parasit.* **48**:123.
     (1954b): *Ann. Trop. Med. Parasit.* **48**:127.
Dassanayake, W. L. P. & Chow, C. Y. (1954): *Ann. Trop. Med. Parasit.* **48**:129.
Datta, S. P. (1967): *Bull. Nat. Soc. India Malaria Mosq. Dis.* **8**:131.
Datta, S. P. & Natarajan, V. (1962): *Bull. Nat. Soc. India Mosq. Dis.* **10**:139.
David, H. L. & Edeson, J. F. B. (1964a): *Proc. Ist Int. Congr. Parasitology* **2**:639.
     (1964b): *Trans. Roy. Soc. Trop. Med. Hyg.* **58**:6.
     (1965): *Ann. Trop. Med. Parasit.* **59**:193.
Davidson, G. (1964): *Riv. Malariol.* **43**:197.
Davidson, G. & Jackson, C. E. (1962): *Bull. Wld Hlth Org.* **27**:303.
Davies, J. B. (1963): *Ann. Trop. Med. Parasit.* **57**:161.
     (1965): *Ann. Trop. Med. Parasit.* **59**:43.
     (1968): *Bull. Wld Hlth Org.* **39**:187.
Davies, J. B., Crosskey, R. W., Johnston, M. R. L. & Crosskey, M. E. (1962): *Bull. Wld
Hlth Org.* **27**:491.
Davis, N. C. (1928): *Amer. J. Hyg.* **8**:457.
     (1931): *Rivista Malariol.* **10**:43.
     (1935): *J. Parasit.* **21**:21.

772   REFERENCES

Davis, T. R. A. (1949): *New Zealand Med. J.* **48**:362.

Davis, A. & Bailey, D. R. (1969): *Bull. Wld Hlth Org.* **41**:195.

Deane, M. P. (1949): "Sôbre a incidência de filária humanas em Manaus, Estado do Amazonas".—Revista do S.E.S.P. 2(3).

Deane, M. P. & Costa, O. R. (1948): Relatório preliminar de experiências com o fim de verificar sua aplicabilidade no contrôle da transmissao da filariose em Belem. Rev. S.E.S.P 2(2).

Deane, L. M. & Damasceno, R. G. (1952): *Rev. Brass. Malariol. D. Trop.* **4**:333.

Deane, L. M., da Rose, E., Rachou, R. G., Martins, J. S., Costa, A., Gomes, H. M. & Carvalho, M. E. (1953): *Rev. Brasil. Malariol. D. Trop.* **5**:17.

Deland, C. M. (1951): (correspondence). *Trans. Roy. Soc. Trop. Med. Hyg.,* **44**:610.

Demarquay, M. (1863): *Gaz. Méd. Paris* **18**:665.

Demos, E. A., Chen, H. H. & Hsieh, H. C. (1954): *J. Formosan Med. Assoc.* **53**:541.

Denecke, K. (1941): *Arch. Schiffs-Tropenhyg.* **45**:609.

Denham, D. A. (1974): *J. Parasit* **60**:642.

Denham, D. A., Dennis, D. T., Ponnudurai, T., Nelson, G. S. & Guy, F. (1971a): *Trans. Roy. Soc. Trop. Med. Hyg* **65**:521.

Denham, D. A., Ponnudurai, T., Nelson, G. S., Guy, F. & Rogers, R. (1971b): *Bull. Wld Hlth Org.* **45**:423.

Dennis, D. T. & Kean, B. H. (1971): *J. Parasit.* **57**:1146.

Deschiens, R., Benex, J. & Yucel, A. (1961): *Ann. Soc. Belge Med. Trop.* **4**:265.

Desowitz, R. S. (1974): The application of a membrane filter concentration method in filariasis surveys in the South Pacific area. WHO/FIL/74.131, 12 pp. (mimeogr.)

Desowitz, R. S. & Hitchcock, J. C. (1974): *Amer. J. Trop. Med. Hyg.* **23**:877.

Desowitz, T. S. & Southgate, B. A. (1973): *Southeast Asian J. Trop. Med. Pub. Hlth* **4**:179.

Desowits, R. S., Saave, J. J. & Sawada, T. (1966): *Ann. Trop. Med. Parasit.* **60**:257.

Desowitz, R. S., Chularerk, P. & Palumbo, N. E (1970): *Southeast Asian J. Trop. Med. Pub. Hlth* **1**:231.

Desowitz, R. S., Southgate, B. A. & Mataika, J. U. (1973): *S. E. Asian J. Trop. Med. Publ. Hlth* **4**:329.

Detinova, T. S. (1962): *World Health Org. Mon. Ser.* **47**:210.

Dhar, S. K., Das, M., et al. (1968): *Bull. Indian Soc. Malaria Comm. Dis.* **5**:79.

Diaz, A. F. (1957): *Bull. Wld Hlth Org.* **16**:676.

Dickerson, C. W. & Tohmpson, P. E. (1966): *J. Parasit.* **52**:1217.

Dickson, J. G., Huntington, R. W. & Eichold, S. (1943): *U.S. Naval Med. Bull.* **41**:1240.

Diesing, S. (1899): *Arch Schiffs-Tropenhyg.* **3**:20.

Dijk, W. J. O. M. van (1958a): *Trop. Geogr. Med.* **10**:21.

      (1958b): *Meded. Dienst. Gezondheid Nederl. Nieuw Guinea.* **5**:58.

      (1959): *Trop. Geogr. Med.* **11**:259.

      (1961): *Trop. Geog. Med.* **13**:143.

      (1963): *Trop. Geog. Med.* **15**:29.

      (1964): *Trop. Geog. Med.* **16**:54.

      (1966): *Trop. Geog. Med.* **18**:53.

Diller, W. F. (1947): *J. Parasit.* **33**:363.

Disney, R. H. L. (1969): *Trans. Roy, Soc. Trop. Med. Hyg.* 63, Correspondence, 292.

      (1970a): *Ann. Trop. Med. Parasit.* **64**:123.

      (1970b): *Ann. Trop. Med. Parasit.* **64**:129.

Disney, R. H. L. & Boreham, P. F. L. (1969): *Trans. Roy. Soc. Trop. Med. Hyg.* **63**:286.

Dissanaike, A. S. (1969a): Control of filariasis in Ceylon. Proc. of Seminar on Filariasis and Immunology of Parasitic Infection and Laboratory Meeting, Singapore. 149–61

      (1969b): The status of research and study of filariasis in Ceylon. Proc. Seminar on Filariasis & Imminitu of Parasitic Infection & Laboratory Demonstration, Singapore. 1968. 210–7

Dissanaike, A. S. & Niles, W. J. (1965): *Ann. Trop. Med. Parasit.* **59**:189.

Dissanaike, A. S. & Niles, W. J. (1967): *J. Helminth.* **41**:291.

Dissanaike, A. S. & Paramananthan, D. C. (1961): *J. Helminth.* **35**:209.

Dissanaike, A. S., Dissanaike, G. A. Niles, W. J. & Surendranathan, R. (1966): *J. Helminth.* **40**:297.

Dissanayake, W. L. P. (1938): *J. Trop. Med. Hyg.* **41**:141.

Diwan Chand, Singh, M. V. & Shrivastava, R. N. (1959): *Indian J. Malariol.,* **13**:163.

Diwan Chand, Singh, M. V. & Pathax, V. K. (1961a): *Indian J. Malariol.* **15**:21.

(1961b): *Indian J. Malariol.* **15**:31.

Diwan Chand, Singh, M. V., Gupta, B. B. & Shrivastava, R. N. (1961c): *Indian J. Malariol.* **15**:39.

Diwan Chand, Singh, M. V., & Shrivastava, R. N. (1961d): *Indian J. Malariol.* **15**:175.

Diwan Chand, Singh, M. V. & Bhaskar, V. K. (1961e): *Indian J. Malariol.* **15**:149.

Diwan Chand, Singh, M. V. & Vyas, L. C. (1962): Indian *J. Malariol.* **16**:269.

Doane, R. W. (1914): *Bull. Entomol. Res.* **4**:265.

Dobbin, J. E., Jr. & Cruz, A. E. (1967): *Rev. Brasil Malariol. D. Trop.* **19**:45.

(1968): *Revta Soc. Bras. Med. Trop.* **2**:9.

Dobrotworsky, N. V. (1967): *Bull. Wld. Hlth. Org.* **37(2)**:251.

Doby, J. M., David, F. & Rault, B. (1959): *Annls Parasit. Hum Comp.* **34**:676.

Dodin, A., Brygoo, E. R., Richard, J. & Moreau, J. P. (1966): *WHO/FIL/*66.61, 19 pp. (mimeogr.)

Do-Doung Thai (1964): *Ceskoslovenska Parasitol.* **11**:33.

Dondero, T. J., Jr. & Ramachandran, C. P. (1972): *Southeast Asian J. Trop. Med. Pub. Hlth.* **3**:25.

Dondero, T. J., Jr., Ramachandran, C. P. & Yusoff, O. (1971a): *Southeast Asian J. Trop. Med. Pub. Hlth,* **2**:503.

Dondero, T. J., Jr., Sivanandam, S. & Lee Chu-Chong (1971b): (Correspondence) *Trans. Roy. Soc. Trop. Med. Hyg.* **65**:691.

Dondero, T. J., Mullin, S. W. & Balasingam, S. (1972): *Southeast Asian J. Trop. Med. Pub. Hlth.* **3**:569.

Donglade, J. H. & Fitzgerald, P. J. (1946): *U.S. Naval Med. Bull.* **46**:193.

Doucet, J. (1950): *Arch. Inst. Scient. Madagascar.* ser. A. 6:83–114.

Doucet, J., Adam, J. P. & Binson, G. (1960): *Ann. Parasit, Hum. Comp.* **35**:391.

Downie, C. G. B. (1966): *J. Roy. Army Med. Cps* **112**:46.

Downs, W. G., Harper, P. A. & Lisansky, E. T. (1947): *Amer. J. Trop. Med.* **27**:Suppl. 3:69.

Dubois, A. (1916): *Bull. Soc. Path. Exot.* **9**:305.

(1917): *Bull. Soc. Path. Exot.* **10**:365.

(1946): *Ann. Soc. Belge Med. Trop.* **26**:109.

(1948): *Ann. Soc. Belge Med. Trop.* **28**:151.

Dubois, A., & Van den Berghe, L. (1948): Diseases of the Warm Climates. Their Clinical Features, Diagnosis and Treatment. Grune & Staratton, New York. 445 pp.

Dubois, A. & Forro, M. (1939): *Ann. Soc. Belge Med. Trop.* **19**:13.

Dubois, A. & Vitale, S. (1938): *Ann. Soc. Belge Med. Trop.* **18**:552.

Dubois, A., Vitale, S. & Birger, Ch. (1939): *Ann. Soc. Belge Med. Trop.* **19**:26.

Dubruel, C. M. E. (1909a): *Bull. Soc. Path Exot.* **2**:355.

(1909b): *Bull. Soc. Path. Exot.* **2**:360.

Duke, B. O. L. (1954a): *Ann. Trop. Med. Parasit.* **48**:349.

(1954b): *Ann. Trop. Med. Parasit.* **48**:416.

(1955a): *Trans. Roy. Soc. Trop. Med. Hyg.* **49**:115.

(1955b): *Ann. Trop. Med. Parasit.* **49**:193.

(1955c): *Ann. Trop. Med. Parasit.* **49**:260.

(1955d): *Ann. Trop. Med. Parasit.* **49**:362.

(1955e): *Ann. Trop. Med. Parasit.* **49**:368.

(1956): *Ann. Trop. Med. Parasit.* **50**:32.

(1957): *Trans. Roy. Soc. Trop. Med. Hyg.* **51**:37.

Duke B. O. L. (1958a): *Ann. Trop. Med. Parasit.* **52**:24.
    (1958b): *Ann. Trop. Med. Parasit.* **52**:123.
    (1959): *Ann. Trop. Med. Parasit.* **53**:203.
    (1960a): *Ann. Trop. Med. Parasit.* **54**:15.
    (1960b): *Ann. Trop. Med. Parasit.* **54**:141.
    (1960c): *Ann. Trop. Med. Parasit.* **54**:147.
    (1961): *Ann. Trop. Med. Parasit.* **55**:447.
    (1962a): *Trans. Roy. Soc. Trop. Med. Hyg.* **56**:271.
    (1962b): *Bull. Wld Hlth. Org.* **27**:629.
    (1962c): *Ann. Trop. Med. Parasit.* **56**:67.
    (1962d): *Ann. Trop. Med. Parasit.* **56**:130.
    (1962e): *Ann. Trop. Med. Parasit.* **56**:255.
    (1963): *Ann. Trop. Med. Parasit.* **57**:82.
    (1964): *Ann. Trop. Med. Parasitol.* **58**:390.
    (1966a): *Ann. Trop. Med. Parasit.* **60**:495.
    (1966): *Trans Roy. Soc. Trop. Med. Hyg.* **60**: Correspondence, 691.
    (1967a): *Ann. Trop. Med. Parasit.* **61**:326.
    (1967b): *Ann. Trop. Med. Parasit.* **61**:200.
    (1968a): *Bull. Wld. Hlth Org.* **39**:137.
    (1968b): *Bull. Wld Hlth Org.* **39**:147.
    (1968c): *Bull. Wld. Hlth Org.* **39**:157.
    (1968d): *Bull. Wld. Hlth Org.* **39**:169078.
    (1968e): *Bull. Wld. Hlth Org.* **39**:179.
    (1968f): *Ann. Trop. Med. Parasit.* **62**:95.
    (1968g): *Ann. Trop. Med. Parasit.* **62**:107.
    (1968h): *Ann. Trop. Med. Parasit.* **62**:164.
    (1968i): *Brit. Med. J.* **4**:301.
    (1970): *Ann. Trop. Med. Parasit.* **64**:421.
    (1972a): *Brit. Med. Bull.* **28**:66.
    (1972b): *Ann. Trop. Med. Parasit.* **66**:163.
    (1972c): Behavioural aspects of the life cycle of *Loa*. in "Behavioural Aspects of Parasite Transmission (Canning, E. U. & Wright, C. A., ed.) 97–105 pp., (Academic Press, New York).
    (1973a): *Ann. Trop. Med. Parasit.* **67**:95.
    (1973b): WHO FIL/WP/73.2. (mimeographed, 7 pp.)
    (1974a): *Trans. Roy. Soc. Trop. Med. Hyg.* **68**:71.
    (1974b): *Ann. Trop. Med. Parasit.* **68**:241.
    (1974c): *Pan Amer. Hlth Org.*, 25–8 pp.
    (1974d): Treatment of onchocerciasis. In "Research and Control of Onchocerciasis in the Western Hemisphere" 46–52 pp.
    (1974e): *Ztschr. Tropenmed. Parasit.* **25**:84.
    (1974f): [Correspondence.] *Trans. Roy. Soc. Trop. Med. Hyg.* **68**:172.
Duke, B. O. L. & Anderson, J. (1972): *Ztschr. Tropenmed. Parasit.* **23**:354.
Duke, B. O. L. and Beesley, W. N. (1958): *Ann. Trop. Med. Parasit.* **52**:274.
Duke, B. O. L. and Hawking, F. (1967): *Trans. Roy. Soc. trop. Med. Hyg.* **61**: Correspondence, 273.
Duke, B. O. L. & Jamison, D. G. (1955): *Trans. Roy. Soc. Trop. Med. Hyg.* **49**:299.
Duke, B. O. L. & Lewis, D. J. (1964): *Ann. Trop. Med. Parasit.* **58**:83.
Duke, B. O. L. & Moore, P. J. (1961): *Ann. Trop. Med. Parasit.* **55**:263.
    (1967): *Trans. Roy. Soc. trop. Med. Hyg.* **61**:614.
    (1974): *Tropenmed. Parasit.* **25**:153.
Duke, B. O. L., & Wijers, D. J. B. (1958): *Ann. Trop. Med. Parasitol.* **52**:158.
Duke, B. O. L., Crewe, W. & Beesley, W. N. (1956): *Ann. Trop. Med. Parasit.* **50**:283.
Duke, B. O. L., Lewis, D. J. and Moore, J. P. (1966): *Ann. Trop. Med. Parasit.* **60**:318.
Duke, B. O. L., Scheffel, P. D., Guyon, J. & Moore, P. J. (1967a): *Ann. Trop. Med. Parasit.* **61**:206.

Duke, B. O. L., Moore, J. P. and De Leon, R. J. (1967b): *Ann. Trop. Med. Parasit.* **61**: 332.

Duke, B. O. L., Moore, P. J. & Anderson, J. (1972): *Ann. Trop. Med. Parasit.* **66**:219.

Dukes, D. C., Gelfand, M., Gadd, K. G., Klarke, V. de V. & Goldsmid, J. M. (1968): Cerebral filariasis caused by *Acanthocheilonema perstans*. *Central African J. Med.* **14**:21

Dunbar, R. W. (1966): *Nature* **209**:597–599.

Dunderdale, G. (1921): *Trans. Roy. Soc. Trop. Med. Hyg.* **15**:190.

Dutta, S. N. & Diesfeld, H. J. (1974): *J. Com. Dis.* **6**:278.

Dutton, J. E. (1901): *British Med. J.* **2(1901)**:612.

Duxbury, R. E. & Sadun, E. H. (1967): *Exp. Parasitol.* **20**:77.

Earl, P. R. (1959): *Ann. N.Y. Acad. Sci.* **77**:163.

Earle, K. V. (1942): *Trans. Roy. Soc. Trop. Med. Hyg.* **35**:235.

East African Medical Journal (1939): *East African Med. J.* **15**:363.

Edeson, J. F. B. (1955): *Trans. Roy. Soc. Trop. Med. Hyg.* **49**:488.

　　　　　(1959a): *Ann. Trop. Med. Parasit.* **53**:381.

　　　　　(1959b): *Ann. Trop. Med. Parasit.* **53**:388.

　　　　　(1962): *Bull. Wld Hlth Org.* **27**:529.

　　　　　(1963): WHO/SEA/Fil/6.

　　　　　(1966): *Proc. 11th Pacific Sci. Congr.* **8**:4.

　　　　　(1972): *British Med. Bull.* **28**:60.

　　　　　(1973): WHO Expert Committee on Filariasis: FIL/WP/73.30, 17 pp.

Edeson, J. F. B. & Buckley, J. J. C. (1959): *Ann. Trop. Med. Parasit.* **53**:113.

Edeson, J. F. B. & Laing, A. B. G. (1959): *Ann. Trop. Med. Parasit.* **53**:394.

Edeson, J. F. B. & Wharton, R. H. (1957): *Trans. Roy. Soc. Trop. Med. Hyg.* **51**:366.

　　　　　(1958a): *Trans. Roy. Soc. Trop. Med. Hyg.* **52**:25.

　　　　　(1958b): *Ann. Trop. Med. Parasit.* **52**:87.

Edeson, J. F. B. & Wilson, T. (1964): *Annual. Rev. Entomology* **9**:245.

Edeson, J. F. B., Wharton, R. H. & Buckley, J. J. C. (1955): *Trans. Roy. Soc. Trop. Med. Hyg.* **49**:604.

Edeson, J. F. B., Hawking, F. & Symes, C. B. (1957): *Trans. Roy. Soc. Trop. Med. Hyg.* **51**:359.

Edeson, J. F. B., Wilson, T., Wharton, R. H. & Laing, A. B. G. (1960a): *Trans. Roy. Soc. Trop. Med. Hyg.* **54**:229.

Edeson, J. F. B., Wharton, R. H. & Laing, A. B. G. (1960b): *Trans. Roy. Soc. Trop. Med. Hyg.* **54**:439.

Edgar, S. A., Beyem H. K. & Mille, R. (1952): *Amer. J. Trop. Med. Hyg.* **1**:1009.

Edghill, II. B. (1961): *West Indian Med. J.* **10**:44.

Edwards, F. W. (1922): *J. Trop. Med. Hyg.* **25**:168.

　　　　　(1922): *Bull. Ent. Res.,* **13**:99.

　　　　　(1923): *Bull. Entom. Res.,* **14**:5.

　　　　　(1924a): *Bull. Entom. Res.,* **14**:351.

　　　　　(1924b): *Ann. Mag. Nat. Hist.,* **14**:568.

　　　　　(1925): *Bull. Entom. Res.,* **15**:257.

　　　　　(1932): Diptera, family Culicidae. *In* P. Wytzman, Genera, Insectorum, Brassels, Fasc. **194**:258.

El Bihari, S. & Ewert, A. (1971): *J. Parasit.* **57**:1170.

El-Dine, K. Z. & Habib, E. (1969): *J. Egypt. Publ. Hlth Ass.,* **44**:481.

Elsbach, E. M. (1937a): *Geneesk. Tijdschr. Nederl.-Indie.* **77**:1036.

　　　　　(1937b): *Geneesk. Tijdschr. Nederl.-Indie.* **77**:1536.

El-Tamami, M. Y. (1960): *J. Egypt. Med. Assoc.* **43**:152.

Engeland, O. (1920): *Arch. Schiffs. Tropenhyg.* **24**:51.

Engeland, O. & Monteufel, P. (1911): *Arch. Schiffs. Tropenhyg.* **15**:721.

Engelhorn, T. D. & Wellman, W. E. (1945): *Amer. J. Med. Sci.,* **209**:141.

Epidemic Prevention Department, Epidemic Prevention Station, Fukien (1959): *Chinese Med. J.* **78**:226.

Erber, M. (1927): *Geneesk. Tijdschr. Nederl.-Indie.*, **67**:318.
Estrada, J. P. & Basio, D. G. (1965): *J. Philipp. Med. Assoc.*, **41(2)**:100.
Ewert, A. (1971): *J. Parasit.* **57**:1039.
Ewert, A. & El Bihari, S. (1971): *Trans. Roy. Soc. Trop. Med. Hyg.*, **65**:364.
Ewert, A. & Singh, M. (1969): *Trans. Roy. Soc. Trop. Med. Hyg.* **63**:603.
Ewert, A., Balderach, R. & El Bihari, S. (1972): *Amer. J. Trop. Med. Hyg.* **21**:407.
Eyles, D. E., Hunter, G. W. III, & Warren, V. G. (1947): *Amer. J. Trop. Med.* **27**:
    203.
Eyles, D. E., Sandosham, A. A., Wharton, R. H. & Sivanan, S. (1962): *Trans. Roy. Soc.
    Trop. Med. Hyg.* **56**:259.
Eyraud, M. & Mouchet, J. (1970): *Cah. O.R.S.T.O.M. Ent. Med. Parasit.*, **8**:69.
Fain, A. (1947a): *Ann. Soc. Belge Méd. Trop.* **27**:25.
    (1947b): *Rev. Zool. Bot. Afr.* **40**:139–50
    (1949): *Rev. Zool. Bot. Afr.* **70**:10.
    (1950): *Rev. Zool. Bot. Afr.* **5**:68, 7:10.
    (1951): *Ann. Parasit. Hum. Comp.* **26**:228.
    (1969): *Ann. Soc. Belge Méd. Trop.* **49**:499.
    (1970): *Ann. Soc. Belge Méd. Trop.* **50**:359.
    (1974): *Ann. Soc. Belg. Méd. Trop.* **54**:195.
Fain, A. & Halot, R. (1965): *Acad. Roy. Sci. Outre-Mer N.S.* **17**:1.
Fain, A. & Maertens, K. (1973): *Bull. Soc. Path. Exot.* **66**:737.
Fain, A., Wéry, M. & Tilkin, J. (1969): *Ann. Soc. Belg. Méd. Trop.*, **49**:629.
Fain, A., Elsen, P., Wéry, M. & Maertens, K. (1974a): *Ann. Soc. Belg. Méd. Trop.*, **54**:5.
Fain, A., Vandepitte, J. & Wéry, M. (1974b): *Ann. Soc. Belg. Méd. Trop.* **54**:121.
Faine, S. & Hercus, C. E. (1951): *Trans. R. Soc. Trop. Med. Hyg.*, **45**:341.
Fairchild, G. B. and Barreda, E. A. (1945): *J. Econ. Ent.* **38**:694.
Famulari, S. (1916): *Malaria e Malat. d. Paesi Caldi* 7:141–5 (*Trop. Dis. Bull.* **8**:519,
    1916).
Fan, P. C. & Hsu, J. (1954): *Chinese Med. J.* (Taipei) **1**:77.
    (1955): *Chinese Med. J.* (Taipei) **2**:151.
    (1957a): *Chinese Med. J.* (Taipei) **4**:35.
    (1957b): *Chinese Med. J.* (Taipei) **4**:81.
    (1957c): *Chinese Med. J.* (Taipei): **4**:137.
Fan, P. C., Hsu, J., Chang, T. L. & Liu, J. C. (1957d): *Chinese Med. J.* (Taipei) **4**:188.
Fan, P. C. & Hsu, J. (1968): *Chinese Med. J.* (Taipei) **15**:54.
Fan, P. C., Wang, Y. C., Liu, J. C. & Khaw, O. K. (1972): *Filariasis in Kinmen (Quemoy)
    Islands, Free China. Joint Meeting of The Amer. Soc. of Trop. Med. and Hyg. and
    The Amer. Soc. of Parasit. Miami Beach, Florida, Nov., 6–10, 1972.*
Fan, P. C., Wang, Y. C. & Liu, J. C. (1973): Epidemiology and treatment of filariasis on
    Kinmen (Quemoy) Islands. *Yonsei Reports Trop. Med.* **4**:184.
Fan, P. C., Wang, Y. C., Liu, J. C. & Hsu, J. (1974a): *Southeast Asian J. Trop. Med.
    Pub. Hlth* **5**:211.
Fan, P. C., Wang, Y. C., Liu, J. C. & Hsu, J. (1974b): *Southeast Asian J. Trop. Med.
    Pub. Hlth* **5**:398.
Farner, D. S. (1944): *U.S. Naval Med. Bull.* **42**:977.
Farner, D. S., & Bohart, R. M. (1945): *U.S. Naval Med. Bull.*, **44**:37.
Farooq, M. & Qutoobdin, M. (1946): *Indian Med. Gaz.* **81**:470.
Faust, E. C., Russel, P. F. & Jung, R. C. (1970): "Clinical Parasitology", 8th Ed. 890
    pp., Lea & Febiger, Philadelphia.
Fawdry, A. L. (1957): *Trans. Roy. Soc. Trop. Med. Hyg.* **51**:253.
Feldman (1904): *Arch. Schiffe-Tropenhyg.* **8**:285.
    (1905a): *Arch. Schiffs-Tropenhyg.* **9**:62.
    (1905b): *Arch. Schiffs-Tropen. Hyg.* **9**:540.
Feng, L. C. (1931a): *Chin. Med. J.* **17**:464.
    (1931b): *Amer. J. Hyg.* **14**:502.
    (1933a): *Chinese Med. J.* **47**:168.

Feng, L. C. (1933b): *Chinese Med. J.* **47**:1214.

               (1934): *Trans. 9th Congr. Far East Assoc. Trop. Med.* **1**:491.

               (1936): *Chinese Med. J.* **50**:Suppl. **1**:345.

Feng, L. C. & Yao, K. F. (1935): *Chinese Med. J.* **49**:794.

Fernando, S. E. (1935): *J. Trop. Med.* **38**:17.

Ferraz. D. M., Mello, A. L., & Rachou, R. G. (1958): *Rev. Bras. Malariol. D. Trop.* **10**: 275.

Ferreira, F. S. da C., Pinto, A. R. & de Almeida, C. L. (1948): *Ann. Inst. Med. Trop. Lisbon,* **5**; 223 pp. Abstracted in *Trop. Dis. Bull.,* **46**; 1105 pp.

Ferreira, F. S. C., Cunha, C. A. C. L., Vieira, R. A. & Matias, M. F. (1965a): *Anais Inst. Med. Trop.* **22**:75.

Ferreira, F. S. C., Matias, M. F., Cunha, C. C. I. & Vieira, R. A. (1965b): *Anais Inst. Med. Trop.* **23**:23.

Ferreira, M. O. & Ferraz, D. M. (1952a): *Rev. Brasil. Malariol. D. Trop.* **4**:65.

                             (1952b): *Rev. Brasil. Malariol. D. Trop.* **4**:413.

Ferreira, M. O., Rachou, R. G., Martins, C. M. & Ferreira Neto, J. A. (1955): *Rev Bras. Malariol D. Trop.* **7**:325.

Field, J. W. (1948): Stud. Inst. Med. Res. F. M. No. 23.

Fife, E. H. Jr. (1971): *Exp. Parasit.* **30**:132.

Figueroa-Marroquin, H. (1974): *Pan Amer. Hlth Org.* 100–4 pp.

Finlay, C. (1882–3): *An. re Acad. de Cien. Med. de la Habana,* **19**:40 (quoted by Mastin, 1888).

Finney, D. J. (1952): Probit Analysis. 2nd Edd., Cambridge Univ. Press.

Finucane, M. I. (1901): *Lancet,* **1**:23.

Fischer. O. (1932): *Arch. Schiffs-Tropen-Hyg.* **36**:Beiheft 1. 7.

Fisher, R. A. & Yates F. (1957): Statistical Tables for Biological, Agricultural and Medical Research. Oliver & Boyd. London, 138 pp.

Floch, H. & Abonnenc, E. (1949): *C. R. Soc. Biol.* **140**:1343.

Floch, H. & Lajudie, P., de. (1947): *Bull. Soc. Path. Exot.* **40**:49.

Flu, P. C. (1911): Filariaonderzoek in Suriname. (cited from Floch et Lajudie, 1947)

               (1918): *Geneesk. Tijdschr. Nederl.-Indie.* **58**:209.

               (1921): *Geneesk. Tijdschr. Nederl.-Indie.* **61**:317.

               (1929): *Geneesk. Tijdschr. Nederl.-Indie.* **69**:975.

Flynn, J. (1903): *Austr. Med. Gaz.* **22**:248.

Flynn, P. D. (1944): *U.S. Naval Med. Bull.,* **42**:1077.

Fontoynont & Leopold Robert (1909): *Soc. Sci. Méd. Madagascar,* A. **6**:63.

Foster, D. G. (1956): *J. Trop. Med. Hyg.* **59**:212.

Foster, R., Pringle, G., King, D. F. & Paris, J. (1969): *Ann. Trop. Med. Parasit.* **63**:95.

Fouques, M., Huet, R. Montangerand, Y. & Rochet, G. (1967): *Med. Trop.* (Marseille) **27**:252.

Fowler, J. L., Warne, R. J., Furusho, Y. & Sugiyama H. (1970): *Amer. J. Vet. Res.* **31**: 903.

Fowler, J. L., Furusho, Y. & Fernau, R. C. (1971): *Southeast Asian J. Trop. Med. Pub. Hlth* **2**:466.

Fraga de Azevedo, J. (1964): *Ann. Inst. Med. Trop.* **21**:312.

Fraga de Azevedo, J., Gandara, A. F. & Ferreira, A. P. (1958): *Anais Inst. Med. Trop.* **15**:235.

Fraga de Azevedo, J., Mouraõ, M. C., Salazar, J. M. C., Tendeiro, J. & Franco, L. T. A. (1960): *Anais Inst. Med. Trop.* **17**:621.

Fraga de Azevedo, J., Pinhõa, R., Meira, M. & Gardette, M. (1969): *Anis Escola Nac. Saude Publ. Med. Trop.* **3**:3.

Francis, E. (1919): *U.S. Hyg. Lab. Bull.* **117**:7.

Franco, O. & Lima, D. M. da S. (1967): *Revta Bras. Malar. D. Trop.* **19**:73.

Franco, L. T. A. & Mendes, A. (1955): *Anis Inst. Med. Trop.* **12**:359.

Franks, M. B. & Stoll, N. R. (1945): *J. Parasit.* **31**:158.

Franks, M. B., Chenoweth, B. M. & Stoll, N. R. (1947): *Amer. J. Trop. Med.* **27**:617.

Fredericks, H. J. & Ramachandran, C. P. (1969): Notes on immunization studies against filarial infections. *Proc. Seminar on Filariasis and Immunology of Parasitic Infections* (Singapore): 103–12 pp.

Freeman, P. (1973): Ceratopogonidae (Biting Midges), in Insects and other Arthropods of Medical Importance, (K. G. V. Smith, ed.) 181–8 pp., British Museum, London.

Freeman, P. & De Meillon, B. (1953): Simuliidae of the Ethiopian Region. 224 pp. London, British Museum (Nat. Hist.)

Frentzel-Beyme, R. (1973): *Zeit. Tropenmed. Parasit.* **24**:339.

Friedheim, E. A. H. (1961): *Ann. Soc. Belge de Med. Trop.* **41**:367.
                      (1962a): *Ann. Trop. Med. Parasitol.* **56**:337.
                      (1962b): *Ann. Trop. Med. Parasit.* **56**:343.
                      (1962d): *Trans. Roy. Soc. Trop. Med. Hyg.* **56**:236.
                      (1962d): *Ann. Trop. Med. Parasitol.* **56**:387.
                      (1963): *J. Trop. Med. Hyg.* (London) **66**:102.

Friedheim, E. A. H. & De Jongh, R. T. (1959): *Bull. Soc. Path. Exot.* **52**:785.
                      (1960): *Bull. Soc. Path. exot.* **53**:43.

Fros, J. (1956): *Documenta Med. Geogr. Trop.* **8**:63.

Fuglsang, H. & Anderson, J. (1973): *Lancet,* Aug. **11**:321.
                      (1974): *Trans. Roy. Soc. Trop. Med. Hyg.* **68**:72.
                      (1974): *J. Helminth.* **48**:93.

Fujisaki, T. (1958): *Nagasaki Igakkai Zasshi,* **33**: (suppl.) 1–77. (in Japanese)

Fujita, K. & Kobayashi, J. (1969a): *Japan. J. Exp. Med.* **39**:481.
                      (1969b): *Japan. J. Exp. Med.* **39**:585.

Fujita, K., Tanaka, H., Sasa, M., Schichinohe, K., Asai, Y. & Kurokawa, K. (1970): *Japan J. Exp. Med.* **40**:67.

Fülleborn, F. (1911): *Arch. Schiffs-Tropenhyg.,* **15**:368.
                      (1912): *Arch. Schiffs-Tropenhyg.* **16**:533.
                      (1913): *Arch. Schiffs-Tropenhyg.* **17** Beih: 1.
                      (1929): Filariosen des Menschen. In Kolle & Wassermann, Handbuch der pathogenen Mikroorganismen. 3 Aufl., VI, 1043–1224 pp.

Gabathuler, M. J. & Gabathuler, A. W. (1947): *East African Med. J.* **24**:188.

Galindo, L., Von Lichtenberg, F. & Baldizon, C. (1962): *Amer. J. Trop. Med. Hyg.* **11**:739.

Galliard, H. (1932): *Bull. Soc. Path. Exot.* **25**:167.
                      (1936a): *Bull. Soc. Med. Chir. Indoch.* **14**:439.
                      (1936b): *Rev. Med. Chir. Fr. d'Extr.-Or.* **14**:439.
                      (1937a): *Bull. Soc. Pathol. Exot.,* **39**:573.
                      (1937b): *Ann. Ecole Med. Phar. Hanoi,* 1935–1937, **1**:53
                      (1938): C. R. Soc. Biol. **128**:1111.
                      (1941): *Rev. Med. Franc. d'Extr.-Orient* **19**:420.
                      (1947): *C. R. Soc. Biol.* **141**:105.
                      (1949): *Bull. Acad. Med.* **122**:149.
                      (1957): *Bull. Wld. Hlth Org.* **16**:601.
                      (1959): *Bull. Soc. Path. Exot.* **52**:578.
                      (1971): *Bull. Soc. Path. Exot.,* **64**:340.

Galliard, H. & Brygoo, E. R. (1955): *Bull. Soc. Path. Exot.* **48**:473.

Galliard, H. & Chabaud, A. G. (1953): *Ann. Parasit. Hum. Comp.* **28**:287.

Galliard, H. & Mille, R. (1949a): *Bull. Acad. Nat. Med.* **133**:83.
                      (1949b): *Bull. Soc. Path. Exot.,* **42**:304.

Galliard, H. & Phiem, N. H. (1939): *Ann. Parasitol.* **17**:193.
                      (1940a): *Rev. Med. Fr. d'Extr.-Or.,* **18**:23.
                      (1940b): *Ann. Ecole Med. et Phar. Hanoi,* **4**:95.

Galliard, H. Huard, P. & Joyeux, B. (1942): *Rev. Med. Fr. d'Extr.-Or.,* **20**:543.

Galliard, H. Huard, P. & Ngu, D. V. (1942): *Ann. Fac. Med. et Phar. Hanoi,* **7**:67; **8**:73.
                      (1947): *Ann. Parasit.* **12**:332.

Galliard, H., Mille, R. & Robinson, W. H. (1949a): *Ann. Parasit. Hum. Comp.* **24**:30.
Galliard, H., Mille, R., & Robinson, W. A. (1949b): *Bull. Soc. Path. Exot.*, **42**:174.
Galliard, H., Brygoo, E. R. & Golvan, Y. (1955): *Ann. Parasit. Hum. Comp.* **30**:481.
Garcia, E. G., Cabrera, B. D. & Lara, E. D. (1968): *J. Philipp. Med. Ass.* **44**:149.
Garms, R. (1973): *Z. Tropenmed, Parasit.*, **24**:358.
Garms, R. and Post, A. (1966): *Z. Tropenmed. Parasit.*, **17**:443.
Garnham, P. C. C. & McMahon, J. P. (1947): *Bull. Entom. Res.* **37**:619.
Garnham, J. C. & Walliker, D. (1965): *Trans. Roy. Soc. Trop. Med. Hyg.*, **59**:672.
Garrat, E. L. (1945): *Trans. Roy. Soc. Trop. Med. Hyg.* **38**:287.
Gasparini, G. (1962): *Arch. Ital. Sci. Med. Trop. Paras.* **43**:635.
          (1964): *Arch. Ital. Sci. Med. Trop. Paras.* **45**:243.
Gault, E. W., Job, G. K. & Webb, J. G. (1960): *Indian J. Malariol.* **14**:633.
Gelfand, H. M. (1955): *Amer. J. Trop. Med. Hyg.* **4**:52.
Gelfand, M. & Bernberg, H. (1959): *Central African J. Med.* **5**:405.
Gelfand, M. & Wessels, P. (1964): *Trans. Roy. Soc. Trop. Med. Hyg.* **58**:552.
Gentilini, M. (1962): Les filarioses pathogènes de l'homme. Leur diagnostic et leur
     traitement actuel. 150 pp. Librairie Arnette, Paris.
Gentilini, M., Pinon, J. M., Niel, G. & Danis, M. (1972): *Bull. Soc. Path. Exot.* **65**:849.
George, M. J. (1963a): *Indian J. Malariol.* **17**:149.
          (1963b): *Indian J. Malariol.* **17**:269.
Gerbert, S. (1937): *Trans. Roy. Soc. Trop. Med. Hyg.* **30**:477.
Gerberich, J. B. & Laird, M. (1966): Annoted bibliography of papers relating to control
     of mosquitos by the use of fish. (Revised and enlarged to 1965). WHO/EBL/66.71
     (mimeogr.) 107 pp.
          (1968): Bibliography of papers relating to the control of
mosquitos by the use of fish. FAO Fisheries Tech. Paper No. 75.
Germain, A., André, L. & Marty, J. (1950): *Bull Soc. Path. Exot.* **43**:283.
Geukens (1950): *Ann. Soc. Belge Méd. Trop.* **30**:1483.
Ghosh, S. M. & Hati, A. K. (1963): *Bull. Calcutta Sch. Trop. Med.* **11**:146.
          (1966): *Bull. Calcutta Sch. Trop. Med.* **14**:9.
Gibbins, E. G. (1939): *East African Med. J.* **15**:378.
Gibbins, E. G. & Loewenthal, L. J. A. (1933): *Ann. Trop. Med. Parasitol.* **27**:489.
Gibson, C. L. (1950): *J. Parasitol.*, **36**:(suppl.) 29.
          (1952): Comparative Morphology of the Skin-inhabiting Microfilariae of
Man, Cattle and Equines in Guatemala. *Amer. J. Trop. Med. & Hyg.* **1**:250
Gibson, C. L. & Dalmat, H. T. (1952): *Amer. J. Trop. Med. Hyg.* **1**:848.
Giglioli, G. (1948a): *Amer. J. Trop. Med.* **28**:43.
          (1948b): *Amer. J. Trop. Med.* **28**:71.
          (1948c): *Medical Dpt. British Guiana.*
Giglioli, G. & Beadnell, H. M. S. G. (1960): *Indian J. Malariol.* **14**:651.
Giglioli, G., Rutten, F. J. & Ramjattan, S. (1967): *Bull. Wld Hlth Org.* **36**:283.
Gillies, M. T. (1958a): *Trop. Dis. Bull.* **55**:713.
          (1958b): *Ann. Trop. Med. Parasit.* **52**:261.
Gillies, M. T. & Wilkes, T. J. (1965): *Bull. Entom. Res.* **56**:237.
          (1969): *Bull. Entom. Res.*, **59**:441.
Glanser, F. (1945): *U.S. Naval Med. Bull.* **44**:21.
Goldman, L., & Ortiz, L. F. (1946): *Arch. Dermatol. & Syphilol.*, **53**:79.
Goldsmith (1899): Tropical diseases in northern Australia. *Trans. 5th Session Inter-
colonial Med. Congr. Australia,* Brisbane 1899:106.
Goldsmid, J. M. (1970): *J. Clin. Path.*, **23**:632.
Goldsmid, J. M., Mahomed, K. & Makanji, H. (1972): *South African Med. J.* **46**:171.
Gomperts, H. C. (1926): *Geneesk. Tijdschr. Nederl.-Indie.*, **66**:598.
Gonsalves, E. P. (1960): *Indian J. Malariol.* **14**:495.
Goodman, A. A., Weinberger, E. M., Lippincott, S. W., Marble, A. & Wright, W. H.
     (1945): *Annals Intern. Med.*, **23**:823.

Gooneratne, B. W. M. (1970): *J. Trop. Med. Hyg.*, **73**:174.
          (1971): (Correspondence) *Trans. Roy. Soc. Trop. Med. Hyg.*, **65**:406.
Gooneratne, B. W. M., Nelson, G. S., Denham, D. A., Furze, H. & Monson, E. (1971): *Trans. Roy. Soc. Trop. Med. Hyg.* **65**:195.
Gordon, R. M. (1955a): *Trans. Roy. Soc. Trop. Med. Hyg.*, **49**:98.
          (1955b): *Trans. Roy. Soc. Trop. Med. Hyg.*, **49**:496.
          (1956): *Ann. Trop. Med. Parasit.* **50**:319.
Gordon, R. M. & Crew, W. (1953): *Ann. Trop. Med. Parasit.* **47**:74.
Gordon, R. M. & Duke, B. O. L. (1955): *Trans. Roy. Soc. Trop. Med. Hyg.*, **49**:299.
Gordon, R. M. & Lumsden, W. H. R. (1939): *Ann. Trop. Med. Parasit.* **33**:259.
Gordon, R. M. & Webber, W. A. F. (1955): *Ann. Trop. Med. Parasit.* **49**:80.
Gordon, R. M., Hicks, E. P., Davey, T. H. & Watson, M. (1932): *Ann. Trop. Med. Parasit.* **26**:273.
Gordon, R. M., Chwatt, L. J. & Joues, C. M. (1948): *Ann. Trop. Med. Parasit.* **42**:364.
Gordon, R. M., Kershaw, W. E., Crewe, W. & Oldroyd, H. (1950): *Trans. Roy. Soc. Trop. Med. Hyg.* **44**:11.
Gordon, R., Ebsary, B. A. & Bennett, G. F. (1973): *Exp. Parasit.* **33**:226.
Grace, A., Grace, F. & Warren, S. (1932): *Amer. J. Trop. Med.* **12**:493.
Granbacka, P. (1973): *Trans. Roy. Soc. Trop. Med. Hyg.*, **67**:150.
Grant, A. M. B. (1933): *Med. J. Australia.* **1**:113.
Gratama, S. (1966): "Onchocerciasis in the South-Eastern territories of Liberia, with studies on the role of *Onchocerca volvulus* and *Wuchereria bancrofti* in the pathogenesis of hydrocele and elephantiasis." 135 pp. Booklet of illustrations and tables. 32 pp. Zwolle: N. V. Uitgeversmaatschappij W. E. J. Tjeenk Willink, Holland.
Gratama, S. (1969): *Trop. Geogr. Med.* **21**:269.
Green, C. A. (1972): *Ann. Trop. Med. Parasit.* **66**:143.
Grenier, P. & Ovazza, M. (1956): *Bull. Soc. Psath. Exot.* **49**:182.
Grenier, P., Hammon, J. & Rickenbach, A. (1955): *Bull. Soc. Path. Exot.* **48**:885.
Grjebine, A. (1955): *Madagascar méd.* **45**:280.
          (1956): *Bull. Wld Hlth Org.* **15**:593.
Grjebine, A. & Brygoo, E. R. (1958): *Mém. Inst. Rech. Scient. Madagascar* Série E. **9**:291.
Gros, H. (1892): *Arch. Méd. Nav.* **57**:365.
Grover, K. K. & Sharma, V. P. (1974): *J. Com. Dis.* **6**:91.
Gubler, D. J. & Bhattacharya, N. C. (1970): *Bull. Calcutta Sch. Trop. Med.* **18**:41.
          (1974): *Am. J. Trop. Med. Hyg.* **23**:1027.
Gubler, D. J., Inui, T. S., Black, H. R. & Bhattacharya, N. C. (1973): *Amer. J. Tropl Med. Hyg.* **22**:174.
Guerin, H. (1924): *Bull. Soc. Path. Exot.* **17**:397.
Guerin, H. & Le Chuiton (1923): *Bull. Soc. Med. Chir. Indoch.*, **110**:399.
Guiteras, J. (1886): *Med. News, N.Y.* **48**:399.
Gujral, J. S. (1958): *Indian J. Malariol.* **12**:101.
Gun Dzyan-Chzhan (1960): *Med. Parasit.* Moscow, **29**:98.
Gunther, F. A. & Blinn, R. C. (1955): Analysis of insecticides and acaricides. Interscience Pub. New York & London, 696 pp.
Guptavanij, P., Harinasuta, C., Sucharit, S. & Vutikes, S. (1971): *Southeast Asian J. Trop. Med. Pub. Hlth* **2**:44.
Guest, M. F. & Coauthors. (1968): *Med. J. Malaya.* **22**:248.
Guest, M. F., Kek, C. L., et al (1966): *Med. J. Malaya.*, **20**:325.
Guest, M. F., Wong, M. M. & Chin, L. Y. (1967): *Med. J. Malaya.* **21**:379.
Guptavanij, P., Harinasuta, C., Sucharit, S. & Vutikes, S. (1971): *Southeast Asian J. Trop. Med. Pub. Hlth* **2**:44.
Guttman, D. (1972): *J. Med. Entom.* **9**:269.

Guzman, R. V. (1933): Incidence of filarial infection among 980 male and female prisoners in Bilibid Prison. *Bull. San Juan de Dios Hospital* No. 7 (quoted by Rozeboom & Cabrera, 1956).

Haga, J. E. & van Edcke, F. J. (1889): *Geneesk. Tijdschr. Nederl.-Indie.,* **29**:109.

Haga, J. E. (1929): *Geneesk, Tijdschr. Nederl.-Indie.,* **69**:763.

Hairston, N. G. & Jachowski, L. A. (1968): *Bull. Wld Hlth Org.* **38**:29.

Hairston, N. G. & De Meilon, B. (1968): *Bull. Wld Hlth Org.* **38**:935.

Halawi, A., Baz, I. & Dawood, M. (1949): *J. Roy. Egypt. Med. Assoc.* **32**:395.

Hamilton, P. J. S., Marshall, T. F. C., Anderson, J. & Fuglsang, H. (1974): Observer variation in clinical onchocerciasis. *Trans. R. Soc. Trop. Med. Hyg.* **68**:187.

Hamon, J. & Dufour, G. (1954): *Bull. Wld. Hlth Org.* **11**:525.

Hamon, J., Burnett, G. F., Adam, J. P., Rickenbach, A. & Grjebine, A. (1967): *Bull. Wld Hlth Org.* **37**:217.

Harinasuta, C. (1969): Epidemiological methods in filariasis *Proc. 3rd S. E. Asian Regional Mtg on Parasit. Trop. Med.* (Singapore) 162–171 pp.

Harinasuta, C., Charoenlarp, P., Guptavanij, P. & Sucharit, S. (1964): *Ann. Trop. Med. Parasit.* **58**:315.

Harinasuta, C., Charoenlarp, P., Sucharit, S., Surathin, K. & Vutikes, S. (1970a): *Southeast Asian J. Trop. Med. Pub. Hlth* **1**:29.

Harinasuta, C., Guptavanij, P., Bell, D. R., Wilson, T., Ramachandran, C. P. & Sivanandam, S. (1970b): *Southeast Asian J. Trop. Med. Pub. Hlth* **1**:152.

Harinasuta, C., Charoenlarp, P., Guptavanij, P., Sucharit, S., Deesin, T., Surathin, K. & Vutikes, S. (1970c): *Southeast Asian J. Trop. Med. Pub. Hlth* **1**:205.

Harinasuta, C., Sucharit, S., Deesin, T., Surathin, K. & Vutikes, S. (1970d): *Southeast Asian J. Trop. Med. Pub. Hlth.* **1**:233.

Harley-Mason, R. J. (1939): *East African Med. J.* **15**:363.

Harper, P. A., Lisansky, E. T. & Sasse, B. E. (1947): *Amer. J. Trop. Med.,* 27:Suppl. No. 3:1.

Harris, B. P. (1940): *Trans. Roy. Soc. Trop. Med. Hyg.* **34**:233.

Harris, J. S. & Summers, W. A. (1945): *Amer. J. Trop. Med.* **25**:497.

Haseeb, M. A., Satti, M. H. & Sherif, M. (1962): *Bull. Wld Hlth Org.* **27**:609.

Hassan, M. Y. bin (1959): *Med. J. Malaya.* **14**:36.

Huard, P. (1941): *Rev. Med. Fran. Extr.-Orient* **19**:768.

Hausermann, W. (1966): *Acta trop.* **23**:365.

Hawking, F. (1939): *Trans. Roy. Soc. Trop. Med. Hyg.* **33**:95.

  (1940a): *Ann. Trop. Med. Parasit.* **34**:107.

  (1940b): *Ann. Trop. Med. Parasit.* **34**:211.

  (1940c): *J. Trop. Med. and Hyg.,* **43**:204.

  (1950): *Trans. Roy. Soc. Trop. Med. & Hyg.* **44**:153.

  (1952): *Brit. Med. J.* **1**:992.

  (1954): *Ann. Trop. Med. Parasitol.,* **48**:382.

  (1955a): *Trans. Roy. Soc. Trop. Med. & Hyg.* **49**:132.

  (1955b): *Pharmacol. Rev.* **7**:279.

  (1957): *Bull. Wld. Hlth. Org.* **16**:581.

  (1958): *Trans. Roy. Soc. Trop. Med. Hyg.* **52**:109.

  (1960): *Ind. J. Malariol.* **14**:567.

  (1962): *Bull. Wld Hlth Org.* **27**:555.

  (1963): *Experimental Chemotherapy* 1:893–912 Acad. Press., New York & London. 1008 pp.

  (1966a): *Experimental Chemotherapy,* **4**:47.

  (1966b): Chemotherapy of filariasis. In: *Progress in Drug Research,* vol. 9, pp. 190–222; Jucker, E. (ed.), Birkhäuser Verlag, Basel & Stuttgart.

  (1967): *Proc. Roy. Soc. Biol.* **169**:59.

  (1973a): Chemotherapy of tissue nematodes, in 'Chemotherapy of Helminthiasis', vol. 1, 437–500 pp., Pergamon Press, Oxford.

Hawking, F. (1973b): The distribution of human filariasis throughout the world. Part two; Asia. WHO/FIL/73:114; 55pp. (mimeogr.)

     (1973c): The distribution of human filariasis throughout the World. Part III. Africa. WHO/FIL/INF/73.3, 34 pp. (mimeogr.)

     (1973d): The distribution of human filariasis throughout the world. Part IV. America (A summary). WHO/FIL/INF/73.2; 4 pp. (mimeogr.)

Hawking, F. & Adams, W. E. (1964): *Soc. Belge Méd. Trop.* **44**:279.

Hawking, F. & Denham, D. A. (1971): The distribution of human filariasis throughout the world. Part 1. The Pacific Region, including New Guinea. WHO/FIL/71.94; 31 pp. (mimeogr.)

Hawking, F. & Joao Marques, R. (1967): *Bull. Wld Hlth Org.* **37**:405.

Hawking, F. & Sewell, P. (1948): *Brit. J. Pharmacol.* **3**:285.

Hawking, F., Sewell, P. & Thurston, J. P. (1950): *Brit. J. Pharmacol.* **5**:217.

Hawking, F., Patanayak, S. & Sharma, H. L. (1966): *Trans. Roy. Soc. Trop. Med. Hyg.* **60**:497.

Hawking, F., Moor, P., Gammage, K. & Worms, M. J. (1967): *Trans. Roy. Soc. Trop. Med. Hyg.,* **61**:674.

Hayashi, S. (1954): *Eisei Dobutsu (Japan. J. Sanitary Zool.)* **4**:(Suppl.) 41. (in Japanese)

     (1955): *Nisshin Igaku* **42**:1.

     (1959): *Japan. J. Parasitol.,* **8**:904.

     (1962): *Japan. J. Expt. Med.,* **32(1)**:13.

Hayashi, S. & Kurihara, T. (1965): *Japan. J. Sanitary Zool.* **16**:29.

Hayashi, S. & Tanaka, H. (1965): *Japan. J. Parasit.* **14**:15.

Hayashi, S., Sasa, M., Kano, R. & Sato, K. (1951): *Nisshin Igaku* **38**:20.

Hayashi, S., Sasa, M., Tanaka, H. & Ishii, S. (1954): *Nihon Ishikai Zasshi* **31**:485.

Hayashi, S., Sato, K. & Osada, Y. (1959): *Japan. J. Parasitol.,* **8**:895.

Hayashi, S., Yamamoto, H. & Kurihara, T. (1965a): *Japan. J. Sanitary Zool.* **16**:34.

Hayashi, S., Kurihara, T. & Saito, K. (1965b): *Japan. J. Sanitary Zool.* **16**:110.

Hayashi, S., Hori, E., Motoyoshi, K., Hirano, S., Fujita, K., Kawai, J. & Motoi, E. (1967): *Japan. J. Parasit.* **16**:278.

Heckenroth, F., Bécuwe, R., Mayan, L. & Leroux, G. (1950): *Bull. Soc. Path. Exot.* **43**:354.

Heim, B. & Callot, J. (1969): *Bull. Soc. Path. Exot.* **62**:722.

Heisch, R. B. (1948): *East African Med. J.* **25**:3.

Heisch, R. B., Nelson, G. S. & Furlong, M. (1959): *Trans. Roy. Soc. Trop. Med. Hyg.* **53**:41.

Heisch, R. B., Goiny, H. H. & Ikata, M. (1956): *Trans. Roy. Soc. Trop. Med. Hyg.* **50**:420.

Helfrich, C. (1860): "Schets eener geneeskundige plaats-beschrijving van de Z. en O.-kust van Borneo.," Geneesk, Tijdschr. Ned.-Ind., **9**:321.

Henrard, C. & Peel, E. (1949): *Ann. Soc. Belge Med. Trop.* **29**:127.

Henrard, C., Peel, E. & Wanson, M. (1946): *Rec. Sci. Méd. Congo Belge* **5**:213.

Herbert, E. W., Meyer, R. P. & Turbes, P. G. (1972): *Mosquito News* **32**:212.

Hernandez Morales, F. & Oliver Gonzalez, J. (1946a): *Puerto Rico J. Pub. Hlth Trop. Med.* **22**:95.

Hernandes Morales, F., Gonzales Barrientos, G. (1946b): *Puerto Rico J. Pub. Hlth Trop. Med.* **22**:99.

Herrman, R. & Genevray, J. (1925): *Bull. Soc. Path. Exot.* **18**:651.

Hertwig, F. & Oberdoerster, F. (1961): *Zeit. Tropenmed. Parasit.,* **12**:41.

Hewitt, R. I., Wallace, W. S., White, E., & Subbarow, Y. (1947a): *J. Lab. Clin. Med.* **32**:1293.

Hewitt, R. I., White, E., Wallace, W. S., Stewart, H. W., Kushner, S., & Subbarow, Y. (1947b): *J. Lab. Clin. Med.* **32**:1304.

Hewitt, R. I., Kushner, S., Stewart, H. W., White, E., Wallace, W. S., & Subbarow, Y. (1947c): *J. Lab. Clin. Med.* **23**:1314.

Hewitt, R. I., White, D. E., Kushner, S., Wallace, W. S., Stewart, H. W., & Subbarow, Y. (1948): *Ann. N. Y. Acad. Sci.* **50**:128.

Hewitt, R., Kenney, H., Chan, A. & Mohamed, H. (1950): *Amer. J. Trop. Med.* **30**:217.

Heydon, G. M. (1931): *Parasitology* **23**:415.

Hicks, E. P. (1932): *Ann. Trop. Med. Parasit.* **26**:407.

Higashi, G. I. & Chowdhury, A. B. (1970): *Immunology* **19**:65.

Higashi, G. I., Dastidar, B. G. & Chowdhury, A. B. (1968): *Bull. Calcutta Sch. Trop. Med.,* **16**:7.

Hinz, E. (1970): *Tropenmed. Parasit.* **19**:245.

Hirakoso, S. (1966a): *Eisei Dobusu (Japan. J. Sanitary Zool.)* **17**:59.

    (1966b): *Eisei Dobutsu (Japan. J. Sanitary Zool.)* **17**:236.

    (1968): *Japan. J. Exp. Med.* **38**:327.

    (1969): *Japan. J. Exp. Med.* **39**:17.

Herakoso, S. & Uchida, M. (1966): *Eisei Dobutsu (Japan. J. Sanitary Zool.)* **17**:196.

Hirata, T. (1939): *Tokyo Ijishinshi* **3137**:1489.

    (1940): *Tokyo Ijishinshi,* **3178**:653.

Hirsch (1886): Handbook of geographical and historical pathology.

Hissette, J. (1931): *Ann. Soc. Belge Méd. Trop.* **11**:45.

    (1932): *Ann. Soc. Belge Méd. Trop.* **12**:433.

Hitchcock, J. C., Jr. (1969): *Proc. New Jers. Mosq. Exterm. Ass.,* **56**:116.

    (1971): *Trans. R. Soc. Trop. Med. Hyg.,* **65**:408.

Hitchcock, J. C., Jr. & Lewis, W. P. (1970): *Trans. Roy. Soc. Trop. Med. Hyg.* **64**:311.

Ho, B. C. & Ewert, A. (1967): *Trans. Roy. Soc. Trop. Med. Hyg.* **61**:663.

Ho Thi Sang & Petithory, J. (1963): *Bull. Soc. Path. Exot.* **56**:197.

Hocking, B. (1967): *Bull. Wld. Hlth. Org.* **37**:323.

Hocking, B. & Hocking, J. M. (1962): *Bull. Wld Hlth Org.* **27**:465.

Hodge, I. G., Denhoff, E., & Vanderveer, J. V. (1945): *Amer. J. Med. Sci.* **210**:207.

Hodgkin, E. P. (1940): *Trans. 10th Congr. Far-East Ass. Trop. Med.* Hanoi, 1938, **2**:617.

Hoeppli, R., & Gunders, A. E. (1962): *Amer. J. Trop. Med. & Hyg.* **11**:234.

Hoeven, J. A. vender (1952): *Docum. Med. Geogr. Trop.* **4**:107.

Hoffmann, C. C. (1930): *Arch. Schiffs Tropenhyg.,* **34**:461.

    (1932): *An. Inst. Biol.* **1**:55.

Hoffman, W. A., Marin, R. A. & Burke, A. M. B. (1932): *Puerto Roco J. Pub. Hlth. Trop. Med.* **7**:321.

Holmes, G. K. T., Gelfand, M., Boyt, W. & McKenzie, P. (1969): *Trans. Roy. Soc. Trop. Med. Hyg.* **63**:479.

Holstein, M. H. (1954): *Org. Mon. Ser.* **9**:172.

Van Hoof, L. (1934): *Trans. Roy. Soc. Trop. Méd. Hyg.* **27**:609.

Van Hoof, L., Henrard, C., Peel, E. & Wanson, M. (1947): *Annls Soc. Belge Méd. Trop.* **27**:173.

Hopkins, C. A. (1952): *Ann. Trop. Med. Parasit.* **46**:165.

Hopkins, C. A. & Nicholas, W. L. (1952): *Ann. Trop. Med. Parasit.* **46**:276.

Hopla, C. E. (1946): *Mosquito News,* **6**:189.

Hori, E. (1960): *Kagoshima Univ. Med. Jour.* **12**:21. (in Japanese)

Horsefall, W. R. (1955): Mosquitoes. Their bionomics and relation to disease. Ronald Press Co. New York; 723 pp.

Howard, R. (1918): *J. Trop. Med. Hyg.* **11**:57.

Hsieh, S. C., Yu-Kun Liu. & Liu, J. (1960): *Chinese Med. J.* (Peking) **80**:166.

Hsu Wei-nan (1958): *Acta Unv. Nanekinensis Sci. Nat.* (2):101 (Abstract in *Chinese Med. J.* **79**:97, 1959)

Hu, M. K., Wong, H. & Li, B. C. (1937): *Chinese Med. J.* **52**:571.

Hu, S. K. M. (1934): *Chinese Med. J.* **48**:1143.

Hu, S. M. K. (1935): *Peking Natural History Bull.* **9**:249.

Huard, P. (1941): *Rev. Med. Fr. Extr. -Or.,* **19**:768.

Hubble, D. R. & Reiff, B. (1967): *Bull. Envir. Contam. Toxicol.* **2**:57.

Huehns, E. R. (1953): *Trans. Roy. Soc. Trop. Med. Hyg.* **47**:549.

Hughens, H. V. (1927): *U.S. Naval med Bull.* **25**:111.

Hughes, M. H. (1952): *West African Med. J.* **1**:16.

Hughes, M. H. & Daly, P. F. (1951): *Trans. Roy. Soc. trop. Med. Hyg.* **45**:243.

Hunter, C. W., III, Ritchie, L. S. & Chang, I. C. (1949): *J. Parasitology* **35**(Suppl):41.

Huntington, R. W., Jr. (1945): *U.S. Naval Med. Bull.* **44**:707.

        (1949): Acute allergic filariasis (mumu) in troops in American Samoa during World War II. *Proc. 7th Pacific Science Congress,* New Zealand.

Huntington, R. W., Fogel R. H., Eichold, S., & Dickson, J. G. (1944): *Yale J. Biol. & Med.* **6**:529.

Husain, A. & Kershaw, W. E. (1971): *Trans. Roy. Soc. Trop. Med. Hyg.* **65**:617.

Hwang, C. H., Kahn, C. M., Lee, C. S., Song, J. S. & Hong (1965): *Korean Central J. Med.* **9**:491.

Hynes, H. B. N., Williams, T. R. & Kershaw, W. E. (1961): *Ann. Trop. Med. Parasit* **55**:197.

Ikeshoji, T. (1971): Oviposition behavior of *Culex pipiens* and the attractants. *in* Sasa, M. (de.), Progress of Medical Zoology, vol. 1, 67–76 pp. (Gakujutsusho Shuppan-kai, Tokyo).

Ikeshoji, T., Hirokoso, S., & Suzuki, T. (1958): *Japan. J. Sanitary Zool.* **9**:302.

Ikeshoji, T., Sasa, M. & Osada, Y. (1959): *Japan. J. Sanitary. Zool.* **10**:188.

Indian Council of Medical Research (1961): Report of the Assessment Committee on the National Filaria Control Programme, India. 116 pp. (New Delhi)

        (1971): Assessment of the National Filaria Control Programme (India), 1961–1970, 156 pp. (New Delhi)

Indrayan, A., Srivastava, R. N. & Bagchi, S. C. (1970): *Indian J. Med. Res.* **58**:1100.

Ingram, R. L. (1954): *Amer. J. Hyg.* **60**:169.

Ishii, A. (1970): *Japan. J. Exp. Med.,* **40**:39.

Ishii, A. & Tanaka, H. (1968): *Japan. J. Parasit.* **17**:509.

Ishii, A., Tanaka, H., Fujita, K., Kamiya, M., Matsuda, H. & Kobayashi, J. (1968): *Japan. J. Parasit.* **17**:402.

Ishii, A., Matsuda, H., Kamiya, M. & Kobayashi, J. (1969): *Japan. J. Parasit.* **18**:1.

Ishizaki, T., Kutsumi, H., Kumada, M. & Komiya, Y., Araki, H., Nozaki, S. & Miyashita, Y. (1960): *Japan. J. Parasit.* **9**:692.

Ishizaki, T., Kutusumi, H., Kumada, M., Hatano, S., Koito, K., Yatabe, T. & Tsujitani, J. (1963): *Japan. J. Parasit.* **12**:82.

Ishizaki, T., Kutsumi, H., Akusawa, M., Kajino, M., Takahashi, H. & Hamada, Y. (1964): *Japan. J. Parasit.* **13**:149.

Islam, N. (1962): *J. Trop. Med. Hyg.* **65**:260.

Ismail, M. M. & Wijayaratnam, Y. (1965): *Ceylon J. Med. Sci.* **14**:36.

Israel, M. S. (1959): *Trans. Roy. Soc. trop. Med. Hyg.* **53**:142.

Iwamoto, I. (1971): *Trop. Med.,* **13**:1. (In Japanese)

Iwamoto, I., Tada, I. & Wonde, T. (1973): *Tropical Med.* (Nagasaki), **15**:36.

Iyengar, M. O. T. (1932): *Indian J. Med. Res.* **20**:671.

        (1933): *Indian J. Med. Res.* **20**:921.

        (1938): *Indian Med. Res. Memoirs* **30**:179.

        (1941): *Indian J. Med. Res.* **29**:677.

        (1949): A report on filariasis in Ceylon (unpublished report quoted by Abdulcader, 1962).

        (1952): *Bull. Wld Hlth Org.* **7**:375.

        (1953): *Bull. Wld Hlth Org.* **9**:731.

        (1954a): Preliminary report on an investigation on filariasis in New Caledonia. Report to South Pacific Commission, Feb. 1954.

        (1954b): Filariasis in New Caledonia. A report on and investigation in Nassirah Village. Report to South Pacific Commission Aug. 25, 1954.

        (1954c): A scheme for filariasis control in Western Samoa (Report to

South Pacific Commission, quoted by Iyengar, 1959).

   (1954d): Distribution of filariasis in the South Pacific Region. South Pacific Comm. Tech. Paper No. 66, 52 pp.

   (1954e): Annoted bibliography of filariasis and elephantiasis. Part 1. Epidemiology of filariasis in the South Pacific Region. South Pacific Comm. Tech. Paper No. 65, 63 pp.

   (1956a): *Ann. Parasitol.* **31**:99;266.

   (1956b): *South Pacific Comm. Tech. Paper* **88**:114.

   (1957a): *South Pacific Comm. Tech. Inf. Circ.* **21**:15.

   (1957b): Annoted bibliography on filariasis and elepahantiasis. Part 3. Symptomatology, aetiology, pathology and diagnosis of filariasis due to *Wuchereria bancrofti* and *W. malayi.* South Pacific Comm. Tech. Paper No. 109: 276 pp., (1959a) suppl. No. 1, 25pp.

   (1959b): Annoted bibliography of filariasis and elephantiasis. Part 4. Treatment. South Pacific Comm. Tech. Paper No. 124: 177 pp.

   (1959c): A review of the literature on the distribution and epidemiology of filariasis in the South Pacific Region. South Pacific Comm. Tech. Paper No. 126, 172 pp. Noumea, New Caledonia.

   (1959d): Filariasis in Netherlands New Guinea. South Pacific Commission Techn. Inf., No. 34.

   (1959e): Filariasis in American Samoa. South Pacific Comm. Techn. Inf. Circ. No. 35.

   (1960a): Annoted bibliography of filariasis and elephantiasis. Part 5. Prophylaxis and control of filariasis due to *Wuchereria bancrofti* and *W. malayi.* South Pacific Comm. Tech. Paper No. 129: 102 pp.

   (1960b): A review of the mosquito fauna of the South Pacific. (Diptera, Culicidae). South Pacific Comm. Tech. Paper No. 130: 102 pp.

   (1965): Epidemiology of filariasis in the South Pacific. South Pacific Comm. Tech. Paper No. 148 183 pp. (mimeogr.) South Pacific Commission, Noumea, New Caledonia.

Iyengar, M. O. T. & Menon, M. A. U. (1955): *Bull. Entom. Res.* **46**:1.

   (1956): Studies on filariasis in New Caledonia. South Pacific Comm. Techn. Inf. Circ. No. 15, March 1956.

Iyenger, M. O. T., de Rook, H. & van Dijk, W.J.O.M. (1959): *Trop. Geogr. Med.,* **11**:287.

Jachowski, L. A., Jr. (1954): *Amer. J. Hyg.* **60(2)**:186.

Jachowski, L. A. Jr & Otto, G. F. (1952): *Amer. J. Trop. Med. Hyg.* **1**:662.

   (1953): *U.S. Naval Med. Res. Inst. Res. Rep.* **869**:

   (1955): *Amer. J. Hyg.* **61**:334.

Jachowski, L. A. Jr., Otto, G. F., & Wharton, J. D. (1950): *J. Parasitol.,* 36(Suppl.): 34.

Jachowski, L. A. Jr., Gonzales-Flores; B. & Lichtenberg, F. V. (1962): *Amer. J. Trop. Med. Hyg.* **11**:220.

Jackson, R. B. (1936): *Chinese Med. J.* **50**:1767.

Jackson, R. E. (1949): *J. Amer. Vet. Med. Assoc.* **115**:17.

Jaffe, J. J. & Doremus, H. M. (1970): *J. Parasit.* **56**:254.

Jamison, D. G. & Kershaw, W. E. (1956): *Ann. Trop. Med. Parasit.* **50**:415.

Jamison, D. G., Kershaw, W. E., Duke, B. O. L. & Fejer, E. A. (1955): *Ann. Trop. Med. Parasit.* **49**:227.

Janssens, P. G. (1952): *Ann. Soc. Belge Med. Trop.* **32**:229.

Janssens, P. G., Van Bogaert, L., Tverdy, G., & Wanson, M. (1958): *Bull. Soc. Path. Exot.* **51**:632.

Jaswant Singh. (1956): *Indian J. Malariol.* **10**:117.

Jaswant Singh & Bhattacharji, L. M. (1944): *Indian Med. Gaz.* **79**:102.

Jaswant Singh & Misra, B. G. (1956): *Indian J. Malariol.* **10**:115.

Jaswant Singh & Raghavan, N. G. S. (1950): *Indian J. Malariol.* **4**:347.

786   REFERENCES

Jaswant Singh & Raghavan, N. G. S. (1957): *Bull. Nat. Soc. India Malaria Mosq. Dis.*
    5:35.
Jaswant Singh, Raghavan, N. G. S. & Krishnaswami, A. K. (1956a): *Indian J. Malariol.*
    10:219.
Jaswant Singh, Krishnaswami, A. K., Raghavan, N. G. S. & Krishnamurthy, B. S.
    (1956b): *Indian J. Malariol.* **10**:239.
Jaswant Singh, Krishnaswami, A. K. & Raghavan, N. G. S. (1956c): *Indian J. Malariol.*
    10:317.
Jayewardene, L. G. (1962): *J. Helminth.* **36**:269.
                    (1963): *Ann. Trop. Med. Parasit.* **57**:359.
Jeffery, W. H. & Maxwell, J. L. (1911): The diseases of China. Philadelphia
Jelliffe, D. B., Jones, P. R. M. & Stroud, C. E. (1962): *Trop. Geogr. Med.* **14**:97.
Jenkins, D. W. (1964): *Bull. Wld Hlth Org.* **30**:(suppl.) 5.
Jirovec, O. & Havlic, O. (1960): *Wiad. Parazyt.* (Warsaw) **6**:81.
Jissette, J. (1938): *Amer. J. Trop. Med.* **18**:Suppl. 58.
Johnson, F. B. (1915): *Southern Med. J.* **8**:630.
Johnson, P. A. G. (1944): *U.S. Naval Med. Bull.* **43**:950.
Johnson, D. S. & Soong, M. H. H. (1963): *Proc. XVI Intern. Congr. Zool.* **1**:246.
Jones, V. E. & Edwards, A. J. (1967): Rare severe toxic effects of mel W (Idiosyncrasy):
    A possible relation to delayed type hypersensitivity. WHO/Fil/67. 70, 6 pp.
Jones, H. L., Jr., Srivastava, P., Shrestha, B. L. & Mack, G. J. (1970): *J. Nepal Med.
    Ass.,* **8**:141.
Joon-Wah, M., Singh, D., Sukoharyono, J. & Sivanandam, S. (1974): *Southeast Asian
    J. Trop. Med. Pub. Hlth.* **5**:226.
Joon-Wah, M., Zaman, V. & Sivanandam, S. (1974): *Amer. J. Trop. Med. Hyg.* **23**:369.
Jordan, P. (1952): *Trans. Roy. Soc. Trop. Med. Parasit.* **44**:207.
            (1953): *East African Med. J.* **30**:361.
            (1954a): *East African. Med. J.* **31**:537.
            (1954b): *J. Trop. Med. Hyg.* **57**:8.
            (1955a): *East African Med. J.* **32**:15.
            (1955b): *Ann. Trop. Med. Parasit.* **49**:42.
            (1955c): *Trans. Roy. Soc. Trop. Med. Hyg.* **49**:271.
            (1955d): *Trans. Roy. Soc. Trop. Med. Hyg.* **49**:460.
            (1956a): *East African Med. J.* **33**:237.
            (1956b): *East African Med. J.* **33**:233.
            (1957): *Central Africa J. Med.* **3**:18.
            (1959a): *Ann. Trop. Med. Parasit.* **53**:42.
            (1959b): *J. Trop. Med. Hyg.* (London) **62**:286.
            (1960a): *Brit. Med. J.* **5178**:1020.
            (1960b): *Ann. Trop. Med. Parasitol.,* **54**:132.
            (1960c): *Indian. J. Malriol.* **14**:353.
Jordan, P. & Goatly, K. D. (1962): *Ann. Trop. Med. Parasitol.* **56**:173.
Jordan, P., Trant, M. H. & Laurie, W. (1956): *Brit. Med. J.* **1**:209.
Joseph, A. (1971): *Indian J. Publ. Hlth* **15**:103.
Joseph, C., & Peethambaran, P. (1963): *Indian J. Malariol.* **17**:33.
Joseph, C. & Prasad, B. G. (1967): *Indian J. Med. Res.* **55**:1259.
Joseph C., Menon, M. A. U. & Nair, G. K. (1960): *Indian J. Malariol.* **14**:663.
Joseph, C., Menon, M. A. U., Unnithan, K. R. & Raman, S. (1963): *Indian J. Malariol.*
    17:311.
Joshi, V. V., Udwadia, F. E. & Gadgil, R. K. (1969): *Amer. J. Trop. Med. Hyg.* **18**:231.
Juminer, B., Diallo, S. & Diagne, S. (1971a): *Arch. Inst. Pasteur Tunis,* **48**:231.
                            (1971b): *Arch Inst. Pasteur Tunis.* **48**:247.
Jung, R. K. (1973): *J. Nepal Med. Assoc.* **11**:155.
Jurgens, A. L. (1932): *Geneesk. Tijdschr. Nederl.-Indie.* **72**:953.
Kachroo, P. & Sharma, J. C. (1958): *Indian J. Malariol.* **12**:253.

Kagan, I. G. (1963): *J. Parasit.* **49**:773.

Kagan, I. G., Norman, L. & Allain, D. S. (1963): *Amer. J. Trop. Med. Hyg.,* **12**:548.

Kalra, N. L., Watal, B. L. & Raghavan, N.G.S. (1967): *Bull. Indian. Soc. Mal. Com. Dis.* **4**:253.

Kanda, T. (1963): *Japan. J. Parasit.* **12**:390. (in Japanese)

Kanda, T. & Ishii, A. (1966): *Jap. J. Trop. Med.* **7**:36.

Kanda, T. & Tasaka, S. (1966a): *Japan. J. Parasit.* **15**:138.
                        (1966b): *Japan. J. Parasit.* **15**:155.

Kanda, T., Kurihara, T. & Kato, K. (1964): *Japan. J. Parasitol.* **13**:70.

Kanda, T., Sasa, M., Kato, K. & Kawai, J. (1967a): *Japan. J. Exp. Med.* **37**:141.

Kanda, T., Tasaka, S. & Sasa, M. (1967b): *Japan. J. Exp. Med.* **37**:149.

Kanda, T., Choi, D.W. & Jyu, S. S. (1974): *Japan. J. Parasit.* **23**:(Suppl.) 53 (Abstract).

Kaneko, K., Saito, K. & Wonde, T. (1973): *Japan. J. Sanitary Zool.* **24**:175.

Kang, S. Y., Ryang, Y. S., Lee, S. H. & Seo, B. S. (1973): *Korean J. Parasit.* **11**:(Suppl). 125 (Abstract).

Kant, L., Sen, S. K. & Puri, B. S. (1956): *Indian J. Malariol.* **10**:199.

Kariadi (1937): *Geneesk. Tijdschr. Nederl.-Indie.,* **77**:912.
       (1938): *Geneesk. Tijdschr. Nederl.-Indie.* **78**:1127.
       (1941): *Geneesk. Tijdschr. Nederl.-Indie.* **81**:107.

Kartman, L. (1946): *J. Parasit.* **32**:91.
            (1953): *J. Parasit.* **39**:571.
            (1954): *Amer. J. Trop. Med. Hyg.* **3**:329.

Katamine, D. (1953): *Nagasaki Igakkai Zasshi* **27**:201. (in Japanese).
            (1962): *Endemic Dis. Bull.* (Nagasaki) **4**:166.
            (1969): *Trop. Med.* (Nagasaki) **11**:1.
            (1970): Studies on the periodicity of microfilaria. In Sasa, M. (ed.) "Recent Advances in Researches on Filariasis and Schistosomiasis in Japan," 123–44 pp. (Univ. Tokyo Press).

Katamine, D., Tamura, Y. & Moriguchi, Y. (1952a): *Nagasaki Igakkai Zasshi* **27**:232 (in Japanese).

Katamine, D., Tamura, Y. Kitamura, S. & Moriguchi, Y. (1952b): *Nihon Hinyokika Gakkai Zasshi* **43**:206 (in Japanese).

Katamine, D., Murakuni, J., Harada, T., Nakabayashi, T. & Suenaga, O. (1967): *Trop. Med.* (Nagasaki) **9**(3):143.

Katamine, D., Imai, J., Tada, I., Sato, A & Otsuji, Y. (1970): On the epidemiological application of skin tests with FPT antigen in endemic areas of bancroftian filariasis. In Sasa, M. (ed.) "Recent Advances in Researches on Filariasis and Schistosomiasis in Japan." 159–68 pp. (Univ. Tokyo Press).

Katamine, D., Aoki, K.,Wada, Y., Sato, A., Tada, I., Fukushima, H., Seo, B. S., Rim, H. J. & Lee, S. H. (1971): *Japan. J. Parasit.* **20**:289.

Katamine, D., Sato, A., Tada, I. & Aoki, Y. (1973): *Japan. J. Trop. Med. Hyg.* **1**:189.

Katiyar, J. C., Chandara, R., Chandra, S., Govila, P., George, P. A. & Sen, A. B. (1973): *Indian J. Med. Res.,* **61**:1087.

Katiyar, J. C., Govila, P., Sen, A. B. & Chandra, R. (1974): *Trans. Roy. Soc. Trop. Med. Hyg.* **68**:169.

Kaul, H. N. & Wattal, B. L. (1968): *Bull. Indian Soc. Malaria Comm. Dis.* **5**:45.

Kenney, M. & Hewitt, R. (1949): *Amer. J. Trop. Med.* **29**:89.

Kerrest, J. M. (1952): *South Pacific Comm. Quarterly Bull.,* **2**:34; *Med. Trop.,* **5**:568.

Kershaw, W. E. (1950): *Ann. Trop. Med. Parasit.* **44**:361.
            (1951): *Ann. Trop. Med. Parasit.* **45**:261.
            (1953): *Trans. Roy. Soc. Trop. Med. Hyg.* **47**:4(Nigeria).
            (1955): *Trans. Roy. Soc. Trop. Med. Hyg.* **49**:143.
            (1961): Report on visit to filariasis endemic areas in Ceylon. WHO/SEA/Fil/2.

Kershaw, W. E. & Duke, B. O. L. (1954c): *Ann. Trop. Med. Parasit.* **49**:340.

788   REFERENCES

Kershaw, W. E. & Nicholas, W. L. (1954): *Ann. Trop. Med. Parasit.* **48**:110.
Kershaw, W. E. & Williamson, J. (1952): *Ann. Trop. Med. Parasit.* **46**:268.
Kershaw, W. E., Zahra, A., Pearson, A. F., Budden, F. H. & Caucki, F. J. (1953a): *Trans. Roy. Soc. Trop. Med. Hyg.* **47**:4.
Kershaw, W. E., Lavoipierre, M. M. J. & Chalmers, T. A. (1953b): *Ann. Trop. Med. Parasit.* **47**:207.
Kershaw, W. E., Keay, R. W. J., Nicholas, W. L. & Zahra, A. (1953c): *Ann. Trop. Med. Parasit.* **47**:406.
Kershaw, W. E., Crew, W. & Beeslay, W. N. (1954a): *Ann. Trop. Med. Parasit.* **48**:102.
Kershaw, W. E., Duke, B. O. L. & Budden, F. H. (1954b): *Trans. Roy. Soc. Trop. Med. Hyg.* **48**:287.
Kershaw, W. E., Chalmers, T. A. & Duke, B. O. L. (1954c): *Ann. Trop. Med. Parasit.* **48**:329.
Kershaw, W. E., Duke, B. O. L. & Budden, F. H. (1954d): *Brit. Med. J.* **2**:724
Kershaw, W. E., Plackett, R. L. & Beesley, W. N. (1955a): *Ann. Trop. Med. Parasit.* **49**:66.
Kershaw, W. E., Beesley, W. N. & Crew, W. (1955b): *Ann. Trop. Med. Parasit.* **49**:114.
Kershaw, W. E., Lavoipierre, M. M. J. & Beesley, W. N. (1955c): *Ann. Trop. Med. Parasit.* **49**:203.
Kershaw, W. E., Duke, B. O. L., Moore, P. J. & Scott-Smith, A. (1955d): *Trans. Roy. Soc. Trop. Med. Hyg.* **49**:6.
Kershaw, W. E., Ross, J. A., & Webber, W. A. F. (1955e): *Trans. Roy. Soc. Trop. Med. Hyg.* **49**:300.
Kershaw, W. E., Deegan, T., Moor, P. J. & Williams, P. (1956): *Ann. Trop. Med. Parasit.* **50**:95.
Kershaw, W. E., Plackett, R. L., Moor, P. J. & Williams, P. (1957): *Ann. Trop. Med. Parasit.* **51**:26.
Kessel, J. F. (1957a): *Bull. Wld Hlth Org.* **16**:633.
       (1957b): *Amer. J. Trop. Med. & Hyg.* **6**:402.
       (1960): *Indian J. Malariol.* **14**:509.
       (1961): The ecology of filariasis. In "Studies in Medical Geography", vol. 2, "Studies in Disease Ecology" Edited by J. M. May. Hefner Publ. Co. New York.
       (1966): *Mosquito News* **26**:490.
       (1967): *Proc. Calif. Mosquito Cont. Assoc.* **35**:17.
       (1971): *Bull. Wld Hlth Org.* **44**:783.
Kessel, J. F. & Massal, E. (1962): *Bull. Wld Hlth Org.* **27**:543.
Kessel, J. F., Thooris, C. C. & Bambridge, B. (1953): *Amer. J. trop. Med. Hyg.* **2**:1050.
Kessel, J. F., Siliga, N., Tompkins, H., Jr. & Jones, K. (1970): *Bull. Wld Hlth Org.*, **43**:817.
Keukenschrijver (1929): *Geneesk. Tijdschr. Nederl.-Indie.*, **69**:308.
Khalil, M. (1935): *J. Egyptian Med. Assoc.* **18**:389.
       (1936): *J. Egyptian Med. Assoc.*, **19**:701.
Khalil, M., Halawani, A. & Hilmy, I. S. (1932): *J. Egypt. Med. Assoc.* **15**:317.
Khrimlyan, A. I. (1965): *Med. Parazit. I parasit. Bolezni* **34**:153.
Khromov, A. S. (1963): *Med. Parazit. I Parazit. Boloezni.* **32**(2):216.
Kim, D. C. (1974): Epidemiological studies of filariasis in inland Korea. 4. Vector determination of filariasis malayi in Yongju area. Abstr., Spring Meeting of Korean Soc. Parasit. 5 p.
Kim, H. K. & Seo, B. S. (1968): *Korean J. Parasit.* **6**:1.
Kim, D. C., Lee, O. Y., Kim, T. W., Han, E. J., Lee, K. W. & Choi, S. H. (1971): *Report NIH, Korea* **8**:147.
Kim, J. S., Lee, W. Y. & Chun, S. L. (1973a): *Korean J. Parasit.* **11**:33.
Kim, D. C., Lee, O. Y., Kim, T. W. & Kwak, J. S. (1973b): *Korean J. Parasit.* **11**:131.
Kindelberger, C. P. (1912): *U.S. Naval Med. Bull.* **6**:464.
King, D. F. (1968): *Ann. trop. Med. Parasit.* **62**:469.
Kire, J. B. (1928): *Trans. Roy. Soc. Trop. Med. Hyg.* **22**:263.

Kirk, R. (1947): *Ann. Trop. Med. Parasit.* **41**:357.
          (1957a): *Bull. Wld Hlth Org.* **16**:485.
          (1957b): *Bull. Wld Hlth. Org.* **16**:593.
          (1960): *Indian J. Malariol.* **14**:387.
Kitamura, S. & Katamine, D. (1953): *'Saishin Kiseichubyogaku,* 7:47, Igaku Shoin Co., Tokyo.
Ktamura, S., Katamine, D., Ohara, R. Arisato, J. & Ueda, H. (1953): *Nihon Ijishimpo,* **1505**:9 (in Japanese).
Kitzmiller, J. B. (1953): *Rev. Brasil. Malariol. D. Trop.* **5**:285.
Kivits, M. (1952): *Ann. Soc. Belge Med. Trop.* **32**:235.
Klokke, A. H. (1961): *Trans. Roy. Soc. Trop. Med. Hyg.* **55**:433.
Klotz, O. (1930): *Amer. J. Trop. Med.* **10**:57.
Knapp, F. W. (1968): *Mosquito News.* **28**:516.
Knapp, F. W. & Rogers, C. E. (1968): *Mosquito News* **28**:535.
Knight, K. L. (1946): *J. Washington Acad. Sci.* **36**:270.
Knipling, E. F. (1959): *Science* **139**:902.
          (1968): The potential role of sterility for pest control. In Labreque & Smith (ed.), 'Principles of Insect Chemosterilization' pp. 7–40, Appleton-Century Crofts, New York.
Knott, J. (1935): *Trans. Roy. Soc. Trop. Med. Hyg.* **29**:59.
          (1938): *Trans. Roy. Soc. Trop. Med. Hyg.* **32**:243.
          (1939a): *Trans. Roy. Soc. Trop. Med. Hyg.* **33**:191.
          (1939b): *Trans. Roy. Soc. Trop. Med. Hyg.* **33**:335.
          (1944): *Trans. Roy. Soc. Trop. Med. Hyg.* **38**:235.
Kobayashi, J., Matsuda, H., Fujita, K., Sakai, T. & Shinoda, K. (1969): *Japan. J. Parasit.* **18**:563.
Korke, V. T. (1927): *Indian J. Med. Res.* **14**:717.
          (1928): *Indian J. Med. Res.* **16**:187.
          (1929a): *Indian J. Med. Res.* **16**:695.
          (1929b): *Indian J. Med. Res.* **16**:1023.
          (1933): *Indian J. Med. Res.* **21**:437.
Kraemer, A. (1903): Die Samoa Inseln.
Krishna Das, K. V., Neelakanta Pillay, N., & Raman, S. (1963): *Indian J. Malariol.* **17**:333.
Krishnamurthy B. S., Ray, S. N. & Joshi, G. C. (1962): *Indian J. Malariol.* **16**:365.
Krishnamurthy, B. S., Kalra, R. L., & Keshavalu, P. G. (1963): *Indian J. Malariol.* **17**: 123.
Krishnaswami, A. K. (1955): *Indian J. Malariol.* **9**:1.
Krishnaswami, A. K., Pattanayak, S. & Raghavan, N. G. S. (1959): *Indian J. Malariol.* **13**:153.
Krishnaswami, A. K., Nair, C. P., Dalip Singh, Bhatnagar, V. N., Mammen, M. L. & Sharma, H. L. (1963): *Indian J. Malariol.* **17**:65.
Kulangara, A. C., & Subramaniam, R. (1960): *Indian J. Med. Research.* **48**:698.
Kume, S. (1957): *Amer. J. Vet. Research* **18**:912.
Kume, S., & Ohishi, I. (1957): *J. Amer. Vet. Med. Assoc.* **131**:476.
Kume, S., Oishi, I. & Nakazawa, K. (1954): *Japan. J. Sanitary Zool.* (Special No.) 54.
Kume, S., Ohishi, I. & Kobayashi, S. (1964): *Amer. J. Vet. Res.* **25**:1527.
          (1968): *Amer. J. Vet. Res.* **28**:975.
Kung Chien-Chang (1959): *Chinese Med. J.* **78**:176.
Kung Chien-Chang, Chang Ch'ao-Lung, Hsu Ai-Na & Sun Pu-Ch'ing (1959a): *Chinese Med. J.* **78**:177.
Kung Yu-Lan & Wang Wen-Cheng (1959): *Chinese Med. J.* **78**:172.
Kurdina, A. A. (1968): *Med. Parazit. I Parazit. Bolezni.,* **37**:351.
Kurihara, T. (1973): *Japan. J. Sanitary Zool.* **24**:73.
Kurihara, T. & S. Hayashi (1965): *Japan. J. Sanitary Zool.* **16**:104.
Kurihara, T. & Oemijati, S. (1974): *Japan. J. Parasit.* **24**:78.

Kurihara, T. & Sasa, M. (1973): *Japan. J. Sanitary Zool.* **24**:79.

Kurihara, T., Sasa, M. & Dhamvanij, O. (1965): *Japan. J. Sanitary Zool.* **16**:239.

Kurihara, T., Hata, K. & Sasa, M. (1973a): *Japan. J. Sanitary Zool.* **24**:83.

Kurihara, T., Sasa, M., Miyamoto, J. & Sato, H. (1973b): *Japan. J. Sanitary Zool.* **24**: 165.

Kuyer, A. (1922): *Geneesk. Tijdschr. Nederl.-Indie.,* **62**:35

Van der Kuyp, E. (1965): Progress achieved in Wuchereriasis bancrofti Control in Surinam. 22 pp., Publicatie No. 8. Surinam: Bureau voor Openbare Gezondheidszorg. (cited in Trop. Dis. Bull. **64**:288)

Labrecque, G. C. & Smith, C. N. (1968; editors): Principles of insect chemosterilization. 354 pp. Appleton-Century-Crofts, New York.

Lacerda, N. B. & Rachou, R. G. (1956): *Rev. Brasil. Malariol. D. Trop.* **8**:437.

Lacour, M. & Rageau, J. (1957): Enquête épidémiologique et entomologique sur la filariose de Bancroft en Nouvelle-Caledonie et dépendences. South Pacific Comm. Tech. Paper No. 110.

Lafont (1905): *Ann. Hyg. Méd. Col.* **8**:497 (Quoted by Brunhes, 1973).

Lagrange, E. (1949): *Ann. Soc. Belge Med. Trop.* **29**:19.

Lagraulet, J. (1971): *Bull. Soc. Path. Exot.* **64**:231.

Lagraulet, J. & Bonnin, P. (1971): *Bull. Soc. Path. Exot.,* **64**:229.

Lagraulet, J. & Thooris, G. (1971): *Bull. Soc. Path. Exot.* **64**:343.

Lagraulet, J., Lebreton, G. & Rit, J. M. (1957): *Bull. Soc. Path. Exot.* **50**:369.

Lagraulet, J., Monjusiau, A. G. M. & Durand. B. (1964): *Méd. Trop.* **24**:566.

Lagraulet, J., Monjusiau, A. G. M. & Dessolle, N. (1966): *Bull. Soc. Path. Exot.* **59**:984.

Lagraulet, J., Baumont, R. & Couland, L. (1967): *Bull. Soc. Path. Exot.* **60**:173.

Lagraulet, J., Pichon, G. & Cuzon, G. (1972a): *Bull. Soc. Path. Exot.* **65**:437.

Lagraulet, J., Pichon, G., Outin-Fabre, D., Stanghellini, A. & Moreau, J. P. (1972b): *Bull. Soc. Path. Exot.* **65**:447.

Lagraulet, J., Barsinas, M. & Fagnaux, G. (1972c): *Bull. Soc. Path. Exot.* **65**:698.

Lagraulet, J., Barsinas, M., Fagneaux, G. & Teahui, M. (1973): *Bull. Soc. Path. Exot.* **66**:139.

Lagraulet, J., Barsinas, M., Fagneaux, G., Merehau, M., Terorotua, R. & Tiaore, D. (1974): *Bull. Soc. Path. Exot.* **67**:73.

Laigret, J. (1929): *Bull. Soc. Path. Exot.* **22**:499.

Laigret, J., Kessel, J. F., Malarde, L., Bambridge, B. & Adams, H. (1965): *Bull. Soc. Path. Exot.* **58**:895.

Laigret, J., Kessel, J. F., Bambridge, B., & Adams, H. (1966): *Bull. Wld Hlth Org.* **34**: 925.

Laing, A. B. G. (1960): *Indian J. Malariol.* **14**:391.

(1961): *Trans. Roy. Soc. Trop. Med. Hyg.* **61**:558 (Corresp.).

Laing, A. B. G. & Wharton, R. H. (1960): Filariasis investigation. *Rep. Inst. Med. Res. Malaya.* 1960–127.

Laing, A. B. G., Edeson, J. F. B. & Wharton, R. H. (1960): *Ann. Trop. Med. Parasit.* **54**:92.

(1961): *Ann. Trop. Med. Parasit.* **55**:86.

Laird, M. (1954): *Bull. Entomol. Res.* **45**:423.

(1955): *Bull. Entomol. Res.* **46**:291.

(1958): *Trans. Roy. Soc. Trop. Med. Hyg.* **52**:291.

(1971): Microbial control of arthropods of medical importance. *In* "Microbial Control of Insects and Mites" (H. D. Burges, ed.), p. 134. Academic Press, New York.

Lambert, S. M. (1928): *Medical J. Australia,* **2**:362.

(1929): *Med. J. Australia* **1**:45.

Lambrecht, F. L. (1971a): *Bull. Entomol. Res.* **60**:513.

(1971b): *S. E. Asian J. Trop. Med. Pub. Hlth.* **2**:222

(1973): Filariasis in the Seychelles Islands and in the British Indian Ocean Territories. (Unpublished Document)WHO FIL/WP/73.3, 10 pp.

Lambrecht, F. L. & Van Someren, E. C. C. (1971): *Southeast Asian J. Trop. Med. Pub. Hlth.* **2**:483

Lämmler, G. & Herzog, H. (1974): *Ztschr. Tropenmed. Parasit.* **25**:78.

Lämmler, G., Saupe, E. & Herzog, H. (1968): *Zschr. Parasitenkunde* **30**:281

Lämmler, G., Enders, B. & Zahner, H. (1969): *Zschr. Parasitenkunde* **32**:254.

Lämmler, G., Herzog. H., Saupe, S. & Schütze, H. R. (1971): *Bull. Wld Hlth Org.* **44**: 751.

Lamotellerie, M. (1972): *Ann. Parasit. Hum. Comp.* **47**:783.

Lampe (1953): *Trop. Dis. Bull.* **50**:785.

Lane, C. (1929): *Lancet,* June 22, 1291–3 pp.

    (1942): *Trans. Roy. Soc. Trop. Med. Hyg.,* **35**:327.

Lang & Noc (1903): *Arch. de Parasitologie* **7**:377

Languillon, J. (1957): *Bull. Soc. Path. Exot.* **50**:417.

Lariviere, M., Diallo, S. & Picot, H. (1966): *Bull. Soc. Afr. Noire.* (Lang. Fr.) **11**:670.

Lartique, J. J. (1967): *Bull. Wld Hlth Org.* **36:** Notes, 491.

Laurence, B. R. (1962): *Proc. Internat. Cong. Entomol.* **11**:127.

    (1963): *Bull. Wld Hlth Org.* **28**:229.

    (1966): *J. Helminth.* **40**:337.

    (1968): *Nature* **219(5154)**:561.

Laurence, B. R. & Simpson, M. G. (1968a): *Trans. Roy. Soc. Trop. Med. Hyg.* **62**:9.

    (1968b): *J. Helminth.* **42**:309.

    (1969): *Trans. Roy. Soc. Trop. Med. Hyg.* **63**:801.

    (1971): *J. Helminth.* **45**:23.

Laven, H. (1957): *Zeitschr. f. indukt. Abstammungs- u. Vererbungslehre* **88**:443.

    (1967): *Nature* (London) **216**:383.

Laveran: (1902): *C. R. Soc. Biol.* **54**:908.

Lavoipierre, M. M. J. (1958a): *Ann. Trop. Med. Parasit.* **52**:103.

    (1958b): *Ann. Trop. Med. Parasit.* **52**:326.

Lavoipierre, M. M. J. & Ho, B. C. (1966): *J. Helminth.* **40**:343.

Laws, E. R., Jr., Sedlak, V. A., Miles, J. W., Joseph, C. R., Lacomba, J. R. & Rivera, A. D. (1968): *Bull. Wld Hlth Org.* **38**:439.

Lazar, M., Lieberman, T. W., Furman, M., and Leopold, I. H. (1968): *Amer. J. Ophthalmol.* **66**:215.

Lazar, M., Lieberman, T. W. & Leopold, I. H. (1970): *Amer. J. Trop. Med. Hyg.* **19**: 232.

Leber, A. (1914): *Arch. Schiffs-Tropenhyg.* **18**:454.

Leber, A. & Prowazek, S. (1911): *Arch. Schiffs-Tropenhyg.* **15**:409.

Leber, A. & Von Prowazek, S. (1914): *Arch. Schiffs-Tropenhyg.* **18**:386.

Lebrun, A. (1954): *Ann. Soc. Belge Méd. Trop.* **34**:751.

Ledentu, G. & Peltier, M. (1937): *Ann. Med. Parm. Colon.* **35**:748.

Lee, C. U. (1926): *Trans. Roy. Soc. Trop. Med. Hyg.* **20**:279.

Lee, D. S., Yoon, H. K., Kim, H. S. & Lee, K. W. (1970): *Korean J. Parasit.* **8**:36.

Lee, K. T. (1961): *Bull. National Inst. Health, ROK.* **4**:107.

Lee, K. T., Kim, S. W., Kong, T. H. & Song, J. S. (1964): *Korean Med. Assoc. J.* (Seoul) **7**:657.

Lee, W. Y. (1969): *Korean J. Parasit.* **7**:153.

Lee, S. H., Kang, S. Y. & Seo, B. S. (1973): *Korean J. Parasit.* **11**:Suppl. 125 (Abstract).

Leger, A. (1912): *Bull. Soc. Path. Exot.* **5**:618.

Léger, Mç (1920): *Bull. Soc. Path. Exot.* **13**:248.

Lèger, M. & Gallen, R. (1914): *Bull. Soc. Path. Exot.* **7**:125.

Leiper, R. T. (1913): *Trans. Roy. Soc. Trop. Med. Hyg.* **6**:265.

Leon, R. J., De (1957a): *Bull. Wld Hlth Org.* **16**:483.

    (1957b): *Bull. Wld Hlth Org.* **16**:523.

Leon, R. J., De & Duke, B. O. L. (1966): *Trans. Roy. Soc. Trop. Med. Hyg.* **60**:735.

Leroy des Barres (1915): *Bull. Méd. Chir. Indoch.* **6**:302.

Lesson, P. (1839): Voyage autour du monde entrepris par ordre du Gouvernement sur la corvette la Conquille. vol. 1: 493–5 pp. (quoted by Iyengar, 1965).

792   REFERENCES

Levine, N. D. & Harper, P. A. (1947): Malaria and other insect-borne diseases in the South Pacific Campaign, 1942–1945. IV. Parasitological observations on malaria in natives and Troops, and on filariasis in natives. *Amer. J. Trop. Med.* **27**:Suppl. No. 3: 119–28 pp.

Lewis, D. J. (1948): *Trans. R. ent. Soc. Lond.* **99**:475.
    (1953a): *Revue Zool. Bot. Afr.* **48**:269.
    (1953b): *Bull. Entom. Res.* **43**:597.
    (1956): *Nature* **178**:98.
    (1957): *Ann. Trop. Med. Parasit.* **51**:340.
    (1958a): *Ann. Trop. Med. Parasit.* **52**:216.
    (1958b): *Simulium domnosum* in the Tonkolili Valley, Sierra Leone. *Proceedings 10th International Congress Entomology* **3**:541.
    (1960a): *Proc. Roy. Ent. Soc. Lond. Ser. B.* **29**:7.
    (1960b): *Bull. Ent. Res.* **51**:95.
    (1960c): *Ann. Trop. Med. Parasit.* **54**:208.
    (1961a): *Proc. Roy. Entom. Soc. Lond. Ser. B.* **30**:107.
    (1961b): *J. Anim. Ecol.* **30**:303.
    (1965): *Ann. Trop. Med. Parasit.* **59**:365.
    (1968): *Trans. Roy. Soc. Trop. Med. Hyg.* **62**:19.

Lewis, D. J. & Duke, B. O. L. (1966): *Ann. Trop. Med. Parasit.* **60**:337.

Lewis, D. J. & Hanney, P. W. (1965): *Proc. Roy. Entom. Soc. Lond. Ser. B.* **34**:12.

Lewis, D. J., & Ibanez de Aldecoa, R. (1962): *Bull. Wld Hlth Org.* **27**:449.

Lewis, D. J., Lyons, G. R. L. & Marr, D. J. M. (1961): *Ann. Trop. Med. Parasit.* **55**: 202.

Lewis, D. J., Disney, R. H. L. & Crosskey, R. W. (1969): *Bull. Entom. Res.* **59**:229.

Lewis, T. (1877): *Filaria sanguinis hominis* (mature form), found in a blood-clot in naevoid elephantiasis of the scrotum. *Lancet,* Sept. **29**:453.

Li Huei-Han (1959a): *Chinese Med. J.* **78**:52.
    (1959b): *Chinese Med. J.* **78**:148.

Li Lei-Shih, Hsiao, Ch'ing-Yen, Ho Yi & K'ung Teh-Lien (1959): *Chinese Med. J.* **78**: 175.

Li, F-P., Hu, H-G., Pen, C-M & Leng, T-I. (1964): Morphological studies of the adult *Brugia malayi* (Brug, 1927) Buckley, 1960 Acta Zool. Sinica **16**:7.

Lichtenberg, F. (1957): *J. Mt Sinai Hospital,* New York, **6**:983.

Lichtenberg, F. & Medina, R. (1957): *Amer. J. Trop. Med. Hyg.* **6**:739.

Lichtenstein, A. (1927): *Geneesk. Tijdschr. Nederl.-Indie.* **67**:742.

Lie, K. J. (1962): *Amer. J. Trop. Med. Hyg.,* **11**:646.
    (1970): *Southeast Asian J. Trop. Med. Pub. Hlth.* **1**:366.

Lie, K. J. & Rees, D. M. (1958): *Proc. Int. Congr. Trop. Med. & Malaria,* Lisbon., **11**: 360.

Lie, K. J. & Sandosham, A. A. (1969): The pathology of classical filariasis due to *Wuchereria bancrofti* and *Brugia malayi* and a discussion of occult filariasis. Proc. 3rd S. E. A. Regional Meeting on Parasit. Trop. Med., Singapore. 125–135 pp.

Lie, K. J., Chow, C. Y., Winoto, R. M. P., Soegiarto & Rusad, M. (1958): *Amer. J. Trop. Med. Hyg.* **7**:280.

Lie, K. J., Soegiarto, C. & Winoto, R. P. M. (1960a): *Berita Kem. Kes.* **9**:18

Lie, K. J. Hudojo, Wijono & Amaliah, S. (1960b): *Indian J. Malariol.* **14**:339.

Lieske, H. (1954): *Biologia Trop.* **2**:37.

Lin, L. C. & Ch'en, K. K. (1958): *Chinese Med. J.* **76**:490.

Lin Liang-chéng, Ch'en Kuei-kuang & Lin Yuan-ch'üan (1959): *Chinese Med. J.* **78**: 446–8.

Lindquist, A. W., T. Ikeshoji, B. Grab, Botha de Meillon & Z. H. Khan (1967): *Bull. Wld. Hlth. Org.* **36**:21.

Little, M. D. & D'Alessandro, A. (1970): *Amer. J. Trop. Med. Hyg.* **19**:831.

Liu, Kusum (1937): *Chinese Med. J.* **52**:579.

Liu, S. Y. (1962): *J. Formosan Med. Assoc.* **61**:391.

Liu, Y-K., Hsieh, S-C., & Tai, T-Y. (1964): *Chinese Med. J.* **83**:17.

Lloyd, R. B. & Chandra, S. N. (1933): *Indian J. Med. Res.* **20**:1197.

Loewenthal, L. J. A. (1934): *Ann. Trop. Med. Parasit.* **28**:47.

(1943): *Ann. Trop. Med. Parasitol.*, **37**:147.

Looss, A. (1904): *Zool. Jahrb., Abt. Syst.,* **20**:549.

Lopdell, J. C. (1953): Filariasis in Western Samoa. Proc. 7th Pacific Sci. Congr., New Zealand (1949).

Lopez-Rizal, L. & Padua, R. G. (1926): *J. Philipp. Is Med. Assoc.* **6**:298.

Low, G. C. (1900): *Brit. Med. J.* **1(1900)**:1456.

(1902): *Brit. Med. J. Jan.* **25**:196.

(1903): *Brit. Med. J.* **1903–I**:722.

(1908): *Lancet,* **1908**:279.

(1927): *Trans. Roy. Soc. Trop. Med. Hyg.* **10**:514.

(1941): *Trans. Roy. Soc. Trop. Med. Hyg.* **35**:197.

Lowman, E. W. (1944): *U.S. Naval Med. Bull.* **42**:341.

Lu, H. C. & Yu, Y. (1959): *Chinese Med. J.* **78**:181.

Lu, H. C., Ma, T. C. & Li, C. P. (1959): *Chinese Med. J.* **78**:180.

Lubran, M. (1950): *British J. Pharmacol.* **5**:210.

Lucasse, C. (1962): *Z. Tropenmed. Parasit.* **13**:404.

Lucasse, C. & Hoeppli, R. (1963): *Z. Tropenmed. Parasit.* **14**:262.

Lucot, J. & Chovet, M. (1972): *Med. Trop.* (Marseille) **32**:523.

Lüders, H. (1937): *Arch. Schiffs. Tropenhyg.* **41**:349.

Lynch, G. W. A. (1905): *Lancet,* **1**:21

Ma, H. C., Yeh, Y. T., Kao, T. F. & Tsap, C. C. (1958): *Acta Microbiol. Sinica* **6**:134.

Ma, H. C., Yeh, Y. C. & Ts'ao, C. C. (1959): *Chinese Med. J.* **78**:173.

Maasch, H. J. (1973): *Z. Tropenmed. Parasit.* **24**:419.

Macdonald, G. (1957): The epidemiology and control of malaria. Oxford Univ. Press, London, 252 pp.

Macdonald, W. W. (1961): *Trans. Roy. Soc. Trop. Med. Hyg.* **55**:306

(1962a): *Ann. Trop. Med. Parasit.* **56**:368.

(1962b): *Ann. Trop. Med. Parasitol.* **56**:373.

(1963a): *Trans. Roy. Soc. Trop. Med. Hyg.* **57**:3.

(1963b): *Ann. Trop. Med. Prasitol.* **57**:452.

(1965): *Proc. Internat. Cong. Entom.* (London) **12**:820.

Macdonald, W. W. & Johnson, M. A. (1962): *Trans. Roy. Soc. Trop. Med. Hyg.* **56**:7.

Macdonald, W. W. & Wharton, R. H. (1963): *Trans. Roy. Soc. Trop. Med. Hyg.* **57**:4.

Macfie, J. W. S. & Corson, J. F. (1922): *Ann. Trop. Med. Parasit.* **16**:465.

Mackerras, M. J. (1958): *Med. J. Australia,* 1958, **21**:702.

Maehata, Y. (1941): *Nagasaki Igakkai Zasshi* **19**:491; 716 (in Japanese).

Mahajan, B. K., Shah, H. H. & Mehta, N. R. (1961): *Indian J. Med. Sci.* **15**:630.

Mahapatra, G. S. (1961): *J. Assoc. Physicians India* **9**:677.

Mahdi, A., Guirguis, S. S., Kolta, S. & Soleit, A. (1963): *J. Egypt. Publ. Hlth Assoc.* **37**:153.

Mahdi, M. A., Mahdi, A. H. & Arafa, M. S. (1969): *J. Egypt. Publ. Hlth Assoc.* **44**:189.

Mahoney, L. E., Jr. & Aiu, P. (1970): *Amer. J. Trop. Med. Hyg.* **19**:629.

Mahoney, L. E., Jr. & Kessel, J. F. (1971): *Bull. Wld Hlth org.* **45**:35.

Malaria Institute of India (1960): Filariasis in India. National Health Problems Series 3, 27 pp. (Delhi).

Maldonado, J. F., Hernandes Morales, F., Fox, I. & Tillet, C. J. (1948): *Puerto Rico J. Pub. Hlth Trop. Med.* **24**:121.

Maldonado, J. F., Hernandes Morales, F., Velez Herrera, V. & Thillet, C. J. (1950): *Puerto Rico J. Pub. Hlth Trop. Med.* **25**:291.

Mamet, J. R. (1968): *Mauritius Inst. Bull.* **6**:119 (quoted by Brengues & Brunhes, 1973).

Mansfield-Aders (1927): *Trans. Roy. Soc. Trop. Med. Hyg.* **21**:207.

Manson, P. (1872): *China Imperial Maritime Customs Medical Reports* **1**:24.
   (1876): *China Imperial Maritime Customs Medical Reports* **10** (July–Sept. 1875): 1.
   (1877a): *Medical Report* 13 & *Customs Gazette* 33 (Jan.–March 1877): 13, Shanghai.
   (1877b): *Chinese Customs Med. Rep.* **2(14)**:1.
   (1877): *Trans. Linn. Soc. London* 2nd Sev. Zoology **11. pt. 10**:367.
   (1878): *Chinese Customs Med. Rep.* **3(No. 14)**:1.
   (1879): *Chinese Customs Med. Rep.* **18**:31.
   (1881): On the periodicity of filarial migration to and from the circulation. *China Imperial Maritime Customs Medical Reports*. 22nd Issue 63–8.
   (1882): Notes on filaria disease. *China Imperial Maritime Customs Medical Reports*. 23rd Issue 1–16.
   (1891): *Filaria sanguinis hominis perstans*. Lancet, 1, 3rd, January.
   (1894): *Brit. Med. J.,* **1**:1186.
   (1896): *Brit. Med. J.,* **2**:1379.
   (1897): *Brit. Med. J.* (1897), **2**:1837.
Manson-Bahr, P. (1941): *Trop. Dis. Bull.* **38**:361.
   (1942): *Trans. Roy. Soc. Trop. Med. Hyg.* **35**:237.
   (1951): *Nature,* Lond., **158**:776.
   (1952): *Doc. Med. Geogr. Trop.* **4**:193.
   (1953a): The pathological and clinical aspects of filariasis. In 'Filariasis in the South Pacific,' (Proc. Conference at Papeete, Tahiti, August-September, 1951'', South Pacific Commission, Noumea, 53–7 pp.
   (1953b): *Nature,* London, **171**:368.
   (1955a): *Trans. Roy. Soc. Trop. Med. Hyg.* **49**:127.
   (1955b): *Trans. Roy. Soc. Trop. Med. Hyg.* **49**:282.
   (1959): *J. Trop. Med. Hyg.* **62**:53 (Pt. 1); 85 (Pt. 2); 106 (Pt. 3); 138 (Pt. 4); 160 (Pt. 5).
Manson-Bahr, P. & Muggleton, W. J. (1952): *Trans. Roy. Soc. Trop. Med. Hyg.* **46**:301.
Manson-Bahr, P. & Wijers, D. J. B. (1972): *Trans. Roy. Soc. Trop. Med. Hyg.* **66**:18.
Maplestone, P. A. (1938): *Indian Med. Gaz.,* **13**:8.
March, H. N., Laigret, J., Kessel, J. F. & Bambridge, B. (1960): *Amer. J. Trop. Med. Hyg.* **9**:180.
Marinkelle, C. J. (1973): *Trop. Geogr. Med.,* **25**:51.
Marinkelle, C. J. & German, E. (1970): *Trop. Geogr. Med.* **22**:101.
Marks, E. N. (1947): Studies on Queensland mosquitoes. Pt. 1. The *Aedes* (*Finlaya*) *Kochi* group with description of new species from Queensland, Bougainville and Fiji. *Univ. Queensland papers,* Dept. of Biology 2/5.
   (1951a): *Ann. Trop. Med. Parasit.* **45**:137.
   (1951b): *Bishop Museum,* **20**:123.
   (1957): *Ann. Trop. Med. Parasit.* **51**:50.
Marr, J. D. M. (1962): *Bull. Wld Hlth Org.* **27**:622.
Marr, J. D. M. and Lewis, D. J. (1964): *Bull. Entom. Res.* **55**:547.
Marshall, C. L. & Yasukawa, K. (1966): *Amer. J. Trop. Med. Hyg.* **15**:934.
Marwah, S. M., Rao, N. S. & Gaur, S. D. (1972): *J. Indian Med. Assoc.* **60**:33.
Mascaro, J. M., Juan, J., Del Valle, R. & Caparros, J. A. (1973): *Medna Cutanea* **7**:165 (abstract in *Trop. Dis. Bull.* **71**:1151).
Massal, E. & Loison, G. (1953): La filariose de Bancroft en Nouvelle-Calédonie. Proc. 8th Pacif. Congr., Manila, 6A: 535–39.
Massequin, A., Taillefer-Grimaldi, J. & Leveuf, J. J. (1954): *Bull. méd. Afr. Occid. fr.* 2, Special number; 141.
Mastin, W. M. (1888): *Ann. Surgery* **8**:321.
Mastrandrea, G. & Sanguigni, S. (1968): *Arch. Ital. Sci. Med. Trop. Parassitol.* **49**:195.
Mataika, J. U. (1965): Filariasis in the Solomon Islands. A survey on Guadalcanal and Florida Islands. *Rep. WHO Seminar on Filariasis,* 6 pp. (mimeographed).

Mataika, J. U., Dando, B. C. & Macnamara, F. N. (1970): Filariasis and arbovirus survey, northern Fiji, 1968–69. A report to the Director of Medical Services, Fiji (mimeogr. 79 pp.).

Mataika, J. U., Dando, B. C., Spears, G. F. S. & Macnamara, F. N. (1971): *J. Hyg., Cambridge*, **69**:273, 297.

Matas, R. (1913): *Amer. J. Trop. Dis. Prev. Med.* **1**:60.

Mathis, C. (1909): *Bull. Soc. Path. Exot.* **2**:144.

Mathis, C. & Leger, M. (1910): *Bull. Soc. Path. Exot.* **3**:142.

Mathis, H. L. & Pant, C. P. (1974): *Southeast Asian J. Trop. Med. Publ. Hlth* **5**:299.

Matsuda, H., Kobayashi, J. & Sakai, T. (1968): *Japan. J. Parasitol.* **17**:221.

Mattingly, P. E. (1962): *Bull. Wld Hlth Org.* **27**:569.

    (1969): The biology of mosquito-borne disease. pp. 184 George Allen & Unwin Ltd., London.

    (1973): Culicidae, in Insects and other Arthropods of Medical Importance (Smith, K. G. V., ed.), 37–108 pp., British Museum. London.

Mattingly, P. F. & Brown, E. S. (1955): *Bull. Entom. Res.* **46**:69.

Mattos, S. S. & Xavier, S. H. (1965): *Rev. Brasil. Malariol. D. Trop.* **17**:269.

Maxwell, J. P. (1921): *Philip. J. Sci.* **19**:257.

Mazzotti, L. (1942): *Rev. Inst. Sal. Enf. Trop.* **3**:223.

    (1948): *Rev. Inst. Salubr. Enferm Trop.* (Mexico), **9**:235.

    (1951a): *Am. J. Trop. Med.* **31**:624.

    (1951b): *Am. J. Trop. Med.* **31**:628.

Mazzotti, L. & Hewitt, R. (1948): *Médicina* (México) **28**:39.

MaCarthy, D. D. (1930): *Trans. Roy. Soc. Trop. Med. Hyg.* **23**:401.

    (1956): *Trans. Roy. Soc. Trop. Med. Hyg.* **50**:66.

    (1959a): *New Zealand Med. J.* **58**:738.

    (1959b): *New Zealand Med. J.* **58**:757.

McCarthy, D. D. & Carter, D. G. B. (1967a): The control of filariasis in Western Samoa: A report to the Medical Research Council of New Zealand. 25 pp.

    (1967b): Filariasis control in Western Samoa. An interim report on an assessment survey—1967. The Medical Research Council of New Zealand, 9 pp.

McCarthy, D. D. & Fitzgerald, W. (1955): *Trans. Roy. Soc. Trop. Med. Hyg.* **49**:82.

McCarthy, D. D. & Fitzgerald, N. (1956): *Trans. Roy. Soc. Trop. Med. Hyg.* **50**:58.

McCarthy, D. D., Simpson, E. & Robati, P. (1962): *New Zealand. Med. J.* **61(355)**:143.

McConnel, E. & Schmidt, M. L. (1973): *Trop. Geogr. Med.* **25**:300.

McCoy, O. R. (1933): *Amer. J. Trop. Med.* **13**:297.

McFadzean, J. A. (1954): *Trans. Roy. Soc. Trop. Med. Hyg.* **48**:267.

McFadzean, J. A., & Hawking, F. (1954): *Brit. Med. J.* **1**:956.

    (1956): *Trans. Roy. Soc. Trop. Med. Hyg.* **50**:543.

McGregor, I. A. & Gilles, H. M. (1960): *Ann. Trop. Med. Parasitol.*, **54**:415.

McGregor, I. A. & Smith, D. A. (1952): *Trans. Roy. Soc. Trop. Med. Hyg.* **46**:403.

McGregor, I. A., Hawking, F. & Smith, D. A. (1952): *Brit. Med. J.* **2**:908.

McKenzie, A. (1925): *Trans. Roy. Soc. Trop. Med. Hyg.* **19**:138.

McLaren, D. J. (1970): *Trans. Roy. Soc. Trop. Med. Hyg.* **64**:191.

    (1972): *Parasitology,* **65**:317.

McLean, J. B. (1910): *Austr. Med. Gaz.* **29**:234.

McMahon, J. P. (1940): *Trans. Roy. Soc. Trop. Med. Hyg.* **34**:65.

    (1951): *Bull. Entom. Res.* **42**:419.

    (1952): *Bull. Entom. Res.* **5**:87.

    (1957): *Bull. Entom. Res.* **5**:76.

    (1967): *Bull. Wld Hlth Org.* **37**:415.

McMahon, J. P., Highton, R. B. & Goiny, H. (1958): *Bull. Wld Hlth Org.* **19**:75.

McMillan, B. (1960): *Trop. Geogr. Med.* **12**:183.

    (1967): *Med. J. Aust.* **1967–2(6)**:243.

    (1968): *Med. J. Aust.* **2(2)**:63.

McNair, P. K., et al. (1949): *U.S. Naval Med. Bull.* **49**: Suppl. 5.
McNaughton, J. G. (1919): *J. Trop. Med. Hyg.* **22**:1.
Meadows, R. (1871): *China Customs Med. Reports.* **1**:35.
Megaw, J. W. A. & Gupta, S. C. (1927): *Indian Med. Gaz.,* **62**:299.
Meillon, B. de (1930): *Bull. Entom. Res.* **21**:185.
    (1957): *Bull. Wld. Hlth Org.* **16**:509.
Meillon, B. de., & Khan, Z. H. (1976a): *Bull. Wld Hlth Org.* **36**:15.
    (1967b): *Bull. Wld Hlth Org.* **36**:169.
Meillon, B. de. & Sebastian, A. (1967a): *Bull. Wld Hlth Org.* **36**:75.
    (1967b): *Bull. Wld Hlth Org.* **36**:168.
    (1967c): *Bull. Wld Hlth Org.* **36**:174.
Meillon, B. de., Sebastian. A. & Khan, Z. H. (1967a): *Bull. Wld Hlth Org.* **36**:7.
      (1967b): *Bull. Wld Hlth Org.* **36**:39.
      (1967c): *Bull. Wld Hlth Org.* **36**:53.
Meillon, B. de., Paing, M., Sebastian, A. & Khan, Z. H. (1967d): *Bull. Wld Hlth Org.*
  36:67.
Meillon, B. de., Hayashi, S. & Sebastian, A. (1967e): *Bull. Wld Hlth Org.* **36**:81.
Meillon, B. de., Grab, B. & Sebastian, A. (1967f): *Bull. Wld Hlth Org.* **36**:91.
Meillon, B. de., Sebastian, A. & Khan, Z. H. (1967g): *Bull. Wld Hlth Org.* **36**:163.
Meira, M. T. V. (1960): *Anais Inst. Med. Trop.* **17**:557.
Menon, K. P. & Iyer, P. V. S. (1936): *Indian J. Med. Res.* **23**:881.
Menon, M. A. U. (1960): *Indian J. Malariol.* **14**:659.
Merlet, Y. (1950): *Bull. Assoc. Med. Nouvelle-Caledonie* **13**:7.
Mesquita, J. F. F. (1959): *Anais Inst. Med. Trop.* **16**: Supl. **6**:488.
Messer, A. B. (1876): *Arch. Méd. Navale (Paris)* **26**:321.
Meyers, F. M. & Kouwenaar, W. (1939): *Geneesk. Tijdschr. Nederl.-Indie.* **79**:853.
Miao, C. W. & Liu, W. T. (1962): *Acta Entomol. Sinica* **11**:363.
Michel, D. A. (1961): *Trans. Roy. Soc. Trop. Med. Hyg.* **55**:52.
Michel, P. (1944): *U.S. Naval Med. Bull.* **42**:1059.
    (1945): *U.S. Naval Med. Bull.* **45**:225.
Militair Geneeskundige Dienst, Hoofdkantoor (1923): *Geneesk. Tijdschr. Ned.-Indie.*
  63:32.
Mille, R., Kessel, J. F., & Beye, H. K. (1949): Filariasis research and control in Tahiti.
  Proc. 7th Pacific Science Congress, New Zealand.
Mille, R., Papa, F. & Delloue, M. (1961): *Bull. Soc. Path. Exot.* **54**:836.
    (1962): *Inst. Pasteur de la Martinique Arch.* **15**:19.
Miller, T. A., Stryker, R. G., Wilkinson, R. N. & Esah, S. (1969): *Mosquito News* **29**:
  688.
Mills, A. R. (1954): *South Pacific Comm. Qrtly. Bull.* **4**:26.
    (1960): *Trans. Roy. Soc. Trop. Med. Hyg.* **54**:597.
    (1969): *Trans. Roy. Soc. Trop. Med. Hyg.* **63**:591.
Minning, W. & McFadzean, J. A. (1956): *Trans. Roy. Soc. Trop. Med. Hyg.* **50**:246.
Mitsui, G., Sakuma, S., Tasaka. S. & Tanaka, H. (1966): *Japan. J. Parasit.* **15**:169.
Miyamoto, J., Kitagawa, K. & Sato, Y. (1966): *Japan. J. Exp. Med.* **36**:211.
Mizutani, K. & Hirakoso, S. (1962): *Japan. J. Sanitary Zool.* **13**:298.
Mizutani, K. & Suzuki, T. (1962): *Japan. J. Sanitary Zool.* **13**:56.
Mochizuki, D. (1911): *Fukuoka Ikadaigaku Zasshi* (Fukuoka) **4**:384.
    (1912): *Igaku Chuo Zasshi* (Tokyo) **10**:4.
Mochizuki, D. & Inoue, S. (1912): *Igaku Chuo Zasshi* (Tokyo) **9**:1505; 1609.
Molser, H. (1939): *Arch. Schiffs-Tropenhyg.* **43**:130.
Momma, K. (1942 a, b): *Dojinkai Zasshi,* **16**:293;302
Money, G. L. (1960): *J. Trop. Med. Hyg.* **63**:238.
Monjusiau, A. G. M., Lagraulet, J., D'Haussy, R. & Göckel, C. W. (1965): *Bull. Wld*
  Hlth. Org. **32**:339.
Montestruc, E. & Bertrand, Ch. (1935): *Bull. Soc. Path. Exot.* **28**:612.
    (1937): *Bull. Soc. Path. Exot.* **30**:695.

Montestruc, E. Blache, R. & Laborde, R. (1950): *Bull. Soc. Path. Exot.* **42**:463.

Montestruc, E., Courmes, E. & Fontan, R. (1960): *Indian J. Malariol.* **14**:637.

Moon, I. J. (1939): *Chosen Igakkai Zasshi (J. Korean Med. Assoc.)* **29**:553; 697; 1426.

Moon, O. R. (1968): *Korean J. Publ. Hlth* **5**:103.

Moorhouse, D. E. & Wharton R. H. (1964): *J. Med. Entom.* **1**:359.

Moraes M. A. P. (1959): *O Hospital* (R. de Janeiro) **56**:869.

Moraes, M. A. P. (1974): Onchocerciasis in Brazil. In 'Research and Control of Onchocerciasis in the Western Hemisphere', *Pan Amer. Hlth Org.*, 122–6 pp.

Moraes, M. A. P. & Chaves, G. M. (1974a): *Bull. Pan Amer. Hlth Org.* **8**:95.

(1974b): *Rev. Inst. Med. Trop. Sao Paulo,* **16**:110.

Moraes, M. A. P. & Dias, L. B. (1972): *Rev. Inst. Med. Trop. Sao Paulo,* **14**:330.

Moraes, M. A. P., Fraiha, H. & Chaves, G. M. (1973): *Bull. Pan American Hlth Org.* **7**:50.

Moreau, J. P. (1965): *Med. Trop.* (Marseille) **25**:486.

Morenas, L. (1929): *Bull. Soc. Path. Exot.* **22**:325.

Morgan, H. V. (1958): *J. Trop. Med. Hyg.* **61**:145.

Morishita, K. (1951): Parasitic diseases in Japan (A Review). *Saishin Kiseichugaku,* Vol. 1, 1–96 pp., Igaku Shoin, Tokyo (in Japanese).

(1960): *Indian J .Malariol.* **14**:363.

Morlan, H. B., McCray, E. M., Jr., Kilpatrick, J. W. (1962): *Mosquito News* **22**:295.

Moty, M. (1892): *Rev. Chir.,* Paris, **12**:1.

Mouchet, R. (1913): *Arch. Schiffs-Tropenhyg.* **17**:657.

Mouchet, J., Grjebine, A. & Grenier, P. (1965): *Entomologie Medicale Cah.* Nos., **3/4**: 67.

Moura Lima, M. & Rachou, R. G. (1959): *Rev. Bras. Malariol. D. Trop.* **11**:573.

Moura Pires, F., Santos David, J. H. & Oliveira E Silva, J. A. A. (1959): *Anais Inst. Med. Trop.* **16**:461.

Mueller, J. C., Mitchell, D. W., Garcia-Monza, G. A., Aguilar, F. J. & Scholtens, R. G. (1973): *Amer. J. Trop. Med. Hyg.* **22**:337.

Muench, H. (1959): Catalytic models in epidemiology. 110 pp. Harvard Univ. Press, Cambridge, Mass.

Mühlens, P. (1926): *Arch. Schiffs-Tropenhyg.* **30**: Beih. 143.

(1932): *Arch. Schiffs-Tropenhyg.* **36**:287.

Muirhead- Thompson, R. C. (1950): *Bull. Entom. Res.* **41**:487.

(1954): *Trans. Roy. Soc. Trop. Med. Hyg.* **48**:208.

(1960): *Indian J. Malariol.* **14**:409.

Mulla, M. S. (1964): *Mosquito News* **24**:212.

Mumford, E. P. & Adamson, A. M. (1933): *Proc. 5th International Congress of Entomology,* 1932, **2**:431.

Murgatroyd, F. & Woodruff, A. W. (1949): *Lancet* **2**:147.

Murray, W. D. (1948): *U.S. Naval Med. Bull.* **48**:327.

Muspratt, J. (1965): *Bull. Wld Hlth Org.* **33**:140.

Myers, W. W. (1881): Observations on *Filaria sanguinis hominis* in South Formosa. *China Maritime Customs Medical Reports,* 21st Issue, 1–25.

(1886): Further observations on *Filaria sanguinis hominis* in South Formosa. *China Imperial Maritime Customs Medical Reports.* 32nd Issue, 1–38.

Nagatomo, I. (1960a, b): *Endemic Dis. Bull.* (Nagasaki Univ.) **2**:296.

(1961): *Endemic Dis. Bull.* (Nagasaki Univ.) **3**:75.

Naidu, C. R. (1962): *Bull. Nat. Soc. India Mal. Mosq. Dis.* **10**:69.

Nair, C. P. (1960): *Indian J. Malariol.* **14**:233.

(1961): *Indian J. Malariol.* **15**:263.

(1962): *Indian J. Malariol.* **16**:47.

(1966): *Bull. Indian. Soc. Malaria Com. Dis.* **3**:198.

(1968): *Anitseptic,* **65**:885.

(1972): *J. Com. Dis.* **4**:97.

Nair, C. P. & Bhatnagar, V. N. (1968): *Antiseptic,* **65**:235.

Nair, C. P. & Chayabejara, S. (1961): *Indian J. Malariol.* **15**:249.
Nair, C. P. & Krishnan, K. S. (1965): *Bull. Indian Soc. Malaria Com. Dis.* **2**:139.
Nair, C. P. & Roy, R. G. (1958): *Indian J. Malariol.* **12**:195.
Nair, C. P. & Roy, A. P. (1959): *Bull. Nat. Soc. India Malaria Mosq. Dis.* **7**:65.
Nair, C. P., Krishnan, K. S. & Roy, R. G. (1959): *Indian J. Malariol.* **13**:117.
Nair, C. P., Roy, R. G. & Joseph, C. (1960): *Indian J. Malariol.* **14**:223.
Nair, C. P., Roy, R. G. & Singh, B. (1971): *Antiseptic.* **68**:403.
Nakagawa, P. Y. & Ikeda, R. M. (1969): Biological control of mosquitoes with larvivorous fish in Hawaii. WHO/VBC/69.173 (mimeographed. 25 pp.).
Nakamura, Y. (1964a): *Endemic Dis. Bull.* (Nagasaki Univ.) **6**:25.
       (1964b): *Endemic Dis. Bull.* (Nagasaki Univ.) **6**:113.
       (1965): *Endemic Dis. Bull.* (Nagasaki Univ.) **7**:142.
Nanda, D. K., Zafar, W., Singh, M. V. & Chand, D. (1960): *Indian J. Malariol.* **14**:157.
Nanda, D. K., Singh, M. V. & Diwan Chand. (1962): *Indian J. Malariol.* **16**:313.
Nanjundiar, K. S. & Jeevandhar Kumar, S. A. (1962): *Bull. Nat. Soc. India Mosq. Dis.* **10**:253.
Napier, L. E. (1944): *Medicine,* **23**:149.
       (1946): The principles and practice of tropical medicine. 659 pp. MacMillan, New York.
Napier, L. E. & Sundar Rao, S. (1940): *Indian J. Med. Res.* **28**:605.
Narayandas, M. G. (1958): *Indian J. Malariol.* **12**:209.
         (1966): *Bull. Indian Soc. Malaria Comm. Dis.* **3**:221.
Narayandas, M. G. & Roy, A. P. (1958): *Indian J. Malariol.* **12**:67.
Neafiie, R. C. (1972): *Amer. J. Clin. Path.* **57**:574.
Nehaul, B. B. G. (1956): *West Indian Med. J.* **5**:201.
Nelson, G. S. (1955): *East African Med. J.* **32**:413.
       (1958a): *Trans. Roy. Soc. Trop. Med. Hyg.* **52**:272.
       (1958b): *Trans. Roy. Soc. Trop. Med. Hyg.* **52**:368.
       (1958c): *Bull. Wld Hlth Org.* **19**:204.
       (1959): *J. Helminth.* **33**:233.
       (1960): *Indian J. Malariol.* **14**:585.
       (1964): Factors influencing the development and behaviour of filarial nematodes in their arthropodan hosts. *In* "Host-Parasite Relationships in Invertrebrate Hosts". (Ed. Dr. A. R. Taylor.) 2nd Symposium of British Society for Parasitology, 75–119 pp.
       (1965): *J. Helminth.* **39**:229.
       (1966): *Helminth. Abstr.* **35**:311.
       (1970): Onchocerciasis. in Dawes, B. (ed.) Advances in Parasitology, vol. 8, pp. 173–226
Nelson, G. S. & Cruikshank, L. M. (1956): Filariasis in Fiji, 1944–1955. *Med. Dept. Fiji,* 50 pp.
Nelson, G. S. & Grounds, J. G. (1958): *East African Med. J.* **35**:365.
Nelson, G. S. & Heisch, R. B. (1957): *Trans. Roy. Soc. Trop. Med. Hyg.* **51**:90.
Nelson, G. S. & Pester, F. R. N. (1962): *Bull. Wld Hlth Org.* **27**:473.
Nelson, G. S., Heisch, R. B. & Furlong, M. (1962): *Trans. Roy. Soc. Trop. Med. Hyg.* **56**:202.
Neppert, J. (1974): *Tropenmed. Parasit.* **25**:454.
Neumann, H. (1944): *J. Trop. Med. Hyg.* **47**:25.
Neumann, E., & Gunders, A. E., (1963): *Amer. J. Ophthal.,* **56**:573.
Neumann, E., Lucasse, C. & Gunders, A. E. (1964): *Amer. J. Opthal.* **57**:217.
Neves, H. A. & Damasceno, R. M. G. (1954): *Rev. Brasil. Malariol. D. Trop.* **6**:367.
Neves, H. A., Rachou, R. G. & Scaff, L. M. (1955): *Rev. Bras. Malariol. D. Trop.* **7**:41.
Newhouse, V. F., Chamberlain, R. W., Johnston, J. G. & Sudia, W. D. (1966): *Mosquito News,* **26**:30.
Newton, W. L. & Wright, W. H. (1956): *J. Parasit.* **42**:246.
Newton, W. L., Wright, W. H. & Pratt, I. (1945): *Amer. J. Trop. Med.* **25**:253.

Ngu, A. V. & Folami, A. O. (1965): *J. Nigerian Med. Assoc.* **2**:160.

Ngu, A. V. & Konstam, P. (1964): *Brit. J. Surg.* **51**:101.

Nicholas, W. L. (1953a): *Ann. Trop. Med. Parasit.* **47**:187.

    (1953b): *Ann. Trop. Med. Parasit.* **47**:309.

Nicholas, W. L. & Kershaw, W. L. (1954): *Ann. Trop. Med. Parasit.* **48**:201.

Nicholas, W. L., Gordon, R. M. & Kershaw, W. E. (1952): *Trans. Roy. Soc. Trop. Med. Hyg.* **46**:377.

Nicholas, W. L., Kershaw, W. E., Keay, W. J. & Zahra, A. (1953): *Ann. Trop. Med. Parasit.* **47**:95.

Nicholas, W. L., Kershaw, W. E. & Duke, B. O. L. (1955): *Ann. Trop. Med. Parasit.* **49**:455.

Nickle, W. R. (1973): *Exp. Parasit.* **33**:303.

Nicolas, C. (1910): *Bull. Soc. Path. Exot.* **3**:737.

Niles, W. J. (1961): *Ann. Trop. Med. Parasit.* **55**:379.

Nnochiri, E. (1964a): *Ann. Trop. Med. Parasit.* **58**:89.

    (1964b): *West African Med. J.* **13**:139.

Noamesi, C. K. (1962): *Bull. Wld Hlth Org.* **27**:620.

    (1964): *Ghana J. Sci.* **4**:44.

    (1966): *Ghana Med. J.* **5**:95.

Noc, F. (1908): *Bull. Soc. Path. Exot.* **1**:369.

Noc, F. & Stevenel, L. (1913): *Bull. Soc. Path. Exot.* **6**:663.

Obeck, D. K. (1973): *J. Parasit.*, **59**: 220.

Obiamiwe, B. A. & MacDonald, W. W. (1971): *Ann. Trop. Med. Parasit.*, **65**:547.

O'Brien, R. D. (1960): Toxic phosphorous esters. 434 pp. Academic Press, New York & London.

O'Connor, F. W. (1922): *Trans. Roy. Soc. Trop. Med. Hyg.* **16**:28.

    (1923): *Res. Mem., Lond. Sch. Trop. Med.*, **4**:57.

    (1937): *J. Trop. Med. Hyg.* **40**:25;42.

O'Connor, F. W. & Beatty, H. A. (1937): *J. Trop. Med. Hyg.*, **40**:101.

    (1938): *Trans. Roy. Soc. Trop. Med. Hyg.* **31**:413.

O'Connor, F. W. & Burke, G. (1929): *Amer. J. Trop. Med.* **9**:143.

O'Connor, F. W. & Hulse, C. R. (1935): *Puerto Rico J. Pub. Hlth Trop. Med.* **11**:167.

Oemijati, S. (1971): *J. Indonesian Med. Assoc.* **21**:149.

Oemijati, S. & Liem Kiat Tjoen (1966): *Proc. 11th Pacific Sci. Congr.* (*Tokyo*), **8**:5.

Oemijati, S. & Partono, F. (1971): *J. Indonesian Med. Assoc.* **21**:67.

Oey Djoen Hoat. (1942): *Geneesk. Tijdschr. Nederl.-Indie.*, **82**:302.

Ogata, K. & Sasa, M. (1955): *Japan. J. Sanitary Zool.* **6**:10.

Ogunba, E. O. (1971): *Ann. Trop. Med. Parasit.* **65**:399.

Oh, H. Y. (1929): *China Med. J.* **43**:16.

Oh, S. N. (1930): *Mansen-no-ikai* **120**:25.

O'Holohan, D. R. & Zaman, V. (1974): *J. Trop. Med. Hyg.* **77**:113.

Okada, Y. (1957): *Kankyo Eisei* (Tokyo). **10**;6.

Okamoto, K., Asechi, S., Nagano, N., Kameko, H. & Shimonuruyu, Y. (1956): *Nihon Ijishimpo* **1672**:35.

Oldroyd, H. (1955): *Trans. Roy. Soc. Trop. Med. Hyg.* **49**:111.

    (1957): The horse-flies (Diptera, Tabanidae) of the Ethiopian region. vol. 3: Subfamilies Chrysopinae, Scepsidinae and Pangoninae and a revised classification. British Museum (Nat. Hist.), London.

    (1973): Tabanidae, in "Insects and other Arthropods of Medical Importance" (K. G. V. Smith, ed.), 195–202 pp., British Museum, London.

Oliver, A. G. & Oliver, J. (1938): *Puerto Rico J. Pub. Hlth Trop. Med.* **14**:18.

Oman, P. W. & Christernson, L. D. (1947): *Amer. J. Trop. Med.* **27**: Suppl. 91.

Omori, N. (1954): On the biology of mosquitoes transmitting bancroftian filariasis. *Rinsho to Kenkyu*, 31 (5); 31.

    (1957): *Nagasaki Igakkai Zasshi Nagasaki Igakkai Zasshi* **32**:1434.

    (1958a): *Nagasaki Igakkai Zasshi* **33**:1045.

800   REFERENCES

Omori, N (1958b): *Yokohama Med. Bull.*, **9**:382.
        (1958c): *Nagasaki Igakkai Zasshi* **33**: suppl. 61.
        (1958d): *Ibid.* 143.
        (1962a): *Endemic Dis. Bull.* (Nagasaki Univ.) **4**:1.
        (1962b): *Bull. Wld Hlth Org.* **27**:585.
        (1965a): *Endemic Dis. Bull.* (Nagasaki Univ.) **7**:29.
        (1965b): *Japan. J. Parasit.* **14**:67.
        (1966): On the role of japanese mosquitoes, especially of *Culex pipiens pallens* in the transmission of bancroftian filariasis. In: Progress of Medical Parasitology in Japan III: 471–507 pp. (Meguro Kiseichukan, Tokyo).
Omori, N. & Wada, Y. (1968): *Tropical Medicine* (Nagasaki) **10**:154.
        (1970): The relation of the natural infection rate of mosquitoes to microfilarial prevalence in inhabitants of villages endemic in bancroftian filariasis in Japan. Recent Advances in Studies on Filariasis and Schistosomiasis in Japan (M, Sasa, ed.), 145–58 pp. (Univ. Tokyo Press).
Omori, N., Kamura, T., Fujisaki, T., Suenaga, O., Kitamura, S., Katamine, D., Era, E. & Fukamachi, H. (1959): *Japan. J. Parasit.* **8**:886.
Omori, N., Suenaga, O. & Nakachi, K. (1962): *Endemic Dis. Bull.* (Nagasaki Univ.) **4**: 194.
Omori, N., Wada, Y., Oda, T. & Nishigaki, J. (1967): *Trop. Med.* (Nagasaki) **9**:97.
Omori, N., Wada, Y. & Oda, T. (1972): Eradication experiment of bancroftian filariasis in the control of vector mosquitoes in Nagate Village, Nagasaki Prefecture. In Yokogawa, M. (ed.), *Research in Filariasis and Schistosomiasis"*, 21–30 pp.; Univ. Tokyo Press.
Ongom, V. L. (1974): *East African Med. J.* **51**:296.
Onori, E. (1963): *West African Med. J.* **12**:3.
Oomen, A. P. (1967): *Trop. Geogr. Med.* **19**:231.
        (1967b): *Ethiop. Med. J.* **5**:159.
        (1969a): *Trop. Geogr. Med.*: **21**:105.
        (1969b): *Trop. Geogr. Med.* **21**:225.
        (1969c): *Trop. Geogr. Med.* **21**:236.
        (1969d): Studies on onchocerciasis and elephantiasis in Ethiopia. De Erven F. Bohn N. V. Haarlem, 115 pp.
Oostburg, B. F. J. (1974): *Scholae Medicinae Tropicae* **41**:7.
Oostingh, R. (1923): *Geneesk. Tijdschr. Nederl.-Indie.* **63**:164.
Oram, R. H. (1958): *Central African J. Med.* **4**:99.
        (1960): *Cental African J. Med.* **6**:144.
Orihel, T. C. (1966): *J. Parasit.* **52**:162.
        (1967a): *J. Parasit.* **53**:376.
        (1967b): *J. Parasit.* **53**:586.
        (1967c): *Amer. J. Trop. Med. Hyg.* **16**:628.
        (1973): *Amer. J. Trop. Med. Hyg.* **22**:596.
Orihel, T. C. & Pacheco. G. (1966): *J. Parasit.* **52**:394.
Otto, G. F. (1958): *J. Parasit.* **44**:1–27.
        (1972): Epizootiology of canine heartworm disease. In Bradley, R. E. (ed.) "Canine Heartworm Disease", 1–15 pp. Univ. Florida, Gainesville.
Otto, G. F. & Maren, T. H. (1947): *Science* **106**:105.
        (1948): *Ann. New York Acad. Sci.* **50**:39.
        (1949): *Amer. J. Hyg.* **50**:92.
Otto, G. F., Brown H. W., Bell, S. D., Jr., & Thetford, N. D. (1952): *Amer. J. Trop. Med. Hyg.* **1**:470.
Otto, G. F., Jachowski, L. A., Jr., & Wharton, J. D. (1953): *Amer. J. Trop. Med. Hyg.* **2**:495.
Outin-Fabre, D., Saugrain, J., Stanghellini, A. & Pichon, G. (1972): *Bull Wld Hlth Org.* **46**:253.
Ouzilleau, F. (1913a): *Annls Hyg. Med. Colon.* **16**:307.

Ouzilleau, F. (1913b): *Bull. Soc. Path. Exot.* **6**:80.
              (1913c): *Bull. Soc. Path. Exot.* **9**:305.
Ovalle, G. (1940): *Rev. Fac. Med. Univ. Nal. Bogotá* **9**:377.
Ovazza, M. (1953): *Bull. Soc. Pathol. Exot.* **46**:575.
Ovazza, M., Ovazza, L. & Balay, G. (1965): *Bull. Soc. Pathol. Exot.* **58**:1118.
Oye, E. van & Peirquin, L (1961): *Bruxelles Med.* **41**:39
Pacheco, G. (1966): *J. Parasit.* **52**:331.
Pacheco, G. & Orihel, T. C. (1968): *J. Parasit.* **54**:1234.
Pacheco, G., Atkins, M. J. & Gurian J. (1972): *J. Parasit.* **58**:275.
Pacheco-Luna, R. (1918): *Amer J. Ophthal.* **3**:805.
Paik, Y. H., Uh, H. B., Huh, L. S. & Yang, Y. J. (1957): *Korean Med. J.* **2**:1175.
Pal, R. & Whitten, M. J. [Edited by]. (1974): The use of genetics in insect control. Elsevier/North-Holland Publishing Company Amsterdam.
Pal, R. Nair, C. P., Ramalingam, S., Patil, P. V. & Ram. B. (1960): *Indian J. Malariol.* **14**:595.
Pampana, E. (1963): A textbook of malaria eradication. Oxford Univ. Press, London 508 pp.
Pan American Health Organization (1974): *Pan Amer. Hlth Org. Sci. Pub.* **298**:154.
Pan American Sanitary Bureau (1950): Bibliografia de onchocercosis. Publication No. 242.
              (1961): Bibliografia de onchocercosis. Suplemento. Publ. varias No. 67.
Pandit, C. G., Ramakrishnan, S. P. & Raghavan, N. G. S. (1963): *Indian J. Malariol.* **17**:1.
Park J. E. (1961): *Indian J. Pub. Hlth.* **5**:114.
              (1962a): *Bull. Nat. Soc. India Mal. Mosq. Dis.* **10**:3.
              (1962b): *Indian J. Med. Sci.* **16**: 604.
Partono, F. & Oemijati, S. (1970): *Southeast Asian J. Trop. Med. Pub. Hlth.* **1**:516.
Partono, F., Cross, J. H., Borahina, Clarke, M. D. & Oemijati, S. (1972a): *Southeast Asian J. Trop. Med. Pub. Hlth* **3**:366.
Partono, F., Hudojo, Oemijati, S., Noor, N., Borahina, J. H., Clarke, M. D., Irving. G. S. & Duncan, C. F. (1972b): *Southeast Asian J. Trop. Med. Pub. Hlth* **3**:537.
Partono, F., Cross, J. H., Purnomo & Oemijati, S. (1973): *Trop. Geogr. Med.,* **25**:286.
Patanayak, S., & Chandrasekhar, A. (1963): *Indian J. Malariol.* **17**: 273.
Patel, T. B. & Paranjpey, P. D. (1958): *Indian J. Malariol.* **12**: 171.
Paterson, H. E. (1964): *Riv. Malar.* **43**:191.
Patterson, J. L. (1878): Fatos relativos a filariose. *Gaz. Med. da Bahia, dez.,* 1878.
Patterson, R. S., Ford, H. R., Lofgren, C. S. & Weidhaas, D. E. (1970a): *Mosquito News,* 30:23.
Patterson, R. S., Weidhaas, D. E., Ford, H. R. & Lofgren, C. S. (1970b): *Science,* (Washington), June 12, **168**:1368.
Pawar, R. G. & Mittal, M. C. (1968): *Indian J. Med. Res.* **56**:370.
Peel, E., and Chardome, M. (1946): *Ann. Soc. Belge Méd. Trop.,* **26**:117.
              (1947): *Ann. Soc. Belge Méd. Trop.* **27**:241.
Peel, E. & Van Oye, E. (1950): *Ann. Soc. Belge. Méd. Trop.* **30**:59.
Peel, E. Mastdagh, M. & Mathieu, J. (1952):   *Ann. Soc. Belge Méd. Trop.* **32**:269.
Pelletier, J. (1912): *Bull. Soc. Path. Exot.* **5**:625.
Perry, W. J. (1949a): *J. Parasit.* **35**:379.
              (1949b): *Amer. J. Trop. Med.* **29**:747.
              (1950): *Amer. J. Trop. Med.* **30**:103.
Pessoa, S. B. & Andradf., Z. A. (1950): *O. Hospital.* **37**:4.
Peters, L., Bueding, E., Valk A. D. Jr., Higashi, A. and Welch, A. D. (1949a): *J. Pharmacol. Exp. Therap.* **95**:212.
Peters, L., Welch, A. D., and Higashi, A. (1949b): *J. Pharmacol. Exp. Therap.* **96**:460.
Peters, W. (1957): *Papua New Guinea Med. J.* **2**:24.
Peters, W. & Cornelius Dewar, S. (1956): *Indian J. Malariol.,* **10**:37.

Petersen, J. J. (1973a): *J. Med. Entom.* **10**:75.
          (1973b): *Exp. Parasit.* **33**:239.
Petersen, J. J. & Willis, O. R. (1970): *J. Econ. Entom.* **63**:175.
          (1972a): *Mosquito News* **32**:226.
          (1972b): *Mosquito News* **32**:312.
Peterson, G. D. (1956): *J. Econ. Entom.* **49**:786.
Pfister, R. (1952): *Bull. Soc. Path. Exot.* **45**:92.
          (1954): *Bull. Soc. Path. Exot.* **47**:408.
Phalen, J. M. & Nichols, H. J. (1908a): *Philipp J. Sci.* **3B**:293.
          (1908b): *Philipp. J. Sci.* **3B**:305.
          (1909): *Philipp. J. Sci.* **4B**:127.
Phelps, R. J. & DeFoliart, G. R. (1964): Nematode parasite of Simuliidae. *Univ. Wisconsin Research Bull.* **245**:78.
Phelps, J. R., Smith, O. A., Carroll, H. H., Washburu, W. A. & Beagley, K. E. (1930): *Naval Med. Bull.* (Washington), **28**:459.
Philippon, B. & Bain, O. (1972): *Cah. O. R. S. T. O. M. Entom. Parasit.* **10**:251.
Picq, J. J. & Roux, J. (1973): *Méd. Trop.* (Marseille,) **33**:451.
Picq, J. J., Coz, J. & Jardel, J. P. (1971): *Bull. Wld Hlth Org.* **45**:517.
Pinhao, R. C. (1961): *Anais Inst. Med. Trop.* (Lisboa). **18**:15.
Pinto, A. R. (1947): Contribuçao para estudos das filariases da Guiné Portuguesa. *Anais Inst. Med. Trop.* (Lisboa), December, 1947.
          (1960): *Anais Inst. Med. Trop.* **17**:817.
Pinto, A. R. & Almeida, C. L. (1947): *Anais Inst. Med. Trop.* **4**:59.
Pipkin, A. C. (1953): *Wuchereria bancrofti* in Micronesia. 8th Pacific Science Congress. Manila Vol. 6 A, 589–605 pp.
Pittman, F. E. (1972): *Amer. J. Trop. Med.* **21**:38.
Poindexter, H. A. (1949): *Amer. J. Trop. Med.* **29**:435.
          (1950): *Amer. J. Trop. Med.* **30**:519.
Polovodova, V. P. (1949): (Determination of the physiological age of female *Anopheles*). Med. Parazit. (Moskow). (in Russian)
Poltera, A. A. (1973): *Trans. Roy. Soc. Trop. Med. Hyg.,* **67**:819.
Polunin, I. (1951): *Med. J. Malaya.* **5**:320.
          (1953): *Med. J. Malaya.* **8**:55.
Ponnampalam, J. T. (1971): *Med. J. Malaya,* **26**:62.
Ponnudurai, T., Denham, D. A. & Nelson, G. S. (1971): *J. Helminth.* **45**:415.
Ponnudurai, T., Denham, D. A., Nelson, G. S. & Rogers, R. (1974): *J. Helminth.* **48**:107.
Postburg, B. F. J. (1974): *Acta Leidensia* **41**:7.
Poynton, J. O. & Hodgkin, E. P. (1938): *Bull. Inst. Med. Res. F. M. S.* **1**:1.
          (1939): *Trans. Roy. Soc. Trop. Med. Hyg.* **32**:555.
Preston, P. G. (1935): *J. Trop. Med. Hyg.* **38**:81.
Pringle, G.; King, D. F. (1968): *Ann. Trop. Med. Parasit.* **62**:462.
Prod'hon, J. (1972): *Cah. O. R. S. T. O. M. ser. Entom. med. et Parasitol.* **10**:263.
Provincial Antifilariasis Station, Shantung (1959): *Chinese Med. J.* **78**:178
Provincial Institute for Control of Filariasis, Shantung & Institute of Parasitic Diseases, Chinese Academy of Medical Science (1959): *Chinese Med. J.* **78**:180.
Puig Solanes, M., Vargas, L., Mazzotti, L. Guevara, R. A. & Noble, B. (1948): Onchocerciasis. Univ. Nac. de México 129 pp.
Putatunda, J. N., & Singh, N. A. (1967): *Bull. Indian Soc. Malaria Com. Dis.* **4**:147.
Puyuelo, R. and Holstein, M. M. (1950): *Méd. Trop.* **10**:395.
Quelennec, G. (1962): *Bull. Wld Hlth Org.* **27**:615.
Quéré, M. A., Basset, A., Larivière, M. and Razafinjato, R. (1963): *Bull. Mém. Fac. Mixte. Méd. Pharm. Dakar.* **11**:238.
Qureshi, A. H. & Bay, E. C. (1969): *Mosquito News* **29**:465.
Rachou, R. G. (1954): *Rev. Brasil. Malariol. D. Trop.* **6**:395.
          (1956): *Rev. Brasil. Malariol. D. Trop.* **8**:268.

Rachou, R. G. (1957a): *Rev. Brasil Malariol. D. Trop.* **9**:79.
   (1957b): *Rev. Brasil. Malariol. D. Trop.* **9**:527.
   (1958): *Rev. Brasil. Malariol. D. Trop.* **10**:277.
   (1960): *Rev. Brasil. Malariol. D. Trop.* **12**:11.
Rachou, R. G. & Deane, L. M. (1954): *Rev. Brasil. Malariol. D. Trop.* **6**:377.
Rachou, R. G. & Ferreira, M. O. (1958): *Rev. Brasil. Malariol. D. Trop.* **10**:391.
Rachou, R. G. & Lacerda, N. B. (1954): *Rev. Brasil. Malariol. D. Trop.* **6**:343.
     (1956a): *Rev. Brasil. Malariol. D. Trop.* **8**:369.
Rachou, R. G. & Scaff, L. M. (1958): *Rev. Brasil. Malariol. D. Trop.* **10**:303.
Rachou, R. G., Ferreira, M. O. & Moura Lima, M. (1954a): *Rev. Brasil. Malariol. D. Trop.* **6**:189.
Rachou, R. G., Deane, L. M., Damasceno, R. G. & Moura Lima, M. (1954b): *Rev. Brasil. Malariol. D. Trop.* **6**:205.
Rachou, R. G., Lacerda, N. B. & Costa, A. (1954c): *Rev. Brasil. Malariol D. Trop.* **6**:407.
Rachou, R. G., Lacerda, N. B. & Santos, D. (1954d): *Rev. Brasil. Malariol. D. Trop.* **6**:409.
Rachou, R. G., Azambuja, C. E. A. & Souza, P. S. (1954e): *Rev. Brasil. Malariol. D. Trop.* **6**:419.
Rachou, R. G. Neves, H. A. & Scaff, L. M. (1955a): *Rev. Brasil Malariol. D. Trop.* **7**:37.
Rachou, R. G., Moura Lima. M., Ferreira Neto, J. A. & Martins. C. M. (1955b): *Rev. Brasil. Malariol. D. Trop.* **7**:51.
Rachou, R. C., Lacerda, N. B. & Barbosa, J. A. (1955): *Rev. Brasil Malariol. D. Trop.* **7**:315.
Rachou, R. G., Villela, A. M., Cruz, A. E. & Carvalho, G. (1956): *Rev. Brasil. Malariol. D. Trop.* **8**:359.
Rachou, R. G., Matta Pires, W. & Mocra Lima, M. (1958a): *Rev. Brasil. Malariol. D. Trop.* **10**:61.
Rachou. R. G., Mello, A. L. & Perraz, D. M. (1958b): *Rev. Brasil. Malariol. D. Trop.* **10**:207.
Radaody-Ralarosy, P. & Guidoni, P. (1940): *Bull. Soc. Path. Exot.* **33**:292.
Raether, W. & Lämmler, G. (1971): *Ann. Trop. Med. Parasit.* **65**:107.
Rageau, J. & Estienne, J. (1959): Enquête sur la filariose à Wallis. 37 pp. Institut Français d'Oceanie, Noumea.
Raghavan, N. G. S. (1951): *Indian J. Malariol.* **5**:203.
   (1956): *Bull. Nat. Soc. India Malaria Mosq. Dis.* **4**:161.
   (1957): *Bull. Wld Hlth Org.* **16**:553.
   (1961): *Bull. Wld Hlth Org.* **24**:177.
Raghavan, N. G. S. & Krishnan, K. S. (1949a): *Indian J. Malariol.* **3**:39.
     (1949b): *Indian J. Malariol.* **3**:249.
Raghavan, N. G. S., & Pattanayak, S. (1963): *Indian J. Malariol.* **17**:285.
Raghavan, N. G. S., Misra, B. G. & Randhagovinda Roy (1952): *Nature* **170**:253.
Raghavan, N. G. S., Singh, D. & Bhatnagar, V. N. (1956): *Indian J. Malariol.* **10**:265.
Raghavan, J. Singh, M. V. & Nanda, D. K. (1957): *Bull. Nat. Soc. India Malaria Mosq. Dis.* **5**:207.
Raghavan, N. G. S., Nair, C. P. & Krishnan, K. S. (1958): *Indian J. Malariol.* **12**:183.
Raghavan, N. G. S., Das, M., Mammen, M. L., et al. (1967a): *Bull. Indian Soc. Mal. Com. Dis.* **4**:318.
Raghavan, N. G. S., Singh, B. Vaid, B. K., Basu, P. G., & Bedi, K. M. S. (1967b): *Bull. Indian Soc. Malaria Com. Dis.* **4**:385.
Rahman N. M. I. & Bhattacharyya, M. N. (1971): *J. Indian Med. Ass.* **56**:363.
Rahman, J., Singh, M. V. & Gujral, J. S. (1957a): *Indian J. Malariol.* **11**:163.
Rahman, J., Singh, M. V. & Nanda, D. K. (1957b): *Bull. Nat. Soc. India Malaria Comm. Dis.* **5**:207.
Rahman, J., Singh, M. V. & Shrivastana, R. N. (1959a): *Bull. Nat. Soc. India Malaria Mosq. Dis.* **7**:53.

Rahman, J., Singh, M. V. & Sharma, K. L. (1959b): *Bull. Nat. Soc. India Malaria Mosq. Dis.* **7**:107.

Rai, K. S. (1969): Status of the sterilemale technique for mosquito control. in "Sterile-male Technique for Eradication or Control of Harmful Insects," pp. 107–14, International Atomic Energy Agency, Vienna, 1969.

Railliet, A. & Henry, A. (1910): *C. R. Soc. Biol.* **68**:248.

Rajagopalan, P. K., Yasuno, M. & Labrecque, G. C. (1973): *Bull. Wld Hlth Org.* **48**:631.

Rajpakse, Y. S. (1974): *J. Trop. Med. Hyg.* **77**:182.

Rakai, I. M., Naserua, J. D., NacNamara, F. N. & Pillai, J. S. (1974): *J. Med. Entom.* **11**:588.

Ramachandran, C. P. (1966): *J. Med. Entom.* **3**:239.

(1969): Human filariasis and its control in West Malaysia. (A mimeographed report to Malaysian Medical Association, 5th Conference of the Public Health Society, Kuala Lumpur, 16 pp.).

(1970a): *Bull. No. 15, Inst. Med. Res.* Kuala Lumpur. 1–39.

(1970b): *Southeast Asian J. Trop. Med. Pub. Hlth* **1**:78.

Ramachandran, C. P. & Dunn, F. L. (1968): *Ann. Trop. Med. Parasit.* **62**:441.

Ramachandran C. P. & Sivanandam, S. (1969): Studies on the transmission of *Wuchereria bancrofti* to animals in the laboratory. *Proc. 3rd S. E. A. Regional Mtg on Parasit. Trop. Med.* (Singapore) 136.

Ramachandran, C. P. & Zaini, M. A. (1968a, b, c): *Med. J. Malaya.* **22**:136, **22**: 198, **22**:323.

Ramachandran, C. P., Edeson, J. F. B. & Kershaw, W. E. (1960): *Ann. Trop. Med. Parasit.* **54**:371.

Ramachandran, C. P., Wharton, R. H., Dunn, F. L. & Kershaw, W. E. (1963): *Ann. Trop. Med. Parasit.* **57**:443.

Ramachandran, C. P., Hoo, C. C. & Bin Omar, A. H. (1964): *Med. J. Malaya* **18**:193.

Ramachandran, C. P., Sandosham, A. A. & Sivandam, S. (1966): *Med. J. Malaya* **20**:333.

Ramachandran, C. P., Cheong, W. H., Sivanandam, S., Abu Hassan Bin Omar & Mahadevan, S. (1970): *Southeast Asian J. Trop. Med. Pub. Hlth.* **1**:505.

Ramachandran, C. P., Dondero, T. J., Jr., Mullin, S. W., Sivanandam, S. & Stevens, S. (1971): *Med. J. Malaya* **25**:273.

Ramachandran, M. (1973): *Indian J. Med. Res.* **61**:864.

Ramakrishnan, S. P. (1962): *Bull. Nat. Soc. India Malaria Mosq. Dis.* **10**:41.

Ramakrishnan, S. P. & Krishnamurthy B. S. (1962): *Indian J. Malariol.* **16**:357.

Ramakrishnan, S. P. & Mohan, B. N. (1959): *Indian J. Malariol.* **13**:189.

Ramakrishnan, S. P., Raghavan, N. G. S., Krishnaswami, A. K., Nair, C. P., Basu, P. C., Dalip Singh & Krishnan, K. S. (1960a): *Indian J. Malariol.* **14**:457.

Ramakrishnan, S. P., Sharma, M. I. D. & Kalra, R. L. (1960b): *Indian J. Malariol.* **14**:545.

Ramakrishnan, S. P., Dalip Singh, Bhatnagar, V. N. & Raghavan, N. G. S. (1961): *Indian J. Malariol.* **15**:255.

Ramakrishnan, S. P., Dalip Singh & Krishnaswami, S. K. (1962): *Indian J. Malariol.* **16**:263.

Ramakrishnan, S. P., Dalip Singh & Raghavan, N. G. S. (1963a): *Indian J. Malariol.* **17**:7.

Ramakrishnan, S. P. Krishnamurthy, B. S., & Singh, N. N. (1963b): *Indian J. Malariol* **17**:119.

Ramalingam, S. C. (1965): The mosquito fauna of Samoa and Tonga and its relation to subperiodic bancroftian filariasis, 172 pp. Ph. D. thesis: Univ. California.

(1968): *Ann. Trop. Med. Parasit.* **62**:305.

(1969): *Med. J. Malaya* **23**:288.

(1973): Vectors of *Wuchereria bancrofti* and *Brugia malayi* in the Southeast Asia Region: Their distribution, biology and control. (WHO mimeogr. doc.) FIL/WP/ 73.31; 32 pp.

Ramalingam, S. & Belkin, N. J. (1964): *Nature* **201**:105.

Ramalingam, S. & Belkin, J. N. (1965): Mosquito studies III. Two new *Aedes* from Tonga and Samoa. Contr. Amer. entom. Inst. **1**:1.

Ramalingam, S., Guptavanji, P. & Harinasuta, C. (1969): "The vectors of *Wuchereria bancrofti* and *Brugia malayi* in South-east Asia.," *Proc. 3rd S. E. A. Regional Mtg on Parasit. Trop. Med.* (Singapore) 172–193 pp.

Ramîrez-Pérez, J. & Vulcano, M. A. (1973): *Arch. Venez. Med. Trop. Parasit. Med.* **5**:375.

Randriambelo, Ph. (1950): *Bull. Soc. Path. Exot.* **43**:247.

Rao, K. N. & Subrahmanyam, D. (1970): *Indian. J. Med. Res.,* **58**:746.

Rao, N. S. N., Murthy, N. S. & Marwah, S. M. (1973): *Indian J. Med. Res.* **61**:943.

Rao, S. S. (1936): *Indian J. Med. Res.* **23**:871.

        (1940): *Indian J. Med. Res.* **28**:609.

        (1942): *Indian J. Med. Res.* **30**:345.

        (1945): *Indian J. Med. Res.* **33**:175.

Rao, S. S. & Iyengar, M. O. T. (1929): *Indian J. Med. Res.* **17**:759.

                      (1932): *Indian J. Med. Res.* **20**:25.

Rao, S. S. & Maplestone, P. A. (1940): *Indian Med. Gaz.,* **75**:159.

Rao, S. S. & Sukhatme, P. V. (1941): *Indian J. Med. Res.* **29**:209.

Rao, T. R. (1974): *J. Com. Dis.* **6**:57.

Raper, A. B. & Ladkin, R. G. (1950): *East African Med. J.* **27**:339.

Raybould, J. N. (1967a): *Ann. Trop. Med. Parasit.* **61**:76.

        (1967b): *Bull. Wld Hlth Org.* **37**:447.

        (1968): *East African Med. J.* **45**:292.

Recio, P. M. (1949): *Acta Med. Philipp.* **6**:47.

Reeling Knap, C. (1930): *Geneesk. Tijdschr. Nederl.-Indie.,* **70**:305.

Reeves, W. C. & Rudnick, A. (1951): *Amer. J. Trop. Med.* **31**:633.

Regester, P. T. (1956; quoted by Barklay, 1965): *J. R. Inst. Publ. Hlth Hyg.* **19**:350.

Reid, J. A. (1953a): *Trans. Roy. Soc. Trop. Med. Hyg.* **47**:84.

        (1953b): *Bull. Entom. Res.* **44**:5.

        (1956): *Ann. Trop. Med. Parasit.* **50**:129.

        (1962): *Bull. Entomol. Res.* **53**:1.

        (1968): *Stud. Inst. Med. Res. Malaya* **31**:520.

Reid, J. A. & Edeson, J. F. B. (1957): Annual Rpt. Inst. Med. Res. Malaya., 1956, 98 pp.

Reid, J. A., Wilson, T. & Ganapathillai, A. (1962): *Ann. Trop. Med. Parasit.* **56**:323.

Renjifo, S. (1949): *An. Soc. Biol.* Bogotá **3**:211.

Renjifo, S. & Orduz, A. (1950): *Rev. Acad. Cien. Exac. Fis. y Matem.* **9(28)**:548.

Rennie, T. (1881): *China Customs Med. Rep.* **2(21)**:50.

Restrepo, M., Latorre, R. & Botero, D. (1962): *Antioquia Med.* (Colombia) **12**:233.

Reynaud, P. H. (1876): *Arch. Med. Navale* **26**:241.

Ridley, D. S. (1956): *Trans. Roy. Soc. Trop. Med. Hyg.* **50**:255.

Ridley, H. (1945): Ocular onchocerciasis including an investigation in the Gold Coast. *Brit. J. Ophthal.* (Monograph Suppl. 10), 58 pp.

Rifaat, M. A., Madhi, A. H., Wassif, S. F. & Morsy, T. A. (1970): *J. Egypt. Publ. Hlth Ass.* **45**:266.

                                       (1971): *J. Egypt. Publ. Hlth Ass.* **46**:200.

Rikugunsho Imukyoku (Bureau of Army Surgeon) (1912): *Gun'idan Zasshi,* **41**:332 (in Japanese).

Rivas, A., Gonzalez, G. L., Zsogon, L., Rasi, E. & Convit, J. (1965): La onchocercosis en Venezuela. *Acta méd. venez.* December, 1965. Suppl. 1. 36 pp.

Rives, M. & Serie, F. (1967): *Méd. Afr. noire* **14**:483.

Rivoalen, A. (1939): *Rev. Med. Fr. Extr.-Or.* **1939**:260.

Roberts, C. J. & Usayi, E. (1971): *Central African J. Med.* **17**:144.

Roberts, C. J., McKeag, A. & Gelfand, M. (1971): *Cental African J. Med.* **17**:101.

Roberts, C. J., Whiteha, J. & Gelfand, M. (1973): *Central African J. Med.* **19**:13.

Roberts, J. M. D., Neumann, E., Göckel, C. W., & Highton, R. B. (1967): *Bull. Wld. Hlth. Org.* **37**:195.

Roberts, R. H. (1970): *Mosquito News* **30**:52.

Robles, R. (1919): *Bull. Soc. Path. Exot.* **12**:442.
Rodenwaldt, E. (1933a): *Mededeel. Dienst. Volksgezondheid Nederl.-Indie.* **22**:44.
         (1933b): *Mededeel. Dienst. Volksgezondheid Nederl.-Indie.,* **22**:54.
         (1934): *Mededeel. Dienst Volksgezondheid. Nederl.-Indie.* **23**:21.
Rodger, F. C. (1957): *Bull. Wld Hlth Org.* **16**:495.
         (1959): *Blindness in West Africa.* H. K. Lewis & Co. Ltd., London. 262 pp.
         (1960): *Amer. J. Ophthal.* **49**:104; 110; 127; 327; 560; 590.
         (1962): *Bull. Wld Hlth Org.* **27**:429.
         (1973): *Trans. Roy. Soc. Trop. Med. Hyg.,* **67**:225.
Rodger, F. C. & Brown, J. A. C. (1957): *Trans. Roy. Soc. Trop. Med. Hyg.* **51**:271.
Rodhain, J. (1943): *Ann. Soc. Belge Méd. Trop.* **23**:91.
         (1952): Les adénolymphocèles du Congo Belge. *Mem. Inst. Roy. Colon. Belge.* 21.
Rodhain, J. & Valcke, G. (1935): *Ann. Soc. Belge Méd. Trop.,* **15**:361.
Rogers, L. (1920): *Brit. Med. J.* **I**:596.
Rohde, K. (1959): *Z. Tropenmed. Parasitol.* **10**:385.
         (1960): *J. Parasitol.* **46**:764.
Rolland, A. (1972): *Trans. Roy. Soc. Trop. Med. Hyg.,* **66**:913.
Romana, C. & Wygodzinsky, P. (1950): *An del Inst. de Med. Regional* **3**:29.
Rombert, P. C., Barbosa, W. & Rocha, R. P. M. (1972): *Revta Patol. Trop.* **1**:107.
Romeo de Léon (1957): *Bull. Wld Hlth Org.* **16**:523.
Romiti, C. (1956): *West Indian Med. J.* **5**:113.
Rook, H. de (1930): *Geneesk. Tijdschr. Nederl.-Indie.* **70**:739.
         (1957a): *Doc. Med. Geogr. Trop.* **9**: 197.
         (1957b): Report of an investigation on filariasis in the Berau region (Inanwatan District, Northwest New-Guinea). South Pacific Com., Tech. paper No. 105, 19 pp.
         (1959): *Trop. Geogr. Med.,* **11**:313.
Rook, H. de & van Dijk, W. J. O. M. (1959): *Trop. Geogr. Med.* **11**:57.
Rosé, G., Biguet, J., Rosé, F. & D'Haussy, R. (1966): *Revue Hyg. Méd. Soc.* **14**:383.
Rose, H. M., Culbertson, J. T. & Molloy, E. (1944): *J. Parasit.* **30**:(Suppl.), 16.
Rosen, D. E. & Bailey. R. M. (1963): *Bull. Amer. Museum Nat. Sci. Hist.,* 126 pp.
Rosen, L. (1953): Mosquito vectors of human filariasis in Oceania. In "Filariasis in the South Pacific," South Pacific Comm. Noumea, 9–14 pp.
         (1954): *Amer. J. Trop. Med. Hyg.* **3**:742.
         (1955): *Amer. J. Hyg.* **61**:219.
Ross, S. G. (1947): *Med. J. Australia* **2**:540.
Rouffiandis, V. (1910): *Bull. Soc. Path. Exot.* **3**:145.
Rousseau, L. (1919): *Bull. Soc. Path. Exot.* **12**:35.
Row, P. (1952): *Med. J. Austr.* **1**:847.
Rowlands, A. (1956): *Trans. Roy. Soc. Trop. Med. Hyg.* **50**:563.
Roy, R. G. & Sharma, G. K. (1960): *Bull. Nat. Soc. India Malaria Mosq. Dis.* **8**:161.
Roy, S. K. & Bose, S. C. (1922): *Indian Med. Gaz.* **57**:281.
Roychowdhury, S. P., Kanan, A. M. & Das, M. (1969): *J. Com. Dis.* **1**:107.
Rozeboom, L. E. & Cabrera, B. D. (1956): *Amer. J. Hyg.,* **63**:140.
         (1963): *Nature* **200** (4909): 915.
         (1964): *J. Med. Entomol.* **1**:18.
         (1965a): *Amer. J. Epidemiol.* **81**:200.
         (1965b): *Amer. J. Epidemiol.* **81**:216.
         (1966): *Acta Med. Philipp.* **3 Ser. 2**:112.
Rozeboom, L. E. & Knight, K. L. (1946): *J. Parasit.* **32**:95.
Rozeboom, L. E., Bharracharya, N. C. & Gilotra, S. K. (1968): *Amer. J. Epidemiol.* **87**:616.
Ruiz Reyes, F. (1949): *Mex. Bull. Epidemiol.* **13**:73.
         (1950): *Medicina (Mexico)* **30**:225.

Ruiz Reyes, F. (1952): *Rev. Méd.* (Mexico) **32**:49.
Saffre (1884): *Arch. Méd. Nav.* **41**:433.
Saito, K. & Hayashi, S. (1967): *Japan. J. Sanitary Zool.* **18**:122.
            (1968): *Japan. J. Sanitary Zool.* **19**:62.
Sakuma, S., Sakuma, M., Sato, Y., Sasa, M. & Kobayashi, J. (1967): *Japan. J. Parasit.* **16**:179.
Salazar Mallen, M. (1974): Onchocerciasis in Mexico. In "Pan American Health Org.: Research and Control of Onchocerciasis in the Western Hemisphere," 112–115 pp.
Salazar Mallén, M. & González Barranco, D. (1971): *Ann. Trop. Med. Parasit.* **65**:393.
Salazar-Mallén, M., González Barranco, D. & Alvarez Fuertes, G. (1962): *Zeitschr. Tropenmed. Parasit.* **21**:213.
Samarawickrema, W. A. (1963): *Bull. Wld Hlth Org.* **27**:637.
            (1967): *Bull. Wld Hlth Org.* **37**:117.
            (1968): *Ceylon J. Med. Sci.* **17**:7.
Sandground, J. H. (1934): On the validity of various species of the genus *Onchocerca* Diesing. In Strong et al. "Onchocerciasis" Cambridge Harvard Univ. Press, 135–72 pp.
            (1936): *Ann. Soc. Belge Méd. Trop.* **16**:273.
            (1938): *Amer. J. Trop. Med.* **18**:Suppl. 91.
Sandosham, A. A. (1964): *Med. J. Malaya.* **18**:137.
Sandosham, A. A. & Sivanadam, S. (1965): *Singapore Med. J.,* **6**:42.
Sandosham, A. A., Wharton, R. H., Warren, M. & Eyeles, D. E. (1962): *J. Parasit.* **48**:489.
Sangage, S. (1967): *Méd. Afrique Noire* **14**:505.
Santiago-Stevenson, D., Oliver-Gonzales, J. & Hewitt, R. I. (1947): *J. Amer. Med. Assoc.* **135**:708.
            (1948): *Ann New York Acad Sci* **50**:161
Santos, D. (1877): Verificacio no Brazil da descoberta de Bancroft, na Australia Progresso Med. Rio de Janeiro 8–11, 95–100 pp.
Sapero, J. J., ; Butler, F. A. (1945): *J. Am. Med. Assoc.* **127**:502.
Saphir (1945): *J. Amer. Med. Assoc.,* **129**:1142.
Sarkar, J. K. (1969): *Trans. Roy. Soc. Trop. Med. Hyg.,* **63**:374.
Sarkies, J. W. R. (1952): *Trans. Roy. Soc. Trop. Med. Hyg.* **46**:435.
Sasa, M. (1944): *Kaigun Gunikai Zasshi (Naval Med. J. Japan).* **33**:90.
            (1962): Distribution of bancroftian filariasis in Japan. "Progress of Medical Parasitology in Japan." Vol. 2: 1–34 (Meguro Kiseichukan, Tokyo) (in Japanese).
            (1963): *Bull. Wld. Hlth. Org.* **28**:437.
            (1966): Epidemiology of human filariasis in Japan. "Progress of Medical Parasitology in Japan," 3:389 (Meguro Kiseichukan, Tokyo).
            (1967): *Bull. Wld Hlth Org.* **37**:629.
            (1969): An introduction to epidemiology and control of filariasis Proc. 3rd S. E. A. Regional Mtg. on Parasit. trop. Med. (Singapore) 89–97 pp.
            (1970): *Nettai* (Tokyo) **5**:89.
            (1972): Observations on some American poeciliid fishes established in polluted waters in Japan and South Asia, with special reference to their use in the control of filaria vectors. in "Research in Filariasis and Schistosomiasis," (ed. by Yokogawa, M) 67–86 pp. Univ. Tokyo Press.
            (1974a): Filariasis in the Americas: a review. In Sasa, M. (ed), "A Symposium on Parasitic Diseases." pp. 3–48, International Medical Foundation, Tokyo.
            (1974b): *Southeast Asian J. Trop. Med. Pub. Hlth* **5**:197.
Sasa, M. & Hayashi, R. (1944): "A new method for the staining of malaria parasites and blood smears for the field use." (in Japanese) Kaigun Gunigakko Hokoku (Rep. Naval Medical School, Japan) **9**:5.
Sasa, M. & Hayashi, S. (1953): Filariasis: (Epidemiology) *Saishin Kiseichugaku,* **7**:1–46, Igaku Shoin, Tokyo.
Sasa, M. & Mitsui, G. (1964): *Japan. J. Exp. Med.,* **34**:17.

Sasa, M. & Tanaka, H. (1972): *Southeast Asian J. Trop. Med. Pub. Hlth* **3**:518.
     (1974): *Japan. J. Exp. Med.* **44**:321.
Sasa, M., Hayashi, S., Sato, K., Komine, I. & Ishii, S. (1951): *Nisshin Igaku* **38**:575 (in Japanese).
Sasa, M., Hayashi, S., Kano, R., Sato, K. Komine, I. & Ishii, S. (1952): *Japan. J. Exp. Med.* **22**:357.
Sasa, M., Tanaka, H., Sato, K., Hayashi, S., Ishii, S., Komine, I. & Kogo, T. (1953): *Nihon Ishikai Zasshi* **30**:609 (in Japanese).
Sasa, M., Hayashi, S., Suzuki, T., Miura, K., Ueno, Y. & Tanaka, H. (1957): *Japan. J. Sanitary Zool.* **8**:5.
Sasa, M., Hayashi, S. & Sato, K. (1959a): *Japan. J. Parasit.* **8**:(suppl.) 14 (in Japanese).
Sasa, M., Hayashi, S., Sato, K., Ikeshoji, T. & Tanaka, H. (1959b): *Japan. J. Exp. Med.* **29**:369.
Sasa, M., Shirasaka, R., Ikeshoji, T., Shimono, O., Hatano, S., Shimagawa, T., Ogawa, H., Yamaoka, K., Honda, M., Hashimoto, T., Koito, K., Harada, M., Yatabe, T., & Seo, T. (1959c): *Japan. J. Parasit.* **8**:880.
Sasa, M., Hayashi, S. & Tanaka, H. (1960): *Indian J. Malariol.* **14**:441.
Sasa, M., Kanda, T., Miura, A. & Yamaguti, N. (1963a): *Japan. J. Exp. Med.* **33**:1.
Sasa, M., Mitsui, G. & Sato, K. (1963b): *Japan. J. Exp. Med.* **33**:47.
Sasa, M., Oshima, T., et al. (1963c): *Japan. J. Exp. Med.,* **33**:213.
Sasa, M., T. Kanda, S. Sakuma, T. Kurihara, K. Saito, A. Miura, E. Motoi, S. Kakegawa, S. Hayashi & K. Matsumoto (1964): *Japan. J. Exp. Med.* **34**:89.
Sasa, M. Kurihara, T. & Harinasuta, C. (1965a): *Japan. J. Exp. Med.* **35**:23.
Sasa, M., Harinasuta, C. Purived, Y. & Kurihara, T. (1965b): *Japan. J. Exp. Med.* **35**:51
Sasa, M., Kurihara, T. Dhamvanij, O. & Harinasuta, C. (1965c): *Japan. J. Exp. Med.* **35**:63.
Sasa, M., Shirasaka, A. & Kurihara, T. (1966): *Japan. J. Exp. Med.* **36**:187.
Sasa, M., Shirasaka, A., Wada, Y. & Kanda, T. (1967): *Japan. J. Exp. Med.* **37**:477.
Sasa, M., Wada, Y., Watanebe, M., Yasuno, M. Hirakoso, S., Shirasaka, A., Umino, T., Kamimura, K. Ishii, A. & Kitago, I., Inatomi, S., Itano, K. & Suguri, S. (1968): *Japan. J. Exp. Med.* **38**:289.
Sasa, M., Kanda, T. Mitsui, G., Shirasaka, A., Ishii, A. & Chinzei, H. (1970): The filariasis control programs in Japan and their evaluation by means of epidemiological analysis of microfilaria survey data. In "Recent Advances in Researches on Filariasis and Schistosomiasis in Japan," 3–72 pp. (Univ. Tokyo Press).
Satchell, G. H. (1950): Report of research expedition to the Cook Islands. Appendix to Rpt. New Zealand Med. Council Expedition to the Cook Islands 1949–1950.
Sato, H. (Hachiro) (1953): Filariasis. Ika Sosho, No. 142, 199 pp. Igakushoin Co. Tokyo (in Japanese).
     (1963): On the treatment of filariasis. in "Progress of Medical Parasitology, Japanese Ed. vol. 2: pp. 101–13, Meguro Kiseichukan, Tokyo.
     (1966): On the treatment of filariasis. in 'Progress of Medical Parasitology in Japan, vol. 3, pp. 513–527. Meguro Kiseichkan, Tokyo.
Sato, H. (Hideki), Okubo, S. Sasa, M., Wada, Y., Motoki, M., Tanaka, H., Yamagishi, H., Okino, T. & Kurihara, T. (1972): *Japan. J. Sanitary Zool.* **23**:113.
Sato, K. (Koji) (1959): *Japan. J. Parasit.* **8**:962.
     (1960): *Japan. J. Parasit.* **9**:22.
Sato, K. (Kumiko) (1969): *Japan. J. Parasit.* **18**:166.
Sato, K., & Sawada, T. (1969): *Japan. J. Exp. Med.* **39**:435.
Sato, S., Takei, K. & Matsuyama, S. (1969): *Japan. J. Parasit.* **18**:21.
Sato, S., Sawada, T., Takei, K. & Sato, K. (1970): An immuno-epidemiological study of filariasis by the intradermal skin test with a purified antigen FST prepared from *Dirofilaria immitis.* in "Recent Advances in Researches on Filariasis and Schistosomiasis in Japan," 191–203 pp. (Univ. Tokyo Press).
Satya Prakash, Charkrabarti, A. K., Pattanayak, S., Dalip Singh, Baboo Ram & Slaich, P. S. (1962): *Indian J. Malariol.* **16**:299.

Saugrain, J. & Outin-Fabre, D. (1972): *Bull. Wld Hlth Org.* **46**:249.

Saunders, G. M. (1941): *Amer. J. Trop. Med.* **21**:481.

Saunders, G. M., Blanco, A. A., & Jordon, W. S. (1946): *U.S. Naval Med. Bull.* **46**: 1242.

Sau-Pheng Kan & Beng-Chuan Ho (1973): *Amer. J. Trop. Med.* **22**:179.

Saussure, P. G. (1890): *Medical News, N. Y.* **56**:704.

Sautet, J. (1949): *Bull. Soc. Path. Exot.* **42**:463.

Sawada, T., Takei, K., Katamine, D. & Yoshimura, O. (1965): *Japan. J. Exp. Med.* **35**: 125.

Sawada, T., Sato, S., Matsuyama, S., Miyagi, H. & Shinzato, J. (1968): *Japan. J. Exp. Med.* **38**:405.

Sawada, T., Sato, K. & Sato, S. (1969): *Japan. J. Exp. Med.,* **39**:427.
           (1970): The further studies on the separation of responsible protein in the skin test antigen FST. in "Recent Advances in Researches on Filariasis and Schistosomiasis in Japan," 169–99 pp. (Univ. Tokyo Press).

Sawyer, T. K. & Weinstein, P. P. (1961): *J. Parasit.* **47**:(Suppl.), 24.
           (1962): *J. Parasit.* **48**:35.
           (1963): *J. Parasit.* **49**:218.

Saxena, R., Iyer, R. N., Anand, N., Chatterjee, R. K. & Sen, A. B. (1970): *J. Pharm Pharmac.* **22**:306.

Scaff, L. M. & Gueiros, Z. M. (1967): *Rev. Brasil. Malariol. D. Trop.* **19**:245.

Schacher, J. F. (1962): *J. Parasit.* **48**:663.
           (1969): *Ann. Trop. Med. Parasit.* **63**:341.
           (1973): *Southeast Asian J. Trop. Med. Pub. Hlth* 336.

Schacher, J. F. & Geddawi, M. K. (1969): *Ann. Trop. Med. Parasit.* **63**:67.

Schacher, J. F. & Sahyoun, P. F. (1967): *Trans. Roy. Soc. Trop. Med. Hyg.* **61**:234

Schacher, J. F. & Sulahian, A. (1972): *Ann. Trop. Med. Parasit.,* **66**:209.

Schacher, J. F., Geddawi, M. K. & Churchill, C. W. (1967): *J. Parasit.* **53**:892.

Schacher, J. F., Sulahian, A. & Edeson, J. F. B. (1969): *Trans. Roy. Soc. Trop. Med Hyg.* **63**:682.

Schacher, J. F., Edeson, J. F. B., Sulahian, A. & Rizk, G. (1973): *Ann. Trop. Med Parasit.* **67**:81.

Schardein, J. L. Lucas, J. A. & Dickerson, C. W. (1968): *J. Parasit.* **54**:351.

Scheepe, F. L. (1935): *Geneesk. Tijdschr. Nederl.-Indie.* **75**:1197.

Schijveschuurder, W. (1927): *Gleneesk. Tijdschr. Nederl.-Indie.* **67**:316.

Schlosser, R. J. (1945): *Amer. J. Trop. Med.* **25**:493.
           (1949): *Amer. J. Trop. Med.* **29**:739.

Schneider, C. R., Blair, L. S., Schardein, J. L., Boche, L. K. & Thompson, L. K. (1968): *J. Parasit.* **54**:1099.

Schneider, J. (1961): *Ann. Soc. Belge Méd. Trop.,* **41**:346.

Schofield, F. D. & Rowley, R. E. (1961): *Amer. J. Trop. Med. Hyg.* **10**:849.

Scott, J. A. (1948): *Amer. J. Trop. Med.* **28**:481.
           (1960): *Indian J. Malariol.* **14**:575.

Scott, J. A. & Macdonald, E. M. (1953): *Exp. Parasit.* **2**:129.

Scott, J. A., Stembridge, V. A. & Sisley, N. M. (1947): *J. Parasit.* **33**:138.

Scott, J. A., Macdonald, E. M. & Olson, L. J. (1958): *J. Parasit.* **44**:507.

Sebai, Z. A., Morsy, T. A. & El-Zawahry, M. (1974): *Castellania.* **2**:263.

Sebastian, A. & Meillon, B. de. (1967): *Bull. Wld Hlth Org* **36**:47.

Seguin (1891): *Arch. Med. Nav.* **55**:81.

Self, L. S. & Tun, M. M. (1970): *Bull. Wld Hlth Org.* **43**:631.

Seligmann, C. G. (1901): *J. Pathol. & Bacteriol.* **7**:308.

Sen, A. B., Chandra, R., Katiyar, J. C. & Chandra, S. (1974): *Indian J. Med. Res* **62**: 1181.

Sen, S. B. & Das, G. C. (1969): *Indian J. Med. Res.* **57**:1745.

Sen, S. B. & Ellappan, S. (1968): *Indian J. Med. Res.* **56**:1535.

Sen, S. K. & Puri, B. S. (1965): *Indian J. Malariol.* **19**:199.

Sen, S. B., Chatierjee, H. & Ramaprasad, S. (1969): *Indian J. Med. Res.* **57**:1738 (S.B.).

Senker, C., Noamesi, G. K. & McRae, T. M. (1973): *Ghana Med. J.* **12**:56.

Senoo, T. (1943): Nihon Kiseichu Gakkai Kiji (Proc. Japan. Soc. Parasit.) **15**:36 (Title only).

Senoo, T. & Lincicome, D. R. (1951): *U.S. Armed Force Med. J.* **2**:1483.

Senviratina, P. (1959): *J. Helminth.* **33**:123.

Seo, B. S. (1965): *Korean J. Parasit.* **3**:139.
        (1966): *Proc. 11th Pacific Sci. Congr.* **8**:11.

Seo, B. S. & Kang, S. Y. (1973): *Korean J. Parasit.* **11**:Suppl. 124.

Seo, B. S. & Lee, J. W. (1973): *Korean J. Parasit.* **11**:61.

Seo, B. S. & Rim, H. J. (1965): The epidemiological studies on the filariasis in Korea I. Filariasis in Cheju-Do (and part island). *WHO Seminar on Filariasis,* Manila.

Seo, B. S. & Whang, K. I. (1974): *Korean J. Parasit* **12**:21.

Seo, B. S., Rim, H. J., Seong, S. H., Park, Y. H., Kim, B. C. & Lim, D. B. (1964): *Korean J. Parasit.* **2**:115.

Seo, B. S., Lim, Y. C. & Rim, H. J. (1965): Distribution and epidemiological studies on the filariasis in Kyungsang-Pukdo. Abstract of 7th Annual Meeting of Korean Society of Parasitology, 12 pp.

Seo, B. S., Rim, H. J., Lim, Y. C., Kang, I. K. & Park, Y. O. (1968): *Korean J. Parasitol.* **6**:132.

Seo, B. S., Cho, S. Y. & Whang, K. I. (1973): *Korean J. Parasit.* **11**: Suppl. 123.

Sérěs (1892): *Arch. Méd. Nav.* **57**:280.

Sergent, E. & Foley, H. (1908): *Bull. Soc. Path. Exot.* **1**:472.

Service, M. W. (1970): *Ann. Trop. Med. Parasit.* **64**:131.

Sery, V., Pham Van Nong, Pham Thi Ngoe & Patova, Marie (1961): *Ceskoslov. Parasit.* (Prague). **8**:391.

Sewell, P. & Hawking, F. (1950): *Brit. J. Pharmacol.* **5**:239.

Shanghai Antischistosomiasis Bureau (1959): *Chinese Med. J.* **78**:49.

Sharma, M. I. D. & Kalra, R. L. (1962): *Indian J. Malariol* **16**:111.

Sharma, V. P. (1974): *J. Com. Dis.* **6**:127.

Sharma, V. P., Patterson, R. S., Grover, K. K. & LaBreque, G. C. (1973): *Bull. Wld Hlth Org.* **48**:45.

Sharp, N. A. D. (1927): *Ann. Trop. Med. Parasit.* **21**:415.
        (1928a): *Trans. Roy. Soc. Trop. Med. Hyg.* **21**:371–96
        (1928b): *Trans. Roy. Soc. Trop. Med. Hyg.* **21**:413.

Shawarby, A. A., Mahdi, A. H., Naguib, K. & Moharram, A. (1965): *J. Egypt Publ. Hlth Assoc.* **40**:267.

Sherlock, I. & Guitton, M. (1967): *Rev. Brasil. Malariol. D. Trop.* **19**:53.

Sherlock, I. A. & Serafin, E. M. (1967): *Rev. Brasil. Malariol. D. Trop.* **19**:373.

Shimono, O. (1961): *Japan. J. Parasitology.* **10**:119.

Shookhoff, H. R. & Dwork, K. G. (1949): *Amer. J. Trop. Med.* **29**:589.

Sice, A. (1927): *Bull. Soc. Path. Exot.* **20**:422.

Silva, D. L. S. & Schacher, J. F. (1959): *Amer. J. Trop. Med. Hyg.* **8**:151.

Silva Araujo, A. J. P. (1877): *Gaz. Med. da Bahia* **2**:492.

Silva Lima, J. da (1878): *Lancet,* March 23, 1878, 440.

Simpson, E. J. S. (1957): *New Zealand Med. J.* **56**:136.

Simpson, M. G. & Laurence, B. R. (1972): *Parasitology* **64**:61.

Simpson, T. W. (1951): *Amer. J. Trop. Med.* **31**:614.

Singh, M. V. (1960): *Indian J. Malariol.* **14**:379.

Singh, B., Basu, P. C. & Raghavan, N. G. S. (1967a): *Bull. Indian Soc. Malaria Com. Dis.* **4**:65.

Singh, B., Basu, P. C., Raghavan, N. G. S. & Bedi, K. M. S. (1967b): *Bull. Indian Soc. Malaria Com. Dis.* **4**:260.

Singh, B., Raghavan, N. G. S., Nagaraj, Kumar & Basu, P. C. (1968): *Bull. Indian Soc. Malaria. Com. Dis.* **5**:108.

Singh, M. V., Rastogi, K. C. & Srivastava, R. N. (1962): *Bull. Nat. Soc. India Mosq. Dis.* **10**:111.

Singh, M. V. Agarwala, R. S. & Srivastava, R. N. (1963a): *Indian J. Malariol.* **17**:279.

Singh, M. V., Agarwala, R. S. & Nawab Singh. (1963b): *Indian J. Malariol.* **17**:295.

Singh, M. V., Agarwala, R. S. Nanda, D. K. (1963c): *Indian J. Malariol.* **17**:297.

Singh, M. V., Rastogi, K. C., Singh, R. P. & Srivastava, V. K. (1963d): *Indian J. Malariol.* **17**:303.

                (1963e): *Indian J. Malariol.* **17**:357.

                (1964):   *Bull. Indian Soc. Malaria Comm. Dis.* **1**: 141.

Sinha, A. P., Nanda, D. K., Singh, M. V. & Diwan Chand. (1959):   *Indian J. Malariol.* **13**:159.

Sinha, V. P. (1967): *Patna J. Med.* **41**:193.

      (1968): *Patna J. Med.* **42**:207.

Sivanandam, S. & Fredericks, H. J. (1966): *Med. J. Malaya* **20**:337.

          (1968): *Med. J. Malaya* **22**:138.

Slee, W. van (1930): *Geneesk. Tijdschr. Nederl.-Indie.* **70**:444.

Smit, A. M. & Zuidema, P. J. (1973): *Ned. Tijdschr. Geneesk.* **117**:1225.

Smith, A. (1955a, b, c, d): *Bull. Entom. Res.* **46**:419; *Ibid,* **46**:437; *Ibid,* **46**:495; *Ibid,* **46**:505.

Smith, A. J. & Rivas, D. (1914): *Amer. J. Trop. Dis.* **2**:361.

Smith, D. E., Wilson, T., Berezancev, Ju. A., Lykov, V., Paing, M., Chari, M. V. & Davis, A. (1971): *Bull. Wld. Hlth Org.* **44**:771.

Smith, E. K. M., Tunks, E. & Tuttle, R. J. (1971): *J. Canadian Med. Ass.* **105**:1315.

Smith, F. R. Jr. (1945): *U.S. Naval Med. Bull.* **44**:719.

Snijders, E. P. (1935): *Nederl. Tijdschr. v. Geneesk.* **79**:3024.

Soetrisno (1940): *Geneesk. Tijdschr. Nederl.-Indie.* **80**:2313.

Soewadji, Prawirohardjo. (1939): *Geneesk. Tijdschr. Nederl.-Indie.* **79**:1691.

Soh, C. T. (1965): Filariasis in Korea, 23–31, pp. in "Review of parasites in Korea," 46 pp. Yonsei Univ. Med. College, Seoul

Soh, C. T. & Kim, D. C. (1974): *Yonsei Reports on Tropical Med.* **5**:104.

Somasundaram, P. (1949): *Indian J. Med. Sci.* **3**:420.

Someren, E. C. C. Van, Teesdale, C. & Furlong, M. (1955): *Bull. Entomol. Res.* **46**: 463.

Someren, V. D. Van & McMahon, J. P. (1950): *Nature,* **166**:350.

Song, J. S. & Lee, K. T. (1964): *Korean J. Parasit.* **2**:125.

South Pacific Commission (1953): Filariasis in the South Pacific. 108 pp.

Southgate, B. A. (1973): *Southeast Asian J. Trop. Med. Pub. Hlth* **4**:172.

        (1974): *Trans. Roy. Soc. Trop. Med. Hyg.* **68**:177.

Soutrisno. (1940): *Geneesk, Tijdschr. Nederl.-Indie.,* **80**:2313–28; 2349.

Souveine, G., Dodin, A., Grjebine, A., & Brygoo, E. R. (1955): *Bull. Soc. Path. Exot.* **48**:669.

Spencer, J. (1962): *J. Trop. Med. Hyg.* **65**:256.

Srivastava, R. N. & Prasad, B. G. (1969): *Indian J. Med. Res.* **57**:528.

Srivastava, S. S. L. (1945): *Indian Med. Gaz.* **80**:94.

Stafford, J. L., Hill, K. L. & de Montaigne, E. L. (1955): *West Indian Med. J.* **4**:183.

Stenhouse, H. M. (1925): *U.S. Nav. Med. Bull.* **22**:1.

Stephens, J. W. W. (1921): *Ann. Trop. Med. Parasitol.,* **14**:341.

Stephens, J. W. W. & Yorke, W. (1920): *Brit. Med. J.* **2**:231.

Steward, J. S. (1937): *Parasitology* **29**:212.

Stoffolano, J. G. Jr. (1973): *Exp. Parasit.* **33**:263.

Stoll, N. R. (1947): *J. Parasit.* **33**:1.

Stone, A. & Rosen, L. (1952): *Proc. Hawaii Entom. Soc.* **14**:425.

        (1953): *J. Wash. Acad. Sci.* **43**:354.

Stone, A., Knight, K. L. & Starcke, H. (1959): A synoptic catalogue of the mosquitoes of the world. 358 pp. Entomological Society of America, Washington.

Strahan, J. H. & Norris, V. H. (1934): *Malayan Med. J.* **9**:44.

Strohschneider, H. (1956): *Amer. J. Trop. Med. Hyg.* **5**:158.

Strong, R. P. (1931): *New England J. Med.* **204**:916.

Strong, R. P. (1934): Onchocerciasis with special reference to the Central American form of the disease. In Strong et al., "Onchocerciasis", 1–132 pp., Harvard Univ. Press.

(1937): *Trans. Roy. Soc. Trop. Med. Hyg.* **30**:487.

(1938): *Amer. J. Trop. Med.* **18**: Suppl. 1.

Strong, R. P., Sandground, J. H., Bequaert, J. C. & Ochoa, M. M. (1934): Onchocerciasis, with special reference to the Central American form of the disease. Harvard Univ. Press, Cambridge, 234 pp.

Stryker, R. G. & Young, W. W. (1970): *Mosquito News,* **30**:388.

Subra, R. (1970): *Cah. ORSTOM. Sér, Ent. Méd. Parasit.* **8**:353.

(1972): *Cah. ORSTOM. Sér. Ent. Méd. Parasit.* **10**:3.

Subra, R. & Mouchet, J. (1968): *Bull. Wld Hlth Org.* **38**:484.

Subramaniam, H. & Temp, M. R. V. (1958): *Indian J. Malariol.* **12**:77.

Subramaniam, H., Ramoo, H. & Sumanam, S. D. (1958): *Indian J. Malariol.* **12**:115.

Subramaniam, R. (1953): *J. Indian Med. Assoc.* **22**:353.

Sucharit, S. & Macdonald, W. W. (1972): *Southeast Asian J. Trop. Med. Pub. Hlth.* **3**:347.

Sucharit, S., Riganti, M. & Harinasuta, C. (1974): *Southeast Asian J. Trop. Med. Pub. Hlth.* **5**:223.

Suganuma, S. (1921): *Nihon Naikagakkai Zasshi* **9**(2).

Suldey, E. W. (1918): *Bull. Soc. Path. Exot.* **11**:61.

Sullivan, T. J. & Hembree, S. C. (1970): *Trans. Roy. Soc. Trop. Med. Hyg.* **64**:787.

Sundaram, R. M., Koteswara Rao, N., Krishna Rao, C., Krishna Rao. P. & Rao, C. K. (1974): *J. Com. Dis.* **6**:290.

Suzuki, T. (1962): *Japan. J. Sanitary Zool.* **13**:311.

(1971): Analytical studies on insecticide resistance. *in* Sasa, M. (ed.), Progress of Medical Zoology, vol. 1, 225–250 pp. (in Japanese), Gakujutsusho Shuppankai, Tokyo.

Suzuki, T. & Mizutani, K. (1962): *Japan J. Exp. Med.* **32**:297.

(1963): *Japan. J. Exp. Med.* **33**:69.

Suzuki, T. & Ogata, K. (1968): "Nihon no eisei gaichu" (Arthropods of medical importance in Japan). Shin Shichosha, Tokyo; 245 pp. (in Japanese).

Suzuki, T. & Sone, F. (1974): *Japan. J. Sanitary Zool.* **25**:251.

Suzuki, T., Mizutani, K., Unimo, T. & Matsunaga, H. (1964a): *Japan. J. Sanitary Zool.* **15**:166.

(1964b): *Japan. J. Sanitary Zool.* **15**:267.

Suzuki, T., Ito, Y. & Harada, S. (1963): *Japan. J. Exp. Med.* **33**:41.

Sweet, W. C. (1924a): *Health* **2**:42.

(1924b): Final Report of the Australian Hookworm Campaign. pt. II. Malaria and filaria survey, Brisbane.

Sweet, W. C. & Dirckze, H. A. (1934): *Ceylon J. Sci.* (D) **3**:177.

Sweet, W. C. & Pillay, V. M. (1937): *Indian Med. Gaz.* **72**:730.

Symes, C. B. (1955): *Trans. Roy. Soc. Trop. Med. Hyg.* **49**:280.

(1960a): *J. Trop. Med. Hyg.* **63**:1.

(1960b): *J. Trop. Med. Hyg.* **63**:31.

(1960c): *J. Trop. Med. Hyg.* **63**:59.

Symes, C. B. & Hadaway, A. B. (1947): *Bull. Entomol. Res.* **37**:399.

Symposium on onchocerciasis (1958): *Trans. Roy. Soc. Trop. Med. Hyg.* **52**:95.

Tabibzadeh, I., Behbehani, G. & Nakhai, R. (1970): *Bull. Wld Hlth Org.,* **43**:623.

Tada, I. & Kawashima, K. (1964): *Japan. J. Parasit.* **13**:427.

Tada, I. & Marroquin, H. F. (1974): *Japan. J. Parasit.* **23**:220.

Tada, I., Sato, A., Katamine, D. & Imai, J. (1970): On the immunologic activity of a refined *Dirofilaria immitis* antigen. In Sasa, M. (ed.) "Recent Advances in Researches on Filariasis and Schistosomiasis in Japan," 205–30 pp. (Univ. Tokyo Press).

Tada, I., Iwamoto, I. & Wonde, T. (1973): *Japan. J. Trop. Med. Hyg.* **1**:13.

Tada, I., Maroquin, H. F. & Takaoka, H. (1974): *Japan. J. Trop. Med. Hyg.* **2**:35.

Tadano, T. (1969): *Japan. J. Sanitary Zool.* **20**:158.
Tadano, T. & Brown, A. W. A. (1967): *Bull. Wld Hlth Org.* **36**:101.
Takaoka, M., Tanaka, H., Kamiya, M. & Shiroma, Y. (1973): *Japan. J. Parasit.* **22**:222.
Takeda, U. Kurihara, T., Suzuki, T., Sasa, M., Miura, A., Matsumoto K., & Tanaka
   H., (1962): *Japan. J. Sanitary Zool.* **13**:31.
Tampi, M. K. (1931): *Puerto Rico J. Pub. Hlth Trop. Med.* **6**:435.
Tamura, Y. (1953): *Nagasaki Igakkai Zasshi* (J. Med. Assoc. Nagasaki) **28**:972.
         (1954): *Nagasaki Daigaku Fudobyo Kenkyusho Gyoseki* (Rep. Endemic
   Diseases Inst., Nagasaki Univ.) **29**:890.
Tanaka, H. (Hidebumi) (1964): *Japan. J. Parasit.* **13**:507.
                        (1965a): *Jikken Dobutsu* (*Bull. Exp. Animals*) **14**:80.
                        (1965b): *Japan. J. Parasit.* **14**:1.
Tanaka, H. (Hiroshi), Chiba, T. & Tanaka, H. (Hidebumi) (1963): *Japan. J. Parasit.*
   12:191.
Tanaka, H., Kobayashi, J., Matsuda, H. & Sasa, M. (1968a): *Japan. J. Exp. Med.* **38**:
   19.
Tanaka, H., Kamiya, M., Fujita, K. & Sasa, M. (1968b): *Japan. J. Exp. Med.* **38**:415.
Tanaka, H., Kobayashi, J., Ishii, A. & Sasa, M. (1969): *Japan. J. Exp. Med.* **39**: 393.
Tanaka, H., Fujita, K., Kobayashi, J., Ishii, A. & Sasa, M. (1970a): Development of
   antibody in cotton rats infected with *Litomosoides carinii*. In Sasa, M. (ed.) "Recent
   Advances in Researches on Filariasis and Schistosomiasis in Japan," 217–30 pp.
   (Univ. Tokyo Press).
Tanaka, H., Fujita, K., Sasa, M., Tagawa, M., Naito, M. & Kurokawa, K. (1970b):
   Japan. J. Exp. Med. **40**:47.
Tanaka, S. (1937): *Taiwan Igakkai Zasshi* (*J. Taiwan Med. Assoc.*) **36**:1815.
         (1938): *Taiwan Igakkai Zasshi* (*J. Taiwan Med. Assoc.*) **37**:515.
T'ang, Chi-Ho, Hsu, Pen-Ch'ien & Chang, Wen-Yi (1959): *Chinese Med. J.* **78**:175.
Tasaka, S. (1965): *Japan. J. Parasit.* **14**:414.
Taufflieb, R. (1955): (Onchocerciasis in Chad) *Bull. Soc. Path. Exot.* **48**:564.
Taylor, A. E. R. (1960a): *Exp. Parasit.* **9**:113.
                  (1960b): *Trans. Roy. Soc. Trop. Med. Hyg.* **54**:450.
Taylor, A. E. R. & Terry, R. J. (1960): *Trans. Roy. Soc. Trop. Med. Hyg.* **54**:33.
Taylor, A. W. (1930): *Ann. Trop. Med. Parasit.* **24**:425.
Taylor, F. H. (1943): Mosquito intermediary hosts of disease in Australia and New
   Guinea. *Common-Wealth of Australia, Dept. Health Service Publication*, 154 pp.
Teischler, H. (1938): *Arch. Schiffs-Tropenhyg.* **9**:421.
Ten Eyck, D. R. (1973): *Amer. J. Epidem.*, **98**:283.
Tesch, J. W. (1937): *Geneesk. Tijdschr. Nederl.-Indie.*, **77**:1434.
Theobald, F. V. (1901): A monograph of the Culicidae of the World. vol. 1:424 pp.
   London.
Thetford, N. D., Otto, G. F., Brown, H. W., and Maren, T. H. (1948): *Amer. J. Trop.
   Med.* **28**:577.
Thézé, J. (1916): *Bull. Soc. Path. Exot.* **9**:464.
Thiraux, A. (1912): *Bull. Soc. Path. Exot.* **5**:438.
Thomas, D. B., Anderson, R. I. & MacRae, A. A. (1973): *Bull. Wld Hlth Org.* **49**:493.
Thomas, T. C. E. (1958): *Ann. Trop. Med. Parasit.* **52**:1.
Thomas, V. (1969): Genetics in control of filariasis. Proc. 3rd S. E. A. Regional Mtg
   on Parasit. Trop. Med. (Singapore) 144–8 pp.
Thomas, V. & Ramachandran, C. P. (1970): *Med. J. Malaya,* **24**:196.
Thompson, K. J., Rifkin, H. & Zarrow (1945): *J. Amer. Med. Assoc.,* **129**:1074.
Thompson, P. E., Boche, L. & Blair, L. S. (1968): *J. Parasit.* **54**:834.
Thooris, G. C., Heuls, J., Kessel, J. F., L'Hoiry & Bambridge, B. (1956): *Bull. Soc.
   Path. Exot.* **49**:1138.
Thorpe, V. G. (1896): *Brit. Med. J.* **2**:922.
                (1898): *Brit. Med. J.* **1**:53.
Tisseuil, J. (1936): *Bull. Soc. Path. Exot.* **29**:47.

814   REFERENCES

(1950): *Bull. Soc. Path. Exot.* **43**:556.
Toffaleti, J. P. & King, W. V. (1947): *J. National Malaria Soc.* **6**:32.
Toufic, N. (1969): *Bull. Soc. Path. Exot.* **62**:728.
Toumanoff, C. (1958): *Bull. Soc. Path. Exot.* **51**:908.
Toumanoff, C., Try, H. T. & Chang, T. L. (1939): *Rev. Med. Fr. Extr.-Or.* **24**:871.
Touzé, M. (1954): *Bull. Soc. Path. Exot.* **47**:284.
Townes, H. (1962): *Proc. Entom. Soc. Washington* **64**:253–62.
(1971): *Ann. Trop. Med. Parasit.* **65**:93.
Trapido, H., D'Alessandoro, A. & Little, M. D. (1971): *Amer. J. Trop. Med. Hyg.* **20**: 104.
Travis, B. V., Vargas, V. M. & Swartzwelder, J. C. (1974): *Rev. Biol. Trop.* **22**:187.
Trent, S. C. (1963): *Amer. J. Trop. Med. Hyg.* **12**:877.
Tribondeau (1900): *Arch. Méd. Nav.* **74**:107.
(1902): *C. R. Soc. Biol.,* Paris, **54**:1419.
(1903): *C. R. Soc. Biol.,* Paris. **55**:996.
Tristan, M., Dodin, A. & Brygoo, E. R. (1963): *Rev. Méd. Madagascar.* **3**:3.
Tsai, Y. H., Grundmann, A. W. (1969): *Proc. Helminth. Soc. Washington,* **36**:61.
Tsai, Y. H., Grundmann, A. W. & Rees, D. M. (1969): *Mosquito News* **29**:102.
Tubangui, M. & Cabrera, B. D. (1948): *Acta Med. Philipp.* **5**:50.
Tulloch, G. S. & Anderson, R. A. (1972): Tetramisole and canine dirofilariasis. *In* Bradley, R. E. (ed.) "Canine Heartworm Disease," 101–4 pp. (Univ. Florida).
Tulloch, G. S., Pacheco, G., Casey, H. W., Bills, W. E., Davis, I. & Anderson, B. A. (1970): *Amer. J. Vet. Res.* **31**:437.
Turner, L. H. (1959a): *Trans. Roy. Soc. Trop. Med. Hyg.* **53**:154.
(1959b): *Ann. Trop. Med. Parasit.* **53**:180.
Turner, L. H. & Edeson, J. F. B. (1957): *Ann. Trop. Med. Parasit.,* **51**:271.
Turner, L. H. & Sodhy, L. S. (1959): *Ann. Trop. Med. Parasit.* **53**:268.
Uemura, S. (1967): *Trop. Med.* (Nagasaki) **9**:24.
Umino, T. (1965a): *Japan. J. Sanitary Zool.* **16**:90.
(1965b): *Japan. J. Sanitary Zool.* **16**:221.
(1965c): *Japan. J. Sanitary Zool.* **16**:282.
(1966): *Japan. J. Sanitary Zool.* **17**:37.
Umino, T. & Suzuki, T. (1964): *Japan. J. Sanitary Zool.* **15**:174.
(1967): *Japan. J. Sanitary Zool.* **18**:144.
Uttley, K. H. (1959): *West Indian Med. J.* **8**:238.
Vadhera, K. K. (1970): *Armed Forces Med. J.,* India, **26**:158.
Vaga, A. C. (1959): *Anais Inst. Med. Trop.* 16, Supl. **6**:452.
Valker, N. J. (1924): *Australian J. Exp. Med. Sci.* **1**:39.
Vanbreuseghen, R. (1950): *Ann. Soc. Belge Med. Trop.* **30**:71.
(1959): *Arch. Venezolanos Med. Trop. Parasit. Med.* **3**:170.
Vargas, L. (1942): *Rev. Inst. Salubr. y Enferm. Trop.* **3**:57.
Varma, B. K. & Sinha, V. P. (1964): *Patna J. Med.* **38**:329.
Varma, B. K., Sinha, V. P. & Dass, N. L. (1960): *Bull. Nat. Soc. India Malaria Comm. Dis.* **8**:149.
Varma, B. K., Dass, N. L., & Sinha, V. P. (1961a): *Indian J. Malariol.* **15**:185.
(1961b): *Indian J. Malariol.* **15**:285.
(1961c): *Indian J. Malariol.* **15**:293.
Varma, B. K., Gupta, B. K. & Sinha, V. P. (1961d): *Bull. Nat. Soc. India Malaria Mosq. Dis.* **8**:113.
Varma, B. K., Prasad, R. M., Dass, N. L. & Sinha, V. P. (1962): *Indian J. Malariol.* **16**: 17.
Varma, B. K., Sinha, V. P. & Dass, N. L. (1964): *Bihar. Ptna J. Med.* **38**:76.
Vasselo, S. M. (1939): *East African Med. J.* **15**:299.
Vedy, J. & Sirol, J. (1973a): *Revue Epid. Méd. Soc. Santé Publ.,* **21**:165.
(1973b): *Revue Int. Trachome,* **50**:47.
Venner, R. B. (1944): *U.S. Naval Med. Bull.* **43**:955.

Vevers, G. M. (1924): *London Sch. Trop. Med. Res. Memoir* **5**:119.

Viala (1909): *Ann. Hyg. Méd. Colon.* **12**:422.

Vickers, W. J. & Strahan, J. H. (1937): "A health survey of the State of Kedah." Kyle Palmer & Co. Ltd., Kuala Lumpur.

Villegas, A. L., Allen, J. H. & Little, M. D. (1972): *Amer. J. Trop. Med. Hyg.* **21**:944.

Vinson, E. (1877): *Arch. Méd. Nav.* **28**:22.

Vivie (1903): *Ann. Hyg. Méd. Col.* **6**:367.

Voelker, J. & Garms, R. (1972): *Z. Tropenmed. Parasit.* **23**:285.

Vogel, E. & Riou, M. (1939): *Ann. Méd. Pharm. Colon.* **37**:430.

Wada, Y., Katamine, D. & Oh, M. Y. (1973): *Japan. J. Trop. Med. Hyg.* **1**:197.

Wagner, W. H. (1956): *Z. Tropenmed. Parasit.* **7**:163.

Wakasugi, M. (1955): *Japan. J. Parasit.* **4**:375.

            (1957a,b): *Japan. J. Parasit.* **6**:211; 397.

            (1958a): *Japan. J. Parasit.* **7**:78.

            (1958b): *Japan. J. Parasit.* **7**:514.

Walker, M. J. (1924): *Austr. J. Exp. Biol. Med. Sci.* **1**:39.

Wallace, C. R. & Screws, R. (1972): Preliminary study of microfilarial embolization after filaricidal therapy. *In* Bradley, R. E. (ed.) "Canine Heartworm Disease," 43–49 pp. (Univ. Florida).

Wang, C. F., Lin, C. L. & Ch'en W. H. (1959): *Chinese Med. J.* **78**:171.

Wang, C. P., Chu, C. H. & Chang, P. H. (1959): *Chinese Med. J.* **78**:179.

Wang, Y. C. & Fan, P. C. (1973): *Southeast Asian J. Trop. Med. Pub. Hlth.* **4**:324.

Wang, Y. H. (1959): *Chinese Med. J.* **78**:180.

Wang, Y. H. & Lu, P. Y. (1959): *Chinese Med. J.* **78**:173.

Wang, Y. S. & Coworkers (1959): *Chinese Med. J.* **68**:174.

Wanson, M. (1949): *Ann. Soc. Belge Méd. Trop.* **29**:73.

            (1950): *Ann. Soc. Belge Méd. Trop.* **30**:667.

Wanson, M. & Peel, E. (1949): *Ann. Soc. Belge Méd. Trop.* **29**:213.

Wanson, M., Courtis, L. & Lebied, B. (1949): *Ann. Soc. Belge Méd. Trop.* **29**:373.

Waring, E. J. (1852): *Indian Ann. Med. Sci.* **5**:1.

Warne, R. J., Tipton, V. J. & Furusho, Y. (1969): *Amer. J. Vet. Res.* **30**:27.

Wartman, W. B. (1944): *Amer. J. Trop. Med.* **24**:299.

            (1947): *Medicine,* **26**:333.

Wartman, W. B. & King, B. G. (1944): *Bull. U.S. Army Med. Dept.* **76**:45.

Wattal, B. L. & Kalra, N. L. (1960): *Indian J. Malariol.* **14**:605.

Wattal, B. L., Kalra, N. L. & Bedi, K. M. S. (1961): *Indian J. Malariol.,* **15**:321.

Wattal, B. L., Bhatnagar, V. N. & Sharma, S. K. (1975): *J. Com. Dis.* **7**:65.

Webber, W. A. F. (1955): *Ann. Trop. Med. Parasit.* **49**:123.

Webber, W. A. F., & Hawking, F. (1955): *Exp. Parasitol.* **4**:143.

Webster, E. H. (1946): *U.S. Naval Med. Bull.* **46**:186.

Webster's Geographical dictionary (1973): G. & C. Merrian Co. Publishers, Springfield, Mass.

Wechsler, Z. (1939): *Schweiz. Med. Wochensch.* **69**:816.

Wegesa, P. (1967a): *Ann. trop. Med. Parasit.* **61**:89.

            (1967b): *Ann. Report East African Institute of Malaria and Vector-Borne Diseases,* 66.

Weidhaas, D. E., Schmidt, C. H. & Seabrook, E. L. (1962): *Mosquito News* **22**:283.

Weidhaas, D. E., Smittle, B. J., Patterson, R. S., Ford, H. R. & Lofgren, C. S. (1973): *Mosquito News,* **33**:83.

Weiner, D. J. & Bradley, R. E. (1972): Serologic changes in primary and secondary infections of beagle dogs with Dirofilaria immitis. In Bradley, R. E. (ed.) "Canine Heartworm Disease," 77–86 pp.

Weinstein, P. P. & Sawyer, T. K. (1961): *J. Para sit.* **47**:(Suppl.), 23.

Welch, H. E. (1960): *Proc. Helminth. Soc. Washington* **27**:203.

            (1962): *Proc. Entomol. Soc. Ontario* **92**:11.

            (1964): *Bull. Wld Hlth Org.* **31**:857.

816   REFERENCES

Welch, H. E. (1965): *Annual Review of Entomology* **10**:275.
Welch, A. D., Peters, L., Bueding, E., Valk, A., Jr., & Higashi, A. (1947): *Science* **105**:486.
Wenceslao, J. M., Oban, E. & Cabrera, B. D. (1972): *Southeast Asian J. Trop. Med. Pub. Hlth* **3**:552.
Wenk, P. & Raybould, J. N. (1972): *Bull. Wld Hlth Org.* **47**:627.
Wenk, P. & Schulz-Key, H. (1974): *Tropenmed. Parasit.* **25**:381.
Werd, H. J. J. M. Van de (1973): *Trop. Geogr. Med.* **25**:307.
Werry, W. B. & McDill, J. R. (1905): *Bull. Bur. Gov. Lab. Biol. Lab.* Manila, P. I., **3**:5.
Wharton, R. H. (1957a): *Ann. Trop. Med. Parasit.* **51**:278.
    (1957b): *Ann. Trop. Med. Parasit.* **51**:422.
    (1959a): *Mosquito News.* **19**:102.
    (1959b): *J. Parasitol.* **45**:513.
    (1959c): *Bull. Wld. Hlth Org.* **20**:729.
    (1959d): *Nature.,* **181**:830.
    (1960a): *Ann. Trop. Med. Parasit.* **54**:78.
    (1960b): *Indian J. Malariology* **14**:375.
    (1962): The biology of *Mansonia* mosquitoes in relation to the transmission of filariasis in Malaya. *Bull. No. 11, Inst. Med. Res.* (Kuala Lumpur) 114 pp.
    (1963): *Zoonoses Res.* **2**:1.
Wharton, R. H. & Omar, A. H. (1962): *Ann. Trop. Med. Parasit.* **56**:188.
Wharton, R. H. & Santa Maria, F. L. (1958): *Ann. Trop. Med. Parasit.* **52**:93.
Wharton, R. H., Edeson, J. F. B. & Laing, A. B. G. (1958a): *Trans. Roy. Soc. Trop. Med. Hyg.,* **52**:288.
Wharton, R. H., Edeson, J. F. B., Wilson, T. & Reid, J. A. (1958b): *Ann. Trop. Med. Parasit.* **52**:191.
Wharton, R. H., Laing, A. B. G. & Cheong, W. H. (1963): *Ann. Trop. Med. Parasit.,* **57**:235.
Wheeling, H. & Hutchison, W. F. (1971): *Japan. J. Exp. Med.* **41**:171.
White, G. B. (1966): *Nature* (London) **216**:383.
    (1971a): *East African Med. J.* **48**:266.
    (1971b): *Trans. Roy. Soc. Trop. Med. Hyg.,* **65**:819.
    (1973): *Bull. Entom. Res.,* **63**:65.
    (1974): *Trans. Roy. Soc. Trop. Med. Hyg.* **68**:278.
White, G. B. & Rosen, P. (1973): *Bull. Entom. Res.* **62**:613.
Whyte, G. D. & Camb, H. (1909): *J. Trop. Med. Hyg.* **12**:175.
Wijetunge, H. P. A. (1967a): *J. Trop. Med. Hyg.* **70**:25.
    (1967b): *J. Trop. Med. Hyg.* **70**:90.
Willesme, J. J. (1959): *Trop. Geogr. Med.,* **11**:237.
William-Olsson, R. (1970): *Acta Trop.* **27**:173.
Williams, E. H. & Williams, P. H. (1966): *East African Med. J.* **43**:208.
Williams, F. M. & Patterson, R. S. (1969): *Mosquito News* **29**:662.
Williams, P. (1960): *Ann. Trop. Med. Parasit.* **54**:439.
    (1961a): *Ann. Trop. Med. Parasit.* **55**:1.
    (1961b): *Ann. Trop. Med. Parasit.* **55**:452.
    (1962a): *Ann. Trop. Med. Parasit.* **56**:149.
    (1962b): *Ann. Trop. Med. Parasit.* **56**:274.
    (1962c): *Ann. Trop. Med. Parasit.* **56**:284.
Williams, R. W. (1968): *WHO Chronicle* **22**:219.
Williams, T. R. (1968): *Trans. Roy. Soc. Trop. Med. Hyg.* **62**:29.
Williams, T. R., Hynes, H. B. N. & Kershaw, W. E. (1964): *Ann. Trop. Med. Parasit.* **58**:159.
Wilson, T. (1950): *Trans. Roy. Soc. Trop. Med. Hyg.* **44**:49.
    (1954): *Ann. Rpt of the Int. Med. Res. Malaya.,* **25**:278.
    (1956): *Trans. Roy. Soc. Trop. Med. Hyg.* **50**:54.

Wilson, T. (1961): *Trans. Roy. Soc. Trop. Med. Hyg.* **55**:107.
    (1962): *Ann. Trop. Med. Parasit.* **56**:191.
    (1969a): *Bull. Wld Hlth Org.,* **41**:324.
    (1969b): *Proc. 3rd S.E.A. Regional Mtg on Parasit. Trop. Med.* (Singapore) 139.
Wilson, T. & Ramachandran, C. P. (1971): *Ann. Trop. Med. Parasit.* **65**:525.
Wilson, T. & Reid, J. A. (1951): "Filariasis.," in "The Institute for Medical Research Kuala Lumpur 1900–1950" No. 25, 209–227 pp.
Wilson, T., Edeson, J. F. B., Wharton, R. H., Reid, J. A., Turner, L. H. & Laing, A. B. G. (1958): *Trans. Roy. Soc. Trop. Med. Hyg.* **52**:480.
Wise, K. S. (1907): *Brit. Guiana Med. Ann.* **135**:40 (quoted by Iyengar, 1967).
    (1908): *Nrit. Guiana Med. Ann.* **35**:35 (quoted by Iyengar, 1957).
    (1909): *J. Trop. Med. Hyg.* **12**:276.
    (1910): *J. Trop. Med. Hyg.* **13**:137.
Wiseman, R. A. (1967): *Trans. Roy. Soc. Trop. Med. Hyg.* **61**:667.
Wolfe, M. S. & Aslamkhan, M. (1968): *Trans. 8th Internt. Congr. Trop. Med. Malaria* (Teheran) 113.
    (1969): *Trans. Roy. Soc. Trop. Med. Hyg.* **63**:147.
    (1971): *Trans. Roy. Soc. Trop. Med. Hyg.* **65**:63.
    (1972): *Amer. J. Trop. Med. Hyg.,* **21**:22.
Wolfe, M. S., Petersen, J. L., Neafie, R. C., Connor, D. H. & Purtilo, D. T. (1974): *Amer. J. Trop. Med. Hyg.* **23**; 361.
Wong, M. M. (1964): *Amer. J. Trop. Med. Hyg.* **13**:66.
    (1969): *Bull. Wld Hlth Org.* **40**:493.
Wong, M. M. & Chong, L. K. (1967): *Med. J. Malaya* **21**:383.
Wong, M. M. & Guest, M. F. (1969): *Trans. Roy. Soc. Trop. Med. Hyg.* **63**:796.
Wongsathuaythong, S., Punyagupta, S., Sirirorasarn, P. & Chularek, P. (1963): *Roy. Thai. Army. Med. J.* **16**:101.
Woodman, H. M. (1948): *East African Med. J.* **25**:95.
    (1949): *Trans. Roy. Soc. Trop. Med. Hyg.* **42**:543.
    (1950): *Trans. Roy. Soc. Trop. Med. Hyg.* **43**:549.
    (1958): *East African Med. J.* **35**:457.
Woodman, H. M. & Bokhari, A. (1941): *Trans. Roy. Soc. Trop. Med. Hyg.* **35**:77.
Woodruff, A. W. (1952): *West African Med. J.* **1**:45.
Woodruff, A. W. & Wiseman, R. (1968): *Exp. Parasit.* **22**:295.
Woodruff, A. W., Choyce, D. P., Pringle, G., Laing, A. B. G., Hills, M. & Wegesa, P. (1966a): *Trans. Roy. Soc. Trop. Med. Hyg.* **60**:695.
Woodruff, A. W., Choyce, D. P., Muci-Mendoza, F., Hills, M. & Petit, L. E. (1966b): *Trans. Roy. Soc. Trop. Med. Hyg.* **60**:707.
World Health Organization (1954): Expert Committee on Onchocerciasis. First Report. WHO Technical Report Series No. 87, 37 pp.
    (1962): Expert Committee on Filariasis (*Wuchereria* and *Brugia* infections) Report Wld Hlth Org. Techn. Rep. Ser. No. 233, 49 pp.
    (1966): WHO Expert Committee on Onchocerciasis. Second Report. WHO Tech. Rep. Ser. No. 335, 96 pp.
    (1967): *Bull. Wld Hlth Org.* **36**:1;163 (collection of 17 papers).
    (1967): Expert Committee on filariasis (*Wuchereria* and *Brugia* infections). Second Report Wld Hlth Org. Techn. Rep. Ser. No. 359, 47 pp.
    (1968): Filariasis. Wld Hlth Statist. Rep. No. 21, 576 pp.
World Health Organization (1971): *Bull. Wld Hlth Org.* **44**:1.
    (1974a): WHO Expert Committee on Filariasis, Third Report. WHO Tech. Rep. Ser. No. 542, 54 pp.
    (1974b): Equipments for vector control. (Second Edition). 179 pp.

World Health Organization: South Pacific Commission, (1968): Second WHO/SPC Joint Seminar on Filariasis. Apia, Western Samoa, 6–12 pp. Aug. Final Report (44 mineographed pp).

World Health Organization & South Pacific Commission (1974): Report on the 4th Joint WHO/SPC Seminar on Filariasis and Vector Control, Apia, Western Samoa. 45 pp.

Worms, M. J. (1972): Circadian and seasonal rhythms in blood parasites. In Canning, E. U. & Wright, C. A. (ed.), "Behavioural Aspects of Parasite Transmission," pp. 53–66; Academic Press, London.

Worms, M. J., Terry, R. J. & Terry, A. (1961): *J. Parasit.* **47**:963.

Wright, F. J. (1972): *J. Trop. Med. Hyg.,* **75**:140.

Wright, J. W. (1971): *Bull. Wld Hlth Org.* **44**:11.

Wright, J. W. & Pal, R. (1967; editors): Genetics of insect vectors of disease, Elsevier Publishing Co., Amsterdam, London, New York. 794 pp.

Wright, R. E. (1934): *Brit. J. Ophthal.* **18**:646.

Wright, R. E., Iyer, P. V. S. & Pandit, C. G. (1935): *Indian J. Med. Res.* **23**:199.

Wright, W. H., & Murdock, J. R. (1944): *Amer. J. Trop. Med.,* **24**:199.

Wu, Chia-chü (1959): *Chinese Med. J.* **80**:190, 1960.

Wu, Y. T. & Huang, Y. S. (1955): *J. Formosan Med. Assoc.* **54**:247.

Yamada, S. (1927): *Sci. Rep. Government Inst. Infectious Diseases* (Tokyo) **6**:559.

Yamagishi, H. (1966): *J. Fac. Sci. Shinshu Univ.* **1**:79.

Yamagishi, H., Nakamura, Y., Wada, Y., Okino, T. & Nakamoto, N. (1966): *Japan. J. Sanitary Zool.* **17**:48.

Yamagishi, H., Okino, T., Nakamoto, N., Nakamura, Y. & Wada, Y. (1967): *Japan. J. Ecology* **17**:206.

Yamaguti, S. (1961): The nematodes of vertebrates, in "Systema Helminthum," vol. 3, Pt. I & II, 1261 pp., Interscience Publishers Inc., New York & London.

Yamamoto, H. (1962): *Japan. J. Sanitary Zool.* **13**:23.
　　　　　　　(1964): *Japan. J. Sanitary Zool.* **15**:245.
　　　　　　　(1965): *Japan. J. Parasit.* **14**:169.

Yamamoto, H. & Hayashi, S. (1965): *Japan. J. Parasit.* **14**:534.
　　　　　　　(1966): *Japan. J. Parasit.* **15**:312.

Yamamoto, H., Hayashi, S., Yasuno, M., Saito, K., Nakamura, Y. & Hirakoso, S. (1966): *Japan. J. Trop. Med.* **7**:44.

Yamamoto, H., Hayashi, S., Hori, E., Otomo, H., Nakamura, Y. & Kawai, J. (1968): *Japan. J. Parasit.* **17**:325.

Yap. L. F., Ramachandran, C. P. & Balasinam, E. (1968): *Med. J. Malaya.,* **23**:118.

Yasuno, M. & Kerdpibule, V. (1967): *Japan. J. Exp. Med.* **37**:559.

Yasuno, M., Hirakoso, S., Sasa, M. & Uchida, M. (1965): *Japan. J. Exp. Med.* **35**:545.

Yasuno, M., Purivethaya, Y. & Harinasuta, C. (1967): *Japan. J. Exp. Med.* **37**:535.

Yen, C. H. (1934): *Lingnan Sci. J.* **13**:607.

Yoeli, M. (1957a): *Trans. Roy. Soc. Trop. Med. Hyg.* **51**:125.
　　　　　　(1957b): *Trans. Roy. Soc. Trop. Med. Hyg.* **51**:132.

Yokogawa, M. (1972 Ed.): Research in filariasis and schistosomiasis. Vol. 2. 261 pp. Univ. Tokyo Press & University Park Press.

Yokogawa, S., Kobayashi, H., Yumoto, Y., Osaka, K., Ro, M. & Yokogawa, M. (1939): *Taiwan Igakkai Zasshi (J. Taiwan Med. Assoc.)* **38**:1452.

Yorke, W., and Blacklock, B. (1917): *Ann. Trop. Med. Parasit.* **11**:127.

York, W. & Maplestone, P. A. (1926): The nematode parasites of vertabrates. 536 pp. Hafner Publishing Co., New York.

Yoshida, C. (1966): *End. Dis. Bull.* (Nagasaki) **8**:127.

Yoshimura, Y. (1912): *Igaku Chuo Zasshi* (Tokyo) **10**:1.

Yoshinaga, F. (1912a): *Igaku Chuo Zasshi* (Tokyo) **9**:2009 (in Japanese).
　　　　　　　(1912b): *Chugai Iho* (Tokyo) **774**:793 (in Japanese).

Yoshinaga, F. & Chosa, H. (1911): *Kyoto Igakkai Zasshi* **8**:114 (in Japanese).

Young, M. D. (1953): *Trans. Roy. Soc. Trop. Med. Hyg.* **47**:346.

Yun, I. S. (1927): *Korean Med. Ass. J.* **76**:326.
Zahner, H. (1974): *Z. Parasitenkunde* **43**:181.
Zaman, V. & Lal, M. (1973): *Trans. Roy. Trop. Med. Hyg.* **67**:610.
Zarrow, M. & Rifkin, H. (1946): *Amer. J. Med. Sci.,* **211**:97.
Zielke, E. (1973): *Z. Tropenmed. Parasit.* **24**:214.
Zimmerman, E. C. (1945): *Proc. Hawaii Acad. Sci.* **19–20**:5.
Zulueta, J. de. (1957): *Bull. Wld Hlth Org.,* **16**:699.